HUMAN LACTATION

Milk Components and Methodologies

CONTENTS

(e) How do the various components of milk interact with each other?

In order to provide answers to these questions an Advisory Committee consisting of Robert G. Jensen, Chair, Stephanie R. Atkinson, Bo Lönnerdal, Margaret C. Neville, Bert Garza and Mary Frances Picciano was founded. This committee organized a Conference on Methodologies in Human Lactation, held in Winter Park, Colorado, August 27-29, 1984. The committee submitted a successful application to the National Institute of Child Health and Human Development to support the conference. Ross Laboratories and Mead Johnson also contributed.

The objectives of this conference were to determine the current status of answers to the above questions and provide a forum where workers in the field of human lactation could exchange information on their endeavors. To facilitate the achievement of these goals, the conference was divided into workshops, each of which discussed a class of milk components or a particular methodological problem. This book represents the outcome of these workshops. In some cases it was possible to achieve a consensus within the workshop and a single article representing the combined viewpoint of the participants was possible. In other workshops, the expertise of the participants was sufficiently diverse that a series of articles was necessary to adequately represent the ideas presented. In both cases we believe that the success of the conference can be measured by the amount of useful information presented in this volume and by the fact that a great need was felt to continue the discussion at a second conference to be held in Oaxaca, Mexico, October 2-6, 1985.

The editors would like to thank the workshop leaders who labored hard to put together cohesive sections on the output of their respective workshops, the participants who contributed to a lively discussion - often until the small hours of the night, and the members of the Lactation Advisory Committee who assisted both in the planning of the conference and the review of these articles. The conference could not have been held without the encouragement and unfailing support of Thorsten Fjelstedt of the National Institutes of Child Health and Human Development. Publication of these proceedings would not have been possible without both the final assistance of Mary Johnson, who organized and copy edited the volume, and the splendid typing of Mimi Radley. Our thanks go also to Dorothy Scally, Jean Rasbach, Valerie Lutes and Diane Honnecke without whose untiring assistance a well organized-conference could not have been achieved. Finally, we gratefully acknowledge the grant (HD-18980) from the National Institute of Child Health and Human Development and grants-in-aid from Ross Laboratories and Mead Johnson. Their support made the conference possible.

Robert G. Jensen
Conference Chairman
July, 1985

PREFACE

Within the last five years the use of human milk in infant feeding has increased enormously and breast milk is now the recommended food for infants up to six months of age. However, studies on lactation and human milk have lagged because of the emphasis on formula feeding and because investigators with the requisite skills have only recently entered the area. Our knowledge, even of the proximate composition of human milk, has been inadequate. This is due in part to a lack of acceptable analytical methods. Although there are many thoroughly tested methods available for the analysis of bovine milk and other body fluids these are not always applicable to human milk. The problem is compounded by the considerable variability in milk composition within a single feed, over the course of a day, between breasts and with the duration of lactation. Further, milk is not a stable homogeneous fluid, but rather a complex mixture of interacting components whose physicochemical properties begin to change as soon as it leaves the breast. All of these characteristics mean that sampling, handling and storage must be carefully done if representative milk analyses are to be obtained. Finally, the parameter of ultimate interest is usually not milk composition *per se* but rather the amount of a particular component transferred from the lactating woman to her infant. This means that the volume of milk secreted in a given time interval must also be measured, usually by indirect means.

These problems were recognized at a 1982 workshop on Milk Banking held at Elk Ridge, MD, under the auspices of the National Institute of Child Health and Human Development where it was concluded that all aspects of the methods used for the analysis of human milk required review. A Committee on Methods was formed with Robert G. Jensen as its chair. A consensus was reached at the meeting that workers in this field needed an opportunity to interact intensively around the following issues:

(a) What is the current status of the sampling and analysis of human milk? Are satisfactory methods available? Can they be used for or applied to small quantities of milk? Are they for field or research applications?

(b) What is a representative sample for each class of milk constituent?

(c) How should the samples be collected and stored to maintain the chemical, physical and biological integrity of each of these constituents?

(d) For which constituents do we need development of new analyses?

Library of Congress Cataloging in Publication Data

Symposium on Methods in Human Lactation (1984: Winter Park, Colo.)
Human lactation.

"Based on the proceedings of a Symposium on Methods in Human Lactation, held August 22-26, 1984, in Winter Park, Colorado"—T.p. verso.
Includes bibliographies and index.
1. Milk, Human—Analysis—Congresses. 2. Milk, Human—Composition—Congresses. 3. Lactation—Congresses. I. Jensen, Robert G. (Robert Gordon), 1926–
II. Neville, Margaret C., 1934– . III. Title. [DNLM: 1. Lactation—congresses. 2. Milk, Human—analysis—congresses. WP 825 S9892h 1984]
QP246.S985 1984 612′.664 85-24419
ISBN 0-306-42111-9

Based on the proceedings of a Symposium on Methods in Human Lactation, held August 22–26, 1984, in Winter Park, Colorado

A Division of Plenum Publishing Corporation
233 Spring Street, New York, N.Y. 10013

Printed in the United States of America

HUMAN LACTATION
Milk Components and Methodologies

Edited by

Robert G. Jensen

University of Connecticut
Storrs, Connecticut

and

Margaret C. Neville

University of Colorado School of Medicine
Denver, Colorado

Plenum Press • New York and London

INTRODUCTION AND OVERVIEW:

PAST, PRESENT AND FUTURE ISSUES IN HUMAN LACTATION RESEARCH

Armond S. Goldman

Division of Immunology and Allergy, Department of Pediatrics, The University of Texas Medical Branch, Galveston, Texas

This conference was the first of a series that will address the problems of research into human lactation and the composition of human milk. For this reason it is important to review the recent history of human lactation and the developments that led to this gathering of leading scientists in the field. In previous centuries, human milk was tacitly accepted to be the principal food for human infants. Substitutes for breast feedings were largely limited to the use of raw cow's milk in comparatively few infants. During the first part of the 20th century, the technology for the commercial processing, storage, and distribution of cow's milk became established. Further, more women entered the workplace making breast-feeding less practical. For these reasons and because of other sociologic pressures, breast-feeding began to be replaced by commercial cow's milk preparations and the frequency of breast-feeding in the USA and other Western societies progressively dropped.

The drop in breast-feeding was abetted by a number of beliefs held by physicians. Many physicians encouraged artificial feedings because they felt more secure with feeding known amounts of a "standard" product. The use of bottle feeding simplified the task for doctors and permitted them to think more scientifically about infant nutrition. Further, the technology existing in the first half of this century did not permit much understanding of the mechanisms of human milk production, of its composition, or even of the volume that was produced during different phases of lactation. Because the volume and composition of cow's milk feedings could readily be measured, cow's milk was deemed to be scientifically superior to human milk for feedings. A further factor was that a marked decline in the morbidity and mortality of infants in this country coincided with a decline in the incidence of breast-feeding. It was, therefore, assumed that human milk and cow's milk were equivalent. In fact, it appeared that cow's milk was a complete replacement for human milk in that the growth of cow's milk fed infants was similar if not indistinguishable from that of breast-fed infants.

Because of the low public interest, the lack of widely accepted knowledge about human lactation, and a preoccupation of most physicians with artificial feedings, organized investigations of human lactation were not encouraged and seldom performed until the last decade. In addition, interest in this subject was obscured by an explosion of scientific developments in cellular-molecular biology and medical technology. It is understandable that many aspiring young scientists were and still are attracted to those highly visible areas. Moreover, because of a paucity of financial support, it is likely that many individuals who would have participated in human lactation studies gravitated to the dairy industry, other attractive biologic sciences, or traditional clinical areas that were professionally secure.

The situation began to change during the past decade as public recognition of the advantages of breast-feeding began to increase. Although the traditional familial support of lactation was absent because of the failure of a generation of women to breast-feed, enlightened members of the public and a few in the medical profession began to encourage breast-feeding by organizing support groups to educate both the public and health care professionals about the uniqueness of human milk. A small nucleus of basic and clinical scientists was established who were able to devote their efforts to studies in this area. Very recently the National Institute of Child Health and Human Development developed special support mechanisms for study of human lactation and the effects of human milk upon the recipient infant.

An outcome of these efforts has been the realization that both the formation and composition of human milk are extremely complex. Consequently it was a recognized that methodologies, originally designed to investigate other systems, must be improved to provide accurate information about human milk. The efforts clearly must be multidisciplinary and this is reflected in the meld of neonatologists, nutritionists, gastroenterologists, immunologists, physiologists, molecular biologists and other scientists who participated in this conference.

What were the important goals for this conference? 1) In addition to summarizing the current state of knowledge and technology in the field, ideas were shared, and cooperative studies arranged between colleagues in several countries. 2) Research priorities were established with respect to investigations of human lactation, the effects of human milk upon the development of mature and immature infants, and the role of human milk in the prevention or amelioration of intestinal and respiratory infections, allergic disorders, and other diseases. 3) These priorities were communicated to National Institute of Child Health and Human Development to provide a background against which the current problems in funding fundamental research in human lactation could be examined.

It is logical that the focus of this first conference was on fundamental methodologic issues in human lactation. The scientific communications at this meeting were intended to provide a foundation for additional international conferences which will examine the physiology of human lactation, the maternal-environmental influences on human lactation, the composition of human milk and the effects of human milk upon the recipient infant. The potential gains from these endeavors should not only advance the science of lactation but also enhance the health of infants and children throughout the world.

SECTION I - MILK VOLUME

WORKSHOP PARTICIPANTS

M. W. Woolridge, Department of Paediatrics, Oxford, UK

N. Butte, Department of Pediatrics, Baylor University, Houston, Texas

K. G. Dewey, Department of Nutrition, University of California, David, California

A. M. Ferris, Department of Nutritional Sciences, University of Connecticut, Storrs, Connecticut

C. Garza, Department of Pediatrics, University of Connecticut, Storrs, Connecticut

R. P. Keller, Department of Physiology, University of Colorado, Denver, Colorado

INTRODUCTION

It is useful to draw the distinction between nutritional research aimed at determining the dietary intake of breast-fed babies in specific situations, and fundamental research into the physiology of lactation. Where estimates of nutrient intake are intended for comparative study, the establishment of uniform methodology is essential. This paper describes the various methods of measurement available for obtaining milk volumes, and it addresses potential methodological differences arising from their use.

METHODS FOR THE MEASUREMENT OF MILK VOLUME INTAKE OF THE BREAST-FED INFANT

M. W. Woolridge
N. Butte
K. G. Dewey
A. M. Ferris
C. Garza
R. P. Keller

INTRODUCTION

The nutrient intake from a breast feed is defined by the product of net volume intake and the average concentration of the specific milk constituent under scrutiny:

$$\text{Net Volume Intake} \times \text{Mean Concentration Constituent X} = \text{Net Intake of Constituent X}$$

Although isolated estimates of nutrient concentration may have their value, net nutrient intake of the individual infant should be uppermost in importance. As such, the measurement of volume intake is central to the estimation of the total nutrient intake, and must be subject to the same rigors of measurement and efforts at standardization as is compositional analysis. Ideally, if estimates are to be rendered as net intake per unit time, the infant's volume intake should be measured over the same period during which composition measurements are made. In this respect, it is difficult to consider volume estimation separately from the need to collect milk samples.

Different methods exist for obtaining milk samples (e.g., total breast expression, manually expressed pre- and post-feed samples, etc.), and different analyses dictate different amounts of sample to be collected. If the volume of sample required is large, it is likely to interfere with subsequent milk intake by the infant; this problem could be overcome by collecting samples on the day after that on which volume measurements are made. Where only small samples are required (e.g., 1-2 ml), collection can be undertaken concurrently with volume estimation.

DEFINING MILK VOLUME

Historically, there have been many ways of defining milk volume in the context of human breast-feeding. Predominantly, the conflict has been between measuring milk volume in terms of the maximum theoretical output of the mother, as estimated by total expression of the breasts, compared to the actual milk intake of the baby, as assessed by direct test weighing of the infant before and after breast feeds. To avoid confusion, it would seem wise to adhere to strict terminology, referring to the former as milk *yield*, and the latter as milk *intake* (see later note on use of the term "volume").

While total expression of the contents of the breasts may be a valid method for estimating the total nutrient content of breast milk, the evidence suggests that the expressed contents are not representative of the milk that a baby takes while being suckled, and so should not be used to derive an estimate of volume intake. Firstly, the natural variability in the pattern of feeding of the demand-fed infant, dictated by his appetite, cannot be modeled adequately by *routine* expression of the breasts. Secondly, many authors have noted that additional milk can be expressed from the breasts after a baby has finished suckling (1,2). An extra 10% can often be expressed after feeding, though values as high as 30% have been reported for a low socioeconomic group of mothers from a traditional rural background (3). Evidence that some of this milk, if not all, is accessible to the baby, is provided by the demonstration that babies at 6 days of age satiate during a feed, leaving milk unconsumed in the breast (4). Anecdotally, (C. Fisher, in a personal comment to MWW) the reverse is also possible. That is, a baby was recorded as consuming 25ml of milk from the breast, after a mother had expressed all she was able to by pumping.

In view of this evidence, we shall limit our discussion of techniques to those which measure, either directly or indirectly, the milk *intake* of the breast-fed baby. Three methods are currently available for estimating the volume (or more strictly the weight) of milk transferred from a mother to her baby:

1. Test Weighing
2. Doppler Ultrasound Human Milk Flowmeter
3. Deuterium Oxide Dilution

Test weighing, despite a number of practical limitations (5-7), remains the reference method for estimating milk intake, both because of its directness, and its proven accuracy when modern integrating electronic balances are used. The other two techniques remain somewhat specialized and are of limited availability to field workers. Further development work and practical study are necessary to demonstrate that these two techniques possess the accuracy and consistency of performance to allow them to be used routinely in the field. However, it should be stressed that each of the three techniques is optimally adapted to making measurements over a different time scale (Table 1).

Despite potential limitations of the two novel methods, there are circumstances where they may be more flexible than test weighing for collecting feed information. These include: at night-time;if the mother travels any distance from her home with her infant; or over long intervals of time (e.g., 2 weeks). The different methods might be better regarded as being complementary, rather than competitive, since the new methods can be used at times (and in situations) in which test weighing either may not be practicable, or its use would introduce such artifact as to compromise its accuracy.

Furthermore, there is little overlap between the time scales to which each method is adapted. Although the range of a method can be extended outside its optimal time scale, it should be appreciated that this may

Table 1. Time Scale or Feed Span, and Optimal Technique for Measurement

Time Span	Purpose			Method
1 sec - 1 min	Instantaneous flow rate measurement			Flow Meter
1 - 5 min	Fractional breakdown of single feeds			Flow Meter or Fractional Test-weighing
5 - 60 min	Complete individual feeds			Testweighing or Flow Meter*
>1hr	Multiple feeds	i.	12 hrs	Testweighing
		ii.	24 hrs (1 day)	Testweighing
		iii.	48-72 hrs (2-3 days)	Testweighing or D_2O dilution*
		iv.	7-14 days	D_2O dilution

* Signifies diminished accuracy on such a time scale of measurement.

incur much greater error. Attempting to validate methods on a time scale other than that to which they are currently adapted can be a self-defeating exercise; and so in general, it is not possible to obtain a quantitative comparison of the three methods.

TEST WEIGHING

Test weighing the infant with an integrating electronic balance, e.g., Sartorius (8,22,36), Mettler (13,21), Toledo (20), or K-Tron (12), must currently be regarded as the reference technique for estimating the milk intake from individual feeds to the nearest 1-2g. Such balances generally have a resolution of 1g or 0.1g, with a maximum error for a test weighing on the order of $\pm$5g (8,9) (as test weighing involves a difference estimate, the error for a single weighing must be doubled.)

Resolution, precision and practical accuracy all describe separate aspects of a balance's performance. The last of these, practical accuracy, includes all possiblé sources of measurement error, including parallax errors in reading a scale, interpolation between scale markings (where applicable), visual integration errors due to movement artifact, and inadvertant misreading and misrecording of weight. These sources of error make an additive contribution to the measurement error variance. The variance is compounded by the cumulative potential errors that may be due to bias and to ignoring "insensible" water loss and "sensible" sweating.

The limitations on accuracy of spring balances are well documented (10,11). Coward (5) has argued that there is an interaction between balance precision, feed frequency and the number of days over which test weighing measurements are made. In view of the day-to-day variation in individual intake, a balance with $\pm$5g accuracy is adequate if measurements are to be made over 4 days. Drewett et al. (12), utilizing the data of other authors, have shown that spring balances have 95% prediction intervals of ±20-40g in use, while the equivalent measure for an electronic balance was ±6.5g. It would appear, therefore, that only the latter balances offer the necessary precision, when one takes account of all practical errors during performance, including bias. The frozen digital display of integrating electronic balances is a crucial practical feature, reducing the potential bias due to analogue interpolation of a moving needle. Certainly, lack of absolute precision in a balance can be compensated for by weighing for longer periods of time, e.g., 4 days. But, it remains the case that the potential for cumulative error and bias with a balance of low resolution and poor precision should not be underestimated or disregarded. In summary, a range of balances is available for making test weighing measurements, from the simplest mechanical balances to sophisticated electronic balances. The latter are of undisputed precision, but of significantly greater cost. While there is a trade-off between balance precision and the number of days over which intake is measured (5), other factors (see below) influence this decision -- suggesting that high precision balances are essential in most instances. A portable, battery--operated balance is now available which is suitable for field use (12).

Rahilly (15) obtained exceptionally accurate test weighing results using, according to Stothers (16), a beam balance. Further tests of practical accuracy under field conditions might prove valuable in locations where funds are limited, or large numbers of balances are called for.

Recently-published data (13) in validation of the technique for measuring milk volume transfer by test weighing the mother rather than the infant (14), suggest that this method is suitable only for population studies. There was a specific overestimate of +25g at each feed, while prediction intervals were on the order of ±73g for a single feed. The technique may still be of value where it is not possible to weigh infants (who, because of their age, are highly active) on the understanding that the activity of the mother is more easily constrained. Alternative strategies for weighing older, more active infants will be discussed below.

Since test-weighing is the method most frequently in use, its methodological considerations will be discussed in more detail than the other two techniques. Table 2 summarizes the practical aspects of the method.

STRATEGIES FOR TEST WEIGHING

Within-feed Determination of the Pattern of Milk Transfer

Test weighing has been used to determine the pattern of milk transfer within a feed, and for cumulated feed totals. The aim of the former approach has been to offer guidelines to the breast-feeding mother regarding the timing and structure of her feeds, i.e., how long or how frequent (17). Two alternative designs exist for examining the pattern of milk flow within a feed: (i) cross sectional weighing, to describe the pattern typical of a population of mother/infant pairs (18), and (ii) fractional test weighing, to establish the pattern of milk transfer for an individual mother/infant pair (17,19). By the former design, feedings of different babies are interrupted and the babies weighed after a specified period of time on either the first or second breast (i.e., one group of babies after 2 minutes of feeding, and further groups after 4 minutes, 7 minutes, etc.) Once interrupted, feeding can continue, but subsequent

Table 2. Summary of Practical Characteristics of Test weighing Method

Accuracy	Electronic balances of proven accuracy (±5g under practical conditions) are less prone to operator bias in use than beam or spring balances. Accuracy of spring balances is poor.
Scope	No reported cultural or ethical reservations concerning the use of test weighing. However, in developing countries, where unscheduled, frequent feeding is the norm, discrete feeds are difficult to define, and test weighing will inevitably disrupt the natural feed routine.
Flexibility	Of limited use at night-time except in Western industrialized societies. During daytime may impair freedom of activity of mother, restricting her to the vicinity of her home, so that she may follow an unrepresentative lifestyle. The availability of battery-operated electronic balances extends the range of use to field studies.
Cost	Electronic balances have a high cost relative to spring balances, but this is changing rapidly.

intake at that feed is not studied, on the premise that interruption is likely to have disturbed the natural pattern of milk transfer. In the second design, individual feeds are interrupted to obtain an intermediate measurement of intake on each breast, the baby is returned to the breast and re-weighed at one (19) or several points later in the feed (17). This method allows definition of the pattern of milk intake for an individual infant, as opposed to that for a population of infants.

The picture of milk transfer suggested by cross-sectional weighing (e.g., 80 to 90% of the milk from a breast taken in 4 minutes) is misleading if used to make clinical recommendations regarding individual feed policies. This is due to a methodological sampling artifact inherent in cross-sectional methods. Babies with a high rate of intake tend to take a large volume of milk and finish feeding early, while babies with a slow rate feed for a longer time and may take a smaller volume. As a result, babies which are fast feeders contribute to early data points (e.g., at 2 and 4 minutes), but are subsequently lost from samples and do not contribute to data points later in the feed (e.g., at 7 and 10 minutes). Furthermore, babies who would naturally complete their intake from a breast after 10 minutes (e.g., at 15 minutes) are interrupted before achieving their final intake, giving an artificially low estimate of total feed volume. The net result of these two effects (i.e., loss of high-intake babies early in the feed, and the curtailed intake of slow feeders) is that the intake curve reaches an artificial plateau early in the feed, giving the impression that babies take little extra milk after the first four minutes of feeding on each breast. In practice, on the order of 95% of babies feeding for longer than 4 minutes will continue to take significant amounts of milk, as can be demonstrated by fractional test weighing (19).

Extrapolations from Shorter Periods of Measurement

The problems of recording milk intake at night are considerable, so that, not surprisingly, researchers have attempted to ascertain the accuracy with which 24-hour intake can be extrapolated from 12-hour intake measurements made during the daytime (2,20), or from single feed totals (21,22). It is clear from the data of Houston et al. (21) that in the first week post-partum, the daily feed pattern is sufficiently homogeneous for 24-hour intake to be estimated from only one or two feeds with quite a high degree of confidence. However, as daytime and night-time patterns of nursing become more disparate (as is often reported to occur in industrialized societies when infants get older, or in developing countries) such estimates will become progressively inaccurate (22).

The same argument applies to the extrapolation of 24-hour intake from 12-hour daytime measurements. Although daytime and night-time intakes may be highly correlated (23), the accuracy of prediction of an individual's intake based on a single estimate may be very low (24). Brown et al. (2), using test weighing, found that in a rural village location, daytime intake varied between 37 to 72% of the 24-hour total. De Carvalho et al. (20), observing that night-time intake was 40% less than daytime intake at one month of age, concluded that for Western babies intakes were too discrepant for a doubling of 12-hour intake to be of value. This situation is exaggerated further by variation between individuals and by marked changes with age (25). It has been shown that a knowledge of the number of feeds (2), and/or their duration (2,24), can improve the accuracy of such estimates. However, there remains the problem of the ease and reliability with which information about night-time nursing patterns can be obtained, particularly in developing countries. Under certain circumstances, 12-hour daytime intake can provide a useful comparative measure, but we suggest that where only 12-hour estimates of intake are available, they should remain as such, and that no transformation be undertaken.

Measurement of Milk Intake over Multiple Days

The converse view is that where a truly representative estimate of an individual's daily intake is required, even a complete 24-hour period may be inadequate. Intra-individual variation in nursing pattern and milk intake from day to day, means that a single day taken at random may be unrepresentative of intake at that age. Using the observed intra-individual variation in 24-hour intake, compared to the level of variation between individuals, it is possible to calculate the number of daily records needed to provide a reliable estimate of intake. Black et al. (26) use a method based on the standard error of mean intake to ascertain whether the measured intake falls within 5% of the "true" intake. Based upon the coefficient of variation (CV) in intake from day to day, 4 days of study would be required for infants with a CV of 10%. Butte et al. (27) found that the mean CV for infants of 1 to 4 months of age was $7.9 \pm 3.6\%$, suggesting that around 3 days of measurement is adequate (limits 1 to 6 days). With highly variable data, the time span required for individual intake estimation may be impractically long (e.g., 10 to 20 days). Furthermore, day-to-day variation in intake, rather than arising simply from errors of time sampling, may be due to actual changes with growth or morbidity, such that intake cannot be considered to be held constant. As a result, a compromise period, on the order of 3 to 5 days, should probably be chosen in advance.

Defining the 24-Hour Period

Where needs dictate that a single 24-hour estimate must suffice, a problem exists as to how to define "24-hour intake." The absolute choice of starting point (e.g., 6:00 a.m., 8:00 a.m., etc.) is completely arbitrary. Because feed times "on demand" are highly variable, some will fall just inside, and some just outside, the 24-hour time window. Once again, for group data this will not matter, as both will occur with equal probability, but for individual estimates such errors may introduce considerable variability.

Of the different sources of intra-individual variation, some can be controlled and some cannot. Variation due to how long either the mother or baby "decides" to devote to feeding on any one day cannot be constrained, but variation due to how feeds fall within a time window can be adjusted to minimize error from this source. This can be done by measuring the "24-hour window" from the end of the feed immediately prior to the allotted 24-hour period (i.e., noting the interfeed interval which straddles the onset of the 24-hour period), and both the interval and feed subsequent to the 24-hour period. Practically, this would be equivalent to taking the two feeds after the 24-hour period (14). The feed total (including the measured feed falling outside the 24-hour period) is then divided by the total time span (i.e., >24 hours), and multiplied by 24, to give an adjusted estimate of 24-hour intake.

It may be argued that such an intake does not actually exist, as the baby must have physically taken either more or less milk. The same criticism would apply to an estimate of 24-hour intake derived as the mean of intake over 2 to 5 days of measurement. If one did not adopt the strategy of using an extended 24-hour period then, strictly speaking, a feed which straddles the 24-hour limits should be interrupted, and the intermediate intake up to that point should be used. However, it is simpler to regard feeds as discrete point events, and feed totals as indivisible.

Measuring intake over multiple consecutive days reduces this problem. The error due to "clipping" or "enclosing" feeds occurs only at the ends of the periods of study, so that measuring over three days would reduce the proportion of such feeds. When measuring over consecutive days, adjusting daily totals is probably undesirable. The reason for this is that information from the same feed would be used to derive two separate daily totals. Against these considerations, it should be said that in many instances adjustments will not be necessary. At high feed frequencies/low feed volumes, such "errors" will be minimal, while at low feed frequencies the nursing pattern tends to conform to a 24-hour clock, determined by the routine of the mother. Knowledge of the typical nursing pattern is useful, as the starting point can be selected to fall in the place where the longest interfeed interval is to be expected.

It is of value to know whether there is one feed during the 24-hour period which is consistently representative of the average feed intake, as has been demonstrated for mean-feed fat concentration by Prentice et al. (28). They have shown, in Keneba, that the first feed after 1300 hours is closest to the 12-hour mean-feed fat concentration. As stressed by these authors, such a relationship would need to be determined for each population under study.

Other Adjustments to Directly Measured Feed Totals

Insensible Water Loss. An estimate of insensible weight loss of 2g/kg/hr may be used as a rough guide (9); so that a 3kg baby might lose 2g during the course of a 20 minute feed. This is close to the practical limits of resolution of test weighing, and so for individual feeds can be ignored. The single proviso should be that, where negative intakes are recorded, although improbable, the measured weight change must be used in calculations (e.g., soon after birth, when a zero intake combined with a 2g IWL would give a measured weight change of -2g). If all negative intakes were considered to be erroneous, and taken as zero, then a correction would be made for low intakes, but not for higher ones.

If intake is measured over 24 hours, then the cumulative effect of insensible water loss on intake may be significant. For a 6kg baby, 24-hour loss will be on the order of 288g, but only a proportion of this will be encompassed and measured by test weighing. With frequent suckling (e.g., 15 minutes every hour) the error could be as high as 72g, but a more typical value would be 32g for a baby feeding for 20 minutes every 3 hours. This error represents a specific underestimate of 4.3% for a 24-hour intake of 750ml. It is reasonable to correct for such an error as it represents a specific bias; the chief problem is to determine the magnitude of correction necessary to fairly represent the ranges of metabolic rate, temperature, humidity and air circulation likely to be encountered. These would need to be assessed for each study location, and would show seasonal variation. We leave it open as to whether such adjustments are made. However, where they are made, we recommend that the amount be specified, and preferably that the uncorrected data also be given. Where no mention of a correction for evaporative water loss is made, the assumption will be that the data represent uncorrected intakes (i.e., as suggested above, averages will include negative weight changes, where "intakes" are recorded as such).

Conversion from weight to volume. Most techniques for estimating milk intake are gravimetric, so that where volume intake is specified, presentation of units in ml should be taken to imply that a conversion from g has been made. Although failure to correct for the density of milk being greater than 1 will result in a 2 to 3% overestimate, this would change with the fat content of the milk taken. As such changes can rarely be taken into consideration, and also because in the majority of published data no such adjustment has previously been made, we suggest that *no* such correction for the density of milk be made. While the semantic error of continuing to refer to milk volume can probably be tolerated, the units in which milk intake is given should accurately reflect the method of measurement, e.g., g for test weighing.

In many studies, the above adjustments will fall under the category of transformations of the data, and so should not affect within-study comparisons. Between-study comparisons will only become more confused by their being applied in some cases and not in others.

Considerations Affecting Number of Weighings

Collecting accurate weight measurements, even with integrating balances, can still be confounded by the activity of the child. Once the child becomes sufficiently mobile to climb off the balance, obtaining a stable measurement can be particularly taxing! Test-weighing the mother is a procedure used specifically to overcome this predicament (6). An alternative procedure developed by Keller and Neville (unpublished) involves suspending the infant in a baby seat in the under-balance weighing position. A programmable balance (Mettler PC24-03) interfaced to a microcomputer (Epson HX-20) allows the rapid, automatic collection of weighings and statistical treatment of the results, as well as the exclusion of deviant results. Four to five months of age is a rough guide as to the age at which more sophisticated methods such as these become necessary.

There is, however, a compromise to be reached between increasing the number of weighings upon which the average is based, versus keeping them to a minimum so that the baby is on the balance for as short a time as possible. Taking the median weight from three cycles of five weighings each, is one of the quickest and mathematically simplest methods. If 2 out of 3 "averages" are identical, the median is automatically one of the identical values. So if the first two "averages" are identical, by definition there is no need to take a third set, allowing the baby to be taken off the balance sooner. Alternatively, using a computer interfaced to the balance can allow evaluation of each point; by this method the weighing can be completed as soon as 3 or 5 satisfactory weights have been obtained.

Thwarting of Data Collection by the Mother

Various efforts can be made to reduce errors caused by either accidental or intentional non-compliance of the mother, but if weighings are carried out unsupervised in the home, by the mother, one must expect that errors will occur. Most are made unwittingly; for example, items of the baby's clothing may be present at one weighing but not at the other, or drapes may brush against the balance pan. There are also instances where a mother may put her baby to the breast for just a couple of minutes, but does not bother to weigh him, as she "knows" her baby was only "sucking for comfort," and so would not have taken any milk! Against these instances, there are a few rare cases where a mother does not wish the true intake of her baby to be known. Where this is the case, she will generally be successful in outwitting most controls or checks (e.g., by including an extra article with the second weighing to give a slightly inflated intake). Alternatively, a mother may wake her infant just prior to the end of the 24-hour period, and give him a quick feed in order to "bump-up" his intake. Such problems have to be accepted as unmeasurable error. To offset such problems, all attempts must be made to ensure that mothers are completely willing participants, and that there is no conflict of interest in providing accurate data.

ADEQUATE DOCUMENTATION OF STUDY POPULATION IN PUBLISHED REPORTS

The ultimate aim of published work is not simply to document typical values and recommendations for the population under study, but to provide results which might be generalized to other populations. This can only be done if sufficient details are documented for the population under study. These include: (i) birth statistics, (ii) breakdown of socioeconomic status (especially educational level), (iii) feed management, nursing policy, typical feed schedules, (iv) enlistment procedure, (v) representation by specialist groups or highly motivated mothers, (vi) drug regimes, pre-, inter- and post-partum.

ALTERNATIVE METHODS TO TEST WEIGHING

Oxford Milk Flowmeter (Nipple Shield and Ultrasound Flow Transducer)

The development of this system was based on the premise that the most accurate statement about the infant's dietary intake from a breast feed could be derived by making simultaneous measurements of the flow and composition of the milk taken by the baby during suckling. Such an approach would allow measurements of intake to be made while allowing for natural variation in feed frequency and duration due to the infant's appetite.

The system is based on a thin latex nipple shield, which was designed to be interposed between mother and infant during feeds and to interfere minimally with normal milk transfer (8,29). A miniature Doppler ultrasound flow transducer has been developed (30, 31), which is embedded in the tip of the shield. An elliptical bellmouth entrance to the transducer constrains the milk to flow through a 1.2 mm lumen between 2 piezo-electric crystals angled at 45° towards the entrance (Figure 1). The frequency of transmitted ultrasound is shifted by reflection off particles transported in the milk (e.g., fat droplets) in direct relation to the velocity of the milk. Processing of the received signal produces an analogue output voltage which defines instantaneous milk flow. Analogue integration of this output yields the cumulative intake (32), which can then be matched to sequential composition data to give a profile of nutrient intake throughout the feed. Table 3 gives a summary of the characteristics of this method.

A battery-operated Doppler processing unit, based on digital flow processing, has been developed to facilitate field studies. This unit has a solid-state memory capable of storing continuous flow data (10-second digital flow counts) over 9 hours (33). To extend its use to 24 hours, the Doppler flow recorder also has an "interval" mode. When the transducer is disconnected, the time interval between feeds is stored in a single location in memory. The memory is assured for one week, and replay is direct to a computer. Software has been developed to integrate digital flow data to provide net volume intake (Figure 2).

In vitro performance of the transducer is satisfactory, producing a linear output from 0-200 ml/minute under continuous flow, and showing an acceptable frequency response under pulsatile flow conditions (31). *In vivo* results have been less satisfactory. The problem stems from the fact that a small error in instantaneous flow measurement will accumulate with time to produce a discrepant final value for volume intake. Further work is required to reduce two main sources of error: (i) reverse milk flow (monitored, but in a non-linear manner), and (ii) passage of air through the transducer (which produces an atypically high signal). Both these problems are potentially surmountable, by either physical or electrical means, but, to date, they remain unresolved.

The system remains the only one available for examining the profile of milk transfer within a feed. As yet, its accuracy is unacceptable for providing cumulative volume intake measurements, and it is unlikely, in the immediate future, to be available as a primary tool for evaluating dietary intake. However, on a more limited basis, it can provide important physiological data, and it can be used to examine the validity of assumptions made by methods currently in field use. For example, composition estimates may be based on the mean composition of expressed pre-feed and post-feed milk samples, assuming linear milk intake over the feed. This assumption is acknowledged as being untenable, but information on the

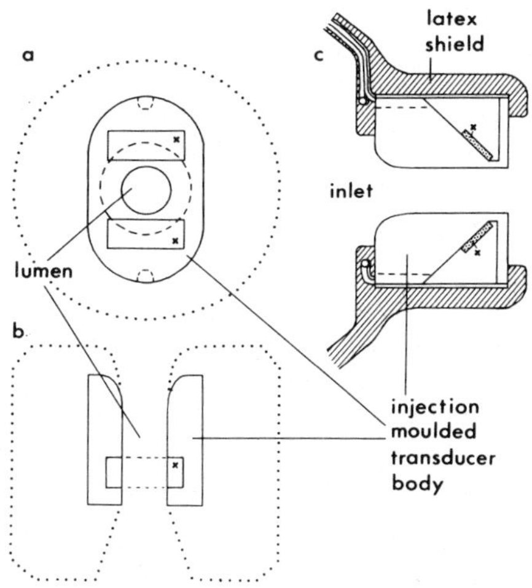

Figure 1. Diagram illustrating injection-molded ultrasound flow transducer.

(a) Cross-section showing flattening of transducer body in one plane, and (b) longitudinal section at minimum width (x indicates position of piezo-electric crystals, dotted outline shows size of prototype (32). (c) Completed miniature flow transducer embedded in latex shield (longitudinal section at maximum width) showing crystals, supply wires and encapsulating sleeve *in situ*.

pattern of milk transfer is required in order to estimate the relative proportions of foremilk and hindmilk consumed. The flowmeter can provide such information for individual subjects, allowing estimates to be adjusted (e.g., 6). Studies are underway to examine the suitability of the portable Doppler flow recorders for field use.

An important property of this system is that the same methodology can be used to obtain composition data. Locating a sampling line behind the nipple shield allows the simultaneous collection of samples of suckled breast milk. The sequential composition estimates can be matched to serial flow data to provide realistic absolute values for nutrient intake. Furthermore, the Doppler recorder automatically logs a complete record of nursing patterns (i.e., feed duration and intervals) which may be used to modify volume estimates obtained by test weighing for shorter periods of time (24).

Deuterium Oxide Dilution Technique

The principle involved in this technique is that a known dose of a tracer (deuterium oxide, D_2O, containing a stable isotope of hydrogen) is given orally to either infant (34) or mother (35). The assumption is that the tracer rapidly becomes uniformly distributed throughout the body fluid compartments. The tracer equilibrates with the saliva, so that removing small amounts of saliva allows one to obtain a representative sample of body water. Over a period of days, dilution of the tracer in the body water can be charted (as additional water is either consumed, metabolized,

Table 3. Summary of Practical Characteristics of Flowmeter Method

Accuracy	Qualitative description of milk flow within a feed - good; determination of individual feed volumes - poor, performance erratic (wide confidence limits); as yet untested for measuring 24-hour intakes.
Scope	Use of the nipple shield system involves the acquisition of a degree of practical skill to ensure normal feeding occurs when the shield is used. Use of the system is likely to be age-restricted, depending upon prior experience of the infant (speculatively 6 to 9 months).
Flexibility	The Doppler flow recorder is battery-operated and portable, allowing the mother to pursue her normal work schedule. Data analysis can be carried out locally, at the nearest center with micrometer facilities.
Cost	Cost of shields, transducers and signal processing equipment is relatively low, e.g., 4 units and 10 transducers are roughly equivalent to the cost of one electronic balance. The microcomputer would be a major capital outlay, but the software can be put on any suitable computer at negligible cost.

or absorbed) and is lost through excretion or evaporation. The Total Body Water (TBW) is estimated either by immediate dilution of the initial dose, or more accurately by extrapolation back to the origin of the exponential dilution curve. The estimated TBW is expressed as a percentage of the body weight, and is presumed to remain constant over the period of study. Changes in body weight, from the beginning to the end of the study, are used to adjust the TBW estimate, and thereby the net water throughput, allowing estimation of the breast milk intake. Table 4 summarizes the characteristics of the method.

Giving the tracer to the infant allows one only to determine fluid intake irrespective of source, and so other sources of water intake must be controlled. This route is not now considered acceptable for estimating the intake of individual infants, primarily because of the difficulties described in the next paragraph (5). Giving the deuterium oxide to the mother means that the dilution curve for both mother and baby must be determined to establish the rate of uptake of breast milk by the baby. Theoretically, the method allows one to estimate the contribution of additional water to intake, but attempts to test this by giving a known amount of supplementary water to exclusively breast-fed babies have not been reported. Dosing the mother is now the preferred strategy for administration, although the infant's TBW must be estimated independently (34).

Butte et al. (36), and Nagy and Costa (37) have discussed possible sources of error. Two of the more significant are likely to be the chemical exchange of isotope with non-aqueous hydrogen within the body, and the physical exchange of water across the skin and lungs (36, 37). Biological fractionation may present a problem, particularly if fluid balance is upset (37), e.g., infants with diarrhea. A further source of

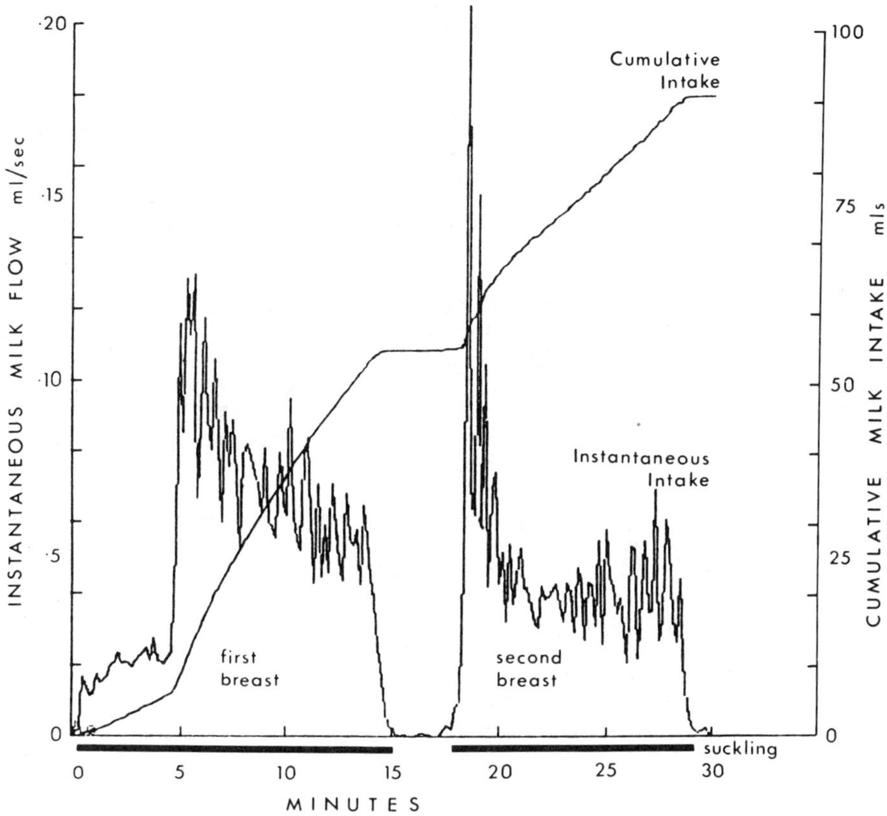

Figure 2. Digital flow profile obtained with miniaturized flow transducer, and Doppler flow recorder (portable signal processing and solid-state memory unit). Computer drawn trace of digital flow data (10-second resolution) logged in memory for a single feed from both breasts. Cumulative intake profile obtained by summation of successive 10-second totals.

possible error relates to the estimation of Total Body Water. Although Coward et al. (34) note that the accurate logging of sampling points is important for accuracy, no recommendations are provided for standardizing measurements of body weight, from which is derived the estimated change in TBW. The validity of the assumptions applied in the derivation of Total Body Water estimates remains a critical aspect of the method.

This remains the only practicable method for measuring intake over a 7 to 14 day period. Although test weighing has been carried out after a 14-day period immediately post-partum, such a period would constitute a considerable imposition on the mother's freedom in later lactation. To date, the dilution technique has only been validated against intermittent 24-hour test weighing or continuous 48-hour test weighing (36).

Table 4. Summary of Practical Characteristics of D_2O Dilution Method

Accuracy	Accuracy moderate - exponential curve fitting has an error of ±10% when sampling is optimally timed over a 14-day period (35). Two-point curve fitting (34) would have a much increased error. Administering the tracer to the infant is unsatisfactory for estimating the milk intake of individuals.
Scope	Milk intake is measured on a time scale which matches that over which growth can be measured. Provides volume information only, composition data must be collected by a separate methodology, and with greater frequency, necessitating additional site visits. Ethical consideration as to whether deuterium oxide can be routinely administered to mothers and/or babies.
Flexibility	Field technology and supervision minimal. Premeasured doses of D_2O are administered, and saliva samples are collected and sealed on site, then dispatched for analysis. Sample analysis highly sophisticated, so that volume intake information is not immediately available on site.
Cost	Mass spectrometer equipment expensive, which means that, for use in overseas studies in developing countries, analysis must be conducted at a technologically sophisticated center.

CONCLUSION

It should be stressed that different practical philosophies lie behind each of the three techniques for determining breast-milk intake; they are not in competition with each other. Selection of one of these depends upon the nature of the study, primarily with regard to the time resolution that is required. Each technique has its limitations, and these must be given due consideration when interpreting the data. An abiding problem remains that comparison between methods is hindered by the fact that they are adapted to different time scales. Although test weighing is the "gold standard" against which new methods are assessed, researchers must remain aware of its limitations. Where it is used as the reference technique, all efforts should be made to ensure that it qualifies as a valid independent variable. Ultimately, it is the needs of the study, its location, the availability of funds, and the ethical and cultural acceptability to the population in question, which influence the choice of method. This calls for critical analysis of the relative merits of each method by any investigator intending to use them.

REFERENCES

1. Hall B. (1975): Changing composition of human milk and early development of an appetite control. Lancet, i, 779.

2. Brown KH, Black RE, Robertson AD, Akhtar NA, Ahmed G, Becker S. (1982): Clinical and field studies of human lactation: methodological considerations. Am J Clin Nutr, 35, 745-756.

3. Khin-Maung-Naing, Tin-Tin-Oo, Kywe-Thein, Nwe-New-Hlaing. (1980): Study on lactation performance of Burmese mothers. Am J Clin Nutr, 33, 2665-2668.

4. Drewett RF, Woolridge MW. (1981): Milk taken by human babies from the first and second breast. Physiol & Behav, 26, 327-329.

5. Coward WA. (1984): Measuring milk intake in breast-fed babies. J Pediatr Gastroenterol Nutr, 3, 275-279.

6. Hartmann PE, Saint L. (1984): Measurement of milk yield in women. J Pediatr Gastroenterol Nutr, 3, 270-274.

7. Ferris AM, Jensen RG. (1984): Lipids in human milk: a review. 1. Sampling, determination and content. J Pediatr Gastoenterol Nutr, 3, 108-122.

8. Woolridge MW, Baum JD, Drewett RF. (1980): Effect of a traditional and of a new nipple shield on sucking patterns and milk flow. Early Hum Dev, 4, 357-364.

9. Hendrickson, EC, Sedeat JM, Neville MC. Insensible water loss in children under one year of age. Acta Paed. Scarel. (In Press).

10. Culley P, Milan P, Roginski C, Waterhouse J, Wood B. (1979): Are breast-fed babies still getting a raw deal in hospital? Br Med J, ii, 891-893.

11. Whitfield MF, Kay R, Stevens S. (1981): Validity of routine test-weighing as a measure of the intake of breast-fed infants. Arch Dis Child, 56, 919-921.

12. Drewett RF, Woolridge MW, Greasley V, McLeod CN, Williams AF, Baum JD. (1984): Evaluating breast-milk intake by test weighing: a portable electronic balance suitable for community and field studies. Early Hum Dev, 10, 123-126.

13. Saint L, Smith M, Harmann PE. (1984): The yield and nutrient content of colostrum and milk of women from giving birth to 1 month post-partum. Br J Nutr, 52, 87-95.

14. Rattigan S, Ghisalberti AV, Hartmann PE. (1981): Breast milk production in Australian women. Br J Nutr, 45, 243-249.

15. Rahilly PM. (1980): Effects of sleep state and feeding on cranial blood flow of the human neonate. Arch Dis Child, 55, 265-270.

16. Strothers JK. (1982): Accuracy of routine clinical test weighing. Arch Dis Child, 57, 810. (Letter).

17. Howie PW, Houston MJ, Cook A, Smart L, McArdle T, McNeilly. (1980): How long should a breast feed last? Early Hum Dev, 5, 71-77.

18. Lucas A, Lucas PJ, Baum JD. (1979): Pattern of milk flow in breast-fed infants. Lancet, ii, 57-58.

19. Woolridge MW, Baum JD, Drewett RF. (1982): Individual patterns of milk intake during breast feeding. Early Hum Dev, 7, 265-272.

20. de Carvalho, Robertson S, Merkatz R, Klaus M. (1982): Milk intake and frequency of feeding in breast fed infants. Early Hum Dev, 7, 155-163.

21. Houston MJ, Howie PW, McNeilly AS. (1983): Factors affecting the duration of breast feeding. 1. Measurement of breast milk intake in the first week of life. Early Hum Dev, 8, 49-54.

22. Neville MC, & Keller R. (1984): Accuracy of single- and two-feed test weighing in assessing 24h breast milk production. Early Hum Dev, 9, 275-281.

23. Whitehead RG, Rowland MGM, Hutton M, Prentice AM, Muller E & Paul A. (1978): Factors influencing lactation performance in rural Gambian mothers. Lancet, ii, 178-181.

24. Williams AF, Greasley V, & Baum JD. Measurement of 24h breast milk intake in infancy. A method for estimating intake from shorter periods of observation. (Unpublished observations).

25. Dewey KG, Lönnerdal B. (1983): Breast milk intake: variations in breast-feeding practices. Am J Clin Nutr, 38, 152-153.

26. Black AE, Cole TJ, Wiles SJ, White F. (1983): Daily variation in food intake of infants from 2 to 18 months. Hum Nutr: Appl Nutr, 37A, 448-458.

27. Butte N, Garza C, Smith EO, Nichols BL. (1984): Human milk intake and growth in exclusively breast-fed infants. J Pediatr, 104, 187-195.

28. Prentice A, Prentice AM, Whitehead RG. (1981): Breast-milk fat concentrations of rural African women. 1. Short-term variations within individuals. Br J Nutr, 45, 483-494.

29. Lucas A, Lucas PJ, Baum JD. (1980): The nipple-shield sampling system: a device for measuring the dietary intake of breast-fed infants. Early Hum Dev, 4, 365-372.

30. How TV, Ashmore MP, Rolfe P, Lucas A, Lucas PJ, & Baum JD. (1979): A Doppler Ultrasound technique for measuring human milk flow. J Med Eng & Technol, 3, 66-71.

31. How TV, Rolfe P, Baum JD. (1980): A Doppler Ultrasound human milk flowmeter: theory and *in vitro* characteristics. In: Rolfe P, ed, Fetal and Neonatal Physiological Measurements. Pitman Medical, 206-219.

32. Woolridge MW, How TV, Drewett RF, Rolfe P, Baum JD. (1982): A method for the continuous measurement of milk intake during breast-feeding. Early Hum Dev, 6, 365-373.

33. McLeod CN, Rolfe P, Burton PJ. (1982): A pocket solid-state recorder for Doppler signals. Ultrasound in Med & Biol, 8, Suppl 1, 126. (Abstract).

34. Coward WA, Sawyer MB, Whitehead RG, Prentice AM, Evans J. (1979): New method for measuring milk intakes in breast-fed babies. Lancet, ii, 13-14.

35. Coward WA, Cole TJ, Sawyer MB, Prentice AM, Orr-Ewing, AK. (1982): Breast milk intake measurement in mixed-fed infants by administration of deuterium oxide to their mothers. Hum Nutr: Clin Nutr, 36C, 141-148.

36. Butte NF, Garza C, Smith EO, Nichols BL. (1983): Evaluation of the deuterium dliution technique against the test-weighing procedure for the determination of breast milk intake. Am J Clin Nutr, 37, 996-1003.

37. Nagy KA, Costa DP. (1980): Water flux in animals: analysis of potential errors in the tritiated water method. Am J Physiol, 238, R454-465.

SECTION II. TOTAL PROTEIN AND NON-PROTEIN NITROGEN IN HUMAN MILK

WORKSHOP PARTICIPANTS

B. Lönnerdal, Department of Nutrition, University of California, Davis, California

L. Hambraeus, Institute of Nutrition, University of Uppsala, Uppsala, Sweden

S. A. Atkinson, Department of Pediatrics, McMasters University, Hamilton, Ontario

P. R. Borum, Department of Food Science and Human Nutrition, University of Florida, Gainesville, Florida

B. L. Larson, Department of Dairy Science, University of Illinois, Urbana, Illinois

INTRODUCTION

The importance of accuracy in the measurement of proteins and other nitrogenous substances in human milk is gaining recognition. From the perspective of infant nutrition, accurate analysis is important both for identification and quantitation of the functional proteins and for estimation of the utilizable nitrogen sources in milk. This information is important for the optimal design of infant formula.

The term "protein" covers a broad spectrum of compounds; the total protein component of breast milk includes caseins, whey proteins, fat globule membrane proteins, immunoglobulins, enzymes, vitamin and mineral binding proteins and even cellular proteins. These proteins have different physicochemical properties, functions and nutritional significance. For this reason, the study of the individual proteins in human milk assumes great importance.

Human milk contains several nitrogenous compounds that may potentially be utilized for protein synthesis (such as peptides, free amino acids and amino sugars), in energy metabolism (such as carnitine and choline) and for amino acid synthesis (such as urea and ammonia). Thus, there is also a need for methods identifying and quantitating the non-protein nitrogen components of human milk. This will provide a basis for assessing their physiological function.

The following papers focus on the currently employed methods for the measurement of nitrogenous substances in milk. They also address the limitations of these methods and the directions for future development of methodology needed to define the complete profile of nitrogen-containing compounds in milk.

METHODS FOR STUDYING THE TOTAL PROTEIN CONTENT OF HUMAN MILK

B. Lönnerdal

There is a recognizable need for the analysis of the protein content of human milk. Several different methods and variations of these methods are used for this analysis; the different methods yield different results. This raises concerns with regard to the physiological significance of such data. The methods each have their advantages and disadvantages, but there has been no general consensus of preferred methodology. This paper discusses the commonly used methods, their validity and the significance of the data obtained.

THE DILEMMMA OF TOTAL PROTEIN ANALYSIS

Since protein is a loosely defined term, the meaning of the "total protein" content of human milk will not only depend upon the method used, but will also depend upon the purpose of the analysis and its physiological interpretation. The method of choice should have advantages and limitations consistent with meeting the purpose of the study. Studies involving the role of protein in human milk evolve from essentially two viewpoints: 1) from a mammary-physiology point of view, i.e., synthesis and transmembrane fluxes of macromolecules, and 2) from an infant nutritional/physiological point of view. This latter role of milk proteins comprises not only a conventional role as the nutrient source of nitrogen and amino acids, but also as a functional role of its protein components, e.g., immunoglobulins and lactoferrin (1).

From a biochemical point of view, protein is defined by size, i.e., polypeptides of molecular weights greater than 6000 (about 50 amino acids). However, from a nutritional point of view, this classification is of minor relevance. Since the nutritional importance of protein is as a source of amino acids and nitrogen, peptides of all sizes as well as free amino acids (and possibly urea) should also be considered. The size definition of protein may, of course, be of relevance from the point of view of mammary gland protein synthesis and translocation.

ANALYSIS OF TOTAL PROTEIN

Sample Handling and Storage

In many instances, e.g., in field work, it is not feasible to analyze the protein content of milk samples immediately. Therefore, the samples will be refrigerated or frozen for some time. For some of the methods of analyzing total protein, this may not have a pronounced effect; however, compartmentalization of proteins may be significantly affected. In addition, some proteins which are detected by enzymatic assays (e.g., lipase) or immunological methods (e.g., lactoferrin) may be reduced in activity/reactivity by storage (2). Two types of reactions are likely to occur with time: a) proteolytic degradation of proteases present in human milk, b) aggregation of proteins caused by freezing. Both these phenomena will give falsely low values for the components being analyzed. Although the extent to which these reactions occur in human milk is largely unknown, there are reports of loss of protein components with storage. It is also known that proteases are present in human milk (3,4); however, protease inhibitors are also present (5,6). Therefore, ideally, milk samples should be as fresh as possible when separated and analyzed. When this is not possible, appropriate controls for the effects of method and duration of storage are necessary.

PRINCIPLES OF ANALYTICAL METHODS

The methods used for total protein analysis can be divided into two major groups: 1) direct analysis, and 2) indirect analysis. The direct analyses include total nitrogen determination by means of Kjeldahl method and total amino acid analysis. These methods, which refer to specific and well-defined components, have been well established and can be used with a high degree of precision to analyze total nitrogen and total amino acid content, respectively. The results from the Kjeldahl analysis are sometimes expressed as "crude protein" by use of various conversion factors (7). However, these factors comprise an approximation which can be misleading, since the fraction of total nitrogen that is of non-protein origin can be substantial and highly variable. This distinction is especially important in the case of human milk.

Consequently, the use of conversion factors is not recommended to express the results obtained from human milk nitrogen analysis. Although amino acid analysis can be recommended as a precise method, this method often underestimates total amino acid content due to difficulties in recovery of tryptophan and cystein from acid hydrolysates.

The indirect methods of protein analyses are all based on certain characteristics of the protein molecule, e.g., tyrosine and phenylalanine content (Lowry), the peptide bond (Biuret), and dye-binding sites (Coomassie-Blue/BioRad, BCA method). Therefore, the choice of protein standard becomes critical since it must relate to the protein to be analyzed. Commonly, a bovine serum albumin (BSA) standard is used. However, this standard yields different results than a human immunoglobulin standard (8). One way to minimize these errors is to use a human milk reference standard which has been analyzed for protein content by means of a complete amino acid analysis. Dialyzed and freeze-dried breast milk protein has been proposed for its convenience as a potential reference standard; however, since several breast milk proteins contain significant carbohydrate moieties which may vary in composition, the weight of such a standard may not truly be representative of milk protein.

ANALYTICAL METHODS IN PRACTICE

Kjeldahl Method

One of the first methods employed for protein analysis was the Kjeldahl nitrogen determination. The nitrogen liberated by digestion with a combination of acids and a catalyst is determined as ammonia colorimetrically or by titration. Although this method previously required large amounts of sample and had very limited capacity for running larger number of samples, it has now been developed to overcome these shortcomings. Sensitive titrators or automatic spectrophotometric instruments have increased the sensitivity substantially to make this method a "micro-Kjeldahl." Because of the higher sensitivity of the analysis, less sample is required (0.5-1.0 ml) and this has made possible the digestion of large numbers of samples (30-60) simultaneously in heating blocks with even heat distribution (7,9). Cautions to be exercised include the tendency of early over-heating at the digestion step, the need of adequate sample size to be significantly above blank values, and the use of proper standards.

It should be emphasized that what is analyzed by this method is <u>nitrogen</u>, not protein. In most foods, protein constitutes the vast majority of total nitrogen, and therefore the well-known conversion factor of 6.25 can be used to multiply nitrogen in order to estimate protein (i.e., 16% of protein is nitrogen). It has previously been found that this conversion factor is not correct for cow's milk; therefore, a factor of 6.38 has been used in this instance. However, this factor is not correct for human milk; an unusually high proportion (20-30%) of nitrogen in human milk is nonprotein nitrogen (NPN) (7,10,11). If a conversion factor were to be used, it should be closer to 5.4-5.6, reflecting the lower than "normal" protein part of total nitrogen. However, the possibility of physiological variations in NPN concentration, of effects of diet on NPN proportion, etc., speaks against the use of such a factor. For example, we have previously shown that a change in the protein concentration of the diet of healthy nursing mothers after only four days significantly alters the concentration of NPN in breast milk (12).

To overcome this problem, the NPN fraction is often separated from the milk and analyzed separately. The NPN is separated by precipitation of the milk proteins with trichloroacetic acid (TCA) or perchloric acid followed by centrifugation. Supernatant (NPN) and pellet (protein) are analyzed for nitrogen separately. Using this method, the protein content of mature human milk was found to be 0.8-0.9% in several groups of women of varied nutritional status (13,14). These results correlated well with results obtained by amino acid analysis (7).

LOWRY METHOD

The advantages of the Lowry method (15) include large capacity, low sample volume, and lack of need for sophisticated equipment. However, this method has at least two drawbacks: a) the assay is subject to spectophotometric interference and b) different proteins have different "color value," i.e., each protein reacts with the color reagent to a different extent (8).

Various approaches have been taken to overcome interference, which is mostly caused by lipid and the presence of cells in milk. Use of a detergent, such as SDS, will disperse lipids and minimize interference (16). Not all laboratories have had success with this procedure for milk, however. Another approach is to separate the lipids and the cells by centrifugation prior to protein analysis. In this procedure, it must be recognized that the lipids do contain protein (fat globule membranes) as do the cells. The relative contribution of protein from these two compartments can be estimated to be <1% (17). Another approach is to extract the lipids with an organic solvent, thereby completely removing this source of interference (18).

The protein standard to be used for the Lowry analysis should be chosen with care. Conventionally, bovine serum albumin has been used for this purpose. This protein, however, has a relatively low color value in the Lowry assay. Preferably, a protein standard should be used which mimics the protein profile of the samples to be assayed. For analysis of human milk, this is a difficult task since human milk is a complex mixture of proteins, and the few pure proteins commercially available would hardly be representative of this complex mixture. It may be better to correlate the bovine serum albumin standard to human milk samples, in which the protein content has been determined by a different method (such as Kjeldahl or amino acid analysis). Problems with the use of a human milk protein standard have been mentioned above.

DYE-BINDING (BIO-RAD) ASSAY

This commercially available protein analysis kit (which is based on binding of Coomassie-blue dye) is often used in many laboratories (19). This method is subject to fewer interferences; however, the above-mentioned problems with varying color value may be even larger in this assay (8). An additional problem in our experience has been the instability of the protein standard provided. This may possibly be overcome by utilizing other types of standards.

BIURET ASSAY

The biuret method, based on the reaction of copper (II) ions with peptide linkages in an alkaline medium, has been widely used for measurement of serum proteins (20). It has a low sensitivity so that milk does not have to be diluted for use. However, there is a high background which cannot be attributed to milk protein and whose origin is currently unknown (21). For this reason, it should not be used for human milk.

BCA PROTEIN ASSAY

There is a new reagent for protein quantitation based on the reaction of bicinchoninic acid (BCA) with copper (I) produced in the presence of protein. It has recently been made available by Pierce Laboratories (22). The assay is simple to use. Recently one laboratory found it to give superior results for both precision and accuracy when compared to the other three colorimetric methods when analyzing milk samples standardized by Kjeldahl analysis (21). However, others have not found this method to yield satisfactory results (23). Validation by other laboratories is suggested.

AMINO ACID ANALYSIS

The most precise way to analyze protein together with its constituent amino acids and peptides is to perform amino acid analysis. However, the low capacity and high cost of this method will exclude it from routine use for human milk protein analysis. It can, though, serve to yield results on a limited number of samples which can subsequently be used as a standard for comparison to results obtained with other methods (7). As usually performed, tryptophan and cystein are not recovered in amino acid hydrolysates, leading to an approximately 3% underestimation of total milk amino acids. If an accurate analysis of these amino acids is desired, tryptophan can be measured by ion-exchange chromatography following base hydrolysis and cystein after performic acid oxidation.

SEPARATION OF MILK PROTEIN CLASSES

The major proteins in human milk can be separated into four major classes: fat globule membranes, casein, whey proteins and cellular proteins. The first step in the separation of these proteins is usually a centrifugation. By using low speed centrifugation (500 x g), milk cells can be sedimented. However, not much is known about the specificity of this method; the pellet found is very loose due to the low centrifugational force. Mature human milk contains few cells; the protein content of this compartment is very low (10,17). However, in colostrum, the cell number can be significantly higher (24).

The milk fat is usually separated by flotation (skimming) at about 5,000 x g. Again, some concern can be raised with regard to the specificity of this procedure -- the flotation layer is comparatively loose and skim milk proteins will be entrapped in this layer. Washing will reduce this problem to some extent (17). In our experience, ultracentrifugation (140,000 x g) has been a very effective method of separating the milk fat (25); a solid "cake" of compacted fat globules is obtained which is easily separated from the infranatant (whey).

Methods currently available for separation of specific milk proteins are discussed in the next paper (24).

REFERENCES

1. Hambreus L, Fransson G-B, Lönnerdal B. (1984): Nutritional availability of breast milk protein. *Lancet*, ii, 167-168.

2. Goldblum, RM, Goldman AS, Garza C, Johnson CA, Nichols BL. (1982): Human milk banking. II. Relative stability of immunologic factors in stored colostrum. Acta Paed Scand, 71, 143-146.

3. Lindberg T. (1979): Protease inhibitors in human milk. Pediatr Res, 13, 969-972.

4. Korycka-Dahl M, Ribadeau-Dumas B, Chene N, Martal J. (1983): Plasmin activity in milk. J Dairy Sci, 66, 704-711.

5. Barkholt-Pedersen V, Keil-Dlouha V, Keil B. (1971): On the properties of trypsin inhibitors from human and bovine colostrum. FEBS Lett, 17, 23-26.

6. Lindberg T, Ohlsson K, Westrom B. (1982): Protease inhibitors and their relation to protease activity in human milk. Pediatr Res, 16, 479-483.

7. Lönnerdal B, Forsum E, Hambraeus L. (1976): The protein content of human milk. I. A transverse study of Swedish normal material. Nutr Rep Int, 13, 125-134.

8. Lönnerdal B, Smith C, Keen CL. (1984): Analysis of breast milk -- current methodologies and future needs. J Pediatr Gastroenterol Nutr, 3, 290-295.

9. Hambraeus L, Forsum E, Abrahamsson L, Lönnerdal B. (1976): Automatic total nitrogen analysis in nutritional evaluations using a block digestor. Anal Biochem, 72, 78-85.

10. Macy IG. (1949): Composition of human colostrum and milk. Am J Dis Child, 78, 589-603.

11. Hytten FE. (1954): Clinical and chemical studies in human lactation. Br Med J, 1, 175-182.

12. Forsum E, Lönnerdal B. (1980): Effect of protein intake on protein and nitrogen composition of breast milk. Am J Clin Nutr, 33, 1809-1813.

13. Lönnerdal B, Forsum E, Hambraeus L. (1976): A longitudinal study of the protein, nitrogen and lactose content of human milk from Swedish well-nourished mothers. Am J Clin Nutr, 29, 1127-1133.

14. Lönnerdal B, Forsum E, Gebre-Medhin M, Hambraeus L. (1976): Breast milk composition in Ethiopian and Swedish mothers. II. Lactose, nitrogen, and protein contents. Am J Clin Nutr, 29, 1134-1141.

15. Lowry OH, Rosebrough NJ, Farr AL. (1951): Protein measurement with the Folin phenol reagent. J Biol Chem, 193, 265-275.

16. Peterson GL. (1977): A simplification of the protein assay method of Lowry et al. which is more generally applicable. Anal Biochem, 83, 346-356.

17. Huston GE, Patton S. Membrane distribution in human milk as revealed by phospholipid and cholestrerol analysis. These proceedings.

18. Patton S, Huston GE. (1984): A procedure for the determination of total protein in human milk. Nutr Rep Int, 30, 1401-1408.

19. Bradford MM. (1979): A rapid and sensitive method for the quantitation of microgram quantities of protein utilizing the principle of protein-dye binding. Anal Biochem, 72, 248-254.

20. Kingsley GR. (1942): The direct biurèt method for the determination of serum proteins as applied to photoelelectric and visual colorimetry. J. Lab Clin Med, 27, 840-845.

21. Keller, RP and Neville MC. (1985): Suitability of four colormetric methods for determination of total problem content of human milk. Fed Proc, 44, 1854.

22. Publication No 23225. Pierce Chemical Company, PO Box 117, Rockford, IL, 61105, U.S.A.

23. Lönnerdal B, Glazier C, Woodhouse LR. Compartmentalization and quantitation of protein in human milk. XIII International Congress of Nutrition. Brighton, U. K. (In press).

24. Paape MJ and Keller M. Determination of numbers and functions of cells in human milk. These proceedings.

25. Fransson G-B, Lönnerdal, B. (1983): Distribution of trace elements and minerals in human and cow's milk. Pediatr Res, 17, 912-915.

DETERMINATION OF SPECIFIC MILK PROTEINS

B. L. Larson

The major families of proteins found in milk bear a strong relationship between species. Many homologous proteins are present, but considerable species difference exists in the relative amounts of specific proteins present. Methods developed for the determination of constituents in milk of one species may not always be applicable to another. For example, direct application of methods developed with bovine milk to the analysis of human milk for determining the nitrogen distribution in the major protein fractions (casein, whey proteins, proteose-peptone, non-protein nitrogen) has led to erroneous values in the literature (1,2). Certain whey proteins in human milk tend to coprecipitate with casein, thereby increasing its apparent content while decreasing that of the whey protein (3,4). Human milk also has a much lower casein content and a higher non-protein nitrogen content that tends to magnify relative errors in isolation procedures. α-Lactalbumin does not precipitate with casein in heated human milk and is included in the proteose-peptone fraction (5). These examples serve to illustrate that caution must be used in applying a general method that was developed for milk of one species to milk of another. Analysis of individual proteins rather than fractions is highly desirable.

Nevertheless, there are many similarities in the milk proteins between species (6). The following discussion concerns those major proteins found in skim milk. The milk protein system most extensively studied is that of the bovine. Homologues of the major families of milk proteins characterized, that differ by varying numbers of amino acids, are being found in the milks of other species (6,7). Genetic variants for many milk proteins exist within a species. The casein family of homologous proteins, first identified in the bovine as single gene products of a related cluster of genes, are α_{S1}-casein, α_{S2}-casein, β-casein and κ-casein. Reliable estimates for their relative concentrations have been reported only for the bovine and similar species (6,8,9) where αS_1-casein and β-casein are present in approximately similar concentrations and together comprise about three-fourths of the total casein. κ-casein and α_{S2}-casein comprise the remainder of bovine casein with approximately similar concentrations.

Care is needed in interpreting studies on casein proteins in other species. Similar Greek letter designations have been used for constituents based on some characteristic in a separation process which may not necessarily correspond to the same homologous bovine protein. This caution is especially true for studies concerning rat milk casein proteins (10,11). Most studies on human milk casein proteins have followed the nomenclature developed for the bovine system.

Table 1. Proteins in Human and Bovine Milk*

	HUMAN	BOVINE
	mg/100 ml	
α-Lactalbumin	250	125
β-Lactoglobulin	0	300
Lactoferrin	175	tr
Lysozyme	45	tr
Serum albumin	50	50
IgA	125	7
IgG	4	45
IgM	3	7
Free secretory component	?	5
Caseins	250	2800
Total protein	900	3500

* Approximate average values summarized from Jenness (1,6) and Blanc (2).
tr trace present
? unknown

The casein proteins (6,12) undergo considerable post-translational modification after synthesis to exist in milk chiefly as a micellar complex along with phosphate, calcium and other minerals and materials (13). Human casein tends to complex with more whey proteins and contains considerably more carbohydrate components and less phosphate than bovine casein (1,2). β-casein is the most studied human casein component (14-16) and is thought to comprise about one-half of the total casein, with κ-casein comprising about one-fifth (17). The presence and status of α_{S1}-casein and α_{S2}-casein in human milk are less certain (6). κ-casein contains about 40% carbohydrate constituents and one phosphate per mol (17). β-casein is present in multiphosphorylated forms (14,16). Potential quantification procedures are complicated by the unphosphorylated form (18) and polypeptides (γ-caseins) derived from β-casein by splitting with plasmin (19).

Although qualitative procedures exist -- such as gel electrophoresis (20,21) -- there are no routine quantitative assay methods available for the individual human casein proteins. Chemical separation methods and column procedures, such as alkylated casein in urea solutions, that have been used for bovine casein are complicated but potentially adaptable (8,9). Quantitative immunological procedures have been slow to develop for various reasons, including a lack of purified preparations and a lack of formation of precipitating antibodies. These shortcomings should be overcome as new immunological techniques are applied and suitable antibodies to the individual casein proteins become available (10).

The characterization of the human casein proteins has been a research area slow in developing, due in small part to the complexity of the human casein system, but primarily to a lack of funding. Significant biofunctions, beyond the availability of important nutrients, have not been ascribed to date for specific casein proteins. In contrast, the isolation and characterization of the bovine-specific casein proteins were accomplished a decade ago (6,22-25). A strong driving force for such studies was the necessity to understand the physiochemical properties of the complex casein system for the commercial utilization of bovine milks. A current developing impetus for identifying individual casein proteins in laboratory animals has been their increasing use as model systems for the study of hormonal control of milk protein gene expression (10,11).

The whey proteins have been far more conducive to the development of quantitative assay methods. Specific biofunctions ascribed to most of them have stimulated research in this area (1,2). Several homologous major whey proteins are present in the milks of all or most species (6), but that does not mean that they have the same structure and behave similarly. Antisera to a protein in the milk of one species does not cross-react with that homologous protein from another species unless the two species are closely related. The approximate concentrations of the major homologous whey proteins in human and bovine milk are summarized in Table 1. α-Lactalbumin and lactoferrin are the major human whey proteins and IgA is the predominant immunoglobulin. Ruminant milk wheys contain the major proteins β-lactoglobulin and α-lactalbumin with IgG as the dominant immunoglobulin. The amounts of these proteins vary widely between species.

Individual whey proteins have been determined by a wide variety of methods summarized in Table 2. Separation procedures using labeled precursors have been useful for determining concentrations and net synthesis of these proteins in secretions both *in vivo* and *in vitro* cell cultures for those proteins synthesized in the mammary secretory cells (α-lactalbumin, β-lactoglobulin, caseins) (9,12,26). Such methods are not applicable to proteins coming into the milk from some other source, such as serum albumin (blood), immunoglobulins (blood, plasma cells), and

Table 2. Milk Protein Determination Methods

METHODS	REFERENCES
Separation -	
Isolation (pH, salts, solvents), column (ion exchange, molecular weight, etc.), use of tracers (^3H, ^{14}C, ^{32}P), milk protein carriers, etc.	(8,9,26,27)
Electrophoresis -	
Moving boundary, paper, acetate, slab, polyacrylamide gel, agarose gel, etc.	(9,17,20,21,27,28)
Immunological -	
Precipitin, Oudin, radial diffusion, radioimmunoassay, immunoelectrophoresis, fluorescent antibody, antibody conjugated enzymes, etc.	(10,28-34)

perhaps lactoferrin whose origin in milk may be from more than one source (1,12). Methods of greatest sensitivity and reliability have been both enzymatic and immunological procedures which also require a small sample size. Relatively simple gel single and double diffusion procedures have been successful with α-lactalbumin, β-lactoglobulin, serum albumin, IgA, IgG1, IgG2, IgM and lactoferrin. Radioimmunoassay procedures are also being widely used for α-lactalbumin and β-lactoglobulin. Other procedures are available as well.

Methods for the determination of enzymes in milk are included in a vast literature (35,36). In bovine milk, several are of commercial importance (phosphatase, lipase, xanthine oxidase, lactoperoxidase). α-Lactalbumin is also readily determined by its specifier role in the lactose synthase reaction (37). Proteins associated with the milk fat globule membrane, which is derived from the plasma membrane surrounding the secretory cell, form another complex family of milk proteins of diverse properties (38). These proteins comprise about 1% of the total milk proteins (39).

REFERENCES

1. Jenness R. (1979): The composition of human milk. Sem Perinatol 3, 225-239.

2. Blanc B. (1981): Biochemical aspects of human milk-comparison with bovine milk. Wld Rev Nutr, 36, 1-89.

3. Lönnerdal B, Forsum E. (1985): Casein content of human milk. Am J Clin Nutr, 41, 113-120.

4. Nagasawa T, Kiyosawa I, Takase M. (1974): Lactoferrin and serum albumin of human casein in colostrum and milk. J Dairy Sci, 57, 1159-1163.

5. Bezkorovainy A, Nichols JH, Sly DA. (1976): Proteose-peptone fractions of human and bovine milk. Internat J Biochem, 7, 639-645.

6. Jenness R. (1982): Inter-species comparisons of milk proteins. In: Fox PF, ed, Developments in Dairy Chemistry. Essex, England: Applied Life Publ Ltd, 87-114.

7. Mercier J-C, Chobert J-M. (1976): Comparative study of the amino acid sequences of the casein macropeptides from seven species. FEBS Lett, 72, 208-214.

8. Davies DT, Law AJR. (1977): An improved method for the quantitative fractionation of casein mixtures using ion-exchange chromatography. J Dairy Sci 44, 213-221.

9. Larson BL, Andersen CR. (1973): Evaluation of milk protein synthesis. In: Kruse PF, Patterson MK, eds, Methods and Applications of Tissue Culture. New York: Academic Press, 589-593.

10. Kaetzel CS, Ray DB. (1984): Immunological characterization with monoclonal antibodies of three major caseins and alpha-lactalbumin from rat milk. J Dairy Sci, 67, 64-75.

11. Rosen JM, Matusik RJ, Richards DA, Gupta P, Rodgers JR. (1980): Multi-hormonal regulation of casein gene expression at the transcriptional and posttranslational levels in the mammary gland. Recent Prog Horm Res, 36, 157-193.

12. Larson BL. (1979): Biosynthesis and secretion of milk proteins: a review. J Dairy Res, 46, 161-174.

13. McMahon DJ, Brown RJ. (1984): Composition, structure and integrity of casein micelles: a review. Dairy Sci, 67, 499-512.

14. Groves ML, Gordon WG. (1970): The major component of human casein: a protein phosphorylated at different levels. Arch Biochem Biophys, 140, 47-51.

15. Nagasawa T, Kiosawa I, Kuwahara K. (1970): Human casein. II. Isolation of human β-casein fraction and human β-casein B. J Dairy Sci, 53, 136-145.

16. Greenburg R, Groves ML, Dower HJ. (1984): Human β-casein amino acid sequence and identification of phosphorylation sites. J Biol Chem, 259, 5132-5138.

17. Yamauchi K, Azuma N, Kobayashi H, Kaminogawa S. (1981): Isolation and properties of human κ-casein. J. Biochem, 90, 1005-1012.

18. Monti JC, Jolles P. (1982): Characterization of a thermosensitive protein from human milk whey. Experientia, 38, 1211-1213.

19. Greenberg R, Groves ML. (1984): Plasmin cleaves human β-casein. Biochem Biophys Res Communic, 120, 463-468.

20. Anderson NG, Powers MT, Tollaksen SL. (1982): Proteins of human milk. I. Identification of major components. Clin Chem, 28, 1045-1055.

21. Swaisgood HE, Larson BL, Kalan EB, Brunner JR, Morr CV, Hansen PMT. (1974): Methods of gel electrophoresis of milk proteins. Champaign, IL: Amer Dair Sci Assoc, 33 pp.

22. Brunner JR. (1981): Cow milk proteins: twenty-five years of progress. J Dairy Sci, 64, 1038-1054.

23. Eigel WN, Butler JE, Ernstrom CA, Farrell Jr HM, Harwalker VR, Jenness R, Whitney RMcL. (1984): Nomenclature of proteins of cow's milk, 5th revision. J Dairy Sci, 67, 1599-1631.

24. Brignon G, Ribadeau-Dumas B, Mercier J-C, Pelissier J-P. (1977): Complete amino acid sequence of bovine α_{S2}-casein. FEBS Lett, 76, 274-279.

25. Grosclaude F, Mercier J-C, Ribadeau-Dumas B. (1970): Structure primaire de la caseine α_{S1}-bovine. Eur J Biochem, 14, 98-107.

26. Groves TDD, Larson BL. (1965): Preparation of specifically labeled milk proteins using bovine mammary cell cultures. Biochim Biophys Acta, 104, 462-469.

27. Lönnerdal B, Forsum E, Hambraeus L. (1976): The protein content of human milk. I. A transversal study of Swedish normal material. Nutr Rpts Internat, 13, 125-134.

28. Laurell C-B. (1966): Quantitative estimation of proteins by electrophoresis in agarose gel containing antibodies. Anal Biochem, 15, 45-52.

29. Kleinberg DL, Todd J, Groves ML. (1977): Studies on human α-lactalbumin: radioimmunoassay measurements in normal human breast and breast cancer. J Clin Endocrinol Metab, 45, 1238-1250.

30. Larson BL, Hageman EC. (1963): Determination of α-lactalbumin in complex systems. J Dairy Sci, 46, 14-18.

31. Leary HL Jr, Larson BL, Nelson, DR. (1982): Immunohistochemical localization of IgG1 and IgG2 in prepartum and lactating bovine mammary tissue. Vet Immuno Immunopath, 3, 509-514.

32. Mancini G, Carbonara AO, Heremans JF. (1965): Immunochemical quantitation of antigens by single radial immunodiffusion. Immunochemistry, 2, 235-254.

33. Fahey JL, McKelvey EM. (1965): Quantitative determination of serum immunoglobulins in antibody-agar plates. J Immunol, 94, 84-90.

34. Forsum E, Lönnerdal B. (1980): Effect of protein intake on protein and nitrogen composition of breast milk. Amer J Clin Nutr, 33, 1809-1813.

35. Shahani K, Kwan AJ, Friend BA. (1980): Role and significance of enzymes in human milk. Amer J Clin Nutr, 33, 1861-1868.

36. Hamosh M, Freed LM, Jones JB, Berkow SE, Bitman J, Mehta NR, Happ B and Hamosh P. Enzymes in human milk. These proceedings.

37. Fitzgerald DK, Colvin B, Mawal R, Ebner KE. (1970): Enzymic assay for galatosyl transferase activity of lactose synthetase and α-lactalbumin in purified and crude systems. Anal Biochem, 36, 43-61.

38. McPherson AV, Kitchen BJ. (1983): Reviews of the progress of dairy science: the bovine milk globule membrane - its formation, composition, structure and behaviour in milk and dairy products. J Diary Res, 50, 107-133.

39. Huston GE and Patton S. Membrane distribution in human milk as revealed by phospholipid and cholesterol analysis. These proceedings.

CHARACTERIZATION OF THE NON-PROTEIN NITROGEN FRACTION OF HUMAN MILK: METHODOLOGICAL CONSIDERATIONS

S. A. Atkinson

INTRODUCTION

The observation that non-protein nitrogen comprises 20 to 25% of total nitrogen in human milk (1-4) but only 3 to 5% in cows' milk (5) has been documented for some time. The major contributors to the non-protein nitrogen fraction of human milk have been identified as peptides, urea, free amino acids, (2,3,6), amino sugars, (7), creatine, creatinine (1,6), uric acid, ammonia (1,3,6), carnitine (8), choline (9), the polyamines (11) and acid-soluble nucleotides (10). However, the nitrogen contained in these components does not account for the total acid-soluble nitrogen content as determined by Kjeldahl analysis following deproteinization (3,6).

Complete characterization of the non-protein nitrogen containing constituents of human milk is important in order to identify those components which may be physiologically significant to the nutrition of the neonate. This paper will provide a critical evaluation of the methods previously applied to characterize and quantitate the non-protein nitrogen components of human milk. It will also suggest future directions for method development and nomenclature of components in this area of human milk biochemistry.

TOTAL NON-PROTEIN NITROGEN (NPN)

Most commonly, the NPN fraction of human milk has been obtained by precipitation of the milk proteins with 12% (w/v) trichloroacetic acid from defatted milk samples (3,4,13), followed by centrifugation. The total acid-soluble nitrogen in the supernatant is then determined by the micro-Kjeldahl technique (14), and the individual components are assayed by specific methods detailed later in this paper. Alternatively, milk has been dialyzed at $5^{o}C$ against changes of deionized water. This was done using cellulose membranes of specific pore size (molecular weight cut-off points of 3500 to 14,000) (15,16). In comparing the two methods, Atkinson (15) found the dialysis procedure to yield lower values for total NPN when the molecular weight cut-off size of pore membranes was 12,000 to 14,000. The percentage of total nitrogen as NPN represented 20.9 $\pm$ 1.9% and 25.1 $\pm$ 2.3%, for the dialyzable and acid-soluble methods, respectively (15). Discrepancies in the NPN measured by Kjeldahl analysis after dialysis versus that obtained by chemical precipitation methods have also been observed in the NPN analysis of cheese whey (17).

UREA

Nitrogen derived from urea has been reported to comprise anywhere from 11 to 52% of NPN in human milk (1,3,5,13). Reported differences in quantitation of urea may be related to the analytical procedures employed: calculation of the urea peak obtained by column chromatography for determination of physiological (free) amino acids in milk (3,18) versus an enzymatic (urease) assay procedure (19). Urea values for human milk derived by both methods were comparable in some studies (3,19), while in another study column chromatography yielded extremely low values (18). Care is required in obtaining good peak separation for urea early in the chromatogram. Urea in milk may also vary directly with the level of circulating urea levels in the plasma of lactating women (6) and with the stage of lactation (3,13). Further systematic evaluation of the contribution of urea to the NPN fraction of human milk is desirable.

PEPTIDES

The peptide fraction of human milk has been estimated to contribute 4 to 5% of the total amino acids (6). The amino acids in this fraction were quantitated in the hydrolyzed supernatant obtained after deproteinization with 5% sulfosalicylic acid (6). Preparative hydrolysis of milk samples for amino acid analysis is generally carried out in 6 N HCl for 22 to 72 hours at 110 to 115°C (15,16), but a procedure using 8 N methanesulfonic acid at 115°C for 48 hours has also been described (6). A comparative study of these methods within one laboratory has not been reported.

Dialysis of human milk samples using a membrane pore molecular weight cut-off of 3500 yielded a NPN representing 10.8 $\pm$ 4.5% of total nitrogen (15). Variation between milk samples for this fraction was great (Range - 4.8 to 17.1% of total nitrogen), likely reflecting the inconsistency of pore membrane sizes in this cut-off range. Nevertheless, comparing these values with those obtained using membranes of 13,000-14,000 molecular weight cut-off (described above), suggests that a fair proportion of the non-protein fraction has a molecular weight of >3500 and is likely comprised of peptides.

FREE AMINO ACIDS

Free amino acids in human milk represent 3 to 5% of the total amino acids (6,20) and contribute 8% (3) to 22% (6) of the nitrogen in the NPN fraction. Generally, delipidated milk is prepared for analysis of amino acids by deproteinization with dry sulfosalicylic acid (50 to 70 mg/ml milk), mixing and centrifugation (3,6). Deproteinization of milk for amino acid analysis has also been done with 10% (w/v) trichloroacetic acid (19,21). In one case this was followed by extraction of the supernatant with diethyl ether for the stated purpose of removing the trichloroacetic acid and minimizing the protein binding that the authors suggest occurs when using sulfosalicylic acid as a precipitant (19). However, the latter method has not been sytematically evaluated against the more frequently employed sulfosalicylic acid precipitation method. By comparing reported free amino acid levels of milk at similar lactational stages using these two methods of precipitation, trichloroacetic acid precipitation (19) yielded similar values for 11 amino acids and lower values for 11 other amino acids, relative to the sulfosalicylic method (3). Clearly, further evaluation of the two methods is required.

AMINO SUGARS

Amino sugars which are components of the oliosaccharides in milk, may make a relatively large contribution to the NPN fraction of human milk. For example, N-acetylglucosamine has been quantitated in milk (7,15,21), and it has been demonstrated that it decreases with progressing lactation (15). The contribution of nitrogen from glucosamine, as it is determined following acid hydrolysis of human milk, would represent approximately 15 to 20% of the total NPN (Atkinson, unpublished observations). However, it is unlikely that the major portion of glucosamine quantitated in this manner is derived from the acid-soluble NPN fraction. In addition to being a major carbohydrate component of glycopeptides (MW~4000)in human milk whey precipitate, N-acetylglucosamine is also a carbohydrate component of glycoproteins (MW>26,000 to 35,000) (8,21). Thus, N-acetylglucosamine and other amino sugars would be distributed among both the acid-soluble and protein-precipitant fractions of human milk. The relative partition of nitrogen-containing sugars between the protein and non-protein fractions of milk has yet to be delineated.

CREATININE AND CREATINE

The levels of creatinine and creatine in human milk are usually determined by a method that addresses the reaction between picric acid and creatinine. This method is based on the technique described by Folin and Wu (22). The analyses yield concentrations of creatinine and creatine in milk which would contribute approximately 2 mg N/dl to the NPN fraction (1). Neville et al. (23) recently obtained a value of about 2 mg/dl for the creatinine content of mature milk.

URIC ACID AND AMMONIA

Nitrogen derived from uric acid and ammonia in human milk each contribute <1% to the NPN (3,6). The level of uric acid is determined by the uricase method adapted from plasma analyses (16). Use of a kit such as the Pierce Uric Acid Rapid Stat Kit (No. 41000, Pierce Chemical Co., Rockford, Ill.) is suggested. Ammonia levels can be determined after steam distillation of the alkalinated milk sample by titration with a dilute HCl solution to a colorimetric (23) or pH endpoint. Alternatively, ammonia levels may be determined on the protein-free, acid-soluble supernatant by standard physiological fluid-amino-acid analysis (3). Proper handling and storage of samples are of extreme importance in preserving the original ammonia concentration of expressed milk.

OTHER NITROGENOUS SUBSTANCES

Polyamines (11) and nucleotides (10,12) have been quantitated in human milk, but their contribution to the NPN would be much less than 1% (12). Choline (9), carnitine (8) and other small nitrogen-containing molecules would also contribute minimally to the nitrogen in the NPN fraction. The methodology for carnitine analysis is discussed elsewhere in this volume.

RECOVERY OF NPN IN HUMAN MILK

Failure to quantitatively recover the total or acid-soluble nitrogen from the calculated nitrogen contribution of the major component parts has been noted by several investigators. Unaccounted nitrogen was reported as 2.3% of total nitrogen by Shahani and Sommers (24). Quantitation of the total amino acid nitrogen, urea nitrogen and glucosamine nitrogen left 9 to 14% of the total nitrogen content determined by Kjeldahl analysis unaccounted for in a more recent study (6). In summing the component parts of the NPN fraction of human milk, Atkinson, et al. (3) quantitatively recovered a maximum of 46% of the NPN based on analysis of free amino acids, urea, uric acid and ammonia. This relatively low calculated recovery of NPN suggested that a major unidentified component might be peptide N which would be part of the acid-soluble supernatant after trichloroacetic acid deproteinization (3). However, Svandberg (6), who directly quantitated the total and free amino acids in the acid-soluble supernatant after protein precipitation, estimated peptide amino acids to be quantitatively similar to the free amino acids. Perhaps, then, the disparity in nitrogen recovery from Kjeldahl analysis or summation of the nitrogen contribution from individually quantitated amino acids may reflect the methodological errors inherent in the measurement of amino acids by ion exchange chromatography. For example, the standard conditions employed for protein hydrolysis vary according to time, temperature and type of acid, which may in turn affect recovery of amino acids such as cystine (25), tryptophan (19,26), glutamine (19), methionine (6) and taurine (27).

In considering another major source of error in quantitating "true" non-protein nitrogen, the analysis of nitrogen-containing oligosaccharides must be addressed. Analysis of N-acetylglucosamine suggested that amino sugars may contribute considerable nitrogen to the NPN fraction (15). However, quantitation of glucosamine and other amino sugars in the acid-soluble supernatant, rather than in the whole milk samples, must be completed before the partition of nitrogen derived from oligosaccharides can be delineated between the protein and non-protein nitrogen fractions of milk.

Finally, I would urge reconsideration of the nomenclature associated with the characterization of nitrogen components of human milk. Obviously, nitrogenous substances such as amino sugars, which physiologically may be considered as "non-protein" or "non-utilizable" nitrogen, will be precipitated with proteins or remain in the retentate following dialysis under the conditions described in this paper. Perhaps the term "non-protein nitrogen" should be replaced with "acid-soluble nitrogen" when referring to nitrogen components in the supernatant following acid precipitation. This approach might also resolve the misconception of assuming "non-protein nitrogen" to be synonymous with "non-utilizable nitrogen." Certainly peptides, amino acids and possibly urea (28,29) in human milk are nitrogen-containing substrates for protein synthesis in the infant.

Clearly, complete characterization and quantitative recovery of the non-protein nitrogen-containing constituents of human milk will have to be achieved before the magnitude of the physiological significance of the various NPN components to the functional and protein requirements of the infant can be addressed.

ACKNOWLEDGEMENT

Dr. Atkinson is supported by a Career Scientist Award from the Ministry of Health of Ontario.

REFERENCES

1. Macy IG. (1949): Composition of human colostrum and milk. Am J Dis Child, 78, 589-603.

2. Lönnerdal B, Forsum E and Hambraeus L. (1976): The protein content of human milk. I. A transversal study of Swedish normal material. Nutr Rept Internat, 13, 125-134

3. Atkinson SA, Anderson GH and Bryan MH. (1980): Human milk: comparison of the nitrogen composition in milk from mothers of premature and full-term infants. Am J Clin Nutr, 33, 811-815.

4. Lemons JA, Moye L, Hall D, Simmons M. (1982): Differences in the composition of preterm and term human milk during early lactation. Pediatr Res, 16, 113-117.

5. Hambreaus L. (1977): Proprietary milk versus human breast milk in infant feeding: a critical appraisal from the nutritional point of view. Pediatr Clin N Am, 34, 17-36.

6. Svanberg U. Gebre-Medhin M, Ljungvist B and Olsson M. (1977): Breast milk composition in Ethiopian and Swedish mothers. III. Amino acids and other nitrogenous substances. Am J Clin Nutr, 30, 499-507.

7. Bezkorovainy A and Nichols JH. (1976): Glycoproteins from mature human milk whey. Pediatr Res, 10, 1-5.

8. Sandor A, Pecsuvac K, Kerner J and Alkonyi I. (1982): On carnitine content of the human breast milk. Pediatr Res, 16, 89-91.

9. Zeisel SH, Stanbury JB, Wurtman RJ, Brigida M, Fierro-Benitez R. (1982): Choline content of mothers' milk in Ecuador and Boston. N Engl J Med, 306, 175-176

10. Johke T. (1963): Acid-soluble nucleotides of colostrum, milk, and mammary gland. J. Biochemistry, 54, 388-397.

11. Sanguansermsri J, Gyorgy P and Zilliken F. (1974): Polyamines in human and cow's milk. Am J Clin Nutr, 27, 859-865.

12. Janas LM and Picciano MF. (1982): The nucleotide profile of human milk. Pediatr Res, 16, 659-662.

13. Hambraeus L, Lönnerdal B, Forsum E and Gebre-Medhin M. (1978): Nitrogen and protein components of human milk. Acta Paediatr Scand, 67, 561-565.

14. Horowitz W, ed. (1965): Milk: total nitrogen. In: Official Methods of Analysis, 10th ed. Washington, D. C.: Association of Official Analytical Chemists, 223.

15. Atkinson SA. (1980): Human milk feeding of premature infants <1.3 kg birthweight: milk analysis and clinical studies during early postnatal life. University of Toronto. (Thesis).

16. Forsum E and Lönnerdal B. (1979): Protein evaluation in growing rats of breast milk and breast milk substitutes with special reference to the content of non-protein nitrogen. J Nutr, 109, 185-192.

17. Rizvi SSH and Josephson RV. (1975): Determination of nonprotein nitrogen content of cheese whey. J Dairy Science, 58, 1521-1523.

18. Rassin DK, Sturman JA and Gaull GE. (1978): Taurine and other free amino acids in milk of man and other mammals. Early Hum Develop, 2/1, 1-13.

19. Harzer G, Franzke V, Bindels JG. (1984): Human milk non-protein nitrogen components, changing patterns of free amino acids and urea in the course of early lactation. Am J Clin Nutr, 40, 303-309.

20. Lemons JA, Reyman D and Moye L. (1983): Amino acid composition of preterm and term breast milk during early lactation. Early Human Develop, 8, 323-329.

21. Nichols JH, Bezkorovainy A and Paque R. (1975): Isolation and characterization of several glycoproteins from human colostrum whey. Biochim et Biophys Acta, 412, 99-108.

22. Folin O and Wu H. (1919): A system of blood analysis. J Biol Chem, 38, 81-110.

23. Neville MC, Keller RP, Seacat J, Casey CE, Allen JC and Archer P. (1984): Studies on human lactation: within feed and between breast variation in selected components of human milk. Am J Clin Nutr, 40, 635-646.

24. Shahani KM and Sommer HH. (1951): The protein and non-protein nitrogen fractions in milk. Methods of analysis. J Dairy Sci, 34, 1003-1009.

25. Moor S. (1963): On the determination of cystine as cysteic acid. J Biol Chem, 238, 235-237.

26. Matheson NA. (1974): The determination of tryptophan in purified proteins and in feeding-stuffs. Brit J Nutr, 31, 393-397.

27. Ebersdabler HF, Greulich HG, Trautwein E. (1983): Determination of taurine in foods and feeds using an amino acid analyzer. J Chromatography, 254, 332-334.

28. Snyderman SE, Holt LE, Dancis J, Roitman E, Boyer A, Bolis ME. (1962): "Unessential nitrogen:" a limiting factor for human growth. J Nutr, 78, 57-72.

29. Heine W, Tiess M, Stople HJ amd Wutzke K. (1984): Urea utilization by the intestinal flora, of infants fed mother's milk and a formula diet, as measured with the N-tracer technique. J Pediatr Gastroentero and Nutr, 3, 709-712.

SECTION III. IMMUNOLOGICAL COMPONENTS OF HUMAN MILK

WORKSHOP PARTICIPANTS

A. S. Goldman, The University of Texas Medical Branch, Galveston, Texas

B. Carlsson, University of Goteborg, Goteborg, Sweden

L. Pickering, University of Texas Medical School, Houston, Texas

M. Keller, U.C.L.A. School of Medicine, Harbor-UCLA Medical Center, Torrance, California

M. J. Paape, USDA/ARS Animal Sci. Inst. MSM Lab, Beltsville, Maryland

INTRODUCTION

During the last few decades, there has been a steady increase in research concerning the nature of the immunologic system in human milk and how the system protects the recipient infant. Investigations of those questions have been hampered because of the complexity of the system (1)

Table 1. Representative Immunologic Components in Human Milk

Bifidus growth factors	Non-antibody proteins and carbohydrates
Complement components	Anti-viral
Enzymes	Anti-bacterial
Lysozyme	Antitoxic
Bile salt stimulated lipase	
Nutrient binders	Antibodies
Lactoferrin	Secretory IgA
B12 binding proteins	IgM
	IgG
Anti-viral lipids	IgD
Anti-enterotoxin glycolipids (gangliosides)	
	Leukocytes
	Neutrophils
	Monocyte-macrophages
	Lymphocytes

(Table 1) and because of the necessity of adapting standard methods or innovating novel ones to study the host resistance factors in human milk.

During the Meadowridge Workshop, the methodologic issues which have posed problems in the investigation of the protective factors in human milk were discussed. These issues included the methods used to identify and investigate the functional capabilities of leukocytes in human milk, the application of immunochemical assays to the measurement of host resistance factors in human milk, the functional assessments of those resistance factors, and directions for future research. A synthesis of these discussions is presented in these papers.

REFERENCE

1. Goldman AS, Goldblum RM. (1984): Protective properties of human milk in nutrition in pediatrics. In: WA Walker, ed, Basic Science and Clinical Application. Little, Brown, and Co., 819-828.

IMMUNOCHEMICAL ASSAYS

A. S. Goldman
B. Carlsson
L. Pickering
M. Keller
M. J. Paape

Immunochemical methods are among the most valuable techniques for detecting and quantitating the protective factors in human milk. There are several important criteria, however, which must be considered in applying these techniques to the measurement of human milk components.

1. The specificity, sensitivity, and reproducibility of the method should be appropriate for the factor to be measured.

2. The standards should apply not only to purified components, but also to the quantitation of the factors in human milk.

3. The method should allow the measurement of the factor in the presence of other components of human milk.

4. The method should detect or quantitate the factor in compartments other than the aqueous phase of human milk.

5. If one wishes to examine the fate of human milk factors in the recipient infant, then the methods should be applicable for the detection of those components in other appropriate biologic fluids.

6. The methods should be readily adapted to laboratories other than that of the originators of the technique.

The most common immunochemical assays which are used for human milk as shown in Table 1. In applying these assays, a number of factors should be taken into consideration. These are discussed in the following sections.

SENSITIVITY-REPRODUCIBILITY OF ASSAYS

The method required to detect or quantitatively measure a factor depends upon the type and quantity of the factor and the research question. For example, if only small amounts of a factor (μg) are present, then a rather sensitive method, such as a solid-phase immunoassay, will be

Table 1. Strenths and Weaknesses of Immunologic Methods Used to Measure Components in Human Milk

METHODS	COMMERCIAL AVAILABILITY	SPECIFICITY[a]	SENSITIVITY[b]	REPRODUCIBILITY[c]
Nephelometry[d]	+++	++	+	+++
Radial immuno-diffusion	+++	++	++	+++
Electroimmuno-diffusion	±	+++[c]	+++	++
Immuno-fluorescence assays	+	+++[c]	++++	++
Enzyme-linked immunoassays	±	+++	++++	++
Radioim-immunoassays[e]	±	+++	++++	+++

[a] Depends upon specificity of antibody detector.
[b] See Table 2 for further information.
[c] Solid phase immunoassays are particularly suited to measure different molecular forms of the same factor.
[d] Turbidity of preparations interferes with measurement.
[e] Monitoring for radioactive contamination is required.

required. The ranges of sensitivity and reproducibility of common methods used to detect one of the components of the immunologic system in human milk, secretory IgA, are listed in Table 2.

THE MOLECULAR FORMS OF THE COMPONENT

The immunologic quantitation of certain factors in human milk is complicated by the simultaneous occurrence of more than one molecular form of the component. This is of particular importance when there are discrepancies in the function of different physical forms of the factor. For example, to measure secretory IgA (a form of IgA which is quite resistant to enzymatic digestion) in the presence of other forms of IgA, a solid-phase immunoassay is required which detects the secretory component bound to IgA (1,2). Other techniques, such as Western Blot methods coupled with labeled antibody detectors, should also prove to be valuable in identifying molecular moietes of proteins in human milk.

Table 2. Comparative Sensitivities and Reproducibilities of Certain Assays Used to Measure Human IgA

ASSAY	SENSITIVITY	REPRODUCIBILITY Coefficient of Variation
Nephelometric assay for total IgA in serum	100 μg/ml	2%
Radial immunodiffusion for total IgA in serum	20 μg/ml	5%
Electrical immunodiffusion for total IgA (5)	8 μg/ml	12%
Fluorescent immunosorbent assay for total and secretory IgA (5)	40 ng/ml	19%
Enzyme-linked immunosorbent assay with competitive inhibition for measuring secretory IgA in serum (6)	31 ng/ml	18%
Enzyme-linked immunosorbent assay for secretory IgA antibodies to type 1 pili from *Klebsiella pneumoniae* (5)	30 ng/ml	21% (same plate) 57% (different plate)

TYPES OF ANTIBODY DETECTORS

Until recent years, antibodies used to detect or quantitate antigens were produced by immunizing laboratory animals, such as rabbits or goats, with the antigens in question. These antisera have proven to be powerful reagents in immunologic research. There have been some drawbacks to their use, however. For example, antisera usually contain antibodies which are directed against several determinants on an antigen as well as against contaminating antigens in the immunizing preparation. This, of course, may be advantageous if the combined effect of several determinants is being investigated. In addition, the antibodies may be distributed in a number of immunoglobulin classes which may thus compete for the same antigenic determinants.

An alternative approach is the utilization of monoclonal antibodies directed against particular epitopes. The use of monoclonal antibodies circumvents the problems brought about by the presence of antibodies in heteroantisera that are directed against antigens other than the component which is to be assayed. The binding kinetics of the antibodies influence the test results. It should be understood that monoclonal antibodies are not useful in assays that require cross-linking, such as precipitation or hemagglutination. These limitations do not apply, however, to more sensitive solid-phase immunoassays. Thus, large quantities of highly specific antibodies of one immunoglobulin class provide considerable advantage in experimental studies. So far, however, only a few investigators have capitalized upon the opportunities to probe and measure human milk factors with monoclonal antibodies. Nevertheless, some studies have already demonstrated the applications of these hybridoma products to the measurement of some of these components (3-5).

STANDARDS

Regardless of the method chosen to quantitate a component, it is imperative that the correct standard be used. In some cases, a purified component will suffice as a standard. In other circumstances (6) human milk, with or without the component, should be used in constructing the standard graphs.

MEASUREMENTS OF FACTORS IN THE PRESENCE OF OTHER COMPONENTS

Although there are comparatively few data concerning this problem, some information is available. As previously mentioned, antibodies to more than one component in heteroantisera will alter qualitative or quantitative measurements. There are also instances where one component may be complexed to another, i.e., some lactoferrin to secretory IgA (7). It is undetermined, however, whether these complexes significantly alter the measurement of either component in the previously discussed assay systems. In addition, the turbidity of human milk precludes the use of certain immunoassays, such as immunonephelometric techniques, in which antigen-antibody aggregates are detected by light scattering (8).

COLLECTION AND PROCESSING PROCEDURES

Some assays may be useful for colostrum where the concentrations of many factors are high, but may not be useful for mature milk where the concentrations are significantly lower.

The time of collection (day versus night), the type of sample (e.g., partial or total collection from a breast), or the presence of bacterial contaminants may affect the composition of the milk specimen. In addition, there are indications that the type of collection container and the time and temperature of storage may affect the concentrations of certain immunologic components that can be detected in human milk. In human milk, secretory IgA antibodies to *Escherichia coli* somatic antigens are absorbed onto the surfaces of polyethylene containers (1). The concentrations of lactoferrin and lysozyme fall by 50% and 40%, respectively, after storage in pyrex or polypropylene at $4^{o}C$ for 24 hours, although the concentration of total SIgA does not change (1). Depending upon the degree and duration of treatment, heating procedures used to reduce microbial contaminants in milk may cause profound reductions (9) or increases (10) in the concentrations of the components. For example, the heating of human milk to $62.5^{o}C$ for 5 to 30 minutes destroys much of the lysozyme, lactoferrin, and secretory Iga (9), whereas those factors are preserved after heating at higher temperatures ($72^{o}C$) for shorter periods (1 to 3 seconds) (10). Extending the heating time (e.g., $72^{o}C$ for 30 seconds), may cause destruction of components (10).

Repeated freezing and thawing of milk samples is also known to denature many of the protein components in human milk, whereas freezing for protracted periods at -20° or -72°C usually preserves the components. If several assays are to be performed on one specimen, then it is best to either perform the measurements simultaneously or divide the specimen into a number of aliquots, which can be individually thawed when needed for analysis.

THE PHYSICAL DISTRIBUTION OF COMPONENTS IN HUMAN MILK

Although it is known that several nutrients are compartmentized in milk (11,12), comparatively little is known about the physical distribution of immunologic components in human milk. There are, however, some clues that suggest that some of these agents may be found in a non-aqueous phase of human milk. Either following centrifugation (13) or brief heating (10), the detectable concentrations of lysozyme and lactoferrin increase as compared to untreated human milk. Further studies of the distribution of these protective factors in human milk are warranted not only to improve the ability to quantify them, but also to understand the biologic function of the components.

In summary, immunochemical assays which have been developed and employed to measure proteins in other human biologic fluids, such as blood, often have to be adapted to quantitate those factors in human milk. Some of the more important methodologic issues include the sensitivity and specificity of the assay, the types of materials used to standardize the assay for use with human milk, the molecular forms of factors that are peculiar to milk, the effect of storage and processing on the components, and the physical distribution of the immunologic components.

ACKNOWLEDGEMENTS

This research was supported by: NICH NO1 HD 22815, NIH-GCRC-RR00425, New Investigator Grant AI-17124-01 from the National Institute of Allergy and Infectious Disease

REFERENCES

1. Goldblum RM, Garza C, Johnson CA, Harrist R, Nichols BL, Goldman AS. (1981): Human milk banking. I. Effects of container upon immunologic factors in mature milk. Nutritional Research, 1, 449-459.

2. Goldblum RM, Powell GK, Van Sickle G. (1980): Secretory IgA in the serum of infants with obstructive jaundice. J Pediatr, 97, 33-36.

3. Kuhn LC, Kraehenhuhl JP. (1983): Monoclonal antibodies to the secreted and membrane domains of the IgA dimer receptor. Annals of NY Acad of Sci, 409, 751-757.

4. Gore ME, Bunnage HJ, McIlhinney RA. (1984): A monoclonal antibody which differentiates between bound and free human secretory component. Eur J Immunol, 14, 344-349.

5. Woodard CS, Splawski JB, Goldblum RM, Denney RM. (1984): IgG antibodies to secretory component in normal human serum. J Immunol, 133, 2111-2115.

6. Keller MA, Heiner DC, Myers AS, Resinger DM. (1985): IgD in human colostrum. Pediatr Res, 19, 122-126.

7. Watanabe T, Nagura H, Watanabe K, Brown WR. (1984): The binding of human milk lactoferrin to immunoglobulin A. FEBS Lett, 168, 203-207.

8. Ritchie RF. (1980): Nephelometric immunoassay. In: Rose N and Bigazzi P, eds, Methods in Immunodiagnostics, 2nd Ed. John Wiley and Sons, Inc.

9. Bjorkesten B, Burman LG, Chateau PD, Fredrikzon B, Gothefors L, Hernell O. (1980): Collecting and banking human milk: to heat or not to heat? BR Medical Journal, 281, 765-769.

10. Goldblum RM, Dill CW, Albrecht TP, Alford ES, Garza C, Goldman AS. (1984): Rapid high temperature treatment of human milk. J Pediatr, 104, 380-385.

11. Lönnerdal B, Stanislowski AG, Hunley LS. (1980): Isolation of a low molecular weight zinc binding ligand from human milk. J Inorganic Biochem, 12, 71-78.

12. Parkash S, Jenness R. (1967): Status of zinc in cow's milk. J Dairy Sc, 50, 127-134.

13. Butte NF, Goldblum RM, Fehl LM, Loftin K, Smith EO, Garza C, Goldman AS. (1984): Daily ingestion of immunologic components in human milk during the first four months of life. Acta Paediatr Scand, 73, 296-301.

DETERMINATION OF NUMBERS AND FUNCTIONS OF CELLS IN HUMAN MILK

M.J. Paape
Margaret Keller

It has been postulated that living leukocytes are an important part of the immunologic system in human milk that serves to protect the mammary gland and the recipient infant. The concentration of these cells in human milk is highest in the first few days of lactation ($1\text{-}3\times10^6$/ml); their numbers gradually fall to less than 1×10^5 /ml over the next 2-3 months (1-3). During the first few weeks of lactation, over 95% of the cells in human milk are leukocytes (1-3). The relative proportion of these cells which are epithelial cells rises to about 80% by 4 to 6 months into lactation (4-6). Because of certain unusual features of these cells, they are difficult to enumerate and categorize. Certain laboratory procedures which are utilized in investigating the numbers and types of these cells will therefore be discussed.

ENUMERATION OF CELLS IN HUMAN MILK

The cells in human milk are difficult to count because of the presence of cell-like particles in the fluid (4,6). These particles (principally milk fat globules) are membrane-bound bodies which originate from the secretory epithelium of the mammary gland by an apocrine process. They contain large amounts of protein, lipids, but no deoxyribonucleic acid (DNA) or other nuclear material. In an effort to define the confounding effect of these particles upon the cell counts in milk, a study (7) was performed on caprine milk to compare methods that depend upon direct visualization of cells to methods that depend upon the detection of DNA (7). Caprine milk is similar to human milk in that it contains many non-cellular particles. Cell counts by the non-DNA methods were considerably higher than those obtained by DNA methods (Table 1). Therefore, only methods that distinguish cells from particles should be used in counting cells in human milk. These techniques are detailed in the Appendix.

The time following nursing that milk is collected may also affect the concentration of cells in the specimen (8). In ruminant milk, cell counts increase to a maximum at 4 hours following nursing. The situation with respect to human milk is uncertain, but it would seem reasonable to collect the samples at a consistent time after nursing, and at a consistent time of day, to avoid potential day-to-night variation. Unless one is interested in the fore-, mid-, or hind-milk, the breast should be emptied with each collection. In addition, the time and temperature of storage of the milk may be important variables (2,3).

Table 1. Comparison of Methods for Enumerating Cells in Milk

METHOD	CELLS x 10^6 /ml
DNA (Spectrophotometric - Indole)	.303[a]
Direct Microscopic (Pyronin Y-Methyl Green Stain)	.340[a]
Fossomatic Cell Counter	.365[a]
Coulter Electronic Counter	.675[b]
Direct Microscopy (Methylene Blue Stain)	.792[b]

Each value represents the mean of 24 determinations run in duplicate on caprine milk samples.

Means with the same superscript letter are not significantly different.

Significance Level $P<.01$
Standard Error $\pm$ .11324

THE IDENTIFICATION OF CELLS IN HUMAN MILK

Because of the unusual morphology of the cells in human milk, it has been difficult to identify them by common procedures which have been applied to the study of leukocytes from peripheral blood. When milk leukocytes are examined by light microscopy, many of them are found to display numerous cytoplasmic vacuoles which are rich in lipids (9). These vacuoles have been identified by transmission electron microscopy to be milk fat globules and casein micelles (9). Because of the presence of these cytoplasmic bodies and the large size of the cells (up to 40 µ in diameter), these cells were once thought to be epithelial cells from the mammary gland. Functional and histochemical studies, however, have shown that these cells are neutrophils and macrophages, in that they adhere and spread on glass. They phagocytize neutral red, carbon and polystyrene particles and microorganisms (10-13), and they contain certain enzymes which are found in those leukocytes but not in epithelial cells (14). It is, therefore, difficult to distinguish epithelial cells, neutrophils and macrophages from one another unless specific histochemical stains or transmission electron microscopy are used. Stains for myeloperoxidase (15) and non-specific esterase (15) are useful for detecting neutrophils and macrophages, respectively, (see Appendix for these methods). With those methods, the relative proportion of leukocytes in human milk during the first few days of lactation are as follows: neutrophils, 45-65%; macrophages, 35-55%; and lymphocytes, 5-10%. Surprisingly few studies of membrane receptors on these milk leukocytes have been published. It is possible that some of these cell populations will be further categorized according to the type and number of their receptor sites. Current fluorescent cell sorting techniques are particularly well suited for those purposes.

Monoclonal antibodies may become important reagents to identify the populations and subpopulations of these cells, but only lymphocytes in human milk have been thoroughly studied with those probes (16,17). Transmission electron microscopy is valuable in identifying the several types of epithelial cells and distinguishing between secretory epithelial cells, macrophages and neutrophils. The ultrastructural features of human milk cells are summarized in Table 2.

METHODS OF SEPARATION AND ENRICHMENT

Cell separation has been a persistent problem in studying human breast milk. Techniques which are standard for peripheral blood cells are not always applicable due to the altered buoyancy of these lipid-rich cells.

Table 2. Ultrastructural Features of Human Milk Leukocytes

CELL TYPES	ULTRASTRUCTURAL FEATURES
LEUKOCYTES	
Neutrophils	Cells with segmented nuclei which are similar to their counterparts in human blood except for abundant fat globules and casein micelles.
Monocytes and Macrophages	Vary from typical blood monocyte to large macrophages (40 μ in diameter) which contain fat globules, casein micelles and other material.
Lymphocytes	Similar to those in peripheral blood.
EPITHELIAL CELLS	
Secretory	Contain abundant cisternae of rough endoplasmic reticulum, lipid droplets, and Golgi apparati producing casein micelles.
Squamous	From galactophores and skin of the nipples. Have typical appearance of squamous cells found in other sites.
Ductal	Often found in 2-4 cell clusters. Display many short microvilli uniformly distributed over the surface. Have tight junctions and remnants of desmosomes.

Adherence to a gelatin-serum substrata by macrophages (14) has been useful for separating macrophages from polymorphonuclear cells and lymphocytes. The technique yields adherent cell preparations that are 87-95% esterase positive and myeloperoxidase negative (e.g., macrophages) and over 95% of cells which are non-specific esterase negative and myeloperoxidase positive (e.g., neutrophils). The total yields of separated cells by this method are, however, comparatively small. Others have successfully adhered milk macrophages to tissue culture plates to study their function (18). Pickering, et al. (13) have prepared cells that are 80% polymorphonuclear by centrifuging the aqueous phase above a Ficoll-Hypaque layer.

Enriching milk-cell populations for the minority lymphocyte population is more difficult. Ficoll-Hypaque (19) separation, which is standard for peripheral blood, yields cell preparations that average only 22-33% lymphocytes (20,21). Parmely, et al. (22) used glass bead columns to deplete macrophages from milk cell preparations and to enrich for lymphocytes. Lymphocyte content varied from 35-80% of the cell preparation.

Richie, et al. (23) have used Percoll gradient centrifugation to provide a lymphocyte-rich population for study. About 75% ± 6% of the prepared cells were lymphocytes and the lymphocyte yield was 81% ± 9%. These preparations of lymphocytes from women 2-5 days postpartum form thermostabile E-rosettes, while peripheral blood lymphocytes do not. Such studies suggest that the T-cell population in milk may represent a selected subset that homes to the mammary gland. Richie, et al. (16) have also used a separation technique that combines Percoll gradient centrifugation and centrifugal elutriation to prepare lymphocytes (82% ± 19% lymphocytes) for T-cell subset analysis. When they examined milk samples within the first week postpartum, the OKT_4/OKT_8 ratio was generally lower in colostrum than in peripheral blood, supporting the hypothesis that the milk T-cell population may be a selected population. Different results have been obtained by Keller, et al. when unseparated cells were examined (17). In these studies, the T-cell subsets were found to be similar in colostrum and peripheral blood. These conflicting data may reflect subset selection by separation techniques or may reflect differences in the populations studied, e.g., days postpartum.

The limited lymphocyte content of human colostrum and milk precludes comparisons of various cell separation techniques on the same specimen, which makes progress difficult. It would be necessary to pool large quantities of milk in order to compare separation techniques. This is generally difficult. Although it is possible to examine unseparated cells for T-cell subset analysis, it would not be possible to study the function of unseparated lymphocytes. Hence, the best method for separation of lymphocytes is an unresolved question and may depend on the particular analysis to be performed.

FUNCTIONAL ASSAYS

Pickering, et al. (13) have found decreased oxidative metabolic activity during phagocytosis of opsonized zymosan particles, and decreased uptake and killing of *Staphylococcus aureus* by milk polymorphonuclear cells. In these studies, the lipid fraction of the milk was found to suppress peripheral blood polymorphonuclear cells and to decrease Fc receptor expression. The effects on respiratory burst and phagocytosis were later shown to be due only to the lipid fraction of colostrum, not that of mature milk. Others (10) have demonstrated that the phagocytic function of unseparated colostral cells was comparable to that of blood leukocytes, but the capacity of colostral cells to kill *Candida albicans* and *Escherchia coli* was significantly less than the ability of peripheral blood phagocytes to do so. Colostrum supernatant did reduce killing of *E. coli* and *C. albicans* by peripheral blood leukocytes, but phagocytic indices were not altered. Discrepancies in results between Ho, et al. (10) and Pickering, et al. (13), concerning phagocytosis, may relate to the use of different bacterial organisms and to whether both macrophages and neutrophils (10), or purified neutrophils (13), were studied. Other studies (11) demonstrate that breast milk phagocytes (macrophages and neutrophils) are equivalent to blood neutrophils in terms of phagocytosis and killing, although the chemiluminescent response is quenched by fat in the milk. Robinson, et al. (12) used a different system to study phagocytosis and the killing of *S. aureus* and *E. coli*; milk cells (both macrophage and polymorphonuclear cells) were opsonized by aqueous defatted milk and blood neutrophils were opsonized in serum. For these two organisms, results were similar for milk cells opsonized with aqueous defatted milk and blood neutrophils opsonized in serum. However, blood neutrophils opsonized in aqueous milk had decreased phagocytosis of *S. aureus*, compared to blood leukocytes opsonized with serum.

Thus, each investigator has studied a different system, which makes comparison and standardization difficult. In studies of the phagocytic function, systems that use colostral macrophages and neutrophils opsonized by aqueous milk may be more physiologic, and hence more representative of what occurs in the gastrointestinal tract of the suckling infant. It may be advantageous to modify assays used traditionally for peripheral blood phagocytes to study milk cells in their natural milieu. This should include examining the effect of alimentary tract secretion upon the function of these cells.

Lymphocyte functional studies have included both blastogenesis and mediator production. Many investigators have demonstrated the lymphocyte blastogenic capability of human milk lymphocytes (1,22,24). Milk cells generally appear to be similar to peripheral blood leukocytes in terms of production of such mediators as interferon (20,25,26) and monocyte chemotactic factor (21). Yields of lymphocytes from colostrum and milk severely limit the functional studies which can be performed. As with the phagocytic studies, few comparisons of results from different laboratories are available to standardize assays.

Steinmetz, et al. (27) used discontinuous Percoll gradients to demonstrate that milk contains cytotoxic leukocytes. The population consisted of lymphocytes and a small portion of the milk macrophages which are less lipid filled. Other studies by their group (28), however, have shown defects in antibody-dependent cellular cytotoxicity by colostral leukocytes and inhibition of peripheral blood cytotoxicity by colostrum. Unlike the studies of polymorphonuclear bactericidal activity, this inhibitory activity was found in both lipid and aqueous fractions. These studies again illustrate the important effect of colostrum constituents on cell function and the importance of determining the effect of the milk milieu upon function. They also illustrate the intrinsic differences between cells in milk and those in peripheral blood.

It should be realized that while some functions of leukocytes in human milk are similar to those in peripheral blood, some functions may be quite limited. For example, recent studies suggest that the response of neutrophils and macrophages in human milk to chemotactic agents may be quite blunted, if not lacking (29). Whether certain functions of these leukocytes in human milk may be unique will require considerable study.

ACKNOWLEDGEMENT

This research was supported in part by grants NICHD NO1 HD 22815, NIH-GCRC-RR00425, and New Investigator Grant AI-17124-01 from the National Institute of Allergy and Infectious Disease.

REFERENCES

1. Ogra SS, Ogra PL. (1978): Immunologic aspects of human colostrum and milk. II. Characteristics of lymphocyte reactivity and distribution of E-rosette forming cells at different times after the onset of lactation. J Pediatr, 92, 550-555.

2. Goldblum RM, Garza C, Johnson CA, Nichols BL, Goldman AS. (1981): Human milk banking. I. Effects of container upon immunologic factors in mature milk. Nutr Res, 1, 449-459.

3. Goldblum RM, Garza C, Johnson CA, Nichols BL, Goldman AS. (1982): Human milk banking. II. Relative stability of immunologic factors in stored colostrum. Acta Paediatr Scand, 71, 143-144.

4. Brooker BE. (1980): The epithelial cells and cell fragments in human milk. Cell and Tissue Res, 210, 321-322.

5. Ho FCS, Wong RLC, Lawton JWM. (1979): Human colostral and breast milk cells. Acta Paediatr Scand, 68, 389-396.

6. Dulin AM, Paape MJ, Berkow S, Hamosh M. Hamosh P. (1983): Comparison of total somatic cells and differential cellular composition in milk from cows, sheep, goats and humans. Fed Proc, 42, 1331.

7. Dulin AM, Paape MJ, Wergin WP. (1982): Differentiation and enumeration of somatic cells in goat milk. J Food Prot, 45, 435-439.

8. Paape MJ, Tucker HA. (1966): Somatic cell content variation in fraction collected milk. J Dairy Sci, 49, 265.

9. Paape MJ, Wergin WP. (1977): Scanning and transmission electron microscopy of polymorphonuclear leukocytes (PMN) isolated from milk. Fed Proc, 36, 1201.

10. Ho PC, Lawton JW. (1978): Human colostral cells: Phagocytosis and killing of *E. coli* and *C. albicans*. J Pediatr, 93, 910-915.

11. Johnson DF, France GL, Marmer DJ, Steele RW. (1980): Bactericidal mechanisms of human breast milk leukocytes. Infect Immun, 28, 314-318.

12. Robinson JE, Harvey BAM, Soothill JF. (1978): Phagocytosis and killing of bacteria and yeast by human milk cells after opsonization in aqueous phase of milk. Brit Med J, 1, 1443-1445.

13. Pickering LK, Cleary TG, Kohl S. (1980): Polymorphonuclear leukocytes of human colostrum. I. Oxidative metabolism and kinetics of killing radiolabeled *Staphylococcus aureus*. J Infect Dis, 142, 685-693.

14. Tsuda H, Dickey WD, Goldman AS. (1984): Separation of human colostral macrophages and neutrophils on gelatin and collagen-serum substrata. Cell Structure and Function, 8, 367-371.

15. Yam LT, Li CY, Crosby WH. (1971): Cytochemical identification of monocytes and granulocytes. Am J Clin Path, 55, 283-290.

16. Richie ER, Steinmetz KD, Meistrich ML, Ramirez I, Hilliard JK. (1982): T-lymphocyte subsets in human colostrum. J Immunol, 129, 1116-1119.

17. Keller MA, Faust J, Rolewic LJ, Stewart D. T-cell subsets in human colostrum. (Paper in preparation).

18. Blau H, Passwell JH, Levanon M, Davidson J, Kohen F, Ramot, B. (1983): Studies on human milk macrophages: effect of activation on phagocytosis and secretion of protaglandin E and lysozyme. Pediatr Res, 17, 241-245.

19. Boyum A. (1968): Separation of leukocytes from blood and bone marrow. Scand J Clin Lab Invest, 21, 77-88.

20. Keller MA, Kidd RM, Bryson YJ, Turner JL, Carter J. (1981): Lymphokine production by human milk lymphocytes. Infect and Immuno, 32, 632-636.

21. Keller MA, Kidd RM, Stewart DD. (1984): PPD-induced monocyte chemotactic factor production by human milk cells. Acta Paediatr Scand, 73, 465-470.

22. Parmely MJ, Beer AE, Billingham RE. (1976): *In vitro* studies of the T-lymphocyte population of human milk. J Exp Med, 144, 358-370.

23. Richie ER, Steinmetz KD, Meistrich ML, Ramirez I, Hilliard HK. (1980): T lymphocytes in colostrum and peripheral blood. Difference in their capacity to form thermostable E-rosettes. J Immunol, 125, 2344-2346.

24. Schlessinger JJ, Covelli HD. (1977): Evidence for transmission of lymphocyte responses to tuberculin by breast feeding. Lancet, 10, 529-532.

25. Emodi G, Just M. (1974): Interferon production by lymphocytes in human milk. Scand J Immunol, 3, 157-160.

26. Lawton JWM, Shortridge KF, Wong RLC, Ng, MH. (1979): Interferon synthesis by human colostral leukocytes. Arch Dis Child, 54, 127-130.

27. Steinmetz KD, Kohl S, Richie ER. (1981): Separation of cytotoxic leukocyte populations of human peripheral blood and colostrum on PVP-silica (Percoll) density gradients. J Immunol Meth, 42, 157-70.

28. Kohl S, Pickering LK, Cleary TG, Steinmetz KD, Loo LS. (1980): Human colostral cytotoxicity. II. Relative defects in colostral leukocyte cytotoxicity and inhibition of peripheral blood leukocyte cytotoxicity by colostrum. J Infect Dis, 142, 884-891.

29. Thorpe LW, Rudloff HB, Goldman AS. Decreased responses of human milk leukocytes to chemotactic factors. (Paper in preparation).

30. Paape MJ, Hafs HD, Synder WW. (1963): Variation of estimated numbers of milk somatic cells stained with Wright's stain or Pyronin Y-methyl green stain. J Dairy Sci, 46, 1211-1216.

APPENDIX: METHODS FOR COUNTING AND IDENTIFYING CELLS IN HUMAN MILK

DNA Staining

Direct Microscopy. One method for counting cells in human milk is as follows. Milk (0.01 ml) is spread onto a circular area (1 cm^2) marked on the upper surface of a clean glass slide (Bellco Glass, Inc., Vineland, NJ 08360, Catalog #5638-01930). The dried milk smears are stained according to a procedure (30) whereby cells are fixed in Carnoy's solution, then are hydrated for 2 minutes each in 50% ethyl alcohol, 30% ethyl alcohol, and distilled water, stained with 0.50% pyronin Y (National Aniline) and 0.30% methyl green (National Aniline) in distilled water, immersed for 20 minutes in N-butyl alcohol, immersed for 3 minutes in N-butyl alcohol, and cleared with two changes of xylene. The slides are kept in the dark to prevent oxidation of the stain until they are examined microscopically with oil immersion. The ocular of the microscope should contain an ocular reticle (Dairy Research Production, Inc., Box 288, Yarmouth, ME 04096). The reticle has a wide and a narrow strip centrally located and perpendicular to each other. Thus, each microscope field is divided into four quadrants to facilitate enumeration of somatic cells. Only cells containing a blue-green nucleus are counted. Cytoplasmic particles stain red with no blue-green nucleus and are not included in the total somatic cell count.

The microscope for the strip-counting procedure is calibrated as follows:

(a) Measure the width of the wide and narrow strips in the reticle with a stage micrometer slide, ruled in 0.1-0.01mm divisions.

(b) A 10X ocular with a 1.8mm oil-immersion objective is preferred. Calculate the strip area. The area of a single strip is equal to the width of the strip times the length of the milk film (11.28 mm). Area of single strip = 11.28mm x D (in mm). Determine the number of single strips in the 0.01 ml milk film by dividing 100 mm^2 (area of 0.01 ml milk film) by the strip area. No. of single strips = 100 mm^2/area of single strip. Convert the number of single strips in 0.01 ml of milk to a 1.0 ml basis by multiplying the number of single strips in 0.01 ml by 100. Determine conversion factors for wide and narrow strips separately for each microscope. The example in Table 3 illustrates this procedure.

Table 3. Illustration of Cell-Counting Technique

Length of Strip (diameter of 1 cm^2 circle) = 11.28mm

Width of wide strip in reticle = .089mm

Equation:

$$\frac{\frac{\text{Total area x dilution factor}}{\text{Area counted}}}{\text{Number of strips counted}} = \text{Conversion factor}$$

Width of narrow strip in reticle = .030mm diameter

Example:

$$\frac{100\text{mm}^2 \text{ x } 100}{11.28\text{mm x } .030\text{mm}} = 29,551$$

Number of strips counted	Strip Size	Conversion Factor
01	Wide	9,961
02	Wide	4,980
03	Wide	3,320
04	Wide	2,490
01	Narrow	29,551
02	Narrow	14,775
03	Narrow	9,850
04	Narrow	7,388

If a technician counts 100 somatic cells in one wide strip, the somatic cell count/ml = 100 x 9,961 = 996,100/ml. The concentration of somatic cells in the sample will determine the number of strips counted and the size of the strip used.

Fossomatic Electronic Cell Counting Procedure. Milk samples are preheated for 15 minutes at 60°C. The sample is taken automatically, mixed with preheated buffer and ethidium bromide dye and is stirred extensively (Foss Electric, Hillerod, Denmark). Part of the mixture is then transferred to a rotating disc which serves as the object plane for the microscope. The mixture on the wheel is illuminated by a xenon arc lamp which excites stained cells to emit fluorescent light. Each cell produces an electrical pulse which is counted and the number of cells/ml is printed after each sample. Only cells containing a nucleus are counted by this technique. Milk cell count standards are available for use with both microscopic and Fossomatic electronic cell counting procedures (Somatic Cell Count Samples (SCCS), 101 William L. Henning Building, the Pennsylvania State University, University Park, Pennsylvania, 16802). The

SCCS sets contain two sample tubes of each dilution: BLANK, LOW, MEDIUM, HIGH. Each sample tube contains about 12 ml. The SCCS cover the range of cell concentrations from approximately 300,000 cells/ml in the LOW dilution to 1,300,000 cells/ml in the HIGH dilution.

Combined Non-Specific Esterase-myeloperoxidase Stain

The procedure is divided into two parts. The first part of the procedure is to detect non-specific esterase in monocytes and macrophages. Fixed smears are incubated for 45 minutes at room temperature in a medium containing 8.9ml of phosphate buffer (.07M,pH 7.6), 0.6ml of hexazotized pararosanilin, and α-naphthyl acetate (Sigma Chemical Co., St. Louis, MO; 10mg/0.5ml ethylene glycol monomethyl ether). The slides are washed, counterstained with 1% methyl green for 1 minute and washed with water. The second part of the procedure is to detect myeloperoxidase in neutrophils. The smears are incubated in 10 ml of Kaplow's benzidine HCl medium containing 4.9mg of sodium cyanide (.01M; final pH adjusted to 6.1 with HCl) for 30 seconds. Non-specific esterase activity is detected by the presence of dark red cytoplasmic granules, whereas peroxidase is found by the presence of blue cytoplasmic granules.

HUMORAL FACTORS IN BREAST MILK THAT PROTECT AGAINST DIARRHEA

L. K. Pickering
S. Kohl
T. G. Cleary

INTRODUCTION

Breast feeding has been shown to have a variable effect on morbidity and mortality from infectious diseases. Most studies suggest that breast feeding is associated with a lower incidence of diarrheal disease, while protective effects against respiratory tract infections and otitis media are less certain (1,2). Several reviewers have summarized the incidence rates of disease in infants who are breast-fed compared to non-breast-fed infants in both industrialized and developing countries (1-3). The strongest evidence for a protective effect of breast feeding in industrialized countries is against diarrheal disease (1). Studies in the United States have been most significant for protection in American Indian and Alaskan infants, in whom the risk of infectious diseases is high. Little information is available concerning the effects of breast feeding on infectious diseases in the disadvantaged urban poor in the United States. Studies of populations in developing countries where infant morbidity and mortality are higher than in industrialized countries show a greater association between breast feeding and a lower incidence of diarrhea (2).

The protective factors in human milk that theoretically modify or prevent infection can be considered under the headings of cells (lymphocytes, monocytes and polymorphonuclear leukocytes), nonspecific factors including all nonantibody factors, and antibodies. Although laboratory studies provide clear biologic evidence that these protective factors are present in human milk, the magnitude of their protective effect *in vivo*, either alone or in combination, is difficult to quantitate. Problems with epidemiologic studies of diarrheal disease conducted to date include failure to identify the causative agents of gastroenteritis, failure to identify protective factors in milk being fed to infants, and lack of correlation of these two categories of information. In many of the older studies, this was not possible since a large number of enteropathogens that currently are recognized causes of diarrhea were not known to be enteropathogens until the late 1970's and 1980's (4,5). In addition, the ability to detect and quantitate protective factors in human milk, and to understand their relation to prevention of disease in animal models and in humans, is in its infancy (6-10). It is probable that the protective factors in human milk, and their relative importance, vary by pathogen and by age of the infant. In this review, we will summarize *in vitro* and *in vivo* studies of nonantibody and antibody protective factors in human milk.

NONANTIBODY PROTECTIVE FACTORS

Several nonantibody protective factors are present in human colostrum and milk. Most of these factors have been shown to be present *in vitro* and their clinical importance remains to be demonstrated in studies of animal models or humans. These factors include the bifidus factor, complement components, lysozyme, nutrient binders such as lactoferrin, lipid factors such as gangliosides, nonantibody proteins and carbohydrate factors.

In Vitro Studies

There is a proliferation of lactobacilli in the intestine of breast-fed infants with subsequent accumulation of short chain fatty acids and other bacterial metabolites. The low protein, phosphate and buffering capacities of milk, plus the bifidus factor, all contribute to the low pH of stools, which is typical in breast-fed infants. This acid environment appears to be antagonistic to the replication of Enterobacteriaceae, including enteropathogens such as some *Escherichia coli*, shigella and salmonella (11-16).

Complement components have been shown to be present at low concentrations in human milk (17). In one study, the bacteriostatic effect of human milk against *E. coli* was not abolished by heating milk to 56°C for 30 minutes, indicating that complement was not responsible for bacteriostasis, since complement is heat labile (18). Conflicting results have been reported in another study, in which the heating of cows' milk destroyed bacteriostatic activity against *E. coli* (19). The role of complement in human milk in the prevention of disease is not known.

Human milk contains about 400 ug/ml of lysozyme, which alone has little or no bacteriolytic activity against *E. coli* (20,21). Reports about the ability of lysozyme to act *in vitro* with IgA to lyse *E. coli* are conflicting (20,22). Lysozyme acts with peroxide and ascorbate to lyse *E. coli* and some salmonella strains (23). The effect of lysozyme in the gastrointestinal tract is unknown.

The content of lactoferrin in human milk is 1 to 6 mg/ml (24). In the presence of antibody and bicarbonate, lactoferrin binds ferric iron and thereby exerts a strong bacteriostatic effect on *E. coli* (18). This effect is overcome by saturating the lactoferrin with iron or by adding citrate, which can bind iron into a citrate-iron complex (24). The *in vitro* growth of *Candida albicans* also is impaired by lactoferrin (25). The activity of this glycoprotein after ingestion into the gastrointestinal tract is unknown. Since lactoferrin in milk is partly unsaturated, it may exert a bacteriostatic action on various organisms by depriving them of iron.

Holmgren, et al. (26) have shown that both the immunoglobulin and nonimmunoglobulin fractions of human milk inhibited bacterial cell adhesion and enterotoxin receptor binding of *Vibrio cholerae* and various *E. coli* isolates in an *in vitro* assay. The strongest effect was seen with the nonimmunoglobulin fraction which inhibited *E. coli* adhesion by binding colonization factor antigen 1 (CFA-1), CFA-2 and K-88 fimbriae. The fraction also inhibited *V. cholerae* hemagglutination as well as binding of cholera toxin and *E. coli* heat-labile enterotoxin (LT) to GM_1 ganglioside. This inhibition of bacterial adherence was thought to be due to a receptor-like glycoprotein or oligosaccharide in milk which prevented bacterial adherence by competition with receptors on target cells (27) Otnaess and

Orstavik (28) found that *E. coli* enterotoxin inhibitory activity in milk could be extracted with a chloroform-methanol mixture, suggesting that this activity was due to a glycolipid.

Gillin, et al. (29) showed that *Giardia lamblia* was rapidly killed by exposure to human milk *in vitro*. The killing did not depend on secretory IgA, but appeared to be due to the bile salt stimulated lipase that is limited to milk of humans and mountain gorillas. Human milk also has been reported to contain several low molecular weight lipids with antiviral activity against nonenveloped viruses (7,9). Inhibition by nonantibody, noninterferon proteins has been found to interfere with the attachment of a broad spectrum of viruses to target cells (30).

In Vivo Studies

Not many *in vivo* studies of nonantibody protective factors have been conducted. In experiments using rabbit intestinal loops, Otnaess and Svennerholm (31) showed that a nonimmunoglobulin, lipid component inhibited fluid secretion by cholera toxin, as well as by *E. coli* LT. They further purified the toxin inhibitory activity from human milk (32) and, using ELISA and rabbit intestinal loop models, showed that the enterotoxin inhibitory compound appeared to be ganglioside-like and resembled the ganglioside GM_1, which is known to be the cell membrane receptor for cholera toxin and *E. coli* LT. Cleary, et al. (33) studied the protective effects of human milk in a suckling mouse model that was challenged with heat stable enterotoxin (ST) of *E. coli*. They demonstrated that human colostrum and milk, and most cow milk specimens (34) contained a factor that protected mice from lethal fluid loss due to *E. coli* ST, and that the factor appeared to be a neutral oligosaccharide.

ANTIBODY MEDIATED MECHANISMS

The major immunoglobulin in all human secretions, including human milk, is secretory IgA. Colostrum contains up to 50 mg/ml. This concentration decreases in mature milk to 10 mg/ml (35,36). This immunoglobulin is not absorbed in significant quantity from the human intestine and therefore presumably acts at the mucosal surface of the intestine (36). Secretory IgA is more resistant to acid degradation and to the proteolytic activity of gut enzymes than is serum IgA, and can be found intact in significant quantities in feces (37). Not only has total IgA in milk been measured, but specific IgA antibodies to many respiratory and gastrointestinal pathogens have been reported. These are summarized in Table 1.

In Vitro Studies

Several reports show that human colostrum and milk contain antibodies to specific bacterial enteropathogens or toxins elaborated by them (Table 1). These antibodies agglutinated common serotypes of *E. coli* and *Salmonella typhimurium* (38,39), were active against both somatic and capsular antigens of *E. coli* (40), and inhibited the induced fluid accumulation in rabbit ileal loops when incubated with *V. cholerae* or *E. coli* enterotoxin (41). Secretory IgA antibody, which neutralized *E. coli* toxin, was shown to be present in milk from undernourished women from Pakistan, but not from healthy women from Sweden (42). Human milk has also been shown to contain secretory IgA cholera toxin and rotavirus antibodies (43), as well as antibodies to somatic antigens of enteropathogenic *E. coli* (44).

Table 1. Antibody in Human Milk to Bacterial Enteric Pathogens

Country (Year Published)	Antibody Activity or Type	Model or Assay Used	Reference
Sweden (1972)	Agglutination of *Escherichia coli*	Indirect hemagglutination	Gindrat et al. (38)
England (1974)	Agglutination of *Salmonella typhimurium*	Agglutination, immunofluorescence	Allardyce et al. (39)
Sweden (1975)	Capsular and somatic antigens of *E. coli*	Indirect hemagglutination, ELISA	Hanson et al. (40)
Guatemala and N. America (1976)	Inhibited fluid accumulation by enterotoxins of *E. coli* and *V. cholerae*	Rabbit ileal loops	Stoliar et al. (41)
Pakistan and Sweden (1976)	Neutralized *E. coli* toxin	Adrenal cell assay, rabbit ileal loops	Holmgren et al. (42)
Costa Rica (1979)	Enterotoxin of *V. cholerae*	ELISA	Simhon et al. (43)
Israel (1979)	*E. coli* somatic antigens	Passive hemagglutination, radial immunodiffusion	Vardinon et al. (44)
Sweden and Pakistan (1981)	Inhibited *E. coli* and *V. cholerae* adhesion and enterotoxin receptor binding	Cell cultures, intestinal epithelium	Holmgren et al. (26)
Ethiopia and Sweden	Antibodies to *E. coli* labile toxin	Adrenal cell assay	Aust-Kettis et al. (45)
Calcutta (1981)	Antibacterial and antitoxin titers noted in sera and milk of convalescent-phase cholera patients	Vibriocidal, indirect hemagglutination, ELISA and neutralization assays	Majumdar et al. (46)
India and Sweden (1982)	Inhibited fluid accumulation and adherence of *V. cholerae*	Adherence to intestinal slices, rabbit ileal loops	Majumdar and Ghose (47)
Ethiopia, Guatemala, Sweden (1982)	*E. coli* somatic antigens	ELISA	Cruz et al. (48)
United States (1984)	Decreased fluid accumulation due to toxins A and B of *Clostridium difficile*.	Yl adrenal cells, suckling mice	Kim et al. (49)

Holmgren, et al. (27,28) showed that human milk and colostrum inhibited *E. coli* and *V. cholerae* adhesion to intestinal epithelium and binding of secreted enterotoxins to specific cell membrane receptors. Part of this inhibitory activity resided in the immunoglobulin fraction; however, the nonimmunoglobulin fraction inhibited both bacterial cell adhesion and enterotoxin binding, usually to a greater extent than did the immunoglobulin fraction. Antibody titers to *E. coli* LT were shown in 33% of milk specimens from Ethiopian women (45). A significant increase in both antibacterial and antitoxin titers was demonstrated in the sera and milk of convalescent-phase cholera patients (46). *V. cholerae* antibacterial and antitoxin titers were significantly higher in colostrum from Indian women than from Swedish women (47). Colostrum from Indian women inhibited adherence of *V. cholerae* to intestinal slices *in vitro* and induced protection against live vibrio challenge in rabbit ileal loops. Malnourished women were able to produce Secretory IgA (SIgA) in milk against E coli somatic antigens in quantities comparable to those observed in well-nourished populations (48).

Milk from 56% of 55 women exhibited neutralizing activity against one or both toxins of *C. difficile* (49). In suckling mice, 65% of milk samples with *in vitro* neutralizing activity against toxin A inhibited fluid accumulation by toxin A, and 65% of milk samples with *in vitro* neutralizing activity against toxin B inhibited fluid accumulation by toxin B. Neutralizing activity against toxin A appeared to reside in the secretory IgA fraction.

Table 2. Antibody to Rotavirus in Human Milk

Country (year published)	Assay	Sample (% positive)	Reference
Canada (1978)	CIE (1)	Colostrum (69%) Milk (19%)	51
South Africa (1978)	IFA	Colostrum (13%)	52
Costa Rica (1978)	ELISA	Colostrum (30%)	56
USA, Guatamala, Costa Rica (1978)	ELISA	Colostrum (100%) Milk (94%)	57
USA (1978, 1979)	RIA	Colostrum (80%) Milk (56%)	54, 55
Australia (1980)	ELISA	Milk and Colostrum (100%)	58
Norway (1980)	IFA NA	Milk (20%) Milk (60%)	53
USA (1980)	ELISA	Colostrum (82%)	59
England (1980)	ELISA	Colostrum (100%)	60
Norway, Ethiopia (1981)	ELISA	Colostrum (86-90%)	28

(1) CIE: counter immunoelectrophoresis, IFA: immunofluorescent assay, ELISA: enzyme-linked immunosorbent assay, RIA: radioimmuno assay, NA: neutralizing assay.

It was not until the 1960's that the neutralizing activity of human milk against viruses was shown to be mediated by immunoglobulin (50). Since then, antibodies to many viral agents have been shown to be present in human colostrum, and in lower dilutions in milk, by various assays. Studies involving detection of antibody in human milk to rotavirus, which is the most common viral cause of diarrhea, are presented in Table 2. In general, as the assays evolved from the least sensitive, such as counter-immunoelectrophoresis (51) and immunofluorescence (52,53), to the more sensitive ELISA and radioimmunoassay (54,55), the detection of antibody to rotavirus in colostrum from women from all over the world became nearly universal (Table 2). The ELISA assay also made it possible to determine that nearly all this activity was in the secretory IgA fraction of colostrum and milk (56-60). Serum IgG antirotavirus activity is capable of being transferred placentally (58). In a study of 92 women from Australia, the only two milk samples which were negative for IgA to rotavirus were obtained from two IgA deficient women (58).

Miotti, et al. (61) showed that milk specimens from women from different geographic locations had IgA antibodies to *G. lamblia*. Using a modified ELISA, Grundy, et al. (62) demonstrated antibodies against *E. histolytica* in 31% of colostral specimens and 14% of sera specimens tested from women living in Kenya. Few women had titers in both milk and serum.

<u>*In Vivo* Studies</u>

Several studies using animal models have shown the protective effect of antibodies in human milk to *E. coli*, *V. cholerae*, and *C. difficile* (Table 1) (41,42,47,49). The significance of these antibodies in protecting human infants from diarrhea is not known. Several epidemiologic studies have shown that human milk protects infants from diarrhea due to specific enteropathogens (Table 3). In the majority of these studies, it is not known whether such protection is mediated by specific immunologic components, nonspecific defense factors or by decreasing exposure to enteropathogens that may contaminate other foods or formula. Nursery outbreaks of diarrhea due to *E. coli* 0111 have been controlled by feeding infants human milk (63). In Guatemala, a lower incidence of *E. coli* colonization and of symptoms associated with enteropathic *E. coli* in breast-fed infants than in bottle-fed infants was found (13).

The number of *E. coli* in stools from breast-fed infants correlated inversely with the concentration of IgA in the milk being consumed (64). However, in studies in which colostrum was successfully used to combat infantile diarrhea caused by *E. coli*, a decrease in the colonization rate after administration of the colostrum could not be demonstrated (65,66). The amount of time that Gambian infants were ill with diarrhea was inversely related to breast milk bacterostatic properties against *E. coli* (67).

In a case control study of 61 episodes of diarrhea due to *V. cholerae* in Bahrain, a significantly higher incidence of cholera in non-breast-fed infants was shown (68). It could not be determined whether the protection was due to protective factors in the milk or to lack of exposure to contaminated bottle feedings. In a prospective study of cholera in Bangladesh, breast milk IgA antibodies did not appear to protect children from colonization with *V. cholerae* 01, but did protect the breast-fed children against symptomatic cholera illness (69).

Table 3. Studies in Which Human Milk Was Shown to Affect Morbidity and Mortality of Specific Enteric Baceteria

Study Location References	Organism	Result	Milk factor(s) Evaluated
Svirsky-Gross (63) (Israel)	*Escherichia coli*	Decreased diarrhea due to *E. coli* 0111	None
Mata and Urrutia (13) (Guatamala)	*E. coli*	Resistance of breast-fed infants to colonization with, and symptoms due to, EPEC.	None
Michael et al. (64) (United States)	*E. coli*	Decreased *E. coli* in stools	IgA
Larguia et al. (66) (Argentina)	*E. coli*	Decreased infantile diarrhea when given therapeutically	None
Rowland et al. (67) (Gambia)	*E. coli*	Protection against Diarrhea correlated with breast milk properties	Unspecified bacteriostatic properties
Gunn et al. (68) (Bahrain, Arabian Gulf)	*Vibrio cholerae*	Higher risk of diarrhea in non-breast-fed infants	None
Glass et al. (69) (Bangladesh)	*V. cholerae*	Less diarrhea in infants fed breast milk containing antibodies	IgA *V.cholerae* antibodies to lipopolysaccharide and cholera toxin
France et al. (70) (United States)	Salmonella	More salmonella in stool of non-breast-fed infants	Neutrophils and macrophages
Stoll et al. (71) (Bangladesh)	Shigella	Shigella diarrhea milder in breast-fed infants	None

France, et al. (70) reviewed histories of 253 infants, less than 12 months old, from whose stools salmonella was identified. Only 5% of the infants involved had ever been breast-fed. Only one infant had been breast-fed near the time of infection, and 27% of the age-matched controls had been breast-fed. An investigation of shigellosis in infants under 2 years of age in Bangladesh (71) showed that the need for hospitalization was significantly less in breast-fed than in non-breast-fed infants (5% vs 19%), as was the requirement for intravenous fluids (16% vs 38%). These results suggest that diarrhea in breast-fed infants may be milder than in non-breast-fed infants.

Multiple types of antibodies to viruses have been detected in milk from animals and humans; however, the role of these antibodies is not entirely clear. Only polio vaccine virus and rotavirus have been shown *in vivo* in humans to be affected by antibody in milk.

Data regarding the role of human milk antibody in preventing or modifying human rotavirus infection are scant. In newborns, breast feeding was associated with a lower rate of neonatal rotavirus infection (22% versus 58%, $p < 0.01$). When infected, breast-fed neonates shed less virus, and it was often clumped (72,73). A similar phenomenon occurs *in vitro* in immune electronmicroscopy when specific antibody causes clumping of viral particles (74). In one of the few convincing studies, breast feeding protected neonates against rotavirus infection (75). The protection was correlated both with antirotavirus secretory IgA and anti-trypsin activity of the mothers' milk (75). Administering high-titer antirotavirus antisera orally to lowbirth-weight infants delayed rotavirus excretion, decreased the amount of excretion, and decreased the severity of the diarrhea (76). In a small study involving older infants, provision of milk to hospitalized children had no effect on rotavirus excretion, but reduced the severity of illness (77). Antirotavirus activity in the milk was not measured. In two immunodeficient children, one with severe combined immunodeficiency and one with agammaglobulinemia, provision of irradiated, lactose-free milk containing antibody to rotavirus seemed to rid the children of their chronic rotavirus excretion and diarrhea (78).

Although protection against *Giardia muris* was transmitted in milk to suckling mice (79,80), a study conducted in humans (81) did not substantiate that finding. The human study was unable to establish clear-cut protection related to human milk anti-*Giardia lamblia* antibodies as measured by immunofluorescence.

SUMMARY

It is uncertain whether the protection by human milk against diarrhea morbidity and mortality extends to all enteropathogens or whether it varies, with greater protection against some agents and less protection against others. The relative role of nonantibody and antibody protective factors in human milk in preventing or modifying diarrhea needs further elucidation.

ACKNOWLEDGEMENT

This research was supported by NIH grant HD-13021

REFERENCES

1. Kovar MG, Serdula MK, Marks JS, Fraser DW. (1984): Review of the epidemiologic evidence for an association between infant feeding and infant health. Pediatrics, 74 (suppl.), 615-638.

2. Jason JM, Nieburg P, Marks JS. (1984): Mortality and infectious disease associated with infant-feeding practices in developing countries. Pediatrics, 74 (suppl), 702-727.

3. Feachem RG, Koblinsky MA. (1984): Interventions for the control of diarrhoeal diseases among young children: promotion of breast feeding. Bull W H O, 62, 271-291.

4. DuPont HL, Pickering LK. (1980): Infections of the gastrointestinal tract. New York: Plenum Publishing Corp.

5. Pickering LK, DuPont HL. (1985): Acute infectious gastroenteritis. In: Pickering LK, DuPont HL, eds, Infectious Diseases of Children and Adults. Menlo Park, CA: Addison Wesley Publishing Company.

6. Goldman AS, Smith CW. (1973): Host-resistance factors in human milk. J Pediatr, 82, 1082-1090.

7. Welsh JK, May JT. (1979): Anti-infective properties of breast milk. J Pediatr, 94, 1-9.

8. Ogra PL, Greene HL. (1982): Human milk and breast feeding: an update on the state of the art. Pediatr Res, 16, 266-271.

9. Goldman AS, Goldblum RM. (1985): Protective properties of human milk in nutrition in pediatrics. In: Walker WA, ed, Basic Science and Clinical Application. Little Brown and Company.

10. Pittard WB. (1979): Breast-milk immunology: a frontier in infant nutrition. Am J Dis Child, 133, 83-87.

11. Beerens H, Romond C, Neut C. (1980): Influence of breast feeding on the bifid flora of the newborn intestine. Am J Clin Nutrit, 32, 2434-2439.

12. Bullen CL, Tearle PV, Stewart MG. (1977): The effect of "humanized" milks and supplemented breast feeding on the faecal flora of infants. J Med Microbiol, 10, 403.

13. Mata LJ, Urrutia JJ. (1971): Intestinal colonization of breast-fed children in a rural area of low socioeconomical level. Ann NY Acad Sci, 176, 93-109.

14. Hentges DJ. (1967): Influence of pH on the inhibitory activity of formic and acetic acids for Shigella. J Bacteriol, 93, 2020-2030.

15. Hanson LA, Winberg J. (1972): Breast milk and defense against infection in the newborn. Arch Dis Child, 47, 845-848.

16. Bullen CL. (1977): The role of pH and buffering capacity of feces in the control of Gram-negative intestinal flora. In: Food and Immunology. XIII Symp Swed Nutrit Foundation, 142-147.

17. Nakajima S, Baba AS, Tamura N. (1977): Complement system in human colostrum. Int Arch Allergy Appl Immunol, 54, 428.

18. Bullen CL, Willis AT. (1971): Resistance of the breast-fed infant to gastroenteritis. Br Med J, 3, 338.

19. Reiter B, Brock JH. (1975): Inhibition of *Escherichia coli* by bovine colostrum and post-colostral milk. I. Complement mediated bactericidal activity of antibodies to a serum susceptible strain of *E. coli* of serotype O111. Immunology, 28, 71.

20. Chandan RC, Shahani KM, Holly RG. (1964): Lysozyme content of human milk. Nature, 204, 706.

21. Adinolfi M, Glynn AA, Lindsay M, Milne CM. (1966): Serological properties of A antibodies to *Escherichia coli* present in human colostrum. Immunology, 10, 517.

22. Heddle RJ, Knop J, Steele EJ, Rowley D. (1975): The effect of lysozome on the complement dependent bactericidal action of different antibody classes. Immunol, 28, 1061-1066.

23. Miller TE. (1969): Killing and lysis of gram-negative bacteria through the synergistic effect of hydrogen peroxide, ascorbic acid and lysozyme. J Bacteriol, 98, 949.

24. Griffiths E, Humphreys J. (1977): Bacteriostatic effect of human milk and bovine colostrum on *Escherichia coli*: importance of bicarbonate. Infect Immun, 15, 396.

25. Kirkpatrick CH, Green I, Rich RR, Schade AL. (1971): Inhibition of growth of *Candida albicans* by iron-unsaturated lactoferrin: relation to host defense mechanisms in chronic mucocutaneous candidasis. J Infect Dis, 124, 539.

26. Holmgren J, Svennerholm A-M, Ahren C: Nonimmune fraction of human milk inhibits bacterial adhesion (hemagglutination) and enterotoxin binding of *Escherichia coli* and *Vibrio cholerae*. Infect Immun 1981; 33:136-141.

27. Holmgren J, Svennerholm A-M, Lindblad M. (1983): Receptor-like glycocompounds in human milk that inhibit classical and El Tor *Vibrio cholerae* cell adherence (hemagglutination). Infect Immun, 39, 147-154.

28. Otnaess AB, Orstavik I. (1981): Effect of fractions of Ethiopian and Norwegian colostrum on rotavirus and *Escherichia coli* heat labile enterotoxin. Infect Immun, 33, 459-466.

29. Gillen FD, Reiner DS, Wang CS. (1983): Human milk kills parasitic intestinal protozoa. Science, 221, 1290-1292.

30. Kumar S, McKerlie ML, Albrecht TE, Goldman AS, Barron S. (1984): A broadly active viral inhibitor in human and animal organ extracts and bodily fluids. Proc Soc Exper Biol Med, 177, 104-111.

31. Otnaess AB, Svennerholm AM. (1982): Non-immunoglobulin fraction of human milk protects rabbits against enterotoxin-induced intestinal fluid secretion. Infect Immun, 35, 738-740.

32. Otnaess AB, Laegreid A, Ertresvag K. (1983): Inhibition of enterotoxin from *E. coli* and *V. cholerae* by gangliosides from human milk. Infect Immun, 40, 563-566.

33. Cleary TG, Chambers JP, Pickering LK. (1983): Protection of suckling mice from heat-stable enterotoxin of *Escherichia coli* by human milk. J Infect Dis, 148, 1114-1119.

34. Cleary TG, Chambers JP, Pickering LK. Protection of suckling mice from heat-stable enterotoxin of *Escherichia coli* by infant formulas. J Pediatr Gastr Nutrit. (In press).

35. Ogra SS, Ogra PL. (1978): Immunologic aspects of human colostrum and milk. I. Distribution characteristics and concentrations of immunoglobulins at different times after the onset of lactation. J Pediatr, 92, 546-549.

36. Ammann AJ, Steihm ER. (1966): Immune globulin levels in colostrum and breast milk, and serum from formula- and breast-fed newborns. Proc Soc Exp Biol Med, 122, 1098.

37. Kenny JF, Boesman MI, Michaels RH. (1967): Bacterial and viral coproantibodies in breast-fed infants. Pediatrics, 39, 202.

38. Gindrat JJ, et al. (1972): Antibodies in human milk against *E. coli* of the serogroups most commonly found in neonatal infections. Acta Paediatr Scand, 61, 587-590.

39. Allardyce RA, Shearman DJC, McClelland DBL, Marwick K, Simpson AJ, Laidlaw RB. (1974): Appearance of specific colostrum antibodies after clinical infection with *Salmonella typhimurium*. Brit Med J, 3, 307-309.

40. Hanson LA, Carlsson B, Ahlstedt S, Svanborg C, Kaijsen B. (1975): Immune defense factors in human milk. Mod Probl Paediatr, 15, 63.

41. Stolier OA, Pelley RP, Kaniecki-Green E, Klaus MH, Carpenter CCJ. (1976): Secretory IgA against enterotoxins in breast milk. Lancet, 1, 1258-1261.

42. Holmgren J, Hanson LA, Carlson B, Linblad BS, Rahimtoola J. (1976): Neutralizing antibody against *E. coli* and *V. cholerae* enterotoxins in human milk from a developing country. Scand J Immunol, 5, 867-871.

43. Simhon A, Yolken RH, Mata L. (1979): S-IgA cholera toxin and rotavirus antibody in human colostrum. Acta Paediatr Scand, 68, 161-164.

44. Vardinon N, Spiner Z, Goldhar J, Kacevman B, Eylan E. (1979): Human milk anti-*E. coli* antibodies: relationship to maternal parity. Eur J Pediatr, 130, 173-180.

45. Aust-Kettis A, Gebre-Medhin M, Habte D, Khosla N, Wadstrom T. (1981): Antibiotics to heat-labile *Escherichia coli* enterotoxins in human milk and sera: a study of Ethiopian and Swedish mothers and their children. Trop Geo Med, 33, 225-230.

46. Majumdar AS, Dutta P, Dutta D, Ghase AC. (1981): Antibacterial and antitoxins in the serum and milk of cholera patients. Infect Immun, 32, 1-8.

47. Majumdar AS, Ghose AC. (1982): Protective properties of anticholera antibodies in human colostrum. Infect Immun, 36, 962-965.

48. Cruz JR, Garcia CB, Gebre-Medhin M, Hofvander Y, Urrutia JJ, Hanson LA. (1982): Studies on human milk III. Secretory IgA quantity and antibody levels against *Escherichia coli* in colostrum and milk from underprivileged and privileged mothers. Pediatrs Res, 16, 272-276.

49. Kim K, Pickering LK, DuPont HL, Sullivan N, Wilkins T. (1984): *In vitro* and *in vivo* neutralizing activity of human colostrum and milk against purified toxins A and B of *Clostridium difficile*. J Infect Dis, 150, 57-62.

50. Michaels RM. (1965): Studies of antiviral factors in human milk and serum. J Immunol, 94, 262-268.

51. Cook DA, Zbitnew A, Dempster G, Gerrard JW. (1978): Detection of antibody to rotavirus by counterimmunoelectrophoresis in human serum, colostrum, and milk. J Pediatr, 93, 967-970.

52. Schoub BD, Protzesky OW, Lecatsas G, Oosthuizen R. (1978): The role of breast-feeding in the prevention of rotavirus infection. J Med Microbiol, 11, 25-31.

53. Otnaess AB, Orstavik I. (1980): The effect of human milk fractions on rotavirus in relation to the secretory IgA content. Acta Path Microbiol Scand Spetc, 88, 15-21.

54. Cukor G, Blacklow N, Capozza F, Panjvani Z, Bedmarek F. (1978): Secretory IgA antibodies to rotavirus in human milk 6-9 months postpartum. Lancet, 2, 631-632.

55. Cukor G, Blacklow NR, Capozza FE, Panjvani ZF, Bednarek F. (1979): Persistence of antibodies to rotavirus in human milk. J Clin Microbiol, 9, 93-96.

56. Simhon A, Mata L. (1978): Anti-rotavirus antibody in human colostrum. Lancet, 1, 39-40.

57. Yolken RH, Wyatt RG, Mata L, Urrutia JJ, Garcia B, Chanock RM, Kapikian AZ. (1978): Secretory antibody directed against rotavirus in human milk - measurement by means of enzyme-linked immunosorbent assay. J Pediatr, 93, 916-921.

58. McLean B, Holmes IH. (1980): Transfer of anti-rotaviral antibodies from mothers to their infants. J Clin Microbiol, 12, 320-325.

59. Palmer EL, Gary GW Jr., Black R, Martin ML. (1980): Antiviral activity of colostrum and serum immunoglobulins A and G. J Med Virol, 5, 123-129.

60. Totterdell BM, Chrystie IL, Banatvala JE. (1980): Cord blood and breast-milk antibodies in neonatal rotavirus infection. Brit Med J, 280, 822-830.

61. Miotti P, Gilman R, Pickering LK, Ruiz-Palacios G, Cleary T, Yolken R. (1984): Serum and milk antibody levels to *Giardia lamblia*. Pediatr Res, 18, 261A.

62. Grundy MS, Cartwright-Taylor L, Lundin L, Thors C, Huldt G. (1983): Antibodies against *Entamoeba histolytica* in human milk and serum in Kenya. J Clin Microbiol, 17, 753-758.

63. Svirsky-Gross S. (1958): Pathogenic strains of *E. coli* (0111) among prematures and the use of human milk in controlling the outbreak of diarrhea. Ann Paediatr, 190, 109-115.

64. Michael JC, Ringenback R, Hottenstein S. (1971): The antimicrobial activity of human colostral antibody in the newborn. J Infect Dis, 124, 445.

65. Gothefors L, Carlsson B, Ahlstedt S, Hanson A, Winberg J. (1976): Influence of maternal gut flora and colostral and cord serum antibodies on the presence of *Escherichia coli* in the feces of the newborn infant. Acta Paediatr Scand, 65, 225-232.

66. Larguia AM, Urman J, Stoliar OA, Ceriani JM, O'Donnell A, Buscuglia JC, Martinez JC. (1977): Fresh human colostrum for the prevention of *E. coli* diarrhea - a clinical experience. J Trop Pediatr Environ Child Health, 23, 289-290.

67. Rowland MGM, Cole TJ, Tully M. (1980): Bacteriostasis of *Escherichia coli* by milk. VI The *in vitro* bacteriostatic property of Gambian mothers' breast milk in relation to the *in vivo* protection of their infants against diarrheal disease. J Hyg, 85, 403-413.

68. Gunn RA, Kimball AM, Pollard RA, Feeley JC, Feldman RA, Dutta SR, Mathew PP, Levine MM. (1979): Bottle feeding is a risk factor for cholera in infants. Lancet, 2, 730-732.

69. Glass RI, Svennerholm A, Stoll BJ, Khan MR, Kossain KMB, Hug MI, Holmgren J. (1983): Milk antibodies protect breast-fed children against cholera. N Engl J Med, 308, 1389-1392.

70. France GL, Marmer DJ, Steele RW. (1980): Breast-feeding and Salmonella infection. Am J Dis Child, 134, 147-152.

71. Stoll BJ, Glass RI, Hug MI. (1982): Epidemiologic and clinical features of patients infected with Shigella who attended a diarrheal disease hospital in Bangladesh. J Infect Dis, 146, 177-183.

72. Totterdell BM, Chrystie IL, Banatvala JE. (1976): Rotavirus infections in a maternity unit. Arch Dis Child, 51, 924-928.

73. Chrystie IL, Totterdell BM, Banatvala JE. (1978): Asymptomatic endemic rotavirus infections in the newborn. Lancet, 1, 1176-1178.

74. Totterdell BM, Banatvala JE, Chrystie IL. (1983): Studies on human lacteal rotavirus antibodies by immuno electron microscope. J Med Virol, 11, 167-175.

75. McLean BS, Holmes IH. (1981): Effects of antibodies, trypsin, and trypsin inhibition on susceptibility of neonates to rotavirus infections. J Clin Microbiol, 13, 22-29.

76. Barnes GL, Hewson PM, McLellan JA, Doyle LW, Knoches AML, Kitchen WH, Bishop RF. (1983): A randomized trial of oral gammaglobulin in low-birth-weight infants infected with rotavirus. Lancet, 1, 1371-1373.

77. Berger R, Hadziselimovic F, Just M, Reigel F. (1984): Influence of breast milk on nosocomial rotavirus infections in infants. Infection, 12, 171-174.

78. Saulsbury FT, Winkelstein JA, Yolken RM. (1980): Chronic rotavirus infection in immunodeficiency. J Pediatr, 97, 61-65.

79. Stevens DR, Frank DM. (1978): Local immunity in murine giardiasis: is milk protective at the expense of maternal gut? Trans Assoc Am Physicians, 91, 268-272.

80. Andrews JS, Jr., Hewlett EL. (1981): Protection against infection with *Giardia muris* by milk containing antibody to Giardia. J Infect Dis, 143, 242-246.

81. Islam A. Stoll BJ, Ljungstrom I, Biswas J, Nazrul H, Huldt G. (1983): *Giardia lamblia* infections in a cohort of Bangladeshi mothers and infants followed for one year. J Pediatr, 103, 996-1000.

FUTURE DIRECTIONS FOR STUDIES OF THE IMMUNOLOGIC SYSTEM IN HUMAN MILK

A. S. Goldman
B. Carlsson
L. Pickering
M. Keller
M. J. Paape

Although many of the techniques which are necessary to define the immunologic system in human milk are at hand, the methodologies which are required to further define the system and investigate the fate and effects of this system upon the recipient infant are still evolving.

1. The leukocytes in human milk will require special attention because of their unusual structures and because of modifications in their functional capabilities. Considerable ingenuity will be required to track the *in vivo* fate of these cells, but that will nevertheless be of considerable importance. Perhaps an adaptation of stable isotope techniques will help in this regard.

2. The compartmentation of immunologic factors in human milk is poorly defined, but such information may be critical to understanding the action of the components of the immunologic system and to identifying those parts of the intestinal tract and respiratory system where the factors are released and where they function.

3. The effect of maternal and environmental factors upon the development of the immunologic system in human milk will undoubtedly be explored in more detail in the next several years. It is known that principal secretory IgA antibodies in human milk originate from lymphoid cells that arise from the entero- and bronchomammary gland pathways, but the extent that these pathways can be manipulated by immunization of the mother to provide a wider spectrum of protective antibodies for the infant is not known. In addition, the transfer of cellular immunity through breast-feeding continues to be a controversial issue that should be explored.

4. The fate and effects of these immune substances and their interactions with the immune system of the infant will undoubtedly be a major focus for future research. One potential approach, which may be particularly fruitful for tracking the fate of the factors, is labelling components with stable isotopes and detecting the labelled factors *in vitro* and *in vivo* by nuclear magnetic resonance. By coupling these types of measurements with immunologic techniques, it should be possible to simultaneously quantify those components which are contributed from the mammary gland and those synthesized by the infant. In that respect, more studies should also be directed to the complex

changes that occur not only during uninterrupted breast-feeding, but also during the weaning and post-weaning periods.

Although the mucosal effects of the defense factors in human milk have been stressed, further attention should also be given to the possible systemic effects of breast-feeding upon the recipient infant.

Thus, it is anticipated that advances in our knowledge regarding the immunologic system in human milk will lead to a better understanding of the manner in which breast-feeding protects the recipient infant, and ways of capitalizing upon those protective mechanisms.

ACKNOWLEDGEMENT

The aid of Susan Kovacevich in the preparation of these manuscripts was greatly appreciated.

The research document herein was supported in part by NIHC NO1 HD 22815, NIH-GCRC-RR00425, New Investigator Grant: AI-17124-01 National Institute of Allergy and Infectious Disease

Section IV. COMPARTMENTATION OF HUMAN MILK

WORKSHOP PARTICIPANTS

G. E. Huston, Department of Neurosciences, University of California, San Diego, La Jolla, California

S. Patton, Department of Neurosciences, University of California, San Diego, La Jolla, California

INTRODUCTION

Human milk is not a homogeneous fluid. Rather, it consists of several compartments, most of which can be separated by differential centrifugation. The fat fraction contributes milk fat globules surrounded by plasma membrane. The cellular compartment contains both white blood cells and mammary epithelial cells. High-speed centrifugation produces a pellet which consists of two layers, a protein pellet and a "fluff" layer. These two papers deal with the separation of these compartments. Related papers on the separation and identification of cells and on the enzyme compartments of the "fluff" layer are found in Sections III and XII, respectively.

ISOLATION OF FAT GLOBULES FROM HUMAN MILK

S. Patton
G. E. Huston

INTRODUCTION

Isolation of milk fat globules, such as for the preparation of the globule membrane (1), is customarily accomplished by centrifugation to collect the globules and by redispersion of them in buffer. Three or four such cycles are usually sufficient to eliminate the other milk constituents and enable one to make further observations on the purified globules. Unfortunately, the structure of milk fat globules is sufficiently fragile that such procedures are of limited value. It has been shown that 85% of the xanthine oxidase and alkaline phosphatase activities are removed from bovine milk fat globules by four successive water washes (2). Moreover, microscopists have called attention to changes in globule membrane structure which transpire spontaneously soon after secretion of the globule from the lactating cell (Ref. 1, p. 299). Such observations stress the importance of using freshly secreted milk and minimum manipulations in order to obtain fat globules with maximum biochemical and structural integrity. We describe a relatively simple method for isolating globules from human milk. The method is based on a single centrifugation through overlying buffer.

MATERIALS AND METHODS

Five ml of freshly collected human milk (uncooled) is placed in a 12-ml round-bottom tube, and 0.25 g of sucrose is added. The tube is gently swirled to dissolve the sucrose. A 9-inch Pasteur-type pipette with a long capillary is placed, capillary end down, in a 15-ml conical centrifuge tube that has been filled with 10 ml of warm (37°C) buffer, saline or water. The sucrose-treated milk is carefully inserted into the open end of the pipette by means of a 6-inch Pasteur-type pipette fitted with a rubber bulb. Transfer of several pipette loads is required, and air bubbles should be avoided. When all the milk has been transferred, the pipette in the tube is lifted so that the tip is just above the milk-buffer interface. It is held there momentarily for drainage, then covered with a finger at the upper end, and removed from the tube in one smooth motion. The tube and contents are centrifuged at 1500 x g and ambient temperature for 20 minutes in a swinging bucket type rotor. The use of a cap or film cover on the tube keeps the surface of the globule layer from drying during centrifugation. The resulting globule layer is transferred to an appropriate dispersing medium with a spatula. Gentle vortex mixing for 1 to 2 minutes is adequate to accomplish resuspension of the globules.

Protein content of globule suspensions was estimated by the method of Lowry et al. (3) using bovine serum albumin as the standard. Turbidity due to lipids was eliminated by extracting the samples with n-butanol following color development. SDS-polyacrylamide gel electrophoresis of globule suspensions and of human milk was accomplished using the procedures of Laemmli (4).

RESULTS AND DISCUSSION

Gel electrophoresis patterns of proteins from globules isolated by our procedure are shown in Figure 1. The globule preparations were from mature milks (greater than 30 days in lactation) of three donors. The three

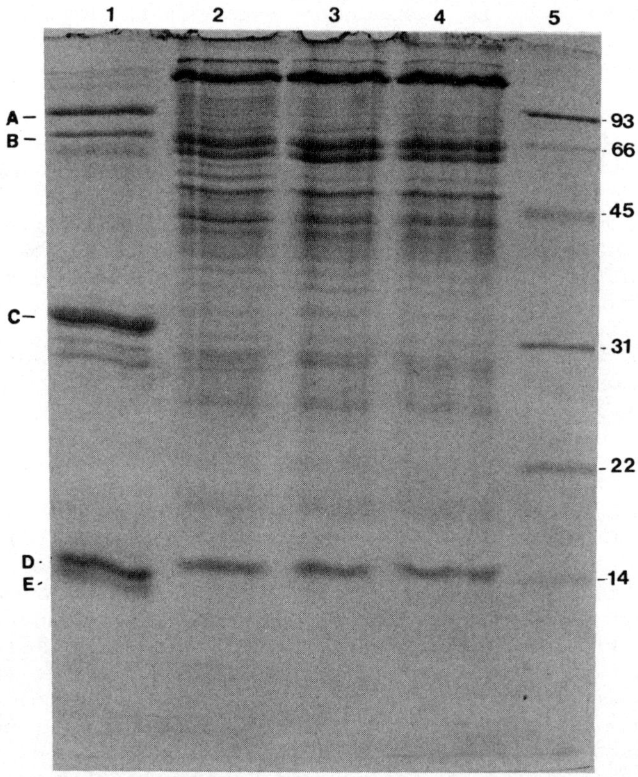

Figure 1. SDS-Polyacrylamide Gel Electrophoresis Patterns of Fat Globules From the Milk of Three Women (Lanes 2-4), of Human Milk (Lane 1), and of Reference Proteins (Lane 5, With $M_r \times 10^{-3}$, as Indicated). Globules were isolated from milk by centrifugation through phosphate buffered salt solution (.025 M phosphate, .15 M saline, pH 7.4). See text for details. Identities of the major (skim) milk proteins are: A-lactoferrin, B-serum albumin, C-βcasein, D-lysozyme, E-α-lactalbumin. Sample loads were 20, 50, and 6 μg of protein for lanes 1, 2-4, and 5, respectively. Samples were heated at 98°C for 2 minutes in SDS-mercaptoethanol-phosphate buffer (pH 7.0). Gel was 12.5% polyacrylamide, 1.5 mm thick, and stained with coomassie blue.

patterns (lanes 2-4) are similar, and they closely resemble the patterns for globules that were prepared by multiple washings as well as the patterns for human milk fat globule membrane that was produced by several methods (data not shown). Comparison of bands for major proteins of human milk (lane 1) with bands for the globules, indicates the absence of skim milk contamination in the globules.

The force of 1500 x g for 20 minutes is more than is needed to spin up all but traces of globules. It produces a skim milk of less than 0.1% lipid. However, such force creates a globule layer that is sufficiently compacted for transfer with a spatula. At lower forces, the cream (globule) layer can be removed with a syringe. For some analytical purposes of either the fat globule or skim milk phases, the most effective separation is to centrifuge in plastic tubes, then freeze the contents, and saw the tubes just below the globule layer.

It is imperative in our method to avoid turbulence and vibration during preparation and centrifugation of tube contents. Scale-up using a 40- or 50-ml centrifuge tube, 25 or 35 ml of buffer, and a 15 ml sucrose-treated (0.75 g) milk sample, yields satisfactory globule separation.

ACKNOWLEDGEMENT

This research was supported by contract NO1-HD-2-2819 from the National Institute of Child Health and Human Development.

REFERENCES

1. Patton S, Keenan TW. (1975): The milk fat globule membrane. Biochim Biophys Acta, 415, 273-309.

2. Zittle CA, Dellamonica ES, Custer JH, Rudd RR. (1956): The fat globule membrane of milk: alkaline phosphatase and xanthine oxidase in skim milk and cream. J Dairy Sci, 39, 528-535.

3. Lowry OH, Rosebrough NJ, Farr AL, Randall RJ. (1951): Protein measurement with the Folin phenol reagent. J Biol Chem, 193, 265-275.

4. Laemmli UK. (1970): Cleavage of structural proteins during the assembly of the head of bacteriophage T4. Nature, 227, 680-685.

MEMBRANE DISTRIBUTION IN HUMAN MILKS

AS REVEALED BY PHOSPHOLIPID AND CHOLESTEROL ANALYSES

G. E. Huston
S. Patton

INTRODUCTION

Milks of the various mammals contain membrane material. Milk fat globules, including those of the human (1), are secreted from the lactating cell by envelopment in membrane (for reviews, 2,3). The various somatic cells in milk (4) are comprised of membranes. There is also ultramicro membrane material in milk. Morton (5) showed that high speed centrifugation of bovine milk produces a sedimenting fraction. He termed this fraction "microsomes," because of its similarities to the classical membrane fraction of that name from cell homogenates. Stewart et al. (6) demonstrated that this fraction of milk is morphologically diverse, as it is comprised of microvilli, flattened sacs and various kinds of membrane-bound vesicles. They designated this the "fluff" fraction because on high speed centrifugation of bovine skim milk, it deposited as a loose layer on top of the casein pellet. The nature and origin of this membrane material has been reviewed (3).

A unique structure to be seen in the so-called fluff fraction is a fat globule with associated cytoplasm from the lactating cell. Wooding et al. (7) drew attention to these fat globules with cytoplasmic crescents. Christie and Wooding (8) demonstrated that these structures in the skim milk phase of goat milk accounted for the lipogenic capability previously detected in such milk (9). These cytoplasmic inclusions normally contain endoplasmic reticulum, among other cell components, so their biosynthetic ability is not surprising. Depending on the relative proportions of fat droplet to cytoplasmic inclusion, such particles will either rise with fat globules, or sediment with the "fluff", on centrifugation. While such fat droplets accompanied by cytoplasm are readily observable in goat (8,10) and human milks (1, also G. E. Huston and S. Patton, unpublished data), they appear to be rare in bovine milk (10).

Thus, it is evident that milks contain membrane material in diverse micro and ultramicro structures. Whether milk membrane has special nutritional merits is not known. However, in infant feeding, it can be conceived as building material for proliferation of intestinal mucosal membrane of the neonate. It can also act as a vehicle, in the case of membrane-bound vesicles, to transport milk or cell components directly (bypassing digestion) into mucosal cells by membrane fusion processes. No doubt digestion products of membranes (such as cholesterol, essential fatty acids, lysophosphatides, oligosaccharides and possibly intact membrane components) benefit the newborn.

For the purposes of analysis, membrane material in milk can be defined in terms of three compartments: milk fat globules, somatic cells, and the skim milk phase (which contains the "fluff" fraction). This division is useful because on relatively gentle centrifugation (about 500 x g) the fat globules with associated membrane rise; the somatic cells sediment, and the fluff material remains suspended in the skim milk. With such a division into globules and skim milk, Patton and associates provided some limited data on membrane distribution in cow and goat milks using phospholipid and cholesterol contents as criteria of membrane. They found that in milks of both species about 60% of the phospholipid is associated with the fat globules and 40% with the skim milk (11). In the skim milks, they observed that 45 to 75% of the phospholipid and unesterified cholesterol were contained in the fluff fraction (6). The somatic cell fraction was not analyzed in those studies.

There have been no attempts to determine the quantities or distribution of membrane in human milks or to characterize the membranes in the fluff or microsomal fraction. We present here schemes for the isolation of the membrane compartments in human milk, observations on membrane distribution in 19 random samples based on phospholipid and cholesterol analyses, and preliminary data on ultrastructure of the fluff fraction.

METHODS

Sampling

Lactation times for the 19 random samples of human milk employed in this study averaged 101 days and ranged from 2 to 448 days. Milk expressions, mainly by hand pump (Egnell or Kaneson), were from single breasts and represented at least a 4-hour accumulation since last nursing. The mean sample volume was 73 ml with a range of 19 to 182 ml.

Fractionation

Preparation of cell, fat globule and skim milk (milk essentially free of fat globules and cells) fractions was initiated within an hour of milking, as follows: 40 ml of milk (but less for 3 samples) was centrifuged at 750 x g and 20-24°C for 20 minutes in a conical tube. The supernatant was decanted quantitatively into a clean centrifuge tube (round bottom) for further fractionation. The small pellet of cells was washed twice by gentle resuspension in 1.5 ml of saline (0.15 M) and recentrifuging. The washed cells were adjusted with water to a volume of 1.5 ml for the purpose of analysis. The cream/skim milk supernatant was centrifuged at 1000 x g and 20-24°C for 15 minutes. The resulting skim milk (lower phase) was removed from under the cream layer with a dispopipette (long capillary) connected to a vacuum via a suction flask. The layer of fat globules was resuspended in warm (37°C) 0.15 M saline by gentle vortexing, made to 40 ml with the saline and centrifuged as before. The saline was removed, as it was for skim milk, and this washing process was repeated twice. The washed globules were resuspended to known volume, one portion in saline, another in distilled water. Portions of all fractions, and the fresh milks, were frozen at -70°C for subsequent analysis.

To determine whether fluff membrane material exists in human milks, we isolated the fraction, as described for bovine milk (6). Skim milk, prepared as described, was centrifuged at 2 to 4°C and 100,000 x g for 3 hours. The material resting on the casein pellet was collected, resuspended in 0.15 M NaCl, resedimented at 2 to 4°C and 100,000 x g for 1 hour and again suspended to a specified volume (1.5 to 2.5 ml) in saline. Fluff was prepared from 16 of the 19 milks, and a portion of each preparation was placed in -70°C storage for subsequent analysis. Several of the fresh fluff isolates were fixed and embedded in a conventional manner for electron microscopy, essentially as for fluff from bovine milk (6). For comparative purposes, fluff also was isolated and processed from goat milk. Sections were viewed in a JEOL 100 B electron microscope.

Analyses

Total lipid was obtained by the Roese-Gottlieb solvent extraction procedure (12), using a 1.0 ml sample and 1.5% addition of NaCl to maximize recovery of phospholipid (13). Following gravimetric quantitation of the lipid, it was dissolved and made to volume (0.5 ml) in 19:1 (v/v) chloroform:methanol. For phospholipid determinations, 100 μl aliquots of this solution were evaporated in duplicate at the origin on a silica gel thin-layer chromatography plate (Merck). The plates were developed with hexane:ethyl ether:acetic acid 50:50:1 (v/v/v) to move triglycerides away from the sample origin, the area which retains the phospholipids. After staining lipids on the developed plate with iodine vapor, the silica gel at the sample origins (including controls) was scraped into ignition tubes and analyzed for phosphorus using Rouser's method (14). Phosphorous was converted to phospholipid by the factor x 25. A 250 μl sample of milk was used to assay total cholesterol by the colorimetric method that uses o-phthalic aldehyde -- See Bachman et al. (15). The reliability of this method was checked against the colorimetric procedure of Sperry and Webb (16).

The method of Lowry et al. (17), as modified by us for application to human milk (18), was used to assay total protein in milk and its fractions. Removal of lipids, the source of a turbidity problem, was not necessary in the analysis of skim milk and fluff fractions. However, the butanol extraction step was required for fat globule samples because of their high lipid-to-protein ratio.

These same assays, with modifications as to sample size, were applied to whole milks, skim milks, washed globules, cell and fluff fractions.

Somatic cells in human milks were determined by the U.S. Public Health Service direct microscopic counting procedure (19) using 10 μl of milk spread over precisely 1 cm^2 on a calibrated glass slide. One μl of 5% sodium caseinate (Fisher Scientific Co., Fair Lawn, NJ) was added to bind the cells to the slide during drying and staining with the methylene blue reagent.

RESULTS

Table 1 summarizes analytical results for the 19 milks and their fractions. As can be seen from the total protein and lipid data, most of the protein went into the skim milk and most of the lipid into the fat globule fraction. The mean value for whole milk phospholipid, 226 μg/ml or 7.3 mg/g of lipid, agrees well with 0.8% of lipid reported by Bitman et al. (20). Somewhat higher levels, 400 μg/ml or 10 mg/g of lipid, were found

Table 1. Lipid, Protein, Phospholipid and Total Cholesterol Contents of Some Human Milks and Fractions Thereof[a]

	Lipid mg/ml	Protein mg/ml	Phospholipid μg/ml	Phospholipid mg/g lipid	Cholesterol μg/ml	Cholesterol mg/g lipid
Milk	30.71±13.7	13.3±4.9	226±92	7.4±2.5	151±54	4.9±3.7
Fat Globules	---	17.9±9.9[b]	---	4.5±1.2	---	4.1±2.2
Skim Milk	1.3 ±1.1	12.7±4.6	44±30	---	40±25	---
Cells	---	0.009[c]	1.2[c]	---	0.31[c]	---
Fluff	---	0.26±0.21[c]	14.4±10[c]	---	5.1±4.0[c]	---

a 19 random samples (mean days of lactation = 101±119), and their fractions, were analyzed (except cells and fluff which are based on 16 samples). Data show standard deviations.

b mg/g of lipid

c per ml of milk

for phospholipid by Hibberd et al. (21). There is considerable variation in the total cholesterol content reported for human milks. Clark et al. (22) and Picciano et al. (23) found approximately 11 mg per 100 ml of milk, and Bitman et al. (20) found a comparable level (0.34% of total lipid). Our results, 15.1 mg/ml of milk (0.49% of total lipid) are somewhat higher than those data, but decidedly lower than the 20.5- and 22-to-35 mg/100 ml of milk reported by Potter et al. (24) and Harzer et al. (25), respectively.

The phospholipid and cholesterol concentrations in the skim milks in comparison to the whole milks, Table 1, provide some evidence of membrane distribution. On average, 19.5% of the phospholipid and 26.5% of the cholesterol are found in the skim milks. These data are probably more reliable than those derived by subtracting concentrations of the two lipids found in fat globules from the whole milk values. We feel that thrice washing of globules may remove membrane lipids as well as wash away smaller globules which have relatively higher phospholipid and cholesterol contents per g of lipid. However, it is clear that no matter which basis of calculation is used, most of the phospholipid and cholesterol of human milk is associated with the fat globules. About one-fourth and one-eighth, respectively, of skim milk phospholipid and cholesterol were recovered in the fluff fraction (see Table 1). These are not precisely quantitative indications of the fluff fraction in the skim milk for reasons discussed below.

From Table 1 it is clear that the contribution of the cell fraction to membrane material is quantitatively insignificant (< 1%). The mean somatic cell count, based on counting 14 of 19 samples, was 869,000 ± 959/ml. This is normal for human milk (4).

Data for phospholipid and cholesterol contents of fluff fractions from the individual milks, Table 2, reveal considerable quantitative variation as well as differences in the proportions of the two skim milk lipids recovered in the fluff. With one or two exceptions, there is good correlation in quantities of the two lipids in the fluff, as would be expected if they occurred in membrane. The mean cholesterol-to-phospholipid weight ratio for these data is 1:2.3.

Regarding the data of Table 2, it should be remembered that removal of fat globules in preparation of the skim milk fractions was not quantitative. Thus, there were variable amounts of phospholipid and cholesterol, associated with residual small globules, which rose to the surface during sedimentation of the fluff fractions. Every skim milk on centrifugation produced a fluff layer, but the size of the layers varied. Because of its flimsy nature and some washing losses, the fluff was not always recovered quantitatively. Nonetheless, we feel that for most of the samples, the data are satisfactory quantitative estimates.

Several samples of fluff were examined in the electron microscope. Membrane-bound vesicles, some of which are electron translucent and others which contain electron diffracting material, appeared characteristic of the fraction, Figure 1 a. A micrograph of the fluff fraction from goat's milk is shown for comparison (Figure 1 b). It too, was rich in vesicles.

Control Data

With the aid of highly purified egg phosphatidylcholine (Supelco Inc., Bellefonte, PA), we evaluated recovery of phosphorus by various aspects of our lipid phosphorus analysis. The phosphorus assay (14), alone or in combination with the thin-layer chromatography step, accounted for 100% of the phospholipid. When the reference phospholipid was dispersed in water at a concentration to approximate whole milk (200 μg/ml), the Roese-Gottlieb extraction procedure recovered an average 87% of the phospholipid.

We wished to check our results for total cholesterol in human milks by another method, because of possible complications presented by plant sterols (26). For this purpose, we chose the procedure of Sperry and Webb (16) which utilizes the specific (Lieberman-Burchardt) color reaction of cholesterol in the presence of acetic anhydride and sulfuric acid. It has been widely employed for many years to determine serum cholesterol. The method was applied both to the lipid unsaponifiable matter and to cholesterol precipitated from the unsaponifiables as the digitonide. Nine human milks were analyzed. Mean data by the procedure of Bachman et al. (15) and by the two Sperry and Webb methods, without and with digitonide isolation, showed respectively: 121 ± 59, 124 ± 54, and 104 ± 49 μg of cholesterol per ml of milk. Agreement between the two methods was close, and although recovery of cholesterol digitonide was not quantitative (84%), it is adequate considering that some loss of product is inevitable in manipulation and washing. Further, following precipitation of cholesterol as the digitonide from the samples of unsaponifiables, there was no Liebermann-Burchardt color generation by substance remaining in (infrantant) solution. Thus, as for bovine milk, the Bachman method is satisfactory for measuring cholesterol in human milk.

Table 2. The Amounts and Proportions of Phospholipid and Cholesterol (Total) in Human Skim Milks Recovered in the Fluff Fraction[a]

	PHOSPHOLIPID			CHOLESTEROL		
Sample: Days in Lactation	Skim	Fluff	% in Fluff	Skim	Fluff	% in Fluff
	μg/ml Milk			μg/ml Milk		
2	125	24.0	19	88	10.8	12
5	119	23.1	19	86	8.9	10
7	94	7.4	8	82	4.2	5
10	81	10.7	13	71	4.3	6
17	25	29.4	100	28	13.8	49
18A	108	20.2	19	58	15.8	27
18B	75	--	--	24	1.1	5
27	84	10.5	13	48	5.0	10
38	53	15.1	28	24	5.0	21
49	19	21.9	100	43	10.4	24
52	24	2.0	8	28	6.8	24
81	--	4.2	--	13	2.9	22
87	8	6.9	86	25	2.6	10
92	38	28.2	74	19	5.5	29
94	16	6.3	39	14	2.8	20
99	34	6.5	19	11	2.1	19
144	28	9.0	32	38	3.3	9
306	63	9.3	15	43	3.6	8
448	44	32.0	73	25	18.0	72
84[b]	58[b]	14.8[b]	26	40[b]	6.7[b]	17

[a] For preparation of the skim milk and fluff fraction, see text. This table includes data for three samples (5, 7 & 18A) not included in the data of Table 1.

[b] Mean Value

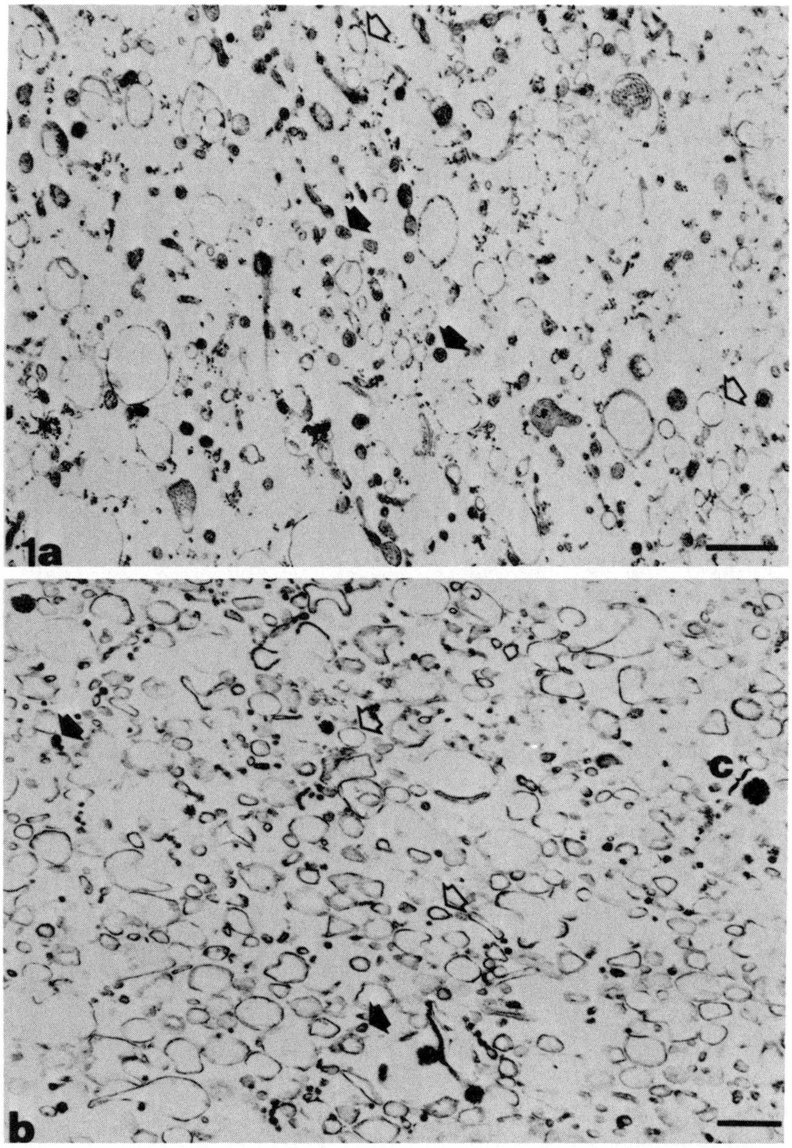

Figure 1. Electronmicrographs.

(a.) UPPER. The membrane, or so-called fluff fraction, of human skim milk showing large electron-transparent vesicles (open arrows) and smaller vesicles containing material which is somewhat electron opaque (solid arrows). Small dark granules are unidentified. Bar (lower right) represents 0.5 μ.

(b.) LOWER. The membrane, or so-called fluff fraction,from goats' skim milk showing large electron-transparent vesicles (open arrows) and smaller electron-opaque vesicles (solid arrows). Dark staining aggregates are casein micelles (C). Bar (lower right) represents 0.5 μ.

DISCUSSION

Our results establish that membrane material, so-called fluff, occurs in the skim milk phase of human milk. On average, we recovered 26% of the phospholipid and 17% of the cholesterol from the skim milks in this fraction. Anderson et al. (27) have reported that mastitic infections elevate the amount of fluff in bovine milks. While the size of this fraction in our human milk samples varied, there was no known mastitis in our donors. Nor was there evidence of such conditions from elevated somatic cell counts in their milks.

From preliminary examination in the electron microscope, the fluff of human milk is comprised in part of membrane-bound vesicles, the contents of which show variations in staining (Figure 1). Apparently such vesicles are carrying proteins, and a number of questions arise on that point. Are they milk proteins or cytoplasmic proteins of lactating or other somatic cells? Are there populations of vesicles carrying only one kind of protein? Such a finding could have important implications for protein transport within the lactating cell. As mentioned earlier, these vesicles and their contents, while not a major milk component, could represent unique nutritional packages for the infant. Our current efforts are to study fluff production, by several donors, throughout lactation and to further characterize the fluff material biochemically and by electron microscopy.

SUMMARY

Nineteen random samples of human milk, representing from 2 to 448 days in lactation, were fractionated into fat globules, somatic cells and skim milks. Phospholipid and cholesterol contents of these milks and fractions were determined and the data used to estimate membrane distribution. Somatic cells accounted for less than 1% of milk membrane material; 20 to 25% was contained in the skim milk, the remainder (greater than 70%) was associated with milk fat globules. A membrane-rich (fluff) fraction, isolated from the skim milks by centrifugation (100,000 x g for 3 hours), represented from 8 to 100% and averaged 26% of the skim milk phospholipids. In the electron microscope, the fluff was seen to contain, among other structures, membrane-bound vesicles. The possible significance of these vesicles in infant nutrition and in protein processing within the lactating cell is discussed in this article.

ACKNOWLEDGEMENTS

We thank J. S. O'Brien and M. Ellisman for use of laboratory facilities, and P. I. Bromberger for making samples available from donors to the University Hospital Milk Bank. This research was supported by NIH Contract NO1-HD-2-2819.

REFERENCES

1. Ferguson DJP, Anderson TJ. (1983): An ultrastructural study of lactation in the human breast. Anat Embryol, 168, 349-359.

2. Saacke RG, Heald CW. (1974): Cytological aspects of milk formation and secretion. In: Larson BL, Smith VR, eds,Lactation, A Comprehensive Treatise, Vol. II. New York, London: Academic Press, 147-189.

3. Patton S, Keenan TW. (1975): The milk fat globule membrane. Biochim Biophys Acta, 415, 273-309.

4. Head JR, Beer AE. (1978): The immunologic role of viable leukocytic cells in mammary exosecretions. In: Larson BL, ed, Lactation, a Comprehensive Treatise, Vol IV. New York, London: Academic Press, 337-364.

5. Morton RK. (1954): The lipoprotein particles in cow's milk. Biochem J, 57, 231-237.

6. Stewart PS, Puppione DL, Patton S. (1972): The presence of microvilli and other membrane fragments in the non-fat phase of bovine milk. Z Zellforsch, 123, 161-167.

7. Wooding FBP, Peaker M, Linzell JL. (1970): Theories of milk secretion: evidence from the electron microscopic examination of milk. Nature, 226, 762-764.

8. Christie WW, Wooding FBP. (1975): The site of triglyceride biosynthesis in milk. Experiementia, 31, 1445-1447.

9. McCarthy RD, Patton S. (1964): Biosynthesis of glycerides in freshly secreted milk. Nature, 202, 347-348.

10. Wooding FBP, Morgan G, Craig H. (1977): "Sunbursts" and "Christiesomes": cellular fragments in normal cow and goat milk. Cell Tiss Res, 185, 535-545.

11. Patton S, Keenan TW. (1971): The relationship of milk phospholipids to membranes of the secretory cell. Lipids, 6, 58-62.

12. Horowitz W, ed. (1975): Official methods of analysis, 13th ed. Washington, D.C.: Association of Official Analytical Chemists, 251-292.

13. Walstra P, De Graaf JJ. (1962): Note on the determination of the phospholipid content of milk products. Neth Milk Dairy J, 16, 283-285.

14. Rouser G, Siakatos AN, Fleischer S. (1966): Quantitative analysis of phospholipids by thin-layer chromatography and phosphorus analysis of spots. Lipids, 1, 85-86.

15. Bachman KC, Lin J-H, Wilcox CJ. (1976): Sensitive colorimetric determination of cholesterol in dairy products. JAOAC, 59, 1146-1149.

16. Sperry WM, Webb M. (1950): A revision of the Schoenheimer-Sperry method for cholesterol determination. J Biol Chem, 187, 97-106.

17. Lowry OH, Rosebrough NJ, Farr AL, et al. (1951): Protein measurement with the Folin phenol reagent. J Biol Chem, 193, 265-275.

18. Patton S, Huston GE. (1984): A procedure for the determination of total protein in human milk. Nutr Rep Int, 30, 1401-1408.

19. Anonymous. (1973): Direct microscopic somatic cell count. United States Public Health Service, Form FD 2400 e. (Rev. 8/73).

20. Bitman J, Wood DL, Mehta NR, et al. (1983): Lipolysis of triglycerides of human milk during storage at low temperatures: a note of caution. J Pediatr Gastroenterol Nutr, 2, 521-524.

21. Hibberd CM, Brooke OG, Carter ND, et al. (1982): Variation in the composition of breast milk during the first 5 weeks of lactation: implications for the feeding of preterm infants. Arch Dis Child, 57, 658-662.

22. Clark RM, Ferris AM, Fey M, et al. (1982): Changes in the lipids of human milk from 2 to 16 weeks postpartum. J Pediatr Gastroenterol Nutr, 1, 311-315.

23. Picciano MF, Guthrie HA, Sheehe DM. (1978): The choloesterol content of human milk. Clin Pediatr, 17, 359-362.

24. Potter JM, Nestel PJ. (1976): The effects of dietary fatty acids and cholesterol on the milk lipids of lactating women and the plasma cholesterol of breast-fed infants. Am J Clin Nutr, 29, 54-60.

25. Harzer G, Haug M, Dieterich I, et al. (1983): Changing patterns of human milk lipids in the course of lactation and during the day. Am J Clin Nutr, 37, 612-621.

26. Ferraina R, Clark RM, Jensen RG. (1984): Sterols in human milk. Fed Proc, 43, 490. (Abstract No. 1201).

27. Anderson M, Brooker BE, Andrews AT, et al. (1974): Membrane material isolated from milk of mastitic and normal cows. J Dairy Sci, 57, 1448-1458.

SECTION V. METHODS FOR THE SAMPLING AND ANALYSIS OF HUMAN MILK LIPIDS

WORKSHOP PARTICIPANTS:

R. G. Jensen, Department of Nutritional Sciences, University of Connecticut, Storrs, Connecticut

J. Bitman, Milk Secretion and Mastitis Laboratory, USDA, Beltsville, Maryland

M. Hamosh, Department of Pediatrics, Georgetown University Medical Center, Washington, DC

M. T. Clandinin, Division of Gastroenterology, Department of Medicine, The University of Alberta, Edmonton, Alberta, Canada

METHODS FOR THE SAMPLING AND ANALYSIS OF HUMAN MILK LIPIDS

R. G. Jensen
J. Bitman
L. Wood
M. Hamosh
M. T. Clandinin
R. M. Clark

INTRODUCTION

The amount of lipids in human milk ranges from 3 to 5% and consists of about 98% triacylglycerol, 1% phospholipid and 0.4% sterols. The lipids are present as emulsified globules with the triacylglycerol core surrounded by a membrane containing phospholipids, cholesterol and other plasma membrane components (1-4). The lipids in their classes and composition are the most variable major component of milk. Lipids contribute approximately 50-60% of the calories; they are carriers of vitamin A, D, E, and K; they provide essential fatty acids (the precursors of prostaglandins); and they supply sterols, phospholipids, and probably other, as yet unidentified, compounds of nutritional importance. In those women who have consumed partially hydrogenated food fats or large amounts of bovine milk lipids, the milk will contain *trans* and positional isomers of unsaturated fatty acids.

Since human milk is food for the neonate, only very small amounts can be diverted to research purposes. Some of the methods we describe for complete lipid analysis were developed for a total volume of 3.5 to 6.0 ml of human milk, sample sizes which are usually available. These methods can be classified as semimicro, in contrast to the macro methods for standard lipid analysis used for bovine milk and to the micro methods used in automated clinical chemistry.

In this paper, we discuss analytical methods for precise determination of milk lipids. In addition to being applicable to small milk volumes, the methods must ensure stability of the lipids during handling, storage and processing. Methods must also maintain the structures of the secreted lipid components.

SAMPLING

The content of lipids in milk varies within a feed, diurnally, in response to diet, and with the stage of lactation (5). To obtain the total lipid content of a feed, the entire contents of one breast should be removed under standard conditions and an aliquot of this analyzed (5). However, there are field conditions in which the complete contents of the breast cannot be obtained. In these circumstances, some investigators have used a weighted average from milk portions collected at the beginning (fore) and end (hind) of nursing; with proper weighting, this procedure provides a content close to the quantities found in entire breast samples (6,7). Neville et al. (8) observed that a single sample taken 2 minutes after let-down gave a population average which was as reliable as a sample taken from the pooled contents of one breast. Either of these sampling procedures is justified when conditions will not allow the emptying of a breast. Whatever procedure is used, it must be rigidly standardized, because according to Hytten (9), the last 12 ml of milk contain considerable amounts of fat.

Measurement of small quantities, <1 ml, of milk can be troublesome, particularly on repeated transfers. The sample should be maintained at about 38°C so that globules will not adhere to the bore of micropipettes. Pipettes with a wire plunger are useful in maintaining repeated delivery of volumes within narrow limits.

Table 1. Protocol for Sample Preparation Prior to the Measurement or Isolation of the Lipids from Human Milk

1. Sample in original container.

   a. Subsample immediately while still warm to test for lipid content or aliquot for storage; *or*

   b. Immediately extract entire sample with solvents containing 0.01% butylated hydroxytoluene and rinse sample container with solvents; or

   c. As soon as possible, heat sample rapidly to 80°C and hold for 1.5 minutes; or

   d. Lyophilize as soon as possible and store at -20 or -70°C

   e. If a, b, c or d cannot be done, go to 2.

2. Storage of sample.

   a. Store at 4°C for a maximum of 72 hours; temper (heat slowly) to 38°C and invert gently several times to mix the cream layer; aliquots may be taken.

   b. Store at -20°C for a limit of 14 days; then proceed as in 2a; since aliquots may not be representative, the appropriate aliquoting should be done before freezing. For analysis, *extract the entire* sample by rinsing container with solvents. The sample can be sonicated for homogenity.

   c. Store at -70°C. Length of storage can be indefinite when containers are flushed with N_2 and closed with a Teflon-sealed screw cap. To thaw, treat as in 2a.

STORAGE

It is important that the milk samples be stored in polypropylene tubes or glass tubes (or vials) with Teflon liners. Caps with bonded paper liners, plastic liners, cork or rubber should not be used because of contaminants which interfere with subsequent thin-layer and gas-liquid chromatography.

After a representative sample has been obtained, further treatment depends upon the information needed. To assist the investigator, Table 1 provides protocols for the preparation of samples prior to the determination or isolation of milk lipids.

The rationale behind the procedures in Table 1 (item 1,a.) is to obtain a representative aliquot before changes caused by lipolysis can occur. The action of lipolytic enzymes can substantially reduce the triacylglycerol content and simultaneously increase the amounts of diacylglycerols, monoacylglycerols and free fatty acids (10). These changes should not affect tests for total lipids, but will alter the amounts of the relevant lipid classes. Immediate extraction, heating to 80°C, or lyophilization and storage at -70°C will minimize or avoid lipolytic activity. Since repeated freezing and thawing increase lipolytic activity (10), these should be avoided by aliquoting to provide individual samples. Milk is tempered to 38°C before sampling for lipids so that the globules will be liquid, and any adhesion to sample bottles, etc., is minimized (11).

The length of storage, at 4°C for 72 hours, was selected because bacterial growth could become appreciable at this point and affect the lipids. Two weeks was chosen for the length of storage at -20°C, because bile-salt stimulated esterase activity lost much of its dependency on bile salts after three weeks at -10°C (13). Lipolysis also has been observed at -20°C, but not at -70°C (10) or -80°C (13,14). Clearly, samples should be extracted within hours after being obtained, but since this is often impossible, storage at -70°C is required for maximum stability. For analysis, the sample should be thawed in warm water to 38°C and then extracted, and the container should be rinsed with the extractant. Tempering is particularly crucial for previously frozen samples in which the emulsion may be disrupted and denatured protein may be present (12). Subsampling of frozen and thawed milk should be avoided.

Lyophilization followed by storage at 4°C for 6 months did not reduce lipase activity or significantly alter the total lipid content or fatty acid composition (15). The phospholipid content was not determined, but in the absence of water and oxygen, oxidative and hydrolytic changes would not be expected. We recommend storage at -20° or -70°C, preferably the latter. While lyophilization produces a sample which has storage stability, the equipment is relatively expensive and the process is lengthy. Reconstitution of samples may also be difficult.

In order to avoid or minimize autoxidation, it is advisable to: a) keep samples cold, b) minimize processing time, c) avoid exposure to air, and d) add antioxidants to the extracting solvents. Butylated hydroxytoluene (BHT) should be added to all solvents at a concentration of 0.01% (100mg/l).

DETERMINATION OF TOTAL LIPID CONTENT

As mentioned, the total amount and the contents of the lipid components vary in response to a variety of conditions. The necessity for proper sampling and identification of the sample cannot be overemphasized. Careful attention to these details would eliminate some of the variables observed in previous studies (16).

The lipid content of human milk can be determined directly on the milk using gravimetric procedures. This can be done with or without destruction of the sample, or it can be done after solvent extraction of the lipids. Analysis of the lipid classes is usually carried out on extracted lipids, while triacylglycerols and cholesterol have been estimated directly. The procedures in recent use are summarized in Table 2 and discussed next.

Table 2. Methods for the Determination and Isolation of Human Milk Lipids

1. Direct

   a. Creamatocrit. Length of fat column in centrifuged hematocrit tube calibrated against lipid obtained by solvent extraction. Requires 75 µl or less (Ref. 16).

   b. Enzymatic. Enzymatic production and measurement of glycerol from acylglycerols. Requires 250 µl (Ref. 22).

   c. Colorimetric. Sulfo-phospho-vanillin. Reaction between triacylglycerols and vanillin at acid pH produces chromogen. Requires 50-100 µl (Ref. 20,27). Not recommended.

   d. Turbidimetric. Determination of optical density after solubilization of protein. Calibrated against lipid obtained by solvent extraction. Requires 50 µl (ref 30).

2. Isolation of lipid by solvent extraction. Lipid measured gravimetrically or densitometrically.

   a. Roese-Gottlieb. Treatment of milk with NH_4OH and extraction with ethanol, diethyl ether and hexane. Requires 1-10 ml (Ref 33).

   b. Mojonnier. Modified Roese-Gottlieb. Special flask used to hasten separation of aqueous and solvent phases (Ref 11).

   c. Modified Folch. Extraction with $CHCl_3$/MeOH, 2/1. Can extract 0.1-10 ml or more (Ref 35).

   d. Erickson-Dunkley. Acidified milk heated with HCl and abs. ethanol. Extracted with hexane. Done on 500 µl (Ref. 37).

   e. Dry column. Milk mixed with Na_2SO_4 and Celite and extracted with CH_2Cl_2/MeOH, 9/1. Can extract 1-10 ml (Ref. 41).

   f. Soaps-Total Lipids. Conversion to and weighing of soaps. (Ref. 43).

Direct Methods

Creamatocrit. The creamatocrit method devised by Lucas et al. (17) has been widely employed (5,6,8,16,18-20). About 75 μl of milk is drawn into a capillary tube sealed at one end and spun in a hematocrit centrifuge. The length of the cream layer (creamatocrit) is measured and calculated as a percentage of the total length of the milk column. Lucas (21) recently studied the effect of temperature on the creamatocrit method, testing it against the Gerber procedure (similar to the Babcock procedure). He found a mean fat content (n=26) of 3.32% with centrifugation at 4°C, 2.73% at 18°C, and 2.45% at 18°C with a previously run centrifuge. Lower contents, 2.99, 2.21 and 2.09%, were obtained after the milks had been pasteurized at 62°C for 30 minutes and centrifuged as before. These values are based on a previously published standardization of the method and illustrate the importance of standardizing the procedure for the specific condition of a particular laboratory. If this is done, the correlation coefficients between the creamatocrit and Gerber methods are high. However, we agree with Lucas (21) that the creamatocrit method must be standardized by each technician using the procedure.

The advantages of the creamatocrit method follow: (1) Preparation of samples is not required. (2) Only a micro-hematocrit or similar centrifuge is needed; the procedure is therefore suitable for field studies. (3) Only 5-15 minutes and 75 μl or less of sample is required. (4) Multiple samples may be run. (5) Frozen or pasteurized samples can be used. The only disadvantages or precautions are, (1) the necessity for standardization in each laboratory for each type of milk sample and each technician, and (2) the failure to function if the cream column is dislocated by the presence of flecks of denatured protein, which may occur in repeatedly frozen samples. When frozen or pasteurized samples are used, the precautions described above are necessary.

Enzymatic Method. This procedure is based on the enzymatic determination of glycerol released from triacylglycerols by saponification or lipolysis. The glycerol is then measured by a coupled reaction in which NADH is produced (18,22-26). Evaluation of the method was described only in reference 26, in which Harzer et al. obtained identical results with this procedure as compared to extraction-gravimetry, using 250 μl of milk. Statistical treatments were not given. With this method, triacylglycerols are measured, but not phospholipids and cholesterol. For routine testing, the procedure is probably acceptable, but proper standardization would be necessary.

Colorimetric. The reaction between vanillin and triacylglycerols at acid pH or the sulfophospho-vanillin reaction for the measurement of serum lipids (27) has been applied to human milk (20,28,29). Lonnderdal et al. (20) checked this method against some others, obtaining similar results. A commercial test kit is available (Boehringer-Mannheim Diagnostics). In using this kit, 50-100 μl of sample is needed, and frozen samples can be analyzed (20). However, a double bond between two carbons is required for the reaction, so the type of fatty acid in the sample could influence the test. For this reason, and because of the relatively large percent variation (10.17%) observed by Lönnerdal et al. (20), this method is not recommended.

Turbidimetry. Nakai and Le (30) developed a turbidimetric procedure for the simultaneous determination of protein and fat in 50 μl of milk. Turbidity caused by fat was measured spectrophotometrically after treatment of the milk with a solution of acetic acid-urea-imidazole. Guthrie et al.

(31) used the method earlier to determine the content of fat in human milk, with apparently acceptable results. The procedure has been checked against other tests by Hundreiser et al. (19), with excellent correlations. The procedure would seem to be acceptable, although Dorea et al. (32) obtained low correlation coefficients when the procedure was compared to the Roese-Gottlieb extraction. However, we do not recommend its use because the creamatocrit method is superior for routine determinations.

Isolation and Measurement of Lipids

With the procedures discussed below (see Table 2, except for item 2.f.) lipids are extracted with solvent mixtures. The solvents are then removed, and the amount of lipid is usually measured gravimetrically. Densitometry has also been employed. Weighing leaves the total lipids available for further separation and analysis.

Roese-Gottlieb and Mojonnier. For measurement of the total amount of lipids, the Roese-Gottlieb extraction is the standard and official method of the Association of Official Analytical Chemists (33). In a slight modification, centrifugation of a specially shaped Mojonnier flask hastens separation of the ethyl ether:petroleum ether extraction mixture from the aqueous:ethanol layer. Ten ml of milk is extracted, but one ml can be used. Mojonnier flasks are available from SGA Scientific, Inc., 735 Broad St., Bloomfield, NJ, 07003. Since NH_4OH is used in this extraction, the ammonium soaps of fatty acids will probably not be recovered in the solvents, and total lipids will be underestimated in samples in which substantial lipolysis has occurred. This also applies to the Mojonnier modification. While this is the recommended procedure for bovine milk, we recommend the modified Folch procedure, described next, for human milk.

Modified Folch. The original Folch extraction with chloroform-methanol was adapted for bovine milk lipids by Timmen et al. (34) and further modified by Clark et al. (35) for human milk. This procedure extracts "all" of the lipids to the extent that recovery can be determined (36). Chloroform, a suspected carcinogen, is one of the extractants, but this can be replaced by dichloromethane (methylene chloride) which is relatively innocuous and is more polar and stable than chloroform. If the sample has been lipolyzed, it should be acidified to pH 2.0 for the reasons described above. Bitman et al. (10) have recently described a modified Folch extraction method which we recommend. It is presented in Table 3.

Erickson-Dunkley Method. In this extraction, developed by Erickson and Dunkley (37) for the recovery of tocopherols from bovine milk, milk is mixed with absolute ethanol and HCl, heated, and the lipids extracted once with hexane. Aitchison et al. (38), Emery et al. (39), and Craig-Schmidt et al. (40) used this technique for extraction of lipid from human milk, but without evaluation. While this extraction probably removes most of the lipids, treatment with HCl cleaves the phosphate ester linkage in the phospholipids, and these will not be extracted as such. Since other satisfactory methods are available, we do not recommend the Erickson-Dunkley procedure.

Dry Column Method. Maxwell et al. (41) described a dry column method for extraction of total lipids from meat and meat products. Later, Marmer and Maxwell (42) reported a similar technique for simultaneous quantitative extraction and separation of neutral and polar lipids from muscle tissue. Compared to the Roese-Gottlieb and modified Folch methods, extraction with the dry column procedure is rapid, problems with emulsions are avoided and a dry extract is obtained. If the sample has been lipolyzed, it should be

Table 3. Method for Modified Folch Extraction of Total Lipids in Human Milk (Bitman et al., 10)

1. After heating to 80°C for 1 minute to inactivate lipases, 1.0 ml of milk is placed in a 50 ml glass test tube with Teflon-lined screw cap containing 18 ml chloroform:methanol (2:1 containing 0.01% butylated hydroxytoluene). Dichloromethane can be substituted for chloroform. Heating can be omitted if a fresh, or frozen and thawed, sample is extracted immediately. If the sample has been lipolyzed, it should be acidified to pH 2.0 before extraction in order to free fatty acid soaps.

2. Homogenize for 30 seconds using a Polytron homogenizer (Brinkmann Instruments, Westbury, NY) or Tekmar homogenizer (Tekmar Co., Cincinnati, OH).

3. Add 6 ml of 0.7% NaCl and invert tube a few times.

4. Centrifuge at 1000 rpm (260 x g) for 10 minutes.

5. Remove upper (methanol/water) phase by suction pipette and discard.

6. Transfer an 8.0 ml aliquot of the lower chloroform phase to a tared (0.0000 place) 15 ml culture tube.

7. Transfer a 3.0 ml aliquot of the chloroform phase to a 4.0 ml amber vial. The lipid in this vial will be used for thin-layer chromatographic separation and gas-liquid chromatographic analysis of fatty acid methyl esters.

8. Evaporate solvent under nitrogen (tube from step 6) and re-weigh. Determine % fat:

   (tube + fat) - tube) x 150 = % fat

9. Add 1 ml of chloroform to the tube and store in freezer under N_2 (-20°C). This will be used to determine neutral lipid and phospholipid classes.

acidified to pH 2.0, so that free fatty acid can be recovered. The procedure will probably replace the modified Folch extraction when comparative recoveries of the lipid classes are documented.

Soaps - Total Lipids. Anderson et al. (43) estimated the quantity of fat in milk with the procedure of Van de Kamer (44). Van de Kamer measured the amount of fat in feces by saponification, acidification, extraction and titration of the resulting free fatty acids. The procedure, almost identical to one employed by Hudson et al. (18), was not developed for human milk and has so many inherent errors, even for the original estimation, that it should not be used for milk, and probably not for feces.

Quantitation of Extracted Lipids. The amount of extracted lipids has been determined by weighing. With the usual analytical balance, this can be done with precision at the level of 10 mg. This means that with careful measurement of volume, the lipid from about 250 µl of milk could be weighed without appreciable variation within a sample. The use of a microbalance could reduce the quantities many fold. Densitometry has been utilized by Anderson et al. (45) who charred milk lipids extracted from 1 ml of milk with H_2SO_4. They used standards of trioleoylglycerol and a sample from pooled human milk. Densitometric analysis, with trioleoylglycerol as a standard, underestimated total milk lipid as compared to gravimetric analysis. There are no apparent advantages over gravimetry, and the sample is destroyed.

<u>Gas-Liquid Chromatography.</u> The total fatty acids in milk can be quantitatively determined by gas-liquid chromatography (GLC), if the extraction solvent contains an appropriate internal standard. The samples should first be analyzed by GLC to establish that the fatty acid selected as an internal standard is not found in significant amounts (>0.1%). The extracted sample is then transmethylated in the presence of an appropriate catalyst. Anhydrous methanolic HCl (10% w/v) or boron trifluoride is suitable, although the latter does not give good yields of shorter chain fatty acids. This method has the advantage that the fatty acid composition is obtained simultaneously. The completeness of esterification must be ascertained. This determination should be considered a secondary method, since it is much simpler to weigh the extracted lipids.

Comparisons of Methods for Total Lipids

Quantitative comparisons of some of these methods have recently been reported by Hundrieser et al. (19), who centrifuged pooled milk into cream and skim milk fraction and prepared 25 samples with a range of 0.5 to 8.0% lipid. The modified Folch, turbidimetric (spectrophotometric) and creamatrocrit techniques were compared to the Roese-Gottlieb (Mojonnier) extraction. There was a high correlation (r=0.977) between the Roese-Gottlieb method and all the other procedures. Lönnerdal et al. (20) have provided additional comparisons of methods for analysis of total milk fat.

The choice of procedures depends on the data needed. For routine and field analyses, the creamatocrit method is the most suitable, but only if properly standardized -- preferably with the Roese-Gottlieb or modified Folch extractions. When fatty acid compositions are required in addition, we use the modified Folch technique, but believe that it may be replaced by the dry column extraction. In our opinion, the Erickson-Dunkley, soap and sulfo-phospho-vanillin methods should not be employed. It is interesting that during the past 7 years, 10 different methods have been used to determine the fat content of human milk, a practice not conducive to uniformity of results.

SEPARATION AND IDENTIFICATION OF LIPID CLASSES

Although there are many classes of lipids in human milk, we will limit our discussion to the triacylglycerols, sterols, phospholipids and fatty acids. These account for about 98+%, 0.4%, and 1.0%, respectively, of the total lipids. The total lipids can be analyzed directly for triacylglycerols, as discussed; cholesterol can be analyzed enzymatically (46), and phospholipids can be analyzed as lipid phosphate multiplied by 25 (16).

The overwhelming amount of triacylglycerol makes it difficult to resolve the other lipid classes. However, the separation into nonpolar (triacylglycerols and sterols) and polar lipids (phospholipids) has been achieved by the dry column extraction previously described (42). Maxwell (personal communication, see reference 42) noted a slight carry-over of triacylglycerol into the polar lipids when bovine milk was extracted, but these were easily separable by thin-layer chromatography (TLC). Bitman et al. (47) resolved the nonpolar and polar lipids by elution of a total lipid extract (Folch) from 5 ml of milk through a silica Sep-Pak cartridge (Waters Associates, Inc., Milford, MA). Hexane:ethyl ether (1:1) was used for the neutral lipids, followed by methanol and chloroform:methanol:water (3:5:2) for the polar lipids.

Separations have been done by TLC with quantitation by densitometry (47,48). Separations have also been done by recovery of the lipid bands from preparative TLC plates followed by appropriate quantitation, usually determination of phosphorous. The phospholipids can be resolved as a class and as phosphatidylcholine, etc., on a single plate (48,49). Bitman et al. (50) separated the phospholipids by thin-layer chromatography with quantitation by densitometry, using a Shimadzu CS-910 Dual Wavelength TLC scanner (Shimadzu Instruments, Inc., Columbia, MD). Hundreiser et al. (51), noting that the determination of small amounts of lipid phosphate in the presence of large quantities of triacylglycerols often results in large variations, applied a colorimetric method used for serum phospholipids to this analysis. In this procedure, a Prussian blue-phospholipid complex is formed. The range of phosphorous concentrations in 39 milk samples was 0.10 to 3.25/dl of milk, with a recovery of 99 to 102%. When compared to a standard acid digestion for lipid phosphate, the correlation coefficient was 0.980. The phosphorous contents are comparable to those previously reported (50). This analysis is easier and less expensive than the other procedures. We are using it to determine the contents of individual phospholipids.

Reported cholesterol contents of milk have varied enormously. This range is due primarily to the nonspecific colorimetric analyses. The method of choice is gas-liquid chromatography. With this procedure, Clark et al. (35) found about 10 mg/dl total cholesterol. Cholesterol has been determined enzymatically (22), but the values obtained were higher (22 mg/dl) than those of Clark et al. (35), casting doubt on the validity of the enzyme method. Ferraina et al. (52) compared the total cholesterol of 15 milk samples measured by three colorimetric methods (LiebermannBurchard, ferric chloride, and o-phthalaldehyde) and two enzymatic test kits (Sigma and Boehringer-Mannheim). The results were individually compared to values obtained by GLC analysis. All determinations were done on the extracted lipids. Least squares and correlation analyses detected significant linear relationships between the five test methods and GLC. Comparison of the regression parameters indicated that both the Liebermann-Burchard and ferric chloride colorimetric assays gave results which varied significantly from those of GLC; this suggests that direct colorimetric procedures are not reliable for the quantitation of human milk cholesterol.

On the other hand, the o-phthalaldehyde-colorimetric assay and the Boehringer-Mannheim colorimetric procedures provided analytical results that were comparable to GLC values. These results were attributed to their greater sensitivities to cholesterol, compared to the Liebermann-Burchard and ferric chloride assays. Both the o-phthalaldehyde and Boehringer-Mannheim procedures require saponification of the samples prior to the analysis of cholesterol. Our data (52) suggest that saponification of the breast milk lipids, as opposed to analysis of the total sample, leads to more accurate estimations of the total cholesterol.

Ferraina et al. (52) and Clark et al. (53) found desmosterol in human milk, but the phytosterols reported by Mellies et al. (54) were not detected. On the gas-liquid chromatographic charts, peaks with the same retention times as some phytosterols were identified by mass-spectrometry as diacylglycerols. The sterols in these studies were isolated by preparative thin-layer chromatography; the sterol and diacylglycerol bands are very close on the plate. The compounds identified by Mellies et al. (54) as phytosterols may have been interfering compounds produced by direct saponification of the milk, or by other unsaponifiables.

Haug and Harzer (55) commented on the high values for cholesterol obtained by enzymatic determination in their laboratory (22). Using a high-performance liquid chromatograhic method for separation, they obtained 19.2 mg/100ml of cholesterol (22.8mg/100ml enzymatically) which is still higher than the quantities found by Clark et al. (53) and Bitman et al. (47). They suggested that the enzymatic procedure overestimates the cholesterol content by 20%. The lower values obtained by GLC (53) and densitometry (47) were attributed to sampling technique. Haug and Harzer (55) also found very small amounts of phytosterols; they identified desmosterol and noted the presence of other sterols.

Kaluzny et al. (56) resolved the lipid classes in bovine adipose tissue with aminopropyl bonded-phase (Bond Elut) columns. Neutral and polar lipids were separated as well as the classes of neutral lipids. The method was rapid and yields were high. It should be applicable to human milk lipids and to the separation of PL classes.

Fatty Acid Analysis of Lipid Constituents

Component fatty acids of human milk lipids are analyzed by gas-liquid chromatography. The only problems here are the use of proper columns for the separation of fatty acids which may have the same retention times, i.e., *cis* and *trans* isomers (57), and the reliable measurement of small quantities (<1%). Milk, unless obtained from vegan donors, will contain varying amounts of *trans* fatty acids which will not be resolved and detected unless suitable columns are used. *Trans* isomers are separable on a 15 m SP-2340 glass or SP-2100 capillary column (Supelco, Inc., Bellefonte, PA) (58). Ackman (59) recommends the use of flexible fused silica wall coated open tubular (WCOT) columns that are bonded with Carbowax 20 M (Supelcowax 10, Supelco, Inc., Bellefonte, PA) as the standard for interlaboratory comparisons. The column provides excellent resolution of long-chain polyunsaturates. Another useful column is the 25 m SP-2100 glass capillary type which provides excellent resolution of fatty acids from 8:0 through very long polyunsaturates. The elution sequence is reliable, and it is suitable for a variety of routine analyses where major and microconstituents are to be quantitated from the same analysis (60).

Small quantities of fatty acids (<1%) are difficult to measure with precision. To avoid this difficulty, Aitchison et al. (30) separated the methyl esters of milk fatty acids into monoenes, dienes, etc., by argentation thin-layer chromatography. The classes and the total fatty acids were analyzed by gas-liquid chromatography. The results were similar, but some *trans* isomers were detected with the class separation that were not found in the total analysis of fatty acids. These could probably be resolved on the newer columns. Aitchison et al. did not report individual amounts for polyunsaturates longer than 18 carbons. Gibson and Kneebone (61) made the same separations, reporting quantities of n-6 and n-3 polyunsaturates. However, Harzer et al. (23) also obtained data on these acids without the argentation thin-layer separation, but probably with less precision. An improved method for separation of fatty acid methyl esters into saturates, monoenes, dienes, etc., by thin-layer chromatography of the methoxy-bromomercuri adducts has been reported (62). It has not been applied to human milk lipids.

Internal standards should be used at two points: they should be added to the extraction solvents, and they should be used just prior to injection of methyl esters into the gas-liquid chromatograph. These are usually odd carbon acids, generally 15:0 or 17:0 for the preinjection standard. Lepage et al. (63) dissolved 9:0, 13:0, and 23:0 in the extraction solvents, although monoacid triacylglycerol would probably have been preferable. Lepage and Roy (64) have devised a method for the direct conversion (transesterification) of the esterified fatty acids in milk to methyl esters, thereby eliminating extraction.

The "real" weights of fatty acids obtained from the internal standards can be used to check recoveries and also to provide gravimetric reports (mg of fatty acid/100 ml of milk) as opposed to normalized reports (each fatty acid as a percent of total fatty acids or wt %). For nutritional purposes, fatty acid data should be given as gravimetric reports (65). These can also be calculated from the total lipid content. Further, if the effects of treatments on fatty acid composition are being compared, then gravimetric data should be used so that valid statistical analyses can be made. Changes in wt% can be caused by normalization to 100%. Marmer et al. (66) noted in their study that 18:0 increased three-fold, yet the wt% decreased. We recommend that fatty acid data be reported both ways or at the very least, the fat content be provided so that weights can be calculated.

SUMMARY

Protocols have been outlined for sample processing prior to the determination or isolation of lipids from human milk. Comparative data for several methods were presented. For routine analysis of fat content, the creamatocrit method is recommended. The Roese-Gottlieb and modified Folch extractions are best for isolation of lipids, with the dry column procedure a possible replacement. Details of techniques for the separation and identification of lipid classes have been discussed, with recommendations for analysis of fatty acids by gas-liquid chromatography. We hope that some standardization of methodologies between laboratories will result from our efforts.

ACKNOWLEDGEMENTS

Some of the research reported in this article was supported in part by Federal funds made available through the provision of The Hatch Act and by NIH Contract NO1-HD-2817.

Scientific Contribution No. 1093, Storrs Agricultural Experiment Station, Storrs, CT 06268

REFERENCES

1. Ruegg M, Blanc B. (1981): The fat globule size distribution in human milk. Biochim Biophys Acta, 666, 7-14.

2. Ruegg M, Blanc B. (1982): Structure and properties of the particulate constituents of human milk: a review. Food Microstructure, 1, 25-47.

3. Baumann DE, Neville MC. (1984): Nutritional and physiological factors affecting lactation. Fed Proc, 43, 2430-2431.

4. Jensen RG, Clark RM, deJong FA, Hamosh M, Liao TH, Mehta R. (1982): The lipolytic triad: human lingual, breast milk and pancreatic lipases: physiological implications of their characteristics in digestion of dietary fats. J Pediatr Gastroenterol Nutr, 1, 243-255.

5. Ferris AM, Jensen RG. (1984): Lipids in human milk: a review. I. Sampling, determination and content. J Pediatr Gastroenterol Nutr, 3, 108-122.

6. Prentice A, Prentice AM, Whitehead RG. (1981): Breast-milk concentrations of rural African women. I. Short-term variations within individuals. Br J Nutr, 45, 483-494.

7. Hartmann PE, Saint L. (1984): Measurement of milk yield in women. J Pediatr Gastroenterol Nutr, 3, 270-274.

8. Neville MC, Keller RP, Seacat J, Casey CE, Allen JC and Archer P. (1984): Studies on human lactation. I. Within-feed and between-breast variation in selected components of human milk. Am J Clin Nutr, 40, 635-646.

9. Hytten FE. (1954): Clinical and chemical studies in human lactation. I. Collection of milk samples. Br Med J, i, 177-179.

10. Bitman J, Wood DL, Mehta NR, Hamosh P, Hamosh M. (1983): Lipolysis of triacylglycerols in human milk at low temperatures: a note of caution. J Pediatr Gastroenterol Nutr, 2, 521-524.

11. Atherton HV, Newlander JA. (1977): Chemistry and testing of dairy products, 4th ed. Westport, Conn: Avi Publishing Company, 38-41.

12. Walstra P, Jenness R. (1984): Dairy chemistry and physics. New York: John Wiley & Sons, 315-317.

13. Hamosh M. (1982): Lingual and breast milk lipases. Adv Pediatr, 29, 33-67.

14. Hamosh M, Berkow S, Bitman J, Fried L, Happ B, Jones JB, Mehta NR, Wood DL, Hamosh P. (1984): Handling and storage of human milk specimens for research. J Pediatr Gastroenterol Nutr, 3, 284-289.

15. Friend BA, Shahani KM, Long CA, Agel EN. (1983): Evaluation of freeze-drying, pasteurization, high-temperature heating and storage on selected enzymes, B-vitamins and lipids of mature human milk. J Food Prot, 46, 330-334.

16. Jensen RG, Clark RM. (1984): Methods of lipid analysis. J Pediatr Gastroenterol Nutr, 3, 296-299.

17. Lucas A, Gibbs JAH, Lyster RLJ, Baum JD. (1978): Creamatocrit: simple clinical technique for estimating fat concentration and energy value of human milk. Br Med J, 1, 1018-1020.

18. Hudson GJ, Gerber H, John PMV. (1979): Creamatocrit procedure versus triacylglycerol analysis. A comparison of methods for the determination of human milk fat in epidemiological studies. J Hum Nutr, 33, 283-287.

19. Hundreiser KE, Clark RM, Jensen RG, Ferris AM. (1984): A comparison of methods for determination of total lipids in human milk. Nutr Res, 4, 21-26.

20. Lönnerdal B, Smith C, Keen CL. (1984): Analysis of breast milk. Current methodologies and future needs. J Pediatr Gastroenterol Nutr, 3, 290-295.

21. Lucas A. (1983): Effect of temperature on creamatocrit method. Br Med J, 287-392.

22. Hibberd CM, Brooke OG, Carter ND, Haug M, Harzer G. (1982): Variation in the composition of breast milk during the first 5 weeks of lactation: Implications for the feeding of preterm infants. Arch Dis Childhd, 57, 658-662.

23. Harzer G, Haug M, Dieterich I, Gentner PR. (1983): Changing patterns of human milk lipids in the course of lactation and during the day. Am J Clin Nutr, 37, 612-621.

24. Butte NF, Calloway DH. (1981): Evaluation of lactational performance of Navaho women. Am J Clin Nutr, 34, 2210-2215.

25. Anonymous. (1980): Triacylglycerols. In: Food analysis. Indianapolis: Boehringer Mannheim Biochemicals, unpaginated.

26. Harzer G, Dieterich I, Haug M. (1984): Effects of diet on the composition of human milk. Ann Nutr Metab, 28, 231-239.

27. Frings CS, Dunn RT. (1970): A colorimetric method for determination of total serum lipids based on the sulfo-phospho-vanillin reaction. Am J Clin Pathol, 53, 89-91.

28. Dewey K, Lönnerdal B. (1983): Milk and nutrient intake of breast-fed infants from 1 to 6 months: relation to growth and fatness. J Pediatr Gastroenterol Nutr, 2, 497-506.

29. Lemons JA, Moye L, Hall D, Simmons M. (1982): Differences in the composition of preterm and term human milk during early lactation. Pediatr Res, 16, 113-117.

30. Nakai S, and Le AC. (1970): Spectrophotometric determination of protein and fat in milk simultaneously. J Dairy Sci, 54, 276-278.

31. Guthrie HA, Picciano MF, Sheehe D. (1977): Fatty acid patterns in human milk. J Pediatr, 90, 39-41.

32. Dorea JG, Horner MR, Bezerra VL, Bongo LA. (1981): Comparison of two methods for determining protein and lipid in human colostrum and milk. Nutr Rep Nutr 24, 985-991.

33. Horwitz W, ed. (1975): Official methods of analysis, 13th ed. Washington, DC: Association of Official Analytical Chemists, 251-292.

34. Timmen H, Dimick PS. (1972): Structure and synthesis of milk fat X. Characterization of the major hydroxy compounds in milk lipids. J Dairy Sci, 55, 919-925.

35. Clark RM, Ferris AM, Fey M, Brown PB, Hundrieser KE, Jensen RG. (1982): Changes in the lipids of human milk from 2 to 16 weeks postpartum. J Pediatr Gastroenterol Nutr, 1, 311-315.

36. Insull W Jr, Ahrens EH Jr. (1959): The fatty acids of human milk from mothers on diets taken *ad libitum*. Biochem J, 72, 27-33.

37. Erickson DR, Dunkley WL. (1964): Spectrophotometric determination of tocopherol in milk and milk lipids. Anal Chem, 36, 1055-1058.

38. Aitchison JM, Dunkley WL, Canolty NL, Smith LM. (1977): Influence of diet on *trans* fatty acids in human milk. Am J Clin Nutr, 30, 2006-2015.

39. Emery WB III, Canolty NL, Aitchison JM, Dunkley WB. (1978): Influence of sampling on fatty acid composition of milk. Am J Clin Nutr, 31, 1127-1130.

40. Craig-Schmidt MC, Weete JD, Faircloth SH, Wickwire MA, Livant EJ. (1984): The effect of hydrogenated fat in the diet of nursing mothers on lipid composition and prostaglandin content of human milk. Am J Clin Nutr, 39, 778-786.

41. Maxwell RJ, Marmer WN, Zubillage MP, Dalikas GA. (1980): Determination of total fat in meat and meat products by a rapid, dry column method. J Assoc Off Anal Chem, 63, 600-603.

42. Marmer WN, Maxwell RJ. (1981): Dry column method for quantitative extraction and simultaneous class separation of lipids from muscle tissue. Lipids, 16, 365-371.

43. Anderson DM, Williams FH, Merkatz RB, Schulman PK, Kerr DS, Pittard III WB. (1983): Length of gestation and nutritional composition of human milk. Am J Clin Nutr, 37, 810-814.

44. Van de Kamer JH. (1949): Rapid method for determination of fat in feces. J Biol Chem, 177, 347-355.

45. Anderson GH, Atkinson SA, Bryan MH. (1981): Energy and micronutrient content of human milk during early lactation from mothers giving birth prematurely and at term. Am J Clin Nutr, 34, 258-265.

46. Gentner PR, Haasemann A. (1979): Methode zur enzymatischen cholesterinbestimmung in milchproben unter verwendung kommerzial erhaltlichen testkombination. Milchwissenschaft, 34, 344-346.

47. Bitman J, Wood LW, Hamosh M, Hamosh P, Mehta MR. (1983): Comparison of the lipid composition of breast milk from mothers of term and preterm infants. Am J Clin Nutr, 38, 300-312.

48. Gentner PR, Bauer M, Dieterich I. (1981): Separation of major phospholipid classes of milk without previous isolation from total lipid extracts. J Chromatogr, 206, 200-204.

49. Haug M, Reinhardt D, Harzer G. (1982): Rapid method for the determination of the phospholipid subclass distribution in human breast milk samples. J Chromatogr, 233, 349-354.

50. Bitman J, Wood DL, Mehta NR, Hamosh P, Hamosh M. (1984): Comparisons of the phospholipid composition of breast milk from mothers of term and preterm infants during lactation. Am J Clin Nutr, 40, 1103-1119.

51. Hundrieser KE, Clark RM, Jensen RG. (1985): Phospholipids in human milk. Am J Clin Nutr, 41, 988-993.

52. Ferraina R, Clark RM, Jensen RG. Methods for the analysis of sterols in human milk. J Pediatr Gastorenterol Nutr. (Submitted).

53. Clark RM, Fey MB, Jensen RG, Hill DW. (1983): Desmosterol in human milk. Lipids, 18, 264-266.

54. Mellies MJ, Burton K, Larsen R, Fixler D, Glueck CJ. (1979): Cholesterol, phytosterols and the polyunsaturated/saturated fatty acid ratios during the first 12 months of lactation. Am J Clin Nutr, 32, 2383-2389.

55. Haug M, Harzer G. (1984): Cholesterol and other sterols in milk. J Pediatr Gastroenterol Nutr, 3, 816-817.

56. Kalzuny MA, Duncan LA, Merritt MV, Epps DE. (1985): Rapid separation of lipid classes in high yield and purity using bonded phase columns. J Lipid Res, 26, 135-140.

57. Hundreisser KM, Clark RM, Brown PB. (1983): Distribution of *trans* octadecenoic acid in the major glycerolipids of human milk. J Pediatr Gastroenterol Nutr, 2, 635-639.

58. Sampugna J, Pallansch LA, Enig MG, Kenney M. (1982): Rapid analysis of *trans* fatty acids of SP-2340 glass capillary columns. J Chromatogr, 249, 245-255.

59. Ackman RG. (1984): The potential of carbowax-20M bonded in flexible fused silica WCOT columns as the standard of interlaboratory comparisons of fatty acids. J Am Oil Chem Soc, 61, 687. (Abstract 206).

60. Chappell JE, Clandinin MT, Salciciole S, Chance GW. (1985): Differences in fatty acid content of human milk from mothers giving birth both prematurely and at term. J Pediatr Gastroenterol Nutr, submitted.

61. Gibson RA, Kneebone GM. (1981): Fatty acid composition of human colostrum and mature human milk. Am J Clin Nutr, 34, 252-257.

62. Sebedio JL, Furguharson TE, Ackman RG. (1982): Improved methods for the isolation and study of the C18, C20 and C22 monoethylenic acid isomers of biological samples: HG adducts, HPLC, $AgNO_3$-TLC/FID, and ozonolysis. Lipids, 17, 469-475.

63. Lepage G, Collet S, Bougle D, Kien LC, Lepage D, Dallaire L, Darling P, Roy CC. (1984): The composition of preterm milk in relation to degree of maturity. Am J Clin Nutr, 40, 1042-1049.

64. Lepage G, Roy CC. (1984): Improved recovery of fatty acid through direct transesterification without prior extraction or purification. J Lipid Res, 25, 1391-1396.

65. Marmer WN, Maxwell RJ, Phillips JG. (1983): Systematic management and analysis of fatty acid data from multiple tissue samples. Lipids, 18, 460-466.

66. Marmer WN, Maxwell RJ, Williams JE. (1984): Effects of dietary regimen and tissue site on bovine fatty acid profiles. J Anim Sci, 59, 109-121.

SECTION VI. ENERGY CONTENT IN HUMAN MILK

WORKSHOP PARTICIPANTS:

N.F. Butte, Department of Pediatrics, Baylor College of Medicine, Houston, Texas

C. Casey, Department of Pediatrics, University of Colorado School of Medicine, Denver, Colorado

K. Dewey, Department of Nutrition, University of California, Davis, California

A. Ferris, Department of Nutritional Sciences, University of Connecticut, Storrs, Connecticut

C. Garza, Department of Pediatrics, Baylor College of Medicine, Houston, Texas

M. W. Woolridge, Department of Pediatrics, University of Oxford, Oxford, United Kingdom

INTRODUCTION

Fat represents approximately 50% of the total energy content and is the most variable of the three major energy-yielding constituents in human milk. The amount of this variability that is experimentally -- rather than biologically -- based is not known. Although there is relatively complete understanding of the physical and chemical processes responsible for *in situ* lipid synthesis and the transfer of dietary and stored fats to the mammary gland, the factors that determine the final concentration of fat, those that account for the diurnal variation of fat concentration, and those that influence the fate of dietary fats (secretion in milk versus deposition in adipose tissue) are defined incompletely (1). The progressive increase in energy content observed in the transition from fore to hind milk may be influenced by the action of oxytocin. In any case, the changes in fat concentration underlie important methodological considerations, because the increase in energy concentration observed as the breast is emptied is not linear (2) and varies at least between individuals and probably among feeding situations. Experimental designs must allow for these influences.

The manner in which the infant influences the energy content of milk is not well understood. Relationships between the maternal capacity for milk production and energy needs dictated by the infant's "growth potential", maintenance needs, and activity remain poorly defined, largely because of methodological constraints on the quantification of relevant measures. Ineffective suckling by the infant results in inadequate emptying of the breast, with subsequent adverse effects on milk production. An infant who obtains inadequate energy often becomes progressively less demanding. Consequently, there may be progressively insufficient stimulation to the breast to counteract the adverse effects of increasing pressure from milk stasis. The outcome is a series of negatively synergistic events: decreased milk production is followed by less effective stimulation which causes a further decrease in milk volume as well as abnormal changes in milk composition due to the premature involution of the mammary gland.

The efficiency with which the infant absorbs nutrients also determines the physiologic fuel values assigned to the major organic constituents of milk. Conventional fuel values (3) (Atwater factors) used to convert the quantities of carbohydrate, fat, and protein into estimates of dietary energy were derived from studies in adults and may not be appropriate when applied to diets of infants, because the efficiency of lactose, protein, and fat absorption may differ substantially between infants and adults (4).

In summary, when the energy content or total yield of energy in human milk is measured, there must also be careful documentation of the physiological state of the lactation process, the environmental variables which may influence composition at the time of sampling, and infant behaviors expected to affect lactation performance. The following two papers discuss methodologies for obtaining representative milk samples and for measuring the energy content of milk.

REFERENCES

1. Garza C, Butte NF. (1984): The effect of maternal nutrition on lactational performance. In: Proceedings of the symposium, Frontiers in Clinical Nutrition. New York: Academic Press. (In Press).

2. Watson MA, Alford ES, Dill CW, Richter RL, Garza C. (1982): Compositional changes during sequential sampling of human milk. Nutr Rep Int, 26, 1105-1111.

3. Davidson S. Passmore R, Brock JF. (1972): Human nutrition and dietetics, 5th ed. Baltimore: Williams and Wilkins Co, 9.

4. Southgate DAT, Barrett IM. (1966): The intake and excretion of caloric constituents of milk by babies. Br J Nutr, 20, 363-372.

SAMPLING MILK FOR ENERGY CONTENT

C. Garza
M. W. Woolridge
N. F. Butte
A. Ferris
C. Casey

Two approaches have been used to obtain milk samples for the estimation of energy content: 1) expression of the contents of one or both breasts at a specified time, or 2) collection of small aliquots of milk at different intervals during a feeding. Factors that must be considered when milk samples are collected for this purpose are: within-day variations in milk composition, interference with the "let-down" reflex, collection of adequate and "weighted" samples of fore and hind milk, maintenance of the breastfeeding pattern, minimized interference with suckling, minimized (either positive or negative) effects on milk synthesis, and the reproducibility of the method.

TWENTY-FOUR HOUR ALIQUOTS

Butte et al. (1) collected milk samples throughout a 24-hour period, in a pattern that mimicked the usual feeding schedule, in order to take into account within-day variations in milk composition. Suckling was maintained throughout each collection period to minimize the interference imposed by the procedure. If milk volume was also studied, the sampling was always done after the test weighing procedure to minimize any effects of the collection method on levels of milk synthesis.

At each feeding during a 24-hour period, the infant was offered one breast and the other breast was emptied. This procedure maximized the likelihood of an effective "let-down" reflex. The breast from which the sample was obtained was not emptied completely. Rather, the mothers were asked not to exceed 15 minutes of pumping and to stop sooner if milk flow was reduced markedly. Throughout successive feeds, alternate breasts were used for feeding and pumping. This permitted samples to be taken from both breasts while maintaining some aspects of the usual feeding pattern. Weighted aliquots of the individual samples collected throughout the day were used to create a 24-hour pool. Mothers were asked not to alter the usual feeding pattern and to offer their infants supplements of human milk that were collected and frozen in advance of the sampling procedure. These supplements were collected in small quantities one to two weeks before the day of sampling to minimize effects on volume of milk production.

Milk samples were obtained by this method to determine the nutrient intake and growth of 45 exclusively breast-fed infants (1). The quantities of milk collected were equivalent to 49 $\pm$ 17% of the daily milk intakes previously determined by test-weighing. The number of samples collected over 24 hours was equal to 90 $\pm$ 22% of the number of feedings recorded during a previous 24-hour test-weighing session.

The degree of interference with the "let-down" reflex and the reproducibility of the method can be assessed only indirectly. Both of these factors are of concern because they influence the representative nature of the sample relative to the infant's usual milk intake. Positive correlations were observed between the volume of milk collected and the energy concentration of the samples (r ranged from 0.33 to 0.43 over 3 successive months of observation, $p<0.05$). When the 24-hour pool was less than 40% of the daily intake determined by test-weighing, the mean energy content was 0.63 $\pm$ 0.09 kcal/g. Pools that represented 40 to 60% of the daily intake had a mean energy density of 0.66 $\pm$ 0.10 kcal/g, and those that represented >60% of the daily intake had a density of 0.68 $\pm$ 0.09 kcal/g.

The reproducibility of the method was not tested rigorously because duplicate pools from the same individual were not obtained within appropriately short intervals. Nevertheless, the method yielded samples with a significant degree of intra-individual consistency in milk composition across the 4 months of observation. The concentrations of total nitrogen, protein nitrogen, lactose, fat, and energy in milks of individual women were significantly correlated to their subsequent monthly values (r ranged from 0.42 to 0.74, $p<0.05$). The r values for fat and energy were approximately 0.65 and 0.62, respectively.

SAMPLING SINGLE FEEDINGS

Abbreviated sampling schemes have been used to obtain samples to predict the energy content of milk produced throughout the day. One or both breasts are emptied at times specified by various protocols (2-4). This approach has been extended to make predictions of 24-hour volumes. Extrapolations from single samples are attractive because of the minimal disruption of breastfeeding patterns. The valid extrapolation of data from a single sample to a 24-hour period, however requires that the volume and caloric content of a single feed be representative of milk production and level of intake for the entire day.

In applying this method, one or both breasts are emptied completely. The time chosen for sampling is usually mid-morning, when the fat content is highest (5). Known variations in the volume and composition of single feeds, however, affect the reliability of these data when they are extrapolated to wider time intervals. Another serious shortcoming in the method is the assumption that the volume of milk obtained reflects the intake of the infant (5).

Studies have compared milk volumes measured at single feedings with those measured over 24 hours. Energy content, however, has been of less interest. Reports of three studies (2-4) have shown that single feed volumes in early lactation correlate well with daily estimates, although each study reported a large unsystematic error within and between subjects. No similar relationships were noted in later stages of lactation (4). Within-day variation in energy contents introduces even greater errors when volume and compositional data from single samples are extrapolated to estimate the caloric content of milk produced over 24 hours.

MULTIPLE SMALL SAMPLINGS

In contrast to techniques based on the total, or nearly total, expression of the contents of one or both breasts, three methods have been developed specifically to avoid interference with normal feeding practices. Such techniques allow concurrent measurements of the volume and composition of milk, rather than independent measurements of volume and composition. Two methods are founded on the premise that representative samples, small enough not to interfere with normal volumes of intake, can be expressed either at mid-feeding (6) or before and after feeding (7). The third method involves the removal of small amounts of milk during suckling (16). Each method attempts to account for the variation in fat content during a feed, in addition to that over the course of the day. In a study of within-feed variation in 10 women, an increase of 4 to 700% was observed in fat content between fore and hind milk (6). The mean increase in fat concentration was twofold. Several patterns of increase were evident in studies in which a number of small samples were taken sequentially until the breast was emptied. The patterns ranged from a gradual, nearly linear increase throughout the entire feeding, to more abrupt increases with continued emptying of the breast (9-12).

The use of mid-feed samples as representations of the total feed was evaluated in 6 women at 2 months lactation (6). The entire contents of both breasts were removed by electric pump, with 5 ml collected separately as a mid-feed sample 2 minutes after milk began flowing into the pump container. The total lipid concentrations in the pooled samples were correlated highly (r=0.89) with the mid-feed values. The means were not significantly different by paired t-test, but the coefficient of variation of the residuals was 28% when mid-feed values were regressed against the values from the pools. This coefficient of variation is much higher than that of the assay for total lipids (6%). The coefficients of variation of the residuals were much lower for protein and lactose (<13%), suggesting that the concentrations of these nutrients in mid-feed samples was reasonably predictive of the concentrations in the entire pool. Results reported by Hytten (9) suggest that if the true mid-feed sample can be obtained, higher correlations can be achieved between the lipid concentrations in the mid-feed sample and the entire breast contents.

Prentice et al. (7) sampled fore and hind milk to obtain samples representative of an entire feeding. This approach was based on data reported by Hytten (9) which suggested that the mean lipid concentration of a pre- and postfeed sample should provide a reasonable approximation of the entire feeding. The nonlinear changes in fat concentration as a feeding progresses and the unreliable assumption that volume transfer is constant (i.e., equal amounts of foremilk and hindmilk are consumed) (8,13) may limit the accuracy and precision of this approach. Hartmann and Saint (14,15) developed an equation to derive mean fat concentrations in a total feeding from samples of fore and hind milk. Confidence and prediction intervals of mean fat concentrations estimated by this equation cannot be assessed easily. In addition to the likely inter- and intra-individual variations, the effects of collection methods on the coefficients of the predictive equation should also be considered. The development of methods to measure instantaneous volume transfer during a feed and to obtain sequential samples of suckled milk simultaneously for compositional analysis is based on the use of a latex nipple shield and flow transducer (13,16). The use of these methods, which have been discussed in Section I, should provide an integrated estimate of caloric intake from serially matched volume and compositional data. Results from the analysis of milk sequentially sampled by manual means during suckling (17) have been compared with results from pre- and postfeed manually expressed samples of milk. Estimates of fat intake by the two methods were significantly different; the results from the sequentially sampled milks were lower.

A potential drawback of the manual method to remove milk during suckling is that milk withdrawal is not flow-related. This issue becomes critical toward the end of a feed when the fat content has risen markedly. Removing milk also affects the rate of milk transfer, and thereby suckling patterns, and it may cause the premature termination of the feed by either mother or infant. The automatic removal of a constant proportion of the milk transferred would avoid such problems and would reflect the average composition of the milk taken by the infant. The flow-related output voltage from an ultrasound flow transducer (13) might be used to drive a sampling system. A simple approximation, however, can be achieved by harnessing the baby's own suction pressure to divert small samples of suckled breast milk into a collecting trap. Such a system is under development.

RECOMMENDATION

No single method can be recommended. The development of an automatic sampling device that would measure milk flow, yet not interfere with feeding, would be ideal. Collecting 24-hour aliquots of milk dissociates determinations of milk composition from those of milk volumes. There are no procedures to validate directly that the milk sampled for compositional analysis represents milk consumed by the infant. The milk, however, represents a weighted aliquot of milk obtained throughout the day in a pattern which mimics the usual feeding schedule. The shortcomings of the single feed approach have been discussed. At best, this method is limited to group estimates, because there are no systematic data on which to base measurements of its precision or accuracy in predicting the caloric content of milk produced throughout the day. Experience suggests that a small midfeed sample may represent the whole feed when group data are of interest. The better the definition or determination of the true mid-feed point, presumably the more representative this sample will be. Large individual deviations in the fat contents, however, indicate that this method is unsuitable for studies in which data are sought for individuals. The non-linear changes in fat concentrations as feedings progress make difficult the recommendation of both midfeed sampling and pre- and postfeed sampling as standard collection methods. The required assumption of a constant volume transfer adds to this difficulty. Therefore, investigators are urged to consider the advantages and disadvantages of each method within the context of specific objectives to identify a method of choice.

REFERENCES

1. Butte NF, Garza C, Smith EO, Nichols BL. (1984): Human milk intake and growth performance of exclusively breast-fed infants. J Pediatr, 104, 187-195.

2. Brown KH, Black RE, Robertson AD, Akhtar NA, Ahmed G, Becker S. (1982): Clinical and field studies of human lactation: methodological considerations. Am J Clin Nutr, 35, 745-756.

3. Houston MJ, Harvie PW, McNeilly AS. (1983): Factors affecting the duration of breast feeding. 1. Measurement of breast milk intake in the first week of life. Early Hum Dev, 8, 49-54.

4. Neville MC, Keller R. (1984): Accuracy of single- and two-feed test weighing in assessing 24 h breast milk production. Early Hum Dev 9, 275-281.

5. Hytten FE. (1954): Clinical and chemical studies in human lactation. Part I-III. Br Med J, 1, 175-182.

6. Neville MC, Keller RP, Seacat J, Casey CE, Allen JC, Archer P. (1984): Studies in human lactation. 1. Within-feed and between-breast variation in selected components of human milk. Am J Clin Nutr, 40, 635-646.

7. Prentice A, Prentice AM, Whitehead RG. (1981): Breast-milk fat concentrations of rural African women. 1. Short-term variations within individuals. Br J Nutr, 45, 483-494.

8. Woolridge MW, Baum JD, Drewett RF. (1982): Individual patterns of milk intake during breast-feeding. Early Hum Dev, 7, 265-272.

9. Hytten FE. (1954): Clinical and chemical studies in human lactation. II. Variation in major constituents during a feeding. Br Med J, 4, 176-179.

10. Forsum E, Lönnerdal B. (1979): Variation in the contents of nutrients of breast milk during one feeding. Nutr Rep Int, 19, 815-820.

11. Emery WB, Canolty NL, Aitchinson JM, Dunkley WL. (1978): Influence of sampling on fatty acid composition of human milk. Am J Clin Nutr, 31, 1127-1130.

12. Watson MA, Alford ES, Dill CW, Richter RL, Garza C. (1982): Compositional changes during sequential sampling of human milk. Nutr Rep Int, 26, 1105-1111.

13. Woolridge MW, How TV, Drewett RF, Rolfe P, Baum JD. (1982): The continuous measurement of milk intake at a feed in breast-fed babies. Early Hum Dev, 6, 365-373.

14. Hartmann PE, Saint L. (1984): Measurement of milk yield in women. J Pediatr Gastroenterol Nutr, 3, 270-274.

15. Saint L, Smith M, Hartmann PE. (1984): The yield and nutrient content of colostrum and milk of women from giving birth to 1 month post-partum. Br J Nutr, 52, 87-95.

16. Lucas A, Lucas PJ, Baum JD. (1980): The nipple-shield sampling system: a device for measuring the dietary intake of breast-fed infants. Early Hum Dev, 4, 365-382.

17. Williams AF, Akinkugbe FM, Baum JD. (1985): A comparison of two methods of milk sampling for calculating the fat intake of breast-fed babies. Hum Nutr: Clin Nutr. 39C, 193-202.

DETERMINATION OF THE ENERGY CONTENT OF HUMAN MILK

C. Garza
N. F. Butte
K. Dewey

Two methods have been used to estimate the energy content of human milk. The heat of combustion is determined directly by experimental calorimetry based on principles developed by Lavoisier and Laplace in the late 1700s (1). Indirect determinations require the application of various conversion factors that relate either the heats of combustion of lactose, protein, and fat, or the physiologic fuel values (2) of these constituents to the proximate analyses of milk.

BRIEF DESCRIPTION OF EXPERIMENTAL CALORIMETRY

Two types of calorimeters are available for the determination of heats of combustion, adiabatic and isothermal (3). Adiabatic calorimeters are designed not to exchange heat with the environment. The increase in the temperature of the calorimeter after the complete combustion of a test substance is used to estimate the heat of combustion of the substance. Isothermal calorimeters are designed with a jacket that maintains a constant temperature. The heat which is transferred to the isothermal jacket is measured to calculate the heat of combustion.

Milk may be combusted either in the liquid state or after it has been dried, preferably lyophilized. When combusted as a liquid, a known amount of an appropriate combustible liquid, e.g., mineral oil, is mixed with a known amount of milk. The mineral oil is used to ensure the complete combustion of liquid milk. Less than 1 g of milk is required for this determination. After the heat of combustion of the mixture is determined, the contribution of heat from the known added material is calculated and subtracted from the total heat produced. The difference represents the heat of combustion of the milk. Alternatively, milk may be lyophilized, formed into a pellet, and then combusted. When lyophilized milk is used, care should be taken that atmospheric moisture is not added inadvertently to the dried milk during the required weighing steps. As in other applications of experimental calorimetry, completeness of combustion must be determined and the heat generated by the material used to initiate combustion must be accounted for in the final estimate of the heats of combustion.

DETERMINATION OF ENERGY CONTENT FROM PROXIMATE ANALYSES

The determination of the heat of combustion from proximate analyses of milk requires the separate determinations of the concentrations of the energy-yielding components in the milk. The common practice is to determine the contents of total fat, lactose, and protein. The caloric equivalents used most often for milk are 5.65 kcal/g protein, 3.95 kcal/g lactose, and 9.25 kcal/g fat (4). The values for protein and fat were derived from bovine milk products. When protein is determined by assays of total nitrogen or acid precipitable nitrogen, the standard practice has been to multiply nitrogen determinations by either 6.25 or 6.38 to convert the determinations to estimates of protein. The sum of the products of the respective concentrations and caloric equivalents represents the gross energy content of milk.

COMPARISON OF DIRECT AND INDIRECT ESTIMATIONS

The energy content of milk samples collected during 24-hour periods at 4 consecutive monthly intervals has been determined both directly and indirectly (5). An adiabatic bomb calorimeter (Parr Instrument, Moline, IL) was used to make the direct determinations. Lactose concentration was determined with the use of an automated analyzer which detects hydrogen peroxide produced from the oxidation of galactose (YSI model 27, Yellow Springs, OH). Fat was determined by a modified Roese-Gottlieb procedure. Protein was estimated from Kjeldahl determinations of total nitrogen and nitrogen in acid precipitable protein. The acid precipitable protein determinations were multiplied by 6.25 to estimate protein. The conversion factors listed in the preceding paragraph were used to estimate the gross energy content of milk from the proximate analyses.

Table 1 compares values derived from proximate analyses with those measured by experimental calorimetry. The agreement between mean values is excellent. Caution, however, must be advised. Figure 1 illustrates the 95% confidence and prediction intervals of the equations which predict directly determined gross heat values from proximate analyses. Prediction intervals represent the confidence bands for individual estimates; confidence intervals pertain to the estimation of means for a group of individuals (6). The 95% prediction intervals at the mean for months 1, 2, 3, and 4 were 15%, 14%, 22%, and 12% of the respective means for each month. The width, or level of uncertainty, in any prediction interval widens as the value moves progressively further from the mean value used as the reference point. Figure 1 illustrates this characteristic. The 95% confidence intervals were approximately 1 to 3% of the mean for each month.

PHYSIOLOGIC FUEL VALUES

In certain studies it may be useful to calculate metabolizable energy based on proximate constituents. To do so, it is necessary to have accurate caloric conversion factors, or "physiologic fuel values," for protein, fat, and carbohydrate. In adults, the standard Atwater factors of 9, 4, and 4 kcal/g of fat, protein, and carbohydrate, respectively, are commonly utilized (7). However, these factors should not be assumed to be correct for the growing infant who is fed human milk.

Table 1. Comparison of measured vs predicted energy contents

Months	Protein[a] cal/g (cv)	Lactose[b] cal/g (cv)	Fat[c] cal/g (cv)	NPN cal/g	A Total[d] cal/g	B Experimental[e] calorimetry (cv)	A/B
1	51(15)	256(4)	335(21)	20*	662*	680(12)	0.97
				3**	645**		0.95
2	50(12)	260(4)	318(20)	18*	646*	643(13)	1.00
				3**	631**		0.98
3	48(11)	263(3)	298(24)	18*	626*	625(15)	1.00
				3**	612**		0.98
4	46(13)	263(4)	322(31)	17*	648*	644(16)	1.01
				3**	634**		0.98

cv: coefficient of variation, NPN: nonprotein nitrogen, PN: protein nitrogen

[a] 5.65 kcal/g applied to PN fraction

[b] 3.95 kcal/g

[c] 9.25 kcal/g

[d] Sum of protein, lactose, fat, and NPN fractions

[e] Values obtained from adiabatic calorimetry

* 5.65 kcal/g, applied to NPN fraction (treated as if all were soluble protein)

** 2.52 kcal/g, applied to NPN fraction (treated as if all were urea).

Among term infants fed untreated human milk at 5-16 days of age, absorption of fat is relatively high (90-95%) (8,9). Preterm infants absorb a somewhat lower percentage of fat in fresh human milk (84-90%) (10,11), and the percentage is reduced as low as 58% when sterilized human milk is fed (10,12). Atkinson et al. suggested that the inactivation of bile salt-stimulated lipase in human milk during sterilization is responsible for reduced fat absorption (10). The percentage of fat absorbed from infant formulas is generally somewhat lower than that absorbed from fresh human milk, although the use of current fat blends of unsaturated and medium chain fatty acids may improve fat absorption from formulas (10).

Because fat contributes 50% or more of the energy content of human milk, the caloric conversion factor utilized to calculate metabolizable energy from fat has a major effect on total calculated energy intake. Based on the reported ranges of fat absorption, this factor would be 8.32-8.74 kcal/g for term infants and 7.77-8.32 kcal/g for preterm infants

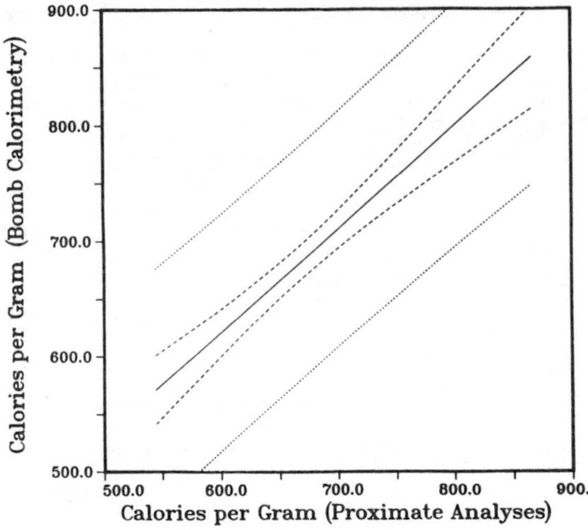

Fig. 1. Prediction of gross caloric content of human milk from proximate analyses - Month 1

fed fresh human milk. If sterilized human milk is used, the fecal excretion of fat should be estimated before using any conversion factor for metabolizable energy, as an absorption of only 58% would decrease the physiological fuel value of fat to 5.37 kcal/g.

Of the three constituents (protein, fat and carbohydrate), the metabolizable energy from carbohydrate in human milk may be the simplest to calculate because net absorption is 97-99% for both term and preterm infants and does not appear to be reduced by heat treatment (8,10). The conversion factor for carbohydrate is, therefore, 3.83-3.94 kcal/g. These calculations do not include potential losses of energy due to malabsorbed lactose reaching the colon, undergoing fermentation, and being absorbed subsequently as volatile fatty acids. The detection of high levels of breath hydrogen in normal breast-fed infants indicates that this is a common occurrence (13,14).

Because a significant proportion of dietary nitrogen is retained by the infant, metabolic studies of energy utilization must consider the percentages of total protein that are absorbed and retained. Among term infants fed fresh human milk at 6 to 9 (15) and 13 to 16 (8) days of age, apparent protein absorption was calculated to be 82-84%, while retention was 52-53%. Preterm infants fed fresh human milk have slightly higher absorption (82-90%) and retention (58-67%) rates (10,16). Both absorption and retention rates were slightly lower when preterm infants were fed sterilized human milk (81-84% and 43-59%, respectively) (10,16). Impaired absorption may be due to unmetabolizable reaction products between lactose and epsilon amino groups which result from heat treatment. Although protein contains approximatly 5.65 kcal/g, only 4.2 kcal/g are available for energy because of the incomplete oxidation of protein to urea in humans. The amount of energy available from protein is reduced further by incomplete absorption and net retention. A single conversion factor is difficult to determine because these factors are influenced by the maturity of the infants and the amounts of dietary protein and metabolizable energy consumed. However, since protein usually provides only 5 to 15% of the calories in human milk, a precise conversion factor is less critical for protein than for fat and carbohydrate.

RECOMMENDATIONS

Experimental calorimetry is recommended as the procedure of choice for the determination of the gross energy content of milk. The value for the heat of combustion obtained experimentally is determined with a high degree of accuracy and precision from measurements which require a small sample of milk. Indirect estimates from proximate analysis are less desirable because at least three different assays are required, each with its own experimental error.

When the energy utilization of infants is a research objective, calculation of metabolizable energy based on proximate constituents should be included in addition to direct measures of energy content from bomb calorimetry. The most sophisticated approach would include metabolic studies to determine the absorption of protein, carbohydrate, and fat, and to calculate metabolizable energy based on those results. However, this rarely is feasible. In most cases, therefore, physiological fuel values should be derived from metabolic studies in which the characteristics, infant age, gestational age, and type and quantity of milk are similar. An accurate estimation of fat absorption is the most critical for deriving caloric conversion factors. Whenever metabolizable energy is reported, however, values for gross energy should be included to facilitate comparisons between studies.

REFERENCES

1. Kleiber N. (1975): The fire of life. Huntington, NY: Robert E. Krieger Publishing Co.

2. Atwater WO, Benedict FG. (1899): Experiments on the metabolism of matter and energy in the human body. Bulletin No. 69. Washington, DC: US Department of Agriculture.

3. Moore WJ. (1965): Physical chemistry, 3rd Edition. Englewood Cliffs, NJ: Prentice-Hall Inc.

4. Watt BK, Merrill AL. (1963): Composition of foods. Agricultural Handbook No. 8. Washington, DC: Agricultural Research Services, USDA.

5. Butte N, Garza C, Smith EO, Nichols BL. (1984): Human milk intake and growth performance of exclusively breast-fed infants. J Pediatr, 104, 187-195.

6. Snedecor GW, Cochran WG. (1967): Statistical methods, 6th Edition. Ames, IA: Iowa State University Press.

7. Southgate DAT, Durnin JVGA. (1970): Calorie conversion factors. An experimental reassessment of the factors used in the calculation of the energy value of human diets. Br J Nutr, 24, 517-535.

8. Southgate DAT, Barrett IM. (1966): The intake and excretion of calorific constituents of milk by babies. Br J Nutr, 20, 363-372.

9. Hanna FM, Navarrete DA, Hsu FA. (1970): Calcium-fatty acid absorption in term infants fed human milk and prepared formulas simulating human milk. Pediatrics, 45, 216-224.

10. Atkinson SA, Bryan MH, Anderson GH. (1981): Human milk feeding in premature infants: protein, fat, and carbohydrate balances in the first two weeks of life. J Pediatr, 99, 617-624.

11. Shaw JCL. (1976): Evidence for defective skeletal mineralization in low-birth-weight infants: the absorption of calcium and fat. Pediatrics, 57, 16-25.

12. Putet G, Senterre J, Rigo J, Salle B. (1984): Nutrient balance, energy utilization, and composition of weight gain in very-low-birth-weight infants fed pooled human milk or a preterm formula. J Pediatr, 105, 79-85.

13. Lifschitz C, Garza C. (1983): Delayed complete functional lactase sufficiency in breast-fed infants. J Pediatr Gastroenterol Nutr, 2, 478-482.

14. Barr RG, Hanley J, Patterson KingsNorth, Woolridge J. (1984): Breath hydrogen excretion in normal newborn infants in response to usual feeding patterns: evidence for "functional lactase insufficiency" beyond the first month of life. J Pediatr, 104, 527-533.

15. Slater JB. (1961): Retentions of nitrogen and minerals by babies 1 week old. Br J Nutr, 15, 83-97.

16. Williamson S, Finucane E, Ellis H, Gamsu HR. (1978): Effect of heat treatment of human milk on absorption of nitrogen, fat, sodium, calcium, and phosphorus by preterm infants. Arch Dis Child, 53, 555-563.

SECTION VII. MEASUREMENT OF ELECTROLYTE AND MACROMINERAL CONCENTRATIONS IN HUMAN MILK

WORKSHOP PARTICIPANTS:

M. C. Neville, Department of Physiology, University of Colorado School of Medicine, Denver, Colorado

R. P. Keller, Department of Physiology, University of Colorado School of Medicine, Denver, Colorado

B. Lönnerdal, Department of Nutrition, University of California, Davis, California

S. Atkinson, Department of Pediatrics, McMaster University, Hamilton, Ontario, Canada

C. L. Wade, Department of Pediatrics, McMaster University, Hamilton, Ontario, Canada

N. Butte, Department of Pediatrics, Baylor College of Medicine, Houston, Texas

P. B. Moser, Department of Food and Nutrition, University of Maryland, College Park, Maryland

MEASUREMENT OF ELECTROLYTE AND MACROMINERAL CONCENTRATIONS IN HUMAN MILK

Margaret C. Neville
Ronald P. Keller
Bo Lönnerdal
Stephanie Atkinson
Carol L. Wade
Nancy Butte
Phylis B. Moser

INTRODUCTION

Understanding the normal and abnormal composition of human milk requires accurate analytical methods suitable for small samples, and specifically adapted to human milk. Ideally, these methods should be inexpensive and should allow the rapid processing of large numbers of samples. Further, knowledge of the variation of the component under study within the feed, diurnally and with the duration of lactation is necessary to formulate a representative sampling regime. This regime should interfere as little as possible with the nursing mother-infant dyad. Finally, samples must be collected and stored in such a way that the normal constituents are not altered. In this report, we will deal briefly with the issues of sample collection, storage and sampling regimens. We will discuss more extensively the currently available analytical techniques for sodium, potassium, chloride, calcium, magnesium, and phosphate in human milk. The forms of calcium in human milk and the approach required to deal with this difficult issue will also be discussed. Before commencing this methodological discussion, we note that it was the firm recommendation of the workshop on minerals and electrolytes that the concentration of these substances in milk be reported in millimoles or mols per liter to facilitate comparison of their concentrations. Such units as mg/dl, g/L or ppm are less useful. The use of mEq is at best confusing; for phosphate, it is incorrect.

SAMPLE HANDLING AND PREPARATION

The most important aspect of milk sampling is the manner in which it is collected. The greatest sources of contamination are probably the perspiration accumulated on the breast and the remaining traces of the infant's saliva. For this reason, the breast should be cleansed with deionized water prior to milk expression. Pump containers, when used, should be acid-washed and rinsed with deionized water. The milk should be stored in acid-washed, mineral-free containers.

Sampling regimes

The timing of sampling for macromineral and electrolyte analysis would appear to be less important than for other milk components, e.g., fat. Thus, Neville et al. (1) found no significant variation in sodium, potassium, chloride, free phosphate, calcium or magnesium through a single feed. Preliminary analyses by the same group suggest significant diurnal variation of most of these components in some women (2). Keenan et al. (3) have observed diurnal variation in sodium and potassium levels in later lactation, an observation supported by Gross et al. (4). There are longitudinal changes in the concentration of most or all of these milk constituents, so attention must be paid to duration of lactation. In addition, mastitis and involutional processes have a profound effect on milk sodium and chloride (1,5,6). For this reason, routine analysis of sodium concentration in milk samples is recommended to rule out these conditions. A suspicion of mastitis or involutional processes should be entertained if the sodium level in the two breasts differs markedly or if, after the first week of lactation, the sodium is greater than 20 mM.

Storage of samples

Macrominerals and electrolytes are among the most stable of milk components so that ordinary care with samples (refrigeration for short-term storage and freezing for long-term storage) should be adequate.

Sample storage is quite another matter if the partition of calcium between the various milk compartments is to be studied (7) or if ionized calcium is of interest (8).

Milk is equilibrated with carbon dioxide in the breast at a pCO_2 of 40 mmHg. This CO_2 is rapidly lost to the air when milk is removed by breast pump or allowed to stand for any period of time. Under such conditions, milk pH rises from a mean around 6.9 to values as high as 7.7 (Allen and Neville, unpublished). Because pH has a profound effect on ionized calcium, for measurement of this constituent it is important to collect and store the sample anaerobically. This is accomplished by manual expression of a small droplet of milk into a glass capillary tube, capping both ends of the tube, and storing it on ice. Such a sample has a pCO_2>30 mmHg, and it maintains a constant pH and ionized calcium for more than 24 hours (8).

Wet ashing, with use of strong acids or bases as digestion agents, reduces the possibility of volatilization when compared to dry ashing (9). Again, contamination must be avoided with meticulous laboratory checks. Sources of contamination include the container, acids, bases, water and airborne particles. The reagents may cause desorption of minerals from the walls of the container. Alternatively, losses may occur due to adsorption to the container. Thus, both blanks and standards must be included with every run. Various acids, acid combinations or bases have been evaluated as digesting agents (10, 11). Concentrated nitric acid (16N) was found to be the most efficacious.

It is possible to assay for Na, K, Ca, and Mg without ashing by using suitable diluents. Neville and Keller (unpublished) diluted breast milk 1:3 with 15 mM LiCl for determination of Na and K by flame photometry. They found overnight incubation in 10% nitric acid containing 0.1% $LaCl_3$ to be suitable for atomic absorption spectrometry of Ca and Mg, if the method of standard additions is used with each sample. Again, careful attention to blanks and purity of reagents is important.

Samples for free phosphate must not be ashed. For total phosphate ashing provides the most straight forward method of breaking down organic phosphates. Chloride can be measured on undiluted samples using potentiometric titration with $AgCl_2$ (12, see below).

Automated methods using either potentiometry or colorimetric procedures are becoming available and usually require considerably less sample preparation. For colorimetric procedures, it is absolutely necessary to remove the milk fat to avoid light-scattering from fat particles. This can be accomplished in the following manner (Keller and Neville, unpublished): The sample is frozen and thawed to break the milk fat globule membranes, thus permitting better consolidation of the lipid during centrifugation. The sample is then centrifuged for 30 minutes at 0^oC at 1500 g in a polyethylene tube. The entire tube and its contents are frozen, then the tube is cut through, just below the fat layer, with a razor blade. The aqueous fraction can be thawed and sampled as needed. If fat-free samples are used, it is important to evaluate the amount of mineral or electrolyte associated with the lipid (see below).

ANALYTICAL METHODS

In no case has a rigorous comparison of the various methods for mineral and electrolyte analysis been published. Thus, it is important that each investigator carefully evaluate the planned techniques. Such an evaluation should include the following: measurements of each constituent under study by two separate methods applied to a group of samples containing a range of concentrations, the use of standard additions to monitor both recovery and matrix effects, and the evaluation of reagents for contamination. Quality controls should be run with each batch of samples to assure run-to-run consistency in analytical methodologies. Use of a reliable standard milk sample would be a desirable further check on the accuracy of the method. Unfortunately, no such sample currently exists for human milk. Lyophilized bovine milk standards are available from the International Atomic Energy Association, Vienna Standard A-11 (dried cow's milk) or National Bureau of Standards, Washington, DC, Sample #1549. Care must be taken with reconstitution of such dried samples to assure homogeneity.

Sodium and Potassium

A survey of the literature reveals a spread of values from 2 to 96.4 mM for sodium and 11.7 to 20 mM for potassium in human milk (13,14). Factors which influence these electrolytes, particularly sodium, include the following: the stage of lactation (early colostrum and weaning milks tend to have high sodium, 7,15-20), gestational stage at delivery (sodium tends to be higher in preterm milk, 15-20) and mastitis (1). In all of these cases, high sodium is thought to be the result of direct passage of ions from the extracellular fluid into the milk via a paracellular pathway which closes during full lactation to form a tight blood-milk barrier (21). At one month of lactation, reported mean sodium values range from 6.6 to 17 mM (Table 1) and mean potassium values from 12 to 15 mM.

Flame photometry and atomic emission spectroscopy on either ashed/-reconstituted or diluted samples are well-established methods for measurement of sodium and potassium, and should be regarded as the standard methods. In general, most authors do not describe the diluent used in their analyses. Atkinson and Wade (unpublished) use lanthanum (2000 ppm) as the diluent for sodium, and cesium (2000 ppm) as the diluent for

Table 1. Sodium and Potassium and Chloride Content of Human Milk at One Month Lactation*

Investigators	N	Sodium (mM)	Potassium (mM)	Chloride (mM)
Dewey and Lönnerdal (15)	20	9.9(6.6)[a]	13.2(1.8)[a]	--
Butte et al. (16)	13	8.0(2.3)[b]	--	--
N Hibberd et al. (14)	10	17.1(15.8)[c]	13.5(2.2)	--
Atkinson et al. (17)	10	10.0(2.0)[b]	15.0(3)[b]	--
Gross et al. (18)	11	8.5(5.9)[c]	15.0(2.3)[c]	13.1(7.6)[e]
Lemons et al. (19)	27	7.0(2.5)[h]	13.0(1.3)[h]	10.5(2.4)[d]
Picciano et al. (24)	26	6.6(2.4)[b]	11.9(2.4)[b]	12.0(2.4)[f]
Schanler and Oh (20)	6	8.8(1.2)[f]	12.5(3.2)[f].	--
Neville and Keller+	12	7.8(2.0)[i]	15.8(1.7)[i]	14.2(4.3)[e]

* Full-term mothers only included; means (S.D.)
\+ Unpublished

Methods

a. Wet ashing with atomic absorption photometry in the emission made.
b. Dry ashing with atomic absorption photometry in emission or absorption made.
c. Dilution of fat free samples followed by atomic absorption photometry.
d. Potentiometric titration (14) with Ag.
e. Colorimetric analysis.
f. Specific ion electrode after oxygen combustion.
g. Flame photometry on nitric acid filtrates.
h. Flame photometry in Lithium containing solution.
i. Ion-selective electrode on fat-free samples.

potassium. Neville and Keller (unpublished) use 15 mM LiCl as the diluent for both. This ion suppresses the effects of ionization enhancement between sodium and potassium and allows both ions to be measured on the same sample. Because sodium and potassium do affect each others flame emission, standards with similar concentrations of sodium and potassium should be used. Serum standards are not satisfactory. Neville, Keller and Atkinson found similar results for the sodium and potassium concentrations of both whole milk and defatted samples (unpublished).

Commercial instruments using ion-selective electrodes have recently become available for measurement of sodium and potassium. These instruments offer rapid analyses which can be performed on diluted or undiluted samples of whole or defatted milk (22, 23). The operating principle is similar to a pH electrode except that the electrodes contain a resin which is sensitive to sodium and potassium and less sensitive to pH. Most instruments include an automatic wash cycle between each reading. (Frequent cleaning with enzyme solutions to remove protein and lipid buildup is important to obtain stable readings.) Milk samples are best diluted 2:1 with deionized water and run with the machine in the urine mode, if such is available. Again, urine rather than plasma standards should be used. Values obtained are similar to those obtained by flame photometry (Atkinson, unpublished; Keller and Neville, unpublished). In establishing this methodology, the intra-assay coefficient of variation was 1.2% for sodium and 1.4% for potassium. The interassay coefficient of variation was 4.2% for sodium and 4.0% for potassium (Atkinson and Wade, unpublished). The limit of sensitivity for sodium in human milk samples using the Radiometer instrument (KNal) was 3 mM.

In the absence of a systematic comparative examination of methods for sodium and potassium in human milk, it is difficult to designate a single method which provides greatest accuracy and precision. Analyses by flame photometry or atomic emission spectrometry, either after wet ashing or LiCl dilution, appear to provide adequate results. Ion-selective electrodes appear to provide a suitable alternative which allows the rapid and inexpensive processing of a large number of samples.

Chloride

Chloride values, determined at one month lactation in various laboratories, are given in Table 1. They vary from 10.5 to 13 mM. The standard method for determination of chloride in biological materials is potentiometric titration with silver (12); this method appears to be satisfactory for human milk. Picciano (24) has used ion-selective electrodes after oxygen combustion in a closed flask to prevent volatilization of chloride.

An automated colorimetric method based on the displacement of thiocyanate from mercuric thiocyanate to react with ferric ions is available (25). Neville and Keller (unpublished) found this method, which requires fat-free milk, to give reasonable correlation with results of potentiometric titration (Figure 1). The colorimetric procedure had an intraassay coefficient of variation of 6% and an interassay coefficient of variation of 9%.

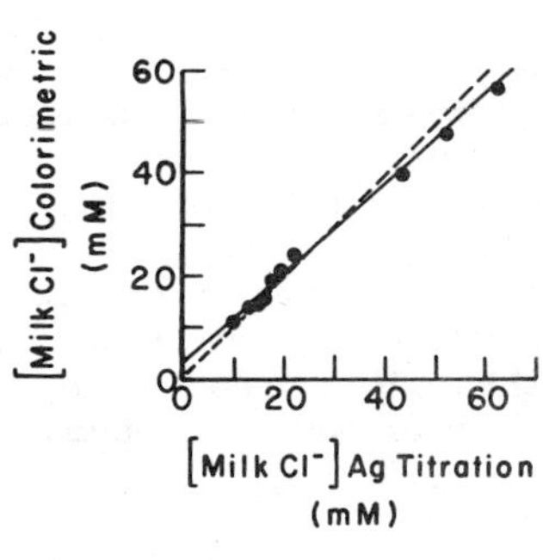

Fig.1. Comparison of chloride analyses in human milk by colorimetric and potentiometric methods (Neville and Keller, unpublished). The best fitting regression line (solid line) through the points has a slope of 0.87 and an intercept of 3.2 mM. r is 1.0 and Sy,x is 1.2 mM.

Calcium

Table 2 shows the values obtained by different investigators for the calcium levels in human milk at about one month lactation. Values ranging from 4.3 to 7.3 mM were obtained in different laboratories using a number of different procedures. Clearly, some standardization is necessary. It is possible in the absence of a reliable human milk standard, that the lyophilized bovine milk standard mentioned above can be used to validate assays.

Most investigators use either wet or dry ashing followed by atomic absorption spectrometry to determine calcium concentrations. With the availability of a rapid, inexpensive, automated colorimetric assay in clinical laboratories (33-35), some investigators have turned to this method, which Neville and Keller have found to give nearly identical values as atomic adsorption spectrometry on *fat-free samples*. The problem is that 10-12% of calcium is associated with the fat fraction (36, Neville and Keller unpublished). The proportion increases with storage at 4°C, and Lönnerdal et al. found that 15-20% of the total calcium was associated with the lipid fraction in samples which had been frozen (7, 38). This means that analysis of fat-free samples tends to underestimate total milk calcium by 5-15%. For nutritional purposes, this is probably unsatisfactory. However,it should be noted that the values for total calcium obtained by Neville and Keller using the colorimetric method are among the highest reported values (Table 2) raising the possibility that ashing procedures can lead to loss of calcium. This possibility should be rigorously tested in every laboratory using such procedures.

Ionized calcium

The methods necessary for the accurate determination of ionized calcium using a calcium electrode system have been described elsewhere (8). Suffice to say here that the measurement requires that the sample be delivered anaerobically to the electrode, that the measurement be made at physiological temperature (37°C), and that the measurement protocol contain adequate procedures to prevent poisoning of the calcium electrode by milk proteins and other components. In the automatic instrument used by Allen and Neville (The Radiometer I-Cal), this was accomplished by the presence of a dialysis membrane between the electrode and the solution, and an automatic wash cycle which removes the milk after brief contact with the electrode system. Standards of appropriate ionic strength must be used and suitable correction for pH is necessary. These conditions are difficult to achieve without an automated analyzer which measures pH and ionized calcium simultaneously.

Forms of calcium in human milk

Although the forms of calcium in serum have been studied in detail, similar data for human milk is limited. Casein in milk has, in general, been considered as a major binding protein for calcium (39). However, in studies in Lönnerdal's laboratory, only 6-10% of total calcium was found to be bound to casein in human milk, compared to 41% in cow's milk (40). Calcium in human milk fat can be studied by separation of the lipids using flotation. In Lönnerdal's experience, ultracentrifugation produces a fat fraction considerably less contaminated by whey proteins than that produced by centrifugation at a lower speed. His group found that 10% of total human milk calcium is bound to the lipid fraction.

Table 2. Calcium, Magnesium and Phosphorus Contents of Milks from Mothers of Term Infants at One Month Lactation*

Reference	Duration of lactation	N	Ca	Mg	P
Butte et al. 1984 (16)	4 wks	13	6.4(1.3)[a]	1.2(0.2)[a]	5.3(0.8)[e]
Hibberd et al. 1982 (14)	29 da	8	4.3(1.2)[i]	1.3(0.4)[b]	--
Atkinson et al. 1980 (17)	27-29 da	7	6.8(1.0)[a]	1.3(0.2)[a]	4.4(0.3)[e]
Gross et al. 1980 (18)	28 da	7	6.2(1.2)[a]	1.0(0.2)[a]	5.1(1.1)[e]
Lemons et al. 1982 (19)	28 da	7	6.6(0.9)[c]	1.1(0.2)[i]	4.5(0.9)[f]
Feeley et al. 1983 (26)	30-45 da	159	6.6(1.6)[d]	1.9(0.5)[d]	4.3(1.2)[d]
Vaughn et al. 1979 (27)	1-3 mo	28	6.4(0.4)[a]	1.2(0.4)[a]	--
Picciano et al. 1981 (24)	1 mo	26	7.2(1.5)[b]	1.2(0.3)[b]	5.0(0.8)[e]
Barltrop & Hillier 1979 (28)	6 wks	12	6.9(1.4)[a]	--	5.2(1.0)[e]
Rajalakshmi et al. 1980 (29)	1-3 mo	77	--	1.2(0.3)[i]	--
Kirksey et al. 1979 (30)	1-3 mo	6	4.7(0.8)[i]	1.2(0.2)[i]	--
Dewey & Lönnerdal 1983 (15)	1 mo	13	6.5(1.2)[b]	1.1(0.2)[b]	--
Greer et al. 1982 (31)	3 wks	18	6.5(1.0)[f]	1.1(0.4)[f]	4.8(0.8)[e]
Winikoff, 1944 (32)	1 mo	48	7.2(1.1)[h]	--	5.2(0.7)[e]
Schanler & Oh, 1980 (20)	22-28 da	6	7.1(1.3)[i]	--	--
Neville & Keller +1984	28 da	12	7.3(1.2)[c]	1.4(0.2)[c]	1.9(0.4)[g]

* All values in mM
\+ Unpublished

Methods

a. Dry ashing plus atomic absorption spectrometry
b. Wet ashing plus atomic absorption spectrometry
c. Colorimetric assay on fat-free milk samples
d. Dry ashing plus emission spectrometry
e. Ashing with colorimetric analysis
f. Automatic analyzer, ashing not specified
g. Colorimetric analysis of inorganic phosphate on fat-free milks
h. Dry ashing with chemical analysis
i. Dilution plus atomic absorption spectrometry

Within this fraction, they separated a putative outer milk fat globule membrane (MFGM) from an inner MFGM and the core lipid material (triglycerides). Using a stepwise solubilization procedure based on addition of detergent (sodium dodecyl sulfate, SDS), the majority of calcium was found in the outer membrane (67±12%). The inner membrane (25±15%) and the triglyceride fraction (8±12%) contained smaller amounts (38). Caution must be used in interpreting these findings because SDS may cause redistribution of calcium.

The distribution of calcium within human whey has been studied by gel filtration and ultrafiltration (7, 37) and with a calcium-sensitive electrode (8). A small but significant amount of calcium was found to be bound to α-lactalbumin in milk (41, 42). The molar ratio of calcium to α-lactalbumin was found to be 1:1, regardless of the duration of lactation or the calcium concentration. The remainder of the calcium ligands were predominantly of low molecular weight. Allen and Neville (8) have analyzed ionized calcium in human milk, taking necessary precautions to avoid changes caused by loss of CO_2 from the samples. Under optimum conditions, 2.8 mmol of ionized calcium per liter was found in early lactation. Their value for total calcium concentration in human milk was 7.2 mmol/L (1), i.e., 39% of total calcium would be in ionized form. About one-half of the total calcium would be expected to be associated with low molecular weight ligands, such as citrate and phosphate (8). Computer modeling using literature-binding constants predicts that one-third of the total calcium is associated with citrate (Allen and Neville, unpublished).

Magnesium

Like calcium, the magnesium content of human milk samples is usually assayed on ashed samples using atomic absorption spectrophotometry (Table 2). The values obtained by these techniques at one month of lactation vary from 1.0 to 1.9 mM. An automated colorimetric procedure, based on the reaction of magnesium ions with calmagnite (43), has been found by Neville and Keller to give similar values to atomic absorption on fat-free milk (Fig. 2). The intra-assay coefficient of variation was 3.5%. Franson and Lönnerdal (7,37,38), as well as Neville and Keller (unpublished), have found that only 1.5 to 2% of the total magnesium in human milk is associated with the lipid fraction. For this reason the colorimetric procedure, which is available in clinical laboratories and can be used on untreated, defatted samples, would seem to offer a satisfactory alternative to atomic absorption.

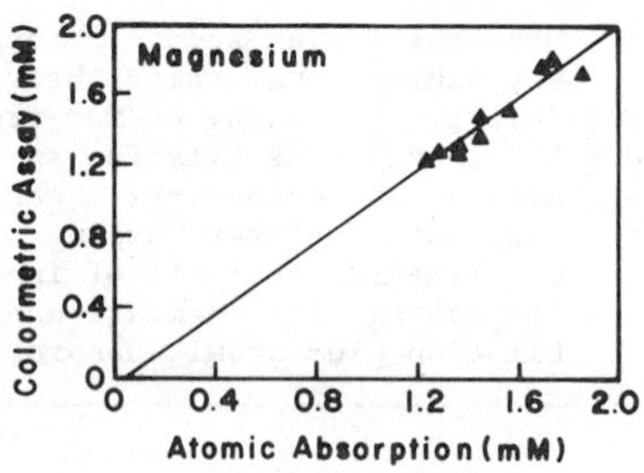

Fig. 2 Comparison of colorimetric and atomic absorption methods for determination of magnesium in human milk (Neville and Keller, unpublished). The constants for the regression lines are: slope, 1.02; intercept, -.05; r, 0.90; $S_{y.x}$, 0.7.

Phosphate

Phosphate is always measured with a variation (44-45) of the Fiske--Subbarow reaction (46), which involves interaction with molybdate in an acid medium to form a blue phosphomolybdate complex. This is measured colorimetrically or spectrophotometrically. As mentioned above, total phosphate must be measured on ashed samples, whereas free phosphate can be measured on fat-free samples. Literature values for total phosphate at one month of lactation vary from 4.3 to 5.3 mM, with about 40% consisting of free phosphate (47).

CONCLUSION

Although macrominerals and electrolytes should be among the easiest milk constituents to measure, a rigorous methodological evaluation does not exist for any of the milk constituents discussed here. In particular, there is a need for critical evaluation of rapid automated assays. Such techniques will be more readily available to investigators in a clinical setting than the traditional methods using ashing with flame or atomic absorption spectrophotometry.

SUMMARY

The current status of methodologies for the determination of calcium, phosphate, magnesium, sodium, potassium and chloride in human milk is reviewed. Within-feed and diurnal variation are minor considerations in developing a sampling regimen for these constituents. For ionized calcium, anaerobic sample handling is necessary. Classical sample preparation involved wet or dry ashing of samples; more recently, many investigators have used simple dilution in various solvents for analysis of sodium, potassium, chloride, calcium and magnesium. No systematic investigation of the relative merits of these techniques has yet appeared. Both flame photometry and ion-selective electrode techniques appear to be satisfactory for sodium and potassium. The standard method for chloride assay is potentiometric titration with silver ions; a colorimetric procedure is available which gives similar accuracy. Atomic absorption spectroscopy is the most commonly used method for calcium and magnesium. Automated colorimetric assays give similar results for fat-free milk. Because the amount of calcium associated with lipid may be as high as 10%, the colorimetric assay for calcium is adequate for whole milk. Total phosphorus must be assayed on ashed samples to release protein-bound phosphate. There is a need for critical evaluation of rapid automated methods for analysis of these milk constituents.

REFERENCES

1. Neville MC, Keller RP, Seacat J, Casey CE, Allen JE, ARcher P. (1984): Studies on human lactation. 1. Within-feed and between breast variation in selected components of human milk. Am J Clin Nutr, 40, 635-646.

2. Neville MC, Archer P, Keller R, Casey C, Hambidge M. (1985): Diurnal variation in human milk volume and composition. Fed Proc, 44, 1675.

3. Keenan BS, Buzek SW, Garza C. (1983): Cortisol and its possible role in regulation of sodium and potassium in human milk. Am J Physiol, 244, 253-261.

4. Gross SJ, Gelb MS, Tomarelli RM. (1981): Composition of breast milk from mothers of preterm infants. Pediatrics, 68, 490-493.

5. Peaker M. (1983): Secretion of ions and water. In: Mepham TB, ed, Biochemistry of Lactation. Amsterdam, New York: Elsevier.

6. Hartmann PE, Kulski JK. (1978): Changes in the composition of the mammary secretion of women after abrupt termination of breast-feeding. J Physiol, 275, 1-11.

7. Fransson G-B, Lönnerdal B. (1983): Effect of freezing on trace element distribution in human and cow's milk. Nutr Res, 3, 845-853.

8. Allen JC, Neville MC. (1983): Ionized calcium in human milk determined with a calcium-selective electrode. Clin Chem, 29, 858-861.

9. Clegg MS, Keen CL, Lönnerdal B, Hurley LS. (1981): Influence of ashing techniques on the analysis of trace elements in biological samples. II. Dry ashing. Biol Trace Element Res, 3, 237-243.

10. Clegg MS, Keen CL, Lönnerdal B, Hurley LS. (1981): Influence of ashing techniques on the analysis of trace elements in animal tissue. I. Wet ashing. Biol Trace Element Res, 3, 107-115.

11. Lönnerdal B, Smith C, Keen CL. (1984): Analysis of breast milk - current methodologies and future needs. J Pediatr Gastroent Nutr, 3, 290-295.

12. Cotlove E. (1964): Determination of chloride in biological materials. Meth Biochem Anal, 12, 277-391.

13. Peitersen B, Bohn L, Andersen H. (1975): Quantitative determination of immunoglobulins, lysozyme, and certain electrolytes in breast milk during the entire period of lactation, during a 24-hour period, and in milk from the individual mammary gland. Acta Paediatr Scand, 64, 709-717.

14. Hibberd C, Brooke O, Carter N, Haug M, Harzer G. (1982): Variation in the composition of breast milk during the first 5 weeks of lactation: implications for the feeding of preterm infants. Arch Dis Child, 57, 658-662.

15. Dewey KG, Lönnerdal B. (1983): Milk and nutrient intake of breast-fed infants from 1 to 6 months: relation to growth and fatness. J Ped Gastroent Nutr, 497-506.

16. Butte N, Garza C, Johnson C, Smith E, Nichols B. (1984): Longitudinal changes in milk composition of mothers delivering preterm and term infants. Early Human Development, 9, 153-162.

17. Atkinson S, Radde I, Chance G, Bryan M, Anderson G. (1980): Macro-mineral content of milk obtained during early lactation from mothers of premature infants. Early Human Development, 41, 5-14.

18. Gross S, David R, Bauman L, Tomarelli R. (1980): Nutritional composition of milk produced by mothers delivering preterm. J Peds, 96, 641-644.

19. Lemons J, Moye L, Hall D, Simmons M. (1982): Differences in the composition of preterm and term human milk during early lactation. Pediatr Res, 16, 113-117.

20. Schanler RJ, Oh W. (1980): Composition of breast milk from mothers of premature infants as compared to breast milk obtained from donors. J Ped, 96, 679-681.

21. Linzell JL, Peaker M. (1974): Changes in colostrum composition and in the permeability of the mammary epithelium at about the time of parturition in the goat. J Physiol (Lond), 243, 129.

22. Sherwin SA, Bruegger BB, Belizle T, Flores O. (1982): A field evaluation of the Beckman system E4 (SE4) electrolyte analyzer. Clin Chem, 28, 1630-1631.

23. Proda L, Simon W. (1970): Determination of potassium concentration of serum using a highly selective liquid membrane electrode. Clin Chem Acta, 29, 289-293.

24. Picciano MF, Calkins E, Garrick J, Deering R. (1981): Milk and mineral intakes of breastfed infants. Acta Paediatr Scand, 70, 189-194.

25. Schoenfield RG, Lewellen C. (1964): A colorimetric method for determination of serum chloride. Clin Chem, 10, 533-539.

26. Feeley R, Eitenmiller R, Jones J, Jr, Barnhart H. (1983): Calcium, phosphorus, and magnesium contents of human milk during early lactation. J Ped Gastroenterology and Nutr, 2, 262-267.

27. Vaughan L, Weber C, Kemberling S. (1979): Longitudinal changes in the mineral content of human milk. Am J Clin Nutr, 32, 2301-2306.

28. Barltrop D, Hillier R. (1974): Calcium and phosphorus content of transitional and mature human milk. Acta Paediatr Scand, 63, 347-350.

29. Rajalakshmi K, Srikantia S. (1980): Copper, zinc, and magnesium content of breast milk of Indian women. Am J Clin Nutr, 33, 664-669.

30. Kirksey A, Ernst J, Roepke J, Tsai T. (1979): Influence of mineral intake and use of oral contraceptives before pregnancy on the mineral content of human colostrum and of more mature milk. Am J Clin Nutr, 32, 30-39.

31. Greer FR, Tsang RC, Levin RS, Searcy JE, Wu R, Steichen JJ. (1982): Increasing serum calcium and magnesium concentrations in breast--fed infants: longitudinal studies of minerals in human milk and in sera of nursing mothers and their infants. J Peds, 100, 59-64.

32. Winikoff D. (1944): Calcium magnesium and phosphorus in the milk of Australian women. Med J Australia, 2, 660-665.

33. Connerly H, Briggs A. (1966): Determination of serum calcium by means of orthocresolphthalein complexes. Am J Clin Pathol, 45, 290-296.

34. Gitelman H. (1967): An improved automated procedure for the determination of calcium in biological specimens. Anal Biochem, 20, 521-523.

35. Sarker B, Chauham V. (1967): A new method for determination of microquantities of calcium in biological materials. Anal Biochem, 20, 155-166.

36. Lönnerdal B, Forsum E. (1985): Casein content of human milk. Am J Clin Nutr, 41, 113-120.

37. Fransson G-B, Lönnerdal B. (1982): Zinc, copper, calcium and magnesium in human milk. J Peds, 101, 504-508.

38. Fransson G-B, Lönnerdal B. (1984): Iron, copper, zinc, calcium and magnesium in human milk fat. Am J Clin Nutr, 39, 185-189.

39. Jenness R. (1979): Comparative aspects of milk proteins. J Dairy Res, 46, 197-210.

40. Fransson G-B, Lönnerdal B. (1983): Distribution of trace elements and minerals in human and cow's milk. Pediatr Res, 17, 912-915.

41. Lönnerdal B, Glazier C. (1983): Calcium binding by human milk α-lactalbumin. Fed Proc, 42, 2266.

42. Murakami K, Andree PJ, Berliner LJ. (1982): Metal ion binding to α-lactalbumin species. Biochemistry, 21, 929-931.

43. Teers RJ, Barnes BA, Butsakis JG, Block DM. (1977): Serum magnesium. A CAP survey-1975. Am J Clin Pathol, 68, 159-161.

44. Daly TA, Eitinghausen G. (1972): Direct method for determining inorganic phosphate in serum with the "centrifichem." Clin Chem, 18, 263-265.

45. Amador E, Urban F. (1972): Simplified serum phosphate analysis by continuous-flow ultraviolet spectrophotometry. Clin Chem, 18, 601-604.

46. Fiske CH, SubbaRow Y. (1925): The colorimetric determination of phosphorus. J Biol Chem, 66, 375-400.

47. Burhaus CW, Smith DN. (1923): The inorganic constituents of human milk with particular reference to racial variations. Am J Dis Child, 26, 303-308.

VIII. MEASUREMENT OF VITAMINS IN HUMAN MILK

WORKSHOP PARTICIPANTS:

M .F. Picciano, Department of Food and Nutrition, University of Illinois, Urbana, Illinois

A. Kirksey, Department of Foods and Nutrition, Purdue University, West Lafayette, Indiana

R. R. Eitenmiller, Department of Food Science, University of Georgia, Athens, Georgia

B. W. Hollis, Department of Nutrition, School of Medicine, Case Western Reserve University, Cleveland, Ohio

C. J. Lammi-Keefe, Department of Nutritional Sciences, University of Connecticut, Storrs, Connecticut

P. R. Borum, Department of Food Science and Human Nutrition, University of Florida, Gainesville, Florida.

INTRODUCTION

Vitamins, which are organic substances, present in minute quantities, and essential to normal metabolism, can be classified into two distinct groups: those which are fat-soluble (vitamins A, D, E and K) and those which are water-soluble (vitamin C, thiamin, riboflavin, niacin, vitamin B-6, folacin, vitamin B-12, biotin and pantothenic acid). Beyond solubility characteristics, there are few other similarities in this group of compounds. With the exception of vitamin C, which is present in milligram quantities in human milk, all other vitamins are present in microgram and sub-microgram quantities. Thus, the analysis of vitamins in human milk, requires highly sensitive and specific techniques.

Our knowledge of the vitamin content of human milk and of factors capable of exerting an influence is meager. That available information has not kept pace with advances in analytical techniques is evident from perusal of the reviews that follow. For example, Dr. Hollis points out that in only one recent study has appropriate methodology been applied to the analysis of vitamin K in human milk (1). Results of the study provide values which are three to five times lower than those of previous reports (2,3) and indicate that milk concentration responds to maternal dietary intake of vitamin K. However, there are no data on milk levels associated with neonatal hemorrhagic disease, and there is evidence that vitamin K deficiency is a clinical reality for newborn breast-fed infants (4).

Presently, adequate methodological approaches are available for the quantification of many vitamins in biological samples, including human milk. A manual of analytical procedures, which can also serve as a reference source for new techniques, has recently been published (5). In general, human milk vitamin assays must involve proper sampling, careful handling and storage procedures, suitable extraction processes and a sensitive and selective detection system. Unfortunately, as is too often the case, there has been the "blind" application of methods for determination of human milk vitamin contents. That is, the validity and the accuracy of assays have not been ascertained. At the very least, recovery experiments should be performed, and ideally two separate methods, based on different principals, should be used to assess validity of the assay.

In future studies, proper evaluation of analytical methods for the accurate and reliable determination of vitamins in human milk should receive highest priority. As is evident from the following reviews, an adequate body of knowledge does not exist to serve as the basis for dietary guidelines to insure optimal vitamin nutrition of either the nursing infant or the lactating woman. Thus, there is also an urgent need for the application of appropriate methods for the determination of human milk vitamins under various conditions (nutritional, environmental, physiological, etc.) that are capable of altering their content, form, distribution and bioavailability.

REFERENCES

1. Haroon Y, Shearer MJ, Rahim S, Gunn WG, McEnery G, Barkhan P. (1982): The content of phylloquinone (vitamin K) in human milk, cows' milk and infant formula foods determined by high-performance liquid chromatography. J Nutr, 112, 1105-1117.

2. Dam H, Dyggve H, Larsen H, Plum B. (1952): The relation of vitamin K deficiency to hemorrhagic disease of the newborn. Adv Pediatr, 5, 129-153.

3. Deodhar AD, Rajakakshmi R, Romankrishnan CV. (1964): Studies on human lactation. III. Effect of dietary vitamin supplementation on vitamin content of breast milk. Acta Paediatr Scand, 53, 42-48.

4. O'Connor ME, Livingston SD, Hannah J, Wilkins D. (1983): Vitamin K deficiency and breast-feeding. Am J Dis Child, 137, 601-602.

5. Augustin J, Klein BP, Becker DA, Venugapal PB. (1984): Methods of vitamin assay, 4th ed. New York: John Wiley and Sons.

ANALYSIS OF WATER-SOLUBLE VITAMINS IN HUMAN MILK: FOLACIN AND VITAMIN B-12

M. F. Picciano

FOLACIN CONTENT OF HUMAN MILK

Folacin, derived from the Latin word for leaf, is a generic term for a family of compounds that function as coenzymes for one-carbon transfer reactions. These coenzymes are essential for biosynthesis of protein, DNA, and RNA -- initial events in cellular division and growth. A high dietary folacin requirement of infants is suggested by their rapid rate of growth. That requirement can be satisfied by exclusive human milk feeding. In recent years, the application of improved techniques to the analysis of folacin in human milk has been accomplished. It is now well recognized that methodological constraints led early investigators to seriously underestimate the folacin content of human milk (1).

The analysis of folacin vitamers in natural products is still not wholly satisfactory. Pteroylglutamic acid (or folic acid, the parent compound) consists of a pteridine ring, para-aminobenzoic acid and a glutamic acid residue. A very large number of derivatives of this compound exist in nature. There are six possible one-carbon substitutes, at least two states of reduction, and up to nine glutamyl residues in gamma peptide linkages that may be present (2). This diversity of folate compounds alone poses problems to the analyst. In addition, folate compounds are present in very low concentration in most biological samples and are labile to heat, light, oxygen and changes in pH (3).

Methods of Folacin Analysis

Methodology for the determination of folacin in biological samples is lengthy and often non-specific. Folacin has been analyzed using the following techniques: chromatography (4-8), direct ultraviolet spectroscopy, fluorimetry, polarography, colorimetry -- after oxidation and reaction with the Bratton-Marshall reagent [N-(1-naphthyl) ethylenediamine dihydrochloride] (9), microbiological assay (10-11), and radiometric assay (12). In studies of human milk, the microbiological assay has been the method of choice because it allows measurement of nanogram quantities of folacin in samples. However, this method suffers from a variety of shortcomings, particularly the length of time required to complete the assay, poor reproducibility of separate assays, and the extreme care that must be taken to avoid erroneously low or high values (3). Radiometric assays for folacin that are based on competitive protein binding also possess the desired sensitivity and offer a significant time advantage.

These assays have other potential advantages because they lack sensitivity to antibiotics and other antimetabolites. However, studies employing radiometric assays for folacin in complex biological samples have yielded variable and inconclusive results (13).

Microbiological assays are not specific for the various forms of folate, but their proper application to human milk does provide a reasonably good estimate of the sum total of folates present. For the quantitative determination of any one biochemical form of folacin, high pressure liquid chromatography holds great promise. Its use to date has been limited because of inadequate sample extraction procedures and lack of sufficiently sensitive and specific detection methods (13).

During the collection of samples and during analysis, it is essential to protect labile folates from destruction by light and oxidation. Ascorbate is the usual antioxidant employed, as it is the most effective on a molar basis, but 2-mercaptoethanol and dithiothreitol have also been employed. Chen and Cooper (14) reported that 1 g ascorbate/L is necessary to adequately protect 5-methyltetrahydrofolic acid, and at this concentration only 20% is lost after 3 hours at 100°C. While Herbert (15) cautioned against employing concentrations of ascorbate greater than 1.5 g/L in the final assay medium, Phillips and Wright (16) reported that concentrations as high as 10 g/L do not alter *L. casei* response curves.

Lactobacillus casei (ATCC 7469), *Streptococcus faecalis* (ATCC 8043) and *Pediocaccus cerevisiae* (ATCC 8081) are the test organisms commonly employed for folacin analysis via microbiological assay. They may be purchased in lyophylized forms from American Type Culture Collection, 12301 Parklawn Drive, Rockville, Maryland, 20852. As shown in Table 1, the growth response of *L. casei* is the broadest, and this is the only microorganism that utilizes 5-methyltetrahydrofolic acid, a principal derivative of folacin in both human and cow milk. Folylpolyglutamates having one to three glutamate residues are utilized by *L. casei*, and this organism partially responds to folylpolyglutamates of chain length greater than three (17). *Streptococcus faecalis* does not respond to folylpolyglutamates with greater than two glutamate residues nor to 5-methyltetrahydrofolic acid. The folacin requirement of *P. cerevisiae* is the most specialized. This organism only responds to reduced monoglutamates except 5-methylated hydrofolic acid. The application of all three microorganisms is useful in the differentiation of the various folate compounds in human milk, thus providing information on the relative proportions of reduced, methylated and non-methylated forms (11).

Most naturally occurring folates exist as folylpolyglutamates. To determine total folacin concentration microbiologically, samples must first be treated with a proteolytic enzyme (gamma-glutamyl-carboxypeptidase or conjugase) to convert the folates to forms that can be used by the test organism. The commonly employed sources of the enzyme are hog kidney and chicken pancreas. Desiccated chicken pancreas is supplied by Difco Laboratories (Detroit, MI) and desiccated hog kidney by Sigma Chemical Company (St. Louis, MO). A diglutamate end product is produced when a sample is treated with the chicken pancreas enzyme, which has a pH optimum of 7.8. Hog kidney conjugase has a pH optimum of 4.5 and yields a monoglutamate end product. Both sources of the enzyme can contain considerable quantities of endogenous folacin, and further purification is recommended (18,19). Since folacin is less stable in acid media, the reaction with hog kidney conjugase is carried out at pH 6.0, where satisfactory recovery has been reported (20). If chicken pancreas conjugase is used, a pH of 7.2 for the reaction medium is recommended (21).

Table 1. Response of *Lactobacillus casei, Streptococcus faecalis* and *Pediococcus cerevisiae* to different monoglutomate forms of folacin *

Form	*L. casei*	*S. faecalis*	*P. cerevisiae*
Folic Acid	+	+	-
Dihydrofolic Acid	+	+	-
Tetrahydrofolic Acid	+	+	+
5-formyltetrahydrofolic Acid	+	+	+
10-formylfolic Acid	+	+	-
10-formyldihydrofolic Acid	+	+	-
5-methyltetrahydrofolic Acid	+	-	-

*Adapted from Blakely RL. The biochemistry of folic acid and related pteridines. New York, NY: American Elsevier Publishing Company, 1969.

L. casei is the only organism suitable for the assay of total folacin content in human milk. Unfortunately, a standard *L. casei* assay does not exist. At each stage of the assay, the possibility of introducing error exists. In general, the assay involves the following: liberation of folacin from its binding proteins, cleavage of folylpolyglutamates, dilution with nutrient medium, sterilization, inoculation, and estimation of *L. casei* growth -- usually turbidimetrically. The use of an internal standard during each stage of the assay is advised. Complete recovery of the internal standard does not assure absolute validity of the assay, since folacin exists in many structural forms in biological samples. However, its use will alert the analyst to conditions of assay which are destructive to the labile folates or to the presence of inhibitors.

In practice, multiple dilutions of sample extracts are assayed. The measured response of the organism to serial dilutions of sample extracts should parallel similar dilutions of the standard solution. Often, a steeper slope is observed for the test materials than for the standard. This phenomenon is described as "positive drift." Possible reasons for the positive drift, proposed by several investigators, include: (a) growth enhancers in sample extracts affecting initial growth rate of bacteria, (b) variable numbers of organisms in the inocula (22), (c) unequal amounts of constituents required for growth of bacteria in final assay tubes (23), (d) incomplete cleavage of folylpolyglutamates (17), and (e) differential response of the organism to different mono- and diglutamate forms (16). The following techniques may be useful in overcoming these difficulties: increasing the incubation time until growth has stopped due to exhaustion of available folate, standardizing the addition of inocula with automatic pipetting devices, providing an excess of constituents required for growth in media, and determining optimal conjugase concentration and incubation time for test materials.

The differential response of *L. casei* to various mono- and diglutamates is the greatest problem. However, recent studies of Phillips and Wright (16) suggest that this problem can be overcome by decreasing the pH of the assay to 6.2, and by increasing the buffering capacity of the medium. At pH 6.2, these authors report equal response of *L. casei* to folic acid, 5-formyltetrahydrofolic acid and 5-methyltetrahydrofolic acid. At pH above 6.2, the response of *L. casei* to 5-methyltertahydrofolic acid was concentration dependent. These authors observed that at the high end of the standard range (0-1.0 ng), the growth response of *L. casei* to 5-methyltetrahydrofolic acid is great enough to produce sufficient lactic acid to cause a drop in the initial pH so that absolute growth after 18-22 hours of incubation is little different from that in folic acid. At the intermediate and low end, observed responses of *L. casei* to 5-methyltetrahydrofolic acid are 70 and 40% of that to folic acid, respectively. Since application of the *L. casei* assay at pH 6.2 has been limited, even the most recent data on the folacin content of human milk likely underestimates the actual quantities present. A detailed description of the principles and procedures of the *L. casei* assays is available (24).

Folacin in Human Milk

It is likely that methodological difficulties are responsible for the wide range of mean values reported for the concentration of folacin in human milk from well nourished women. Complete descriptions of analytical schemes and conditions of sampling and storage are not always furnished by investigators. However, a number of generalizations can be made. Folacin in human milk is present at considerably greater concentrations than reported by early investigators (1). Recent reports provide a range of mean values from 26 to 141 ug folacin /L milk (25-31). Most, but not all, investigators report approximately half of human milk folacin to be present as folylpolyglutamates (25-27,29,31). The application of differential microbiological assays to the study of human milk folacin indicates that folylpolyglutamates of three and greater glutamic acid residues and 5-methyltetrahydrofolic acid are the predominant forms in human milk (32). A positive relationship ($r = 0.71$) exists between the concentration of folate-binding proteins and milk folacin concentration (33). This quantitative relationship is unique to milk. In other tissues, the folate-binding capacity comprises a small fraction of total folate content.

Only in a severe deficiency does maternal folacin status bear a relationship to milk content. There is evidence for an increased dietary folacin requirement during lactation in both animals and humans (34,35). Additionally, lactation alone is reported to produce maternal folacin deficiency (36). When dietary inadequacy is severe enough to cause maternal megaloblastic anemia and a decline in milk folacin activity, supplemental folacin is utilized by the mammary gland in preference to hemopoietic tissues (34). However, when maternal blood folacin concentrations are within the acceptable range, oral administration of folacin will cause elevations in blood concentrations, but not in milk content (26,27,29).

Sampling techniques do influence the measurement of human milk folacin. Results from longitudinal studies indicate that human milk folacin activity increases as lactation advances (26,27,29). Ek (30) noted that during weaning, the concentration of milk folacin declines. The measurement of human milk folacin activity may also be influenced by the stage of lactation and the time of sample procurement during the day or within a feeding. Smith et al. (29) observed higher folacin activity in hindmilk compared to foremilk samples and in milk samples collected in the evening compared to those collected earlier in the day.

Further research is indicated to elucidate the role of the many forms of folacin in human milk. A functional relationship between the folacin pattern of human milk and human milk folate-binding proteins may exist. A search for folate polyglutatmate synthetase in the mammary gland may prove worthwhile in defining the mechanism by which folylpolyglutamates appear in human milk. It is important that future investigators employ the improved techniques for the analysis of folacin and pay due attention to sampling and handling procedures in order to provide results which reflect the actual levels of folacin and the many folate derivatives in human milk.

VITAMIN B-12 CONTENT OF HUMAN MILK

Vitamin B-12 is a collective term for a group of compounds commonly referred to as cobalamin. The major portions of the vitamin B-12 molecule are the corrin nucleus (containing cobalt) and the base (5-6 dimethylbenzimidazole) which is linked to the nucleus via D-1-amino-2-propanol. The parent compound is cyanocobalamin. Other cobalamins are hydroxycobalamin, aquocobalamin, nitritocabalamin, 5-deoxyadenosylcobalamin and methylcobalamin in which the designated moieties substitute for the cyanide group. The latter two forms of cobalamins are known to be coenzymatically active in humans (37). Vitamin B-12 is required for normal hemopoiesis and neurological integrity.

In the recent literature, there are a number of reports of vitamin B-12 deficiency in human-milk-fed infants of vegan or malnourished mothers (38,39). These reports suggest that vitamin B-12 in human milk is seriously diminished when the lactating woman is deficient in this vitamin. However, because of limitations in methodology, there is scant information on the vitamin B-12 content of human milk from well-nourished women, and the possible factors exerting an influence. Sandberg and associates (40) carefully evaluated extraction procedures prior to their analyses (by *Euglena gracilis*) of vitamin B-12 activity in human milk. They reported that human milk contains two cobalamin binders, the R type or cobalophilin and transcobalamin II. The R type was found to be dominant and in considerable excess of the vitamin. These authors also provide convincing evidence for the need to release cobalamin from, and to destroy the R binder prior to, assay. Failure to do so will yield falsely low results via bioassay (41,42) or radioisotope dilution procedure (43). Their analyses of 19 mature human-milk samples provided a mean value of 0.97 ug cobalamin per liter of milk (range: 0.33 to 3.2 ug/L). The milk of ten mothers receiving 5 to 100 ug of supplemental cyanocobalomin was similar in vitamin B-12 content to milk from unsupplemented mothers. Chromatographic analyses of pooled samples from both groups of mothers revealed that methylcobalamin was the principal form of native cobalamin in human milk with 5-deoxyadenosylcobalamin the next most abundant form. Small amounts of hydroxycobalamin and cyanocobalamin were likewise noted.

There is some indication that vitamin B-12 is high in colostrum (41). However, since proteolytic digestion was not employed in this study, the apparent elevation may only indicate that the vitamin is more easily extracted from colostrum than from milk. Sandberg et al. (40) noted that transcobalamin II was highest in milk from mothers in late lactation (7-15 months) and that observed concentrations in these milk samples exceeded those common to sera.

There is an urgent need for the application of improved assay techniques to the study of human milk vitamin B-12 content. Milk concentrations associated with development of deficiency in breast-fed infants are not known with any degree of certainty. The functional significance of the high concentration of R-type binder in human milk is likewise unknown. This protein in gastric juice has been implicated in the development of vitamin B-12 deficiency (44).

ACKNOWLEDGEMENT

This work was supported in part by USDA/SEA grant #5901-0410-9-0306 and the Illinois Agricultural Experiment Station.

REFERENCES

1. Macy IG. (1949): Composition of human colostrum and milk. Am J Dis Child, 78, 589-603.

2. Kisliuk RL. (1981): Pteroylpolyglutamates. Mol and Cell Biochem, 39, 331-345.

3. Baugh CN, Krumdiek CL. (1971): Naturally occurring folates. Ann NY Acad Sci, 186, 7-28.

4. Scott JM. (1980): Thin-layer chromatography of pteroylmonoglutamates and related compounds. In: McCormick DB, Wright LD, eds, Methods in enzymology. New York, NY: Academic Press, 437-443.

5. Reif VD, Reamer JT, Grady LT. (1977): Chromatographic assays for folic acid. J Pharm Sci, 66, 1112-1116.

6. Reed LS, Archer MC. (1976): Separation of folic acid derivatives by high-performance liquid chromatograph. J Chromatogr, 121, 100-103.

7. Reingold RN, Picciano MF, Perkins EG. (1980): Separation of folate derivatives by *in situ* paired-ion high-pressure liquid chromatography. J. Chromatogr, 190, 237-240.

8. Day BP, Gregory JF. (1981): Determination of folacin derivatives in selected foods by high-performance liquid chromatography. J Agr Food Chem, 29, 374-377.

9. Hashmi M (1973): Assay of vitamins in pharmaceutical preparations. New York, NY: Wiley-Interscience.

10. Scott JM, Ghanta V, Herbert V. (1974): Trouble free microbiologic serum and red cell folate assays. Am J Med Technol, 40, 125-134.

11. Bird OD, McGlohon VM. (1972): Differential assays of folic acid in animal tissues. In: Kavanagh F, ed, Analytical microbiology, Vol. 2. New York, NY: Academic Press, 409-437.

12. Waxman S, Schreiber C. (1980): Determination of folate by use of radioactive folate and binding proteins. In: McCormick DB, Wright LD, eds, Methods in enzymology. New York, NY: Academic Press, 468-483.

13. Gregory JF. (1985): Folacin: Chromatographic and radiometric assays. In: Augustin J, Klein B, Becker D, Venugopal B, eds, Methods of vitamin assay, 4th ed. New York, NY: John Wiley and Sons, 473-496.

14. Chen TS, Cooper RG. (1979): Thermal destruction of folacin: effect of ascorbic acid, oxygen, and temperature. J Food Sci, 44, 713-716.

15. Herbert V, Fisher B, Koontz BJ. (1961): The assay and nature of folic acid activity in human serum. J Clin Investigation, 40, 81-91.

16. Phillips DR, Wright AJA. (1982): Studies on the response of *Lactobacillus casei* to different folate monoglutamates. Brit J Nutr, 47, 183-189.

17. Tamura T, Shin YS, Williams MA, Stokstad ELR. (1972): *Lactobacillus casei* response to pteroylpolyglutamates. Anal Biochem, 49, 517-521.

18. Iwai K, Luttner PM, Townnies G. (1964): Blood folic acid studies. VII. Purification and properties of folic acid precursors of human erythrocytes. J Biol Chem, 239, 2365-2369.

19. Tamura T, Romero JJ, Watson JE, Gong EJ, Halsted CH. (1981): Hepatic folate metabolism in the chronic alcoholic monkey. J Lab Clin Med 97, 654-661.

20. McMartin KE, Vivayotha V, Tephyl TR. (1981): High-pressure liquid chromatography separation and determination of rat liver folates. Arch Biochem Biophys, 209, 127-136.

21. Eigen E, Shockman GD. (1963): The folic acid group. In: Kavanagh F. ed., Analytical microbiology. New York, NY: Academic Press, 431-488.

22. Streter AM, O'Neill BJ. (1969): Effect of incubation time on the *L. casei* bioassay of folic acid in serum. Blood, 34, 216-221.

23. Temperley IJ, Horner N. (1966): Effect of ascorbic acid on the serum folic acid estimation. J Clin Pathology, 19, 43-45.

24. Keagy PM. (1985): Folacin: Microbiological and animal assays. In: Augustin J, Klein B, Becker D. Venugopal B, eds, Methods of vitamin assay, 4th ed. New York, NY: John Wiley and Sons, 445-472.

25. Areekful S, Vongyuthitham M, Yamarat P, Sunthornthom S. (1978): Folic acid and folic acid binding proteins in milk. J Med Assoc Thailand, 61, 81-86.

26. Tamura T, Yoshimura Y, Arakawa T. (1980); Human milk folate and folate status in lactating mothers and their infants. Am J Clin Nutr, 33, 193-197.

27. Butte NF, Calloway DH. (1981): Evaluation of nutritional performance of Navaho women. Am J Clin Nutr, 34, 2210-2215.

28. Cooperman JM, Dweck HS, Newman LJ, Garbarino C, Lopez R. (1982): The folate in human milk. Am J Clin Nutr, 36, 576-580.

29. Smith AM, Picciano MF, Deering RH. (1983): Folate supplementation during lactation. Maternal folate status, human milk folate content, and their relationship to infant folate status. J Pediatr Gastroenterology Nutr, 2, 622-628.

30. Ek J. (1983): Plasma, red cell, and breast milk folacin concentrations in lactating women. Am J Clin Nutr, 38, 929-935.

31. Eitenmiller RR, Bryan WD, Khalsa IK, Feeley RM, Barnhart HM. (1984): Folate content of human milk during early lactational stages. Nutr Res, 4, 391-397.

32. Brown CM, Smith AM, Picciano MF. (1984): Forms of human milk folacin and variation pattern. Fed Proc, 43, 491.

33. Selhub J. Arnold R, Smith AM, Picciano MF. (1984): Milk folate binding protein (FBP): a secretory protein for folate? Nutr Res, 4, 181-187.

34. Metz J. (1970): Folate deficiency conditioned by lactation. Am J Clin Nutr, 23, 843-847.

35. Nelson MM, Evans HM. (1946): The beneficial effects of synthetic pteroylglutamine acid on lactation. Arch Biochem, 13, 265-275.

36. Nelson MM, Evans HM. (1948): The effect of succinylsulphathiazole on pteroylglutamine deficiency during lactation in the rat. Arch Biochem, 18, 153-159.

37. Herbert V. (1984): Vitamin B-12. In: Present knowledge in nutrition, 5th ed. Washington, DC: The Nutritional Foundation, Inc., 347-364.

38. Higginbottom MC, Sweetman L, Nyhan WL. (1978): A syndrome of methylmalonic aciduria, homocystinuria, megaloblastic anemia and neurologic abnormalities in a vitamin B-12 deficient breast-fed infant of a strict vegetarian. N Engl J Med, 299, 317-323.

39. Srikantia SG, Reddy V. (1967): Megaloblastic anemia of infancy and vitamin B-12. Br J Haemat, 13, 949-953.

40. Sandberg DP, Begley JA, Hall CA. (1981): The content, binding and forms of vitamin B-12 in milk. Am J Clin Nutr, 34, 1717-1724.

41. Samson RR, McClelland DBL. (1980): Vitamin B-12 in human colostrum and milk. Acta Pediatr Scand, 69, 93-99.

42. Department of Health and Social Security. (1977): The composition of mature human milk. London: Her Majesty's Stationery Office.

43. Thomas MR, Kawamoto J, Sneed SM, Eakin R. (1979): The effects of vitamin C, vitamin B-6 and vitamin B-12 supplementation on the breast milk and maternal status of well nourished women. Am J Clin Nutr, 32, 1679-1685.

44. Herzlich G, Drivas G, Herbert V. (1982): Abnormal binder with high specificity for cobalamin at pH 8 in gastric juice of patients with pernicious anemia: production by pancreatic enzymes. Clin Res, 30, 283.

ANALYSIS OF WATER-SOLUBLE VITAMINS IN HUMAN MILK: VITAMIN B-6 AND VITAMIN C

A. Kirksey
S.A. Udipi

INTRODUCTION

Vitamin B-6 and vitamin C are water-soluble, light-sensitive vitamins which exist in human milk in more than one biologically active form. The vitamins differ substantially in their physical and chemical properties and show distinct differences in their concentrations in milk in response to different levels of vitamin intake. Vitamin B-6 appears to pass readily into milk without any apparent regulation of its concentration, in contrast to vitamin C, which reaches saturation in the milk of well-nourished women. Factors such as length of gestation and stage of lactation also affect vitamin B-6 and vitamin C composition of human milk in different ways. The concentration of vitamin B-6 has been observed to be low, whereas the concentration of vitamin C is high in milk from women who deliver prematurely, compared to values for women who deliver at term.

Reasonable uniformity should be maintained in the conditions under which milk samples are obtained for vitamin analyses. These include the degree and method of extraction of milk from the breast and the interval between collection of the sample and the previous feed. Furthermore, if the nutritional needs of infants are to be based on the composition of milk from well-nourished mothers, an attempt should be made to assess whether the mother is in fact well-nourished. This paper will focus both on methodology and on the factors which may influence the concentrations of vitamin B-6 and vitamin C in human milk. The vitamins will be discussed separately.

VITAMIN B-6

Vitamin B-6 is the recommended generic descriptor for all 3-hydroxy-2-methylpyridine derivatives: pyridoxine (PN), pyridoxal (PL), pyridoxamine (PM), and their phosphorylated derivatives -- pyridoxal phosphate (PLP) and pyridoxamine phosphate (PMP). These forms are interconvertible *in vivo* (1). These vitamers occur in foods in the free form or bound to protein, carbohydrate or other non-protein compounds. The interaction between B-6 vitamers and proteins or amino acids and the factors affecting the bioavailability of vitamin B-6 from foods, including the effects of processing and storage, were reviewed recently by Gregory and Kirk (2). Differences in bioavailability of the B-6 vitamers have not been demonstrated conclusively; therefore, total vitamin B-6 content of foods, including human milk, is commonly used in evaluating nutritional quality.

Sampling and Storage of Milk

The percent distribution of the five B-6 vitamers found in human milk is shown in Table 1. The vitamers are stable to heat, acid, alkali and light with the exception of the aldehyde forms (PL, PLP), which are unstable to light, especially in neutral and alkaline media (3). Approximately 90% of the B-6 vitamers in milk are present as PL and PLP (Table 1); therefore, light sensitivity is an important consideration in both the handling and storage of milk samples prior to analysis for vitamin B-6. Milk samples for vitamin B-6 analysis should be collected and stored frozen (-20°C) in amber-colored or light-protected vials. Subdued light or yellow light (incandescent or fluorescent) should be used in the laboratory where milk is prepared for storage or analysis of vitamin B-6 (4). Long-term stability of total vitamin B-6 in frozen human milk has been observed in our laboratory (unpublished data). No significant changes were observed in total vitamin B-6 content of human-milk samples which were protected from light and stored at -30°C for more than two years.

Previous work from this laboratory (5) showed that vitamin B-6 content was not significantly different in fore or hind milk or in milk collected from the right or left breast. Also, diurnal variation in vitamin B-6 content of milk was minimal for women who did not take vitamin B-6 supplements. Consequently, the time of collection of milk samples from unsupplemented women does not appear to be an important variable. The

Table 1. Percent distribution of B-6 vitamers in human milk.

Vitamer	RPLC N=80	Ion-exchange HPLC 1 N=2	Ion-exchange HPLC 2 N=12
	% total vitamin B-6		
PL	82.8	81.4	76.8
PLP	6.2	12.5	23.2
PM	5.2	0.6	ND
PMP	1.4	1.9	ND
PN	4.4	3.6	Trace

[1]Coburn, Mahuren (7)

[2]Vanderslice et al. (8)

ND = not detected

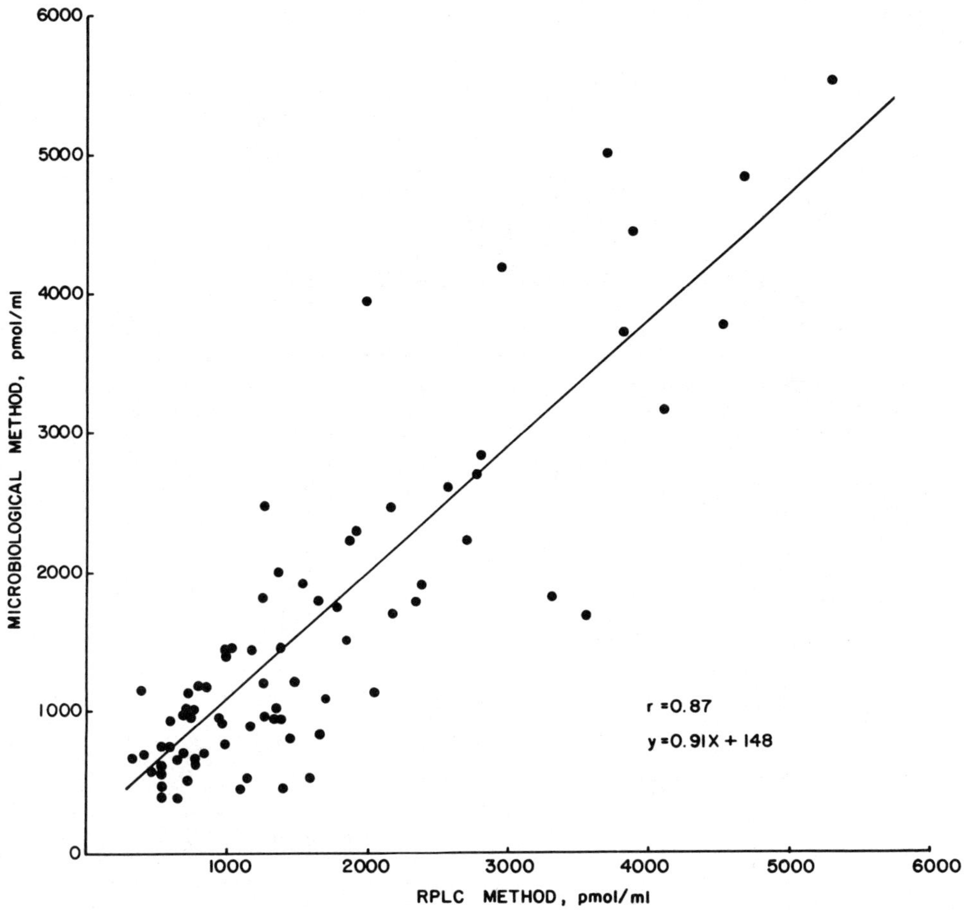

Figure 1. Total B-6 concentration in human milk samples analyzed by RPLC and microbiological (*S. uvarum*) methods. Mean values were 1636 and 1683 pmol/ml for RPLC and microbiological assays, respectively.

significant effects of vitamin B-6 supplementation on diurnal variation in vitamin B-6 levels of milk and the implications for milk sampling will be discussed in a subsequent section.

Methods and Analysis

The microbiological method using *S. uvarum* is widely accepted for the estimation of total vitamin B-6 content in foods, including human milk. Since the yeast grows only on the free forms of the vitamin, hydrolysis of samples is necessary to release the vitamin from phosphate and protein. Most cultures of *S. uvarum* grow with approximately equal efficiency in response to PL, PN and PM; however, some cultures show a lower growth response for PM (80%) compared to PN or PL (6). This does not pose a problem in the analysis of milk with *S. uvarum*, since milk contains low levels of PM.

Recent advances in ion-exchange high performance liquid chromatography (HPLC) have led to the separation of individual vitamers in milk: PN, PL, PM, and PLP and PMP (7,8). HPLC methods have been shown to be accurate and reliable for the measurement of a wide range of vitamin B-6 concentrations (7,9). Our laboratory recently developed reverse-phase liquid chromatography (RPLC) for B-6 vitamer analysis in milk (10). The results of this method compared well with the vitamer distribution reported from the use of two ion-exchange HPLC methods (Table 1). When RPLC is compared to ion-exchange HPLC methods for B-6 vitamer analysis, the former is potentially faster, simpler and less expensive. Analysis of total vitamin B-6 in 80 human-milk samples in our laboratory showed an acceptable correlation (r=0.86) between RPLC and a microbiological method using *S. uvarum* (Figure 1). The latter method is more cumbersome than the chromatographic procedure; it relies on stability of the culture, and it depends upon the organism being equally sensitive to each form of the vitamin. RPLC is accurate and reliable and can now be considered an alternative to microbiological methods for analysis of vitamin B-6 in human milk.

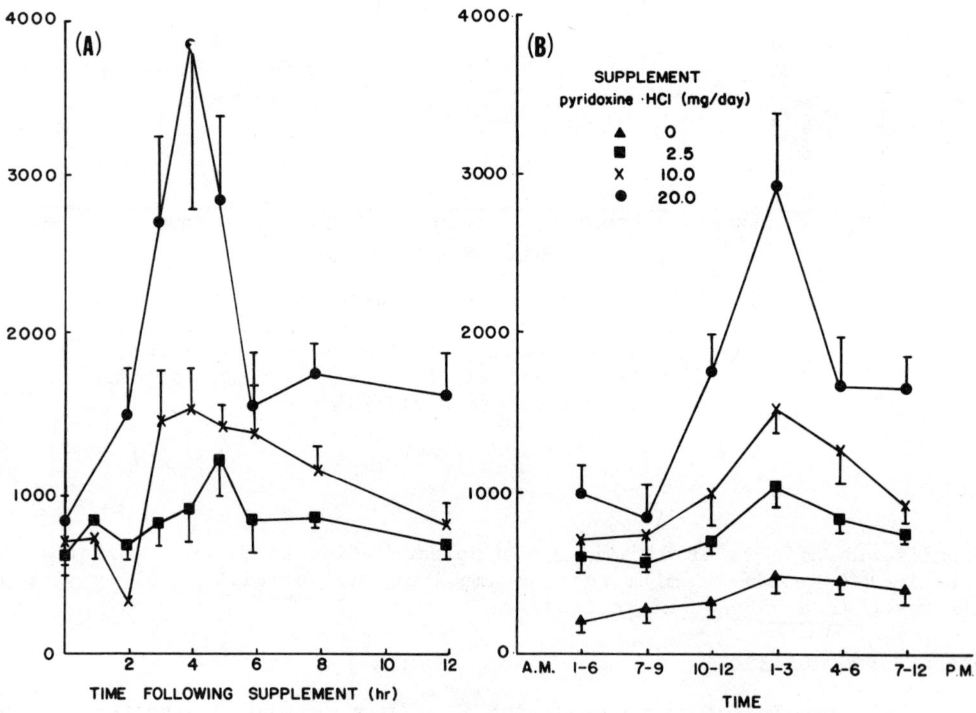

Figure 2. Vitamin B-6 concentration in milk during: (A) two 12-hour periods on consecutive days following PN.HCl supplementation, and (B) two 24-hour periods on consecutive days for women supplemented with different levels of PN.HCl N = 6 per group. Vertical bars represent mean ± SEM.

Table 2. Influence of different levels of intake of vitamin B-6 on the concentrations of vitamin B-6 in milk.

Intake of Vitamin B-6			Vitamin B-6 Concentration in Milk		
PN.HCl Suppl	Diet	(Diet + Supplements)			
mg/day	mg/day	mg/day	μg/l	μg/g[d] protein	μg/[e] 100 Kcal
0	2.0±0.1[a]	2.0±0.1[b]	93±8[b]	7±1[b]	12±1[b]
2.5	1.9±0.1	4.4±0.1[b]	192±16[c]	14±2[c]	25±2[c]
10.0	1.6±0.1	11.3±0.2[b]	247±25[c]	18±2[c]	33±3[c]
20.0	1.7±0.5	21.1±0.4[b]	413±45[c]	30±4[b]	55±5[b]

[a] Mean ± SEM; n = 6 per group.

[b] Significantly different ($p<0.05$) from means of all other groups.

[c] Significantly different ($p<0.05$) from means of nonsupplemented and 20.0 mg supplemented groups.

[d] 15 μg vitamin B-6/g protein recommended (RDA, 1980).

[e] 35 μg vitamin B-6/100 Kcal minimum recommendation (Am Acad Pediat, Committee on Nutrition, Pediat 1976, 57, 278).

Concentration of Vitamin B-6 in Milk

Currently available information concerning levels of vitamin B-6 in human milk is based on data from seven published investigations (5, 11-16). These studies show that the vitamin B-6 content of human milk is influenced by vitamin B-6 nutritional status (13,14), vitamin B-6 intake (5, 11-15), stage of lactation (13,15) and use of certain drugs (14,16). Because of these factors, especially vitamin B-6 intake, investigators do not agree regarding a normal/adequate level of vitamin B-6 in human milk for the human infant.

Table 3. Comparison of two methods for the estimation of vitamin B-6 intakes of breast-fed infants.

Supplement PN HCl	No. of 24-Hour Periods of Measurement	Milk Intake	Methods for Estimation of Vitamin B-6 Intakes of Infants[c]	
			Estimate of Milk Volume Intake	
			Test weighing	850 ml/24-Hour (assumed)
mg/day		ml/day	mg/day	mg/day
0	6	667±48[a]	0.06±0.01	0.06±0.01
2.5	11	664±52	0.12±0.02	0.10±0.02
10.0	8	799±58	0.22±0.02	0.17±0.02[b]
20.0	18	720±47	0.28±0.03	0.18±0.02[b]

[a]Mean ± SEM.

[b]Significantly different ($p<0.05$) from mean of test weighing method.

[c]Milk volume at each feeding/24-hour. X vitamin B-6 concentration (μg/ml) at each feeding/24-hour.

<u>Influence of Vitamin B-6 Intake.</u> Vitamin B-6 levels in human milk respond rapidly to changes in vitamin B-6 intake. Karlin (11) observed that within one hour after intramuscular injections of PN were given to five lactating women, the level of vitamin B-6 in milk rose to six times the initial level. The highest concentration, ten times the original level, was reached 3 hours after the injection. After 24 hours, the concentration was more than three times the base level and did not return to the original level until 5 to 7 days later. Similar findings were obtained following oral administration of PN (11).

In our laboratory (17,18), the vitamin B-6 level in human milk was found to increase in response to small doses of vitamin B-6 contained in prenatal supplements. Approximately 5 hours after lactating women took oral supplements of 10 or 20 mg PN.HCl, vitamin B-6 levels in milk doubled or tripled, reaching about 1500 and 3800 pmol/ml, respectively (Figure 2). Approximately 12 hours later, levels of vitamin B-6 were elevated only slightly compared to the initial concentration. These findings indicated the importance of obtaining milk samples at each feeding throughout a 24-hour period from women who take vitamin B-6 supplements, if true infant intakes are to be estimated.

Figure 2 also shows the influence of no supplement and of different levels of vitamin B-6 supplements on the concentrations of vitamin B-6 in milk obtained at each feeding during two consecutive 24-hour periods. A peak in vitamin B-6 concentration was observed in the early afternoon in milk from women who took supplements of vitamin B-6, whereas concentration changes were minimal in milk from nonsupplemented women. Subjects who took no vitamin B-6 supplements had a mean level of vitamin B-6 of 376±33 pmol/ml milk, compared to levels of 777±64, 1258±102 and 1671±180 pmol/ml milk for women supplemented daily with 2.5, 10.0 and 20.0 mg PN.HCl, respectively (Table 2). In individuals, the maternal intake and the level of vitamin B-6 in milk were positively correlated (r=.80). The vitamin B-6/protein and vitamin B-6/Kcal ratios were significantly lower in milk of mothers who took no vitamin B-6 supplement or ≤2.5 mg PN.HCl/day than in the milk of mothers who received 10.0 or 20.0 mg PN.HCl The ratios were below the currently accepted standards.

In the past, vitamin B-6 intakes of infants were often calculated from a single milk sample and an assumed milk output of 850 ml/day. We found that vitamin B-6 intakes of breast-fed infants calculated in this way, or by test-weighing, were similar for infants whose mothers took no PN.HCl supplements or less than 2.5 mg/day (Table 3). The assumed-volume method for estimation of vitamin B-6 intake was based on the vitamin B-6 concentration in milk samples obtained at one early morning feeding. Therefore, vitamin B-6 intake was underestimated for infants of mothers who took 10.0 and 20.0 mg PN.HCl/day because the midafternoon peak in vitamin B-6 concentration which followed supplementation was not included. This method may be suitable for estimation of vitamin B-6 intakes of infants whose mothers take no supplement or no more than 2.5 mg PN.HCl/day. However, intakes will probably be underestimated when larger supplements are taken by the mother.

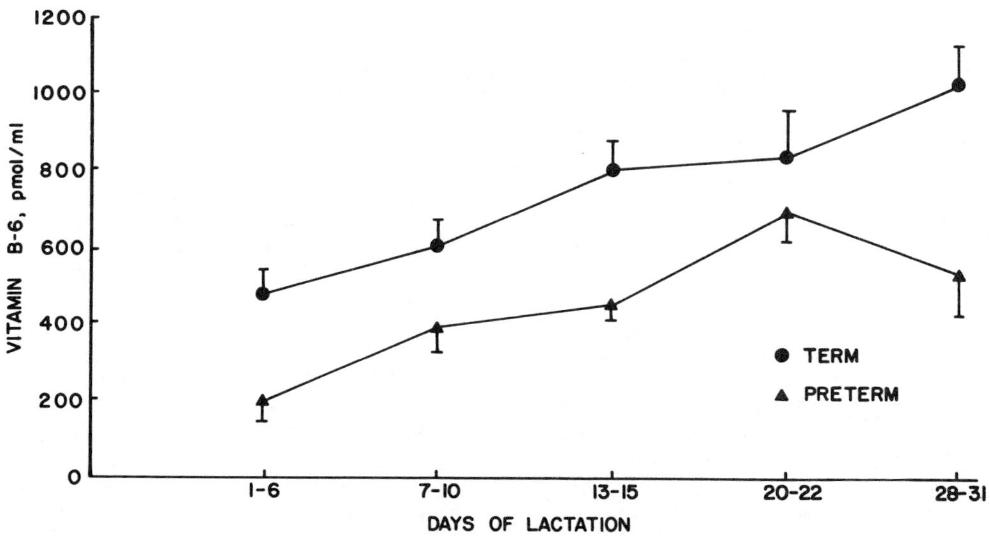

Figure 3. Vitamin B-6 content of term and preterm milk from mothers supplemented with 5-10 mg PN.HCl/day. Vertical bars represent mean ± SEM.

Elevated levels of vitamin B-6 in milk were observed following oral supplementation, whereas extremely low levels paralleled low intakes of the vitamin. In this laboratory, West and Kirksey (5) observed less than 50 μg vitamin B-6/l in the milk of a subject whose intake of vitamin B-6 was estimated to be only 1.5 mg/day. Thus, less than 4% of this woman's daily intake of vitamin B-6 appeared in her milk, an amount that was inadequate for her infant. These data indicated that the mammary gland is unable to concentrate vitamin B-6 in milk when the intake of the vitamin is inadequate. This conclusion is supported by data from rat experiments. Following a short period (6 days) of vitamin B-6 deficiency during lactation in the rat, the vitamin B-6 content in milk decreased to less than 20% of control values (19). The short period of dietary inadequacy only slightly decreased vitamin B-6 concentrations in liver tissue and did not alter it significantly in muscle tissue. The failure of these tissues to supply vitamin B-6 to milk when vitamin B-6 intake was inadequate, supports our postulates that the mammary gland does not concentrate the vitamin and that milk levels can be an early indicator of impending vitamin B-6 inadequacy.

Influence of Stage of Lactation. Roepke and Kirksey (13) observed that the vitamin B-6 content in milk of women whose intake of the vitamin was greater than 2.5 mg/day increased from 65±12 pmol/ml in colostrum at 3 days postpartum to 231±28 pmol/ml in transitional milk at 14 days post-partum and then to 914±120 pmol/ml in mature milk at 4 to 6 weeks of lactation. Also, Karlin (11) reported that during the first few days of lactation, human milk contained only 59 to 119 pmol vitamin B-6/ml and noted that the levels rose to 595 pmol/ml in mature milk of nonsupplemented women at 4 weeks lactation. Thomas et al. (15) reported that levels of vitamin B-6 in human milk at 5 to 7 days postpartum (762 pmol/ml) were lower than values for mature milk at 43 to 45 days (1214 pmol/ml) when no supplements were taken. Values reported by these investigators at 5 to 7 days were higher than those reported by Karlin (11) or Kirksey and West (5) for 1 to 3 days of lactation. The vitamin B-6 content in mature human milk was not significantly affected by the stage of lactation; values were 1525±184 and 1476±351 pmol/ml at 3 and 7 months lactation, respectively (12).

Concentrations of vitamin B-6 were significantly lower in both term and preterm milk at 1 to 6 days of lactation when compared to values at later stages of lactation. Levels of vitamin B-6 in preterm milk were significantly lower than those in term milk throughout the first month of lactation (Figure 3). Vitamin B-6 supplementation of preterm mothers did not significantly affect concentrations of the vitamin in colostrum and transitional milk (20). Presently, no explanation can be given for the extremely low levels of vitamin B-6 in preterm milk in spite of adequate maternal intake of the vitamin. These findings emphasize the need for vitamin B-6 supplementation of preterm infants who are fed their mothers' milk during the neonatal period.

The ratio of vitamin B-6 concentration in milk to that in maternal plasma was less than 1.0 in colostrum at 3 days of lactation, whereas at 6 weeks the ratio exceeded 7.0 (13,17). This finding suggests that the mammary gland has a greater ability to concentrate vitamin B-6 in later lactation than at earlier stages. The ratio of vitamin B-6/protein (μg/g) increased from ≤1.0 at 3 days lactation to >15 at 6 weeks and later stages of lactation. This relationship is important in infant nutrition since vitamin B-6 needs are known to increase with increments in dietary protein. During early lactation when the levels of vitamin B-6 in milk are low, infants appear to be protected by high concentrations of the vitamin in their blood. Levels of vitamin B-6 in cord serum are 2- to 3-fold those in maternal serum at delivery (13,14).

Influence of Vitamin B-6 Nutritional Status. Vitamin B-6 nutritional status appears to influence significantly the vitamin B-6 content in human milk. This is supported by the finding (13) that maternal nutritional status, assessed by the level of vitamin B-6 in maternal serum at 5 months of gestation, was significantly correlated (r=0.51) with the level of vitamin B-6 in milk at 14 days postpartum.

Roepke and Kirksey (13) observed that levels of vitamin B-6 in maternal serum as well as in milk at 3 and 14 days postpartum were significantly lower in mothers whose infants had unsatisfactory Apgar scores (<7) at 1 minute after birth. These data strongly suggest that the vitamin B-6 nutritional status is poorer in mothers whose infants had low Apgar scores than in mothers whose infants received acceptable ratings.

Previous long-term use (>36 months) of oral contraceptives was associated with low levels of vitamin B-6 in maternal serum, cord serum, and milk (14). Levels of vitamin B-6 in milk were not significantly different in the early postpartum period (3 days) among women grouped according to oral contraceptive use, but at 14 days postpartum the levels of vitamin B-6 in milk were significantly lower for long-term oral contraceptive users (161 pmol/ml) than short-term users (292 pmol/ml) or nonusers (388 pmol/ml). This finding raises questions about the adequacy of vitamin B-6 in milk of long-term oral contraceptive users.

VITAMIN C

Vitamin C (1-threo-2,3,4,5,6-pentahydroxy-1-hexenoic acid-1-lactone) exists in two biologically active forms: ascorbic acid (AA), which is the more stable reduced form, and dehydroascorbic acid (DHAA), the reversible oxidized form. Munks et al. (21) observed that DHAA accounted for approximately 11% of the total vitamin C in human milk. However, prevention of oxidation of the vitamin during expression and collection of milk is difficult. L-AA undergoes oxidation slowly to DHAA which is then converted to 2,3 diketogulonic acid (2,3 DKGA) and to other metabolites which are physiologically inactive. The rate of oxidation of AA depends on many factors including temperature, light, presence of oxidizing enzymes or of certain metallic ions which act as catalysts to the metabolic process (22).

Methods of Analysis

The interconvertibility of AA and DHAA by oxidation and reduction is widely used in the analysis of vitamin C. Methods based on reactions of AA measure only this form of the vitamin, but a subsequent estimation following the reduction of any DHAA which is present allows determination of the sum of both forms of the vitamin (22). Various methods used in the analysis of vitamin C are summarized in Table 4. Microautomated procedures have been developed to facilitate the rapid analyses of large numbers of samples. By far the greatest proportion of published procedures for vitamin C analyses are concerned with different ways of oxidizing AA.

2,6 Dichlorophenol-Indophenol Method. Among the various oxidants for AA analysis [2,6 dichlorophenol-indophenol (2,6 DCPIP), ferric salts, bromine, iodine and N-bromo-succinimide], 2,6 DCPIP is the most widely used. It can be used in the visual titration of acidic solutions of AA

Table 4. Methods for vitamin C analysis.

I. Chemical Methods Based On:

A. Oxidation of ascorbic acid (Oxidants used: 2,6-dichlorophenol indophenol, N-bromosuccinimide, ferric salts, bromine or iodine).

B. Reactions of ascorbic acid.
   1. Measurement (244 nm) in hydrochloric acid- potassium chloride buffer.
   2. Measurement (265 nm) before and after treatment with ascorbic acid oxidase.
   3. Measurement after treatment with reagents such as diazotized 4-methoxy-2-nitroaniline and alkali.

C. Reactions of dehydroascorbic acid.
   1. Measurement (fluorescence at 427 nm) of the quinoxalinyl. lactone formed by condensed DHAA with o-phenyldiamine.
   2. Polarography.

D. Reactions of 2,3-diketogulonic acid.
   1. Measurement (520-540 nm) of the chromogen formed by treatment with 2,4-dinitrophenylhydrazine.

II. Gas Liquid Chromatography.

III. High Performance Liquid Chromatography.

A. Ion-exchange.

B. Reverse-phase.

Detectors used: UV and amperimetric. Measures only ascorbic acid.

(22,23); however, the 2,6 DCPIP method has been adapted photometrically toimprove the precision and to eliminate the inaccuracy due to the difficulty in visually judging a rapidly disappearing end point (23). The procedure, although simple, has drawbacks. The sample itself may have excessive color and may contain other reducing substances, such as sulphur dioxide, tannins, cysteine, certain metallic ions, etc. EDTA has been used to avoid interference by metallic ions; however, no methodological adaptation has satisfactorily prevented interference by compounds such as thiosulfate, sulfite and ferrous, cuprous or stannous salts which react rapidly with indophenol (23).

Dinitrophenylhydrazine Method. This method is based upon spectrophotometric measurement of the chromogen formed by the coupling of 2,4 dinitrophenylhydrazine (DNPH) with the ketonic groups of oxidized AA (24). AA must be oxidized to DHAA before coupling with DNPH can occur. A widely used oxidizing reagent for AA is Norit (charcoal), which also serves as a clarifying agent. Measurable chromogen formation from nonascorbic substances is avoided by dilution of the extract, carrying out the coupling reaction at a low temperature (37°C), and by running a parallel sample blank for each sample (22). The DNPH method can be used to determine either AA, DHAA, and DKGA collectively, or AA and DHAA separately (22,25).

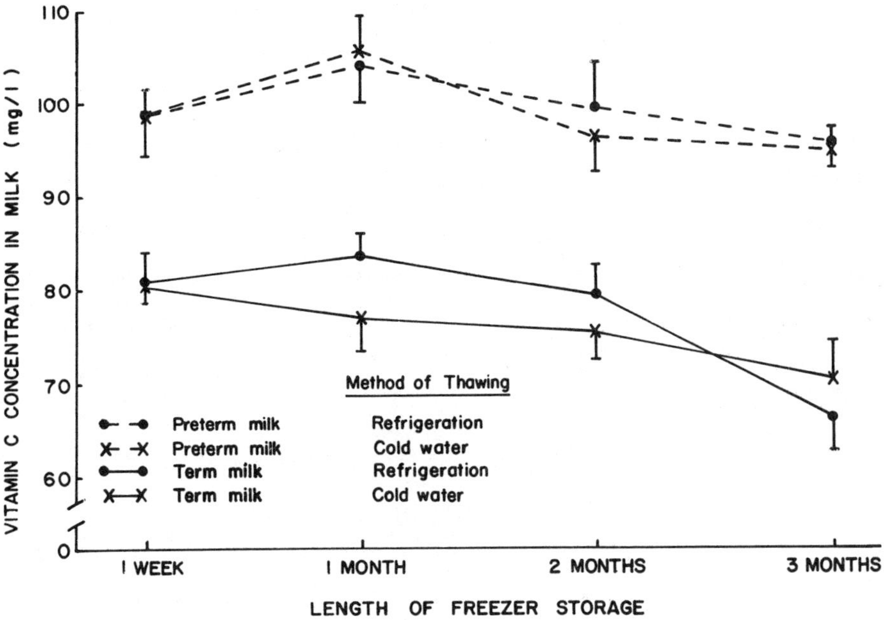

Figure 4. Effects of length of freezer storage and method of thawing on the vitamin C concentration in milk from mothers of term and preterm infants. Vertical line indicates SE.

Other Methods. In addition to the spectrophotometric methods currently used for AA analysis, other analytical methods such as fluorometry are available (22). AA has also been estimated by use of gas liquid chromotography and high performance liquid chromotography (22). Ion pair and reverse phase HPLC methods (26-29) have been developed for AA determination in milk with the use of amperometric or ultraviolet (UV) detectors. However, these methods do not detect DHAA, which is a physiologically active form of vitamin C and important in nutrition. DHAA can be detected with a chemiluminescent reagent which requires a reductant, although the sensitivity for DHAA is lower than for AA (22).

Preparation of Samples for Analysis

In general, samples to be analyzed for vitamin C should not be stored. If immediate analysis is not possible, an extracting solution (for example, 4% metaphosphoric acid) should be added to the milk sample as soon as possible after collection, and then this mixture should be frozen

Table 5. Effects of length of refrigerator storage on vitamin C concentration in human milk.

Length of Refrigeration Storage	Vitamin C Concentration in Milk
HOURS	mg/1
0	118.8 ± 8.2^{a}
4	114.5 ± 9.8^{a}
8	$109.0 \pm 10.6^{a,b}$
18	$107.1 \pm 15.3^{a,b}$
24	92.3 ± 12.0^{b}

[a,b]Means within the same column with different superscripts differ significantly ($p<0.05$).

immediately. Addition of an extracting-stabilizing solution may restrict losses of vitamin C to 5% or less (22). Dilution and stabilization of samples are of particular importance for samples which are collected in the field and which may require several hours to transport to a laboratory. The extent of dilution of samples varies from 1:5 (22) to 1:50 (23). In this laboratory, a 1:20 dilution of milk samples is used.

Most analytical procedures for vitamin C require clear solutions of protein-free filtrates, usually prepared by dilution of the sample with acids such as metaphosphoric acid (3 to 6%). Other acids which may be used are acetic acid, trichloroacetic acid or oxalic acid. Samples which are freeze dried can lose vitamin C very rapidly (22); therefore, the use of this procedure for sample preparation is not recommended.

Ascorbic acid in solution is sensitive to light, hence extraction and analysis should be performed in subdued light. Storage of milk in clear glass vials and exposure to light result in a total loss of vitamin C within 3 hours (30).

Storage of Samples. Bank et al. (31), in this laboratory, observed that the vitamin C concentration of milk that was frozen immediately after collection and stored at -20°C in amber vials did not change significantly until after 2 months of storage (Figure 4). Between 2 and 3 months of freezer storage, a significant decrease was observed in vitamin C levels of samples which were not stabilized with acid prior to freezing. However, this decrease was not observed in milk from mothers who delivered preterm infants (Figure 4).

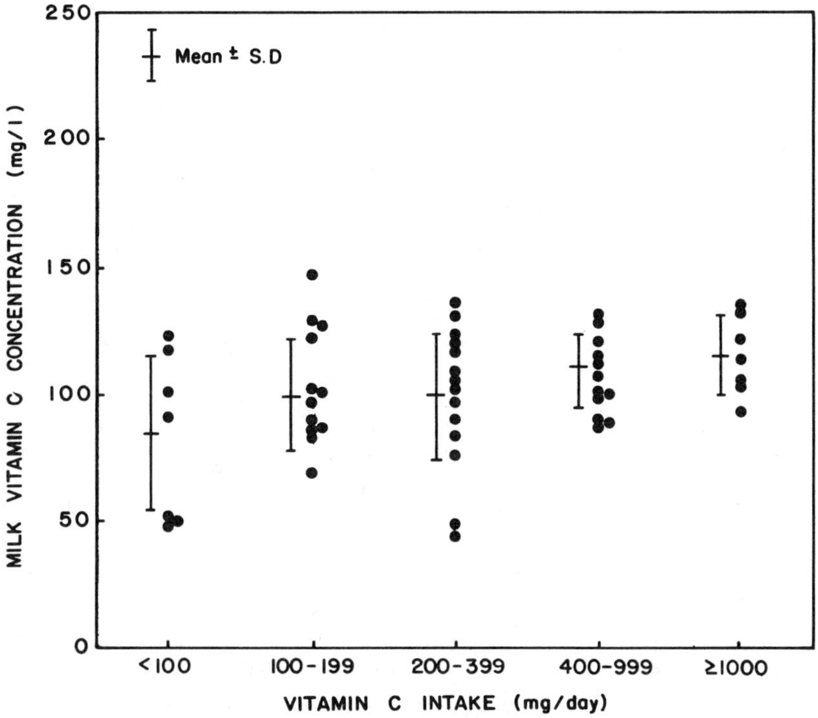

Figure 5. Vitamin C concentrations in milk in relation to different levels of vitamin C intake.

The vitamin C concentration in milk samples measured immediately after collection and at 4, 8, 18, and 24 hours of refrigeration (31), showed a decrease of 22% after 24 hours of refrigeration (Table 5). This was in agreement with findings of Selleg and King (32), who observed an average loss of 27% in the vitamin C concentration of samples stored in a refrigerator for 18 hours. Vitamin C concentration was similar in frozen samples that were thawed either in a refrigerator overnight or by immersing the sample in cold water (Figure 4). Vitamin C content of milk which was frozen for one month, thawed, and then refrigerated for 2 hours was not significantly different from the level of vitamin C determined immediately after thawing (31). For laboratory analysis, it may be convenient to thaw samples overnight in a refrigerator.

Effects of Supplementation

Studies in developing countries indicate that the vitamin C concentration in breast milk of undernourished mothers can be increased by ascorbic acid supplementation (33,34). In a recent study, Bates et al. (35) reported that an increase in vitamin C intake from 34 to 103 mg/d by undernourished women in a West African rural community was parallelled by

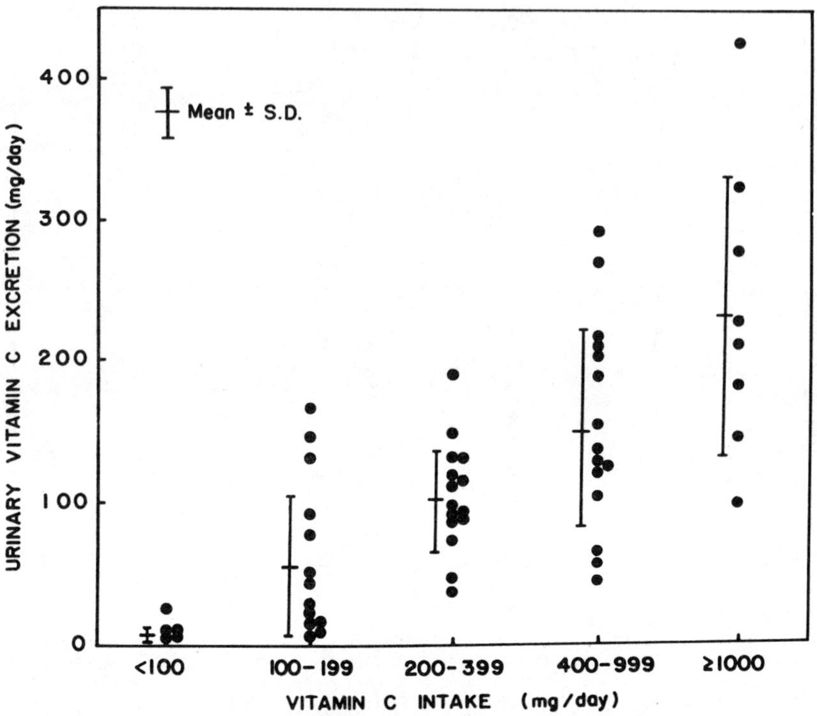

Figure 6. Urinary excretion of vitamin C in relation to different levels of vitamin C intake.

increased vitamin C levels in their breast milk. At the higher levels of vitamin C intake, the vitamin concentration in milk approached a plateau. Sneed et al. (36) observed that the vitamin C levels in milk from unsupplemented American women of low socioeconomic status were not significantly different from those in milk from women supplemented with 90 mg ascorbic acid/day.

In this laboratory (37), supplementation of 25 lactating, well-nourished women with 90, 250, 500 or 1000 mg/day did not significantly affect the vitamin C levels in their milk (Figure 5). However, urinary excretion of the vitamin increased significantly and parallelled the level of ascorbic acid supplementation (Figure 6). Similar findings from other studies in this laboratory (unpublished) showed that vitamin C concentration in milk did not vary significantly among women taking 0, 50, 100 or 200 mg ascorbic acid supplements daily from 1 to 8 months of lactation. These findings suggested that saturation is reached at low vitamin C intake and that a regulatory mechanism in the mammary gland controls the concentration of vitamin C in milk.

Diurnal Variation

Munks et al. (21) found that the vitamin C content of human milk fluctuated during the day, with the lowest concentration usually observed at 2 or 10 p.m. However, Sneed et al. (36) reported that concentrations of vitamin C in milk were significantly lower in the morning before ascorbic acid supplements were taken and that the concentration increased about 12 hours after supplementation.

Byerley and Kirksey (37) observed fluctuations in the levels of vitamin C in milk at different feedings throughout the day; however, the differences were not statistically significant at any time interval examined. This was confirmed by further work in this laboratory (unpublished data). Only 7 of 31 mothers studied from 4 weeks to 8 months of lactation showed consistent diurnal variation in vitamin C concentrations during a 24-hour period. Concentrations of vitamin C in milk from most mothers usually did not exceed 150 to 160 mg/l, and during the day concentrations fluctuated from 50 to 70 mg/l. Three women occasionally had vitamin C concentrations in milk between 175 and 240 mg/l at a particular feeding. However, at other feedings or at different stages of lactation, these women did not exhibit high concentrations of vitamin C in their milk.

Since vitamin C concentrations do not appear to differ significantly during a 24-hour period, it should be possible to use a single sample instead of a 24-hour collection for the estimation of vitamin intakes of infants. Mean vitamin C concentration in samples of early morning milk was similar to that for samples collected throughout a 24-hour period from women between 4 weeks and 8 months of lactation (unpublished data). However, regression analysis indicated that vitamin C concentrations in milk samples obtained at an early morning feeding were not good indicators of the concentration in a pooled 24-hour collection. The mean concentration of vitamin C in early morning samples differed approximately 20 to 35% from the mean in 24-hour pooled samples.

Vitamin C concentrations in milk obtained at an early morning feeding were with $\pm$15 mg/l of the mean value for 24-hour samples in 30 to 40% of these mothers. In contrast, 35 to 80% of the milk samples obtained at 1300 $\pm$1.5 hours were within $\pm$15 mg vitamin C/l of the mean for samples obtained throughout a 24-hour period. Vitamin C concentrations in samples obtained at the first feed after 1300 hours differed by 13 to 21% from the mean for 24-hour pooled samples. Thus, it appears that in situations where collection of milk samples throughout a 24-hour period is not possible, a single sample collected at 1300 hours, or between 1300 and 1450 hours, could be used.

Maturation Changes in Vitamin C Concentration of Milk

Selleg and King (32) reported variation in the vitamin C concentration of colostrum; however, the mean was comparable to that of mature milk. Munks (21) observed an increase in vitamin C concentrations from days 1 to 3 postpartum, but concentrations on day 3 postpartum were similar to those observed on days 6 to 10 (72 mg/l). Vitamin C concentration of milk expressed between 68 and 360 days postpartum was lower (52 mg/l) than on days 6-10. These findings agree with those of Macy (38) who reported that the vitamin C concentration of milk collected on days 1 to 5 and 6 to 10 postpartum was similar and that the concentration decreased between 15 days and 15 months of lactation. Thomas et al. (15) observed no significant differences in the vitamin C concentration in milk obtained on days 5 to 7 and that obtained 43 to 45 days postpartum. Findings from this laboratory (20) indicated that milk obtained from mothers who delivered term or preterm infants was significantly lower in vitamin C concentration on days 1 to 6 postpartum compared to days 13 to 15. Results from these studies indicate the need for further studies of maturational changes in vitamin C levels of human milk.

CONCLUSIONS

Future studies on the vitamin B-6 and vitamin C content of human milk should be designed to take into account: 1) the nutritional status of the lactating mother, 2) the quantity, frequency of use and time of supplementation, 3) time of milk sampling, particularly in relation to vitamin intake (diet and/or supplements), 4) protection of milk samples from light during handling and storage, 5) protein concentration of milk relative to the level of vitamin B-6, 6) use of oral contraceptives or other drugs which may interfere with the normal function of vitamins, and 7) stage of lactation and postconceptual age of infant.

ACKNOWLEDGEMENTS

This research was supported in part by USDA/SEA grant No. 59-2182-0-1-492-0. Paper No. 10096 of Purdue University Agricultural Experiment Station, West Lafayette, IN 47907

REFERENCES

1. Brin M. (1978): Chemistry, absorption, metabolism, catabolism and toxity. In: Human vitamin B-6 requirements. Washington DC: Natl Acad Sci, 1-20.

2. Gregory JF, Kirk JR. (1981): The bioavailability of vitamin B-6 in foods. Nutr Rev, 39, 1-8.

3. Gregory JF, Kirk JR. (1978): Vitamin B-6 in foods: assessment of stability and bioavailability. In: Human vitamin B-6 requirements. Washington DC: Natl Acad Sci, 72-77.

4. Ang CYW. (1979): Stability of three forms of vitamin B-6 to laboratory light conditions. J Assoc Off Anal Chem, 62, 1170-1173.

5. West KD, Kirksey A. (1976): Influence of vitamin B-6 intake on the content of the vitamin in human milk. Am J Clin Nutr, 29, 961-969.

6. Polansky M. (1980): Microbiological assay of vitamin B-6 in foods. In: Methods in vitamin B-6 nutrition. Washington DC: Natl Acad Sci, 21-44.

7. Coburn SP, Mahuren JD. (1983): A versatile cation-exchange procedure for measuring the seven major forms of vitamin B-6 in biological samples. Anal Biochem, 129, 310-317.

8. Vanderslice JT, Brownlee SG, Maire CE, Reynolds RD, Polansky M. (1983): Forms of vitamin B-6 in human milk. Am J Clin Nutr, 37, 867-871.

9. Gregory JF, Kirk JR. (1981): Determination of vitamin B-6 compounds by semiautomated continuous-flow and chromatographic methods. In: Leklem JE, Reynolds RD, eds, Methods in vitamin B-6 nutrition. New York: Plenum Press, 149-170.

10. Hamaker B, Kirksey A, Borschel M. (1983): Distribution of B-6 vitamers in milk of pyridoxine-supplemented mothers determined by high performance liquid chromatography (reverse phase). Fed Proc, 42, 1329.

11. Karlin R. (1959): Effet d'un enrichissement en pyridoxine sur la teneur en vitamin B-6 du lait de femme. Bull Soc Chim Biol, 41, 1085-1091.

12. Kirksey A, West KD. (1978): Relationship between vitamin B-6 intake and the content of the vitamin in human milk. In: Human vitamin B-6 requirements. Washington DC: Natl Acad Sci, 238-251.

13. Roepke JLB, Kirksey A. (1979): Vitamin B-6 nutriture during pregnancy and lactation. I. Vitamin B-6 intake, levels of the vitamin in biological fluids, and condition of the infant at birth. Am J Clin Nutr, 32, 2249-2256.

14. Roepke JLB, Kirksey A. (1979): Vitamin B-6 nutriture during pregnancy and lactation. II. The effect of long-term use of oral contraceptives. Am J Clin Nutr, 32, 2257-2264.

15. Thomas MR, Kawamoto J, Sneed SM, Eakin R. (1979): The effects of vitamin C, vitamin B-6, and vitamin B-12 supplementation on the breast milk and maternal status of well-nourished women. Am J Clin Nutr, 32, 1679-1685.

16. Kirksey A, Groziak S. (1984): Maternal drug use: Evaluation of risks to breast-fed infants. Wld Rev Nutr Diet, 43, 60-79.

17. Kirksey A, Roepke JLB, Styslinger LM. (1980): The vitamin B-6 content in human milk. In: Methods in vitamin B-6 nutrition. Washington DC: Natl Acad Sci, 269-288.

18. Styslinger LM, Kirksey A. (1985): Effect of different levels of vitamin B-6 supplementation on vitamin B-6 in human milk and on vitamin B-6 intake on the breastfed infant. Am J Clin Nutr, 41, 21-31.

19. Felice JH, Kirksey A. (1981): Effects of vitamin B-6 deficiency during lactation on the vitamin B-6 content of milk, liver and muscle of rats. J Nutr, 111, 610-617.

20. Udipi SA, Kirksey A, West K, Giacoia G. (1983): Comparison of vitamin C, vitamin B-6, folacin and protein levels in full-term and pre-term milk. Fed Proc, 42, 920.

21. Munks B, Robinson A, Williams HH, Macy IG. (1945): Human milk studies XXV. Ascorbic acid and DHascorbic acid in colostrum and mature human milk. Am J Dis Child, 70, 176-180.

22. Cooke JR, Moxon RED. (1981): The detection and measurement of vitamin C. In: Cobinsell JN, Hornig DH, eds, Vitamin C (Ascorbic Acid). London: Applied Science Publishers, 167-198.

23. Roe JH. (1961): Appraisal of methods for the determination of l-ascorbic acid. Ann Ny Acad Sci, 92, 277-283.

24. Roe JH, Kuether CA. (1943): The determination of ascorbic acid in whole blood and urine through the 2,4-dinitrophenylhydrazine derivative of dehydroascorbic acid. J Biol Chem, 147, 399-407.

25. Roe JH, Mills MB, Oesterling MJ, Damron CM. (1948): The determination of diketo-l-gulonic acid, dehydro-l-ascorbic acid, and l-ascorbic acid in the same tissue extract by the 2,4-dinitrophenylhydrazine method. J Biol Chem, 174, 201-208.

26. Heiliger F. (1980): Ascorbic acid analysis by LCEC. Current Separations, 2, 5.

27. LCEC Application Note No. 22. Bioanalytical System Inc., West Lafayette, Indiana.

28. Sood SP, Sartori LE, Wittmer DP, Haney WG. (1976): High-pressure liquid chromatographic determination of ascorbic acid in selected foods and multivitamin products. Anal Chem, 48, 796-798.

29. Pachla LA, Kissinger PT. (1976): Determination of ascorbic acid in foodstuffs, pharmaceuticals and body fluids by liquid chromatography with electrochemical detection. Anal Chem, 48, 364-367.

30. Malin JD. (1975): Folic acid. Wld Rev Nutr Diet, 21, 198-222.

31. Bank MR, Kirksey A, West K, Giacoia G. (1985): Effects of storage time and temperature of folacin and vitamin C content in milk from mothers of full-term and preterm mothers. Am J Clin Nutr, 41, 235-242.

32. Selleg I, King CG. (1936): The vitamin C content of human milk and its variation with diet. J Nutr, 11, 599-606.

33. Doedhar AD, Rajalakshmi R, Ramakrishnan C. (1964): Effect of dietary vitamin supplementation on vitamin contents of breast milk. Acta Paediatr, 53, 42-48.

34. Gopalan C, Belavada B. (1961): Nutrition and lactation. Fed Proc, 20, 177-184.

35. Bates CJ, Prentice AM, Prentice A, Lamb WH, Whitehead RG. (1983): The effect of vitamin C supplementation on lactating women in Keneba, a West African rural community. Int J Vit Nutr Res, 53, 68-76.

36. Sneed SM, Zane C, Thomas MR. (1981): The effects of ascorbic acid, vitamin B-6, vitamin B-12 and folic acid supplementation on the breast milk and maternal nutritional status of low socioeconomic lactating women. Am J Clin Nutr, 34, 1338-1346.

37. Byerley LO, Kirksey A. (1985): Effects of different levels of vitamin C intake on the vitamin C concentration in human milk and the vitamin C intakes of breast-fed infants. Am J Clin Nutr, 41, 665-671.

38. Macy IG. (1949): Composition of human colostrum and milk. Am J Dis Child, 78, 589-603.

ANALYSIS OF WATER-SOLUBLE VITAMINS IN HUMAN MILK: THIAMINE, NIACIN, RIBOFLAVIN, BIOTIN AND PANTOTHENIC ACID

R. R. Eitenmiller

THIAMINE

Methods for the analysis of thiamine in foods include the thiochrome procedure and a microbiological assay using *Lactobacillus viridescens* ATCC 7469. The two methods usually give comparable results (1,2), and both procedures have been applied to human milk. The thiochrome method is based on the oxidation of thiamine to thiochrome by alkaline ferricyanide with subsequent fluorometric detection of the thiochrome. Manual and semi-automated thiochrome procedures are described in the AOAC *Official Methods of Analysis*, 13 ed. (Sec 43.024-43.030, Sec 43.031-43.034) (3).

The *L. viridescens* assay was described by Diebel et al. in 1957 (4). This assay has become a reliable and sensitive method for thiamine quantitation from complex matrices. The organism requires intact thiamine and responds to phosphorylated forms of the vitamin. A mutant strain has been isolated that does not respond to thiamine pyrophosphate. The potential appearance of this mutant necessitates the use of a phosphatase treatment during the extraction of thiamine from food samples (2).

Values for the thiamine content of human milk are presented in Table 1. Feeley et al. (5), in a study of the thiamine, riboflavin and niacin content of human milk during early lactational stages, found that thiamine levels increased rapidly during the first 30 days of lactation. Milk at 4 to 7 days postpartum contained 5.5 µg/100 ml, increasing to 13.9 µg/100 ml in the mature milk (>30 day postpartum). This value compares closely to the thiamine level of 16 µg/100 ml reported in 1977 in Great Britain (6). The *L. viridescens* assay was used by Feeley et al. (5), whereas the thiochrome procedure was used in the British study demonstrating the strong agreement between the two methods (6). The values are in close agreement with earlier reports by Macy and Kelly (7).

NIACIN

Several methods are currently available for the determination of niacin in foods, biological fluids and pharmaceuticals. A routine chemical procedure is based on the classical Konig reaction in which nicotinic acid reacts with cyanogen bromide to form colored complexes that are measured colorimetrically. Microbiological assay is accomplished using *Lactobacillus plantarum* ATCC 8014. Semiautomated continuous-flow techniques have been successfully applied to the cyanogen bromide method for niacin

Table 1. Thiamine, Niacin and Riboflavin content of human milk.

		μg/100 ml		
	Time Postpartum	Thiamine	Niacin	Riboflavin
Macy and Kelly (7)	> 30 days	14	183	37
British Study (6)	> 30 days	16	230	31
Feeley et al. (5)	4 to 7 days	5.5	76	50
	10 to 14 days	10.5	224	53
	30 to 45 days	13.9	219	50

(3,8), and in many laboratories microbiological assay procedures have been partially automated. The semiautomated method for niacin in food products gives results comparable to those of the microbiological and manual colorimetric methods (8). Procedures for both the colorimetric and microbiological methods are given in the AOAC (3) (Sec 43.044-051 and Sec 43.150 and Sec 43.155-158).

While the colorimetric procedure should be useful for quantitation of niacin in human milk, recent studies have relied on the *L. plantarum* assay (5,6). Feeley et al. (5) found that niacin levels increased rapidly during the first two weeks of lactation and then stabilized. Feeley et al. reported niacin levels of 219 μg/100 ml at the mature stage (Table 1). This value compared closely to the niacin level of 230 μg/100 ml reported in Great Britain in 1977 (6). Macy and Kelly (7) reported a niacin content of 183 μg/100 ml (7).

RIBOFLAVIN

Commonly accepted riboflavin methods include a fluorometric procedure (AOAC, Sec. 43.039-43.042) (3) and a microbiological procedure using *Lactobacillus casei* ATCC 7469 (AOAC, Sec. 43.139-43.147) (3). Another microorganism, *Streptococcus zymogenes* ATCC 10100, has been used for quantitation of riboflavin in human milk (6).

Studies by Feeley et al. (5) on the riboflavin content of human milk were completed using *L. casei* as the assay organism. Results of this study showed the riboflavin content of the milk to be constant over the first month of lactation (Table 1). Riboflavin levels reported by Feeley et al. (6) were higher for mature milk than those reported in Great Britain (6) (50 μg/100 ml compared to 31 μg/100 ml). The large difference in riboflavin levels noted in the two studies is likely due to differences in responses of the assay organisms used in the respective studies. *Streptococcus zymogenes*, which was used in the British study, has not been routinely used in the analysis of riboflavin content in foods. Macy and Kelly (7) reported a value of 37 μg/100 ml for mature milk using a fluorometric procedure.

BIOTIN

The accepted procedure for biotin quantitation in foods follows the method of Skeggs (9) using *Lactobacillus plantarum* ATCC 8014 as the assay organism. This assay has been used in several recent studies on the biotin content of human milk (6,10,11). Data from these studies is given in Table 2. Some variation exists in the biotin levels reported by various researchers. Goldsmith et al. (10) reported biotin levels of 0.07 μg/100 ml for early transitional (3 to 8 days postpartum), 0.32 μg/100 ml for transitional (10 to 14 days postpartum), and 0.5 μg/100 ml for mature milk (30 to 45 days postpartum).

Another study (6) on samples collected in five separate locations in Great Britain, but all transported to one laboratory for analysis, reported large geographical differences with mean values ranging from 0.52 μg/100 ml in one area to 1.13 μg/100 ml in another area. A mean of 0.72 μg/100 ml was reported for samples from each of the other three locations, resulting in an overall average of 0.76 μg/100 ml. These mean values were determined on pooled samples of mature milk collected 14 to 63 days postpartum. Hood and Johnson (11) found that the biotin content increased rapidly between day one and day seven, from 0.30 to 0.68 μg/100 ml, followed by an increase to 1.25 and 1.27 μg/100 ml at days 49 and 70, respectively. The fact that these values are much higher than the results reported in other studies could be due to geographical location and/or differences in diet.

Milk samples used by Goldsmith et al. (10) were from earlier postpartum periods (30 to 45 days) than those used in other studies. Macy (12) reported biotin levels of 0.06 μg/100 ml in colostrum (one to five days postpartum) and 0.35 μg/100 ml in transitional milk (six to 12 days postpartum). These values are similar to those reported by Goldsmith et al.; however, Macy (12) reported a higher level of 0.81 μg/100 ml for mature milk. Macy's value for biotin in mature milk was determined from milk collected 15 days to 15 months postpartum. Since Hood and Johnson (11) indicated that the biotin content of human milk continued to increase with duration of lactation, the variation in literature values is not surprising.

Table 2. Biotin content of human milk.

	Time Postpartum	μg/100 ml
Macy (12)	< 5 days	0.06
	6 to 12 days	0.35
	15 days to 15 months	0.81
British Study (6)	> 30 days	0.72
Hood and Johnson (11)	49 days	1.25
	70 days	1.27
Goldsmith et al. (10)	3 to 8 days	0.07
	10 to 14 days	0.32
	30 to 45 days	0.50

PANTOTHENIC ACID

While a variety of methods exist for the analysis of pantothenic acid (13), most recent studies on the pantothenic acid content of foods have utilized a microbiological procedure using *Lactobacillus plantarum* ATCC 8014 (14) or a radioimmunoassay (RIA) developed by Wyse et al. (15) in 1979. The RIA method was shown to be an acceptable alternative to the microbiological assay (16).

As is true for many micronutrients in human milk, the literature does not present a clear indication of the pantothenic acid content. In 1981, Johnston et al. (17) reported a mean pantothenic acid content of 0.67 mg/100 ml for mature human milk collected from 1 to 6 months postpartum from 22 donors. This level is considerably higher than most published values. For example, USDA Handbook 8-1 (18) and the 1977 report of the extensive British study (6) gave values of 0.22 mg/100 ml and 0.26 mg/100 ml, respectively, for the pantothenic acid content of mature human milk. Other investigators (19,20,21) reported mean pantothenic acid levels of approximately 0.2 mg/100 ml.

Johnston et al. (17) reported a significant positive correlation between the pantothenic acid in the diet of the mother the day before milk samples were collected and the pantothenic acid content of the milk. They attributed the higher pantothenic acid content of the milk reported in their study to the higher pantothenic acid intakes, prior pantothenic acid status of the donors, and differences in assay methodology.

Since 1981, two studies have been completed on the pantothenic acid content of human milk. Eitenmiller (unpublished) studied the pantothenic acid content of early lactational milk, and Song et al. (22) determined the effect of pantothenic acid status on the content of the vitamin in human milk. Eitenmiller, using the *L. plantarum* assay and the routine double enzyme treatment with alkaline phosphatase and pigeon liver preparation, found that total pantothenic acid content was constant throughout the first month of lactation. A numerical, but nonsignificant, downward trend was present in the data (0.40 mg/100 ml at 10 to 14 days postpartum and 0.35 mg/100 ml at 30 to 45 days postpartum). Of the total pantothenic acid content, 83% was in the free form (0.29 mg/100 ml at the mature stage).

The RIA procedure and the double enzyme extraction using purified pantetheinase was used by Song et al. (22). These authors found that 85-90% of the vitamin was in the free form. This value agrees with the results of Eitenmiller (unpublished) and shows the importance of the double enzyme treatment in obtaining valid information on the pantothenic acid content of human milk. Song et al. (22) found low, but significant, correlations with the pantothenic acid content of fore and hind milk samples ($r = 0.49$ and 0.53, respectively) and estimated maternal dietary intake. These authors reported a total pantothenic acid level of 0.26 mg/100 ml at 12 weeks postpartum. This level is somewhat lower than that found by Eitenmiller and considerably lower than that reported by Johnston et al. (17). The relatively small difference noted between the values of Song et al. (22) and Eitenmiller is possibly due to differences in response of the microbiological and RIA methods. The higher value for pantothenic acid in mature milk (of 0.67 mg/100 ml) reported by Johnston et al. (17) remains difficult to explain.

REFERENCES

1. Hankin L, Squires S. (1960): An evaluation of the *Lactobacillus viridescens* assay for thiamine. Appl Microbiol, 8, 209-211.

2. Pearson WN. (1967): Thiamine. In: Gyorgy P, Pearson WN, eds, The Vitamins, Vol 7. New York: Academic Press, 53-94.

3. Association Official Analytical Chemists. (1980): Official Methods of Analysis, 13 ed. Arlington, VA.

4. Deibel RH, Evans JB, Niven CF, Jr. (1957): Microbiological assay for thiamin using *Lactobacillus viridescens*. J Bacteriol, 74, 818-821.

5. Feeley RM, Eitenmiller RR, Jones JB, Barnhart HM. (1982): Niacin, riboflavin, thiamin, mineral and ash contents of human milk. Institute of Food Technologists Annual Meeting. Las Vegas, NV. (Abstract).

6. Department of Health and Social Security. (1977): The composition of human milk. London: Her Majesty's Stationery Office.

7. Macy I, Kelly H. (1961): Human milk and cow's milk in infant nutrition. In: Kon SK, Cowie AT, eds, Milk: The Mammary Gland and Its Secretion. New York: Academic Press, 265-304.

8. Egberg DC. (1979): Semiautomated method for niacin and niacinamide in food products: collaborative study. J Assoc Off Anal Chem, 62, 1027-1030.

9. Skeggs HR. (1963): Biotin. In: Kavanagh F, ed, Analytical Microbiology. New York: Academic Press, 421-443.

10. Goldsmith SJ, Eitenmiller RR, Feeley RM, Barnhart HM, Maddox FC. (1982): Biotin content of human milk during early lactational stages. Nutr Res, 2, 579-583.

11. Hood RL, Johnson AR. (1980): Supplementation of infant formulations with biotin. Nutr Reports International, 21, 727-731.

12. Macy IG. (1949): Composition of human colostrum and milk. Am J Dis Child, 78, 589-603.

13. Bird OD, Thompson RQ. (1967): Pantothenic Acid. In: Gyorgy P, Pearson WN, eds, The Vitamins, Vol 7. New York: Academic Press, 209-241.

14. Skeggs HR, Wright LD. (1944): The use of *Lactobacillus arabinosus* in the microbiological determination of pantothenic acid. J Biol Chem, 156, 21-26.

15. Wyse BW, Wittwer C, Hansen RG. (1979): Radioimmunoassay for pantothenic acid in blood and other tissues. Clin Chem, 25, 108-111.

16. Walsh, JH, Wyse BW, Hansen RG. (1980): A comparison of microbiological and radioimmunoassay methods for the determination of pantothenic acid. J Food Biochem, 3, 175-189.

17. Johnston L, Vaughan L, Fox HM. (1981): Pantothenic acid content of human milk. Am J Clin Nutr, 34, 2205-2209.

18. Posati LP, Orr ML. (1976): Composition of Foods. Dairy and egg products, raw processed, prepared. United States Department of Agriculture Handbook, 8-1.

19. Schmidt V. (1950): Content of pantothenic acid and alanine in human milk. Int J Vitam Nutr Res, 22, 21-26.

20. Karlin R. (1957): Recherches sur les vitamines dans le lait de femme ll. Teneur en acide pantothenique. Variations au cours de la lactation. Soc Biol Compt Rend (Paris), 151, 1521-1524.

21. Pellegrini DY, Chiari G. (1955): La determinazione microbiologica dell' acido pantothenico. Int J Vitam Nutr Res, 26, 32-35.

22. Song WO, Chan GM, Wyse BW, Hansen RG. (1984): Effect of panto thenic acid status on the content of the vitamin in human milk. Am J Clin Nutr, 40, 317-324.

ANALYSIS OF FAT-SOLUBLE VITAMINS IN MILK: VITAMINS D AND K

B. W. Hollis

INTRODUCTION

The assessment of fat soluble vitamins in native milk has been an area of research spanning several decades (1-13). Early studies designed to determine the fat soluble vitamin content of milk were based on either colorimetric reactions (1-3,8,9), or bioassay (5,7). Later studies designed to quantitate these compounds in milk involved high-performance liquid chromatography (HPLC) and/or competitive protein-binding analysis (CPBA) (4,6,10-13).

The complexity of current methods for assessing the various fat soluble vitamins in native milk varies greatly, primarily due to great variances among the respective concentrations of the vitamins in this fluid. Vitamins A and E are relatively easy to quantitate in milk by using direct ultra-violet (UV) absorption following HPLC, since they occur in microgram/ml (10^{-6}) amounts (4,13). Vitamin K_1 (phylloquinone) can also be quantitated in native milk using direct UV absorption following HPLC; however, large sample sizes and significant preparative chromatography are required because vitamin K is present in native milk in the nanogram/ml (10^{-9}) range (6). The most difficult of the fat soluble vitamins to quantitate in native milk is undoubtedly vitamin D. Vitamin D and its major metabolite, 25-hydroxyvitamin D (25-OH-D), occur in native milk in the picogram/ml (10^{-12}) range (10,11). This low concentration of vitamin D in milk prohibits its direct quantitation by UV absorption and necessitates the use of CPBA for final quantitation. However, prior to CPBA quantitation of vitamin D or 25-OH-D in milk, HPLC must be employed to ensure sample purity. This process eliminates the chance of spurious results in the CPBA. In the past, such results have occurred due to non-specific interferences (14).

In this paper I will describe the appropriate procedures involved in obtaining valid measurements of vitamins D and K in native human milk. These methods are quite involved and require the use of both HPLC and/or CPBA. However, "shortcuts" in the analysis of these compounds in milk will result in spurious results with questionable validity.

MATERIALS AND METHODS

Sample Collection

The following requirements are recommended to ensure meaningful data from samples to be analyzed. The milk sample should be from at least a total breast-expression, preferably collected with an electric pump. The sample should then be stored at a minimum of -20°C. Upon thawing, the sample should be violently shaken to ensure homogeneous mixing prior to subsampling for analysis.

Variables

Variables known to affect the vitamin status of milk include maternal diet, maternal drug intake, lactational stage and, in the case of vitamin D, subject race. It is good practice to know all of the above prior to analysis and subsequent reporting of results.

Vitamin D Analysis

Compounds. ($1\alpha,2\alpha$ - ^3H)-Vitamin D_3 (12.3 Ci/mmol) was obtained from The Radiochemical Center (Amersham, Arlington Heights, IL). (26,27-^3H)-25-OH-D_3 (90 Ci/mmol) and (26,27-^3H)-25-OH-D_2 (90 Ci/mmol) were gifts from Drs. R.L. Horst, T.A. Reinhardt (Ames, Iowa), and J.L. Napoli (Dallas, TX). Vitamins D_2, D_3 (Sigma, St. Louis, MO), 25-OH-D_3 (Upjohn Col, Kalamazoo, MI) and 25-OH-D_2 (Drs. Horst and Reinhardt) were obtained to serve as standards in the forthcoming procedures.

Solvents. HPLC grade methanol, methylene chloride, chloroform, ethyl acetate, hexane, isopropanol and acetonitrile were purchased from Fisher Scientific (Pittsburgh, PA). All other reagents used in the procedure were of reagent grade unless otherwise noted.

Milk Extraction. The milliliters of whole milk were placed in a 50-ml screw-top glass centrifuge tube. To each milk sample were added 1,000 cpm of the following radioactive standards for monitoring the analytical recoveries of the assay: (^3H)-vitamin D_3; (^3H)-25-OH-D_2 and (^3H)-25-OH-D_3. After vortex-mixing of the milk samples, the lipids were extracted using potassium carbonate: ethyl acetate. To accomplish this extraction, 0.17 milk volume of saturated potassium carbonate was added to each sample and mixed well. Next, 0.8 milk volume of distilled water was added, mixed well, and followed by the addition of 3 milk volumes of ethyl acetate with further mixing. The samples were then centrifuged at 1,000 x g for 5 minutes at 20°C. This was followed by removal of the upper organic phase by aspiration. Three additional milk volumes of ethyl acetate were reintroduced to each sample, and the procedure was repeated. The organic phases were combined and dried under N_2 in preparation of the alkaline backwash.

Alkaline backwash. The organic residue from the extraction procedure was resuspended in 2.5 ml of methylene chloride. The methylene chloride solution was then mixed with 5 ml of 0.2 M Na_2HPO_4 (pH 10.5). Following mixing, 5 ml of a mixture of chloroform: hexane (5:1, v/v) was added with further mixing. The samples were then centrifuged at 1,000 x g for 5 minutes at 20°C. This was followed by removal of the lower organic phase by aspiration. The organic layer was then dried under N_2 and stored in isopropanol at -20°C.

Preparative chromatography. Silica Sep-Pak preparative chromatography cartridges (Waters Associates, Milford, MA) are used to eliminate some contaminating lipids and also to separate vitamin D from 25-OH-D (Fig. 1). If the organic extracts have been stored in isopropanol, they should again be brought to complete dryness under N_2. The Sep-Pak cartridges are prepared and equilibrated by eluting 3 ml methanol, 4 ml isopropanol and, finally, 7 ml hexane. The samples are applied to the Sep-Pak in 0.25 ml x 2 washes of 25% methylene chloride in hexane. The cartridges are then eluted under vacuum with a Sep-Pak cartridge rack (Waters Assoc.). The following sequence is used: 9 ml hexane (discard), 3 ml 7% ethyl acetate in hexane (discard), 15 ml 7% ethyl acetate in hexane (vitamins D_2 and D_3), 2.5 ml 15% ethyl acetate in hexane (discard), and 9.5 ml 3% isopropanol in hexane (25-OH-D_2 and 25-OH-D_3). The fractions collected are dried under N_2 in preparation for further chromatography.

The vitamin D fraction is further purified using a silica Bond Elut cartridge (Analytichem International, Harbor City, CA). The Bond Elut columns are prepared and equilibrated by eluting with 4 ml 20% isopropanol in methylene chloride and 5 ml 0.2% isopropanol in methylene chloride. The vitamin D fraction is applied to the Bond Elut cartridge in 0.125 ml x 2 washes of 0.2% isopropanol in methylene chloride. The cartridges are then eluted under vacuum using the Sep-Pak cartridge rack with the following sequence: 2 ml 0.2% isopropanol in methylene chloride (discard) and 8 ml 0.2% isopropanol in methylene chloride (vitamin D). The collection is dried under N_2 and stored in isopropanol at -20°C until further analysis.

The 25-OH-D fraction eluted from the Sep-Pak cartridges was further purified on a column (0.7 x 12 cm) of Sephadex LH-20 (Pharmacia, Piscataway, N.J.) developed in and eluted with hexane: chloroform: methanol (9:1:1, v/v), as previously described (11).

The 25-OH-D fraction (containing both 25-OH-D_2 and 25-OH-D_3) from this chromatographic system was collected, dried under N_2, and stored at -20°C in isopropanol until further analysis.

High-performance liquid chromatography. Final purification of vitamins D_2, D_3, 25-OH-D_2 and 25-OH-D_3, prior to quantitation by competitive protein binding assay (CPBA), was performed using various HPLC systems. Normal-phase HPLC was performed using a 0.4 x 25 cm Zorbax-Sil column (Dupont, Wilmington, Del.). Reverse-phase HPLC was carried out using a 0.4 x 25 cm Vydac-ODS column (Separations Group, Hisperia, CA) on a Beckman Model 344 high-performance liquid chromatograph.

The vitamin D fraction from the Bond Elut cartridge was purified further, using two separate HPLC systems (Fig. 1). The first system was normal-phase and was developed in hexane: methylene chloride: isopropanol (49.75: 49.75: 0.5, v/v), with a flow rate of 2 ml/min (15). Vitamins D_2 and D_3 coeluted on this system, with their retention time being approximately 8 minutes. The vitamin D peak from this system was collected and applied to the final HPLC system (reverse-phase), which separated vitamin D_2 from vitamin D_3. This system was developed in acetonitrile: chloroform (95:5, v/v), with a flow rate of 1.75 ml/min. Under these conditions, vitamin D_2 eluted at approximately 10 minutes, while vitamin D_3 eluted at approximately 12 minutes. The fractions containing vitamin D_2 and D_3 were collected independently, dried under N_2, and suspended in absolute ethanol for assay and recovery estimates. The 25-OH-D fraction from the Sephadex LH-20 was purified by HPLC, using a single normal-phase chromatographic

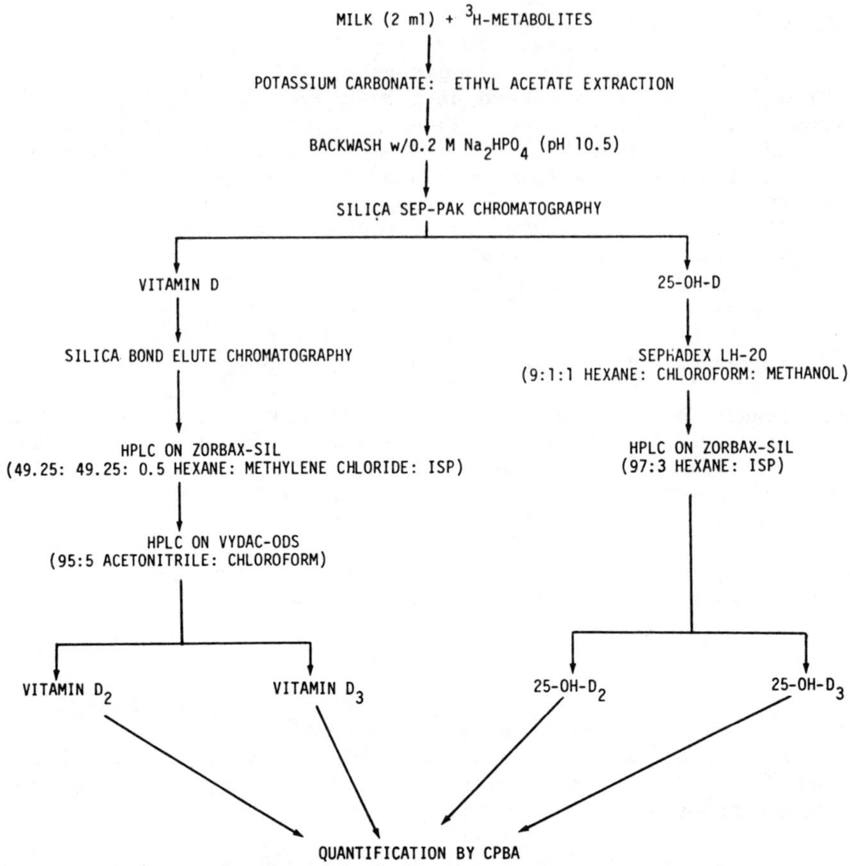

Figure 1. Schematic of the purification and ultimate quantification steps used for the assay of vitamins D_2, D_3, 25-OH-D_2 and 25-OH-D_3 in human milk.

system developed in hexane: isopropanol (97:3, v/v), with a flow rate of 2ml/min. This system separates 25-OH-D_2 from 25-OH-D_3; these compounds have retention times of approximately 8.5 and 10.5 minutes, respectively, under these conditions. These two fractions were collected independently, dried under N_2, and suspended in absolute ethanol for assay and recovery estimates.

Competitive protein binding analysis. Vitamins D_2, D_3, 25-OH-D_2 and 25-OH-D_3 were quantitated by CPBA using previously described procedures (11). Briefly, these assays utilized the rat plasma vitamin D-binding protein that was diluted 1:35,000 in 0.05 of borate buffer (pH 8.4) containing 0.02% gelatin. Each assay mixture was placed into 12 x 75-mm borosilicate glass tubes and consisted of: (1) 0.5 ml of 1:35,000 rat plasma diluted in buffer (above); (2) standard vitamin D_2, 2D3, 25-OH-D_2, 25-OH-D_3 or unknowns in 25 μl of ethanol; and (3) 5,000 cpm of (^{3}H)-25-OH-D_3 in 25 μl ethanol. However, addition of this final component to the assay tubes was delayed due to the use of nonequilibrium conditions (11). For the vitamin D_2 and D_3 assays, a 24-hour preincubation was used prior to the addition of (^{3}H)-25-OH-D_3, which was permitted to incubate for an additional hour before separation of bound and free sterol. The

Table 1. Vitamins D_2, D_3, 25-OH-D_2 AND 25-OH-D_3 in human milk samples.[a]

		Sterol (pg/ml ± SD)			
Subject Treatment	Sample No.	VITAMIN D_2	VITAMIN D_3	25-OH-D_2	25-OH-D_3
Vitamin D (10 g day/4 wks)	2	152 ± 40	99 ± 9	101 ± 7	238 ± 116
Vitamin D (10 g day/3 mon)	2	56 ± 6	124 ± 37	48 ±15	297 ± 121
Vitamin D (60 g day/2 wks)	1	2,670	120	127	100
Pre UV Exposure	2	51 ±20	115 ± 84	101 ± 42	151 ± 81
Post UV Exposure[b]	2	43 ± 19	2,800 ± 1,294	131 ± 43	203 ± 34

[a] Source: Hollis (11).
[b] Samples were obtained 48 hours following the subjects' exposure to 1.5 minimal erythema irradiation.

25-OH-D_2 and 25-OH-D_3 assays were performed in a similar fashion, but for only a 2-hour preincubation prior to the addition of tracer. Bound sterol was separated from free sterol using dextran-coated charcoal, as previously described (11).

The standard curve range for vitamins D_2, D_3, 25-OH-D_2 and 25-OH-D_3 was 0.02-0.4, 0.01-0.25, 0.01-0.05, and 0.01-0.05 ng, respectively. The entire assay procedure is depicted in Fig. 1. Data generated from an assay procedure of this type if listed on Table 1.

Calculations. Final concentrations of each sterol can be calculated by hand from a standard curve constructed from plotting cpm (^{3}H)-25-OH-D_3 bound vs. standard concentration. Alternatively, the standard curve data may be transformed and calculated using a logit/log transformation (16). The amount of unknown per tube is then corrected for dilution and final recovery, with the results expressed in picograms per millimeter of milk.

Vitamin K Analysis

Vitamin K_1 (phylloquinone) in native milk should be assessed as previously described (6).

DISCUSSION

Only in the last few years has the vitamin D content of human milk been adequately defined (10,11). Prior to this work, bioassay data existed which roughly defined the antirachitic properties of human milk (7), but (as with most bioassay data) the variability was large. The primary reason for the delay in defining the vitamin D content of milk was a lack in acceptable technology. Until CPBA coupled with HPLC became available, the task of defining the actual vitamin D content of milk was impossible. Hollis et al. (10) demonstrated that vitamin D and its major metabolites 25-OH-D, 24, 25-$(OH)_2$-D and 1,25-$(OH)_2$-D were all present in human milk. However, it appears that only vitamin D and 25-OH-D are quantitatively important in human milk. Under normal circumstances, 25-OH-D accounts for about 80% of the total antirachitic activity in human milk. It is also true that the 25-OH-D content of milk is very difficult to alter because 25-OH-D levels in plasma tend to be very stable. However, it is possible to elevate significantly the amount of parent compound, vitamin D, in milk. This elevation can be accomplished either by dietary increases in vitamin D or ultraviolet phototherapy (11,17). In fact, we have observed a case where human milk had potentially toxic amounts of vitamin D due to the mother's huge dietary supplementation (18).

The literature is very sparse concerning the vitamin K content of human milk. Dam et al. (5) first reported the vitamin K content of human milk. Their study was based on a curative bioassay in chicks. As with most bioassays, the results obtained by Dam et al. varied widely from sample to sample. Furthermore, the relevance of the values obtained in this study are doubtful because the vitamin K compound used to standardize the bioassay was menadione, which is not a naturally occurring form of vitamin K. Based on the above bioassay data, Dam et al. (5) found human milk to contain 15 µg phylloquinone/liter.

Haroon et al. (6), using HPLC, have provided direct ultraviolet quantitation of phylloquinone in human milk. They found human milk to contain 2.5 µg/liter phylloquinone, far less than that reported by Dam et al. (5). Further, Haroon et al. (6) found human colostrum and cows' milk to contain 2.3 and 4.9 µg/liter phylloquinone, respectively.

The methods that Haroon et al. (6) used to quantitate and identify vitamin K appear to be quite sound, but, like vitamin D analysis, very cumbersome. Briefly, their analysis involved extracting a 5-20 ml milk sample using the method of Folch et al. (19). The sample was further purified using preparative column chromatography, semipreparative HPLC and, finally, UV quantitation following analytical HPLC. Vitamin K isolated in this fashion was further identified using direct probe mass spectrometry. This study also demonstrated the ability of maternal oral supplementation of vitamin K to increase the amount of that compound present in the milk.

Appropriate methods for the analysis of any substance in milk should be well conceived and tested prior to the reporting of data. This will help avoid the propagation of inaccurate studies, such as those reported for vitamin D sulfate (8,9). Vitamin D sulfate in human milk was supposed to be the answer to the question of why breast-fed infants rarely suffered from rickets (9). These studies based their quantitation of vitamin D sulfate on an insensitive and very nonspecific colorimetric assay procedure. In fact, vitamin D sulfate likely does not exist in human milk (12), and even if it did, it has been shown to be biologically inactive (20). This report about vitamin D sulfate clouded the pediatric literature for more than a decade.

ACKNOWLEDGEMENT

This work was supported in part by Grant HD-16510 and Research Career Development Award HD-000479 from the NIH. I gratefully acknowledge Pamela Woodruff for the typing of this manuscript.

REFERENCES

1. Kon SK, Mawson EH. (1950): Human milk. Wartime studies of certain vitamins and other constituents. Med Res Council Spec Rep Ser No. 269. London: His Majesty's Stationery Office.

2. Medhin-Gebre M, Vahlquist H, Hofvander Y, Uppsall L, Vahlquist B. (1976): Breast milk composition in Ethiopian and Swedish mothers. I. Vitamin A and β - carotene. Am J Clin Nutr, 29, 441-451.

3. Quaife ML. (1947): Tocopherols in milk: their chemical determination and occurrence in human milk. J Biol Chem, 169, 513-514.

4. Jansson L, Akesson B, Holmberg L. (1981): Vitamin E and fatty acid composition of human milk. Am J Clin Nutr, 34, 8-13.

5. Dam H, Glavind J, Larsen EH, Plum P. (1942): Investigations into the cause of the physiological hypoprothrombinemia in newborn children. IV. The vitamin K content of women's milk and cow's milk. Acta Med Scand, 112, 210-216.

6. Haroon Y, Shearer MJ, Rahim S, Gunn WG, McEnery G, Barkhan P. (1982): The content of phylloquinone (vitamin K_1) in human milk, cows' milk and infant formula foods determined by high-performance liquid chromatography. J Nutr, 112, 1105-1117.

7. Harris RS, Bunker JW. (1939): Vitamin D potency of human breast milk. Am J Publ Health, 29, 744-747.

8. Sahashi Y, Suzuki T, Higaki M, Ansano T. (1967): Metabolism of vitamin D in animals. V. Isolation of vitamin D sulfate from mammalian milk. J Nutr Sci Vitaminol, 13, 33-36.

9. Lakdawala DR, Widdowson EM. (1977): Vitamin D in human milk. Lancet, i, 167-168.

10. Hollis BW, Roos BA, Draper HH, Lambert PW. (1981): Vitamin D and its metabolites in human and bovine milk. J Nutr, 111, 1240-1248.

11. Hollis BW. (1983): Individual quantitation of vitamin D_2, vitamin D_3, 25-hydroxyvitamin D_2 and 25-hydroxyvitamin D_3 in human milk. Anal Biochm, 131, 211-219.

12. Hollis BW, Roos BA, Draper HH, Lambert PW. (1981): Occurrence of vitamin D sulfate in human milk whey. J Nutr, 111, 384-390.

13. Chappel JE, Francis T, Clandinin MT. (1983): Vitamin A and E content of human milk at early stages of lactation. Fed Proc, 42, 920.

14. Osborn TW, Norman AW. (1977): A 25-hydroxycholecalciferol-like compound in milk as determined by specific competitive binding radioassays. In: Norman AW, ed, Vitamin D: Biochemical, Chemical and Clinical Aspects Related to Calcium Metabolism. Berlin: deGruyter, 523-525.

15. Hollis BW, Pittard WB. (1984): Evaluation of the total fetomaternal vitamin D relationships at term: evidence for racial differences. J Clin Endo Metab, 59, 652-657.

16. Chard T. (1978): An Introduction to Radioimmunoassay and Related Techniques. N.Y.: North-Holland, 440.

17. Greer FR, Hollis BW, Cripps DJ, Tsang RC. (1984): Effects of maternal ultraviolet B irradiation on vitamin D content of human milk. J Pediat, 105, 431-433.

18. Greer FR, Hollis BW, Napoli JL. (1984): High concentrations of vitamin D_2 in human milk associated with pharmacologic doses of vitamin D_2. J Pediat, 105, 61-64.

19. Folch J, Rees M, Stanley GHS. (1957): A simple method for the isolation and purification of total lipids from animal sources. J Biol Chem, 226, 497-509.

20. Reeve LE, DeLuca HF, Schnoes HK. (1981): Synthesis and biological activity of vitamin D_3-sulfate. J Biol Chem, 256, 823-826.

ANALYSIS OF FAT-SOLUBLE VITAMINS IN HUMAN MILK

VITAMINS E AND A

C. J. Lammi-Keefe
P. R. Borum
F. M. Verda

INTRODUCTION

The analysis of the fat-soluble vitamins in human milk can currently be accomplished with relative ease, sensitivity and precision with high performance liquid chromatography (HPLC). HPLC has permitted the separation and quantitation of closely related isomers and/or metabolites while allowing recovery of sample components. It is the method of choice for prospective studies involving the quantitation of the fat-soluble vitamins in human milk.

There is still much to be learned about the factors that may influence the levels of vitamins E and A in breast milk. Because information is incomplete at the present time, the recommendations for sampling, handling and storage, and analysis are conservative. Until new data are available, the following recommendations may serve as guides to researchers and those individuals who are handling human milk for banking purposes.

SAMPLING

Because the amounts of milk lipids are variable and change during a feeding, diurnally, and in response to diet and stage of lactation, it is recommended that samples for analysis of fat-soluble vitamins be taken under standard conditions, as outlined by Ferris and Jensen (1) and discussed in a separate workshop of this conference (2). In brief, a 24-hour sample from both breasts would represent the ideal. The total content of one breast is the minimum acceptable sample, and, when possible, the pooled total-breast collection from both breasts at an a.m. and p.m. sampling would be preferable to the single sampling. Because it simulates the suckling infant and can most completely empty the breast, the Egnell electric breast pump (Egnell, Inc., Cary, IL) is the instrument of choice for collecting milk. There is a correlation between total tocopherol and lipid content of mature milk (3,4,5); therefore, standard sampling conditions that control for lipid content (e.g., total-breast emptying) should be ensured.

Among the variables that may influence levels of fat-soluble vitamins in human milk are lactational stage, gestational age, and maternal diet and supplements (6). Data from our laboratory demonstrate that stage of lactation clearly is a factor that affects α-tocopherol levels of breast

Table 1. Alpha-tocopherol content of breast milk at 2 and 16 weeks postpartum (μg/100 mls)

Subject	2 weeks	16 weeks
1	711.4	498.8
2	1042.9	349.4
3	804.7	444.6
4	399.8	233.2

milk (Table 1). Between 2 and 16 weeks postpartum α-tocopherol decreased. Linear decreases in milk vitamin A also have been observed between the first and sixth weeks of lactation (7).

Maternal serum retinol was correlated with retinol in human milk, indicating an influence of maternal diet on levels of vitamin A in breast milk (8). This relationship between milk A and maternal diet is similar to that reported by Hollis (9) for milk vitamin D.

The importance of controlling for the above factors during sampling is apparent. Additionally, mothers should be screened for absence of medical risks (or pathologies should be noted) and use of medications known to interfere with lactation should be recorded (1).

STORAGE AND HANDLING OF SAMPLES

Samples may be stored in glass or polypropylene bottles, protected from light. Teflon-lined caps are recommended. Milk samples to be stored should be placed on dry ice immediately and transferred to a -70°C freezer until analysis. Because the lipid-soluble vitamins exhibit surprising stability, duration of storage may not be a critical problem at -70°C; however, storage stability studies have not been performed.

In preparation for extraction and analysis, milk samples should be quickly and completely thawed at about 40°C, and they should be thoroughly swirled to ensure complete mixing of fat and aqueous fractions prior to aliquot transfer. The mixing step should be repeated between removing aliquots.

EXTRACTION AND ANALYSIS

Vitamin E

Methods of analysis for vitamin E have included colorimetry, fluorometry, GLC, and, most recently, HPLC. The popular colorimetric methods present problems with specificity (10) and reproducibility (11), and the TLC (12) or combined thin-layer/gas chromatographic methods (13) are complex. The only satisfactory method for the measurement of tocopherols in food is HPLC, which is sensitive and reproducible, allowing the separation of α-tocopherol and its isomers.

Milk samples for vitamin E analysis by HPLC may be extracted by using a one-step n-hexane extraction, as detailed by Jansson (3), or by using a modified Folch procedure (14,15). The advantage of the one-step procedure is its speed. However, the advisability of expressing tocopherol content in terms of total polyunsaturated fatty acids (16), warrants the use of the latter procedure. Other extraction methods that probably extract nearly total lipids (e.g., Roese-Gottlieb and dry column methods) presumably also could be used (17). Total lipid before injection is determined gravimetrically. The lipid extracted with either procedure can be solubilized in hexane and injected directly into the HPLC without further fractionation for vitamin E quantitation (3,18). Use of the modified Folch procedure obviates the necessity of two separate extractions to quantitate total lipid (and P/S ratio) and vitamin E. In general, extraction of 4.0 to 5.0 ml milk samples usually provides adequate lipid for both quintuplicate 10 μl injections into the HPLC and lipid for total fatty acid determinations (18).

Table 2 shows the HPLC operating conditions that have been successful in our hands for separation and quantitation of the tocopherol isomers in a milk extract obtained using the modified Folch procedure. Each run can be completed in approximately ten minutes. These operating conditions allow separation of the four tocopherol isomers, though only α- and γ-tocopherol have been present in sufficiently large amounts to permit quantitation.

Quantitation is accomplished by constructing a standard curve of isomer concentration vs. ratio of integrated peak areas of the external standard, α-tocopherol acetate, and the isomer. The regression formula derived from regression analysis for each curve can be used to quantitate the vitamin E in milk samples. Because we are working with small volumes, we make an assumption regarding lipid density in order that lipid concentration can be determined. For our calculations, we assume that the lipid density is 0.91 g/cc (19).

Precision is 95% for the determination of α-tocopherol by this method, and the detection level for α-tocopherol is approximately 30 μg/100 ml milk, more than 10-fold lower than the amount found in mature breast milk.

Table 2. HPLC operating conditions for separating tocopherol isomers

Instrument:	Varian Model 5000 Liquid Chromatograph
Column:	Alltech-NH2, (25 cm x 4.6 mm)
Solvents:	n-hexane:2-propanol (98:2)
Flow rate:	2.0 ml/min
Detector:	UV, 290 nm
Absorbance Range:	0.01

Use of this system provides the added safety advantage that elution with di-isopropyl ether (20) is avoided. Di-isopropyl ether may also contain peroxides, which can be absorbed on the columns, destroying tocopherols during chromatography (21).

Vitamin A

Vitamin A is present in human milk as retinol, retinyl esters and, as its precursor, β-carotene (8,22). While the established spectrophotometric and Carr-Price colorimetric procedures may be used to determine total retinoids, resolution of these requires lengthy chromatographic procedures (23). Furthermore, the carotenoid pigments, which may be substantial in human milk (8,24) and, to a lesser degree, vitamin D of milk, interfere with the Carr-Price colorimetric procedure. Vitamin A in milk may also be determined by fluorometry (25), but that procedure requires saponification, which can cause extensive degradation of retinoids (26). Interference from unrecognized fluorescent substances is also a possibility (25).

HPLC has gained in popularity for the analysis of retinoids due to stability of retinoids on HPLC columns, sensitivity and resolution, rapidity of analyses, and ability to separate not only the isomers (26), but retinoids of different oxidative states. Methods have been reported that use HPLC to quantitate vitamin A as retinol or retinyl palmitate in foods and infant formulas (27) and as retinyl palmitate and β-carotene in cows' milk (25). However, there are no published methods for resolving and determining retinol, retinyl esters and β-carotene in human milk. Landen (27) reports a reverse-phase HPLC method for quantitating vitamin A in formulas. That method involves fractionation of the vitamins from the lipid material with high performance gel permeation chromatography followed by quantitation of retinol, retinyl esters and β-carotene using non-aqueous reverse-phase HPLC.

Following the schema described by Landen (27), a specific method for quantitating vitamin A in human milk would entail: (a) organic extraction for removal of lipids from milk, (b) semipreparative chromatography for lipid removal and fractionation of the retinoids and carotenoids (Sep-Pak cartridges may be useful for this step), and (c) resolution of the retinol, retinyl esters and β-carotene by HPLC, followed by quantitation using direct UV or fluorometric analysis.

SUMMARY

Recommended methods for the analysis of vitamins E and A in human milk have been outlined. Guidelines for sampling to ensure a representative sample and for handling and storage to minimize loss of activity are also detailed. The HPLC method described for the analysis of tocopherol is precise and can be used with ease. Total lipid extracts can be analyzed directly by HPLC. Resolution of the four tocopherol isomers can be achieved, though alpha- and gamma- are the predominant isomers in human milk. The recommended method for vitamin A is direct analysis by HPLC following extraction from the milk, removal of other lipids, and partial purification of the vitamin.

REFERENCES

1. Ferris AM, Jensen RG. (1984): Lipids in human milk: a review. 1. Sampling, determination and content. J Ped Gastroenterol Nutr, 3, 108-122.

2. Woolridge MW, Butte N. et al. Methods for the measurement of milk volume intake of the breast-fed infant. (These proceedings).

3. Jansson L, Akesson B, Holmberg L. (1981): Vitamin E and fatty acid composition of human milk. Am J Clin Nutr, 34, 8-13.

4. Harris PH, Quaife ML, O'Grady P. (1952): Tocopherol content of human milk and of cow's milk products used for infant feeding. J Nutr, 46, 459-466.

5. Lammi-Keefe CJ, Moffat PA, Ferris AM, Clark RM, Jensen RG. (1985): Alpha-tocopherol and total lipid contents of milk at 2, 6, 12, and 16 weeks postpartum. Fed Proc, 44, 1855.

6. Lammi-Keefe CJ, Jensen RG. (1984): Fat-soluble vitamins in human milk. Nutr Rev, 42, 365-371.

7. Chappell JE, Francis T, Clandinin MT. (1982): Vitamin A and E content of human milk at early stages of lactation. Fed Proc, 42, 920.

8. Butte NF, Calloway DH. (1981): Evaluation of lactational performance of Navajo women. Am J Clin Nutr, 34, 2210-2215.

9. Hollis BW. Analysis of fat-soluble vitamins in milk: determination of vitamins D and K. (These proceedings).

10. Kobayashi H, Kanno C., Yamauchi K. Tsugo T. (1975): Identification of α-, β-, γ-, and ∂-tocopherols and their contents in human milk. Biochim Biophys Acta, 380, 282-290.

11. Taylor SL, Lamden MP, Tappel AL. (1976): Sensitive fluorometric method for tissue tocopherol analysis. Lipids, 11, 530-538.

12. Stowe HD. (1963): Separation of β- and γ-tocopherol. Arch Biochim Biophys, 103, 42-44.

13. Lovelady HG. (1973): Separation of individual tocopherols from human plasma and red blood cells by thin-layer and gas-liquid chromatography. J. Chromatogr, 85, 81-92.

14. Folch J, Lees M, Sloan-Stanley GH. (1957): A simple method for the isolation and purification of total lipids from animal tissue. J Biol Chem, 226, 497-509.

15. Clark RM, Ferris AM, Fey M, Brown PB, Hundrieser KE, Jensen RG. (1982): Changes in the lipids of human milk from 2 to 16 weeks postpartum. J Pediatr Gastroenterol Nutr, 1, 311-315.

16. Bieri JG, Tolliver TJ, Catignani GL. Simultaneous determination of α-tocopherol and retinol in plasma and red cells by high pressure liquid chromatography. Am J Clin Nutr, 32, 2143-2149.

17. Lammi-Keefe CJ, Jensen RG. (1984): Lipids in human milk: a review. 2. Composition and fat-soluble vitamins, J Ped Gastroenterol Nutr, 3, 172-198.

18. Verda FM. (1984): Analysis of tocopherol in human milk. M.S. Thesis. Storrs, CT: University of Connecticut.

19. Mulder H, Walstra P. (1974): The milk fat globule. Wageningen, the Netherlands: Centre Agricultural Publications and Documents.

20. Jansson L, Milsson B, Lindgren R. (1980): Quantitation of serum tocopherols by high-performance liquid chromatography with fluorescence detection. J Chromatogr, 181, 242-247.

21. Manz U, Philipp K. (1981): A method for the routine determination of tocopherols in animal feed and human foodstuffs with the aid of high performance liquid chromatography. Internat J Vit Nutr Res, 51, 342-348.

22. Moore T. (1957): The transfer of vitamin A from mother to offspring. In: Moore T, ed, Vitamin A. London: Elsevier, 245-257.

23. Roberts AB, Nichols MD, Frolik CA, Newton DL, Sporn MB. (1978): Assay of retinoids in biological samples by reverse-phase high-pressure liquid chromatography. Canc Res, 38, 3327-3332.

24. Gebre-Medhin M, Vahlquist A, Hofvander Y, Upsall L, Vahlquist B. (1976): Breast milk composition in Ethiopian and Swedish mothers. I. Vitamin A and B-Carotene. Am J Clin Nutr, 29, 441-451.

25. Thompson JN, Hatina G, Maxwell WB. (1980): High performance liquid chromatographic determination of vitamin A in margarine, milk, partially skimmed milk, and skimmed milk. J Assoc Off Anal Chem, 63, 894-898.

26. Frolik CA, Olson JA. (1984): Extraction, separation, and chemical analysis of retinoids. In: Sporn MB, Roberts, AB, Goodman DS, eds, The retinoids, Volume 1. New York: Academic Press, 181-233.

27. Landen WO. (1982): Application of gel permeation chromatography and nonaqueous reverse phase chromatography to high performance liquid chromatographic determination of retinyl palmitate and α-tocopherol acetate in infant formulas. J Assoc Off Anal Chem, 65, 810-816.

SECTION IX. GROWTH FACTORS IN MILK

WORKSHOP PARTICIPANTS

W. R. Kidwell, Laboratory of Pathophysiology, National Cancer Institute, Bethesda, MD

Y. W. Shing, Departments of Biological Chemistry and Surgery, The Children's Hospital and Harvard Medical School, Boston, MA

F. H. Morriss, Jr., Departments of Pediatrics and of Obstetrics, Gynecology, and Reproductive Sciences, Medical School, University of Texas Health Science Center, Houston, TX

INTRODUCTION

A number of growth factors have been detected in human milk. It has been presumed that these factors are physiologically relevant to the mother or the baby. A critical examination of the attempts to date to demonstrate physiological roles lends support to this postulate for some of the growth factors, but their precise roles are by no means certain.

This presentation reviews the approaches that have been utilized in attempts to answer questions of physiological relevancy for those growth factors that have been well characterized in milk (paper by Morriss). In addition, it includes a description of a number of growth factors that have recently been detected in and (in some cases) highly purified from human milk (papers by Shing et al. and by Kidwell et al.).

In assessing the significance of the presence of growth factors in milk, several important concepts and cautions were formulated. As an example, a new set of growth factors, so-called transforming growth factors or TGFs, was detected using NRK cells, which are exquisitely sensitive to TGFs. These activities were only detected when NRK cell growth was measured in suspension cultures. The point illustrated here is that the detection of new growth factors may be dependent on the assay of milk or milk fractions using special cell types or using cells grown in special environments.

A second major point that emerged, dealt with the quantitation of milk growth factors. Evidence is presented for synergistic interactions between different types of growth factors. Such interactions present a possible pitfall for experimenters who attempt to quantitate a specific growth factor by performing a bioassay of whole milk with and without a neutralizing antiserum. In the case of synergism between growth factors, this type of assay can lead to overestimates in the amount of growth factor present in a milk sample. Underestimates of milk growth factors have also been observed in bioassays of unfractionated milk. These appear to be due to complexing of the growth factor with other milk constituents or to inhibitory substances in milk. A further complexity of growth factor assays in unfractionated milk is seen when more than one milk factor produces the same biological response, e.g., DNA synthesis or anchorage independent growth. Examples are presented in which subfractionation of milk must be accomplished before a particular milk growth factor can be quantitated by a bioassay or even by a radioreceptor assay.

The latter observations emphasize the need for the development of selective immunoassays for the individual milk growth factors. This obviously can only be achieved following extensive growth factor purification.

It is apparent from a review of the literature that the most important need, from a physiological standpoint, is the unequivocable demonstration that the milk factors do act on the mother (breast cells) or the baby (multiple tissue targets). This concept raises several important issues that have not been adequately considered, and it reemphasizes others that are more obvious. Which test systems are appropriate for determining human relevancy? Are there species specificities which preclude the use of certain animal model systems? If some human milk growth factors are found to be inactive in animal model systems, what tests can be ethically and safely performed on human infants? This point is not as moot as one might think, since MDGF1-like activities from mouse and rat sources have different potencies when tested on rat and mouse mammary cells in primary culture.

The last point also leads to a further issue bearing on physiological relevancy, a need for specifying the types of cells that respond to a particular milk growth factor. The possibility that a milk growth factor acts on the mammary epithelium can be tested with human mammary epithelium as explants or isolated epithelium in culture systems that are currently well developed.

METHODS FOR INVESTIGATING THE PRESENCE AND PHYSIOLOGIC ROLE OF GROWTH FACTORS IN MILK

F. H. Morriss, Jr.

Milks of several species have been found to stimulate *in vivo* growth of gastrointestinal tissues, to promote *in vitro* replication of cultured cells, to contain assayable hormones that are known to promote growth, or to contain other substances that are shown to promote growth. In general, such growth-promoting characteristics are more pronounced in colostrum than in mature milk. The biologic significance of growth-promoting activities in colostrum and mature milks is not yet clear. It is not known whether the factors in milk that possess the capacity to stimulate cell proliferation: (a) influence growth of the mammary tissue, (b) promote growth of cells within or comprising the intestines of the recipient neonate, or (c) are absorbed from the neonatal gut, enter the circulation of the neonate, and exert an effect upon enteric or other target organs.

Table I provides a summary of important observations of potential or demonstrated growth-promotion in milk. The table is in a format that permits comparison of human and non-human milks. Evidence has been gathered by: (a) assay in milk or a hormone or other substance that is known or demonstrated to have growth-promoting effects, (b) demonstration that milk or a milk fraction stimulates *in vitro* growth of cells or tissues, and (c) demonstration that milk or a milk fraction stimulates *in vivo* growth of tissues or organs in recipient animals.

Evidence gathered using several of these methods supports the hypothesis that epidermal growth factor (EGF) is an important growth factor in human milk. EGF (or β-urogastrone) has been measured in human milk by both radioreceptor assay (3) and radioimmunoassays (1,2). The concentration of EGF is many-fold greater in precolostrum, colostrum, and mature milk than it is in serum. The EGF concentration decreases rapidly from colostrum to transitional milk; this appears to be a dilutional effect. No diurnal variation has been detected. Mature milk from mothers who gave birth prematurely contains approximately the same EGF concentration found in mature milk from mothers who gave birth at term gestation.

EGF stimulates the growth of various cells or organs in culture, including fetal mouse duodenal mucosal cells (33), and it causes cell proliferation *in vivo*, including rat and mouse gastrointestinal mucosa (34,35). Importantly, the mitogenic activity of human milk that stimulates DNA synthesis by human fibroblasts in cell culture may be significantly, but not completely, blocked by the addition of antibodies to human EGF (21). Further, Read et al. found that the concentration of EGF required to promote significant increases in protein or DNA synthesis by L6, 3T3-L1,

Table 1. Some milk constituents or activities that may promote growth *in vitro* or *in vivo*

Constituent/Activity	Reported to be present in or a property of*	
	Human Milk	Non-human Milk
A. Hormones and other substances with growth-promoting potential assayed in milk		
1. Epidermal growth factor (β-urogastrone)	1,2,3	3,4
2. Insulin	3,5	3,6
3. Thyroxine	7,8,9	10
4. Cortisol	11,12,13	14,15,16
5. LHRH	17	18
6. Human milk growth factors I, II, & III	19,20	
7. Mammary derived growth factor I	21a	
8. Transforming growth factors	21a	
B. Demonstrated *in vitro* effect on growth of cells or tissues		
1. Epidermal growth factor (β-urogastrone) a) antibodies to EGF block mitogenic effect of milk	21	
2. Purified human milk growth factor III (5000-6000 mol. wt.)	19,20	
3. Mammary derived growth factor I	21a	
4. Transforming growth factors	21a	
5. Lactoferrin	22	22
6. Colony stimulating factor (240,000-250,000 mol. wt.)	23	
7. *Bifidobacterium* bifidum growth factors A and B	24,25,26,27	25
C. Demonstrated *in vivo* effect on growth of tissues or organs		
1. Rapid increase in mass of intestinal mucosa in *suckled vs. fasted* newborn animals	28,29	
2. Increased mass of intestinal mucosa secondary to hypertrophy and hyperplasia in *suckled vs. formula-fed* newborn animals	30,31	
3. Increased concentration of and synthesis of DNA in intestines of *colostrum-fed versus mature-milk-fed* newborn animals	32	

* Numbers refer to references, which are representative rather than exhaustive.

and T47D cells *in vitro* is much greater than that found in human colostrum or milk (3). Thus, while EGF is present in high concentrations in human colostrum and milk, and while human milk is a mitogen for certain cells *in vitro* -- an effect which can be significantly blocked by antibodies to EGF, human milk appears to possess additional growth-promoting activity.

Seeking to identify the agent(s) responsible for the balance of mitogenic activity of human milk on several cell lines in culture, Read et al. assayed human milk for insulin by radioimmunoassay (3). Insulin was present in colostrum at concentrations 30 times that in human serum; after the third postpartum day, the insulin concentration in human milk was reduced, but still several-fold that in serum, and it did not decline further. However, as had been found with EGF, the concentration of insulin in colostrum and milk was less than that required to stimulate significant increases in protein and DNA synthesis in several cell lines *in vitro*.

Thyroxine is present in human and primate milks (7,8,9,10). In colostrum the concentration of thyroxine is low; the concentration increases by the first week postpartum, and it gradually declines thereafter. While the principal effect of thyroxine in the developing human infant is maturational rather than mitogenic, there is a body of evidence that supports the notion that the thyroxine present in human milk affords some protection to breast-fed infants with congenital hypothyroidism (8,36). There also is intriguing evidence in several species suggesting that suckling promotes TRH release in the lactating mammal and that TRH concentration in turn increases in the milk of a suckled female and remains biologically active in her milk and in the neonatal stomach (37). Whether neonatal gastrointestinal absorption of TRH obtained from milk is responsible for the increased levels of TSH reported in suckled infants, when compared with age-matched weaned infants, remains speculative.

Cortisol is present in relatively high concentration in mammary secretions during late gestation and in colostrum (13). The concentration declines rapidly by the second postpartum day and remains low thereafter. It has been postulated that one role of cortisol in milk is to control the transport of fluids and salts in the gastrointestinal tract of infants (13). On the other hand, it is possible to postulate a role for milk glucocorticoids in the growth of the pancreas of the suckled neonate. In the suckling rat pup administration of hydrocortisone at physiological doses produces both hyperplasia and hypertrophy of the pancreas (38). This effect is opposite to that which glucocorticoids have on somatic growth and on cellular proliferation in the liver, heart, kidneys, and adrenals of immature rats. Moreover, the hyperplastic effect on the pancreas is lost after weaning. There is some evidence that the growth of the pancreas proceeds more rapidly in colostrum-fed newborn animals than in mature milk-fed littermates (*vide infra*).

Somewhat surprisingly, LHRH is present in milk in high concentrations (17,18). Whether ingested LHRH in milk promotes release of gonadotropins, which in turn play some role in growth processes, is still only speculative. The presence of TRH and LHRH in milk raises the question of whether these, or indeed other, substances of hypothalamic origin play a role in the infant's hypothalmic-pituitary axis and possibly modulate neonatal hormone responses that affect growth (*vide infra*).

Klagsbrun and his co-workers have isolated and characterized three polypeptides in human colostrum and milk which have been called human milk growth factors I, II, and III (19,20). Factor III has a molecular weight of 5000-6000; this polypeptide stimulates DNA synthesis and cellular proliferation in cultured fibroblasts and epithelial cells. Human milk growth factor III has many properties that suggest that it is EGF. Bovine colostrum possesses similar growth-promoting activity, but cannot sustain the long-term growth of cultured fibroblasts (39). Klagsbrun has subsequently shown that addition of fibronectin, an adhesion-promoting factor that is very low in concentration in bovine colostrum relative to serum, permits long-term growth of fibroblasts to be supported by bovine milk (40). The issues of whether human milk contains fibronectin and, if so, whether it exerts any influence on growth in the recipient infant, are presently only speculative.

Kidwell and his colleagues have detected two additional classes of growth factors in human milk (21a). Mammary-derived growth factor I, a 62,000 molecular weight protein with $P_I = 4.8$, stimulates mammary cells and rat kidney cells *in vitro* to synthesize extracellular matrix proteins, including collagen. Several transforming growth factors have also been detected, one of which is EGF. These factors stimulate the growth of normal rat kidney and mouse mammary tumor cells in soft agar.

Lactoferrin, a substance known to contribute to the protective effect that milk bestows upon its recipients against microorganisms, recently has been isolated from human and bovine milks and has been shown to be an essential growth factor for human B- and T-lymphocytes (22). Neither other human cell lines tested nor mouse lymphocytes could be supported in lactoferrin-enriched medium. Thus, lactoferrin in human milk may promote the viability of human lymphocytes in milk or of gut-derived lymphocytes in the suckled neonate.

Human milk has been reported to contain a large molecular weight (240,000-250,000) polypeptide growth factor that stimulates proliferation and differentiation of colony-forming granulocytic macrophage progenitor cells in bone marrow cultures *in vitro* (23). The biologic role of this factor, which is not present in bovine milk, has not been determined.

For thirty years it has been recognized that human and other milks contain one or more factors that promote the selective growth of *Bifidobacterium bifidum* in the intestines of breast-fed infants (24,25,26). This acid-producing organism lowers the pH of the gut of the human-milk-fed infant and thus retards the growth of more harmful bacteria such as *E. coli*, bacteriodes, and clostridium. Recently, this activity has been shown to be associated with two distinct peaks (A and B) separable by HPLC, but not further characterized (27). Milk growth factors such as lactoferrin, colony-stimulating factor, and *Bifidobacterium bifidum* growth factors A and B, appear to exert their growth effects not on cells of the recipient infant *per se*, but to act upon cells and organisms important in host defense mechanisms; in this manner, milk growth factors and host defense factors clearly overlap.

A third, and important, method for studying growth factors in milk is to study the *in vivo* growth of neonatal subjects that have received colostrum or milk. The seminal work in this area was performed by Widdowson and her colleagues (28,29), who observed striking increases in the mass of the intestinal mucosa of suckled newborn piglets and rabbits compared to littermates that were fasted for 24 hours after birth. Subsequently, Heird et al. compared suckled beagle dogs with littermates that were fed an artificial formula which provided comparable energy and protein intakes (30). They showed that enteric mucosal mass was 75% greater; DNA content was 56% greater, and protein content was 93% greater in dogs that suckled for 24 hours than in newborn dogs just after birth. There was no increase, however, in these parameters in the artificially fed dogs when compared with the newborn dogs.

Both cellular hyperplasia and hypertrophy contributed to the colostrum-associated intestinal growth during the initial 24 hours after birth. Sucrase-specific activity, but not other disaccharidase activities, were decreased in the intestinal mucosa of suckled dogs. In a preliminary report, Schwarz and Heird showed that the rapid growth of enteric mucosal growth in suckled dogs was limited to the first 24 hours after birth; after 3 days, there were no differences in growth, although there were differences in lactase and alkaline phosphatase activities (31).

To remove the possibly confounding effects of mode of feeding and nutritional equivalency, Berseth et al. tube-fed equicaloric amounts of rat colostrum or mature rat milk to rat pups for 40 hours after birth (32). Both groups demonstrated increases in the weights of stomach and intestine, when compared to animals at birth, but there was no difference detected in organ weight between the colostrum-fed and mature-milk-fed rat pups, when sacrificed at 41 hours of age. However, both the concentration of DNA and the rate of synthesis of DNA in the intestines were greater in rats fed colostrum than in those at birth or those fed mature milk. Interestingly, the rate of ^{3}H-thymidine incorporation into DNA in the pancreas was greater in colostrum-fed than in mature-milk-fed pups. This observation suggests a blood-borne effect of some colostrum-associated growth factor, rather than solely a direct action on enteric mucosal cells in contact with milk in the lumen of the gut. These investigators have preliminarily reported that serum gastrin levels are elevated in newborn beagle dogs that are fed bitch colostrum for the first 48 hours after birth, but not in littermates fed an artificial formula. This raises the possibility that enhanced release of endogenous gastrin is a mediator for the rapid gut growth in colostrum-fed newborn animals (41).

Finally, a review of growth factors *in* milk should acknowledge that milk may differentially influence the growth of target tissues in the suckled infant by provoking an endogenous hormonal response that is different from that provided by the ingestion of a proprietary formula. In a series of papers, Aynsley-Green and colleagues have described the hormonal responses to human milk feedings over the first several weeks of life, in term and pre-term infants (42-46). Included in their observations are different endocrine responses to breast versus bottle feedings (44). Bottle-fed neonates had significant changes in plasma concentrations of a group of hormones including insulin and enteroglucogon, two agents that promote growth, whereas breast-fed neonates did not. While these specific observations do not explain the growth effects produced by colostrum ingestion compared with formula ingestion, they do suggest that the developmental biology of the newborn mammal is tied to the mammary secretions of the species in complex ways.

REFERENCES

1. Beardmore JM, Lewis-Jones DI, Richards RC. (1983): Urogastrone and lactose concentrations in precolostrum, colostrum, and milk. Pediatr Res, 17, 825-828.

2. Moran JR, Courtney ME, Orth DN, et al. (1983): Epidermal growth factor in human milk: daily production and diurnal variation during early lactation in mothers delivering at term and at premature gestation. J Pediatr, 103, 402-405.

3. Read LC, Upton FM, Francis GL, Wallace JC, Dahlenberg GW, Ballard FJ. (1984): Changes in the growth-promoting activity of human milk during lactation. Pediatr Res, 18, 133-139.

4. Byyny RL, Orth DN, Cohen S, Doyne ES. (1974): Epidermal growth factor: effects of androgens and androgenic agents. Endocrinology, 95, 776-782.

5. Cevreska S, Kovacev VP, Stankovski M, Kalamares E. (1975): The presence of immunologically reactive insulin in milk of women during the first week of lactation and its relation to changes in plasma insulin concentration. God Zb Med Fak Skopje, 21, 35-38.

6. Beck NFG, Tucker HA. (1978): Mammary arterial and venous concentration of serum insulin in lactating dairy cows. Proc Soc Exp Biol Med, 159, 394-396.

7. Sack J, Amado O, Lunenfeld B. (1977): Thyroxine concentration in human milk. J clin Endocrinol Metab, 45, 171-173.

8. Tenore A, Parks JS, Bongiovanni AM. (1977): Relationship of breast feeding to congenital hypothyroidism. In: Chiumello G, Laron Z, eds, Recent Progress in Pediatric Endocrinology. London: Academic Press, 213-221.

9. Koldovsky O, Krulich L, Tenore A, Jumawan J, Horowitz C, Lau H. (1980): Effect of triiodothyronine injection on levels of triiodothyronine and thyroid-stimulating hormone in sera and milk of lactating rats and in sera of their sucklings; precocious development of jejunal-disaccharidases in the sucklings. Biol Neonate, 37, 103-108.

10. Montalvo JM, Wahner HW, Christie RJ. (1976): Triiodothyronine and thyroxine levels in the milk of humans and primates. Program of American Endocrine Society, A91.

11. Payne DW, Peng LH, Pearlman WH. (1976): Corticosteroid-binding proteins in human colostrum and milk and rat milk. J Biol Chem, 251, 5272-5279.

12. Rosner W, Beers PC, Awan T, Khan MS. (1976): Identification of corticosteroid-binding globulin in human milk: measurement with a filter disk assay. J Clin Endocrinol Metab, 42, 1064-1073.

13. Kulski JK, Hartmann PE. (1981): Changes in the concentration of cortisol in milk during different stages of human lactation. Aust J Exp Biol Med Sci, 59, 769-778.

14. Gwazdauskas FC, Paape MJ, McGilliard ML. (1977): Milk and plasma glucocorticoid alterations after injections of hydrocortisone and adrenocorticotropin (39714). Proc Soc Exper Biol Med, 154, 543-545.

15. Kesler DJ, Peterson RC, Erb RE, Callahan DJ. (1976): Concentrations of hormones in blood and milk during and after induction of parturition in beef cattle with dexamethasone and estradiol-17 β. J Anim Sci, 42, 918-926.

16. Patterson JY, Linzell JL. (1971): The secretion of cortisol and its mammary uptake in the goat. J Endocrinol, 50, 493-499.

17. Sarda AK, Nair RM. (1981): Elevated levels of LRH in human milk. J Clin Endocrinol Metab, 52, 826-828.

18. Baram T, Koch Y, Hazum E, Fridkin M. (1977): Gonadotropin-releasing hormone in milk. Science, 198, 300-302.

19. Klagsbrun M. (1978): Human milk stimulates DNA synthesis and cellular proliferation in cultured fibroblasts. Proc Natl Acad Sci USA, 75, 5057-5061.

20. Shing YW, Klagsbrun M. (1984): Human and bovine milk contain different sets of growth factors. Endocrinology, 115, 273-282.

21. Carpenter G. (1980): Epidermal growth factor is a major growth-promoting agent in human milk. Science, 210, 198-199.

21a. Kidwell W.D, et al. Mammary derived growth factors in human milk. (These proceedings).

22. Hashizume S, Kuroda K, Murakami H. (1983): Identification of lactoferrin as a essential growth factor for human lymphocytic cell lines in serum-free medium. Biochem Biophys Acta, 763, 377-382.

23. Sinha SK, Yunis AA. (1983): Isolation of colony stimulating factor from human milk. Biochem Biophys Res Commun, 114, 797-803.

24. Gyorgy P. (1953): A hitherto unrecognized biochemical difference between human milk and cow's milk. Pediatrics, 11, 98-107.

25. Gyorgy P, Kuhn R, Rose CS, Zilliken F. (1954): Bifidus Factor II. Its occurrence in milk from different species and in other natural products. Arch Biochem Biophys, 48, 202-207.

26. Beerns H, Romond C, Neut C. (1980): Influence of breast-feeding on the bifid flora of the newborn intestine. Am J Clin Nutr, 33, 2434-2439.

27. Ashoor SH, Monte WC. (1983): High performance liquid chromatographic determination of Vifidobacterium bifidum growth factors in human milk. J Assoc Off Anal Chem, 66, 135-139.

28. Widdowson EM, Colombo VE, Artavanis CA. (1976): Changes in the organs of pigs in response to feeding for the first 24 hours after birth. II. The digestive tract. Biol Neonate, 28, 272-281.

29. Hall RA, Widdowson EM. (1979): Response of the organs of rabbits to feeding during their first days after birth. Biol Neonate, 35, 131-139.

30. Heird WC, Schwarz SM, Hansen IH. (1984): Colostrum-induced enteric mucosal growth in beagle puppies. Pediatr Res, 18, 512-515.

31. Schwarz SM, Heird WC. (1981): Further studies of colostrum-stimulated enteric mucosal growth. Pediatr Res, 15, 546. (Abstract).

32. Berseth CL, Lichtenberger LM, Morriss FH. (1983): Comparison ot the gastrointestinal growth-promoting effects of rat colostrum and mature rat milk in newborn fats *in vivo*. Am J Clin Nutr, 37, 52-60.

33. Beaulieu J-F, Calvert R. (1981): The effect of epidermal growth factor (EGF) on the differentiation of the rough endoplasmic reticulum in fetal mouse small intestine in organ culture. J Histochem Cytochem, 29, 765-770.

34. Johnson LR, Guthrie PD. (1980): Stimulation of rat oxynitic gland mucosal growth by epidermal growth factor. Am J Physiol, 238, G45-G49.

35. Malo C, Menard D. (1982): Influence of epidermal growth factor on the development of suckling mouse intestional mucosa. Gastroenterology, 83, 28-35.

36. Bode HH, Vanjonack WG, Crawford JD. (1978): Mitigation of cretinism by breast feeding. Pediatrics, 62, 13-16.

37. Strbak V. Alexandrova M, Macho L, Ponec J. (1980): Transport of ^{3}H-TRH from plasma to rat milk: accumulation and slow degradation in milk and presence of unaltered hormone in gastric content of pups. Biol Neonate, 37, 313-321.

38. Morisset J, Jolicoeur L. (1980): Effect of hydrocortisone on pancreatic growth in rats. Am J Physiol, 239, G95-G98.

39. Klagsbrun M. (1980): Bovine colostrum supports the serum-free proliferation of epithelial cells but not of fibroblasts in long-term culture. J Cell Biol, 84, 808-814.

40. Steimer KS, Packard R, Holden D, Klagsbrun M. (1981): The serum-free growth of cultured cells in bovine colostrum and in milk obtained later in the lactation period. J Cell Physiol, 109, 223-234.

41. Berseth CL, Lichtenberger LM, Bayley HS, Morriss FH. (1982): Role of endogenous gastrin in mediating colostrum-stimulated gut growth. Pediatr Res, 16, 156A. (Abstract).

42. Lucas A, Bloom SR, Aynsley-Green A. (1978): Metabolic and endocrine events at the time of first feed of human milk in preterm and term infants. Arch Dis Child, 53, 731-736.

43. Aynsley-Green A, Lucas A, Bloom SR. (1979): The effects of feeds of differing composition on entero-insular hormone secretion in the first hours of life in human neonates. Acta Paediatr Scand, 68, 265-270.

44. Lucas A, Blackburn AM, Aynsley-Green A, Sarson DL, Adrian TE, Bloom SR. (1980): Breast vs. bottle: endocrine responses are different with formula feeding. Lancet, i:1267-1269.

45. Adrian TE, Lucas A, Bloom SR, Aynsley-Green A. (1983): Growth hormone response to feeding in term and preterm neonates. Acta Paediatr Scand, 72, 251-254.

46. Aynsley-Green A. (1983): Hormones and postnatal adaptation to enteral nutrition. J Pediatr Gastroenterol Nutr, 2, 418-427.

DETECTION OF THREE GROWTH FACTORS, HMGF I, HMGF II, AND HMGF III IN HUMAN MILK

Y. W. Shing
S. Dai
M. Klagsbrun

The physiological function of milk is to provide substances that are important for nutrition, development, and growth of the mammalian newborn. The composition of milk has been well documented. Among the constituents of milk are lipids, proteins, carbohydrates, minerals, vitamins and trace elements. Aside from these nutrients required for growth, there is evidence that human milk is a source of growth factors (1-4). In 1978, Klagsbrun developed an assay for the measurement of growth factor activity in human milk (1). The assay was based on the ability of milk samples to stimulate both DNA synthesis and cell division in confluent monolayers of

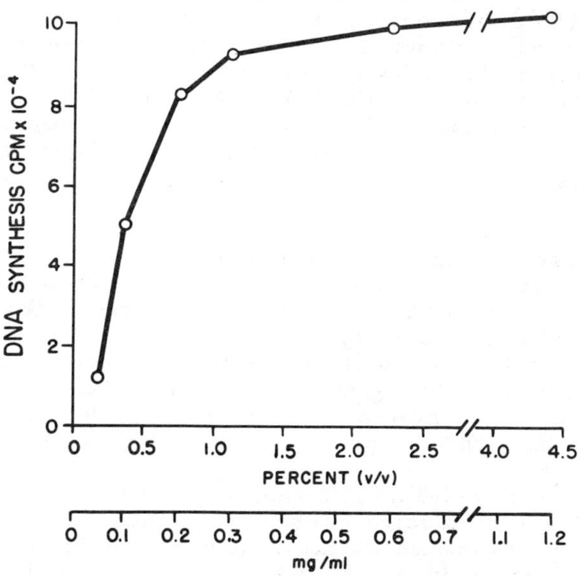

Figure 1. Growth factor activity in human milk. Human milk obtained about 1 month postpartum was centrifuged to remove fat and cells. Growth factor activity was measured by testing the ability of varying concentrations of human milk to stimulate DNA synthesis in 3T3 cells.

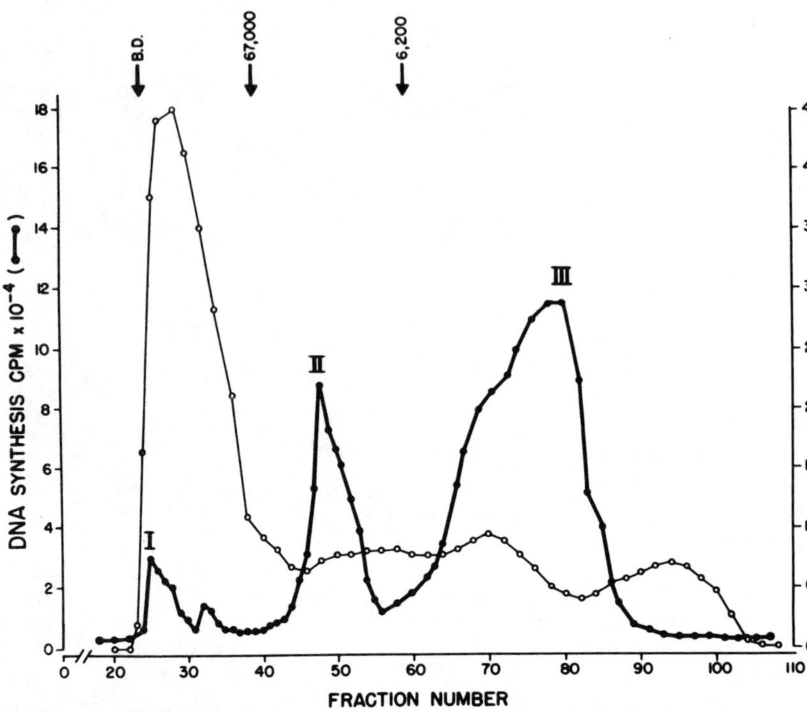

Figure 2. Gel filtration chromatography of human milk. Defatted acellular milk (100 ml) was acidified to pH 4.3, and the precipitate formed was removed by centrifugation. The supernatant fraction was lyophilized. About 1.5 g of protein dissolved in 20 ml of equilibration buffer was applied to a Sephadex G-100 column (5cm x 90cm) equilibrated with 0.1 M NaCl and 0.01 M sodium acetate, pH 4.3. Fractions (18 ml) were collected, measured for absorbance at 280 nm, and tested for the ability to stimulate DNA synthesis in 3T3 cells.

quiescent fibroblasts. Figure 1 shows the dose-dependent stimulation of DNA synthesis in cultured cells by human milk. Half-maximal stimulation was obtained with about 0.5% (vol/vol) of defatted milk in the culture medium. The growth factor activity of human milk declined as the lactation period progressed. Although growth factor activity could still be detected 6 months after birth, it was generally higher in the first month after birth. Human milk can be stored as whole milk or defatted milk at -20°C for at least 6 months without appreciable loss of growth factor activity.

The growth factor activity in human milk can be resolved into 3 peaks by Sephadex G-100 gel filtration (Figure 2). These three peaks of growth factor activity are designated as human-milk growth factors (HMGF) I, II, and III in descending order of molecular weight (4). The relative activities of HMGF I, II, and III vary from batch to batch, but in general they account for about 5, 20, and 75%, respectively, of the total growth factor activity found in the supernatant fraction of the acidified milk. However, with some individual samples, it has been found that HMGF III accounts for more than 95% of the total growth factor activity. The molecular weights of human-milk growth factors I, II, and III can be

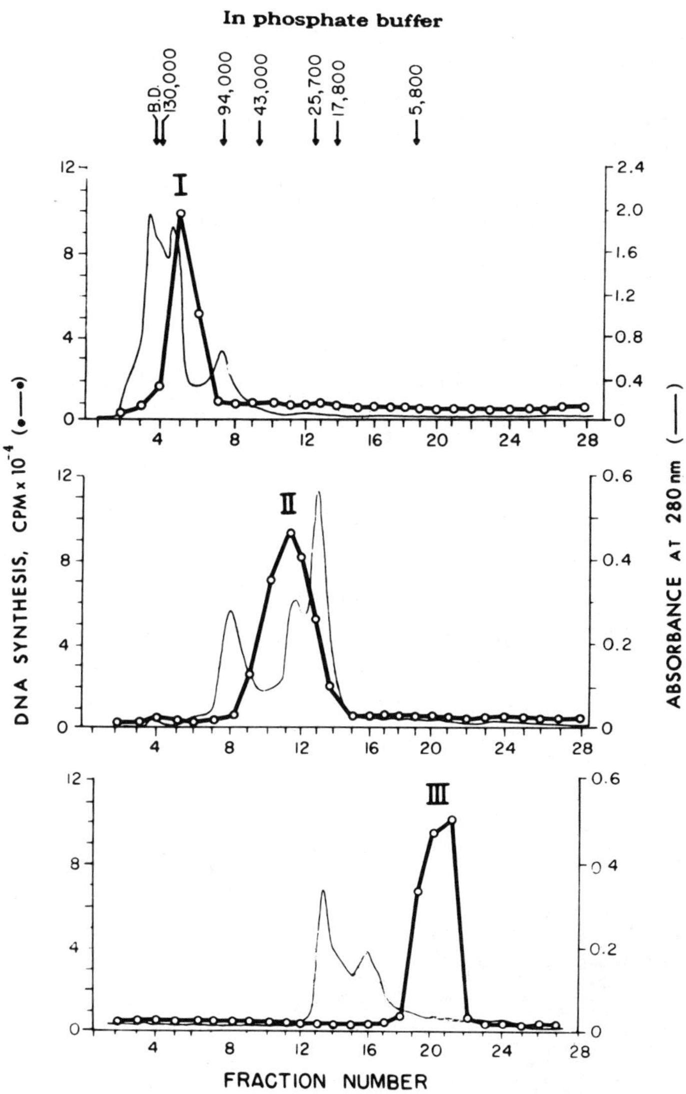

Figure 3. Analysis of human-milk growth factors I, II, and III by means of HPLC size-exclusion columns. HMGF samples were prepared by Sephadex G-100 gel filtration as shown in Figure 2. About 8, 4, and 2 mg of HMGF I (top), II (center), and III (bottom), respectively, were resuspended in 100 μl of equilibration buffer and analyzed on TSK 2000 size-exclusion columns equilibrated with 0.1 M ammonium sulfate and 0.05 M potassium phosphate, pH 7.0, at a flow rate of 1 ml/min. Fractions (0.85 ml) were collected, dialyzed against deionized distilled water, and tested for the ability to stimulate DNA synthesis in 3T3 cells.

determined more accurately by high-performance liquid chromatography (HPLC) on size-exclusion column (Figure 3). Under the nondenaturing condition using phosphate buffer, HMGF I, II, and III have molecular weights of about 110,000, 32,000, and 6,000 respectively. When the chromatography is carried out under the denaturing condition using 6 M guanidine HCl (Figure 4, left panel), the molecular weights of HMGF I and II reduce to about 36,000 and 14,000, respectively. The molecular weight of HMGF III appears to be unchanged by the presence of guanidine. Thus, HMGF I and II, but not HMGF III, either form aggregates or are bound to a large molecular weight carrier. In addition, the biological activities of both HMGF I and II are eliminated by 5 mM dithiothreitol, while that of HMGF III is not adversely affected by this reducing agent (Figure 4, right panel).

Human-milk growth factor III can be purified to homogeneity by a combination of acid precipitation, gel filtration, anion-exchange chromatography, and size-exclusion HPLC (4). A single band with a molecular weight of about 6,000 is evident on SDS polyacrylamide gel electrophoresis after visualization with a silver stain (Figure 5). Purified HMGF III stimulates DNA synthesis in 3T3 cells in a dose-dependent manner (Figure 5). Half-maximal stimulation occurred at a concentration of about 25 ng/ml.

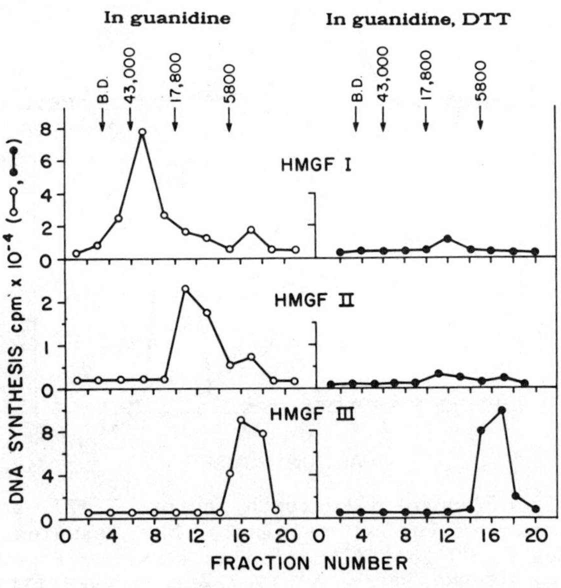

Figure 4. Analysis of human-milk growth factors using HPLC size-exclusion columns in the presence of guanidine-HCl and dithiothreitol. HMGF I, II, and III prepared by Sephadex G-100 gel filtration (Figure 2) were analyzed on TSK 3000 size-exclusion columns equilibrated with 0.02 M 2-(N-morpholino ethane sulfonic acid, pH 6.5, in the presence of 6 M guanidine-HCl (left panel) and 6 M guanidine-HCl plus 5 mM dithiothreitol (right panel). Fractions (0.85 ml) were collected, dialyzed against deionized distilled water, and tested for the ability to stimulate DNA synthesis in 3T3 cells.

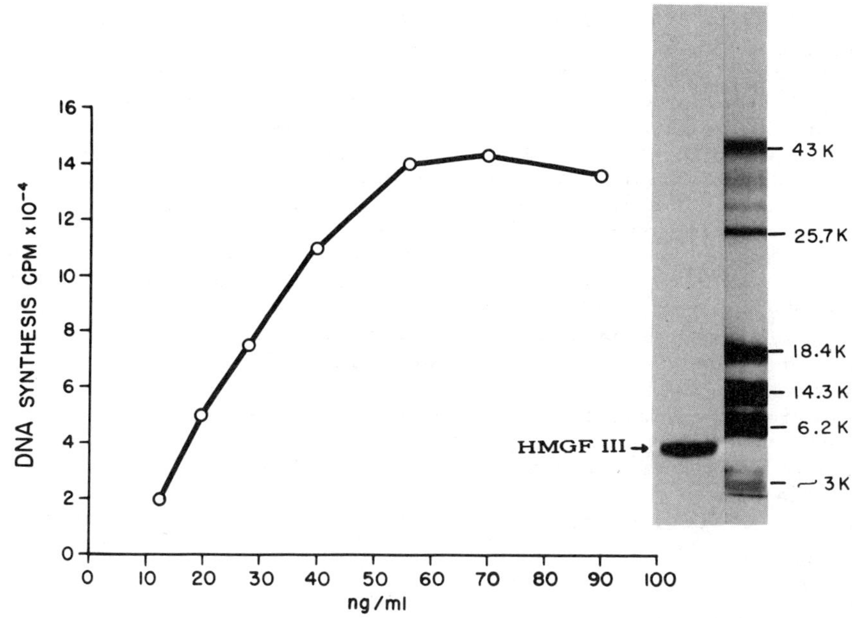

Figure 5. Dose-dependent stimulation of DNA synthesis by purified human-milk growth factor III. Various concentrations of a homogeneous preparation of HMGF III were tested for the ability to stimulate DNA synthesis in 3T3 cells. The homogeneity of the purified HMGF III sample was demonstrated by the single band developed with a silver stain on the polyacrylamide gel. Molecular weight standards (Bethesda Research Labs): 400 ng/protein (ovalbumin, alpha-chymotrypsinogen, beta-lactoglobulin, lysozyme, bovine trypsin inhibitor, and insulin).

HMGF III has a molecular weight of about 6,000 and an isoelectric point between 4.4 and 4.7 (4). It migrates close to mouse EGF on both SDS-polyacrylamide gel and size-exclusion HPLC in the presence of guanidine and dithiothreitol (5). These structural characteristics, along with Carpenter's finding that about 70% of the growth factor activity in human milk can be neutralized by antibody directed against human epidermal growth factor (3), strongly suggest that HMGF III is probably a form of epidermal growth factor (EGF). EGF has been well known as an inhibitor of gastric acid secretion (6) and has been used to promote healing of ulcers (7). A similar activity in human milk would be of physiological interest, since it would suggest that defined macro-molecular factors in human milk are capable of having an effect on the gastrointestinal tract of the human infant.

We have tested the anti-ulcer activity of human-milk growth factor III on mouse duodenum. Duodenal ulcers were induced in male mice by 2 subcutaneous injections of cysteamine-HCl (350 mg/kg), the second injection being given 7 hours after the first. The mice were randomly divided into groups of about 12. Ten minutes prior to each cysteamine injection, groups of mice were pretreated with subcutaneous injections of either saline (10 mg/ml), atropine sulfate (10 mg/ml), or HMGF III in various concentrations (0.5, 2, 8, 32, and 128 mg/kg). Twenty four hours after the first cysteamine injection, the mice were sacrificed by rapid cervical dislocation, and their duodena were removed. The duodena were opened along the anti-mesenteric side and examined under a dissecting microscope for mucosal lesions. The incidence of mucosal lesions was determined in each group. The severity of ulcers was assessed using the score system of Smith (8): 0 - normal, 1 - superficial mucosal erosion, 2 - hemorrhagic ulcer, and 3 - perforation. The ulcer index was calculated by adding the severity score to the incidence of duodenal ulcer multiplied by 2 (9). Table 1 demonstrates that pretreatment of mice with HMGF significantly reduces the incidence and severity score of cysteamine-induced duodenal ulcers. Figure 6 shows that the ulcer index is decreased in a dose-dependent manner when the mice are pretreated with increasing concentrations of HMGF III. In these experiments, partially purified HMGF III (obtained from Sephadex G-100 column) was used because not enough pure growth factor was available to treat the large number of mice. Therefore, there is no conclusive proof as yet that it is the growth factor that prevents ulcers. However, the

Table 1. Incidence and severity score of duodenal ulceration induced by cysteamine in mice

Pretreatment with two subcutaneous injections of:	Number of Mice	Duodenal Ulcers	
		Incidence (%)	Severity Score
Saline 10 ml/kg	16	62.50	1.52 ± 0.33
Atropine sulfate 10 mg/kg	11	18.18	0.36 ± 0.24
HMGF III (mg/kg)			
0.5	12	66.67	1.51 ± 0.33
2	12	58.33	1.14 ± 0.31
8	12	33.33	0.83 ± 0.37
32	11	18.18	0.32 ± 0.22
128	12	16.67	0.33 ± 0.22

The severity scores are expressed as means $\pm$ S.E.M.

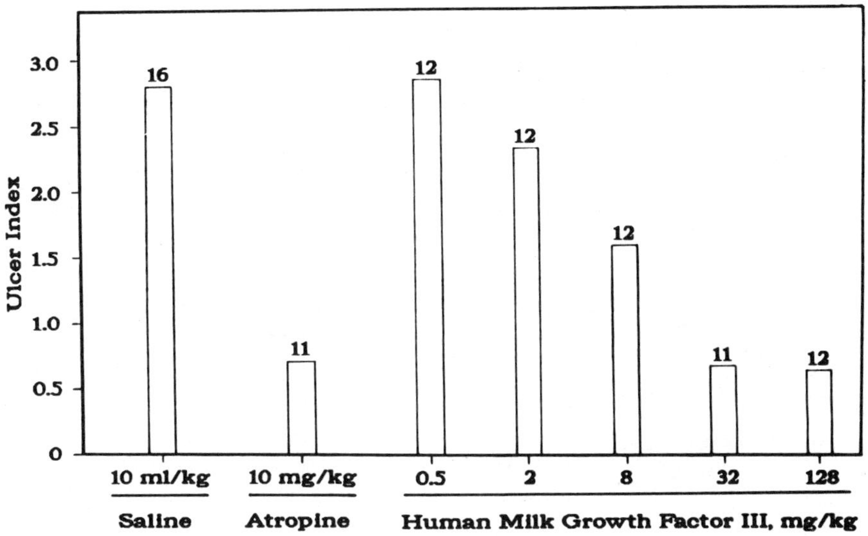

Figure 6. Effects of human-milk growth factor III on cysteamine-induced duodenal ulcers in mice. Duodenal ulcers were induced by two injections of cysteamine. Ten minutes prior to each cysteamine injection, groups of mice were pretreated with either saline, atropine or HMGF III in various concentrations. Numbers on the bar represent the number of animals in each group. The ulcer index was calculated by adding the arithmetic mean of the severity score in a group and the incidence of duodenal ulcer multiplied by 2.

structural similarities of HMGF III to human urine-derived EGF (urogastrone), a well known anti-ulcer reagent (10), strongly suggests that it is the growth factor that is responsible for the anti-ulcer effect. HMGF III was given to mice subcutaneously rather than orally, because subcutaneous administration is a much more efficient technique for growth factor delivery. However, the stability of HMGF III to exposure to pH 1 (11) and the presence of trypsin inhibitor in human milk (12) make it plausible that this growth factor could survive transport through the gastrointestinal tract. Thus the anti-ulcer effect of HMGF III might be one of the protective mechanisms that human milk is postulated to have for the breast-fed infant.

REFERENCES

1. Klagsbrun M. (1978): Human milk stimulates DNA synthesis and cellular proliferation in cultured fibroblasts. Proc Natl Acad Sci USA, 75, 5057.

2. Hirata Y, Orth, DN. (1979): Epidermal growth factor (urogastrone) in human fluids: size heterogeneity. J Clin Endocrinol Metab, 48, 673.

3. Carpenter G. (1980): Epidermal growth factor is a major growth-promoting agent in human milk. Science, 210, 198.

4. Shing YW, Klagsbrun, M. (1984): Human and bovine milk contain different sets of growth factors. Endocrinology, 115, 273.

5. Shing YW, Klagsbrun M. (1984): Isolation of growth factors from human milk. In: Sato G, Sirbasku D, Barnes D, eds, Methods in Molecular and Cellular Biology, Vol 1. New York: Alan R. Liss, 159.

6. Bower JM, Camble R, Gregory H, Gerring EL, Willshire IR. (1975): The inhibition of gastric acid secretion by epidermal growth factor. Experientia, 31, 825.

7. Gregory H, Bower JM, Willshire IR. (1977): Urogastrone and epidermal growth factor. In: Kastrup IW, Nielsen JH, eds, Growth Factors. London: Pergamon Press, 75.

8. Smith JA. (1983): The effect of atropine, cimitidine and FPL 52694 on duodenal ulcers in mice. Eur J Pharmacol, 88, 215.

9. Szabo S. (1978): Animal model: cysteamine-induced acute and chronic duodenal ulcer in the rat. Am J Pathol, 93, 273.

10. Hollenberg MD. (1979): Epidermal growth factor-urogastrone, a polypeptide acquiring hormonal status. Vit Horm, 37, 69.

11. Klagsbrun M, Shing Y. (1984): Growth promoting factors in human and bovine milk. In: Guroff G, ed, Growth and Maturation Factors, Vol 2. New York: John Wiley & Sons, 161.

12. Laskowski M Jr, Laskowski M. (1951): Crystalline trypsin inhibition from colostrum. J Biol Chem, 190, 563.

MAMMARY DERIVED GROWTH FACTORS IN HUMAN MILK

W.R. Kidwell
M. Bano
K. Burdette
I. Lococzy
D. Salomon

INTRODUCTION

Milk is known to contain a variety of polypeptide growth factors and hormones, such as insulin (1), EGF (2), fibroblast growth-promoting activities (3) and bone marrow colony stimulating factors (4). To this list we now add four new growth-factor species that appear, on the basis of their chemical, physiochemical and biological properties, to be distinct from any of the known milk-derived growth factors. One factor, MDGF1, is a 62,000 MW acidic protein which stimulates mammary cell growth at picomolar concentrations and greatly amplifies their production of collagen and laminin, components of the extracellular matrix (5). The activity is heat stable, is unaffected by dithiothreitol, but is inactivated by trypsin (5). Due to the presence of interfering components, this activity can currently only be quantitated in milk following subfractionation. A second class of factors is the so-called transforming growth-factor activity, or TGF. Fractionation of milk by isoelectric focusing has revealed the presence of at least four TGF species, one of which is EGF, a known component of milk and colostrum (2). The combined non-EGF activity of milk can be quantitated without fractionation of milk by the addition of neutralizing amounts of anti-EGF serum.

The function of MDGF1 might be to promote the growth of the mammary epithelium, since mammary epithelial cells are responsive to MDGF1 whether cultivated as isolated cells or whole mammary glands. The function of the TGFs is unknown, but it is probable that TFGs have a physiological role, since they have been detected in normal as well as neoplastic tissues (6,7,8,9). In this sense, the name TGF is a misnomer, even though these factors promote the growth of normally *anchorage-dependent* cells in an *anchorage-independent* state. It is this characteristic, the stimulation of growth in the absence of cell attachment to substratum, a general phenotypic property of transformed cells, that originally led to the naming of such activities as transforming growth factors. Once the physiologic role of TGFs is known, it will be necessary to rename them more appropriately.

MATERIALS AND METHODS

MDGF1 was purified to apparent homogeneity by isoelectric focusing and high performance liquid chromatography. Details of the purification are published elsewhere (5). The protein was iodinated according to Johnson and Thorell (10). Attempts to quantitate the amount of the factor in milk were based on the ability of milk to inhibit the binding of ^{125}I-MDGF1 to membrane receptors. These studies were performed by the addition of 10 ng iodinated growth factor (2×10^5 cpm per 10 ng) to 2.5 μg A431 cell membranes that were bound to microtiter wells (published procedures were followed) (11). Bioassays of MDGF1 activity were performed by incubating isolated normal mouse mammary ducts and alveoli in a serum-free growth medium to which 2 μCi/ml ^{14}C proline (Amersham, 256 mCI/mM) was added. Following three days of incubation at 37°C, the amount of label incorporated into collagen and into total cell protein was determined. Details of the methods for cell isolation and cultivation and the estimation of collagen and non-collagen labeling have been described previously (12,13).

Transforming growth-factor assays

Approximately 2×10^3 NRK (clone 49F), mouse mammary tumor cells, were placed in 0.5 ml suspension of 0.3% agar in Dulbecco's modified Eagle's medium containing 15% fetal calf serum, 2mM glutamine and antibiotics (14). This suspension was layered over 0.5 ml of 0.6% agar in microtiter plates in the same medium. After the top layer had solidified, aliquots of milk, or fractions derived therefrom by isoelectric focusing, were placed on top of the cell suspension.

Five days later 0.2 ml nitroblue tetrazolium (50 mg/ml phosphate buffered saline) was added, and the cells were stained overnight before the growing colonies were quantitated with an Artek electronic colony counter (14). The size discriminator was set so that colonies of fewer than 10 cells were not counted. NRK cells, normal rat kidney cells, are exquisitely sensitive to TGFs (6).

Isoelectric focusing

Milk was centrifuged for 30 minutes at 20,000 x g at 4°C and the lipid layer removed and discarded. The supernatant fluid was dialyzed overnight at 4°C against 10 volumes of water in 3500 molecular weight cutoff tubing. Material which precipitated was removed by centrifugation as described above. The sample was mixed with Buffalite (pH 3-10, Pierce Chemicals) in a 0-30% sucrose gradient and focused at 1000 V for 16 hours at 4°c in an LKB focusing apparatus (model 110). Three ml fractions were collected and the pH measured. Then they were dialyzed (as described above) to remove the ampholytes, and lyophylized to dryness. The residue was dissolved in one ml growth medium containing 15% fetal calf serum. Aliquots were tested for collagen synthesis-stimulating activity or transforming growth-factor activity, as described.

Materials

Human EGF was obtained from Amgen, Inc. It was produced in bacterial-carrying expression vectors containing the human EGF gene. In our hands, the product was equipotent to authentic mouse EGF in competing for ^{125}I-EGF binding to EGF receptors on A431 membranes. Anti-human EGF antiserum was a gift of C. Savage, Temple University, Philadelphia, PA. Fifty μl of a 1:500 dilution of the antiserum was sufficient to neutralize 10 ng of human

EGF as determined in a radioreceptor assay with labeled EGF. Human milk was obtained from the Milk Bank, Georgetown University. It was collected asceptically from healthy women who were non-smokers, non-drug users, and not on medication. The donors were judged to be free of hepatitis and tuberculosis. Milk was collected from individual donors no earlier than two weeks postpartum. It was stored at -20°C until assayed, unless otherwise stated. Colostrum, collected on day four, was supplied by M. Neville, University of Colorado.

RESULTS

MDGF1 Activity

The most characteristic activity of MDGF1 is its ability to promote collagen synthesis by NRK cells and mammary ducts and alveoli in primary culture. This activity was originally detected in milk that had been fractionated by isoelectric focusing (5). The activity was predominantly localized in the pH 4.8 fraction (5). An attempt was made to quantitate the activity in various samples of milk and colostrum by estimating the effects of milk on the differential amplification of collagen synthesis in NRK cell cultures. Very little differential stimulation of [^{14}C] proline incorporation into collagen was observed when aliquots up to 100 μl milk per ml growth medium were added to the cell cultures. In fact, some collagen synthesis-inhibiting activity was detected at high milk concentrations with three of four milk samples tested, and with colostrum. That milk contains considerable collagen synthesis-stimulating activity (MDGF1 activity) is shown in Figure 1. Milk was isoelectrically focused, and an aliquot of the recovered fractions, equivalent to 100 μl of milk per ml medium, was tested in the collagen synthesis assay. The major peak of activity was localized at pH 4.8, as previously noted. The degree of stimulation of collagen synthesis seen with this fraction was at least 600% above that of control cultures. That is about ten times as much stimulation as was produced by an equivalent amount of unfractionated milk.

Since MDGF1 has now been purified to apparent homogeneity (5), we attempted to quantitate the amount of this factor in different milk samples, based on the ability of milk to inhibit the binding of MDGF1 to cell receptors (5). The factor was iodinated and added with or without 50 μl milk to dishes on which A431 membranes had been absorbed (5). We found that receptor binding was reduced by the presence of milk, but there was no dose-response relationship. There was about the same degree of inhibition of ^{125}I-MDGF1 binding by 10, 25, and 50 μl of milk (34, 36, and 44%, respectively). This result was very surprising since MDGF1 had previously been found to bind with high affinity and high selectivity to A431 membrane receptors; $K_d = 10^{-10}$M, by Scatchard analysis (5). These latter observations indicated that milk must be subfractionated before MDGF1 quantitation is possible. Consequently, four different milk samples were isoelectrically focused, and aliquots of the pH 4.8 fraction were analyzed for collagen synthesis-stimulating activity. An aliquot equal to 100 μl of milk was tested. The degree of differential stimulation of ^{14}C-proline incorporation into collagen ranged from 2.5- to 12-fold the level of collagen synthesis in the control cell cultures, an average value being six-fold. This procedure is time consuming and may be improved upon by radioimmunoassays for MDGF1 which we plan to develop, providing we are successful in generating specific antibodies against the factor.

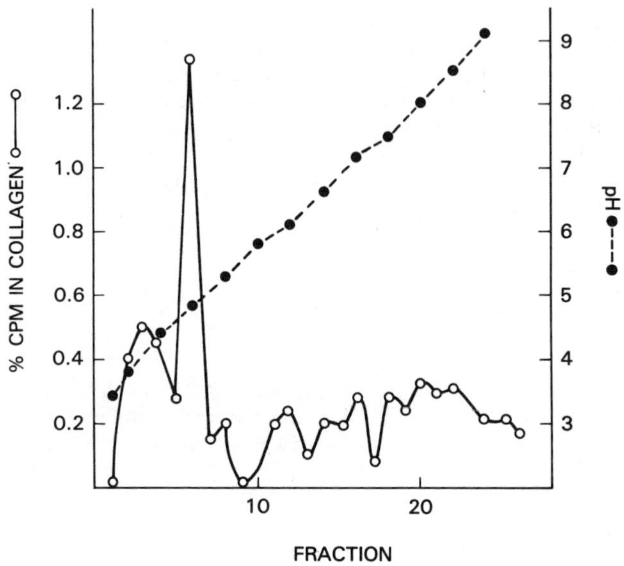

Figure 1. Collagen synthesis-stimulating activity (MDGF1) detected in milk fractionated by isoelectric focusing. Milk was focused and the fractions collected, dialyzed and assayed for activity, as described in text.

Transforming Growth-Factor Assays

TGF assays were performed by assessing the ability of aliquots of milk to stimulate the growth of NRK cells in soft agar. Activity was readily detectable with as little as 5 μl of unfractionated milk (Figure 2). With no milk added, there was no growth of the cells in agar. NRK cells were utilized in most experiments because of their exquisite sensitivity to TGFs (6). The milk samples were also tested using normal mammary ducts and alveoli plated in soft agar, but these cells did not grow. Rather, they became highly keratinized and died within ten days of plating in agar. However, a mouse mammary tumor cell line which did not grow in soft agar in the absence of milk, responded well when milk was added (results not shown). One requirement for TGF responsivity might be cell immortality, insofar as growth in soft agar is concerned.

The growth of the NRK cells in soft agar was not linearly related to the milk concentration (Figure 3). In fact, one milk sample (donor 3) gave a positive response at low milk concentrations, but higher amounts were inhibitory. The non-linear response was not surprising, since an isoelectric focusing of milk revealed the presence of at least four fractions (pI 3.9, 4.6, 6.6, and 7.0), which stimulated NRK cells to grow in soft agar (Figure 3). The pI 4.6 fraction is probably EGF, since EGF reportedly has a pI of about 4.5 (16).

A direct demonstration that human EGF has some TGF activity is presented in Figure 4. Cells were plated in soft agar with and without human EGF or milk. After five days of incubation, the colonies growing in soft agar were stained and counted. Photographs of oscilloscope displays from the colony counter are shown in Figure 4. Figure 4c is the control

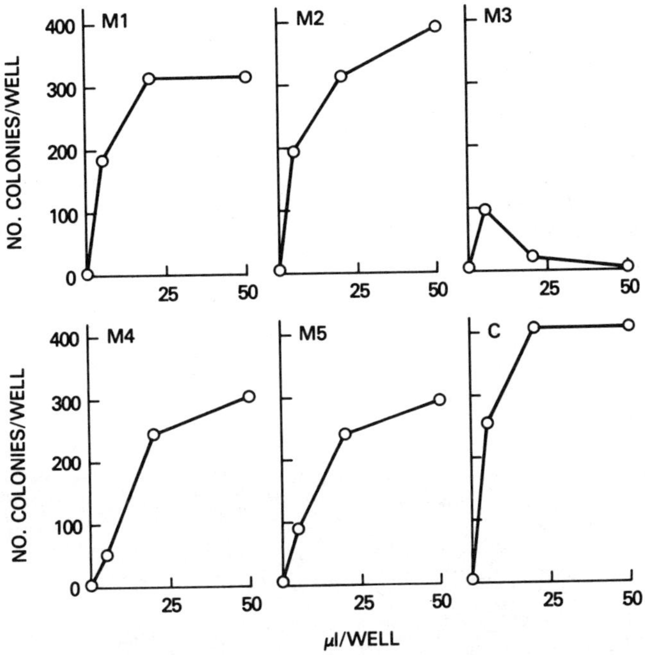

Figure 2. TGF activity of unfractionated milk. Aliquots of milk and colostrum were tested for their ability to stimulate growth of NRK cells in soft agar. M1 - M5 represent milk samples from five different donors. Sample C is a four-day colostrum.

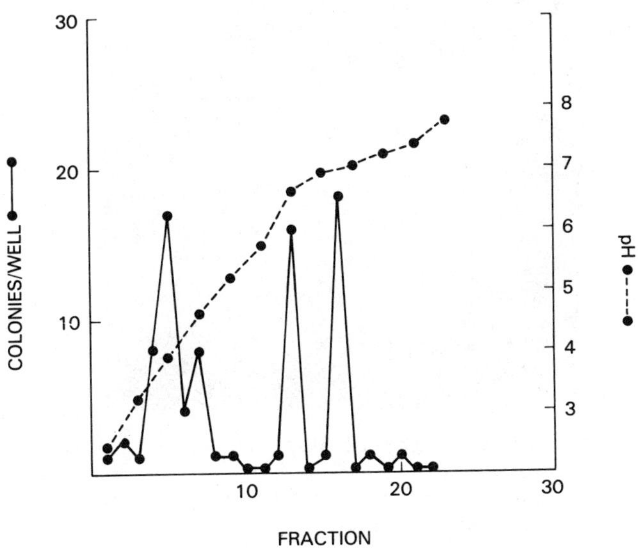

Figure 3. Multiple TGF species detected in milk following isoelectric focusing.

culture with neither milk nor EGF added. Figure 4a is the culture with 5 ng/ml human EGF added, and figure 4b is the culture which had been supplemented with 25 μl of milk (Donor 2). As is readily apparent, the EGF was much less active than the whole milk (456 vs 51 colonies per well with milk and EGF, respectively). Although the milk sample was not analyzed, the reports of the upper limit of milk EGF concentration indicate that 25 μl milk would contain no more than 2.5 ng of EGF (2). Dose response curves with human EGF indicated that maximal effects on NRK cell growth in soft agar were produced at 0.5 ng EGF/ml, with no inhibitory effects seen at concentrations up to 50 ng/ml (not shown).

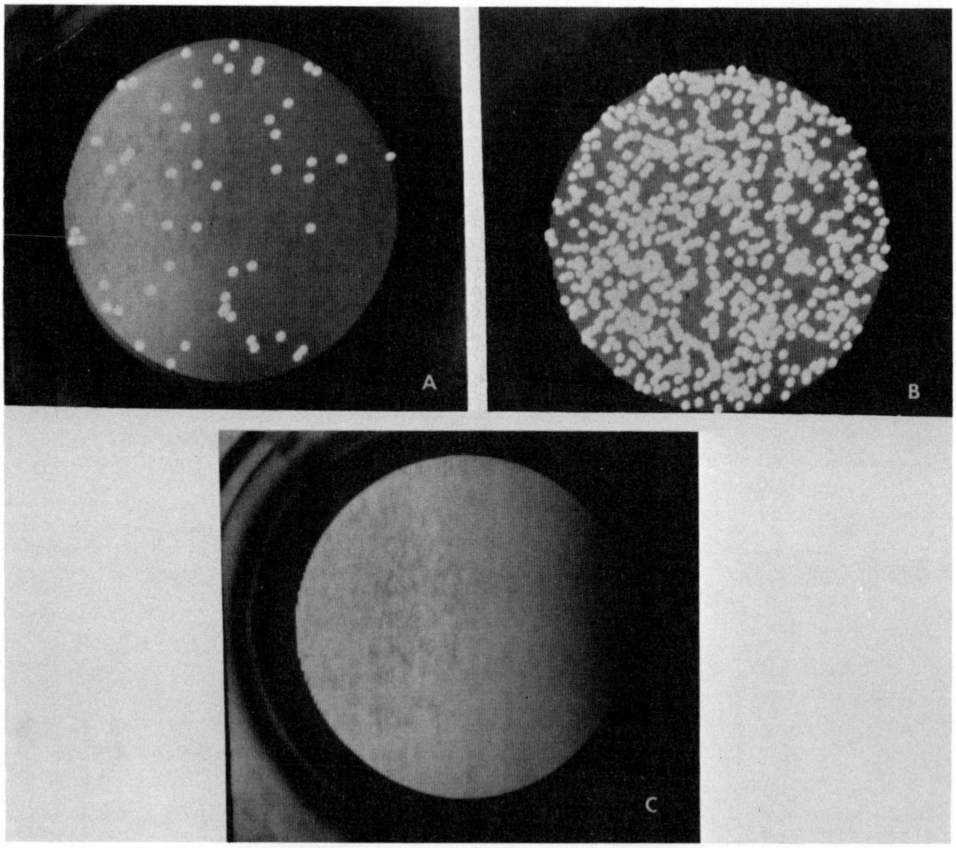

Figure 4. TGF activity of unfractionated milk or pure human EGF. Colonies were stained and counted five days after plotting cells in soft agar.

A. EGF-supplement (5ng/ml).
B. Unfractionated milk supplement (25 μl)
C. Control buffer supplement.

Table 1. Effect of anti-human EGF antiserum on the TGF activity of unfractionated milk

Sample	Antiserum	NRK Colonies/Well*
M2, 50μl	0	119,131
M2, 50μl	50μl	78, 76
None	50μl	3, 3

*Replicate Values.

Attempts were made to estimate the non-EGF TGF activity of milk, without the necessity for isoelectric focusing. Fifty μl of milk was assayed for soft agar growth-promoting activity with and without the addition of anti-human EGF antiserum (Table 1). The latter was sufficient to neutralize 10 ng EGF as estimated from radioreceptor assays. The anti-EGF antiserum alone (50 μl of 1:500 dilution) had no direct stimulatory effect on NRK cell growth in soft agar, but it reduced by 1/3 the number of colonies that formed in response to 50 μl of milk. The magnitude of the anti-EGF antiserum effect was somewhat surprising, since the amount of colony growth stimulation seen in the EGF region of the isoelectric focusing experiment (Figure 3) was only 14% of the total TGF activity of all the fractions. These results suggest that there might be a synergistic effect of EGF on the activity of the other TGF species of milk. This is likely, in fact, because the potency of the individual TGF peaks is much less than anticipated, based on the total TGF activity of unfractionated milk. Also, a potentiation of certain TGF species by mouse EGF has been previously reported(18).

While the total non-EGF TGF activity in milk can be estimated as described above, quantitation of the individual TGF species requires fractionation before assaying. Two milk samples, M1 and M2, have been compared for the relative amounts of the different TGF activities. Ten ml of milk were isoelectrically focused and the activity in the different pH regions analyzed. Aliquots of the milk fractions equivalent to 100 μl of milk were tested for colony growth-promoting activity. As shown in Table 2, the relative amount of TGF activity in the four peaks was not constant, indicating the presence of variable amounts of the individual TGF species in the two milk preparations. The four TGF species were also tested for possible synergism. Each factor was tested separately, and all four were combined in one assay. As seen in Table 3, a greater than additive effect was produced when all four factors were added to the NRK cell cultures.

The isoelectric focusing experiment of Figure 3 revealed not only the presence of multiple TGF species, but it also showed that the TGF activity of whole, unfractionated milk was greater than the sum of the individual TGF activities. As mentioned, these results are consistent with a synergistic interaction of the TGFs. A second possibility is that the TGFs are inactivated during fractionation. While this has not been tested for the individual TGF activities, the stability of total TGF activity of unfractionated milk has been assessed. A comparison was made of the activity of a milk sample that had been stored at -20°C and assayed

Table 2. Relative amounts of the four TGF species in 100 μl equivalents of milk

TGF Species	Colonies/Well		M2/M1*
	M1	M2	
pH 3.9	26	17	0.65
pH 4.6	34	8	0.23
pH 6.6	75	16	0.21
pH 7.0	34	18	0.53

*M1 and M2 refer to milk samples from Donors 1 and 2, respectively. Average values of triplicate assays are given. The number of colonies per well varied by less than 5% for the triplicates.

immediately after thawing, or stored an additional two weeks at 4°C before assaying. Also, the effects of repeated freezing and thawing on activity were determined. No significant differences in activity were observed for any of the samples. Thus, the TGF activity of unfractionated milk is quite stable.

DISCUSSION

Five different milk samples and one colostrum sample have been evaluated for the relative amounts of two different types of growth factors that we have discovered in milk. One of these, MDGF1, is present in variable amounts in the different samples. We show that quantitation of this activity can, at present, only be performed after isoelectric focusing, because of interfering substances in milk. This factor is believed to be synthesized by the mammary epithelium and may have a growth regulatory function on the producing tissue (13). However, cell types other than mammary cells are responsive to MDGF1, and its effects, if any, on neonates have not yet been tested because of the limited quantities available.

A second type of activity, named transforming growth-factor activity because of the ability to confer an anchorage-independent growth phenotype on normally anchorage-dependent cells (15), has been found in variable amounts in milk. Milk TGF is resolvable into four different species on the basis of molecular charge. One of these has been identified as EGF, since anti-human EGF antiserum significantly reduces total TGF activity of milk.

Analysis of milk TGF activities, individually and in combination, has shown that milk TGFs can interact cooperatively in facilitating anchorage-independent growth. This is also suggested from the observation that anti-EGF anti-serum reduces the TGF activity of milk more dramatically than one would anticipate on the basis of the amount of TGF activity detected in

Table 3. Synergistic effects of milk TGFs

Each TGF species was assayed separately (100 μl milk equivalents) and in combination. Colonies were stained and counted ten days after plating the cells in soft agar. The fractions were prepared by isoelectric focusing of 10 ml of milk sample M1.

Fraction	Colonies/Well*
pI 3.9	32
pI 4.6	43
pI 6.6	88
pI 6.6	36
Sum of the four fractions individually assayed	159
All four fractions assayed in combination	295

*Samples were assayed in triplicate and agreed within 5% of each other.

the isoelectric focusing position of EGF. Consequently, the most appropriate assessment of the TGF activity of milk may be the direct determination of the TGF activity of whole milk, rather than a quantitation of individual species, although the abundance of the various TGFs does vary in two milk samples that were tested.

Whether the milk TGFs we have detected are physiologically important to either the neonate or the mother is not known. It is likely that TGFs play some role(s) in normal processes, and they have been detected in a number of normal tissues and body fluids (6,7,8,9). Three activities that apparently interact synergistically have been extracted from platelets (8). It has been suggested that they are important for wound healing (19). Milk TGFs might be active in facilitating the proliferation of gut epithelium in the neonate. Questions about the function(s) of both the TGF activities and MDGF1 will require that large amounts of these factors be purified and tested for effects *in vivo* -- a goal that we are pursuing.

SUMMARY

Recent attention has focused on the presence of growth factors in milk and their possible physiological roles. We have detected two new classes of growth factors and report here on their abundance, stability, methods of assay and synergistic effects on cultured cells. One activity, MDGF1, stimulates mammary cell division and basement membrane collagen biosynthesis. The second activity class, TGFs, promotes anchorage-independent growth of certain testor cells. This latter class consists of at least four species that are resolvable on the basis of molecular charge. Variable amounts of these two types of activity are present in milk from a number of donors.

REFERENCES

1. Cevreska S, Kouacev VP, Stankovski M, Kalamares E. (1975): The presence of immunologically reactive insulin in milk of women during the first week of lactation and its relation to changes in plasma insulin concentration. God 26 Med Fak Skopje, 21, 35-38.

2. Carpenter G. (1980): Epidermal growth factor is a major growth-promoting agent in human milk. Science, 210, 198-199.

3. Sting YW, Klagsbrun M. (1984): Human and bovine milk contain different sets of growth factors. Endocrin, 115, 273-282.

4. Sinha SK, Yanis AA. (1983): Isolation of colony stimulating factor from human milk. Biochem Biophys Res Commun, 114, 797-803.

5. Bano M, Salomon DS, Kidwell WR. Purification of mammary derived growth factor MDGF1, from human milk and human mammary tumors. J Biol Chem, 260, 5745-5752.

6. Todaro G, Delarco JE, Frgling C, Johnson PA, Sporn MB. (1981): Transforming growth factors (TGFs): properties and possible mechanism of action. J Supramol Struct Mol Biochem, 15, 287-301.

7. Brown KD, Blakeley DM. (1984): Transforming growth factors: sources, properties, and possible roles in normal and malignant cell growth control. Biochem Soc Trans, 12, 168-173.

8. Childs CB, Proper JA, Tucker RF, Moses HL. (1982): Serum contains a platelet-derived transforming growth factor. Proc Natl Acad Sci USA, 79, 5312-5316.

9. Assoian RK, Komoriya A, Meyers CA, Miller DM, Sporn MB. (1983): Transforming growth factor β in human platelets. Identification of a major storage site, purification and characterization. J Biol Chem, 258, 7155-7160.

10. Thorell JI, Johansson BG. (1971): Use of lactoperoxidase for the radioidonation of proteins. Biochem Biophys Acta, 251, 363-369

11. Kimball ES, Warren TC. (1984): Epidermal growth factor (EGF) binding to membranes immobilized in microfiler wells and estimation of EGF-related transforming growth factor activity. Bioch Biophys Acta, 771, 82-88.

12. Kidwell WR, Bano M, Salomon DS. (1984): Growth of normal mammary epithelium on collagen in serum-free medium. In: Sirbasku DA, Barnes DW, Sato GH, eds, Methods for Serum-Free Culture of Cells of the Endocrine System. Growth of Mammary Cells on Collagen in Serum-Free Medium. New York: Alan R. Liss, Inc., 105-126.

13. Bano M, Zwiebel JA, Saloman DS, Kidwell WR. (1983): Isolation and characterization of a collagen synthesis stimulating activity from rat mammary adenocarcinomas. J Biol Chem, 258, 2729-2735.

14. Zwiebel JA, Davis M, Kohn E, Saloman DS, Kidwell WR. (1982): Anchorage -independent growth conferring factor production by rat mammary tumor cells. Cancer Res, 42, 5117-5125.

15. Delarco JE, Reynolds R, Curlberg K, Engle C, Todaro GJ. (1980): Sarcoma growth factor from mouse sarcoma virus-transformed cells. J Biol Chem, 225, 3685-3690.

16. Hollenberg MD. (1979): Epidermal growth factor - urogastrone, a polypeptide acquiring hormonal status. Vitamin Horm, 37, 69-110.

17. Starkey R. Orth DN. (1977): Radioimmunoassay of human epidermal growth factor (urogastrone). J Clin Endocrinol Metab, 45, 1144-1150.

18. Anzio MA, Roberts AB, Smith JM, Sporn MB, De Larco JE. (1983): Sarcoma growth factor from conditioned medium of virally transformed cells is composed of both type α and type β transforming growth factors. Proc Natl Acad Sci USA, 80, 6264-6268.

19. Sporn MB, Harris GD. (1981): Proliferative diseases. Amer J Med, 70, 1231-1235.

SECTION X. TRACE ELEMENTS

WORKSHOP PARTICIPANTS

C. E. Casey, University of Colorado Health Sciences Center, Denver, Colorado

R. R. Howell, University of Texas Medical School, Houston, Texas

B. Lönnerdal, University of California, Davis, California

P. B. Moser, University of Maryland, College Park, Maryland

M. F. Picciano, University of Illinois, Urbana, Illinois

S. V. Rumball, Massey University, Palmerston North, New Zealand

INTRODUCTION

There is currently a great deal of interest in trace elements in human milk, as evidenced by the recently completed WHO/IAEA study in which levels of 24 different elements were measured in 550 milk samples from 7 countries. Part of this interest arises from the growing recognition of clinical disorders due to trace element imbalances, and the realization that although only small amounts of the elements may be required, nonetheless one cannot assume that intakes will always be adequate. The nutritionally essential trace elements, zinc, copper, iron, selenium, iodine and fluorine, are of greatest practical interest and, to date, the most studied. They are, therefore, the most emphasized in the first paper. However, the general principles discussed apply to analysis of any trace element. Two additional papers deal with the important problem of trace-element binding in milk.

PRINCIPLES OF TRACE ELEMENT ANALYSIS AND NOTES ON SOME IMPORTANT ELEMENTS

C. E. Casey
R. R. Howell
B. Lönnerdal
P. B. Moser
M. F. Picciano
S. V. Rumball

Although literature values are available for the concentrations in human milk of a large number of both essential and non-essential trace elements, the effects of such factors as duration of lactation and diet are documented for only a few of the more abundant essential elements (e.g. iron, copper, selenium, zinc). The recent history of measurement of some of the metallic elements in blood suggests that one should be hesitant in accepting early reports of values for the minor elements, unless the report contains independent evidence of its accuracy or until levels can be confirmed using newer analytical techniques with greater sensitivity and lower limits of detection.

Almost all of the trace elements of nutritional or environmental interest can now be measured with reasonable to very good precision and accuracy. Even with excellent analytical technology, however, the problem of sample contamination remains the greatest source of analytical error. Contamination is a problem with all trace element work, but it is especially so with human milk because of the low intrinsic levels of many elements, as well as the liquid matrix, and the unavoidable exposure to possible contamination, from skin and air, during collection. Thus, great care must be taken at all stages of sample collection, preparation and analysis.

SAMPLE COLLECTION

Procedures

The rules for collection of human milk for trace element analysis are the same as for any other type of sample: minimize contamination and check all possible exogenous sources of the element. Mothers should be asked to bathe on the day of collection and not to use any deodorants, powders or creams. This is particularly important if zinc is to be analyzed, as many such preparations may contain high concentrations of this element. Immediately prior to milk collection, mothers should rinse the breast with deionized water. As long as containers are washed appropriately, there seems to be little difference between collections done by manual expression or pump, so the choice of method will depend largely on practical considerations. There are no special storage requirements for samples to be analyzed for total trace element content. Freezing is most widely used and a domestic freezer which maintains -20°C is adequate. Containers must be water-tight or small samples may dessicate; checks should be made that there is no loss or gain of element from the storage container. If milk is to be freeze-dried prior to shipping or analysis, the process should be checked for contamination.

Variation

Variations in trace element content due to the sampling protocol have received only limited systematic study. Some women, but not all, showed differences of up to 50% in the concentration of zinc between milk samples taken from the two breasts (1). No significant within-feed variations have been reported for trace elements, except for two studies which showed that iron increased during a feed (2,3). Some workers, but not others, have reported significant diurnal variations for iron (2-5), copper (2,4,5), and zinc (2,4-6). Diurnal variations were not found in manganese (7), selenium (8,9), or fluorine (10). Many of these studies included only small numbers of women and no late night or early morning milk samples. For a number of milk constituents, both the normal levels and the strength of within-feed and diurnal patterns may vary widely among women (5,11-13), and results from few subjects may not be generally applicable.

For most of the essential trace elements, the major determinant of concentration is the duration of lactation. The effect is most marked for zinc, which may fall as much as ten-fold in the first week (14), and then continue to decline less precipitously for the remainder of lactation (6,14-17). Concentrations of copper, iron, manganese, selenium and fluorine have all been reported to decline with duration of lactation, the changes being particularly marked in the first 1-2 months (6,7,9,14-16, 18-24). Conversely, levels of chromium do not appear to change with progressing lactation (25, 26). Other elements have not been investigated for this source of variation.

ANALYSIS

Preparation

The method of sample preparation should be chosen according to the element(s) to be measured and the analytical technique. Again, the methodology used should be carefully checked for both adventitious loss or gain of element. Unless one is specifically interested in the distribution among milk fractions, analyses should be done on whole milk. There is evidence to show that a high and variable proportion of elements like iron, copper, and zinc may be associated with the fat and pellet after centrifugation (27). Removal of protein by precipitation may also cause loss of elements that are bound to protein or left in trapped whey (28).

Minimizing sample pretreatment reduces the risk of contamination and permits the use of very small sample sizes. Use of the graphite furnace in atomic absorption spectrophotometry allows simple dilution for many elements; most other techniques require some pretreatment to remove the organic matrix, especially the fat. Wet digestion with a variety of acids is only suitable for a few elements (e.g. iron, selenium), as it is difficult and expensive to obtain acids of sufficient purity for many of the minor elements. Conversely, dry ashing in a muffle furnace (to 450°C) is inappropriate for elements with a low boiling point, such as selenium or arsenic. Both of these methods require sample sizes of at least 2 - 5 ml for adequate precision, but they do allow the sample to be concentrated. Low temperature ashing (to 120°C) in an oxygen plasma under reduced pressure is suitable for most elements, including those with low boiling points, but is inefficient with sample sizes of greater than 500 µl. Specific aspects of the complex matrix of milk may need to be considered in specific situations, e.g., interaction with calcium in the analysis of chromium by isotope dilution mass spectrometry.

Analytical technique

The choice depends on the element(s) of interest. It must be remembered that many elements are present in human milk in comparatively low concentrations, so the usefulness of a given technique may be restricted by detection limits. The most common, and currently most practical, analytical technology is atomic absorption spectrophotometry, both from considerations of cost and the range of elements which can be measured. Zinc, copper and iron can be analyzed by flame atomic absorption after pretreatment of samples. Electrothermal atomization (graphite furnace) expands the capabilities of atomic absorption spectrophotometry to permit determination of almost all metallic elements likely to be of interest, with reasonable to very good precision and in small sample sizes (14). Selenium, arsenic and mercury can also be measured by atomic absorption with suitable adaptation such as hydride generation or Zeeman background correction.

Atomic absorption spectrophotometry, however, suffers the limitation of being a single element technique, and it can be slow. Other spectrometric methods, including inductively coupled plasma and X-ray fluorescence, permit simultaneous determinations of a large number of elements. Unfortunately, at present, detection limits are too high for the measurement of most elements at the levels of occurrence in human milk. Thus, the application of these methods to the analysis of trace elements in human milk is currently restricted to zinc, copper, iron, and some of the non-essential elements, such as rubidium, occurring at higher concentrations (29).

Both neutron activation analysis and mass spectrometry give very good results for a wide range of elements, but they cannot yet be regarded as routine methods. Neutron activation has been widely used in the last few years for analyses of human milk, especially in Europe, but mostly in laboratories where research is predominantly in analytical methodologies rather than human lactation *per se* (30). For many of the elements of nutritional and toxicological interest (including, for example, chromium, nickel, lead, cadmium), the detection limits are too high for human milk. Mass spectrometry is capable of measuring a larger number of elements with a high degree of precision and reliability. It is currently too slow and expensive for routine analysis of the large numbers of samples generated by most studies of human lactation, but it is useful for proving analyses obtained by other techniques (26). Improvements in technology, including sample introduction techniques and software, should make mass spectrometry more widely accessible in the near future.

Specific details of methodologies depend on the element being measured and the type of analytical equipment used; further details of techniques for some specific elements are given below. The references given in this section are by no means exhaustive, and a more extensive list of references to methods which have been used for various elements is given in Table 1.

Table 1. Trace Elements in Human Milk

Element	Concentration[a]	Method[b]	References[c]
Zn	2 - 4 μg/ml	FAAS, GFAAS, ICP, NAA, XRF	4-6,13-17,19,23,24 29,30-36
Cu	0.2 - 0.6 μg/ml	FAAS, GFAAS, ICP, NAA, XRF	4-6,14-16,18,19,23 24,29,31-34
Fe	0.3 - 0.8 μg/ml	FAAS, ICP NAA, XRF	3-6,19,20,29,30,32 33
Mn	2 - 7 ng/ml	GFAAS, NAA	7,14,21,30,31,33,34
Se	9 - 40 ng/ml	AAS: GF,F, hydride; NAA, GC-EC, Fluo	8,9,22,30,31,33 37-42
Cr	0.3 ng/ml	GFAAS	25,26
I	30 - 500 ng/ml	NAA, ISE, Colo	36,43-46
F	9 - 11 ng/ml	ISE, Colo	10,45,47,48
As	0.5 ng/ml	NAA	31,34
Br	1.8 μg/ml	ICP	29
Cd	0.2 ng/ml	GFAAS, NAA	31
Co	0.2 - 3 ng/ml	NAA	30,31,33
Cs	2 - 74 ng/ml	NAA	30
Hg	1 ng/ml	NAA	30,31,33
Mo	12 ng/ml	NAA	34
Ni	16 ng/ml	GFAAS, ICP	49
Pb	18 ng/ml	GFAAS	49
Rb	1 - 6 μg/ml	NAA	30
Sb	0.2 - 3 ng/ml	NAA	30,31,33
Sc	0 - 0.8 ng/ml	NAA	30
V	0.14 ng/ml	NAA	31

a Concentrations at 1 month postpartum for Zn, Cu, Fe, Mn, Cr; all others pooled milk from 1 to 10 months.

b FAAS: flame atomic absorption spectrophotometry; GFAAS: graphite-furnace atomic absorption spectrophotometry; ICP: inductively coupled plasma; NAA: neutron activation analysis; XRF: X-ray fluorescence; hydride: hydridegeneration atomic absorption spectrophotometry; GC-ED: electron capture gas chromatrography; ISE: ion-specific electrode; Fluo: fluorimetry; Colo: colorimetry.

c Published methods; not necessarily a complete list.

Proving the Analysis

A major problem with any technique for analyzing trace elements in biological samples is that of proving the accuracy of the method, especially for some of the "newer" essential elements. Standard procedures include determination of detection limits, analytical precision, and proof of the lack of significant contamination. The internal consistency of the method may be shown by use of recoveries and standard additions. However, the need for an outside proof of accuracy is underscored by the very wide range of values reported from different laboratories, analyzing the same material, for the concentration of an element like copper, which has few analytical complications (50).

For some of the more routinely measured elements, such as iron, zinc, copper and selenium, analysis of a suitable reference material may provide adequate proof of the accuracy of the method. For less commonly measured elements, proof of accuracy should include analysis of reference materials, and ideally, independent confirmation of levels in some samples, or a stock human milk, by another laboratory using a different technique.

A suitable reference material is one which contains the elements in similar concentrations to those in human milk, and importantly for some techniques (including those involving extensive sample preparation and graphite furnace atomic absorption), a similar matrix. There are currently two standard reference materials available for milk analyses, both made from bovine milk:

(i) IAEA Reference Material A-11: from the International Atomic Energy Agency (Analytical Quality Control Services, Laboratory Seibersdorf, P.O. Box 1000, A-1400 Vienna, Austria). Reference values are given for calcium, chloride, copper, iron, mercury, potassium, manganese, sodium, phosphorus, rubidium, strontium, zinc and for SR^{90} and Cs^{137}. There may be problems with homogeneity of this material. IAEA also produced a freeze-dried human milk (HM-1) as a quality control for their collaborative study on the elemental composition of human milk, but this may no longer be available.

(ii) NBS Standard Reference Material 1549: from the National Bureau of Standards (Office of Standard Reference Materials, US Department of Commerce, National Bureau of Standards, Washington, D.C. 20234). This material is certified for calcium, cadmium, chloride, chromium, copper, mercury, iodine, potassium, magnesium, manganese, sodium, lead, selenium, sulphur, and zinc. Additional values are given for "information only" for silver, aluminum, arsenic, bromine, cobalt, iron, fluorine, molybdenum, phosphorus, rubidium, antimony, silicon, and tin.

REPORTING RESULTS

Because of the technical difficulties involved in trace element analysis, all reports of results (including those for more "common" elements such as iron, zinc, and copper) should include some indication of the reliability of the methodology used: contamination checks, analytical precision, and most importantly, reference material values or other checks of accuracy.

Because of the strong influence of duration of lactation on the concentration of many elements, milk samples or results should not be pooled over a wide time span (<1 months post-partum: weekly; >1 month post-partum: monthly), unless it has been shown that longitudinal variation is not important. In all cases, duration of lactation should be explicitly stated. Other maternal parameters, such as diet or geographical location, can have a significant influence on concentration of elements such as selenium, iodine, fluorine, and some non-essential elements. These parameters should be reported.

Because of the use to which reports are normally put, it is recommended that concentrations always be reported in terms of milk volume (molarity or per ml). If weight of liquid milk is used (g), information on specific gravity should be provided to allow conversion. There has been a tendency for some laboratories, especially those using neutron activation analysis, to report levels per unit dry weight. This type of report is not very useful for practical purposes and makes comparisons with other reports difficult.

NOTES ON SOME SPECIFIC ELEMENTS

Zinc and Copper

Significant diurnal variation has been reported by some workers, but not by others (2,4-6). Krebs et al. (35) analyzed zinc levels in 699 milk samples collected from 48 women over a total of 29 days, and found no significant variation due to time of day or time during feed. They concluded that for group studies, a sample collected at any feed during the day and at any stage during the feed would reflect the average concentration over the whole 24 hours. However, the duration of lactation, or time post-partum, does exert a significant effect on the concentrations of zinc and copper. It has been a consistent finding that as lactation progresses, the levels of both these elements in breast milk decline (2, 4-6,14-19,29,32,51-54).

Depending on the type of analytical equipment used, samples may simply be diluted prior to analysis, or pretreated to remove the organic matrix; both wet and dry digestion techniques have been used successfully. Zinc and copper are most commonly analyzed by atomic absorption spectrophotometry, but a very wide variety of methods has been used to measure these elements in human milk, including both flame and graphite furnace atomic absorption, as well as inductively coupled plasma, neutron activation, X-ray fluorescence, mass spectrometry and colorimetry. Generally good agreement is achievable between methods. Figure 1 shows results for zinc concentrations as measured by atomic absorption and X-ray fluorescence in the same milk samples in Dr. Howell's laboratory (29). Concentrations of both elements are high enough that detection limits are not a problem. Techniques like X-ray fluorescence present advantages of minimum sample preparation, rapid turnover and simultaneous analysis of both zinc and copper (and other elements), making this a particularly useful method for routine analysis of large numbers of samples. Table 2 summarizes some of the information in the literature for zinc and copper concentrations in human milk. It shows the relatively consistent values among the different laboratories for samples collected at the same post-partum interval, and it shows the consistent finding of declining concentrations of both elements with duration of lactation.

Selenium

There are obvious geographic differences in selenium levels of human milk, which are closely linked to variations in dietary selenium intake.

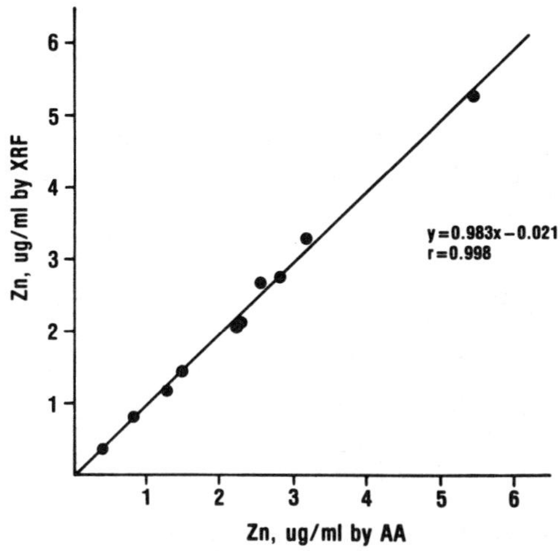

Figure. 1. Comparison of zinc concentrations in 10 individual milk samples measured by X-ray fluorescence spectrophotometry (XRF) and atomic absorption spectrophotometry (AA). (From Ref. 29, with permission.)

There is a sharp fall in milk selenium concentration during the first weeks of lactation, declining from very high levels in colostrum to a plateau in mature milk by one month (8,9,22,37-39,41). There appears to be no effect of time of day (8,9), but hind milk contained greater concentrations of selenium than fore milk in samples of mature milk (9). Because of geographic and individual variations in milk content, the population of lactating women used for sample collection must be well defined. Ideally, estimations of maternal dietary selenium intake should be made at the time of milk collection to detect a possible relationship between maternal selenium intake and milk content.

Samples for selenium analysis may be stored for some time at -20°C with little effect. However, if localization of the element is to be investigated, including analysis of activity of the enzyme glutathione peroxidase, in which form 25% of milk selenium is estimated to be present (55), optimum storage conditions must be determined. Picciano is currently investigating the effect of storage time and temperature on human milk glutathione peroxidase activity, and, until the results of this study are available, it is recommended that milk samples for analysis of selenium and glutathione peroxidase activity be stored at -20°C immediately after collection.

The techniques most commonly used for selenium determination in human milk are fluorimetry utilizing diaminonaphthalene (8,22,39-41), instrumental or radiochemical neutron activation analysis (22,42), graphite furnace atomic absorption (37), and hydride generation atomic absorption spectrophotometry (38). Although these methods have been widely employed, they all suffer from various drawbacks. Most of the methods require prolonged sample digestion and extensive extraction and purification steps. The fluorimetric technique is complicated by interference from co-extractants and poor precision at the low levels found in human milk. Neutron activation analysis and isotope dilution mass spectrometry have the required sensitivity for selenium determination in human milk, but are not

Table 2. Zinc and Copper in Human Milk

Investigator	Time postpartum	Zn µg/ml	Cu µg/ml	Reference
Picciano, Guthrie (1976)	6 - 12 weeks	1.68	0.24	5
Vaughan et al. (1979)	1 - 3 months	1.6	0.43	19
	4 - 6 months	1.05	0.33	
Vuori, Kuitunen (1979)	4 weeks	2.5	0.47	15
	11 - 13 weeks	1.1	0.32	
	23 - 25 weeks	0.49	0.17	
Kirksey et al. (1979)	day 3	4.61		6
	day 14	3.12		
	1 - 3 months	2.04		
	5 - 7 months	0.93		
Butte, Calloway (1981)	1 month	2.8	0.3	52
Picciano et al. (1981)	1 month	2.21	0.21	32
	2 months	2.08	0.20	
	3 months	1.93	0.21	
Moser, Reynolds (1983)	1 month	2.6	0.48	51
	3 months	1.3	0.37	
	6 months	1.1	0.28	
Feeley et al. (1983)	4 - 7 days	5.2	1.04	4
	10 - 14 days	4.1	0.93	
	30 - 45 days	2.9	0.84	
Dewey, Lönnerdal (1983)	1 month	1.80	0.25	23
	2 months	1.39	0.23	
	4 months	0.77	0.20	
	6 months	0.54	0.20	
Dewey et al. (1984)	≧7 months	0.40	0.17	24
Krebs et al. (1984)	1 month	2.65		53
	9 months	0.67		
Casey et al. (1985)	1 - 2 days	9.79	0.50	14
	3 - 4 days	6.75	0.53	
	5 - 7 days	5.39	0.62	
	8 - 14 days	4.28	0.53	
Howell et al. (1985)	1 - 4 days	7.74	0.77	54
	5 - 8 days	6.27	0.79	
	17 - 20 days	3.71	0.62	
	61 - 64 days	2.45	0.68	

readily available to many laboratories. The preferred atomic absorption method for human milk analysis is hydride generation, which utilizes the chemical reduction of selenium to hydrogen selenide (38). This is a very sensitive method, but it may be complicated by interference in the reduction step by several common cations yielding systematic negative error. Smith et al. (9) have used the recently developed technique of electron-capture gas chromatography to measure selenium in milk (56). This procedure is based on the reaction between Se(IV) and 4-nitro-o-phenylenediamine to form piazselenoles which can be extracted into organic solvents. Subjecting the organic extract to gas chromatography overcomes interference from organic co-extractants, which is the principal limitation of the fluorescence method. The limit of detection of this method is approximately 0.5 pg Se, permitting determination of selenium in sample volumes of 200 - 500 μl human milk.

Mean values for selenium in human milk of 10 ng/ml or less have recently been reported for mature milk from New Zealand (40), Finland (37), and Belgium (38), countries known to have low dietary selenium intake for adults. In contrast, higher mean values have been reported for mature milk from Germany, 28.3 ng/ml (42), the United States, 16.3 ng/ml (9), and Japan, 18 ng/ml (22).

Manganese

The manganese concentration of human milk does not appear to vary significantly within a feed or diurnally (7). Stastney et al. (7) found a decline in milk manganese between 1 and 3 months postpartum. Vuori (21) reported that levels declined from 2 weeks to 2 months postpartum, then changed little up to 6 months of lactation. Unlike iron, copper and zinc, manganese levels in human milk may be influenced by the level in the maternal diet or blood (Picciano, unpublished observations). Vuori et al. (57) observed a significant correlation between maternal intake and the concentration of manganese in milk. This direct relationship was evident even as milk manganese levels declined with progressing lactation.

Manganese is most commonly measured by graphite furnace atomic absorption spectrophotometry (7,14,21) or by neutron activation analysis (30,31,33,34). For graphite furnace analysis, milk samples may be predigested by ashing in a muffle furnace (7,21), or diluted and applied directly to the graphite tube with standard additions (14). Concentrations of manganese in human milk obtained from 1 to 3 months postpartum, as measured by these two methods, are in the order of 3 - 8 ng/ml (7,14,21, 30,31,33,34). Mean values outside this range (6,19) may reflect contamination of samples or analytical difficulties. However, additional work is needed to determine whether the manganese content of human milk is a reflection of the maternal intake or whether it is maintained within a narrow range, as is the case for other essential trace elements.

Iodine and Fluorine

Both elements are believed to be present in milk predominantly as the anions, iodine (I^-) and fluoride (F^-), and most analytical techniques utilize this property. Iodine and fluorine can be accurately determined by microchemical procedures which require 1 - 5 ml milk (58,59). Recently, ion-selective electrodes have been developed for the assay of these two elements; the electrodes have high sensitivity, and both the ionized form of the element and total content can be determined (45,47,60). The iodine electrode may respond non-specifically to other ionized groups, such as sulfydryl groups. Human milk contains about

180 ng/ml (1.3 μM) iodine, but a high degree of variation is evident. The concentration of fluorine is approximately 7 - 11 ng/ml (0.5 μM). Stage of lactation does not appear to have a strong effect on iodine or fluorine concentrations; however, maternal intake appears to influence milk levels of both elements (10,45-48).

CONCLUSION

Almost all trace elements are known to be present in human milk, but for many there is very little further information available. Even for the nutritionally essential element molybdenum, there have been few reports of the normal range of concentrations and no studies of variability. This has been due in part to the lack, in the past, of analytical techniques with sufficient sensitivity to accurately measure the low concentrations normally present in human milk. The past 10 to 15 years have seen the commercial development of analytical equipment (e.g., graphite furnace atomic absorption spectrophotometry, mass spectrometry) with considerably lowered detection limits. Coupled with a growing appreciation of the necessity for rigid control of contamination, this has permitted considerable improvement in the reliability of reported values for many elements. At the same time, the accepted normal level of elements such as chromium (25,26) and manganese (7,14) has been decreased by an order of magnitude. The continuing improvement of analytical methodologies will permit more detailed investigation of many elements, both nutritionally essential (e.g., molybdenum), and those suggested as essential for animals but not yet proven to be essential for humans, such as silicon and vanadium.

REFERENCES

1. Neville MC, Keller RP, Seacat J, Casey CE, Allen JC, Archer P. (1984): Studies on human lactation: 1. Within-feed and between-breast variation in selected components of human milk. Am J Clin Nutr, 40, 635-646.

2. Picciano MF. (1978): Mineral content of human milk during a single nursing. Nutr Rep Internat, 18, 5-10.

3. Fransson G-B, Lönnerdal B. (1980): Iron in human milk. J Pediatr, 96, 380-384.

4. Feeley RM, Eitenmiller RR, Jones JB, Barnhart H. (1983): Copper, iron, and zinc contents of human milk at early stages of lactation. Am J Clin Nutr, 37, 443-448.

5. Picciano MF, Guthrie HA. (1976): Copper, iron and zinc content of mature human milk. Am J Clin Nutr, 29, 242-254.

6. Kirksey A, Ernst JA, Roepke JL, Tsai T-L. (1979): Influence of mineral intake and use of oral contraceptives before pregnancy on the mineral content of human colostrum and of more mature milk. Am J Clin Nutr, 32, 30-39.

7. Stastny D, Vogel RS, Picciano MF. (1984): Manganese intake and serum manganese concentrations of human milk-fed and forumula-fed infants. Am J Clin Nutr, 39, 872-878.

8. Millar KR, Sheppard AD. (1972): α-Tocopherol and selenium levels in human and cow's milk. N Z J Sci, 15, 3-15.

9. Smith AM, Picciano MF, Milner JA. (1982): Selenium intakes and status of human milk and formula fed infants. Am J Clin Nutr, 35, 521-526.

10. Spak CJ, Hardell LI, de Chateau P. (1983): Fluoride in human milk. Acta Paediatr Scand, 72, 699-701.

11. Macy IG, Nims B, Brown M, Hunscher HA. (1931): Human milk studies VII. Chemical analyses of milk representative of the entire first and last halves of the nursing period. Am J Dis Child, 42, 569-589.

12. Nims B, Macy IG, Brown M, Hunscher HA. (1932): Human milk studies. IX. Variations in the composition of milk at four hour intervals during the day and night. Am J Dis Child, 43, 828-844.

13. Neville MC, Archer P, Casey CE, Hambidge KM. (1985): Diurnal variation in human milk volume and composition. Fed Proc, 44, 1675.

14. Casey CE, Hambidge KM, Neville MC. (1985): Studies in human lactation: zinc, copper, manganese and chromium in the first four weeks of lactation. Am J Clin Nutr, 41, 1193-1200.

15. Vuori E, Kuitunen P. (1979): The concentrations of copper and zinc in human milk. A longitudinal study. Acta Paediatr Scand, 68, 33-37.

16. Moran JR, Vaughan R, Stroop S, Coy S, Johnston H, Greene HL. (1983): Concentrations and total daily output of micronutrients in breast milk of mothers delivering preterm: a longitudinal study. J Pediatr Gastroenterol Nutr, 2, 629-634.

17. Butte NF, Garza C, Johnson CA, O'Brien Smith E, Nichols BL. (1984): Longitudinal changes in milk composition of mothers delivering preterm and term infants. Early Hum Develop, 9, 153-162.

18. Hambidge KM. (1976): The importance of trace elements in infant nutrition. Curr Med Res Opin, 4, Suppl. 1, 44-53.

19. Vaughan LA, Weber CW, Kemberling SR. (1979): Longitudinal changes in the mineral content of human milk. Am J Clin Nutr, 32, 2301-2306.

20. Siimes MA, Vuori E, Kuitunen P. (1979): Breast milk iron -- a declining concentration during the course of lactation. Acta Paediatr Scand, 68, 29-31.

21. Vuori, E. (1979): A longitudinal study of manganese in human milk. Acta Paediatr Scand, 68, 571-573.

22. Higashi A, Tamari H, Kuroki Y, Matsuda I. (1983): Longitudinal changes in selenium content of breast milk. Acta Paediatr Scand, 72, 433-436.

23. Dewey KG, Lönnerdal B. (1983): Milk and nutrient intake of breast-fed infants from 1 to 6 months: relation to growth and fatness. J Pediatr Gastroenterol Nutr, 2, 497-506.

24. Dewey KG, Finley DA, Lönnerdal B. (1984): Breast milk volume and composition during late lactation (7-20 months). J Pediatr Gastroenterol Nutr, 3, 713-720.

25. Kumpulainen J, Vuori E. (1980): Longitudinal study of chromium in human milk. Am J Clin Nutr, 33, 2299-2302.

26. Casey CE, Hambidge KM, Neville MC. (1984): Chromium in human milk from American mothers. Br J Nutr, 52, 73-77.

27. Fransson G-B, Lönnerdal B. (1983): Distribution of trace elements and minerals in human and cow's milk. Pediatr Res, 17, 912-915.

28. Lönnerdal B, Smith C, Keen CL. (1984): Analysis of breast milk: current methodologies and future needs. J Pediatr Gastroenterol Nutr, 3, 290-295.

29. Palma PA, Seifert WE, Caprioli RM, Howell RR. (1983): X-ray fluorescence spectrometry in the analysis of trace elements in human milk. J Lab Clin Med, 102, 88-94.

30. Clemente GF, Ingaro G, Santaroni GP. (1982): The concentration of some trace elements in human milk from Italy. Sci Total Environ, 24, 255-265.

31. Kosta L, Byrne AR, Dermelj M. (1983): Trace elements in some human milk samples by radiochemical neutron activation analysis. Sci Total Environ, 29, 261-268.

32. Picciano MF, Calkins EJ, Garrick JR, Deering RH. (1981): Milk and mineral intakes of breast-fed infants. Acta Paediatr Scand, 70, 189-194.

33. Iyengar GV, Kasperek K, Feinendegen LE, Wang YX, Weese H. (1982): Determination of Co, Cu, Fe, Hg, Mn, Sb, Se, and Zn in milk samples. Sci Total Environ, 24, 267-274.

34. Dang HS, Jaiswal DD, Wadhwani Cn, Somasunderam S, Dacosta H. (1983): Infants with a congenital anomaly and the concentration of Mo, As, Mn, Zn and Cu in the mother's milk. Sci Total Environ, 27, 43-47.

35. Krebs NF, Hambidge KM, Jacobs MA, Mylet S. (1985): Zinc in human milk: diurnal and within feed patterns. J Pediatr Gastroenterol Nutr, 4, 227-229.

36. Department of Health and Social Security, (1977): The composition of mature human milk. Report on Health and Social Subjects No. 12. London: HMSO.

37. Kumpulainen J, Vuori E, Kuitunen P, Makinen S, Kara R. (1983): Longitudinal study on the dietary selenium intake of exclusively breast-fed infants and their mothers in Finland. Internat J Vit Min Res, 53, 420-426.

38. Robberecht H, Roekens E, Deelstra H, Van Caille-Bertrand M, Clara R. (1985): Longitudinal study of the selenium content in human breast milk in Belgium. Acta Paediatr Scand, 74, 254-258.

39. Shearer TR, Hadjimarkos DM. (1975): Geographic distribution of selenium in human milk. Arch Environ Health, 30, 230-233.

40. Williams MMF. (1983): Selenium and glutathione peroxidase in mature human milk. Proc Uni Otago Med Sch, 61, 20-21.

41. Hadjimarkos DM, Shearer TR. (1973): Selenium in mature human milk. Am J Clin Nutr, 26, 583-585.

42. Lombeck I, Kasperek K, Bonnermann B, Feinendegen LE, Bremer HJ. (1978): Selenium content of human milk, cow's milk and cow's milk infant formulas. Europ J Pediatr, 129, 139-145.

43. Etling N, Padovani E, Gehin-Fouque F, Tato L. (1983): Iodine and thyroid hormone levels in serum and urine of full-term newborn infants. Helv Paediatr Acta, 38, 117-122.

44. Gushurst CA, Mueller JA, Green JA, Sedor F. (1984): Breast milk iodide: reassessment in the 1980s. Pediatrics, 73, 354-357.

45. Backer-Dirks O, Jongeling-Eijnhoven JMPA, Flissebaalje TD, Gedelia I. (1974): Total free and ionic fluoride in human and cow's milk as determined by gas-liquid chromatography and the fluoride electrode. Caries Res, 8, 181-186.

46. Bruhn JC, Franke AA. (1983): Iodine in human milk. J Dairy Sci, 66, 1396-1398.

47. Esala S, Vuori E, Helle A. (1982): Effect of maternal fluorine intake on breast milk fluorine content. Br J Nutr, 48, 201-204.

48. Ekstrand J, Spak C-J, Falch J, Afseth J, Ulvestad H. (1984): Distribution of fluoride to human breast milk following intake of high doses of fluoride. Caries Res, 18, 93-95.

49. Camara Rica C, Kirkbright GF. (1982): Determination of trace concentrations of lead and nickel in human milk by electrothermal atomization atomic absorption spectrophotometry and inductively-coupled plasma emission spectroscopy. Sci Total Environ, 22, 192-201.

50. Kosta L. (1980): Reference samples for trace elements in biological materials and associated analytical problems. In: Elemental analysis of biological materials. Technical Report Series No. 197. Vienna: IAEA, 317-345.

51. Moser PB, Reynolds R. (1983): Dietary zinc intake and zinc concentrations of plasma, erythrocytes, and breast-milk in antepartum and postpartum lactating and nonlactating women: a longitudinal study. Am J Clin Nutr, 38, 101-108.

52. Butte NF, Calloway DH, Van Duzen JL. (1981): Nutritional assessment of pregnant and lactating Navajo women. Am J Clin Nutr, 34, 2216-2228.

53. Krebs NF, Hambidge KM, Jacobs MA, Oliva-Rasbach J. (1985): The effects of a dietary zinc supplement during lactation on longitudinal changes in maternal zinc status and milk zinc concentrations. Am J Clin Nutr, 41, 560-570.

54. Howell RR, Palma PA, Seifert WE, Caprioli RM. Longitudinal changes in human milk regarding serum trace metals. In: Howell RR, Morriss FH, Pickering LK, eds, Human Milk and Infant Nutrition. Springfield, Illinois: Charles C. Thomas. (In press).

55. Hojo Y. (1982): Selenium concentration and glutathione peroxidase activity in cow's milk. Biol Tr Elem Res, 4, 233-239.

56. McCarthy TP, Brodie B, Milner JA, Bevill RF. (1981): Improved method for selenium determination in biological samples by gas chromatography. J Chromat, 225, 9-16.

57. Vuori E, Makinen SM, Kara R, Kuitunen P. (1980): The effects of the dietary intakes of copper, iron, manganese and zinc on the trace element content of human milk. Am J Clin Nutr, 33, 227-231.

58. Stolc V, Nemeth S. (1961): Microestimation of iodine in milk. J Dairy Sci, 44, 2187-2193.

59. Dixon EJ. (1970): Determination of microgram amounts of fluoride with zirconium and solochrome cyanine R. Analyst, 95, 272-277.

60. Bruhn JC, Franke AA. (1978): An indirect method for the estimation of the iodine content in raw milk. J Dairy Sci, 61, 1557-1560.

TRACE ELEMENTS IN HUMAN MILK: STRUCTURAL ASPECTS

S.V. Rumball
E.N. Baker

INTRODUCTION

In recent years, research concerning the trace elements iron, copper and zinc in human milk has been concentrated in the following areas:

(a) measurement of total trace element concentrations (1),
(b) measurement of relative amounts of each trace element in the various milk compartments (2,3),
(c) separation and identification of specific metal-ligand complexes (2,4,5,6), and
(d) theoretical calculations on the distribution of metals among the various ligands present in milk (7).

Underlying the research areas of (b), (c) and (d) is the recognition that iron, copper and zinc will be found in milk in a variety of different forms. Trace elements such as these are present in milk almost entirely in bound form, rather than as free ions, the ligands being generally either proteins or low molecular weight ligands such as organic acids, amino acids and sugars. The distribution of the metals among the ligands present in human milk is controlled by metal concentrations, ligand concentrations, pH and ionic strength. The strength with which these ligands bind different metals, however, also depends critically on their three-dimensional structures.

BIOAVAILABILITY OF TRACE ELEMENTS

Interest has arisen in the form of iron, copper and zinc in human milk in response to observations concerning differences in availability of these metals between bovine and human milks (8,9). Bioavailability of a trace element is a function of both the amount and the chemical form ingested, as well as of the conditions prevailing in the gastrointestinal tract. Absorption of trace elements occurs in the small intestine, generally by penetration of neutral low molecular weight complexes into the intestinal cell. In this case the complex must release its metal ion inside the cell, so that the metal can be subsequently incorporated into proteins. In contrast, it has been suggested that iron from milk may be absorbed directly in protein-bound form (10,11).

Although conditions in the gastrointestinal tract differ from those in milk with regard to pH, local concentrations of metals and ligands, presence of proteolytic enzymes, etc., much can be learned about these processes by identifying and characterizing the various metal-ligand complexes in milk.

METAL-PROTEIN COMPLEXES

Milk metal-protein complexes can be classified in terms of their origins and functions. Some of the proteins present in milk are derived from the blood, while others are synthesized in the mammary gland. Some have the function of catalysis (enzymes), while others are involved in metal transport or storage; these roles may be relevant to the presence of the protein in blood, or in the mammary gland, or in milk. On the other hand, where binding of metals to proteins is weak, this may not have any specific functional significance, but may be merely a consequence of the effects that the availability of metal-binding groups have on the protein and of the appropriate concentrations of metal and protein.

As far as the bioavailability of trace elements is concerned, the most useful classification depends on the strength of binding and the nature of the binding site(s). Two classes should be differentiated:

(i) Metalloproteins (including metalloenzymes). In these compounds the metal ion is tightly bound and is an integral part of the protein. The stereochemical constraints of a protein molecule are such that it can present chemical groups (e.g., the side-chains of amino acids such as histidine, cysteine, tyrosine, methionine, aspartic and glutamic acids) in a particular geometrical arrangement, suited to the binding of a particular metal ion. These are then specific binding sites. Bioavailability of the metal in this case would depend mainly on susceptibility of the protein to denaturation in the gastrointestinal tract with subsequent release of the metal.

(ii) Metal-associated proteins. In these, metal ions are bound much more loosely than in metalloproteins, probably to some of the many functional groups residing on the protein exterior. These are likely to be able to bind a variety of metal ions, and thus provide non-specific binding sites. Bioavailability of metals in this form would be influenced by denaturation, by the presence of other ligands able to compete successfully for the (weakly) bound metal, and by local metal ion concentrations, which may be such that the metal simply dissociates.

Proteins in human milk which have been identified as loci of iron, copper and zinc include xanthine oxidase (1,6), alkaline phosphatase (1,6), casein (1,2), serum albumin (2) and lactoferrin (3). Of these, casein can bind iron, copper and zinc, and serum albumin can bind copper, and possibly zinc. In both cases, binding is weak and apparently non-specific; the metals can probably be removed by other chelating agents. On the other hand, the other three proteins have specific sites for certain metals: xanthine oxidase for two molybdenum and eight iron atoms (which are important for its enzymatic activity), alkaline phosphatase for four zinc atoms (two essential for enzymatic activity and two fulfilling a structural role) and two magnesium atoms, and lactoferrin two iron atoms. These metals are strongly bound and not easily removed.

LOW MOLECULAR WEIGHT METAL-LIGAND COMPLEXES

Low molecular weight species in milk with the ability to bind metals include organic acids, amino acids, sugars and peptides. At present, citrate and glutamate have been identified as copper ligands (4), and citrate as a zinc ligand (4,5). Other ligands such as picolinate have been postulated (12), and milk contaminants (e.g., salicylic acid in aspirin) are also potential ligands.

INVESTIGATION OF METAL-LIGAND COMPLEXES BY X-RAY DIFFRACTION

In order to fully understand the structure and function of the metal--ligand complexes in human milk, it is important that the environment of the metal be known, i.e., that the identity and geometrical arrangement of the metal-binding groups be known, together with (in metal-protein complexes) the location of the metal-binding sites within the protein tertiary structure.

The technique of X-ray diffraction has proved invaluable in providing definitive information about the detailed arrangement of atoms within molecules. The essential requirements for an X-ray structure analysis are: that the material be isolated or synthesized pure, that single crystals of the compound can be grown, that they diffract well, and that they are stable to irradiation.

The methods of structure determination by X-ray diffraction are well established, although they differ in detail for "small molecule" and macromolecular complexes. Given automated equipment for measuring the X-ray diffraction data (an X-ray diffractometer), a single crystal structure analysis of a low molecular weight complex may be completed in a few days to a few weeks. For a protein structure analysis the time is likely to be much longer (one to five years) because far more data must be collected, crystals are less stable, and isomorphous heavy atom derivatives must be prepared as part of the technique of structure determination. (These are generally prepared by non-specific binding of heavy metal ions or complexes to the protein in its crystalline state. This is possible because protein crystals typically contain 50% liquid, and small molecules and ions can be diffused into the crystals, to bind to the protein, without disturbing the relative orientations or positions of the protein molecules.) On the other hand, the complete 3-dimensional structures of very complex molecules can be determined in this way and precise information on metal binding sites obtained.

STUDIES ON LACTOFERRIN

Here we use lactoferrin as an illustration of some of the complexities of a metal-binding protein system, and of the objectives of structural research.

Lactoferrin is a glycoprotein present in human milk whey. It binds two moles of iron per mole of protein in the presence of bicarbonate. These iron atoms are bound tightly into specific binding sites. It can also bind a number of other metal ions, mostly into the iron sites (if not already occupied by iron), but sometimes into non-specific sites (13,14). There is controversy as to whether lactoferrin binds zinc (15,2). In human milk, only about 5% of the lactoferrin normally has iron bound.

The role of lactoferrin in milk is presently under investigation. It has been suggested that it has a bacteriostatic role by binding free iron so tightly into its vacant iron-binding sites that bacteria are deprived of essential iron (16). While lactoferrin has been shown to inhibit the growth of certain micro-organisms *in vitro* it is less certain whether it has this effect *in vivo*. It may also be involved in absorption of iron by donation of iron to specific receptors at the brush border membrane in the small intestine (10). Other hypotheses suggest it protects against excess iron absorption by binding iron in the duodenum (17) or regulates iron absorption (11). There is speculation that other metal-lactoferrin complexes may form in the duodenum and so promote absorption of these metals (18). One of the key points in the above discussion is the apparent resistance of lactoferrin, in both the iron-free and iron-saturated form, to destruction by gastric acidity or proteolytic activity (11,19). Again, this probably depends on structure.

In order to fully characterize the structure of human milk lactoferrin, its amino acid sequence has been determined (20), and an X-ray analysis of its three-dimensional structure is in progress (21). In the latter work, problems have been experienced with crystal variability, but full sets of data for the native protein and one derivative have been measured, which should allow the determination of the structure in the near future.

The structural determination of lactoferrin will provide details of the iron-binding sites (ligands, geometry, the role of bicarbonate), and their location within the protein tertiary structure. This should give insight into the way in which lactoferrin can both bind iron and release it as required, and into its resistance to proteolysis (11,19,22). Lactoferrin can also be crystallized with other metal ions (e.g., Cu^{2+}) in place of iron, so that the binding of these can also be studied. In the future, it is hoped that comparisons will be made on the structure of human lactoferrin with bovine lactoferrin, although at present, difficulties have been experienced in growing suitable crystals of the bovine protein. Information about the conformation of the protein in the two species might help explain reported differences in susceptibility to proteolysis of human and bovine lactoferrins (22).

SUMMARY

In order to understand the bioavailability of trace elements in human milk, the form in which the element is present both in milk and in the duodenum needs to be known. Details of the molecular structures of the metal-ligand complexes present can be obtained by X-ray diffraction, providing the material can be isolated pure (or synthesized, in the case of a low molecular weight ligand), and subsequently crystallized. X-ray diffraction studies of the Fe-lactoferrin complex are underway.

REFERENCES

1. Lönnerdal B, Keen CL, Hurley LS. (1981): Iron, copper, zinc and manganese in milk. Ann Rev Nutr, 1, 149-174. (And references therein).

2. Lönnerdal B, Hoffman B, Hurley LS (1982): Zinc and copper binding proteins in human milk. Amer J. Clin Nutr, 36, 1170-1176.

3. Fransson GB, Lönnerdal B. (1980): Iron in human milk. J Pediatr, 90, 380-384.

4. Martin MT, Licklider KF, Brushmiller JG, Jacobs FA. (1981): Detection of low molecular weight copper(II) and zinc(II) binding ligands in ultrafiltered milks - the citrate connection. J Inorg Biochem, 15, 55-65.

5. Lönnerdal B, Stanislowski AG, Hurley LS. (1980): Isolation of a low molecular weight zinc binding ligand from human milk. J Inorg Biochem, 12, 71-78.

6. Fransson G-B, Lönnerdal B. (1984): Iron, copper, zinc, calcium and magnesium in human milk fat. Am J Clin Nutr, 39, 185-189.

7. May PM, Smith GL, Williams DR. (1982): Computer calculation of zinc(II)-complex distribution in milk. J Nutr, 112, 1990-1993.

8. Sandström B, Cederblad A, Lönnerdal B. (1983): Zinc absorption from human milk, cow's milk, and infant formulas. Am J Dis Child, 137, 726-729.

9. Saarinen U, Siimes MA. (1979): Iron absorption from breast milk, cow's milk, and iron-supplemented formula: an opportunistic use of changes in total body iron determined by hemoglobin, ferritin, and body weight in 132 infants. Pediatr Res, 13, 143-147.

10. Cox TM, Mazurier J, Spik G, Montreuil J, Peters TJ. (1979): Iron binding proteins and influx of iron across the duodenal brush border. Evidence for specific lactotransferrin receptors in the human intestine. Biochim Biophys Acta, 588, 120-128.

11. Brock JH. (1980): Lactoferrin in human milk: its role in iron absorption and protection against enteric infection in the newborn infant. Arch of Dis Child, 55, 417-421.

12. Evans GW, Johnson PE. (1980): Characterization and quantitation of a zinc-binding ligand in human milk. Pediatr Res, 14, 876-880.

13. Ainscough EW, Brodie AM, Plowman JE. (1979): The chromium, manganese, cobalt and copper complexes of human lactoferrin. Inorg Chim Acta, 33, 148-153.

14. Ainscough EW, Brodie AM, Plowman JE, Bloor SJ, Loehr JS, Loehr TM. (1980): Studies on human lactoferrin by electron paramagnetic resonance, fluorescence, and resonance Raman spectroscopy. Biochem, 19, 4072-4079.

15. Blakeborough P, Salter DN, Gurr MI. (1983): Zinc binding in cow's milk and human milk. Biochem J, 209, 505-512.

16. Bullen JJ, Rogers HJ, Leigh L. (1972): Iron-binding proteins in milk and resistance to Escherichia coli infection in infants. Brit Med J, i, 69-75.

17. DeVet BJCM, Van Gool J. (1974): Lactoferrin and iron absorption in the small intestine. Acta Med Scand, 196, 393-402.

18. Quarterman J. (1983): Milk, lactoferrin and heavy-metal absorption. Proc Nutr Soc, 42, 45A.

19. Spik G, Brunet B, Mazurier-Dehaine C, Fontaine G, Montreuil J. (1982): Characterization and properties of the human and bovine lactotransferrins extracted from the faeces of newborn infants. Acta Paediatr Scand, 71, 979-985.

20. Metz-Boutigue M-H, Jolles J, Mazurier J, Schoentgen F, Legrand D, Spik G, Montreuil J, Jolles P. (1984): Human lactotransferrin: amino acid sequence and structural comparisons with other transferrins. Eur J Biochem 145, 659-676.

21. Baker EN, Rumball SV. (1977): Crystallographic data for human lactoferrin. J Mol Biol, 111, 207-210.

22. Brines RD, Brock JH. (1983): The effect of trypsin and chymotrypsin on the in vitro antimicrobial and iron-binding properties of lactoferrin in human milk and bovine colostrum. Unusual resistance of human apolactoferrin to proteolytic digestion. Biochim Biophys Acta, 759, 229-235.

METHODS FOR STUDYING TRACE-ELEMENT BINDING LIGANDS IN HUMAN MILK

B. Lönnerdal

INTRODUCTION

The growing infant is dependent on an adequate intake of trace elements for growth and optimum health. To achieve an adequate intake requires that the diet contain an ample supply of the element, and that a certain proportion of this supply is absorbed for utilization by the infant. The first question to be resolved is the matter of assessing supply (dietary intake). Methods have been developed and documented for collecting representative breast-milk samples, analyzing trace elements and assessing volume ingested by the infant (see other chapters of this book). The remaining question will be the degree to which ingested trace elements are utilized by the infant. The bioavailability of a trace element is determined both by endogenous factors and by composition of the diet. Among the endogenous factors, are the development of the gastrointestinal tract (acid secretion, biliary and pancreatic function, and mucosal function -- such as pinocytosis), and the trace element status of the infant. Iron, for example, is known to be better absorbed from a subject with a poor iron status than when iron status is good (1). The composition of the diet is known to have a pronounced effect on the bioavailability of several trace elements. The relative contribution of factors stimulating or inhibiting trace element uptake in the small intestinal mucosa will determine the net absorption of the element.

The absorption of several trace elements from human milk has been shown to be superior to absorption from other infant foods, such as cows' milk and soy formulas. Absorption studies have been performed on iron in human infants (2,3), zinc in human adults (4,5) and zinc and copper in suckling animal models (6,7). The high concentration of lactoferrin, a specific iron-binding protein in human milk, has been suggested to be a major factor underlying the high bioavailability of iron from human milk. The low concentration of casein in human milk, as well as the difference in its physical characteristics, has been suggested as being responsible for the high bioavailability of zinc and copper from human milk (6,7). The phytate content of soy may negatively affect the absorption of iron (8), zinc (4,6) and copper (7) from soy formula. In conclusion, it is apparent that the factors that bind trace elements in human milk and other infant foods are important determinants of bioavailability.

The isolation and identification of ligands that bind trace elements in human milk have been areas of controversy due to methodological errors, lack of control experiments and conceptual mistakes. While most experimental techniques can identify potential binding ligands, it is important to recognize that any change in pH, ionic strength, temperature, ligand concentration and CO_2 concentration can alter the *in vivo* distribution of trace elements among their ligands. The following presentation will discuss some of the major methods used.

GEL FILTRATION CHROMATOGRAPHY

In principle, this separation procedure is a very "mild" method. The ionic strength and pH of the buffer used can be chosen so that the conditions of separation are very similar to those conditions *in vivo*, i.e., in human milk. The calcium ion concentration is also important since deletion of Ca^{++} from the buffer can lead to disaggregation of casein micelles, and this can result in a change in the elution position for casein (9). As the binding strength between a trace element and its ligand is affected by the ionic strength, pH, and temperature, changes in these parameters may obscure the results.

The trace elements can be detected following chromatography either by analyzing the native element with atomic-absorption spectrophotometry or by using a radioactive tracer. Radioisotopes are available for most trace elements, and since most of them are gamma-emitters, sensitivity can be increased significantly. The very small amount of element added is not likely to change any equilibria within the milk; however, it should be emphasized that the isotope is added extrinsically. It should not be taken for granted that this extrinsic tag is distributed among ligands in a manner similar to the distribution of the native (cold) element. For example, it is known that molybdenum in xanthine oxidase is available but not exchangeable (10). It has also been shown that radioiron added to human milk is not distributed among the iron-binding ligands in the same pattern as native iron, but is grossly over-represented in the lactoferrin compartment (11). It can be predicted that an element such as selenium cannot be added extrinsically, since at least some of the selenium is covalently bound to proteins and amino acids (12). Although other elements, such as zinc, copper and manganese, do equilibrate with the native elements (6,13-14), appropriate experiments are always required to validate the method.

Regardless of the method of detection utilized, it is essential to ascertain that the amount of element applied to the column is recovered in the eluant. Many gel matrices contain small but significant amounts of residual negative charges. These charges can successfully compete with ligands in the milk and cause poor recovery (15), with the result that weaker ligands may show a low degree of binding, or no binding at all. A more severe consequence, however, is that the gel filtration column acts as an ion-exchanger. Any change in ionic strength, such as introduction of a sample, may cause elution of the element, possibly now bound to another ligand (or salts) or redistributed among ligands. Different approaches have been used to overcome this complication: a) chemical treatment of the gel to remove the charges (15), b) saturation of the charges with trace elements, bound or in free form, such as pre-running the column with liver homogenate (16), or c) "swamping" the system by adding the trace element to the running buffer (17). It should be noted that "masking" gel charges with trace-element/ligand complexes does not eliminate the problem. As stated above, this gel still acts as an ion-exchanger, and these ligands can be eluted by small changes in ionic strength and/or pH. The so-called "modified-gel chromatography," i.e., Hummel and Dreyer's method of adding a base-line concentration of an element (18), can be a useful tool when studying the *capacity* of various ligands in milk to bind trace elements. However, this does not reflect *in vivo* binding of trace elements to ligands; the use of this method will result in binding to even the weakest ligands present in the fluid studied. Trace elements (by definition) are not in abundance *in vivo*, i.e., only the strongest ligands and those present in high concentration will successfully compete for the element. As a final note of caution, it is necessary to demonstrate that an isolated trace-element/ligand complex elutes at a position identical to the elution position of the element found for human milk. When documenting this position, consideration should be given to the relative size and concentration of the sample and the ligands after radial dilution on the column, as these factors play a role in reproducibility.

ION-EXCHANGE CHROMATOGRAPHY

Some groups, after initial purification of a trace-element/ligand complex by gel filtration, have proceeded further using ion-exchange chromatography. Since the association constant for the complex studied is dependent on temperature and ionic strength, it can be predicted that this separation method, which is based on elution with either an increased salt concentration or a change in pH, can introduce misinterpretations. In addition, it is important that the sample introduced to the column is of the same pH and ionic strength as the running buffer; i.e., the sample has to be dialyzed against this buffer with possible changes from *in vivo* conditions. Again, proper control experiments, such as elution profiles before and after dialysis, are required.

The elution of the ligand from the column is achieved by changing the running buffer. By necessity, both the binding of the element to the ligand and the binding of the ligand to the column are gradually decreased. In addition, cation exchangers can bind trace elements themselves, which may be eluted. One example of this is the simultaneous elution of lactoferrin and its tightly bound iron from a cation exchanger, CM-Sephadex, at the same position as zinc which was non-specifically bound to the ion-exchanger (19). If proper control experiments are not run, this could lead to the mistaken conclusion that zinc binds to lactoferrin in milk (20).

DIALYSIS

The distribution of trace elements bound to macromolecules, such as proteins, and to low molecular weight ligands, can be determined by equilibrium dialysis. However, caution should be exercised since, a) the membrane may contain trace elements (which could be removed by EDTA treatment), b) the dialysis buffer and the temperature used may change the equilibrium in the milk (as discussed previously), or c) the presence of impermeant ions on one side of the membrane may limit transfer of permeant ions across the membrane (the Donnan effect).

ULTRACENTRIFUGATION

This method has been used to a limited extent. In our experience, ultracentrifugation is a very mild method for separation of milk ligands such as casein micelles, cells and fat globules (21). Since it is based on sedimentation/flotation, only the size (sedimentation coefficient)/density of the compartments should determine the separation, and no changes in physical equilibria are introduced. However, there are some reports of charge redistribution (22). This method may serve as a useful tool in an introductory separation of ligands.

ULTRAFILTRATION

Membranes with pores of varying sizes can be used to separate trace-element/ligand complexes of different sizes. Although mild in nature (only pressure is used), the molecular weight cut-off points are not accurate enough to make this an analytical tool, but rather a preparative method. There have been some recent reports of poor recovery of trace elements from some ultrafiltration membranes with low molecular weight cut-offs, emphasizing the need for preliminary recovery experiments. As mentioned above for dialysis, ultrafiltration is subject to Donnan effects.

COMPUTER MODELING

In theory, the distribution of trace elements among binding ligands is determined by the concentrations of the trace element and the various competing ligands, the concentrations of other divalent cations, the binding constants of the ligands, temperature and pH. This concept has been utilized by several investigators to calculate what the distribution should be *in vivo* (23-25). However, several criteria for the use of computer modeling may not be fulfilled. First, all binding ligands in the milk need to be identified. Second, the binding constants of these ligands for each element must be known. Third, this approach is valid only for trace elements which exchange freely among ligands. For example, no investigator has entered ATP (or ADP) into the equations; this may at least in part be responsible for the prediction that citrate binds Mg^{2+} in human milk (26). In fact, ATP is a well-known binder of magnesium, and we have shown that these two compounds co-elute by gel filtration of human milk (unpublished observations). The second criteria, the lack of knowledge of binding constants for some ligands, is exemplified by casein, which is a heterogeneous population of micelles consisting of several polypeptide subunits. Finally, trace elements are integral parts of some enzymes and may be physically entrapped within the fat globule membranes (27), in micelles, or in cells. In conclusion, this method has so far had limited value, but can be used in less complicated systems, such as milk diffusates (23). Complex formations can be predicted by computer modeling and compared to experimental results. With increased knowledge about individual components in human milk, this approach may become even more valuable.

SUMMARY

The factors that bind trace elements in human milk and other infant food are important determinants of trace element bioavailability. It is therefore essential to develop methods to further isolate and characterize the trace-element/ligand complexes in human milk. Such knowledge will enable investigation of their individual and combined effects on intestinal uptake processes. Trace-element binding ligands are commonly isolated by gel filtration chromatography, ion-exchange chromatography, dialysis, ultracentrifugation and ultrafiltration. These techniques can be important investigative tools, provided caution is taken to avoid ligand re-distribution, non-specific absorption and contamination. Computer modeling is a theoretical method to determine trace element distribution; it should be valuable as a companion to experimental techniques.

REFERENCES

1. Hallberg L. (1981): Bioavailability of dietary iron in man. Ann Rev Nutr, 1, 123-147.

2 McMillan JA, Oski FA, Lourie G, Tomarelli RM, Landaw SA. (1977): Iron absorption from human milk, simulated human milk, and proprietary formulas. Pediatrics, 60, 896-900.

3. Saarinen UM, Siimes MA, Dallman PR. (1977): Iron absorption in infants: high bioavailability of breast milk as indicated by the extrinsic tag method of iron absorption and by the concentration of serum ferritin. J Pediatr, 91, 36-39.

4. Casey CE, Walravens PA, Hambidge KM. (1981): Availability of zinc: loading tests with human milk, cow's milk, and infant formulas. Pediatrics, 68, 394-396.

5. Sandstrom B, Cederblad A, Lönnerdal B. (1983): Zinc absorption from human milk, cow's milk and infant formulas. Dis of Child, 137, 726-729.

6. Sandstrom B, Keen CL, Lönnerdal B. (1983): An experimental model for studies of zinc bioavailability from milk and infant formulas using extrinsic labeling. Am J Clin Nutr, 38, 420-428.

7. Lönnerdal B, Bell JG, Keen CL. Copper absorption from human milk and infant formulas: effects of copper and zinc concentrations. In: Proceedings of the Fifth International Symposium on Trace Element Metabolism in Man and Animals (1984). Aberdeen, Scotland. (In press).

8. Morch TA, Cook JD. (1981): Factors affecting the bioavailability of dietary iron. Cereal Foods World, 26, 667-672.

9. Pepper L, Farrell HM Jr. (1982): Interactions leading to formation of casein submicelles. J Diary Sci, 65, 2259-2266.

10. Johnson JL, Hainline BE, Rajagopalan KV. (1980): Characterization of the molybdenum cofactor of sulfite oxidase, xanthine oxidase and nitrate reductase. J Biol Chem, 255, 1783-1786.

11. Fransson G-B, Lönnerdal B. (1983): Distribution of added ^{59}Fe among various fractions of human and cos'w milk. Naringsforskning, 27, 108.

12. Young VR, Nahapetian A, Janghorbani M. (1982): Selenium bioavailability with reference to human nutrition. Am J Clin Nutr, 35, 1076-1088.

13. Lönnerdal B, Bell JG, Keen CL. Copper absorption from human milk, cow's milk and infant formulas using a suckling rat model. Am J Clin Nutr. (In press).

14. Lönnerdal B, Keen CL, Hurley LS. (1985): Manganese binding proteins of human and cow's milk. Am J Clin Nutr, 41, 550-559.

15. Lönnerdal B, Hoffman B. (1981): Alkaline reduction of dextran gels and crosslinked agarose to overcome nonspecific binding of trace elements. Biol Trace Elem Res, 3, 301-307.

16. Cousins RJ, Smith KT. (1980): Zinc-binding properties of bovine and human milk *in vitro*: influence of changes in zinc content. Am J Clin Nutr, 33, 1083-1087.

17. Martin MT, Licklider KF, Brushmiller JG, Jacobs FA. (1981): Detection of low molecular weight copper (II) and zinc (II) binding ligands in ultrafiltered milks -- the citrate connection. J Inorg Biochem, 15, 55-65.

18. Hummel JP, Dreyer WJ. (1962): Measurement of protein-binding phenomena by gel filtration. Biochim Biophys Acta, 63, 530-532.

19. Lönnerdal B, Hoffman B, Hurley LS. (1983): Zinc and copper binding proteins in human milk. Am J Clin Nutr, 38, 420-428.

20. Ainscough EW, Brodie AM, Plowman JE. (1980): Zinc transport by lactoferrin in human milk. Am J Clin Nutr, 33, 1314-1315.

21. Fransson G-B, Lönnerdal B. (1983): Distribution of trace elements and minerals in human and cow's milk. Pediatr Res, 17, 912-915.

22. Schachman HK. (1959): Ultracentrifugation in Biochemistry. New York: Academic Press, 225.

23. Holt C, Dalgleish DG, Jenness R. (1981): Calculation of the ion equilibria in milk diffusate and comparison with experiment. Anal Biochem, 113, 154-163.

24. May PM, Smith GL, Williams DR. (1982): Computer calculation of zinc (II) complex distribution in milk. J Nutr, 112, 1990-1993.

25. Holt C, Jenness R. (1984): Interrelationship of constituents and partition of salts in milk samples from eight species. Comp Biochem Physiol, 77A, 225-282.

26. Holt C. (1981): Zinc binding ligands in milk: both arguments err seriously. J Nutr, 111, 2240-2242.

27. Fransson G-B, Lönnerdal B. (1984): Iron, copper, zinc, calcium and magnesium in human milk fat. Am J Clin Nutr, 39, 185-189.

SECTION XI. ENZYMES IN HUMAN MILK

WORKSHOP PARTICIPANTS

M. Hamosh, Department of Pediatrics, Georgetown University Medical Center, Washington, D.C.

C. E.Isaacs, Institute for Basic Research in Mental Retardation, Staten Island, New York

O. Hernell, Department of Pediatrics, University of Umea, Sweden

INTRODUCTION

M. Hamosh

The workshop on "Enzymes in Human Milk" led to the following recommendations:

1) Uniform methods of specimen collection and storage should be used.

2) Reliable assay systems should be used and data should be presented either per ml/milk or per 24-hour milk volume.

3) The following topics should be investigated:

   A. Compartmentalization of the enzymes in human milk.

   B. Comparison between the activity and the subcellular distribution of enzymes in fresh and frozen milk.

   C. The effect of other milk components on enzyme activity.

Since the enzymes in human milk may act in the mammary gland, in milk or in the infant, studies should be designed to evaluate the site of action of these enzymes. When milk enzymes are considered to function in the infant (either in the digestive system or after absorption from the gut), it is important to demonstrate that these milk enzymes remain active in the digestive system of the newborn.

Of major importance is the standardization of the assay systems used for quantification of the level of activity of the enzymes in human milk, which will enable comparison of data generated in different laboratories.

ENZYMES IN HUMAN MILK

M. Hamosh
L. M. Freed
J. B. Jones
S. E. Berkow
J. Bitman
N. R. Mehta
B. Happ
P. Hamosh

The most recent reviews on the enzymes in human milk are those of Jenness (1), Shahani, et al. (2), Blanc (3) and Jenness (4). The first lists only the names of 27 enzymes detected in human milk, without giving any information about their level of activity. The second review, which lists 22 enzymes, compares activity levels of the enzymes in human and bovine milk and discusses briefly their potential significance. Most of the studies cited in the latter review were carried out in the 50's and 60's when the methods were much less sensitive then they are now. We have listed the enzymes described by Shahani (2) in Table 1, which also gives the reference dates. Several points should be emphasized: (a) All activity levels are compared to the "gold standard" -- bovine milk. (b) The enzymes are listed in alphabetical order without any attempt to classify them according to potential function. Shahani et al. made several important comments: "There is no uniformity among the assay procedures, substrates used or activity units expressed for the same enzyme, reported by different workers. Consideration must be given to standardizing these parameters so that activities reported by various workers can be readily compared. Calculation of specific activities in terms of moles substrate per minute per standard amount of milk could be of value." Both Jenness (1) and Shahani et al. (2) emphasize that there is little information about the biochemical and physiological function of these enzymes. Blanc (3) lists 34 enzymes in human milk, whereas the more recent review of Jenness (4) compares the activity of 13 enzymes in human and bovine milk. In general, careful evaluation of the methods used in the more recent studies (the last 5 to 6 years) indicates that more sensitive assay procedures are generally used, but there still is no uniformity in the methods and timing of milk collection. The use of more sensitive assay techniques has led to the recent detection of enzymes that could not be quantitated previously in human milk. Examples of such enzymes are neuraminidase, which can be measured by using a ^{3}H labeled C_8-analog of N-acetylneuraminic acid (7), rather than the commonly used periodic acid thiobarbituric acid assay. In Table 2 we have listed a few of the recently studied enzymes, and where data are available, have tried to classify them according to their potential function in the lactating mammary gland, in milk or in the development of the newborn infant.

Table 1. Enzymes in Human Milk

ENZYME	RELATIVE ACTIVITY*	REFERENCE DATE
ATP-ase		1963
Ala-aminotransferase	x23	1962
Aldolase	x400	1962
α-Amylase	x5	1971
β-Amylase	x25	1962
Arylesterase	x400	1963
Asp-aminotransferase	1/4	1962
Catalase	x10	1963
Cholinesterase	x10	1963
Gluc-6.phosph.isomerase	x9-16	1962
β-Glucuronidase	x2	1968
LDH	x20-30	1964,1967
Lactose Synthetase	x3.5	1969
Lipase	x10	1972
Lysozyme	x10	1964
Malate dehydrogenase	x3000	1964,1967
Peroxidase	x1-5	1963,1972
Phosphatase-acid	1/100	1962
Phosphatase-alkaline	same	1958,1962
Protease	1/40	1956,1963
RNA-ase	x5	1964,1970
Xanthine oxidase	1/3.5 1/10	1960,1976

*Relative enzyme activity compared to that in bovine milk.
From Shahani et al., (1980): A.J.C.N., 33,1861-1868.

MAMMARY GLAND FUNCTION

Although some milk enzymes have no known function in milk, they reflect the physiological changes occurring in the mammary gland during lactation.

Phosphoglucomutase

Phosphoglucomutase (PGM) catalyzes the production of glucose-1-phosphate, the first intermediate in the pathway of synthesis of the galactose moiety of lactose. Phosphoglucomutase (.-D-glucose-1,6-bisphosphate:.D-glucosel-phosphate phosphotransferase) is the product of three loci: PGM1, PGM2, and PGM3. In most tissues, PGM1 isozymes account for 85 to 95% of the total PGM activity, PGM2 for 2-5% and PGM3 for 1-2%. In erythrocytes PGM1 and PGM2 are found in equal amounts, while PGM3 is absent. The PGM patterns in human milk are different and independent from those in the erythrocytes and can be explained on the basis of a distinct PGM4 locus (5). Recent studies show that in the human non-lactating mammary gland, PGM activity is due to PGM1 and PGM2. These isozymes are not present in milk, indicating a switch-off of the PGM1 and PGM2 genes and a simultaneous switch-on of the PGM4 gene. This switch is reversible and is probably dependent on hormonal activation of lactation (5). The recent

Table 2. Functions of Enzymes in Human Milk

ENZYME	FUNCTION	REFERENCE DATE
Antiproteases	Prevent proteolytic activity in mammary gland. Protect bioactive proteins (enzymes, immunoglobulins) from hydrolysis in milk and in the intestine of the newborn.	1979, 1982
α-Amylase	Facilitates digestion of polysacharides (in milk, formula and beikost) by the infant.	1982
Lipase, bile salt stimulated	Hydrolysis of fat in the intestine of the newborn. Bactericidal activity.	1953, 1974, 1984
Lipase, serum stimulated	Regulates long chain triglyceride, phospholipid and cholesterol concentration in milk.	1974, 1984
Sulfhydryl Oxidase	Catalyzes oxidation of SH groups: possible role in maintaining structure and function of proteins containing disulfide bonds.	1978, 1984
Lysozyme	Bactericidal	1972, 1982
Peroxidase	Bactericidal, present in milk leukocytes.	1982

study of Cantu and Ibarra (5) is the first report of a distinct gene for awidely distributed protein being functionally restricted to the lactating mammary gland, since no evidence of its activity has been found in other tissues previously studied.

Galactosyltransferase

This group of enzymes catalyzes the synthesis of the heteropolysaccharide moieties of complex carbohydrates. One of the best known galactosyltransferases is UDP-galactose: N-acetylglucosamine galactosyltransferase, a membrane-bound enzyme responsible with α-lactalbumin for lactose synthesis. This enzyme has been purified from various animal and human body fluids, but, with the exception of the amino acid and carbohydrate content of the bovine milk enzyme, no information on its structure is available. Recent studies show that galactosyltransferases from human amniotic and ascites fluids have similar isoelectric focusing patterns, whereas the milk enzyme is less negatively charged (6). The study suggests that the milk enzyme contains less sialic acid, possibly as a result of the neuraminidase activity in human milk (7) and that the electrophoretic difference between the enzyme in milk and in other body fluids is of post-ribosomal rather than genetic origin.

Alkaline Phosphatase

Alkaline phosphatase is located on the luminal surface of the epithelial cells of the ducts and acinar glands. The enzyme is released into milk as part of the plasma membrane during the formation of milk fat globules. The high levels of the enzyme in colostrum and intermediate milk

milk may be due to the sudden activation of the milk secretory mechanism. Although the enzyme was purified from bovine milk about ten years ago (8) it has only recently been characterized in human milk (9,10). The conclusions reached by two groups of investigators differ as to the nature of the enzyme in milk. Whereas one group (9) suggests that functional, antigenic and structural analysis indicate that the milk enzyme is the same protein species as that of adult human liver, the data reported by the second group (10) suggest that the milk enzyme is a mixture of isozymes similar to bone and liver alkaline phosphatase.

Plasminogen Activator

Plasminogen activator is another enzyme without a known function. Although the enzyme was first reported in milk in 1952 (11), it has only recently been characterized (12,13). The purified enzyme has a molecular weight of 86,000 and was shown to be antigenically different from urokinase, a well-characterized plasminogen activator isolated from urine. Inhibition of activity by DFP (diisopropylflurophosphate) indicates that serine is at the active site, similar to earlier findings for urokinse.

Lactate Dehydrogenase

As seen for many enzymes in milk, lactate dehydrogenase activity is highest in colostrum and decreases as a function of lactation. Recent studies suggest that in addition to changes in enzyme concentration, there is also a change in isozyme pattern from an LD-5 maximum in colostrum to an LD-1 maximum in transitional milk (14). The patterns for colostrum and transitional milk differ from that of maternal serum for which LD-2 and LD-3 are the main isozymes. The LD molecule consists of four subunits of two different kinds designated H (heart muscle) and M (skeletal muscle). Five different combinations of these subunits are possible which correspond to LD-1 through LD-5. Cardiac muscle is richest in LD-1 and liver in LD-5. During the early stages of lactation, therefore, a change occurs in the isozyme spectrum of the milk enzyme. This alteration in mammary enzyme as a function of lactation is especially interesting in the view of the fact that the LDH isozyme pattern of each organ is considered to be unique.

Lipoprotein lipase

Lipoprotein lipase regulates the uptake of circulating triglyceride-fatty acids, cholesterol, and phospholipids by the lactating mammary gland (15-17). LPL has a central role in providing the lipid constituents of milk. In the mammary gland, LPL is located both in the endothelium (its site of activity) and in the alveolar cells, the site of its synthesis.

The extreme variations in enzyme levels in the milk of different species (18) suggest either species differences in the mechanism of milk secretion or a possible relationship between damage to the mammary cells and the state of development of the offspring, i.e., the pressure applied to the mammary gland during suckling (17). Since expression of milk with the aid of a breast pump might cause some rupture of alveolar cells, we compared the levels of LPL activity in milk expressed from one breast by pumping, to the enzyme activity present in milk that drips spontaneously from the opposite breast (19). Our study showed that LPL levels were lower in pumped than in drip milk. This would suggest that leakage of enzyme from ruptured cells is probably not the mechanism of its release into milk.

The enzyme has no known function in milk or in the newborn, but has been implicated in hydrolysis of milk triglycerides and in the release of free fatty acids in human (20) and bovine milk (21) during storage.

MILK ENZYMES IMPORTANT IN NEONATAL DEVELOPMENT

Proteolytic Enzymes and Antiproteases in Human Milk

Human milk contains both proteolytic enzymes and protease-inhibiting activity; the net proteolytic activity will therefore depend upon the quantitative interaction of the two enzyme groups. The nature of the proteolytic activity in human milk is unknown (22). Recent studies indicate caseinolytic activity and elastase-like activity to be present, but no trypsin or chymotrypsin-like activity was detected (23). It is possible that leucocytes are the source of the elastase-like activity in human milk. Although the presence of protease inhibitors in human milk was reported about 30 years ago (24), their nature and amounts have been carefully investigated only recently (23, 25). The recent studies show that α-1-antichymotrypsin and α-1-antitrypsin are the main protease inhibitors in human milk. As measured by electroimmunoassay, the level of α-1-antichymotrypsisn in day-one colostrum was higher (133%) than in normal serum. Other anti proteases, such as inter-α-trypsin inhibitor, α-2-antiplasmin, α-2-macroglobulin, antithrombin-III, or antileucoprotease could also be detected, but amounted only to traces. Although concentrations were much higher in colostrum and decreased sharply in transitional and mature milk, all milk specimens had demonstrable protease-inhibiting activity. These studies also show that one third of the colostrum specimens studied (18 out of a total of 53 samples) had no detectable protease-inhibiting activity in spite of the presence of immunoreactive protease inhibitors; furthermore, caseinolytic activity was present in all these colostrum specimens. The data suggest that the α-1-antitrypsin might have been inactivated.

The very high concentration of α-1-chymotrypsin in colostrum suggests that it may be synthesized in the mammary gland. The authors (23) emphasize that no other biological fluids contain such high levels of α-1-antichymotrypsin, with the possible exception of seminal plasma.

The physiological function of protease inhibitors in human milk is not clear at present. We may postulate that they protect the mammary gland from local proteolytic activity by leucocytic and lysosomal proteases during different stages of differentiation and lactogenesis or during pathogenic conditions such as mastitis; they may prevent the proteolytic breakdown of other enzymes and proteins in milk (and may thus be important in milk banking), and last but not least, they may affect the absorption of milk proteins (immunoglobulins) in the newborn.

Furthermore, the presence of antiproteases would facilitate the delivery of compensatory digestive enzymes (lipase and α-amylase) in an active form from milk to the infant. It was recently suggested that the antitryptic and antichymotryptic activity of human milk might prevent the absorption of endogenous and bacterial proteases in infants and thereby contribute to the passive protection of extraintestinal organs, such as the liver (26). The high concentration of antiproteases in colostrum coincides with the period of greatest transfer of non-immunoglobulin protein from the intestine to the systemic circulation of the newborn (27).

Follow-up studies of the infants of mothers with and without milk protease-inhibiting activity, however, failed to show any difference (such as nutritional problems or increased susceptibility to infection) between the two groups (23). Although this single study of full-term infants does not show a direct beneficial effect of inhibition of the proteolytic activity in the milk, a large body of information supports the concept that the newborns of many species benefit from the transfer of macromolecules from maternal milk. In the human, in whom maternal antibodies are acquired *in utero* (28), breast milk immunoglobulins are also transported across the intestine into the circulation of the newborn infant (29,30). This transfer is even more important in species which acquire maternal immunoglobulins only postnatally from colostrum and milk (cows, sheep, horses and pigs) or both prenatally and postnatally (rats and mice) (28,30). Protease inhibitors in porcine colostrum (32,33) have been shown to increase the efficiency of absorption of undergraded colostrum proteins in the intestine of the newborn pig, probably by inhibiting gastrointestinal proteolysis (32). The delivery of growth factors (34) and hormones (35) in active form from human milk to the newborn infant may also depend on the antiprotease activity of human milk.

Sulfhydryl Oxidase

Sulfhydryl Oxidase is another enzyme present in human milk and in the milk of other species (36-38) that might function in milk and in the gastrointestinal system of the newborn infant. The enzyme is present in colostrum as well as in mature milk. Sulfhydryl oxidase catalyzes the oxidation of sulfhydryl groups, using O_2 as oxidant and producing, in equimolar quantities, H_2O_2 and the corresponding disulfide. The enzyme has a broad specificity, acting on both small thiol compounds and proteins, and might be essential for the activity of proteins whose structure and function depend upon intact disulfide bonds (36,37). The role of the enzyme could involve maintenance of structural and functional integrity of milk proteins, enzymes and immunoglobulins. Furthermore, recent reports that this enzyme is stable at low pH (38) suggest that it might retain activity during passage through the stomach and might function in the intestine of the newborn, where it could be instrumental in the uptake of macromolecules by altering the physical state of the intestinal mucus-diffusion barrier (38). Details on the compartmentalization of this enzyme in human milk and on the effect of milk storage on its activity are presented in Dr. Isaac's article.

γ-Glutamyltransferase Activity

γ-Glutamyltransferase activity is high in human colostrum and although its activity decreases thereafter, considerable amounts of enzyme are present in transitional and mature milk (39,40). The enzyme catalyzes the transfer of the γ-glutamyl group, the receptors differing according to the source of γ-glutamyl transferase (the renal enzyme utilizes different amino acid and peptide receptors from the milk enzyme). In addition to kidney, appreciable amounts of γ-glutamyltransferase are present in liver, pancreas, and prostate tissues as well as breast cyst fluid (39). It has been suggested (39) that the enzyme is localized in the Golgi apparatus and that it plays a role in the endo and/or exocytotic transport of proteins. Indeed in milk the enzyme is also associated with the membrane fraction of skim milk (Isaacs, this workshop). The high levels of γ-glutamyltransferase in the serum of newborn infants have been attributed to absorption of the intact enzyme from breast milk (40).

Peroxidase

Peroxidase in human milk was earlier considered to be lactoperoxidase (41), whereas a recent study establishes that the activity in milk is derived from milk leucocytes and is thus a myeloperoxidase (42). The distinction between a true secretory peroxidase (lactoperoxidase) and a peroxidase derived from leuckocytes (myeloperoxidase) is important because the two enzymes have different structures (single polypeptide chains of molecular weight 77,000-79,000 vs. two subunits and molecular weight 118,000-144,000, respectively). Both enzymes catalyze the oxidation of thiocyanate ions to products with bacteriostatic activity; however, only myeloperoxidase catalyzes the oxidation of the chloride ion. The products of the latter reaction only have bactericidal activity. It is interesting that bovine milk and human saliva have potent lactoperoxidase activity (42). The difference in the nature and source of human milk peroxidase between the earlier and more recent investigators can be attributed to the different methods used, the second group (42) employing more sensitive assay techniques.

Lysozyme

Lysozyme catalyzes the hydrolysis of the β. (1-4) linkage between N-acetylglucosamine and N-acetylmuramic acid in bacterial cell walls. The enzyme lyses mostly gram positive and few gram negative bacteria; it is a major component of the human-milk whey fraction and has been shown to play a role in the antibacterial activity of human milk. The lysozyme of human milk is composed of 130 amino acid residues and has a molecular weight of 14,400 daltons. Although its sequence exhibits considerable homology with the lysozymes of chicken egg-white (43), recent studies show a marked difference in the tertiary structure of the two proteins, resulting in greater organization and hydrophobicity of the human milk protein (44). Lysozyme and α-lactalbumin of human milk seem to be derived from a common ancestral molecule because of identical amino acids in 49 positions (45).

Although not related to the topic of "Enzymes in Human Milk," it is worth noting that another antimicrobial agent in human milk, lactoferrin, was recently shown to be highly resistent to proteolysis, both in its iron-free (apolactoferrin) and iron-containing forms (46,47). Because native milk lactoferrin is largely free of iron, it can withhold iron from, and thus retard the *in vitro* growth of, microorganisms (48). The marked susceptibility of bovine milk lactoferrin to proteolysis led the investigators (46) to suggest that the unusual resistance of human apolactoferrin to proteolysis may reflect an evolutionary development designed to permit its survival in the intestine of the infant.

Similar studies (47) do not support a bacteriostatic role for the vitamin B12 binding protein of human milk. It was earlier suggested that the highly unsaturated vitamin B12 binding protein might exert a bacteriostatic action by making the vitamin unavailable to bacteria that require it (49).

Xanthine Oxidase

Xanthine oxidase is a major component of the milk fat globule membrane in bovine milk (1,2). It has been suggested that the enzyme has a function in the secretion of milk fat droplets, possibly changing the fluidity of the plasma membrane by peroxidizing membrane-associated lipids (50). The very low levels of xanthine oxidase in human milk suggest major differences in the composition of the milk fat globule membrane and possibly in the mechanism of secretion of fat globules into the milk of these two species.

COMPENSATORY DIGESTIVE ENZYMES IN HUMAN MILK

We have left the bile salt stimulated lipase and α-amylase of human milk for the end of our presentation, chiefly because our laboratory is currently engaged in studies of these enzymes, which have a compensatory digestive function in the newborn infant.

α-Amylase

The newborn infant has adequate levels of lactase, an intestinal brush border enzyme that hydrolyzes lactose, the main carbohydrate of human milk. α-amylase, the chief polysaccharide digesting enzyme, is, however, not developed at birth. Even in full-term infants, α-amylase in the duodenum amounts to only 0.2-0.5% of the adult level (52). Human milk contains 0.5-1.0 g/dl oligosaccharides (1); in addition, many breast-fed infants receive glucose polymers or starch from infant formulas or beikost, given often as supplements. For the digestion of glucose polymers, the infant depends upon salivary amylase (51), glucoamylase (52), and the amylase of human milk (53,54).

Since the preterm infant is even more dependent upon extrapancreatic enzymes than the term newborn, we have recently measured the α-amylase levels in the milk of mothers of premature infants (54). The aim of our study was, in addition, to determine whether enzyme activity levels change as a function of length of pregnancy and lactation and, if α-amylase were present, to assess whether it could retain activity after passage through the stomach. The results of this study are presented in Table 3. The

Table 3. Compensatory Polysaccharide Digestive Enzymes α-Amylase in Human Milk

Ontogeny	Present after term and preterm (26-36 weeks) delivery.
Site of Action	Stomach and Intestine
pH Optimum	5.5 - 7.5
Stability	Stable at pH 5-9 Relatively stable at pH 3.0 (75% activity retained during 2 hours). Inactivated at pH 2.0 (10% activity retained during 10 minutes).
Isozyme	Salivary type
Effect of Storage	Full activity retained at -20°C and -70°C.
Function	Digestion of Polysaccharides

data show that α-amylase is present in the milk of mothers of preterm infants and that activity is highest in colostrum in both preterm and term mothers. However, because of the marked increase in milk volume during the transition from colostrum to mature milk, the total amount of amylase received by the infant remains constant, or it declines only slightly during the first six weeks of lactation. Human milk α-amylase has a broad pH optimum range of 4.5-7.5 and loses only little activity during incubation for 2 hours at pH 3.0. These studies show that hydrolysis of polysaccharide could start in the stomach (the postprandial pH of milk-fed infants is in the range of 5.0-6.0) and that the enzyme is stable in the conditions encountered in the stomach and small intestine. The level of α-amylase activity is 10-60 times higher in milk than in normal human serum (53).

We have recently extended the study of α-amylase in human milk to answer the following questions: Is there any change in the α-amylase levels between the first 6 weeks of lactation and the following 6 weeks in the milk of mothers of premature and term infants? Is enzyme activity affected by prolonged storage at -20°C and -70°C? What is the nature of mammary amylase? The studies now in progress show that the level of α-amylase remains almost constant in milk during the first 12 weeks of lactation, that the enzyme is stable during storage at either -20° or -70°, and that more than 95% of milk α-amylase is of the "salivary" type rather than the "pancreatic" type. It is of interest that little or no α-amylase activity is detected in fresh milk from cow, sheep, goat, or swine assayed under the same conditions as those used for measuring human milk amylase (54). The bile salt stimulated lipase (Table 4) found only in milk of humans and gorillas is another example of a digestive enzyme in milk which makes its appearance late in the evolutionary continuum.

During the past 50 years, there has been an increasing tendency to introduce solid foods to the infant's diet as early as the first month of life (55). Such early addition of starch might be well tolerated in breast-fed infants because of high intestinal levels of α-amylase provided by the human milk. Indeed, this assumption is supported by observations in Egypt of a lack of digestive disturbances in breast-fed infants offered starch-containing foods early, which occurs particularly among the poor (2).

Many commercially available infant formulas contain corn syrup or tapioca starch. These oligosaccharides are added not only for their caloric value, but also to assure adequate shelf life and physical stability of the formula. Furthermore, one of the first supplemental foods given infants is rice cereal, a food high in starch content.

The results of our study indicate that the small preterm infant may benefit from its own mother's milk, not only because of the nutritional values, but also because of the biologic activity of preterm milk. Furthermore, the high α-amylase activity in the milk of mothers of preterm infants suggests that starch-containing supplements could be well tolerated by breast-fed premature infants.

Bile Salt Stimulated Lipase

Fat digestion requires adequate lipase activity and bile salt levels, the former for the breakdown of triglyceride, the latter for emulsification

Table 4. Compensatory Digestive Lipases in the Newborn

	LIPASE IN GASTRIC ASPIRATES	HUMAN MILK BILE SALT STIMULATED LIPASE
Origin	Lingual serous glands Gastric mucosa	Mammary gland (Human & gorilla)
Ontogeny	Present from 24 weeks gestation	Present after term & pre-term (26-36 wks) delivery
Site of Action	Stomach (duodenum)	Intestine
Characteristics:		
pH Optimum Stability	3.0 - 6.0 >2.2	7.0 - 9.0 >3.5
Rate	MCT > LCT FA unsaturated > saturated	MCT = LCT Water soluble esters
Reaction Products	FFA, DG, MG	FFA, glycerol
Bile Salts	20 - 40% stimulation	Obligatory
Mol. Wt.	46,000 - 48,000	90,000 - 125,000
Function	Hydrolysis of 50 - 70% of ingested fat	Hydrolysis of 30-40% of milk fat

MCT - Medium chain triglyceride, LCT - Long chain triglyceride, FA - Fatty acids, FFA - Free fatty acids, DG - Diglyceride, MG - Monoglyceride, Mol. Wt. - Molecular Weight

of fat prior to and during lipolysis. In the newborn, and especially the premature infant, both pancreatic lipase activity and bile salt concentrations are low (51). The newborn depends on two alternate lipases for fat digestion. Of special importance is intragastric lipolysis where lingual and gastric lipases compensate for low pancreatic lipase. The breast-fed infant depends on an additional compensatory mechanism for fat digestion -- the bile salt stimulated lipase of human milk, an enzyme found to date only in the milk of primates (57). Lingual and gastric lipases, hydrolyze triglycerides in the stomach to free fatty acids and partial glycerides; these reaction products compensate for low bile salts by emulsifying the lipid mixture. Hydrolysis of milk fat involves first the penetration of lingual lipase into the milk fat globule and partial hydrolysis of the core triglyceride (58). This process is then completed in the intestine by the bile salt stimulated lipase of human milk. The combined activity of these two enzymes can lead to complete hydrolysis of dietary fat, and thus can effectively substitute for low levels of pancreatic lipase (Table 4). The properties of human milk bile salt stimulated lipase are fully compatible with activity in the intestine of the newborn. The enzyme is stable at low pH (thus is not inactivated in the stomach) and remains active in the intestine for at least two hours (59). Its lack of substrate specificity and complete hydrolysis of glyceride to free fatty acids and glycerol suggest efficient hydrolysis of triglycerides and various esters (such as retinyl palmitate, the main component of vitamin A) (60). The milk lipase, which amounts to 1% of total milk protein, is immunologically identical to a protein present in the human pancreas, suggesting that this lipase is a pancreatic protein that in primates (human and gorilla) is secreted also by the lactating mammary gland (60). The synthesis of this lipase in the human mammary gland is, however, independent of pancreatic function, since we found normal levels of the enzyme in milk produced by a woman with cystic fibrosis and pancreatic insufficiency (61). The marked stability of this enzyme (years at -80°C), and the fact that it is secreted in equal amounts in drip milk (19) (the main form of banked milk in several countries), indicate that frozen (but not heated) banked milk might contain sufficient lipase activity. Bile salt stimulated lipase is the main reason that the fat in fresh human milk is absorbed to a greater extent than the fat in boiled human-milk or in infant formulas (62).

An additional function of the bile salt stimulated lipase of human milk might be the hydrolysis of bacterial lipids. A recent report, that human milk is bactericidal to Giardia organisms, suggests that the latter is the result of hydrolysis of bacterial lipids by the bile salt stimulated lipase of human milk (63).

Our recent studies on the lipases in human milk have centered on the following questions: Are there differences in the levels of lipase and esterase (BSSL and BSSE) activity in human milk both as a function of length of pregnancy and length of lactation? What is the effect of repeated freezing and thawing on lipase activity? Could a difference in dependence upon bile salts in certain milks explain the link between free fatty acid levels in milk and breast-milk jaundice? Our data (19) show that bile salt stimulated lipase was present in all the milk specimens studied; activity was almost constant and did not change with length of gestation or with length of lactation; the activity range was 20-35 units/ml milk. Lipase activity is tested by the hydrolysis of long chain triglyceride ([^{3}H]-triolein) substrate, whereas the esterase activity is quantitated with the water soluble substrate p-nitrophenyl acetate (19). Each milk specimen was tested for lipase activity in the presence and absence of sodium taurocholate. Lipase activity showed absolute dependence on bile salts; less than 5% of the specimens had a trace of activity (0.75 U/ml) when incubated without bile salt. Bile salt stimulated esterase (BSSE) activity was also present in all the specimens of milk studied. Studies on the effect of storage temperature (important for milk banking) (56) and on the effect of freezing and thawing (69) show that the lipolytic activity is remarkably stable, whereas the esterolytic activity is more labile during storage at +4 C°, and -10°C, gradually losing its bile salt dependence. Furthermore, there are differences in the extent of bile salt dependence among milk specimens from different mothers; in some, esterolytic activity retains full dependence upon bile salts ("stable" milks), whereas in other specimens the esterase activity becomes bile salt independent ("unstable" milks). Whether this bile salt independent esterase is identical to the "unstimulated lipase" linked with the development of breast-milk jaundice (64) remains to be established.

Our studies have also shown that the lipase and esterase activities, as well as the bile salt-independent esterolytic activity, are all associated with the same protein (58).

The esterolytic activity is markedly affected by detergents and amphiphylic substances such as free fatty acids; thus, a variety of milk components can affect the level of esterolytic activity as well as its dependence upon bile salts. The lipolytic activity is, however, much less affected by these changes and should be used as the only measure of bile salt stimulated lipase in human milk.

Our recent studies show that although both BSSL and LPL are not activated during repeated freezing and thawing of human milk (65), there is a progressive rise in the level of FFA during storage (higher at -20°C than at -70°C) (66).

The milk fat globule is almost completely resistent to lipolysis, as long as its structure remains intact. The freezing and thawing of milk may disrupt the membrane and allow a greater access of milk lipases to the triglyceride contained within the core of the fat globule.

ACKNOWLEDGEMENT

The authors' studies are supported by NIH Contract HD-2-2816.

REFERENCES

1. Jenness, R. (1979): The composition of human milk. Seminars in Perinatology, 31, 225-239.

2. Shahani KM, Kwan AJ, Friend BA. (1980): Role and significance of enzymes in human milk. Am J Clin Nutr, 33, 1961-1968.

3. Blanc B. (1981): Biochemical aspects of human milk - comparison with bovine milk. World Rev Nutr Dietetics, 36, 1-89.

4. Jenness R. (1982): Interspecies comparison of milk proteins. In: Fox DF, ed, Developments in Dairy Chemistry, chapter 3. Essex: Applied Science Pub.

5. Cantu JM, Ibarra B. (1982): Phosphoglucomutase: evidence of a new locus expressed in human milk. Science, 216, 639-640.

6. Gerber AC, Kozdrowski I, Wyss SR, Berger EG. (1979); The charge heterogeneity of soluble human galactosyltransfrases isolated from milk, amniotic fluid and malignant ascites. Eur J Biochem, 93, 453-460.

7. Schauer R, Veh RW, Wembler M. (1976): Demonstration of a neuramidinase activity in human blood serum and human milk using a modified, radioactively labeled α-Glycoprotein as substrate. Hoppe-Seyler's Z. Physiol Chem, 357, 559-566.

8. Linden G, Mazeron P, Michalowski JB, Alois C. (1974): Alkalin phosphatase du lait de vache. I. Purification et proprietes molecularies. Biochim Biophys Acta, 358,82-90.

9. Hamilton TA, Gornicki SZ, Sussman HH. (1979): Alkaline phosphatase from human milk. Biochem J, 177, 197-201.

10. Worth GK, Retallack RW, Gutteridge DH, Jeffries M, Kent J, Smith J, Smith M. (1981): Serum and milk alkaline phosphatase in human milk. Clin Chim Acta, 115, 171-177.

11. Astrup T, Sterndorff I. (1953): A fibrinolytic system in human milk. Proc Soc, Exp Biol Med, 84, 605-608.

12. Yamamoto J, Horie N, Okamoto U. (1980): Enzymatic properties of milk plasminogen activator in relation to synthetic chromogenic substrates. Thormb Res, 18, 263-266.

13. Okamoto U, Horie N, Nagamotsu Y, Yamamoto J. (1981): Plasminogen activator in human early milk: its partial purification and characterization. Thrombos Haemostos, 45, 121-126.

14. Patil KP, Rangnekar NR. (1983): Lactate dehydrogenase and its isoenzymes in human milk - a preliminary study. Clin Chem, 29, 1568-1570.

15. Scow RO, Blanchette-Machie EJ, Mendelson C, Hamosh M, Zinder O. (1975): Incorporation of dietary fatty acids into milk triglycerides: mechanism and regulation. In: Modern problems in pediatrics, Vol. 14. Basel: Karger.

16. Hamosh M, Clary TR, Chernick SS, Scow RO. (1970): Lipoprotein lipase of adipose and mammary tissue and plasma triglyceride in pregnant and lactating rats. Biochim Biophys Acta, 210, 473-482.

17. Hamosh M. (1981): Physiological role of milk lipases. In: Lebenthal E, ed, Textbook of gastroenterology and nutrition in infancy. New York: Raven Press, 473-482.

18. Hamosh M. Hamosh P. (1983): Lipoprotein Lipase: its physiological and clinical significance. Molec Asp Med, 6, 199-289.

19. Mehta NR, Jones JB, Hamosh M. (1982): Lipases in preterm human milk ontogeny and physiologic significance. J Pediatr Gastroenterol Nutr, 1, 317-326.

20. Castberg HB, Hernell O. (1975): Role of serum stimulated lipase in lipolysis in human milk. Milchwissenschaft, 30, 721-724.

21. Jensen RG, Pitas RE. (1976): Milk lipoprotein lipase. a review. J Dairy Sci, 59, 1203-1214.

22. Heyndrickz GV. (1963): Further investigations of the enzymes in human milk. Pediatrics, 31, 1019-1030.

23. Lindberg T, Ohlsson K, Westrom B. (1982): Protease inhibitors and their relation to protease activity in human milk. Pediatr Res, 16, 479-483.

24. Storrs AB, Hull ME. (1956): Proteolytic enzymes in human and cow's milk. F Dairy Sci, 39, 1097-1103.

25. Lindberg T. (1979): Protease inhibitors in human milk. Pediatr Res, 13, 969-972.

26. Udall JN, Bloch KJ, Walker WA. (1982): Transport of proteases across neonatal intestine and development of liver disease in infants with α-1-antitrypsin deficiency. Lancet, 1, 1441-1443.

27. Udall JN, Pan K, Fritze L, Kleinman R, Walker WA. (1981): Development of gastrointestinal mucosal barrier. The effect of age on intestinal permeability to macromolecules. Pediatr Res, 15, 241-244.

28. Ogra PL. (1979): Ontogeny of the local immune system. Pediatrics, 64, 765-774.

29. Ogra SS, Weintraub D, Ogra PL. (1977): Immunological aspects of human colostrum and milk. Fate and absorption of cellular and soluble components in the gastrointestinal tract of the newborn. J. Immunol, 119, 245-248.

30. Iyengar L, Selvaraj RJ. (1972): Intestinal absorption of immunoglobulins by newborn infants. Arch Dis Child, 47, 411-414.

31. Kraehenbuhl JP, Campiche MA. (1969): Early stages of intestinal absorption of specific antibodies in the newborn. J Cell Biol, 42, 345-365.

32. Carlsson LCT, Westrom BR, Karlsson BW. (1980): Intestinal absorption of proteins by the neonatal piglet fed on sow's colostrum with either natural or experimentally eliminated trypsin-inhibiting activity. Biol Neonate, 38, 309-320.

33. Westrom BR, Svendsen J, Karlsson BW. (1982): Protease inhibitor levels in porcine mammary secretions. Biol Neonate, 42, 185-194.

34. Moran JR, Courtney ME, Orth DN, Vaughan R, Coy S, Mount CD, Sherell BJ, Greene HL. (1983): Epidermal growth factor in human milk: dairy production and diurnal variation during early lactation in mothers delivering at term and at preterm gestation. J Pediatr, 103, 402-405.

35. Hamosh M. (1984): The biologic function of human milk in neonatal development. In: Colon AR and Ziai M, eds, Pediatric Pathophysiology. Boston, MA: Little Brown and Co. (In Press).

36. Janolino VG, Sweisgood HE. (1975): Isolation and characterization of sufhydryl oxidase from bovine milk. J Biol Chem, 250, 2532-2538.

37. Clare DA, Blakistone BA, Sweisgold HE, Horton HR. (1981): Sulfhydryl oxidase - catalyzed conversion of xanthine dehydrogenase to xanthine oxidase. Arch Biochem Biophys, 211, 44-47.

38. Isaacs CE, Pascal T, Wright CE, Gaull GE. (1984): Sulfhydryl oxidase in human milk: stability of milk enzymes in the gastrointestinal tract. Pediatr Res, 18, 532-535.

39. Brinkley F, Wiesemann ML, Groth DP, Powell RW. (1975): Glutamyl transferase: a secretory enzyme. FEBS Lett, 51, 168-170.

40. Patil KP, Rangnekar NR. (1982): Glytamyltransferase activity in human milk. Clin Chem, 28, 1724-1725.

41. Gothefors L, Marklund S. (1975): Lactoperoxidase activity in human milk and in saliva of newborn children. Infect Immun, 11, 1210-1215.

42. Moldoveanu Z, Tenovuo J, Mestecky J, Pruitt KM. (1982): Human milk peroxidase is derived from milk leukocytes. Biochim Biophys Acta, 718, 103-108.

43. Bezkorovainy, A. (1977): Human milk and colostrum proteins: a review. J Dairy Sci, 60, 1023-1037.

44. Dubois T, Guillard R, Prieels JP, Perraudin JP. (1982): Comparisons between the folding of reduced hen-egg white lysozyme and that of reduced human milk. Biochemistry, 21, 6516-6523.

45. Dayhoff MD. Atlas of protein sequence and structure. Vol 5, Suppl. 2. Washington, DC: National Biomedical Research Foundation.

46. Brincs RD, Brock JH. (1983): The effect of trypsin and chymotrypsin on the *in vitro* antimicrobial and iron binding properties of lactoferrin in human milk and bovine colostrum. Biochim Biophys Acta, 759, 229-235.

47. Samson RR, Mirtle C, McClelland BDL. (1980): The effect of digestive enzymes on the binding and bacteriostatic properties of lactoferrin and vitamin B_{12} binder in human milk. Acta Pediatr Scand, 59, 517-523.

48. Bullen JJ, Rodgers HJ, Leigh L. (1972): Iron binding proteins in milk and resistance to Escherichia coli infections in infants. Br Med J, 1, 69-75.

49. Ford JE. (1974): Some observations on the possible nutritional significance of vitamin B_{12} and folate binding proteins in milk. Br J Nutr, 31, 243-257.

50. Mather IH, Keenan TW. (1983): Function of endomembranes and the cell surface in the secretion of organic milk constituents. In: Mepham TB, ed, Biochemistry of Lactation. Amsterdam: Elsevier Science Publ, 231-283.

51. Zoppi G, Andreotti G, Pajno-Ferrara F, Njai DM, Gaburro D. (1972): Exocrine pancreas function in premature and full-term neonates. Pediat Res, 6, 880-886.

52. Kelly JJ, Alpers OH. (1973): Properties of human intestinal glucoamylase. Biochim Biophys Acta, 315, 113-120.

53. Fridhandler L, Berk JE, Montgomery KA, Wang D. (1974): Column chromatographic studies of isoamylases in human serum, urine and milk. Clin Chem, 20, 547-555.

54. Jones JB, Mehta NR, Hamosh M. (1982): α-amylase in preterm human milk. J Pediatr Gastroenteral Nutr, 1, 43-48.

55. Lee PC, Nord KS, Lebenthal E. (1981): Digestibility of starches in infants. In: Textbook of Gastroenterology and Nutrition in Infancy. New York: Raven Pres, 233-243.

56. Hamosh M. (1982): Lingual and breast milk lipases. Adv Pediatr, 29, 33-67.

57. Freudenberg E. (1953): Die Frauenmilch-Lipase. Basel, Karger.

58. Patton JS, Rigler MW, Liao TH, Hamosh P, Hamosh M. (1982): Hydrolysis of triacylglycerol emulsions by lingual lipase - a microscopic study. Biochim Biophys Acta, 712, 400-407.

59. Hernell O. (1975): Human milk lipases. III. Physiological implications of the bile salt stimulated lipase. Eur J Clin Invest, 2, 267-272.

60. Hernell D, Blackberg L. (1983): Bile salt stimulated lipase of human milk and lipid digestion in the neonatal period. J Pediatr Gastroenterol Nutr, 2, S242-S247.

61. Hamosh M, Bitman J, Wood DC, Mehta NR, Welch JM, Osher AB, Jones JB, Hamosh P. (1982): Human milk in cystic fibrosis: composition and enzyme content. Pediatr Res, 16, 164A.

62. Alemi B, Hamosh M, Scanlon JW, Hamosh P. (1981): Fat digestion in very low birth weight infants: effect of addition of human milk to low birth weight formula. Pediatrics, 68, 484-488.

63. Gillin FD, Reiner DS, Wang CS. (1983): Human milk kills parasitic intestinal protozoa. Science, 221, 1290-1292.

64. Poland RL, Schultz GE, Garg G. (1980): Human milk lipase activity associated with breast milk jaundice. Pediatr Res, 14, 1238-1242.

65. Bitman J, Wood L, Mehta NR, Hamosh P, Hamosh M. (1983): Lipolysis of triglycerides of human milk during storage at low temperatures: a note of caution. J Pediatr Gastroenterol Nutr, 2, 521-524.

66. Berkow SE, Freed LM, Hamosh M, Bitman J, Wood DL, Happ B, Hamosh P. (1984): Lipases and lipids in human milk: effect of freeze-thawing and storage. Pediatr Res, 18, 1257-1262.

LIPASE AND ESTERASE ACTIVITIES IN HUMAN MILK

O. Hernell
L. Bläckberg

INTRODUCTION

Two different lipases have been described in human milk (1). A serum-stimulated (lipoprotein) lipase (LPL) is present in low and variable concentrations and is not known to have any useful function in milk or in the gastrointestinal tract of the breast-fed infant (2). Its physiological substrate is the triglyceride-rich plasma lipoproteins, but it can hydrolyze other substrates, e.g., p-nitrophenyl esters. Thus, it has an esterase activity (3).

The major lipase in human milk is the bile salt-stimulated lipase (BSSL) (1,4). This lipase has been purified and characterized (5,6). It has a low substrate specificity, i.e., it is a non-specific lipase. This is true both with respect to the chemical structure of the substrate and to its physical state (7). Thus, it has been shown to hydrolyze long-and short-chain triglycerides (8,9), diglycerides, 1(3)- as well as 2-monoglycerides (10), cholesteryl esters (11), retinyl esters (12) and p-nitrophenyl esters (7,8,13). It hydrolyzes emulsified substrates [e.g., milk (14) and other long-chain triglycerides] as well as micellar substrates (e.g., monoglyceride-bile salt micelles) and soluble substrates (e.g., p-nitrophenyl acetate) (7). All these activities are enhanced by bile salts. Against soluble substrates and against tributyrin, BSSL has some activity even in the absence of bile salts; against long-chain triglycerides it is completely inactive without bile salts (8). The reason for this difference is not yet understood.

Recently it was reported that when milk is stored at -10°C, the activity against p-nitrophenyl acetate becomes less dependent on bile salts (15). Another interesting observation was that the bile salt-stimulated esterase (p-nitrophenyl acetate as substrate) and lipase (emulsified long-chain triglycerides as substrate) activities did not vary in parallel in milk under various conditions. Thus, the bile salt-stimulated esterase, in contrast to the lipase activity, decreased as a function of length of gestation and lactation, and it was suggested that the bile salt-stimulated esterolytic activity develops earlier than the lipase activity (15). This is, however, somewhat contradicted by the observation made by Wardell et al. (16) who found that the two activities strongly correlated to one another.

Using human milk as both the source of enzyme and substrate, Hall and Muller (17) observed two patterns of bile salt-stimulated lipase activity. One group of milks gave the same high activity with both unpurified and purified glycine-conjugated bile salts. The other group gave lower activity with purified than with unpurified bile salts. The activities of the low-activity milks assayed with purified bile salts could be increased following storage at -20°C, sonication or the preparation of an acetone-ether powder in some cases reaching the maximal activity obtained with the unpurified bile salt preparation. These procedures, however, had no effect on the activity of the high-activity milks. The results could be compatible with a heterogeneity of bile salt-stimulated lipases in human milk.

Although we have previously suggested that there is only one bile salt-stimulated lipase in human milk and that the lipase and esterase activities reside in one enzyme molecule, the recent results (15,17) had reopened the question of the number of lipases and esterases in human milk. In the present study we give further evidence that our previous conclusions remain valid.

RESULTS AND DISCUSSION

Incorporation of Diisopropylfluorophosphate into Milk Proteins

BSSL, in contrast to LPL, is inhibited by the organophosphate diisopropylfluorophosphate (DFP) (2,5). When human milk protein, after incubation of whole milk with an excess of radiolabeled DFP, was separated on gel electrophoresis, there was no evidence that any protein, except BSSL, had been labeled with the inhibitor (Figure 1). Thus, it is not likely that human milk contains significant amounts of another esterase with a serine residue in the active site and with a molecular weight different from BSSL.

Inhibition of Bile Salt-stimulated Lipase and Esterase Activities by Antibodies

In none of six samples of mature milk, obtained from different mothers of infants born at term, could lipase activity be detected in the routine BSSL-assay in the absence of bile salt. Addition of 10 mM bile salt gave activities within the normal range. When the lipase activity was determined, after preincubation of the milk samples with rabbit antibodies raised against purified BSSL (5), no activity could be detected in the presence of bile salt (Table 1).

As expected, a significant esterase activity, i.e., against p-nitrophenyl acetate, was recorded in all samples in the absence of bile salt, although the activities were increased by bile salt. Independent of bile salt, however, activity could not be detected in any of the samples after incubation with antibodies against purified BSSL (Table 1).

The results are strong evidence that there is only one major bile salt-stimulated lipase and one major bile salt-stimulated esterase activity in human milk and that these reside in the same enzyme molecule. Therefore, it is difficult to understand, at least on the molecular level, how one activity can develop before the other (15) and how different milks can contain enzyme species with different activation mechanisms (17). A more likely explanation is, perhaps, that the optimal conditions under which the respective activities are recorded may vary. The results obtained can of course not rule out the possibility that human milk can contain comparatively low activities of molecularly different lipases and esterases stimulated or not stimulated by bile salts, e.g., activities too low to make a significant contribution to activities recorded in the assays used.

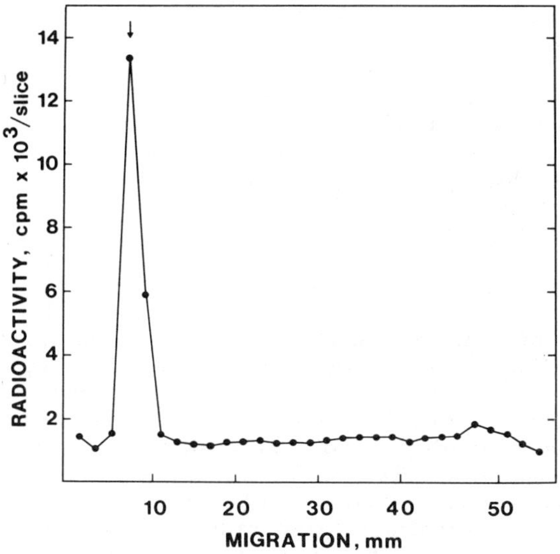

Figure 1. Incorporation of [^{3}H]-diisopropylfluorophosphate into human milk proteins. 25 µl of human milk was mixed with an excess of radio-labeled diisopropylfluorophosphate. After 30 minutes incubation at 37°C, the mixture was subjected to dodecylsulfate polyacrylamide gel electrophoresis. The gel was sliced in 2 mm slices from which radioactivity was eluted and counted in a scintillation counter (5). The arrow indicates the position of purified bile salt stimulated lipase run on a parallel gel.

Table 1. Bile salt stimulated lipase activity and esterase activity in human milk

Activity* Recorded	Without Bile Salt: No Preincubation	Without Bile Salt: Preincubation with Antibodies	With Bile Salt: No Preincubation	With Bile Salt: Preincubation with Antibodies
Lipase	n.d.	---	21.6±6.6	n.d.
Esterase	1.3±0.3	n.d.	7.6±1.3	n.d.

*Lipase activity was determined with an emulsion of long-chain triglycerides as substrate, as described (5), in the absence and presence of 10 mM sodium taurocholate. Esterase activity was determined against p-nitrophenyl acetate. This assay mixture contained in a total volume of 100 µl: 50 µl 0.1 M sodium phosphate buffer, pH 7.5, 0.3mM sodium cholate, when indicated, and milk. The reaction was initiated by the addition of 200 µl of 1 mM p-nitrophenyl acetate. The assay was performed in microtiter plates (Flow Lab Inc., Inglewood, CA), which were read on a Titertek Multiscan with a 405 nm filter. Preincubation with antibodies was performed as follows: the respective milk sample was mixed (1:1, vol/vol) with an immunoglobulin fraction (10 mg/ml) prepared from a rabbit antiserum to purified human milk BSSL. After incubation for 4 hours at 4°C, the respective enzyme activities were determined. Values are expressed as µ mol fatty acid or p-nitrophenol, respectively, released per minute and ml milk, and are mean ± SD of one sample from each of six different donors. Non-detectable activities are indicated with n.d.

For instance, it should be noted that, although active against p-nitrophenyl acetate (3), LPL did not contribute to this activity. Because LPL and BSSL do not crossreact immunochemically (18), this can be deduced from the fact that no activity was recorded after inhibition with antibodies (Table 2). The lack of contribution to the recorded esterase activity is explained by the fact that in comparison with BSSL, LPL is present in much lower amounts in human milk (1,15), and that its activity against p-nitrophenyl acetate is only a few percent of its optimal activity against emulsified substrates (3).

Effect of Detergents on the Esterase Activity

The effect of bile salts and other detergents on the esterase activity in human milk is illustrated in Figure 2. The milk sample used hydrolyzed p-nitrophenyl acetate in the absence of bile salt; but again, the activity was enhanced about 5-fold by the primary bile salt sodium cholate. Interestingly, the same degree of stimulation was obtained with sodium deoxycholate (a secondary bile salt), Triton X-100 (a non-ionic detergent), and with sodium dodecylsulfate (Figure 2). Since activation of BSSL against emulsified long-chain triglyceride is specific for primary bile salts (14), it is obvious that the esterase activity does not share the same specificity. In fact, it is detergent-stimulated rather than bile salt-stimulated. Whether the effect recorded is due to an effect on milk, on the substrate, or to a direct effect of the detergent on the enzyme protein is not known. It should be noted, however, that the same nonspecific effect is also seen with purified BSSL, (Blackberg and Hernell, unpublished). Furthermore, the presence of sodium deoxycholate, which in itself cannot activate BSSL, lowers the molar requirement of sodium taurocholate for activation (7); this in fact, might be the explanation of why Hall and Muller (17) found an impure bile salt preparation to be more effective as an activator for some milks.

Table 2. Serum-stimulated (lipoprotein) lipase activity in human milk

Sample	Lipase activity (μmol x min $^{-1}$ x ml^{-1})		
		20% serum (v/v)	
	Without Serum	No Preincubation	Preincubation with antiserum
1-6	0.02±0.01	0.20±0.12	
6	0.04	0.40	0.02

Lipase activity was determined by an assay designed for lipoprotein lipase with Intralipid as substrate (24) in the presence and absence of 20% serum. Values are expressed as μmol fatty acid released per minute and ml milk, and are mean ± SD of the six milk samples analyzed (1-6). The milk with the highest activity (sample 6) was chosen for an antiserum experiment. It was mixed with equal volume of rabbit antiserum to purified bovine milk lipoprotein lipase. After incubation at 4°C for 4 hours, activity was determined, as above, in the presence of serum.

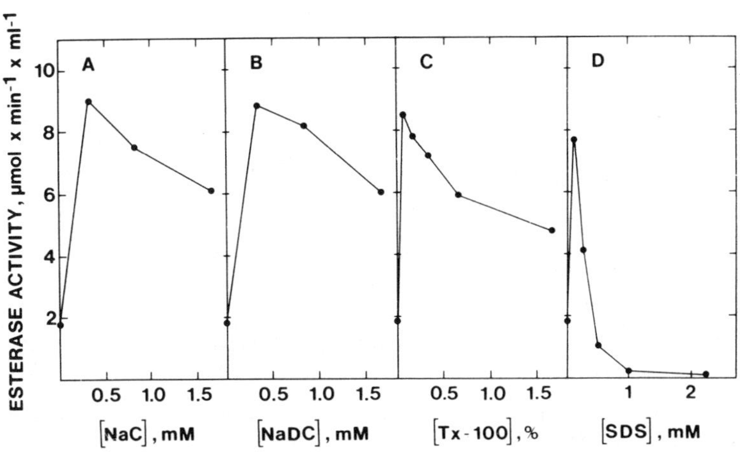

Figure 2 Effect of different detergents on the esterase activity in human milk. Esterase activity was determined as described in Table 1 with the addition of the different detergents to the concentrations indicated. The detergents were: A) sodium cholate (NaC), B) sodium deoxycholate (NaDC), C) Triton X-100 (Tx-100), and D) sodium dodecylsulfate (SDS).

Effect of Time and Temperature of Storage on the Esterase Activity

When milk samples from five mothers were stored at 4°C for 10 days, the esterase activity recorded in the presence of bile salt remained fairly constant, but the activity recorded without bile salt increased, i.e., it seemed as if the esterase activity was less influenced by addition of detergent to the assay system (Figure 3). This is an observation partly in agreement with others (15,19). In contrast, when the samples were stored at -20°, no such effect could be seen, not even after the samples had been frozen and thawed up to four times (Figure 4). Hamosh (19) reported the same general effect when samples were stored at -10°C or -20°C as when they were stored at 4°C, but the effect was abolished when samples were stored at -80°C. In fact, she found 2 groups of milks, i.e., one stable group which did not lose activity during storage and which retained almost complete bile salt dependence, and one unstable group in which a greater loss of activity occurred during storage, as well as marked loss of bile salt dependency. In view of the fact that the BSSL activity is very stable (the purified enzyme can be stored for months at 4°C or -20°C), and that both the esterase and the lipase activities are inhibited by DFP, a rapid loss of the esterase activity is not what one would expect. Wardell et al. (16) did not find any systematic tendency for lipase or esterase activities to increase or decrease when milk samples were stored at 25°C, 4°C, or were subjected to freezing and thawing, although they noticed wide fluctuations in the activities recorded.

It seems reasonable to believe that both the lipase and the esterase activities are fairly stable when milk samples are stored. However, in light of our observation of the nonspecific detergent effect on the esterase activity (Figure 2), it seems probable that physical-chemical alteration of milk during storage, i.e., release of amphiphilic

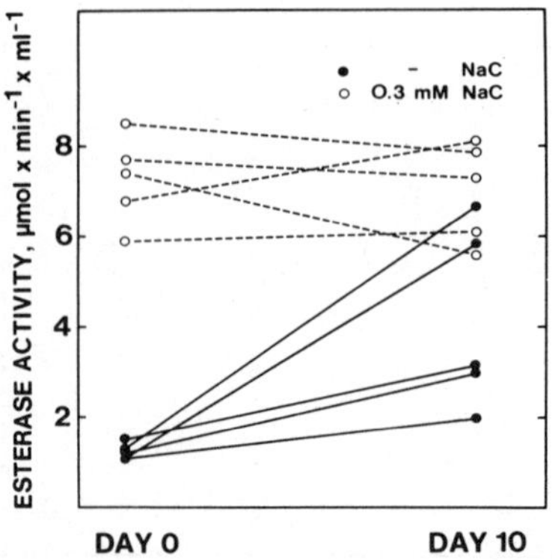

Figure 3 Effect of storage at 4°C on the esterase activity in human milk. Esterase activity was determined as in Table 1, in the presence and absence of 0.3 mM sodium cholate (NaC) in fresh milk samples and after 10 days storage at 4°C.

compounds such as fatty acids (20,21), will reduce the bile salt concentration required for optimal activity in the assay. In fact, concentrations above optimal may even cause inhibition and reduce the magnitude of the activity recorded (Figure 2). Because determination of the lipase activity with emulsified long-chain triglyceride as the substrate (5) is less influenced by such effects, and hence more reproducible, this assay is to be preferred in routine clinical work.

Lipoprotein Lipase Activity in Human Milk

The LPL activity in human milk varies, but it is generally much lower than the BSSL activity (1,15). LPL preferentially hydrolyzes long-chain triglycerides, and for optimal activity it needs a co-factor, apolipoprotein CII. It is, however, also active against milk triglycerides in the absence of its cofactor, although the rate of hydrolysis is low. We found that there was a strong correlation between the LPL activity in human milk and the release of free fatty acids during storage at 4°C. No such correlation was observed with the BSSL activity (20). This is probably due to the compartmentalization of enzyme, substrate and activator: BSSL being mainly in skim milk rather than associated with the milk fat globule substrate (1), while the activator is secreted with the bile (14). Such so-called spontaneous lipolysis is a problem with bovine milk, since fatty acids released into the milk may cause rancidity. Due to the much lower LPL activity, this problem should be less serious when human milk is stored.

To what extent LPL contributes to hydrolysis of milk triglycerides in the gastrointestinal tract of the breast-fed newborn has not been settled. Due to the low activity in human milk and the probable lack of optimal concentrations of co-factor, it is unlikely that the contribution should be of any significance. Furthermore, LPL, in contrast to BSSL, is not stable in gastric contents of newborn infants (Figure 5).

It has been shown that there is a correlation between so-called breast-milk jaundice and the concentration of free fatty acids in the milk consumed. Since the release of fatty acids into the milk during storage correlates with the LPL activity (20), it is not surprising that a correlation between breast-milk jaundice and lipase activity has also been

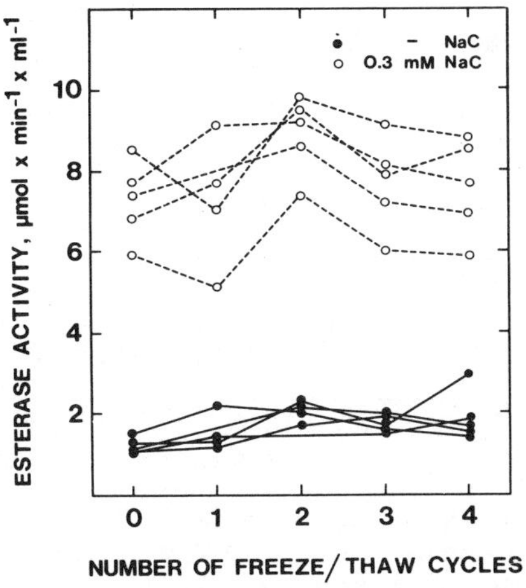

Figure 4 Effect of freezing and thawing on the esterase activity in human milk. Esterase activity was determined as in Table 1 in fresh milk samples and after up to four freeze/thaw cycles. The total time of storage was 10 days, and the temperature was -20°C. After each thawing the samples were immediately frozen again.

reported (22). The nature of this lipase activity has, however, been questioned (19,22,23). Therefore, we determined the LPL activity in the same six milk samples in which BSSL and esterase activities were determined. Low but significant activities were recorded in the absence of activating co-factor (serum) in five of the samples (Table 2). The activities increased about 10-fold when serum was added to the assay mixtures. The sample with the highest activity (sample 6) was from the mother of an infant with breast-milk jaundice. After preincubation of this sample with antibodies raised against bovine milk LPL (18), at least 95 percent of the serum-stimulated activity had been lost (Table 2). It should be noted that in the same sample, antibodies directed towards purified BSSL caused inhibition of all the BSSL and esterase activities (Table 1). This observation, that antibodies directed toward purified BSSL and LPL inhibit virtually all lipase and esterase activities, even in milk of a mother of a breast-milk jaundiced infant, strongly supports the view that there is no other major lipolytic enzyme in human milk.

CONCLUSIONS

Since antibodies directed toward purified human milk BSSL and bovine milk LPL together inhibited virtually all of the lipase and esterase activities in human milk, the possibility of any third lipolytic activity of quantitative or qualitative importance in human milk could be ruled out. Furthermore, only one protein, corresponding to BSSL, incorporated radiolabeled DFP, a commonly used esterase inhibitor.

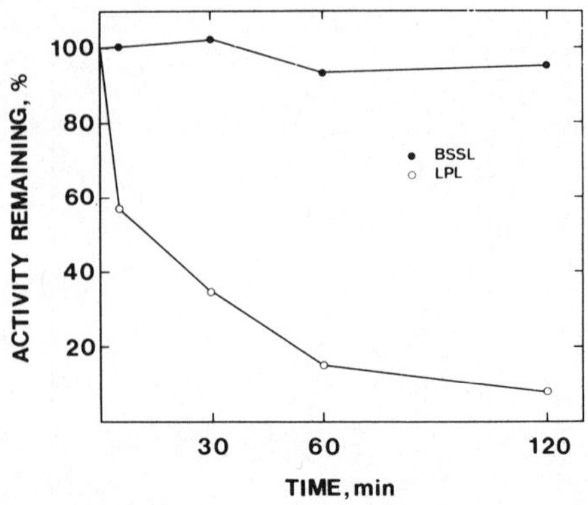

Figure 5 Stability of milk lipases in gastric content. Gastric content was taken from an infant 60 minutes after a meal. It was centrifuged for 20 minutes at 5,000 x g. The clear infranatant was used for the experiment. Human milk was mixed (1:1) with the gastric content infranatant and incubated at 37°C. At the times indicated, samples were withdrawn and assayed for BSSL and LPL activity, as described in Tables 1 and 2, with 10 mM NaTC and 20% serum, respectively. The activities are expressed as a percent of that of a milk sample incubated with 0.9% NaCl instead of gastric content.

Bile salt had no specific effect on the esterase activity recorded in human milk, but the activity was enhanced in a nonspecific way by both various bile salts and other types of detergents. This probably explains why the stimulatory effect of bile salt can be lost upon storage of the milk, i.e., it is known that during storage, lipolysis occurs in the milk, and it is reasonable to believe that fatty acids and other components of amphiphilic character can substitute for bile salts. Therefore, it is evident that the esterase activity recorded in human milk can vary considerably, depending on the assay conditions and on the conditions under which the milk has been collected and stored. It is much safer and more relevant from a physiologic point of view to quantitate the lipase content by determination of the lipase activity against long-chain triglyceride. This activity is fairly constant, reproducible and easy to determine by use of a radiolabeled substrate.

SUMMARY

Diisopropylfluorophosphate, a commonly used esterase inhibitor, was incorporated into only one human milk protein. This protein had a molecular weight corresponding to the bile salt stimulated lipase, the major human milk lipolytic enzyme. Antibodies raised against the pure enzyme inhibited all bile salt stimulated lipase (emulsified long-chain triglyceride as substrate) and all recorded esterase (soluble p-nitrophenyl acetate as substrate) activity, stimulated or not by bile salts. This proves that there is only one bile salt stimulated lipase and that the esterase activity recorded in human milk, whether stimulated by bile salts or not, resides in the same molecule. In fact, the esterase activity was stimulated in a nonspecific way by detergents rather than specifically by bile salts, which might explain why the bile salt effect may be lost during storage of milk. When samples of human milk were simultaneously preincubated with antibodies against bile salt stimulated lipase and lipoprotein lipase (the other lipase known to be present in human milk), virtually all lipase activity was lost. Thus, there is no evidence of a third lipolytic activity of qualitative or quantitative importance in human milk.

ACKNOWLEDGEMENTS

We are grateful to Mrs. Else-Britt Lundstrom for skillful technical assistance and to Mrs. Rebecca Ankener for preparing the manuscript. Support by grants from the Swedish Medical Research Council (19X-05708), the Swedish Baby Food Fund for Nutritional Research, the Medical Research Council of the Swedish Life Insurance Companies and the Medical Faculty, University of Umea is gratefully acknowledged.

This paper was presented while one of us (O.H.) was a post doctoral international research fellow sponsored by a Fogarty International Fellowship (1 F05 TW03521-01), and by grants from the Swedish Medical Research Council, the Henning and Johan Throne Holst's Foundation, the Sweden-America Foundation and Pfrimmer/Meda AB.

REFERENCES

1. Hernell O, Olivecrona T. (1974): Human milk lipases. I. Serum-stimulated lipase. J Lipid Res, 15, 367-374.

2. Hernell O, Blackberg L, Olivecrona T. (1981): Human milk lipases In: Lebenthal E, ed, Textbook of Gastroenterology and Nutrition in Infancy. New York: Raven Press, 347-354.

3. Egelrud T, Olivecrona T. (1973): Purified bovine milk (lipoprotein) lipase: activity against lipid substrates in the absence of exogenous factors. Biochim Biophys Acta, 306, 115-127.

4. Freudenberg E. (1953): Die Frauenmilch-lipase. Basel: S. Karger.

5. Blackberg L, Hernell O. (1981): The bile salt stimulated lipase in human milk. Purification and characterization. Eur J Biochem, 116, 221-225.

6. Wang C-S. (1980): Purification of human milk bile salt-activated lipase by cholic acid-coupled sepharose 4B affinity chromatography. Anal Biochem, 105, 398-402.

7. Blackberg L, Hernell O. (1983): Further characterization of the bile salt stimulated lipase in human milk. FEBS Lett, 157, 337-341.

8. Hernell O, Olivecrona T. (1974); Human milk lipase II. Bile salt stimulated lipase. Biochim Biophys Acta, 369, 234-244.

9. Wang C-S, Kuksis A, Manganaro F, Myher JJ, Downs D, Bass HB. (1983): Studies on the substrate specificity of purified human milk bile salt activated lipase. J Biol Chem, 258, 9197-9202,

10. Hernell O, Blackberg L. (1982): Digestion of human milk lipids: Physiologic significance of *sn*-2 monoacylglycerol hydrolysis by bile salt stimulated lipase. Pediatr Res, 16, 882-885.

11. Blackberg L, Lombardo D, Hernell O, Guy O, Olivecrona T. (1982): Bile salt stimulated lipase in human milk and carboxyl ester hydrolase in pancreatic juice. Are they identical enzymes? FEBS Lett, 136, 284-288.

12. Fredrikzon B, Hernell O, Blackberg L, Olivecrona T. (1978): Bile salt stimulated lipase in human milk: evidence of activity *in vivo* and of a role in the digestion of milk retinol esters. Pediatr Res, 12, 1048-1052.

13. Wang C-S. (1981): Human milk bile salt activated lipase: Further characterization and kinetic studies. J Biol Chem, 256, 10198-10202.

14. Hernell O. (1975): Human milk lipases. III. Physiological implications of the bile salt stimulated lipase. Eur J Clin Invest, 5, 267-272.

15. Mehta NR, Jones JB, Hamosh M. (1982): Lipases in preterm human milk. Ontogeny and physiologic significance. J Pediatr Gastroenterol Nutr, 1, 317-326.

16. Wardell JM, Wright AJ, Bardsly WG, D'Souza SW. (1984): Bile salt stimulated lipase and esterase activity in human milk after collection, storage, and heating: Nutritional implications. Pediatr Res, 18, 381-386.

17. Hall B, Muller DR. (1983): Studies on bile salt stimulated lipolytic activity in human milk. II. Demonstration of two groups of milk with different activities. Pediatr Res, 17, 716-720.

18. Hernell O, Egelrud T, Olivecrona T. (1975): Serum-stimulated lipases (lipoprotein lipases). Immunological crossreaction between the bovine and the human enzymes. Biochim Biophys Acta, 381, 233-241.

19. Hamosh M. (1982): Lingual and breast milk lipases. Adv Pediatr, 29, 33-67.

20. Castberg H, Hernell O. (1975): Role of serum-stimulated lipases in lipolysis in human milk. Milchwissenschaft, 30, 721-724.

21. Wardell JM, Hill CM, D'Souza SW. (1981): Effect of pasteurization and of freezing and thawing human milk on its triglyceride content. Acta Paediatr Scand, 70, 467-471.

22. Poland RT. (1981): Breast milk jaundice. J Pediatr, 99, 86-88.

23. Hernell O. (1982): Breast milk jaundice. J Pediatr, 101, 311-312.

24. Bengtsson G, Olivecrona T. (1981): Lipoprotein lipase: modification of its kinetic properties by mild tryptic digestion. Eur J Biochem, 113, 547-554.

MILK ENZYME FUNCTION: EFFECTS OF COMPARTMENTATION AND STORAGE CONDITIONS ON SULFHYDRL OXIDASE AND γ-GLUTAMYL TRANSPEPTIDASE

C. E. Isaacs

INTRODUCTION

Huston and Patton (1) have shown that human milk components are distributed in several compartments which can be separated by differential centrifugation. In my studies, I have been concerned with the distribution of enzymes between the skim milk membranes and the milk fat globule membranes. The former creates a "fluffy layer" of small vesicles above a firmer pellet containing casein and other proteins, after long-term centrifugation of human milk. The latter surround the milk fat globules and are at least partially removed with the fat fraction after low speed centrifugation. Many milk enzymes are bound to either the skim milk membranes or the milk fat globule membranes (2) and are, therefore, compartmentalized within the fluid phase of milk. Both the skim milk membrane and the milk fat globule membrane have been shown to originate from the plasma membrane material (a mixture of true plasma membrane and fused Golgi membrane) at the apex of the mammary secretory cells (2,3). However, despite their common origin, there are significant compositional and biochemical differences between the two membrane fractions (2,4).

Compartmentation is potentially a means to control the function of milk enzymes both in the milk and in the gastrointestinal tract. Enzymes may be separated from molecules that can stimulate activity, e.g., bovine milk galactosyltransferase and phosphatidyl choline (5,6), and they can be separated from potential inhibitors, e.g., xanthine oxidase and folate compounds (7,8,9,10). They can also be maintained in close proximity to other macromolecules producing synergistic effects as postulated by Moldoveneau et al., e.g., peroxidase, secretory IgA and lactoferrin (11). Disruption of normal milk compartmentation by some storage methods may inappropriately activate milk enzymes. For example, Hamosh et al., postulated that storage of human milk at -20°C leads to hydrolysis of triglycerides by milk lipase (12) because the triglyceride substrate becomes accessible to the enzyme.

Sulfhydryl oxidase (SOX) and γ-glutamyltranspeptidase (GGT) are membrane-bound enzymes (2) that have been found in the milk of all species tested (13). SOX catalyses the net synthesis of disulfide bonds (14) and GGT is involved in glutathione metabolism (15). In the present study, our intent was (a) to determine whether there is enzymatic heterogeneity among the skim milk membrane fractions which have been shown to be morphologically heterogeneous (16), and (b) to study the effects of different storage conditions on the membrane distribution of SOX and GGT. To this end the skim milk membranes were fractionated and the distribution of SOX and GGT studied.

METHODS

Human milk samples were obtained through the La Leche League of Staten Island, and informed consent was obtained. All of the experiments were done using milk from one mother, thereby eliminating possible individual variation.

SOX activity was measured as previously described using dithiothreitol (13). GGT (EC 2.3.2.2) was measured by the method of Griffith and Tate (17) with p-nitroanilide as substrate at 25°C.

Milk was fractionated by centrifuging whole milk at 4,000 g for 30 minutes at 4°C. The 4,000 g infranatant was then centrifuged at 100,000 g for 90 minutes. The 100,000 g supernatant was then centrifuged at 150,000 g for 16 hours.

RESULTS AND DISCUSSION

Fractionation of Fresh Human Milk

Following centrifugation at 4,000 g, 95% of SOX activity remained in the skim milk phase of fresh human milk (Table 1). When the skim milk was centrifuged at high speed (100,000 g, 90 min), 80% of SOX was found in the supernatant and approximately 15% in what would usually be designated in the "microsomal" fraction. When the 100,000 g supernatant was centrifuged at 150,000 g overnight, three distinct fractions were obtained. These were a supernatant, a fluffy membrane layer between the supernatant and the pellet, and the pellet. SOX was found primarily in the pellet, with a significant amount in the fluffy layer. This suggests that human milk SOX is a membrane-bound enzyme which is attached to the skim milk membranes.

GGT had a different milk membrane distribution than SOX (Table 1). After a 4,000 g centrifugation, less than half of the GGT activity was found in the skim milk, indicating that a substantial amount of GGT was bound to the MFGM. GGT not in the lipid fraction was found primarily in the 100,000 g supernatant, and, unlike milk SOX, is therefore not equivalent to a "microsomal" enzyme. When the 100,000 g supernatant was fractionated, almost all of the remaining GGT was found in the fluffy layer. There was a significant loss of both SOX and GGT activity following the 150,000 g separation. This may be due to separation of the enzymes from their membranes, which results in decreased stability. These results indicate that human milk GGT is a membrane-bound enzyme which is primarily found in the milk fat globule membrane and fluffy layer of the skim milk membrane fraction.

Thus, though both are bound to milk membranes, SOX and GGT are compartmentalized differently. Milk fat globule membranes appear to be the primary site of GGT, but appear to have very little SOX activity. Small amounts of both SOX and GGT are pelleted at 100,000 g. This may represent a "microsomal" membrane fraction or nonspecific association of some of the skim milk membrane with pelleting caseins. The distribution of SOX and GGT within the SMM fraction is also different. SOX is distributed mainly in the 150,000 g pellet and GGT in the fluffy layer. Therefore, while there is 6-7 times more GGT than SOX activity in the fluffy layer, there is 4-5

Table 1. Fractionation of SOX and GGT from Fresh Human Milk[a]

Fraction	SOX u/ml	Total SOX units	% Yield	GGT u/ml	Total GGT units	% Yield
Whole milk	0.30	1.52	100	1.41	7.10	100
4,000 g Infranatant	0.38	1.45	95.4	0.77	3.23	45.5
100,000 g Supernatant	0.38	1.21	79.6	0.70	2.22	31.3
150,000 g Supernatant	0.05	0.08	4.9	0.05	0.07	0.9
150,000 g Fluffy layer	1.40	0.13	8.6	9.18	0.80	11.6
150,000 g Pellet	1.46	0.30	19.7	0.34	0.07	1.0

[a] One unit of SOX activity is expressed as μmol SH oxidized/min. One unit of GGT activity is expressed as μmol p-nitroaniline released/min.

times more SOX in the pellet. The significance of this compartmentation of milk membrane-bound enzymes in terms of *in vivo* function in the milk or in the gut of the neonate is not known.

Fractionation of Human Milk Stored at 4°C

The concentration of SOX in human milk stored at 4°C for 7 days was the same as in fresh milk (Table 2). The membrane distribution of SOX following centrifugation at 4,000 g and 100,000 g was also unaltered. Following centrifugation at 150,000 g, the supernatant and pellet had the same SOX distribution as in fresh milk, but there was an increased level of SOX in the fluffy layer.

GGT activity in milk stored at 4°C was decreased 30% when compared to the activity found in fresh milk (Table 2). The compartmentation of the remaining GGT was the same after storage at 4°C as in fresh milk. However, there was a 3-fold elevation of GGT activity in the fluffy layer. This increased activity could be due to either increased production of the fluffy layer membrane fraction or to the alteration of its membrane structure during storage at 4°C. In the latter case, the number of enzyme molecules would be constant, but activity would be increased. Conversely, an altered membrane structure may result in decreased loss of enzyme activity by preventing the separation of SOX and GGT from the milk membrane. Membrane alteration could be accomplished by the action of milk proteases or lipases.

Storage at 4°C appeared to have no effect on the total milk activity of some milk membrane enzymes (SOX), but appeared to lead to the inactivation of others (GGT). However, these results indicate that even when the total concentration per ml of milk is unchanged, the level of enzyme activity in different membrane fractions can be affected.

Table 2. Fractionation of SOX and GGT from Human Milk Stored at 4°C

Fraction	SOX u/ml	Total SOX units	% Yield	GGT u/ml	Total GGT units	% Yield
Whole Milk	0.30	2.25	100	0.97	7.28	100
4,000 g Infranatant	0.24	1.80	80	0.54	4.05	55.6
100,000 g Supernatant	0.23	1.70	75.6	0.38	2.85	39.1
150,000 g Supernatant	0.02	0.05	2	0.01	0.03	0.4
150,000 g Fluffy layer	0.81	0.77	34.2	2.30	2.40	33
150,000 g Pellet	1.91	0.41	18.2	0.36	0.08	1.1

Fractionation of Human Milk Stored at -20°C

Storage of milk at -20°C did not decrease SOX activity (Table 3). The membrane distribution of SOX was also the same as in fresh milk. However, the amount of SOX present in the fluffy layer was substantially increased, as in milk stored at 4°C.

GGT stored at -20°C followed a pattern similar to that in milk stored at 4°C (Table 3). GGT activity was lost during storage, but the fluffy layer had increased GGT activity. The enzyme was still associated with the fat fraction.

There appear to be no differences, in terms of the stability and compartmentation of milk membrane-bound enzymes, between storage at 4°C and -20°C. The increased activity of both SOX and GGT in the fluffy layer occurs at both temperatures. This indicates that even at -20°C, some processes, whether enzymatic or physical in nature, remain active. Hamosh et al. (14) have shown that human milk lipases remain active at -20°C, but not at -70°C, and suggest that banked human milk be stored at -70°C [but see Hernell and Blackberg (18)]. The results presented here provide support for this suggestion. Lipases are probably not the only milk enzymes that remain active at -20°C, and thus banked human milk may be significantly altered in terms of both its macromolecular content and its nutritional quality.

SUMMARY

The human milk membrane-bound enzymes sulfhydryl oxidase (SOX) and γ-glutamyl transpeptidase (GGT) have different compartmentation patterns. The major GGT fraction was in the milk fat globule membranes, whereas SOX was found primarily in the skim milk membranes. The skim milk membranes are themselves heterogenous, both morphologically and, as we have shown here, biochemically. The fluffy layer had significantly more GGT than SOX, whereas the 150,000 g pellet had greater SOX than GGT activity.

Table 3. Fractionation of SOX and GGT from Human Milk Stored at -20°C

Fraction	SOX u/ml	Total SOX units	% Yield	GGT u/ml	Total GGT units	% Yield
Whole Milk	0.33	1.96	100	1.09	8.18	100
4,000 g Infranatant	0.32	1.79	91.3	0.55	4.13	50.5
100.000 g Supernatant	0.31	1.53	78.1	0.42	3.15	38.5
150,000 g Supernatant	0.05	0.07	3.6	0.004	0.01	0.1
150,000 g Fluffy layer	1.15	0.41	20.9	1.95	2.26	27.6
150,000 g Pellet	1.40	0.28	14.3	0.36	0.07	0.9

SOX was more resistant to inactivation than GGT during storage at 4°C and -20°C. In fact, SOX activity remained unchanged during storage. Storage at both 4°C and -20°C yielded increased SOX and GGT activity in the fluffy layer fraction of the skim milk membranes. This implies that even at -20°C banked human milk is being altered.

ACKNOWLEDGEMENT

I wish to thank the La Leche League of Staten Island for providing us with human milk samples. I also wish to acknowledge the work of Ann Parese in preparing this manuscript.

REFERENCES

1. Huston GE, Patton S. Membrane distribution in human milk as revealed by phospholipid and cholesterol analysis. (These proceedings).

2. Kitchen BJ. (1974): A comparison of the properties of membranes isolated from bovine skim milk and cream. Biochim Biophys Acta, 356,257-269.

3. Plantz PE, Patton S. (1973): Plasma membrane fragments in bovine and caprine skim milks. Biochem Biophys Acta, 291, 51-60.

4. Patton S and Keenan TW. (1971): The relationship of milk phospholipids to membranes of the secretory cell. Lipids, 6, 58-61.

5. Mitranic MM, Boggs JM, Moscarello MA. (1983): Modulation of bovine milk galactosyltransferase activity by lipids. Jour of Biol Chem, 258, 8630-8636.

6. Blanc B. (1981): Biochemical aspects of human milk - comparison with bovine milk. Wld Rev Nutr Diet, 36, 1-89.

7. Lewis AS, Murphy L, McCalla C, Fleary M, Purcell S. (1984): Inhibition of mammalian xanthine oxidase by folate compounds and amethopterin. Jour Biol Chem, 259, 12-5.

8. Antony AC, Utley CS, Marcell PD, Kolhouse JF. (1982): Isolation, characterization, and comparison of the solubilized particulate and soluble folate binding proteins from human milk. Jour Biol Chem, 257, 10081-10089.

9. Hansen SI, Holm J, Lyngbye J, Pedersen TG, Svendsen I. (1983): Dependence of aggregation and ligand affinity on the concentration of the folate-binding protein from cow's milk. Arch Biochem Bioph, 226, 636-642.

10. Colman N, Hettiarachchy N, Herbert V. (1981): Detection of a milk factor that facilitates folate uptake by intestinal cells. Science, 211, 1427-1429.

11. Moldoveanu Z, Tenuovuo J, Pruitt KM, Mansson-Rahemtulla B, Mestecky J. (1983): Antibacterial properties of milk: IgA-peroxidase-lactoferrin interactions. Ann N.Y. Acad Sci, 409, 848-850.

12. Hamosh M, Freed LM, Berkow SE, Bitman J, Wood DL, Hamosh P. (1984): Lipases and lipids in human milk: Effect of freeze-thawing and storage. Fed Proc, 43, 491.

13. Isaacs CE, Pascal T, Wright CE, Gaull GE. (1984): Sulfhydryl oxidase in human milk: stability of milk enzymes in the gastrointestinal tract. Pediatr Res, 18, 532-535.

14. Janolino VG, Swaisgood HE. (1975): Isolation and characterization of sulfhydryl oxidase from bovine milk. J Biol Chem, 250, 2532-2538.

15. Tate SS, Meister A. (1981): γ-Glutamyltranspeptidase: catalytic, structural and functional aspects. Mol Cell Biochem, 39, 357-368.

16. Stewart PS, Puppione DL, Patton S. (1972): The presence of microvilli and other membrane fragments in the non-fat phase of bovine milk. Z Zellforsch, 123, 161-167.

17. Griffith OW, Tate SS. (1980): The apparent glutathione oxidase activity of a γ-glutamyltranspeptidase. J Biol Chem, 255, 5011-5014.

18. Hernell O, Blackberg L. Lipase and esterase activities in human milk. (These proceedings.)

SECTION XII. CARBOHYDRATES, AMINO ACIDS, METABOLIC INTERMEDIATES, AND ALL OTHER NUTRIENTS

WORKSHOP PARTICIPANTS:

P. R. Borum, Department of Food Science and Human Nutrition, University of Florida, Gainesville, FL

S. A. Atkinson, Department of Pediatrics, McMaster University, Hamilton, Ontario, Canada

A. M. Ferris, Department of Nutritional Sciences, University of Connecticut, Storrs, CT

L. Hambraeus, Institute of Nutrition, University of Uppsala, Sweden

M. C. Neville, Department of Physiology, University of Colorado Health Science Center, Denver, CO

T. A. Picone, Pediatric Nutrition, Ross Laboratories, Columbus, OH

"Carbohydrates, amino acids, metabolic intermediates, and all other nutrients" indicates a heterogenous grouping of nutrients that includes those nutrients with well-characterized levels of requirements and functions, as well as those with only postulated functions and possible requirements in human milk. Methods of analysis for these nutrients, with adequate sensitivity and accuracy, in the matrix of human milk are essential to many investigations concerning the physiology of lactation, nutrient composition of milk, and functions of milk constituents. Suggested methods for analysis of glucose, lactose, free amino acids, carnitine, and citrate in human milk samples are discussed with the caveat that more research is needed to improve these methods.

CARBOHYDRATES, AMINO ACIDS, METABOLIC INTERMEDIATES, AND ALL OTHER NUTRIENTS

P. R. Borum
S. A. Atkinson
A. M. Ferris
L. Hambraeus
M. C. Neville
T. A. Picone

INTRODUCTION

This heterogenous grouping of nutrients is extremely interesting due to the many potential functions and requirements that may be met by its members. Some of these nutrients have been termed "conditionally essential nutrients" because, although exogenous sources of these nutrients are not required by healthy adults, exogenous sources may be required under certain physiological conditions, such as enzymatic immaturity during the neonatal period.

CARBOHYDRATES

Two of the most important carbohydrates in human milk are lactose and glucose. There are several methods for the determination of lactose and glucose in milk. High performance liquid chromatography methods, using a Waters carbohydrate analysis column (Waters Associates, Melford, Massachusetts 01757) and an 82:18 acetonitrite/water solvent system, are used to separate sugars which are then quantified by area-under-the-curve measurements of a set of known lactose standards. This HPLC method is available for standardization of other methods. The glucose oxidase method (1) is accurate, simple to perform and requires relatively inexpensive supplies and instrumentation.

Boehringer-Mannheim Biochemicals sells a kit based on the enzymatic breakdown of the carbohydrate into the following components:

1) Lactose + H_2O $\xrightarrow{\text{B-galactosidase}}$ Glucose + B-galactose

2) B-galactose + NAD + $\xrightarrow[\text{dehydrogenase}]{\text{B-galactose}}$ galactonic acid + $NADH^+$ H^+.

The NADH formed in the second reaction is stoichometric with lactose, and its absorbance is measured at 340 nm. This method gives good results, but is considered more tedious to perform and requires more expensive reagents than the glucose oxidase method. An automatic analyzer is available from Yellow Springs Instrument Company (Yellow Springs, Ohio

45387, YSI model 27 Industrial Analyzer). The instrument uses galactose oxidase immobilized on a membrane (for lactose measurements) or immobilized glucose oxidase (for glucose measurements) in the presence of oxygen to catalyze the production of hydrogen peroxide that is quantitated with an amperometric electrode. Whole milk is diluted 1:60 and a 24 microliter aliquot is used. The YSI instrument allows a large number of samples to be analyzed in a short period of time. The accuracy of this procedure is excellent as determined by standardization using HPLC. Long chain polysaccharides were not found to interfere with the assay (Neville and Keller, unpublished).

Human milk contains large quantities of heterogenous oligosaccharides either free or combined with protein. Although a considerable amount of work has been devoted to determining the structure of these oligosaccharides (see references 2 and 3 for examples), very little information on their overall contribution to the carbohydrate content of milk has become available since the pioneering studies of Grummanprez and Montreuil in the early sixties (4,5).

FREE AMINO ACIDS

Free amino acids in milk have been investigated since the early 1960's (6,7,8,9) and documented to be a large proportion of the non-protein nitrogen component of both preterm and term milk (10). Analysis of the free amino acid composition of milk has been useful in determining whether or not mothers with chronic illnesses should breast-feed their infants (11).

There are many indications that human lactation studies concerned with both mammary gland physiology and infant nutrition will require accurate quantitation of the free amino acid profiles of human milk. At the present time, satisfactory methods are being used in several laboratories, but there is no published method that can be identified as a reference method. As with the analysis of many compounds in milk, application of unmodified plasma methods for free amino acid profiles gives unacceptable results with milk samples.

Preparation of the milk sample immediately after collection is important if the purpose of the analysis is to quantitate glutamine, glutamic acid, cystine, or tryptophan. An example of one possible method of sample preparation is given in Appendix A. In addition to acid precipitation of proteins and removal of lipid by ultracentrifugation used in this method, ultrafiltration can also be used for deproteinization and delipidation. Care must be taken to avoid the introduction of any contaminants leached from the ultrafiltration membranes.

Sample size, pH, and ionic strength can greatly alter the initial portion of the aminogram. Since this portion contains amino acids, such as taurine, that are of critical importance in many human lactation studies, greatest care is needed to insure the complete resolution of each peak during the chromatography.

Taurine is a free amino acid in milk which is of special interest in many investigations. Most commonly used chromatographic procedures result in elution of taurine, phosphoethanolamine, and urea in the same general area of the chromatogram, and special procedures are required to insure that these three peaks are completely resolved. Chromatographic parameters must be customized for each instrument and may require slight modification when new lots of buffers are used. There are concentration errors in some lots of calibration mixtures, and, therefore, the results derived from a new lot should be carefully compared to results obtained from the previous lot.

The introduction of integrators has greatly speeded up the calculations from a chromatographic run, but it is still necessary to determine if the proper integration parameters were used for each individual chromatogram before acceptance of the calculations performed by the integrator. The quantitation of the amino acids has traditionally used ninhydrin.

Although ninhydrin is still frequently used, it is being replaced by more sensitive techniques. There has been a great deal of success recently in performing amino acid analysis of protein hydrolysates on various HPLC systems. However, applications of many of these methods for physiological amino acid profiles have remained unsatisfactory. In many respects the modern amino acid analyzers are HPLC instruments specially designed for amino acid analysis. It appears that the complexity of physiological samples may require these dedicated instruments.

The expected increase in need for free amino acid analyses of milk in many types of research and the highly complex nature of the methods dictate that a major emphasis be given to improvement of these methods.

METABOLIC INTERMEDIATES

Carnitine is found in the milk of all species tested and may be an essential nutrient for the newborn. The concentration of total carnitine in human milk appears to vary with duration of lactation (12). The presently used enzymatic assay (13) is accurate but tedious. There are many steps in the assay that are subject to the introduction of artifacts. Carnitine analysis of milk is more difficult than the carnitine analysis of other biological fluids. Appendix B presents a method for carnitine analysis of milk samples that has an intrassay coefficient of variation of 6.2%. Work is needed to simplify this procedure.

Citrate and other Krebs cycle intermediates are important metabolic intermediates in milk. Citrate in milk can be measured with a commercially available kit (Citric Acid Test -- Combination kit, Boehringer-Manheim Biochemicals, Indianapolis, Indiana 46250) that utilizes citrate lyase to convert citrate to oxaloacetate and acetate. The oxaloacetate and its decarboxylation product, pyruvate, are reduced to malate and lactate with malate dehydrogenase and lactate dehydrogenase. The amount of NADH oxidized is measured spectrophotometrically at 340 nm. The assay requires 40 microliters of fat free milk.

Amino sugars, such as glucosamine, galactosamine and lactosamine, can be measured chromatographically, but much work needs to be done on the methodology. There is currently a great void in the literature.

Choline, ethanolamine, isoantigens, polyamines, nucleotides, urea cycle intermediates, prostaglandins, drugs, environmental toxins, and many other substances can be quantitated in human milk, but, in general, the methods for analysis need improvement. Craig-Schmidt and her colleagues appear to have used acceptable methods for measurement of prostaglandins (14).

DISCUSSION

Recent investigations have greatly improved the methods of analysis for the many different types of substances in this grouping of all other nutrients. However, even for many substances routinely analyzed in physiological fluids other than milk, improved sensitivity and accuracy in the matrix of human milk are needed for most methods presently available.

ACKNOWLEDGEMENT

This research was supported in part by NIH Contracts No. NO1-HD-2-2818 and NO1-HD-2-2808.

REFERENCES

1. Beach EF, Turner JJ. (1958): An enzymatic method for glucose determination in body fluids. Clin Chem, 4, 462.

2. Yamashita K, Tachibana Y, Kolsata A. (1977): Oligosaccharides of human milk. J Biol Chem, 252, 5408 - 5411.

3. Prieto PA, Smith DF. (1984): A new sialylolesosaccharide from human milk: isolation and characterisation using anti-oligosaccharide antibodies. Arch Biochem Biophys, 229, 650-656.

4. Ebner KE, Schanbacher FL. (1974): Biochemistry of lactose and related carbohydrates. In: Larson BL, Smith VR, eds, Lactation, Vol 2. New York: Academic Press, 77-113.

5. Grummanprez L, Montreuil J. (1975): Isolement et etude des proprietes physicochimibues d'oligosaccharides du lait du femme. Biochimie, 57, 695-701.

6. Armstrong MD, Yates KN (1963): Free amino acids in milk. Proc Soc Exp Brol Med, 113, 680-683.

7. Ghadimi H, Tecora P. (1963): Free amino acids of different kinds of milk. Am J Clin Nutr, 13, 75-81.

8. Svanberg V, Gebre-Medhin M, Ljungqvist B, Olsson M. (1977): Breast milk composition in Ethiopian and Swedish mothers III. Amino acids and other nitrogeneous substances. Am J Clin Nut, 30, 499-507.

9. Wurtman JJ, Sernstrom JD (1979): Free amino acid, protein, and fat contents of breast milk from Guatemalan mothers consuming a corn-based diet. Early Human Devel, 3, 67-77.

10. Lemons JA, Reyman D, Moye L. (1983): Amino acid composition of preterm and term breast milk during early lactation. Early Human Devel, 8, 323-329.

11. Gahl WA, Rizzo WB. (1983): Normal free dibasic amino acids in breast milk of a woman with cystinuria. New Eng J Med, 309, 1388-1389.

12. Sandor A, Pecsuvac K. Kerner J, Alkonyi I. (1982): On carnitine content of the human breast milk. Ped Res, 16, 89-91.

13. Cederblad G, Lindstedt S. (1972): A method for the determination of carnitine in the picomole range. Clin Chim Acta, 37, 235-243.

14. Craig-Schmidt MC, Weeke JD, Faircloth SA, Wickwire MA, Livant EJ. (1984): The effect of hydrogenated fat in the diet of nuring mothers on lipid composition and prostaglandin content of human milk. Am J Clin Nutr, 39, 778-786.

APPENDIX A

Sample Preparation for Amino Acid Analysis

1. Disassociate free amino acids that may be bound to proteins by adding 80 μl of fresh milk to an equal volume of 0.5% sodium dodecylsulfate and incubating at room temperature for 15 minutes.

2. Denature protein by adding 100μl of 10% sulfosalicylic acid.

3. Adjust pH of the sample to the appropriate pH for injection by adding 140 1 of 0.5M LiOH (pH needed will vary with instrument and chromatography procedure).

4. Precipitate denatured proteins by spinning at 2000xg for 15 minutes in a refrigerated centrifuge.

5. Store supernatant at -70°C until day of assay.

6. On the day of assay, thaw sample and remove any remaining denatured protein and fat particles by spinning at 100,000xg for 5 minutes in an Airfuge.

7. Fluid should be taken from the layer below the fat layer and above the denatured protein pellet and applied to the column.

APPENDIX B

Method for Carnitine Analysis of Milk Samples

Principle. Acetylcarnitine and acylcarnitine are hydrolyzed by alkaline hydrolysis. The total carnitine is measured by incubation of the sample with ^{14}C-acetyl CoA and carnitine acetyltransferase. The radioactive acetylcarnitine is separated from the unreacted radioactive acetyl CoA using a Dowex 2x8 anion exchange column. The radioactive acetylcarnitine fraction is quantitated by counting in a liquid scintillation counter.

Sample Preparation. Keep milk on ice and deliver to the laboratory as soon a possible after collection. Sample may be stored at -20°C in plastic containers for at least 21 days with no detectable loss of carnitine.

Assay Procedure.

1. Prepare in quadruplicate, standards of L-Carnitine within the range of 1.25 to 15 nmoles.

2. Assay samples in triplicate.

3. Hydrolyze short chain and long chain esters of carnitine by combining 100 1 of milk sample, 125µl distilled deionized H_2O and 25 1 of 1N KOH and incubating at 50°C for 30 minutes.

4. Denature and precipitate protein by adding 750µl of 0.6M perchloric acid and spinning at 2000xg for 15 minutes.

5. Remove fatty acid particles and small particles of denatured protein by filtering through 0.2 micron Gelman Acrodisc filters.

6. Adjust the pH and ionic strength by adding 500µl of the filtrate to tubes containing phenol red and adding 4N KOH until the solution turns bright pink. Store at 4°C overnight to allow formation of potassium perchlorate crystals. Spin at 2000xg for 15 minutes to precipitate the crystals.

7. Determine the carnitine concentration of the sample by adding 100 µl of the prepared sample to 100 µl of Ingredient mixture containing 2 volumes of 50uCi/150ml ^{14}C-Acetyl CoA, 1 volume of 0.1mM acetyl CoA, and 1 volume of 24mM N-ethylmaleimide in 1M potassium phosphate buffer pH7.0. Add 40 µl of a suspension of carnitine acetyltransferase (approximates 25 units/ml) to each tube at 30 second intervals and incubate at 37°C for exactly 30 minutes. Remove 200 µl of each reaction mixture and place on a 35 mm Dowex 2-X8 column in a 5-3/4 inch Pasteur pipet. Wash each column with two 500 µl aliquots of deionized H_2O and count the elutant in a scintillation counter.

8. Calculate the carnitine concentration of the sample using the L-Carnitine Standard Curve.

LIST OF CONTRIBUTORS AND PARTICIPANTS

Stephanie A. Atkinson, Department of Pediatrics, McMaster University, 1200 Main Street West, Hamilton, Ontario M9A 4R1

E. N. Baker, Department of Chemistry, Biochemistry and Biophysics, Massey University, Palmerston North, New Zealand

M. Bano, Laboratory of Pathophysiology, National Cancer Institute, Bethesda, MD 20205

Susan E. Berkow, Department of Pediatrics, Georgetown University Medical Center, Washington, DC 20007

Joel Bitman, Milk Secretion and Mastitis Laboratory, USDA, Beltsville, MD 20705

Lars Bläckberg, Department of Physiological Chemistry, University of Umeå, S-901-85, Sweden

Peggy R. Borum, Department of Food Science and Human Nutrition, University of Florida, Gainesville, Florida 32611

K. Burdette, Laboratory of Pathophysiology, National Cancer Institute, Bethesda, MD 20205

Nancy Butte, Department of Medicine and Pediatrics, Baylor College, 1200 Moursund Avenue, Houston, TX 77030

Barbara Carlsson, University of Goteburg, Goteburg, Sweden

Clare E. Casey, Departments of Pediatrics and Physiology, University of Colorado Health Sciences Center, Denver, CO 80262

M. Thomas Clandinin, Division of Gastroenterology, Department of Medicine, The University of Alberta, Edmonton, Alberta, T6G 2G3

Thomas G. Cleary, Department of Pediatrics, University of Texas Medical School at Houston, Houston, TX 77030

Soter Dai, Department of Biological Chemistry and Surgery, The Children's Hospital and Harvard Medical School, Boston MA 02115

Kay Dewey, Department of Nutrition, University of California, Davis, CA 95616

Ronald R. Eitenmiller, Department of Food Science, University of Georgia, Athens, GA 30602

Ann M. Ferris, Department of Nutritional Sciences, University of Connecticut, U-17, Storrs, CT 06268

Thorsten A. Fjellstedt, NICHHD, Room 7C17, Landow Building, 7910 Woodmont Avenue, Bethesda, MD 20205

Lois M. Freed, Department of Pediatrics, Georgetown University Medical Center, Washington, DC 20007

Cutberto Garza, Department of Pediatrics, Baylor College of Medicine, Childrens Nutrition Research Center, Medical Towers Building, 6608 Fannin, Suite 601, Houston, TX 77030

Armond S. Goldman, Division of Immunology and Allergy, Department of Pediatrics, University of Texas Medical Branch, Galveston, TX 77550

K. Michael Hambidge, Department of Pediatrics, University of Colorado Health Sciences Center, 4200 East Ninth Avenue, Box C233, Denver, CO 80262

Leif Hambraeus, Institute of Nutrition, Box 551, University of Uppsala, Uppsala, Sweden

Margit Hamosh, Department of Pediatrics, Georgetown University Medical Center, Washington, DC 20007

Paul Hamosh, Department of Physiology and Biophysics, Georgetown University Medical Center, Washington, D.C. 20007

Lars A. Hanson, Department of Immunology, University of Goteberg, Goldhedsgaton 10-413,46, Goteborg Sweden

Barbara Happ, Community Human Milk Bank, Georgetown University Medical Center, Washington, DC 20007

Olle Hernell, Department of Pediatrics, University of Umeå, S-901 85 Umeå, Sweden

Bruce W. Hollis, Department of Nutrition, School of Medicine, Case Western Reserve University, Cleveland, OH 44106

Rodney R. Howell, Department of Pediatrics, University of Texas Health Science Center at Houston Medical School, P.O. Box 20708, Houston, TX 77025

Gail E. Huston, University of California at San Diego, School of Medicine, Neuroscience M-008, La Jolla, CA 92093

Charles E. Isaacs, Institute for Basic Research, 1050 Forest Hill Road, Staten Island, NY 10314

Robert G. Jensen, Department of Nutritional Sciences, University of Connecticut, Storrs, CT 06268

Jay B. Jones, Department of Clinical Chemistry, Geisinger Medical Center, Danville, PA

Margaret Keller, Department of Pediatrics, UCLA School of Medicine, Harbor-UCLA Medical Center, Los Angeles, CA 90502

Ronald P. Keller, Department of Physiology, C240, University of Colorado School of Medicine, 4200 East Ninth Avenue, Denver, CO 80262

William R. Kidwell, Laboratory of Pathophysiology, National Cancer Institute, Bethesda, MD 20205

Avanelle Kirksey, Department of Foods and Nutrition, Purdue University, West Lafayette, IN 46907

Michael Klagsbrun, Departments of Biological Chemistry and Surgery, The Children's Hospital and Harvard Medical School, Boston MA 01225

Steve Kohl, Program on Infectious Diseases and Physical Microbiology, University of Texas Medical School at Houston, Houston, TX 70030

Carol Lammi-Keefe, Department of Nutritional Sciences, University of Connecticut, Storrs CT 06268

Bruce L. Larson, University of Illinois, Department of Dairy Science , 1207 Gregory, Urbana, IL 61801

I. Lococzy, Laboratory of Tumor Immunology and Biology, National Cancer Institute, Bethesda, MD 20205

Bo Lönnerdal, Department of Nutrition, University of California, Davis, CA 95616

Nitin R. Mehta, Department of Pediatrics, Georgetown University Medical Center, Washington, DC 20007

Frank. H. Morriss, Jr., Departments of Pediatrics and of Obstetrics, Gynecology and Reproductive Sciences, Medical School, University of Texas Health Science Center, Houston, TX 77030

Phyllis B. Moser, Department of Food and Nutrition, University of Maryland, College Park, MD

Margaret C. Neville, Deptartment of Physiology, C240, University of Colorado School of Medicine, 4200 East Ninth Avenue, Denver, CO 80262

Max J. Paape, U.S. Department of Agriculture, Agriculture Research, Animal Science Institute, Beltsville, Maryland 20705

Stuart Patton, University of California at San Diego, School of Medicine, Neuroscience M-008, La Jolla, CA 92093

Mary Frances Picciano, Division of Foods and Nutrition, Division of Nutritional Sciences, College of Agriculture, The University of Illinois, 905 S. Goodwin Avenue, Urbana, IL 61801

Larry K. Pickering, University of Texas Medical School at Houston, 6431 Fannin Street, Houston, TX 77030

Thomas A. Picone, Ross Laboratories, Pediatrics and Nutrition, 625 Cleveland Avenue, Columbus, OH 43216

Sylvia B. Rumball, Massey University, Department of Chemistry, Biochemistry and Biophysics, Palmerston North, New Zealand

D. Salomon, Laboratory of Tumor Immunology and Biology, National Cancer Institute, Bethesda, MD 20205

Yuen W. Shing, Departments of Biological Chemistry and Surgery, The Children's Hospital and Harvard Medical School, Boston MA 02115

Shobha A. Udipi, Department of Foods and Nutrition, Purdue University, West Lafayette, IN 46907

Francesca M. Verda, Department of Nutritional Sciences, University of Connecticut, Storrs, CT 06268

C.L. Wade, Department of Pediatrics, McMaster University, Hamilton, Onterio, Canada

Michael W. Woolridge, John Radcliffe Hospital, Department of Pediatrics, Headington, Oxford, University of Oxford, Oxford, OX3 90U, United Kingdom

INDEX

HUMAN LACTATION 2

Maternal and Environmental Factors

HUMAN LACTATION 2

Maternal and Environmental Factors

Edited by

Margit Hamosh

Georgetown University Medical Center
Washington, D.C.

and

Armond S. Goldman

University of Texas
Galveston, Texas

Plenum Press • New York and London

Library of Congress Cataloging in Publication Data

International Workshop on Maternal-Environmental Factors in Human Lactation (1986: Oaxaca, Mexico)
Human lactation 2.

"Proceedings of an International Workshop on Maternal-Environmental Factors in Human Lactation, held January 15-19, 1986 in Oaxaca, Mexico"—T.p. verso.
Includes bibliographies and index.
1. Breast feeding—Congresses. 2. Breast feeding—Cross-cultural studies—Congresses. 3. Lactation—Congresses. 4. Mothers-Nutrition—Congresses. I. Hamosh, Margit. II. Goldman, Armond S. III. Title. IV. Title: Human lactation two. [DNLM: 1. Breast Feeding—congresses. 2. Lactation—congresses. 3. Milk, Human—congresses. WP 825 I613h 1986]
RJ216.I58 1986 363.8′2 86-20537
ISBN 0-306-42389-8

Proceedings of an International Workshop on Maternal-Environmental Factors in Human Lactation, held January 15-19, 1986, in Oaxaca, Mexico

A Division of Plenum Publishing Corporation
233 Spring Street, New York, N.Y. 10013

Printed in the United States of America

PREFACE

The International Workshop on human lactation dedicated specifically to the topic of Maternal and Environmental Effects on Lactation represents the recent progress of research in human lactation. Only four years ago it was clear that we do not yet have sensitive research techniques specifically adapted to the study of human milk. This need was addressed by an NIH convened workshop in 1982, the concensus being that appropriate methods have to be developed for the study of the composition of human milk. The progress in the development of these techniques was the subject of the second workshop on human lactation, dedicated specifically to "Milk Components and Methodologies." The workshop was held in Colorado in 1984 and resulted in the publication of the first volume in the series of "Human Lactation." At the Colorado meeting it was readily apparent that considerable progress has been made in the development of sensitive techniques able to quantitate the bioactive components of human milk (enzymes, growth factors, immuno-protective agents) as well as the macro, micro and trace elements. At the Colorado workshop it became clear that these workshops greatly benefit the research of human lactation by enhancing communication and collaboration among the investigators in the field. As a result it was decided to have a future workshop about a year later on the topic of "Maternal-Environmental Effects on Human Lactation", and I was charged with chairing it. Of course this meant that funds as well as an appropriate location had to be found for the next workshop. The first task was attended by submitting a conference grant to the National Institutes of Health as well as asking for grants-in-aid from private industry. Luckily we were successful and received an NIH conference grant as well as generous contributions from Ross Laboratories from Mead Johnson Nutritional Division and from Brystol-Meyers International Group. We are deeply grateful to the National Institutes of Health specifically the Institute for Child Health and Human Development and to the above listed infant formula companies for their financial help.

As to the location of the workshop, for several reasons I wanted it to be in Oaxaca, Mexico. Why Mexico? First, it would provide the opportunity for a good exchange of ideas and practical information with our immediate neighbors to the south, as well as with other countries in Central America. And, indeed the workshop had participants not only from Mexico, but also from Costa Rica, Honduras, and Guatemala. The second reason was the gracious offer of Drs. Salvador Villalpando-Hernandez and Samuel Flores-Huerta from the Social Security Hospital, Mexico City, Mexico, who attended the Colorado meeting, to help with the local organization. The third reason was purely personal. I thought it would be wonderful to have the workshop in a city not only a jewel in itself, but in addition, located between the old Mixtec and Zapotec civilizations of Mitla and Monte Alban. In fact, the Temple of the Dancers erected at Monte Alban some 2,500 years ago, seems to have been a hospital or school of medicine, according to the opinion of scholars who have studied its intricate carvings. Indeed where could one find a better place for a workshop on human lactation, than one which probably has the oldest carvings of a pregnant woman in the Western hemisphere!

The workshop was originally scheduled to start on October 6th, but had to be postponed because of the severe earthquake that hit Mexico City at the end of September. Although the hospital in which Drs. Villalpando-Hernandez and Flores-Huerta work, was completely destroyed, they were unharmed and proceeded undaunted with the local preparations. We all owe them a debt of gratitude for the excellent local organization of this workshop.

The workshop specifically addressed the recommendations generated by the Surgeon General's Conference on breast feeding, namely the benefits (nutritional, immunologic, and other) and contraindications (assessment of drugs and xenobiotics) of breast feeding. Because of the rising incidence of premature delivery, the workshop also addressed the specific topic of "Preterm Milk." The different topics of the conference were presented at 6 workshops, each preceded by a plenary lecture that gave a "State of the Art" overview of the subject, followed by several shorter lectures on recent and ongoing research in the field. The 6 workshops covered the following subjects:

1. Ethnic-Cultural Effects On Human Lactation.
2. Effect of Duration of Pregnancy and Lactation Upon Composition of Human Milk.
3. Lactation Performance.
4. Effects of Maternal Nutrition on Human Lactation.
5. Drugs and Toxins in Human Milk.
6. Host Defense Factors in Human Milk.

In additon we had an excellent poster presentation in which much new material was presented.

The conference was opened by the key note address of Professor Lars Hanson on the topic "Breast Feeding in Reality," an elegant and stimulating lecture that set the tone for the entire conference.

I would like to thank all the participants for making this an outstanding conference. We all started early and ended "early" (in the wee hours of the morning!) and in the process learned a great deal. Thanks are due to the Lactation Advisory Committee Members for their help in planning the conference. I especially want to thank Professor Armond Goldman, Vice-Chair of the conference, for his input in planning the meeting and for going to Oaxaca in the summer of 1985 to locate the wonderful accomodations that we enjoyed so much during the meeting. Special thanks are due to Dr. Homero Hernandez-Montes for his expert supervision of all visual aids and to Mrs. Luz Maria Luna Landeros for her expert secretarial work. Our deep gratitude to Dr. Thorsten Fjellstedt from the National Institute of Child Health and Human Development for his tireless efforts in promoting research on human lactation and for his enthusiasm, encouragement and support throughout the planning of this workshop.

The end of the conference was also the starting point for the editorial process of this book. I want to thank all workshop leaders, professors Hambraeus, Atkinson, Hartmann, Lonnerdal, Wilson and Pickering for reviewing all the manuscripts.

We are all thankful to the Mayor of Oaxaca the Hon Dr. Jorge Iturribaria-Bolanos and to the members of the City Council the Hons C. Moreno Lopez, A. Calvo Cuervo, J. Suarez, M. Gonzalez, R. Garcia, P.

Águilar, L. Castameda Melgoza, V.J. Arias Cruz, J. Lopez Luna, A.V. Garcia, A. Zarate Vazquez, E. Hernandez Vargas, C. Hempshire Franco, and P. Wooldridge Fernandez, for conferring upon the organizers of the meeting the honor of "Distinguished Visitor of the City of Oaxaca." It was a wonderful session in the beautiful town hall, highlighted by the moving address of the Honorable Perla Wooldrich Fernandez on the immortality of the bond between mother and infant as contrasted to the short lived glory of even the greatest empires!

The historical background of the city, its people and its customs, and especially the role of the reboso, the traditional local garment, in the life of the Oaxacan woman was vividly described by Dr. Ester Bonilla from the University of Oaxaca.

Last, but not least, the conference would certainly not have been the success it was without the organizing skill of my husband, Professor Paul Hamosh, who generously contributed his expertise, time and patience to the detailed planning of the conference. My thanks also go to my daughters Tamar and Leora, who gave generously of their summer vacation time for the initial organizing of the conference and the final editorial work, respectively.

May, 1986

Margit Hamosh
Conference Chair
Washington

CONTENTS

SECTION III

LACTATION PERFORMANCE

SECTION IV

EFFECTS OF MATERNAL NUTRITION ON HUMAN LACTATION

SECTION V

DRUGS AND TOXINS IN HUMAN MILK

SECTION VI

HOST DEFENSE FACTORS IN HUMAN MILK

SECTION VII

POSTER PRESENTATION

BREAST FEEDING IN REALITY

L.Å. Hanson, I. Adlerbert, B. Carlsson, Fehmida Jalil, J. Karlberg, B.S. Lindblad, L. Mellander, Shaukat R. Khan, Rafia Hasan, A.Kaleem Sheiku and T.Söderström

Departments of Clinical Immunology, Pediatrics and Anatomy
University of Göteborg, Sweden

Departments of Pediatrics and of Social and Preventive Pediatrics
King Edward Medical College, Lahore

Department of Psychology
Punjab University, Lahore, Pakistan

and Department of Pediatrics, Karolinska Institute
Stockholm, Sweden

INTRODUCTION

The decline in breast feeding during the last few decades seen first in the developed and then in the developing countries is not as unique in history as often believed. We tend to think that previously mothers always breast-fed, but we are rather repeating history. The authorities in Sweden became aware of the slow population growth during the eighteenth and nineteenth centuries through the Central Bureau of Statistics founded in 1749. It was obvious that this slow growth was due to a very high infant mortality, which was around 200 promill from 1750-1800. In local areas it remained even around 400 promille up to about 1830. According to the registries of the priests in each parish and the continuous reporting to the authorities by the provincial doctors the infant mortality was due mainly to gastroenteritis and was inversely related to the frequency of breast feeding (1,2). In some quite distinct areas in Sweden and Finland artificial feeding was predominant. Here infant mortality was high. The babies were mostly fed undiluted cow's milk through a cow horn which could not be cleaned and was stinking so that the doctor knew already when he entered a home that there was an artificially fed baby.

The reasons for the mothers not to breastfeed were local traditions and socio-economical factors. The poor mothers and also the farmer's wives often had to leave their infants to work outside the home and there was in fact an inverse relationship between the frequency of breast feeding and the mothers' workload, just as is seen today e.g. in Pakistan (Table 1).

Table 1. Correlation between daily burden of work and length of lactation period in three population groups in Lahore, Pakistan.

Area	No. of mothers	r	p value
Mud hut	21	- 0.76	<0.01
City slum	20	- 0.60	<0.01
Elite	19	- 0.71	<0.01

The importance of breast feeding was realized, among others by Carl von Linné (3) and the authorities managed via the provincial doctors, well trained midwives and the clergy to inform about the advantages of breast feeding and improved hygiene. As a result of that and other activities infant mortality decreased to around 85 promille at 1900 and the population increased from 1.7 million in 1750 to 5.0 million in 1905. The birth rate remained rather unchanged and the decreasing infant mortality was the main factor behind this increase (2). One reason for the success could be the relatively good educational level: at the year 1800 about 90 per cent of the Swedish population could read. Schools became compulsory in 1842.

These observations clearly illustrate the role of breast feeding as one among several factors of great importance for health and survival of the young child. In developing countries today, we see again a similar situation as in Sweden 150-250 years ago. A poor, uneducated, under-nourished mother with a heavy workload cannot easily manage to breast-feed, even if she knew she should. Her socio-economic situation and lack of supportive network, especially in the big city slums, work against successful breast feeding. By unfortunate and efficient advertisements about artificial feeding she is rather influenced not to breast-feed. Actually, 42% of the mothers from a low socio-economic group in Pakistan knew the name of at least one infant formula brand (4).

However, infants do not stay healthy only by being breastfed. Under the hygienic conditions that many mothers and infants live in poor societies breastfeeding alone may not be enough to prevent repeated infections.

There are numerous reports demonstrating that breast feeding can protect against infections, especially gastroenteritis, and according to some studies also against infections in the respiratory tract (5,6,7). However, in other studies it has not been obvious that breast feeding is protective (5,6). The reason may be the design of the studies and various methodological differences, but there could also be other substantial factors. This became clear to us during an extensive prospective study of infants in a poor community in Lahore, Pakistan. Although the number of episodes of diarrhoea and upper as well as lower respiratory tract infections related to house and educational standard (Table 2), they did not relate to the duration of breast feeding. Does this indicate that breast feeding does not protect against infections, or could there be other explanations?

Table 2. Multiple regression analysis of the total number of episodes for a certain type of infection from birth up to 24 months of age for 910 children living in a slum area in Lahore, Pakistan. A significant value for a certain infection shows an increased number of episodes for a lower house standard and educational level respectively.

Dependent variables	Independent variables	
Total number of episodes of	House standard	Education level
diarrhoea	$p < 0.05$	$p < 0.001$
upper respiratory infection	$p < 0.05$	$p < 0.0001$
lower respiratory infection	$p < 0.0001$	n.s.

n.s. = not significant

This review will bring up two factors which we feel are important in this context, and which are usually disregarded. The first is the fact that babies are rarely exclusively breast-fed in developing countries, and the second is that there may be such a heavy exposure to infectious agents that it can overcome the host defence also of the breast-fed infant.

THERE ARE HARDLY ANY EXCLUSIVELY BREAST-FED INFANTS IN DEVELOPING COUNTRIES

In Lahore, as in many other communities, the incidence of breast feeding has been declining. In 1983, 73% of the infants were breast-fed and given extra water during the first month of life. There was a continuous decline in breastfeeding during the following months. In a detailed follow up of the feeding patterns of infants in the slums of the city of Lahore and a village outside in 1984-85, cross-sectional analyses showed that just 20% were given "only breast milk" at one month of age (Fig. 1). On further analysis all but 4 of the 50 infants in this group used a soother, which was never washed. Furthermore, other foods or fluids than breast milk may in fact have been given, as discussed further below. By 2 months of age no more than 12% of the infants were "exclusively" breast-fed. The others were given buffalo milk via bottle as well (31%), extra water (42%) or bottle milk only (12%). During the following months, a few more infants were given water than buffalo milk, in addition to the breast milk. Only 3% were still "exclusively" breast-fed at 6 months. The reason for weaning was usually "insufficient milk production", but there was also an inverse relationship to the mother's daily burden of work (Table 1).

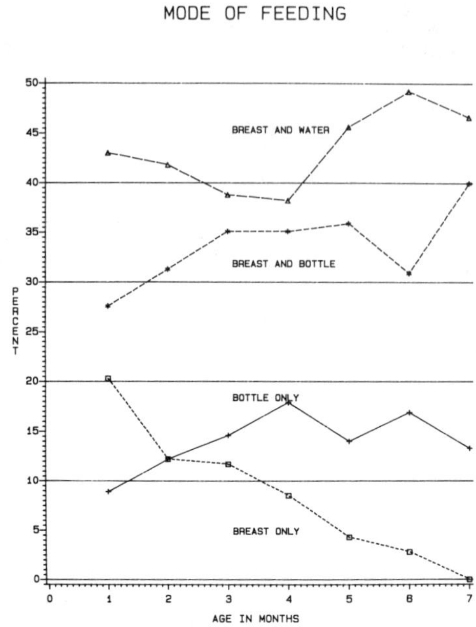

Fig. 1. Cross-sectionally analyzed percentages of feeding patterns in 285 infants followed from birth. They come from four different areas in and around Lahore in Punjab, Pakistan, a village, a mud hut area, the old city slum and an elite group, cf Table 3.

Infants in developing countries reported to be breast-fed are presumably not exclusively breast-fed in most instances. According to social anthropologists, who during their studies lived with families in such countries in many parts of the world, breast-fed babies are usually given extra food by various members of the family (8). This food is sometimes chewed first and most likely contaminated with various micro-organisms. Furthermore, extra fluid is given, especially in hot climates. Again, this fluid is most probably often contaminated as has been illustrated i.a. by studies in the Gambia (9).

Colostrum is regarded unsuitable as food for the newborn in many societies, for instance in China, Pakistan and Turkey. Table 3 shows what is given to the newborns instead of colostrum in a village outside Lahore, in the mud hut slum, in the old city slum and in a privileged group in Lahore. Many of the neonates in the village and the mud hut area were given sugar water, or a herb concoction (rosewater, anis, cardemum, etc. extracted for several years before use). In the city slum and in the privileged group it was common to feed honey. A few were given a laxative. These various materials are most probably contaminated with microbes, for instance honey has been reported to occasionally carry spores for Clostridium botulinum, possibly causing sudden death in infancy (10). The fluids and foods provided instead of colostrum were given with spoon, by hand, bottle or other means (Table 4). Again it is obvious that this could provide further microbial contamination, especially in surroundings where the hygiene is poor as further discussed below. It cannot be excluded that the 9 infants dying of neonatal septicemia, or the 2 of acute and 5 of chronic diarrhoea in the slum areas of Lahore during one stage of the study (Table 5) were infected via these fluids/foods given instead of colostrum.

Table 3. Fluids and foods given to infants before the start of breast feeding in three populations from Lahore and one from a village outside of Lahore

Area	Total no.	Herb concoction	Honey	Laxative	Sugar water	Saline
Village	87	65*	2	-	18	-
Mud hut	82	38	6	4	36	-
City slum	72	4	69	1	5	-
Elite	44	-	28	1	2	13

* = no. of infants. One infant can have obtained none or several of the indicated materials.

Table 4. Means of giving fluids and foods to infants before start of breast feeding (%) (Lahore, Pakistan)

Area	Total no.	Spoon	Hand	Bottle	Other means
Village	87	32.1	5.7	8.0	54.0
Mud hut	82	65.8	7.3	10.9	17.0
City slum	72	13.8	79.1	2.7	18.0
Elite	44	25	29.5	45.4	-

Table 5. Causes of neonatal deaths (Lahore, Pakistan)

Area	No. of births	No. of deaths						
		Sepsis	Acute diarr.	Chronic diarr.	Resp. inf.	Menin-gitis	Teta-nus	Sudden death
Village	119	2			6			
Mud hut	107	4	1		1			1
City slum	108	3	1	5	1	1	1	
Elite	44							
% of total number of deaths (N=27)		30	6.7	16.7	26.7	3.3	3.3	3.3

TIME AT ONSET OF BREAST FEEDING

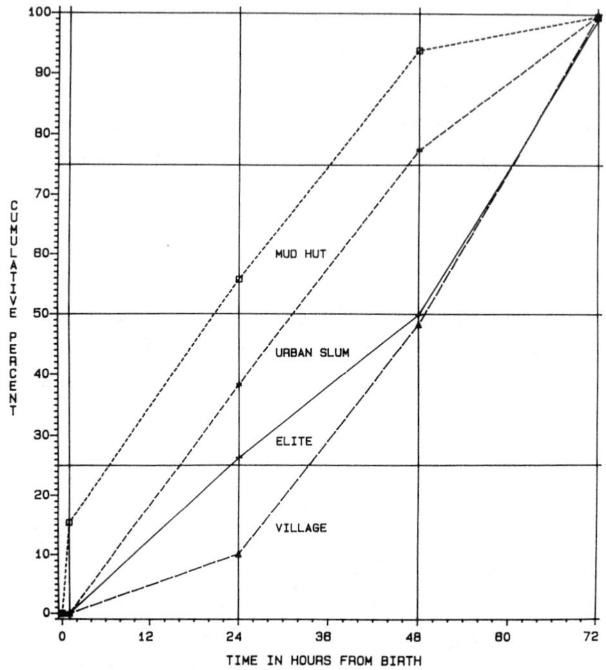

Fig. 2. Age at onset of breast feeding during the first three days of life among 285 infants in the four areas investigated, see legend fig. 1.

Breast feeding started only slowly among these infants as shown in figure 2. In the mud hut area 15% had in fact initiated breast feeding at one hour after birth, but at 48 hours about 50% of the newborns in the village and elite groups had not yet received breast milk. At 72 hours of life all of those to be breast-fed were given breast milk.

Recent studies by our group, as well as by others, have suggested that extra fluid is not required by the fully breast-fed baby even in a hot and dry climate (11). Therefore, it should be possible to rely on complete breast feeding. Doing so might substantially reduce the microbial exposure of the breast-fed infant and prevent the infections, which can appear during breast feeding in areas with heavy microbial contamination as shown i.a. by Mata et al in their studies of the infants of Santa Maria Cauqué in Guatemala (12). In fact, few studies of breast feeding in a developing country may have been performed in exclusively breast-fed infants. This may help explain why some studies have had problems showing protection against infections by breast feeding (5).

The early supplementation of the breast-fed infant by various formulas, fluids and foods is known to expose it to a number of micro-organisms, especially using the bottle (9,13,14)). Delaying the introduction of such material and relying on complete breast feeding for the first four-six months of life might further decrease the risk of infection.

MICROBIAL EXPOSURE IN THE MILIEU OF THE BREAST-FED INFANT

Breast feeding diminishes the exposure of the baby to the microbes of other fluids and foods. Still, the risk of infection persists, since the environment surrounding the breast-fed infant in a developing country is often heavily contaminated. This was demonstrated by a comparative analysis of the situation in a village outside of Lahore, the mud hut area around the city, and the old city slum. The study was performed in 1984 and in each area, 1,000 families were interviewed.

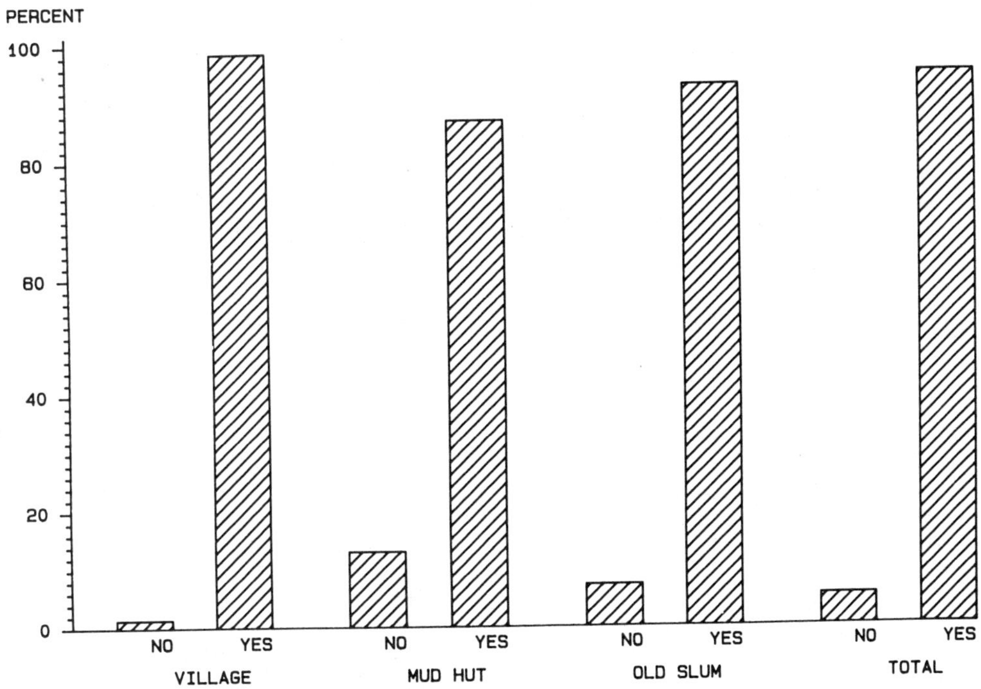

Fig. 3. Percentage of families with animals living in the same quarters. In each of the three areas studied for this parameter 1000 families were interviewed.

The hygienic situation was illustrated by the fact that in the village and slums animals lived in the same quarters as the family in around 90 per cent of the population (Fig. 3). The water supply was mostly shared with other families (Fig. 4), as were the lavatories, if they existed.

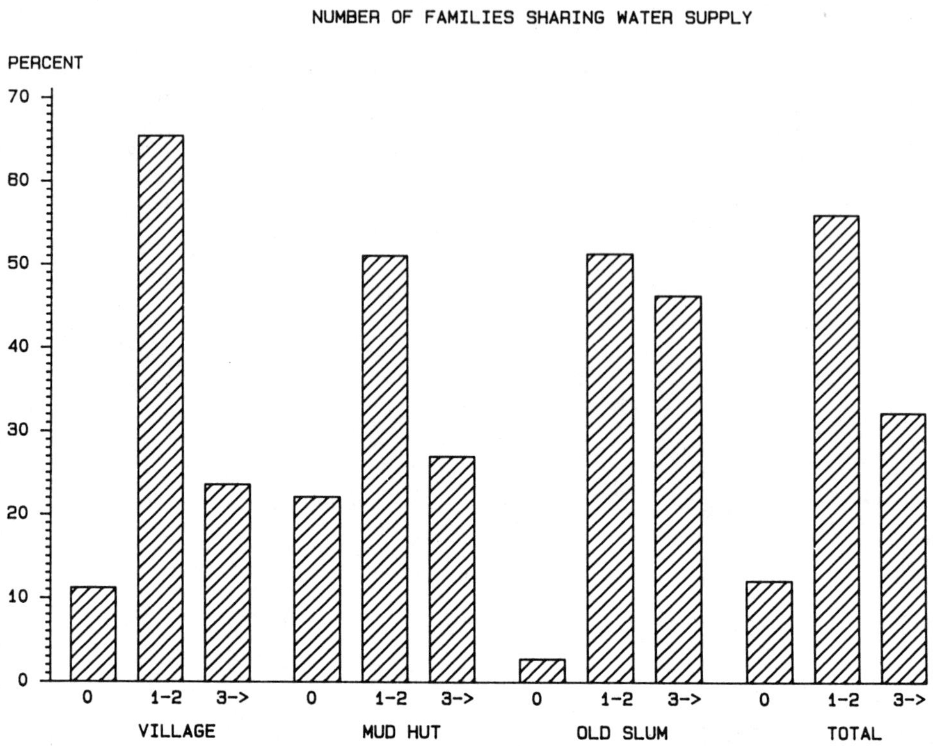

Fig. 4. Percentage of families with shared water supply. In 1000 families were included.

One striking illustration of the hygienic situation came from the question of what the families did with their garbage. In the village, the garbage was almost always left outside the house, whereas in the mud hut area, 83 % left all garbage, including children stools, in the mud hut using it to fill out the marshy land the huts are built on (Fig. 5). In the old city slum, in contrast, 68% used a refuse dump while the remainder left the garbage outside the house. Open sewage drains were seen in 63% in the village and in 98% in the city slum. In the mud hut area there were no drainage or sewage systems at all. Living under such circumstances with no or limited facilities for hygiene, such as washing of hands and breast nipples, it is obvious that microbial exposure must be heavy, even for a fully breast-fed baby.

Another striking illustration of the high prevalence of potential pathogens in this society appeared from a study of the intestinal colonization by aerobic enterobacteria in 40 newborns delivered in a hospital in Lahore. As many as one third of the neonates had E.coli causing mannose-resistent hemagglutination of human red blood cells which could imply that these strains carry CFA/I, or E 8775 adhesins, often found to be associated with enterotoxin production. Further studies using specific antisera have suggested that this hemagglutinin may be a yet unrecognized E.coli structure, possibly involved in colonization.

It was remarkable that the frequency of diarrhoeal infections was higher during the first months of life than later during the first and second year ($p<0.0001$, Table 6). This presumably shows the heavy microbial exposure in the milieu of the infants almost from birth onwards. Also upper and lower respiratory tract infections were more common during the first than the second year (Table 6). The number of

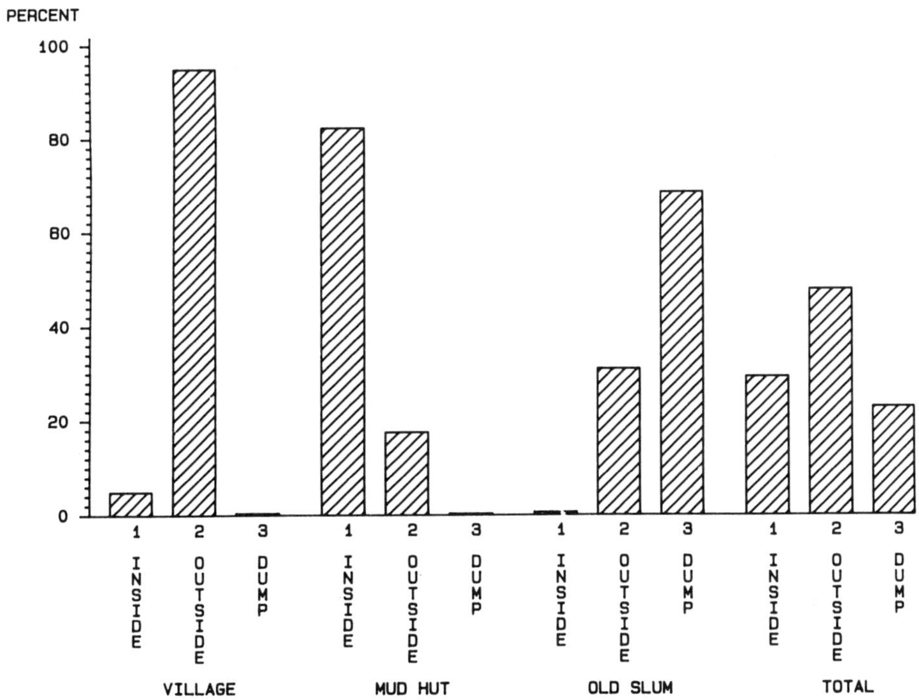

Fig. 5. The mode of disposal of garbage in percentage of the 1000 families interviewed in each of three areas.

infections related to the socio-economic level of the family (Table 2). This is demonstrated in figs 6a and 6b showing a strong relation between number of episodes of diarrhoea and educational level of the parents ($p<0.001$) and number of episodes of lower respiratory infections and house standard ($p<0.0001$). The frequency of the respiratory infections was almost as high as that of diarrhoea illustrating that microbial exposure of the respiratory tract is heavy also, often causing disease.

Table 6. Percent of infants in a city slum having at least one period with a given infection during a three months period. All of the 910 longitudinally followed infants were observed during each interval

Age interval in months	Diarrhoea	Upper respiratory infection	Lower respiratory infection
00-03	17.2	14.1	13.8
03-06	14.4	14.9	15.1
06-09	13.7	13.5	14.7
09-12	13.4	13.2	13.2
12-15	12.3	11.8	11.3
15-18	10.6	11.5	11.6
18-21	9.3	10.4	9.9
21-24	9.2	10.7	10.2
chi-square	(p<0.0001)	(p<0.0001)	(p<0.0001)

p-values are given for the comparison of the frequency of infections early and late in the observation period.

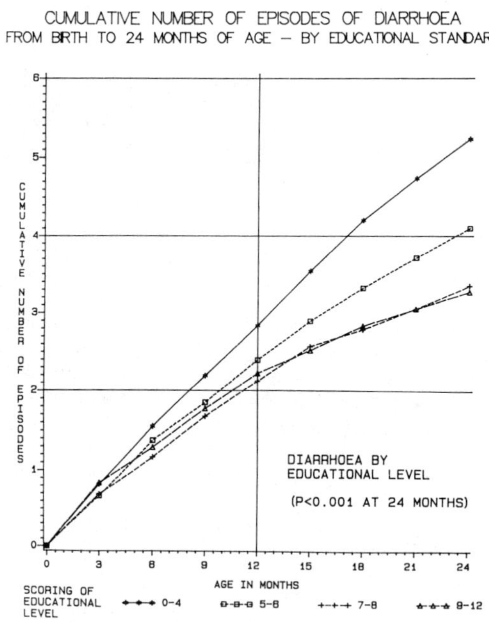

Fig. 6a. Mean of cumulative numbers of episodes of diarrhoea up to a certain age for 910 longitudinally followed children from a slum area in Lahore, Pakistan. The material is divided in four equal groups according to the educational level of the parents which is scored from lowest level (scores 0-4) up to highest level (9-12). At 24 months of age there is a striking difference, p<0.0001, between the the number of episodes in relation to the educational level, cf Table 2.

One factor of possible importance for the appearance of respiratory infections could be contamination of the dust in and outside the living quarters by gram-negative bacteria of animal and human fecal origin. Endotoxin-containing dust can cause symptoms on inhalation (15). Malaise, dyspnoe, possible catabolic and mitogenic effects, etc. could arise from

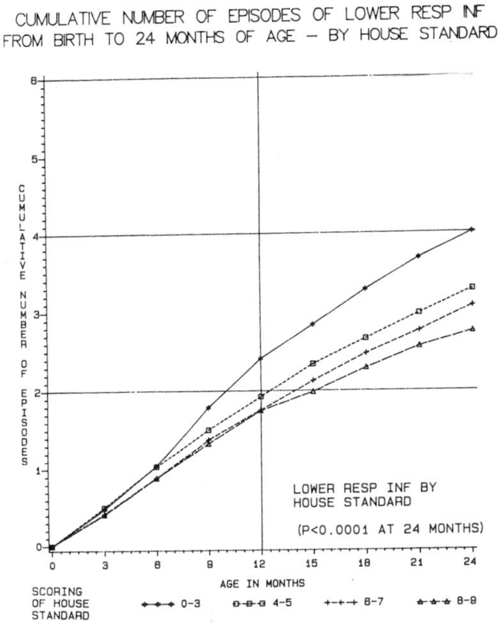

Fig 6b. Similar analysis as in fig. 6a on the same sample but for lower respiratory tract infection and house standard (scores 0-3=lowest, and 8-9=highest standard). At 24 months of age there is a significant difference, $p<0.001$, between the number of episodes in relation to the house standard, cf Table 2.

the pulmonary endotoxin exposure. With human and animal stool being abundantly present in the milieu, this problem could be important and should be investigated. It could even be considered that the rapid increase of mucosal secretory IgA antibodies to E.coli O antigens during the first few weeks of life of Pakistani infants (16) could be due to respiratory tract, as well as intestinal tract exposure to endotoxins.

Against this background, illustrating a sanitary situation which may represent the condition for many infants in the developing world, it is not surprising that the host defense provided by breast feeding can be insufficient. This is a strong argument for exclusive breast feeding and the improvement of the sanitary situation of these infants and their parents. This requires better education of the parents and further detailed epidemiological research to define in detail the relevant factors and provide a basis for optimal intervention strategies.

REFERENCES

1. U.-B. Lithell, Breastfeeding and reproduction. Studies in marital fertility and infant mortality in 19th century Finland and Sweden, Acta Universitatis Upsaliensis. Studia Historica Upsaliensis. Vol. 120 (1981).
2. A. Brändström, The loveless mothers. Acta Universitalis Umensis, Umeå Studies in the Humanities 62 (1984) (In Swedish, with English summary).
3. C. von Linné, C. Amman som styvmoder, (Nutrix Noverca). Uppsala (1752).
4. Fehmida Jalil, B. Forsberg, U. Hellgren and B. S. Lindblad, Infant feeding habits in poor families and infant formula marketing in the city of Lahore, Pakistan, Paediatric J. 1. 95 (1983).
5. M. G. Kovas, M. K. Serdula, J. S. Marks, D. W. Fraser, Review of the epidemiologic evidence for an association between infant feeding and infant health, Pediatrics 74, (suppl) 615 (1984).
6. J. M. Jason, P. Nieburg, J. S. Marks, Mortality and infections disease associated with infant-feeding practices in developing countries, Pediatrics 74 (suppl), 702 (1984).
7. L. Å. Hanson, P. Brandtzaeg, Mucosal Immunity in: R. T. Stiehm , ed., "Immunological Diseases in Infants and Children", Saunders, New York, 3 ed (1986).
8 D. Raphael, F. Davis. "Only Mothers Know. Patterns of Infant Feeding in Traditional Cultures", Greenwood Press, Westport, Conn. (1985).
9 M. G. M. Rowland, R. A. E. Barrell and R. G. Whitehead, Bacterial contamination in traditional Gambian weaning foods, Lancet I, 136 (1978).
10. S. S. Arnon, Infant botulism, Ann. Rev. Med. 31, 541 (1980).
11. S. G. Almroth, Water requirements of breast-fed infants in a hot climate, Am. J. Clin. Nutr. 31, 541 (1980).
12. L. J. Mata, "The Children of Santa Maria Cauqué: A prospective field study of health and growth," The MIT Press, Cambridge, Massachusetts and London (1978).
13. G. Stinzing, R. Möllby, and D. Habte, Enterotoxi genic Escherichia coli and other enteropathogens in paediatric diarrhoea in Addis Ababa, Acta Paediatr. Scand. 71: 279 (1982).
14. G. Stinzing and R. Möllby, Colonization of the upper jejunum by enteropathogenic and enterotoxigenic Eschericha coli in paediatric diarrhoea. Acta Paediatr. Scand. 71: 457 (1982).
15. R. Rylander, K. Andersson, L. Belin, G. Berglund, R. Bergström, L. Å. Hanson, M. Lundholm and I. Mattsby, Sewage worker's syndrome, Lancet II: 478 (1976).
16. L. Mellander, B. Carlsson, F. Jalil, T. Söderström and L.Å. Hanson, Secretory IgA antibody response against Escherichia coli antigens in infants in relation to exposure. J. Ped. 107, 430, 1985.

CROSS-CULTURAL DIFFERENCES IN LACTATIONAL PERFORMANCE

Andrew Prentice, Alison Paul, Ann Prentice, Alison Black, Tim Cole and Roger Whitehead

Dunn Nutrition Unit
Milton Road
Cambridge, UK
and
Keneba
The Gambia

INTRODUCTION

In 1974 the Dunn Nutrition Unit began parallel studies of lactational performance in the rural village of Keneba, The Gambia and in the affluent university city of Cambridge, England. Our interest was focussed on lactation by the fact that infants in The Gambia entered a period of severe weight faltering at 2-3 months of age when compared to standard growth curves[1], and that this faltering started before the introduction of weaning foods and before infectious diseases became common in the children. Waterlow[2,3] reviewed a number of other studies from developing countries and concluded that they all showed a similar pattern of faltering growth in the second or third month of life. When viewed in the light of Whitehead's calculations that on average the amount of breast-milk produced by a well-nourished mother should be sufficient to support her infant for 4-6 months, this growth faltering in the developing world suggested that such children were receiving insufficient breast-milk even in the first few months of life[4,5]. This conclusion was reinforced by the published data on milk intakes which showed a striking difference between the reported values for exclusively breast-fed infants from affluent and developing countries at 3 months of age (Figure 1). Although it was recognised that many of the very high values were obtained from professional wet-nurses such values encouraged the belief that mean outputs in excess of 1 litre per day should be easily achievable in well-fed women.

Studies of maternal diets from many areas of the developing world also showed that lactating women had energy intakes which were exceptionally low compared to the WHO/FAO recommendations[25,26]. These low intakes seemed an obvious explanation for the apparent difference in lactational performance, particularly since animal nutritionists and farmers had known for many years that there is a direct relationship between maternal food intake and milk production in many species.

In this paper we will argue on the basis of our extensive studies in two nutritionally disparate communities and by reviewing other recent studies from throughout the world that these initial impressions were in

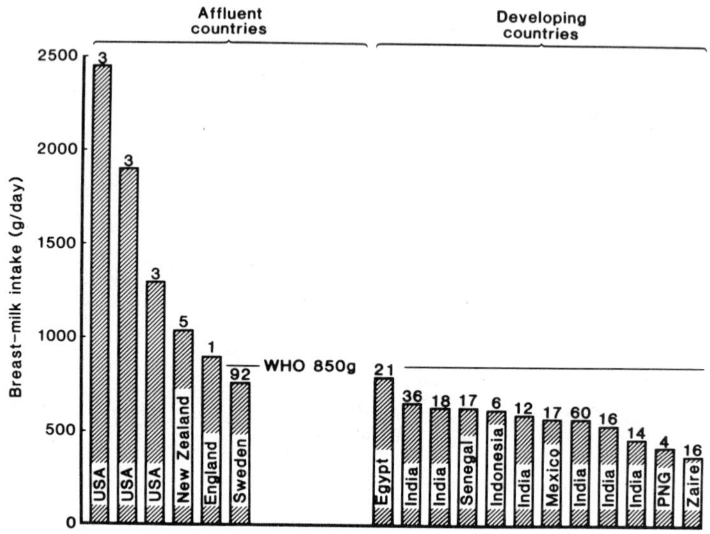

Fig. 1. Pre-1975 data on breast-milk intakes at 3 months of age. Compiled from refs 6-24.

fact misleading and that, except in the most severe nutritional circumstances, breast-milk production in the developing world is not limited by an inadequate substrate supply but rather is controlled by the characteristics of the mother-infant pair in much the same way that it is when maternal nutrition is adequate.

LACTATION IN THE GAMBIA AND UK

Keneba

Keneba is broadly representative of many communities in the developing world. Subsistence farming provides a diet which is marginally adequate for survival in the presence of the added stresses of infection and a heavy agricultural work load at certain times of year. A "hungry" season occurs during the rains when the previous year's harvest has been exhausted and body fat stores are used to buffer the effects of these lean periods.

Women start lactation following a pregnancy in which weight gain and fat deposition are suboptimal and in which nutritionally mediated intra-uterine growth retardation results in average birth weights below 3.0 kg with a high proportion of low-birth-weight (<2.5 kg) babies[27,28]. The severity of these effects depends on the month of conception due to the seasonal fluctuations in energy balance, but preparation for lactation can never be considered ideal.

All women in Keneba breast-feed for at least 18 months and usually for more than two years. If all children survive mothers lactate about 8-10 times during their reproductive span, but this number may be much larger if some lactations are curtailed by the death of an infant. Failure to establish and sustain lactation only ever occurs when babies are born very prematurely (<1 kg). Genuine demand feeding is practised with feed frequencies of 14-18 feeds per 24 hours in early lactation and more frequent feeding when infants are ill or require comforting. The total time spent breast-feeding varies from 230 minutes/day (16%) in early lactation to 175 minutes/day (12%) in late lactation. Infants sleep with

Table 1. Maternal Characteristics in Gambia and U.K.[a]

	Keneba	Cambridge
Age (y)	26	28
Parity	4.9	1-2
Weight (kg)	51.0 (48.1 - 53.1)	56.7
Height (m)	158.1	162.7
Weight/height^2	20.4 (19.3 - 21.3)	21.3
% body fat	21.5 (18.6 - 24.5)	28.2
Pregnancy fat gain (kg)	0 (-4.9 - +3.3)	3.5
Infants' birth weight (kg)	2.9 (2.75 - 3.05)	3.4

[a] Mean values with seasonal variation in parentheses for Keneba

Table 2. Breast-Milk Volume Data Sets

Gambia : 12-hour test-weighings

n = 4430 from 350 children

No. of lactations per mother	n
1	69
2	69
3	40
4	5
Total	= 183 mothers

Recorded by fieldworkers from 07.00 - 19.00.
Mothers studied monthly for 18 months.

Gambia : 24-hour test-weighings

n = 95 from 95 mother/infant pairs

Recorded by fieldworkers from 19.00 - 19.00.
Overnight measurements in mothers' houses.

Cambridge: 96-hour test-weighings

n = 318 from 48 mother/infant pairs.

Self-recorded by mothers at home.
Maximum duration 9 months.

their mothers throughout lactation and accompany them almost everywhere except during the farming season when older infants are left in the care of nursemaids for up to 8 hours. Breast-feeding in Keneba can therefore probably be considered to be representative of natural, unrestricted lactation.

Great care was taken to cause as little disruption to the pattern of lactation as possible during test-weighing measurements which were performed at monthly intervals for each mother up to 18 months post-partum between 1976 and 1982. Most measurements were over a 12 hour period, but a smaller number of 24 hour measurements were also made. The characteristics of the study mothers and the details of the test-weighing data sets are given in Tables 1 and 2.

Weaning foods are traditionally introduced at a median time of 3.5 months in Keneba, but throughout the period of these studies all infants received a dietary supplement between 3 and 12 months of age. In the younger children this tended to replace the home produced weaning foods and was not given in addition to them.

Further details of Keneba, the study methodology, and maternal food intake and anthropometry have been published elsewhere[25,27,29].

Cambridge

Subjects in the Cambridge study were self-selected volunteers classified as 14 from social class I, 20 from social classes II + IIINM, 12 from social class IIIM and 2 from social classes IV and V[30]. The distribution was therefore heavily biased towards well educated, highly motivated and affluent women and it is most unlikely that there was any financial constraint on the quantity of food eaten although food choice may have been constrained. A few subjects admitted to some restrained eating during lactation but this was neither serious nor widespread[31].

Most women in Cambridge followed a flexible-schedule or semi-demand feeding pattern but, although night feeds were given, the babies did not sleep with their mothers. Mean feed frequencies were only 5-6 per 24 hours. Two-thirds of the women maintained exclusive breast-feeding for 4 months, but this had decreased to only 5 mothers by 6 months and 1 at 7 months.

Test-weighing was performed by the mothers themselves over continuous 96-hour periods each month until the child was weaned. The time of introduction and quantity of weaning foods were recorded. Details of the mothers and the test-weighing data set are given in Tables 1 and 2 and further details of the methods and maternal food intake have been published[31].

Early Child Growth in Keneba and Cambridge

Figure 2 illustrates the profound difference in early child growth in the two communities. The inappropriateness of the NCHS standards[32] for use with modern breast-fed babies is illustrated by the initial positive and then negative deviance of the Cambridge babies[33,34]. Values for Keneba babies are for the seasons combined and illustrate that the babies are born small but grow parallel to the NCHS standards in the first 2-3 months of life before entering a period of severe weight faltering. At 12 months they average 75-80% weight-for-age depending on the time of year. Prior to our medical interventions in Keneba and its neighbouring villages mortality in the under-5's was greater than 50% and a high proportion of this was related to malnutrition[35].

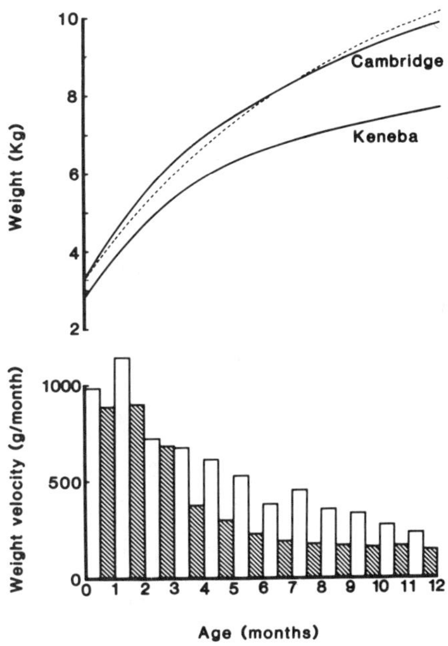

Fig. 2. Early growth of infants in Keneba and Cambridge. All values are from boys. Keneba data represents seasons combined. Dotted line is NCHS standard. Open columns:Cambridge. Hatched columns:Keneba.

Statistical Analysis

All statistical analyses were performed using the GENSTAT statistical package.

EVIDENCE AGAINST THE NUTRITIONAL LIMITATION THEORY

Food Intake and Milk Volumes in Keneba and Cambridge

The dietary energy intake of each lactating woman was measured by direct weighing over 50 days per year in Keneba and over 4 days per month in Cambridge. Dietary energy is taken as representative of total food intake in both communities. In Keneba this is valid for the major nutrients including protein but not for various micronutrients including vitamins A, B_2 and C together with calcium and iron.

Energy intakes in Cambridge varied from 2400 kcal/day in early lactation to 2160 kcal/day after 7 months with an average of 2320 kcal/day. These intakes are lower than the recommendations of 2500, 2700 and 2750 kcal/day by NRC[36], WHO/FAO[37] and DHSS[38], but since they represent the voluntary intake of healthy, successfully lactating women in the absence of dietary constraints such intakes must be considered adequate for women with low levels of physical activity[39]. Very similar levels of energy intake have been observed in a recent study from Houston, Texas[40].

In Keneba the pattern of energy intake during lactation was complex since it varied both with stage of lactation and season of the year. After the first 3 months of lactation the average energy intake was 1700-1800 kcal/day in the dry season and as low as 1200 kcal/day during August and September. The pattern in early lactation was similar but with an

Table 3. Tabulated Test-Weighing Results from Keneba and Cambridge

	Age (months)	n	Milk intake[a] (g)	No. of feeds	Intake per feed (g)
Keneba[b] (12-hr)	1	56	327 ± 91	6.8	48
	2	255	372 ± 105	6.8	55
	3	304	377 ± 117	6.4	59
	4	290	312 ± 115	5.7	55
	5	284	304 ± 113	5.6	54
	6	262	302 ± 114	5.6	54
	6-9	808	304 ± 125	5.6	54
	9-12	731	286 ± 124	5.3	54
	12-15	705	296 ± 140	5.1	58
	15-18	735	257 ± 155	4.7	55
Keneba[c] (24-hr)	1	7	649 ± 113	12.9	50
	2	8	705 ± 183	13.2	53
	3	6	782 ± 168	10.7	73
	4	10	582 ± 169	13.3	44
	5	17	643 ± 149	13.8	47
	6-9	16	607 ± 131	11.3	54
	9-12	16	594 ± 180	12.1	49
	12-18	15	633 ± 141	10.3	61
Cambridge (96-hr ÷ 4)	2	48	741 ± 142	6.2	120
	3	47	785 ± 168	5.8	135
	4	48	783 ± 176	5.4	145
	5	42	717 ± 207	5.0	143
	6	45	588 ± 206	4.5	131
	7	38	493 ± 216	4.0	123
	8	31	342 ± 228	3.2	107
	9	19	328 ± 292	3.1	106

[a] Means ±1 S.D.
[b] Corrected to represent average season, average parity (5) and equal sex distribution.
[c] Sexes and seasons combined. Average parity varies by age group.

additional 100-200 kcal/day consumed when food was plentiful. Since body fat stores were used to subsidise dietary intake during the lean season the resultant amount of energy available to the mother remained relatively constant throughout the year. However, competition for nutrients between the mammary glands and other maternal organs would still have been greatest during the lean season since maternal energy expenditure was highest at this time[27,41].

Compared with the WHO/FAO recommended intakes the energy intakes observed in Keneba seem impossibly low. However, a more realistic comparison is with the Cambridge mothers in which case the average deficit throughout the year was 27%. Many other studies from developing countries report similarly low levels of food intake in lactating women[42] and although it seems likely that many of these have underestimated energy intakes there can be no doubt that intake is constrained and in some cases

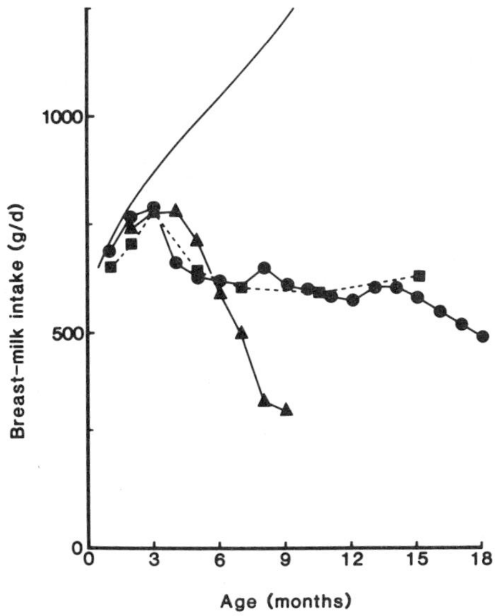

Fig. 3. Breast-milk intake in Keneba and Cambridge. Triangles:Cambridge. Circles:Keneba 12-h data x 2. Adjusted to parity 1.5 and averaged over wet and dry seasons. Squares:Keneba 24-h data. Unadjusted for parity (mean 4.9) and averaged over wet and dry seasons. Upper solid line represents WHO/FAO recommended energy intake converted to milk equivalents.

severely so. The seasonal loss of up to 50% of their body energy reserves in lactating women provides adequate proof of this in Keneba.

In the light of such different energy and nutrient intakes there is a remarkable similarity in breast-milk production in the two communities. Average milk intakes calculated from the 3 complete data sets are shown in Figure 3 and given in detail in Table 3. Values from Keneba and Cambridge can be directly compared up to 3 months of age since only a small proportion of children have received weaning foods by this age. This comparison shows identical milk volumes at peak lactation in the two communities (Cambridge = 785 g; Keneba 24-hr = 782 g; Keneba 12-hr (adjusted to equivalent parity as Cambridge) = 784 g). Since the Keneba values are somewhat disadvantaged by representing both harvest and lean seasons combined and by representing the intake of smaller babies (e.g. boys 5.99 kg vs 5.40 kg) it can safely be concluded that milk production in Keneba was at least as good as in Cambridge at peak lactation. Nutrient availability could therefore only be limiting if the genetic potential for milk production is actually higher in Gambian than in English women.

A comparison of milk composition in Keneba with standard UK or Cambridge values is presented in Table 4. Although there are small seasonal variations in the concentration of certain milk components including the proximates in Keneba the average composition was very similar in the two communities. Exceptions to this were the low levels of certain water-soluble vitamins which reflected the low maternal plasma levels in the Gambian women and which could be rectified by supplementation with the individual vitamins in question[46,47]. The levels of most of the immunoproteins studied were significantly higher in milk from the Gambian

Table 4. Comparison of Milk Composition in The Gambia and U.K.[a]

		Gambia	U.K.	Gambia as % U.K.
Proximates[b]	Energy (kcal/dl)	70	70	100
	Protein (g/dl)	1.32	1.34	99
	Fat (g/dl)	4.2	4.2	100
	Lactose (g/dl)	7.7	7.4	104
Vitamins[c]	Thiamin (μg/ml)	0.16	0.16	100
	Riboflavin (μg/ml)	0.21	0.31	68
	Vitamin B6 (μg/ml)	0.12	0.06	200
	Nicotinic acid (μg/ml)	1.13	2.30	49
	Vitamin B12 (ng/ml)	0.16	0.10	160
	Folic acid (ng/ml)	38	52	73
	Biotin (ng/ml)	9.0	7.6	118
	Pantothenic acid (μg/ml)	2.0	2.6	78
	Vitamin C (mg/dl)	3.4	3.8	88
Immunoproteins[b]	Lactoferrin (mg/dl)	318	216	147
	IgA (arb.mg/dl)	46	37	123
	IgG (mg/dl)	6.5	2.8	236
	IgM (mg/dl)	4.6	2.4	194
	C3 (mg/dl)	1.9	1.2	158
	C4 (mg/dl)	2.4	0.9	259
	Lysozyme (mg/dl)	4.1	4.0	101

[a] Compiled from refs 43, 44 and 45.
[b] All values from 0-3 months post-partum.
[c] U.K. values from 0-3 months; Gambian values from 0-18 months post-partum.

mothers[45,48], which may be in response to the higher prevalence of infections in both the mothers and children.

As in the case of milk volume it can reasonably be concluded that, with the exception of a few micronutrients, milk composition is not compromised by the low level of food intake in Keneba.

Seasonality of Lactational Performance

Breast-milk production decreased during the wet season in Keneba. This is illustrated in the top portion of Figure 4 which represents all stages of lactation combined. Analysis of the full 12-hour data set reveals a higher seasonal variation in older children, but this is partly accounted for by the fact that these older children tend to be left at home during the day when their mothers work in the fields. The 24-hour data revealed that in the wet season they received a higher proportion of their daily intake during the night as indicated in Table 5. In the younger children there was a peak-to-trough difference in milk intakes of 22% in the 12-hour data which could not be accounted for by a diurnal redistribution of intakes (Table 5). The decrease in total intake was caused both by a decrease in the feed frequency and in the intake per feed.

Figure 4 illustrates the similarity between the seasonal changes in milk output, maternal energy intake and maternal fat stores as measured by D_2O dilution. We initially interpreted these findings with caution since

Table 5. Effect of Season on Diurnal Feeding Patterns in Keneba[a]

	Age (months)		
	0-6	6-12	12-18
<u>Dry Season</u>			
Milk intake	52.3	58.6[b]	57.0[c]
No. of feeds	53.4	55.2	50.9
Duration	56.7	52.7	52.6
Intake/feed	97.8	110.7	109.6
	(20)	(12)	(7)
<u>Wet Season</u>			
Milk intake	50.9	45.9[b]	42.6[c]
No. of feeds	51.5	48.4	45.0
Duration	53.0	45.9	42.3
Intake/feed	99.8	95.1	98.2
	(29)	(19)	(8)

[a] Values are for daytime (07.00-19.00) as % of total.
[b] $p < 0.05$; [c] $p < 0.01$ for wet vs dry difference.

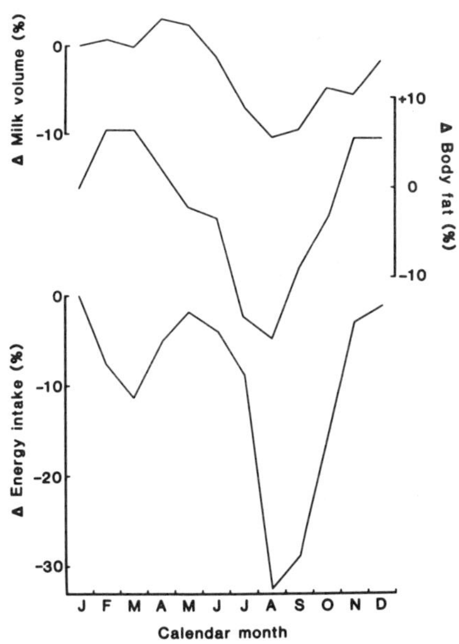

Fig. 4. Seasonal variation in milk intake, maternal energy intake and body fat stores in Keneba. Milk volume: All stages of lactation combined. Body fat: Calculated from total body water by D_2O dilution. Energy intake: Measured by direct-weighing over 4 days per month in an average of 85 women per month. Rains occur from June to October.

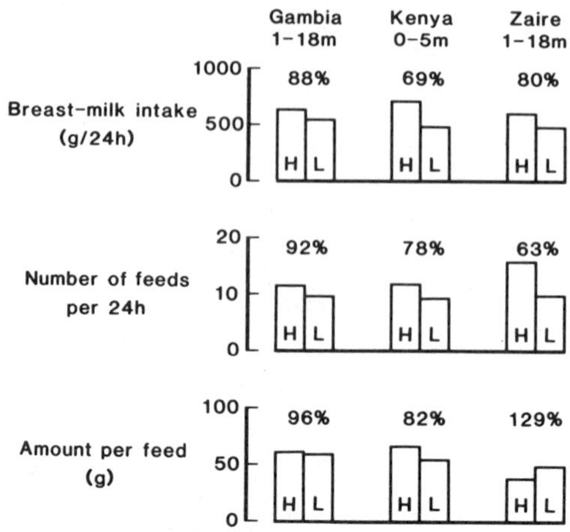

Fig. 5. Seasonality of milk intake in 3 African countries.
Compiled from refs 49 and 50.
H = harvest; L = lean.

it was apparent that a number of other changes occurred during the wet season which might have been the cause of the fall in milk intake by the children. The subsequent publication of similar seasonal effects on milk production from Kenya[49] and Zaire[50], where the lean season decrease in milk output and maternal food intake appeared to be less complicated by concurrent changes in infant or maternal morbidity, seemed to provide additional strong evidence for an association with maternal energy restriction. However, as shown in Figure 5 the decrease in milk output in these studies was associated with a larger decrease in the number of feeds than in the intake per feed and it is therefore possible that the reduced milk production resulted from behavioural changes forced upon the mothers by time-consuming and arduous farm work. Indeed in the Kenyan study the time spent feeding per 12 hours observation in the lean season was only 61% of that in the harvest season in the 0-5 month age group[51]. It is possible therefore that nutritional limitation was not the cause of the seasonal decline in lactational performance in these studies.

The need for an alternative to the maternal energy restriction theory was emphasised in Keneba by the fact that maternal dietary supplementation (see below), which removed the wet season decrease in food intake, had no effect on the seasonal pattern of milk production.

An alternative explanation could be that the suppression of milk synthesis is mediated by the infant's appetite. Appetite in turn will be affected by many factors but perhaps most importantly by illness. Figure 6 illustrates the similarity between the seasonal increase in the prevalence of diarrhoea in children from 0-18 months and the decrease in milk intake. Diarrhoea has the greatest growth suppressing impact of all disease categories in Keneba[52] and is associated with anorexia in addition to its effects on decreasing nutrient absorption. Other infections might have an equally great anorectic effect even though their effect on growth is less pronounced than diarrhoea since they only influence nutrient intake. Diseases such as respiratory tract infections, otitis media and others which also have an increased incidence in the wet season, may also be important in suppressing the demand for and hence production of breast-milk. Such observations are consistent with the suggestion that it is the infant which is down-regulating its own milk intake.

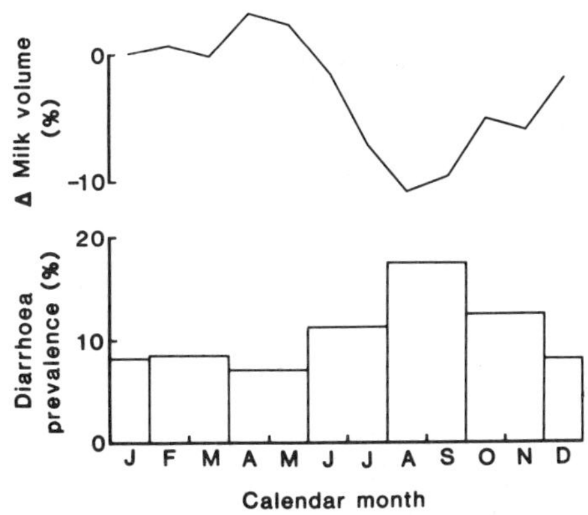

Fig. 6. Seasonal variation in milk intake and prevalence of diarrhoea in Keneba. Prevalence of diarrhoea recorded as % of days ill according to maternal history. Averaged over 0 - 18 months.

Figures 7 and 8 illustrate examples of the seasonal pattern of milk intake, infection and growth in children from Keneba. In both of these examples milk intake averaged approximately the mean plus 2 standard deviations for the community until the rainy season when the intake decreased by 3 and 2 standard deviation units respectively. Morbidity, recorded when mothers brought their infants to a free daily clinic, increased dramatically during the wet season and appeared to precede or at least coincide with the decrease in milk intake. Both of these infants lost weight as a result of the combined impact of infection, anorexia and a decreased breast-milk intake. Data from a third infant is shown in Figure 9 in order to illustrate the fact that decreases in milk intake do not only occur in the wet season. This infant decreased its intake during two rainy seasons but also in the middle of the dry season when it was about 300 days old. Although there was a cluster of infections at this time they do not appear to precede the decrease in milk intake.

Inspection of the data from all the other lactations studied leads to three main conclusions: a) the pattern of seasonal decreases in milk intake is variable from child to child and is sometimes absent in children who survive a wet season without major episodes of infection; b) decreases in milk intake are usually, but not always, associated with clusters of infection, and c) that there is sufficient evidence to suggest that the combination of illness-induced anorexia and altered breast-feeding patterns cause the observed seasonal decrease in milk output and that it is unnecessary to invoke nutritional limitation in the mother as a causative factor.

Dietary Supplementation and Lactational Performance

The most satisfactory way to test the hypothesis that the low levels of energy intake consumed by lactating women in many areas of the developing world are limiting to milk production is to correct the energy deficit by maternal supplementation and to observe the effect. In Keneba we supplemented all lactating women (n = 130) over a 12 month period and compared their milk output retrospectively with the milk output data collected from all women in the previous year (n = 120). The supplement consisted of a nutritionally balanced combination of groundnut-based

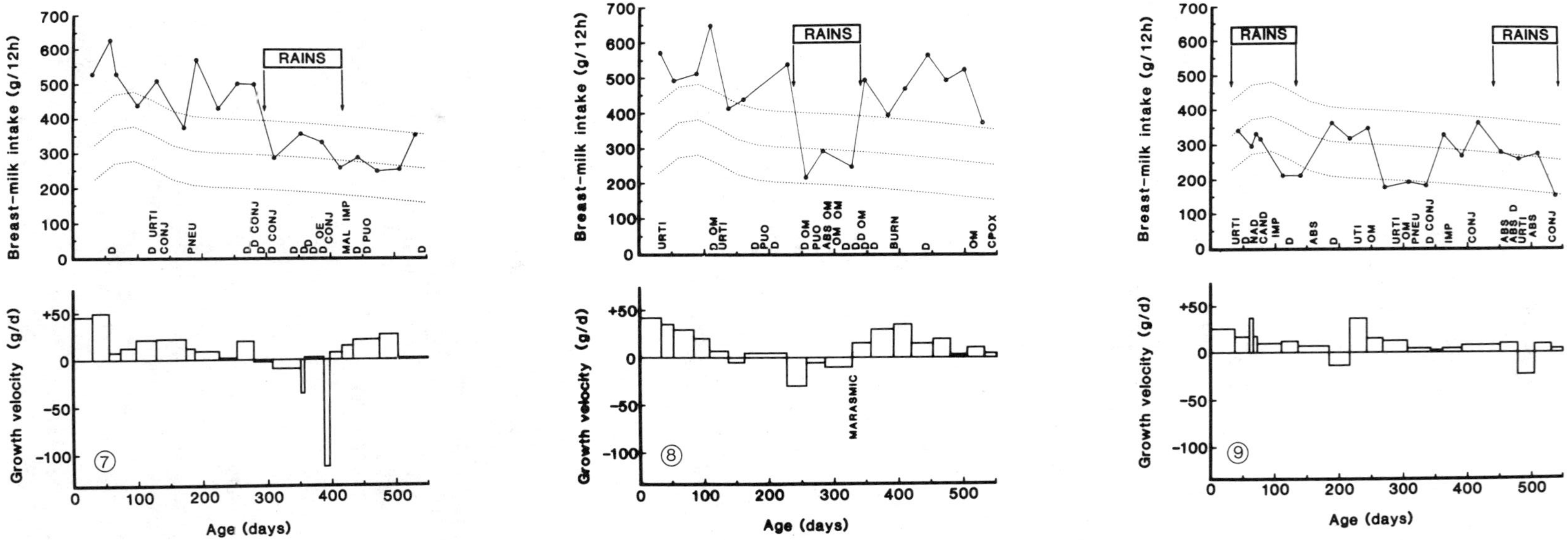

Figs. 7, 8 and 9. Examples of seasonal variation in milk intake, infection and growth in individual children in Keneba. Dotted lines represent the smoothed community mean milk intake (± 1 S.D.) for sexes and seasons combined.
ABS=abscess; BURN=burn; CAND=oral candidiasis; CONJ=conjunctivitis; CPOX=chicken pox; D=diarrhoea; IMP=impetigo; MAL=malaria; NAD=child ill but nothing abnormal detected; OE=otitis externa; OM=otitis media; PNEU=pneumonia; PUO=pyrexia of unknown origin; URTI=upper respiratory tract infection; UTI=urinary tract infection.

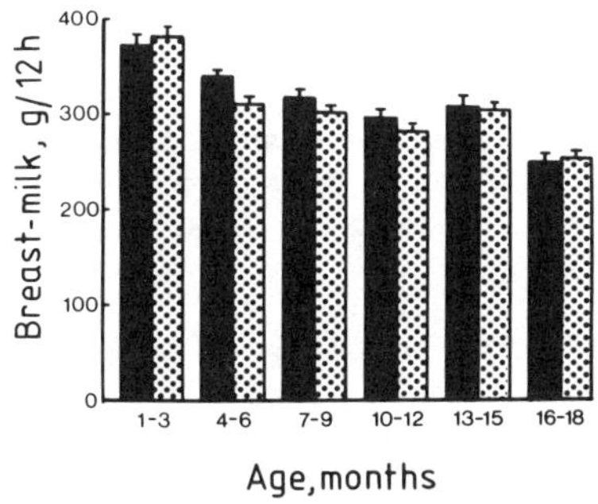

Fig. 10. Effect of dietary supplementation on breast-milk output in Keneba. Solid bars: unsupplemented women, May 1978 - April 1979 (n = 120). Stippled bars: supplemented women, May 1979 - April 1980 (n = 130).

biscuits and a vitamin-fortified tea drink and was provided under strict supervision on a daily basis. The net increase in energy intake after allowing for a slight replacement of the home diet was 723 kcal/day yielding a gross intake of 2291 kcal/day[44,53,54]. Although this new level of energy intake was still lower than international recommendations for lactating women it exactly matched the observed intakes of the Cambridge women and can therefore be considered adequate.

Figure 10 demonstrates that the supplement had no effect on milk output and this remained the conclusion, however the data were subdivided for analysis. For instance, supplementation did not increase milk output during the rainy season, in women with a previous history of low outputs or low energy intakes, or of women with a low W/H^2 index. The supplement did raise milk nitrogen by 7% ($p < 0.01$), but had no effect on total energy content since an increase in breast-milk fat concentration (+7.9%, NS) was offset by a decrease in milk lactose (-7.6%, $p < 0.01$). The milk vitamin content was improved for those vitamins for which the supplement provided a significant proportion of the recommended daily intake.

A number of other field trials of dietary supplementation have been conducted in developing countries[19,23,24,55-60]. Most of these studies had an inadequate methodological design and must be interpreted with caution. However, recent reviews have concluded that none of these provide convincing evidence of a positive effect of dietary supplementation on milk output[61,62,63]. It is important to note that this is in direct contrast to our own[28] and other studies of prenatal supplementation which almost universally have a beneficial effect on birth outcome in the developing world[64,65].

With the benefit of hindsight our interpretation of these supplementation findings is that under the dietary conditions prevalent in the communities studied milk secretion was not quantitatively limited by substrate availability prior to supplementation and that no effect should therefore have been expected. However, in spite of this lack of effect on the main outcome variable of interest (i.e. milk production) our studies demonstrated profound changes in the hormonal and energy substrate profiles of the lactating women. These changes have been interpreted as indicating a relaxation of the competition between the mammary secretory cells and the remainder of the mother's body with the result that the mother herself benefitted from supplementation[53]. It has been suggested that the decrease in serum prolactin levels and the shortening of the period of post-partum amenorrhoea observed when women were supplemented is one manifestation of this reduced competition for nutrients and that the very high prolactin levels observed in lactating women in most developing countries result from the need of the infant to suckle vigorously and often in order to obtain as much milk as the child of a well-nourished mother[66]. This hypothesis requires testing, but for the purposes of the present discussion the important conclusion is that the infants in Keneba did obtain as much milk as those in Cambridge even if they had to suckle more frequently and for longer to achieve it.

Milk Production in Mothers of Twins

Well-nourished women who breast-feed twins are able to respond to the increased demands of their infants by producing approximately twice as much milk as mothers with singleton children[67]. We have measured the milk intake of 3 sets of twins in Keneba. The average milk intakes in the first year of life (with range) of two of these sets of twins were 1205 (980-1480) g/24 hours and 1250 (1040-1660) g/24 hours. These values were predicted from 12 hour measurements, but were confirmed by single 24 hour measurements. Milk intake of the third set of twins was very low initially but stabilised after 9 months at about 900 g/24 hours. The mother of this set was of parity 9 and had delivered prematurely in hospital following a difficult delivery. The babies were given milk formula from birth by the hospital staff and this may have accounted for the poor start to her lactation. Although she never produced twice as much milk as other mothers her milk output in the second year represented 2 standard deviations above the community average. Orr-Ewing has observed similarly high intakes by twins in Papua New Guinea[68].

The ability of these mothers to synthesise extra milk in response to the high demands of their twins provides further evidence to suggest that milk output in mothers of singletons in the developing world is not usually limited by substrate availability.

Milk Production in Women with Dysfunctioning Breasts

It has often been suggested that malnutrition at the time of puberty or during the period when mammary secretory cells proliferate in early pregnancy may result in suboptimal breast development and function in women in the developing world, and that this may explain the previously assumed low levels of milk production. However, in Keneba we have studied women with severe unilateral breast dysfunction as evidenced by extremely abnormal milk composition from the affected breast and virtual cessation of suckling by the infant[69]. Figure 11 illustrates the milk intake of 2 infants of one such mother. The evidence for unilateral breast dysfunction is shown in the lower half of the figure which demonstrates that milk sodium levels were 10-15 times higher than in the unaffected breast. The upper half of the figure shows that milk production by this mother was perfectly normal indicating that her unaffected breast had doubled its output in order to compensate. A second subject is illustrated in Figure 12. In this case breast function reverted to normal in the second of the two lactations studied. This appeared to make no difference to her milk output. The other subjects with unilateral breast dysfunction gave similar results indicating that there is ample spare capacity for milk production even in women such as those studied who were subjected to suboptimal nutrition during early life and pregnancy.

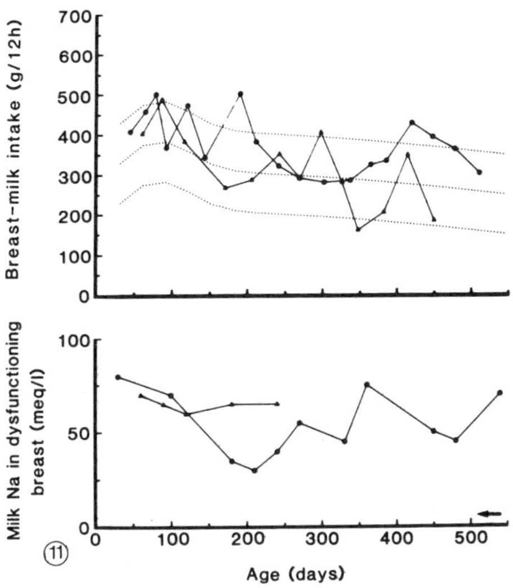

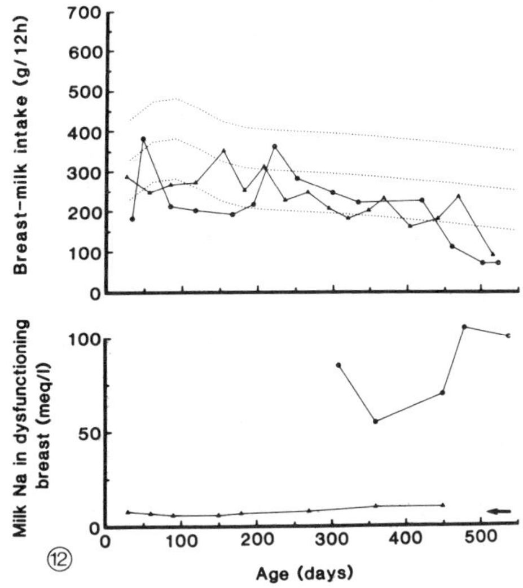

Figs. 11 and 12. Breast-milk output over successive lactations in women with unilateral breast dysfunction.
Dotted lines represent the smoothed community mean milk intakes (± 1 S.D.) for sexes and seasons combined.
Arrow indicates normal milk sodium concentration.

Within Country Comparisons of Lactational Performance

Cross-country comparisons such as those between The Gambia and England may be criticised on the basis that observed differences are difficult to attribute to any particular cause when there are so many cultural and environmental variables to be considered. Such criticism is less

Table 6. Within Country Studies of Nutritional or Cultural Influences on Milk Output [g/day (n)]

	Stage post-partum	Urban rich	Urban poor	Rural poor
China	0-6m	707 (80)	784 (58)	779 (64)
Guatemala	3m[a]	653 (28)	548 (30)	686 (27)
Philippines	3m[a]	320 (20)	639 (32)	622 (28)
Zaire	3m[a]		588 (99)	356 (57)
India	4m	650 (2)	740 (36)	
Egypt	1-4m	880 (12)	793 (9)	
India		"Well fed"	"Poorly fed"	
	3m	583	665	
	6m[a]	705	858	
Kenya		High W/H[b]	Low W/H	
	2-3m	783 (17)	738 (16)	

a Some children receiving supplementary food.
b W/H = Weight/height.

pertinent in this instance since we are stressing the similarities rather than the differences between the two communities; indeed it is remarkable that lactational performance is so similar given the disparity in the cultural, nutritional and environmental influences on breast-feeding.

A number of studies comparing lactational performance in affluent and under-privileged groups within the same country are summarised in Table 6. Interpretation of some of these studies is difficult. This is particularly true for the WHO Collaborative Study on Breast-Feeding[71] since results are not presented separately for exclusive and non-exclusive breast-feeders. However, the overall impression is that, with the exception of Zaire, there is little evidence to suggest that poor rural mothers produce less breast milk than their urban counterparts. The 6% difference between the high W/H and low W/H group in the Kenyan study may be mediated through a difference in their infants' size and may not necessarily reflect an influence of maternal nutrition.

Differences in Lactational Performance between Affluent and Developing Countries - a Reappraisal Based on Recent Studies

In addition to our own studies in Keneba and Cambridge there have been many other studies of lactational performance throughout the world in the past decade. The results of these new studies are summarised in Figure 13 for infants at 3 months of age. This data shows a completely different pattern to the older data summarised in Figure 1 and now supports the conclusion that nutrient limitation is not inhibiting milk production in women in most areas of the developing world.

The differences between the old and the new data are probably methodological. The recent studies have taken care to be non-selective in their subject recruitment when studying women in affluent societies and reveal a consistent average milk output of about 750 g/day in exclusively breast-fed infants at 3 months of age. The exception to this was the Australian study which employed test-weighing of the mother rather than the baby as is more usual and may have contained an element of selection since the subjects were all members of a Breast-feeding Mothers Association. In the developing country studies much greater care has been taken not to disturb the traditional pattern of demand feeding or to impose psychological stresses on the mother-infant pair by performing the studies in a metabolic ward or on a scheduled feeding basis as was the case in many of the earlier studies. When such precautions are taken the mean milk intakes at 3 months of age in the developing world appear to be indistinguishable from those measured in developing countries.

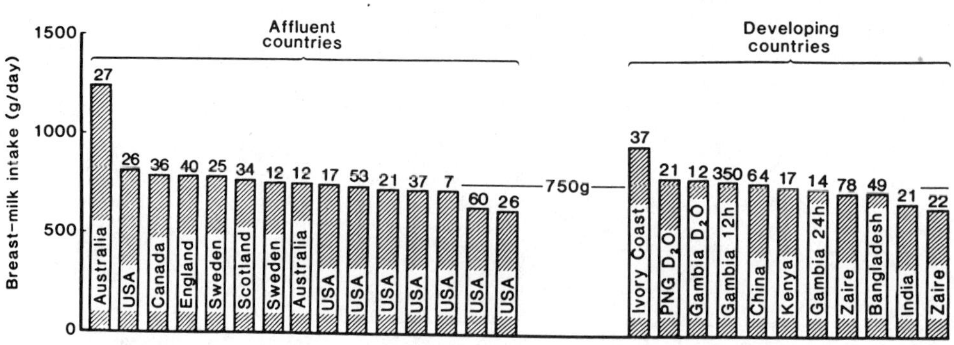

Fig. 13. Post-1975 data on breast milk intake at 3 months of age. Compiled from refs 39, 49, 50, 68, 70 and 72-90.

Evidence from Animal Studies

Almost all studies of the relationship between milk output and either food intake at the whole body level, or substrate supply to the mammary gland, have used species bred for exceptionally high milk yields (e.g. cows and goats) or species with large, rapidly growing litters which demand very large quantities of milk (rabbits, rats and mice). These studies demonstrate a proportional relationship between blood flow or substrate supply to the mammary gland and milk synthesis, and it is readily demonstrated that restriction of glucose, amino acid or fatty acid supply to the gland inhibits milk output[91,92]. However, due to the slow growth rate of their young, primates and humans in particular have much lower energy requirements for milk synthesis than most species when expressed as a proportion of the mothers' usual energy intake. In addition women have proportionately larger fat deposits than many species and can therefore develop the alternative strategies of increasing their food intake or drawing from their body stores, or a combination of the two, in order to meet the additional energy demands of lactation. It is therefore probably quite inappropriate to extrapolate the results of most animal studies to humans. For instance, the observation that when fasted the milk yield of goats falls to 50% of the fed level within 8-16 hours[91] is not consistent with our studies of women who fast during Ramadan[93], or with studies of short-term caloric restriction in lactating women[81]. This is perhaps not surprising since the women were able to remain normoglycaemic. This would presumably maintain adequate substrate for lactose synthetase which is the probable rate-controlling process in milk synthesis.

For the reasons indicated above it is likely that animal studies intended to identify the threshold of energy intake in humans below which lactational performance will start to deteriorate will have to be performed in primates. We are only aware of one such study which demonstrated in baboons that restriction of energy intake to 80% of the *ad lib* intake had no effect on milk output. Restriction to 60% of the *ad lib* intake reduced milk output by less than 5% in weeks 1-3 post-partum but this increased to a 37% reduction in output by weeks 9-10. Energy restriction had no effect on the proximate composition of the milk[94]. In comparison women in Keneba would be close to the 80% restriction level compared to the '*ad lib*' Cambridge controls, and therefore lie well within the range in which energy saving adaptations can spare lactational performance.

CONTROL OF MILK OUTPUT IN WELL-NOURISHED AND UNDER-NOURISHED MOTHERS

On the basis of the evidence presented above we have concluded that milk production is not limited by substrate availability or by the secretory capacity of the breast in either Cambridge or The Gambia. However, the rate of milk synthesis must be controlled in order to match maternal production with infant demand in early lactation, and after peak lactation milk synthesis must be down-regulated by an unknown mechanism since milk production fails to match the increasing needs of the infant. The size and structure of the Keneba and Cambridge data set provides a unique opportunity to investigate the factors controlling lactational performance.

Patterns of Milk Production: Within-Child, Within-Mother and Within-Family Similarities

As indicated in Table 2 the 12-hour test-weighing data set from Keneba contains information from 350 different lactations with an average of 12.6 monthly measurements per lactation. Sixty-nine mothers were studied over two consecutive lactations, 40 additional mothers over three lactations,

Table 7. Constancy of Milk Production Within Child, Within Mother and Within Family - Analysis of Variance

Within vs between children[a]	F	df	p
Milk intake	8.72	349, 4052	< 0.001
No. of feeds	5.18	349, 4052	< 0.001
Intake/feed	6.60	349, 4052	< 0.001
Within vs between mothers[a]	F	df	p
Milk output	3.79	182, 159	< 0.001
No. of feeds	2.25	182, 159	< 0.001
Output/feed	3.49	182, 159	< 0.001
Within vs between mother/daughter pairs[a,b]	F	df	p
Milk output	3.44	12, 13	< 0.02
Within vs between sister/sister pairs[a,b]	F	df	p
Milk output	1.18	18, 20	NS

[a] After adjustment for stage of lactation and season of the year.
[b] After adjustment for parity.

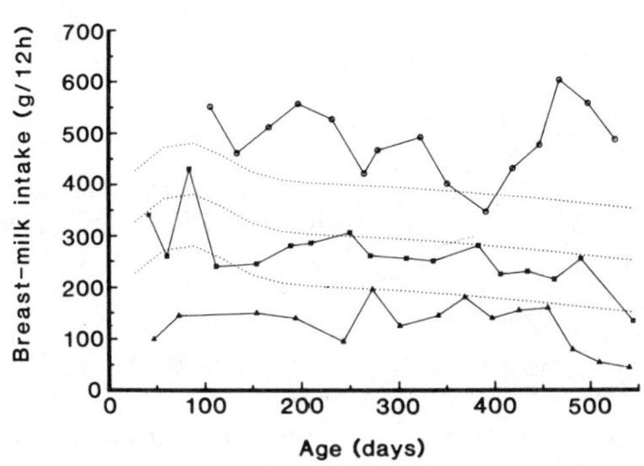

Fig. 14. Examples of infants from Keneba with consistently high, average and low milk intakes.

and five mothers over four lactations. The data set also includes information from 17 pairs of mothers who were full-sisters and even from 13 mother/daughter pairs who were lactating within the study period (i.e. from lactating grandmothers).

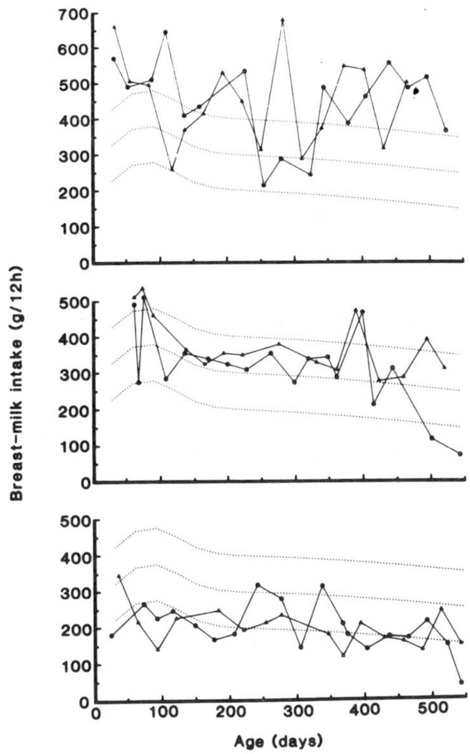

Fig. 15. Examples of mothers from Keneba with consistently high, average and low milk outputs over 2 successive lactations.

Analysis of variance performed after adjustment for changes due to stage of lactation and season of the year demonstrated that each child tended to have a characteristic level of milk intake compared to other children throughout lactation ($F = 8.72$, $p \ll 0.001$, Table 7). Examples of infants from different mothers with consistently high, average and low milk intakes are shown in Figure 14. The differences in total intake between children were caused by a combination of differences in the number of feeds and in the intake per feed which both tended to remain ranked for a given child.

Analysis of variance also indicated that different mothers had a characteristic level of milk output in successive lactations (Table 7) and that maternal factors therefore contributed to the differences between children. Once again the differences in total intake were related both to the number of feeds and to feed size. Examples of women with high, average and low milk outputs are shown in Figure 15 and further examples of the constancy of milk production within individual women have appeared in Figures 11 and 12. Figures 14 and 15 both illustrate a general tendency for children with large intakes to have more variable intakes.

We have attempted to investigate whether genetic factors influence a mother's milk output by analysing the results from mother/daughter and sister/sister pairs. Figure 16 and Table 7 show a strong correlation between the milk outputs of mothers and daughters after correction for the effect of parity ($r = +0.66$, $p < 0.02$). A similar association should have been observable between the sisters but was not apparent. However, the

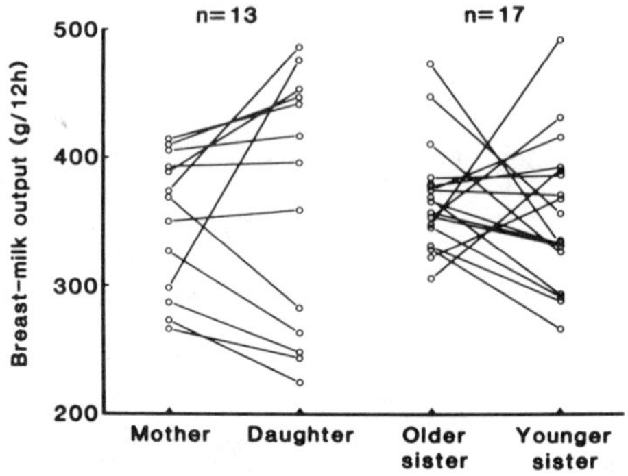

Fig. 16. Breast-milk outputs of mother/daughter and sister/sister pairs in Keneba. Values represent each woman's characteristic volume derived by averaging up to 50 measurements per subject after adjustment for stage of lactation, season and parity.

within sister-pair variance for milk output was exactly the same as the within mother-daughter variance and failure to reach significance in the analysis of variance was caused by the unusual homogeneity of the sister-sister data which resulted in an equally small between pair variance. It is probably fair to conclude, therefore, that we have strong evidence that the phenotype variance in Keneba consists of a combination of genotype variance and environmental effects as would be expected on the basis of studies in dairy cattle. We have insufficient milk composition data from the mother-daughter and sister-sister pairs to look for associations in milk quality, but in cows milk composition is a more strongly inherited trait than milk volume indicating that an association could be expected[95].

Infant Factors Regulating Milk Intake

It has been known for many years that there is feedback control between an infant's demand for and the mother's supply of breast milk. As early as the 1920's it was demonstrated that milk output can be increased by placing another infant on the breast or by stripping the breast at frequent intervals[6,82,96] and that this can be demonstrated at any time after delivery[97]. However, the full importance of the infant in determining both short-term and long-term differences in its own milk intake has only recently been appreciated[98].

It is reasonable to assume that an infant's appetite and hence suckling intensity will be related to its nutritional requirements for maintenance and growth, and that appetite will be periodically suppressed by episodes of infection and weight loss, and progressively suppressed by the introduction of weaning foods as the infant grows older. We have investigated the relative importance of each of these variables in Keneba and Cambridge by multiple regression analysis in which an infant's maintenance and growth requirements are represented by its current weight and its weight velocity respectively.

Correlation coefficients for the two communities are tabulated in Tables 8 and 9. In comparing correlations between Keneba and Cambridge it should be remembered that the within-subject variance for milk output has a coefficient of variation of only 10% in Cambridge where measurements were

Table 8. Factors Correlated with Infants' Milk Intake in Keneba

	Months of lactation		0-2	2-4	4-6	6-9	9-12	12-15	15-18
Infant factors	Birth weight	r	0.34[a]	0.28[a]	0.27[a]	0.24[a]	0.22[a]	0.24[a]	0.16
		df	178	240	225	226	202	195	183
		t	4.8	4.5	4.2	3.7	3.2	3.4	2.1
	Current weight (between children)	r	0.49[a,d]	0.48[a,d]	0.44[a]	0.37[a]	0.39[a]	0.39[a]	0.38[a]
		df	114	276	273	292	256	243	230
		t	6.0	9.2	8.2	6.9	6.8	6.6	6.3
	Current weight[b] (within children)	r	-	-0.12[d]	0.02	0.07	0.12	0.15[a]	0.18[a]
		df	26	223	210	440	380	372	399
		t	-	-1.8	0.3	1.50	2.4	2.9	3.6
	Weight velocity	r	0.55[a,d]	0.31[a,d]	0.23[a]	0.04	0.13	0.25[a]	0.07
		df	116	198	181	189	173	163	151
		t	7.0	2.8	3.2	0.5	1.7	3.3	0.9
Maternal factors	Height[c]	r	0.21	0.13	0.16	0.11	0.05	-0.04	0.02
		df	117	199	182	190	174	163	151
		t	2.3	1.9	2.2	1.6	0.7	-0.5	0.2
	Weight[c]	r	0.24[a]	0.20[a]	0.20[a]	0.13	0.10	0.12	0.11
		df	117	199	182	190	174	163	151
		t	2.7	2.8	2.7	1.9	1.3	1.6	1.3
	Weight/height^2	r	0.15	0.11	0.08	0.07	0.12	0.17	0.05
		df	117	199	182	190	174	163	151
		t	1.8	1.5	1.0	0.9	1.5	1.9	0.4
Others	Feeding frequency (between children)	r	0.04	0.28[a]	0.31[a]	0.15[a]	0.24[a]	0.27[a]	0.26[a]
		df	139	261	264	278	256	235	216
		t	0.5	4.6	5.2	2.5	3.9	4.4	4.0
	Feeding frequency[b] (within children)	r	-	0.12	0.14	0.16[a]	0.08	0.15[a]	0.16[a]
		df	13	206	195	386	322	310	286
		t	-	1.8	2.0	3.2	1.5	2.7	2.7

[a] $p < 0.01$
[b] Within-child analysis performed on all children providing more than one pair of variables in each age group.
[c] All correlations with maternal anthropometry become non-significant when adjusted for child weight and weight velocity.
[d] Age adjusted within each age group to allow for rapid growth.

Table 9. Factors Correlated with Infants' Milk Intake in Cambridge

	Months of lactation	2-3	3-4	4-5	5-6	6-7
	df	43	44	39	35	32
<u>Infant factors</u>	Birth weight	0.48[c]	0.47[c]	0.31[a]	0.18	0.10
	Current weight	0.68[c]	0.62[c]	0.39[b]	0.07	0.01
	Weight velocity	0.29[a]	0.27	0.06	-0.23	-0.05
<u>Maternal factors</u>	Height	0.09	0.18	0.07	-0.01	0.16
	Weight	0.01	0.06	-0.01	-0.15	0.04
	Weight/height^2	-0.14	-0.23	-0.22	-0.25	-0.13
	Parity	-0.08	0.02	0.17	0.24	0.08
	Social class	-0.42[b]	-0.47[c]	-0.52[c]	0.51[c]	-0.23
	Energy intake	0.35[a]	0.41[b]	0.51[c]	0.43[b]	0.45[b]
<u>Others</u>	Feeding frequency	0.02	0.01	0.26	0.58[c]	0.75[c]
	Weaning food intake	-0.22	-0.33[a]	-0.68[c]	-0.87[c]	-0.91[c]

[a] $p < 0.05$; [b] $p < 0.01$; [c] $p < 0.001$.

made over 96 hours (i.e. 8 x 12) compared to 20% in Keneba where single 12 hour estimates were used. An equivalent biological correlation would therefore be expected to yield a higher correlation in the Cambridge data set.

Birth weight (BW) was significantly correlated with milk intake up to the 5th month of lactation in Cambridge and up to the 15th month in Keneba when analysed on a between child basis. However, this effect was entirely accounted for by the infant's current weight (CW) which was itself correlated with birth weight (e.g. in Keneba between-child CW vs BW by age groups: r = 0.76, 0.65, 0.59, 0.55, 0.54, 0.55, 0.58). Step-wise multiple regression of the Cambridge data set revealed that when current weight was in the regression birth weight had a negative influence on milk intake (-121 g milk/kg BW at 2 months). Dewey has reported a similar relationship[84]. Similarly, a within-child analysis of the Keneba data also revealed that current weight tended to be negatively correlated with milk intake up to 4 months of age (Table 10). We believe that this apparent negative impact of birth weight on milk intake in the first few months is an artefact caused by a small number of babies being born well below their genetic potential due perhaps to placental insufficiency. These babies may demand large milk intakes to allow rapid catch-up growth as they cross centiles during the first few months of life, and thus explain the negative association with birth weight.

Between-child analysis of the effect of an infant's current weight in determining its milk intake showed strong positive correlations in both communities. The correlation decreased rapidly in Cambridge as the amount of weaning food received by the infant became the major determinant of milk intake. Similar findings have been observed in Hungary, Sweden, Guatemala and the Philippines[71] and in the USA[84]. In Keneba the association between milk intake and current weight remained highly significant throughout lactation (t values in excess of 6.0). The slopes of these regressions are given in Table 10. This finding is consistent with results from Zaire[71] although the Kenyan study failed to demonstrate a strong relationship[51]. It is probable that the close correlation remains until late lactation in The Gambia and Zaire because the introduction of weaning foods is not associated with a conscious decision to start the process of weaning the infant from the breast as is the case in many countries.

The strong correlation between milk intake and a baby's current weight explains the frequently observed difference in intake between boys and girls. In both the Cambridge and Keneba data sets a baby's milk intake is strongly correlated with its sex with girls having lower intakes. However, this can be completely accounted for by the differences in weight between the sexes.

The within-child analysis in Keneba demonstrated a steady change from a negative correlation at 2-4 months, as discussed above, to a significant positive correlation after 9 months of age. This positive correlation appears at the time when children are most susceptible to infections and to the growth faltering impact of these infections during the wet season. The correlation indicates that small fluctuations in weight within children are associated with corresponding changes in milk intake although the relationship might not be causal since both of these factors will be influenced by periods of anorexia.

Weight velocity was rather weakly correlated with milk intake in Cambridge in the first age group (r = +0.29) and much more strongly correlated in Keneba (r = +0.55). In Keneba the measurements in the first age group were clustered towards the end of the age range and are therefore similar in timing to the Cambridge values. The correlation disappears fatness were not correlated with milk output at any age in Cambridge. In Keneba maternal weight and height were correlated with milk output, but these correlations disappeared when child weight was introduced into the regression demonstrating that the high intakes were caused by large women tending to have large babies. Maternal weight/height^2, measured at 6 weeks post-partum, was not correlated with milk production in any age group. This lends further support to the conclusion that poor maternal nutritional status does not limit milk output until a certain threshold is reached and that this threshold is lower than conditions normally observed in most developing countries.

In Cambridge there was a strong association between social class and milk output with high social class mothers producing most milk. Step-wise multiple regression indicated that, after child weight, social class accounted for more of the variance than any other factor in the 2-3 and 3-4 month age groups. It is difficult to explain this correlation in early lactation especially since the high outputs of high social class mothers were due to an increased volume per feed and not to a change in the number of feeds. The effect may be a result of subtle influences on lactational performance such as increased motivation and confidence. The correlation with social class increased as lactation progressed owing to the fact that lower social class mothers introduced weaning foods at an earlier stage and sustained lactation for a shorter period. This finding is consistent with a national survey in the U.K.[100].

In Cambridge maternal energy intake was weakly correlated with milk output in early lactation and more strongly correlated later. However, it is not possible to distinguish cause and effect, and it cannot necessarily be concluded that a high level of energy intake stimulates lactation. Figure 4 illustrates the close cross-sectional correlation between maternal energy intake and milk output in Keneba which we have concluded is coincidental. This correlation makes it extremely difficult to perform even a between-mother analysis and as in the Cambridge analysis it would still not be possible to distinguish cause from effect. Based on our earlier conclusions we would not expect to observe a correlation since the possible effect of a low maternal energy intake would be buffered by the mother's fat stores assuming that these had not been exhausted.

The Effect of Feeding Frequency on Milk Intake

The most striking difference between breast-feeding in Keneba and Cambridge was in the difference between demand and scheduled feeding. It is argued that the high feed frequency usually observed in communities practising natural breast-feeding in the developing world is necessary firstly for the infant to obtain sufficient milk when there is competition for limited substrate between maternal tissues and milk synthesis, and secondly in order to sustain lactation for long periods.

Between-child analysis showed no correlation between feed frequency and milk intake in the very early stages of lactation. This may reflect the fact that, with the exception of children of very high parity mothers, all babies receive adequate milk in the first 2 or 3 months of life to achieve their genetic potential for growth, and that feeding frequency is unimportant at this stage. In Cambridge the correlation between milk intake and feed frequency rises sharply after the fifth month but this merely reflects the fact that some mothers have partially weaned their babies from the breast by this stage. In Keneba there is a significant positive correlation between feed frequency and milk intake at all ages after 2 months. The within-child analysis in Keneba also revealed positive correlations in the 6-9, 12-15 and 15-18 month age groups indicating that individual children who increased their feed frequency during the given

Table 10. Relationship Between a Child's Weight and Milk Intake - Regression Slopes[a,b]

	Between child analysis		Within child analysis	
Age group	Slope	t	Slope	t
0-2m[c]	78	6.0	-248	-1.30
2-4m[c]	54	9.2	-63	-1.83
4-6m	38	8.2	6	0.25
6-9m	27	6.9	25	1.50
9-12m	29	6.8	42	2.39
12-15m	31	6.6	53	2.93
15-18m	30	6.3	43	3.58

a Slopes represent grams of breast-milk per 12 hours per kg body weight.
b See Table 8 for numbers in each group.
c Age adjusted within each age group.

after 6 months in Keneba, but then reappears in the 9-12 and 12-15 month age groups. This is consistent with the within-child analysis of current weight and once again may reflect the effects of infection, anorexia and weight loss in the wet season.

In the first few weeks of life a mother's capacity to produce milk usually exceeds her baby's demands as evidenced by breast engorgement and leakage. This was as evident in Keneba as it was in Cambridge. It therefore appears likely that the observed correlations with weight velocity were caused by fast growing babies demanding and receiving more milk rather than by the babies of inherently good lactators growing faster. However, a possible contributory explanation for the very high correlation in Keneba concerns the effect of parity. Primiparous mothers deliver small babies and have relatively high milk outputs, while mothers of very high parity produce babies of average size but have low milk outputs and their children exhibit poor growth in the first few months[99]. The relative importance of genetic potential and breast-milk availability in determining growth in the first few months of life require further study, particularly since a baby's attained weight at 3 months is very highly correlated with its weight at 18 months even in an environment such as Keneba where infections during the intervening 15 months might be expected to minimise any association. In Keneba the correlations between current weight in subsequent age groups and weight at 3 months are: 0.93, 0.83, 0.80, 0.80 and 0.76.

Maternal Factors Influencing Milk Output

It was demonstrated above that individual women had characteristic levels of milk production. Including child weight in the analysis demonstrated that 20% of the between-mother variance was due to the tendency of women to have either large or small children. A further 20% of the variance was accounted for by maternal parity which also has an important influence on milk composition as discussed elsewhere in this volume[99].

Correlations between milk intake and other maternal factors which may influence it are shown in Tables 8 and 9. Maternal weight, height or periods also increased their milk intake. As for the within-child relationships with weight and weight velocity, this is probably a seasonal effect, reflecting the fact that a child showing catch-up growth in the recovery phase after an infection will suckle vigorously and often.

Since feed frequency is one of the few variables influencing lactational performance which can be altered it is important to know whether the observed relationship with milk intake is causal. We have previously demonstrated that mothers in both Cambridge and Keneba who have high milk outputs in early lactation are aware of this since they delay the introduction of weaning foods. It is therefore possible that the relationship between feed frequency and milk volume in Keneba is caused by the fact that mothers with high milk outputs offer less weaning food to their babies and hence maintain a higher breast-feeding frequency. However, this is somewhat unlikely since most of the variance between women with high and low milk outputs is caused by differences in feed volume rather than in feed frequency, and a causal effect therefore remains possible and should be tested by a controlled intervention study.

The Effect of Weaning Foods on Milk Intake

In Cambridge the introduction of weaning foods is associated with a conscious decision to begin the weaning process and almost all mothers had completely stopped breast-feeding within a few months of first introducing alternatives to breast-milk. This accounts for the high correlations in Table 9.

In Keneba women expect to introduce weaning foods from the second or third month onwards, but also expect to continue breast-feeding for two years or more, and their intention is therefore that the weaning foods should supplement and not replace breast-milk. The extent to which this was achieved is difficult to analyse since all the infants received an institutionalised supplement from 3 to 12 months of age in an unsuccessful attempt to reverse their growth faltering at this age. However, close inspection of the 12-hour data in Figure 3 shows a sharper than expected decline in milk intake between months 3 and 4 when supplementation commenced, and a rise in milk intake in months 13, 14 and 15 after the institutionalised supplementation ceased perhaps indicating an inhibitory effect. We are currently studying the relationship between the manner and timing of supplementation and any suppressive effect on milk intake, and intend to delay the introduction of the Keneba supplement in order to test whether peak milk output is sustained for longer.

CONCLUSIONS

On the basis of these results from two communities representing diverse nutritional states we conclude that the processes controlling lactational performance are remarkably similar and that the same control mechanisms will be revealed in most other communities if sufficiently detailed studies are carried out. We also conclude that there is a strong drive towards milk production in lactating women, often to the detriment of maternal tissues, and that even the low dietary intakes observed in most countries in the developing world do not fall below the threshold at which lactational performance is compromised. It is important to stress, however, that the fact that low energy intakes do not seem to inhibit lactation should not be used to argue that such intakes are optimal or even adequate, since the effect of the combined stresses of low intakes and the demands of lactation on the mother herself must be considered.

ACKNOWLEDGEMENTS

We would like to thank the many people who have assisted us over the years with these studies particularly Lamin Colley, Andy Coward, Bakari Dibba, Frances Foord, Melanie Hutton, Ramou Jagne, Isatou Jammeh, Bakari Kanteh, Elizabeth Muller, Sue Roberts, Mike Rowland, Lamin Tarawalli, Laurence Villard, Mike Watkinson, and Marjorie Roberts for preparing the manuscript. Above all we thank Pa Alkali Minte and the mothers of Keneba and Cambridge for their patient and enthusiastic cooperation.

AP is supported by Bristol Myers International who also provided a travel grant to AP and AMP for this Symposium.

REFERENCES

1. Whitehead, R.G. Some quantitative considerations of importance to the improvement of the nutritional status of rural children. Proc. R. Soc. Lond. B. 199: 49-60 (1977).
2. Waterlow, J.C. and Rutishauser, I.H.E. Malnutrition in man. In: Early Malnutrition and Mental Development. Cravioto, J., Hambraeus, L. and Vahlquist, B., eds. Swedish Nutrition Foundation Symposia No. XIII. Almqvist and Wiksell, Stockholm: 13-26 (1974).
3. Waterlow, J.C. Observations on the suckling's dilemma - a personal view. J. Hum. Nutr. 35: 85-98 (1981).
4. Whitehead, R.G. and Paul, A.A. Infant growth and human milk requirements: a fresh approach. Lancet ii: 161-163 (1981).
5. Whitehead, R.G., Paul, A.A. and Cole, T.J. How much breast milk do babies need? Acta Paed. Scand. Suppl. 299: 43-50 (1982).
6. Macy, I.G., Hunscher, H.A., Donelson, E. and Nims, B. Human milk flow. Am. J. Dis. Child. 39: 1186-1204 (1930).
7. Morrison, S.D. Human milk. C.A.B. Tech. Publ. 18. Commonwealth Agricultural Bureaux, Slough (1952).
8. Hoobler, B.R. The effect on human milk production of diets containing various forms and quantities of protein. Am. J. Dis. Child. 14: 105-112 (1917).
9. Deem, H.E. Observations on the milk of New Zealand women. Arch. Dis. Child. 6: 63-70 (1931).
10. Chilver, J.E. and McCance, R.A. The food intake and growth records of a baby reared on breast milk. Nutrition 21: 199-205 (1967).
11. Wallgren, A. Breastmilk consumption of healthy full-term infants. Acta Paed. Scand. 32: 778-790 (1944).
12. Hanafy, M.M., Morsey, M.R.A., Seddick, Y., Habib, Y.A. and El Lozy, M. Maternal nutrition and lactation performance. J. Trop. Pediatr. 18: 187-191 (1972).
13. Rajalakshmi, R. Reproductive performance of poor Indian women on a low plane of nutrition. Trop. Geog. Med. 23: 117-125 (1971).
14. Rao, K.S., Swaminathan, M.C., Swarup, S. and Patwardhau, V.N. Protein malnutrition in South India. Bull. WHO 20: 603-639 (1959).
15. Senecal, J. Alimentation de l'enfant dans les pays tropicaux at subtropicaux. Cour. Centr. Int. Enfance 9: 1-22 (1959).
16. Blankhart, D.M. Measured food intakes of young Indonesian children. J. Trop. Pediatr. 8: 18-21 (1962).
17. Venkatachalam, P.S., Susheela, T.P. and Rao, P. Effect of nutritional supplementation during early infancy on growth of infants. J. Trop. Pediatr. 13: 70-76 (1967).
18. Martinez, C. and Chavez, A. Nutrition and development of infants in poor rural areas. 1. Consumption of mothers milk by infants. Nutr. Rep. Internat. 4: 139-149 (1971).
19. Karmarkar, M.G., Rajalakshmi, R. and Ramakrishnan, C.V. Studies on

human lactation. 1. Effect of dietary protein and fat supplementation on proteins, fat and essential amino acid contents of breast milk. Acta Paed. Scand. 52: 473-480 (1963).

20. Devadas, R.P. and Murthy, N.K. Nutrition of the preschool child in India. Wld. Rev. Nutr. Diet. 27: 1-33 (1977) (quoting Devadas, R.P. 1971)).
21. Gopalan, C. Studies on lactation in poor Indian communities. J. Trop. Pediatr. 4: 87-97 (1958).
22. Jansen, A.A.J., Luyken, R., Malcolm, S.H. and Willems, J.J.L. Quantity and composition of breast milk in Biak Island (Neth. New Guinea). Trop. Geog. Med. 2: 138-144 (1960).
23. Holemans, K. and Martin, H. Etude de l'allaitment maternel et des habitudes alimentaires de sevrage chez les indigenes du Kwango. Ann. Soc. Belge Med. Trop. 34: 915-923 (1954).
24. Holemans, K., Lambrechts, A. and Martin, H. Etude qualitative et quantitative du lait des femmes indigenes du Kwango (Congo Belge). Rev. Med. Liege 9: 714-723 (1954).
25. Prentice, A.M. Variations in maternal dietary intake, birthweight and breast-milk output in The Gambia. In: Maternal Nutrition during Pregnancy and Lactation. Aebi, H. and Whitehead, R.G., eds. Hans Huber Publishers: Bern: 167-183 (1980).
26. WHO/FAO. Energy and protein requirements. WHO Tech. Rep. Series No. 724. Geneva: WHO (1985).
27. Prentice, A.M., Whitehead, R.G., Roberts, S.B. and Paul, A.A. Long-term energy balance in child-bearing Gambian women. Am. J. Clin. Nutr. 34: 2790-2799 (1981).
28. Prentice, A.M., Whitehead, R.G., Watkinson, M., Lamb, W.H. and Cole, T.J. Prenatal dietary supplementation of African women and birthweight. Lancet i: 489-492 (1983).
29. Dunn Nutrition Unit. Maternal and child nutrition. Publications 1974-1984. Prentice, A.M. ed. Dunn Nutrition Unit, Cambridge, U.K. (available on request).
30. Offices of Population Censuses and Surveys. Classification of occupations 1970. HMSO: London (1970).
31. Black, A.E., Wiles, S.J., Paul, A.A. and Cole, T.J. The nutrient intakes of pregnant and lactating mothers of good socioeconomic status in Cambridge, UK: some implications for recommended daily allowances of minor nutrients. Br. J. Nutr. in press.
32. Hamill, P.V.V. NCHS growth curves for children, birth to 18 years. US Department of Health, Education and Welfare publ. No. PHS 78-1650. National Centre for Health Statistics, Hyattsville, MD. (1977).
33. Whitehead, R.G. and Paul, A.A. Human lactation, infant feeding, and growth: secular trends. In: Nutritional Needs and Assessment of Normal Growth. Gracey, M. and Falkner, F., eds. Raven Press: New York: 85-121 (1985).
34. Whitehead, R.G. and Paul, A.A. Growth charts in the assessment of infant feeding practices in the western world and in developing countries. Early Hum. Dev. 9: 187-207, (1984).
35. Billewicz, W.Z. and McGregor, I.A. A birth-to-maturity longitudinal study of heights and weights in two West African (Gambian) villages 1951-1975. Annals Hum. Biol. 9: 309-320 (1982).
36. NRC. Recommended dietary allowances. 9th revised edition. National Academy of Sciences, National Research Council. Washington, DC (1980).
37. WHO/FAO. Energy and protein requirements. WHO Tech. Rep. Ser. No. 522, WHO, Geneva (1973).
38. DHSS. Recommended daily amounts of food energy and nutrients for groups of people in the United Kingdom. Rep. Health Soc. Subj. No. 15, HMSO, London (1979).
39. Prentice, A.M., Coward, W.A., Davies, H.L., Murgatroyd, P.R., Goldberg, G.R., Black, A.E., Sawyer, M., Ashford, J. and Whitehead, R.G. Unexpectedly low levels of energy expenditure in healthy women. Lancet i, 1419-1422 (1985).

40. Butte, N.F., Garza, C., Stuff, J.E., Smith, E.O'B. and Nichols, B.L. Effect of maternal diet and body composition on lactational performance. Am. J. Clin. Nutr. 39: 296-306 (1984).
41. Roberts, S.B., Paul, A.A., Cole, T.J. and Whitehead, R.G. Seasonal changes in activity, birth weight and lactational performance in rural Gambian women. Trans. Roy. Soc. Trop. Med. Hyg. 76: 668-678 (1982).
42. Prentice, A.M. Adaptations to long-term low energy intake. In: Energy Intake and Activity. Alan R. Liss Inc., New York: 3-31 (1984).
43. DHSS. The composition of mature human milk. Rep. on Health Soc. Subj. No. 12. HMSO, London (1977).
44. Prentice, A.M., Roberts, S.B., Prentice, A., Paul, A.A., Watkinson, M., Watkinson, A.A. and Whitehead, R.G. Dietary supplementation of lactating Gambian women. I. Effect on breast-milk volume and quality. Hum. Nutr.: Clin. Nutr. 37C: 53-64 (1983).
45. Prentice, A., Prentice, A.M., Cole, T.J., Paul, A.A. and Whitehead, R.G. Breastmilk antimicrobial factors of rural Gambian mothers. 1. Influence of stage of lactation and maternal plane of nutrition. Acta Paed. Scand. 73: 796-802 (1984).
46. Bates, C.J., Prentice, A.M., Watkinson, M., Morrell, P., Sutcliffe, B.A., Foord, F.A. and Whitehead, R.G. Riboflavin requirements of lactating Gambian women: a controlled supplementation trial. Am. J. Clin. Nutr. 35: 701-709 (1982).
47. Bates, C.J., Prentice, A.M., Prentice, A., Lamb, W.H. and Whitehead, R.G. The effect of vitamin C supplementation on lactating women in Keneba: a West African rural community. Int. J. Vit. Nutr. Res. 53: 68-76 (1983).
48. Prentice, A., Prentice, A.M., Cole, T.J. and Whitehead, R.G. Determinants of variations in breast milk protective factor concentrations of rural Gambian mothers. Arch. Dis. Child. 58: 518-522 (1983).
49. van Steenbergen, W.M., Kusin, J.A., van Rens, M., de With, K. and Jansen, A.A.J. Lactation performance. In: Maternal and Child Health in Rural Kenya. van Ginneken, J.K. and Muller, A.S., eds. Croom Helm, London: 153-165 (1984).
50. Hennart, Ph. and Vis, H.L. Breast-feeding and post-partum amenorrhoea in Central Africa. 1. Milk production in rural areas. J. Trop. Paediat. 26: 177-183 (1980).
51. van Steenbergen, W.M., Kusin, J.A. and van Rens, M.M. Lactation performance of Akamba mothers, Kenya. Breast feeding behaviour, breast milk yield and composition. J. Trop. Paediat. 27: 155-161 (1981).
52. Rowland, M.G.M., Cole, T.J. and Whitehead, R.G. A qualitative study into the role of infection in determining nutritional status in Gambian village children. Br. J. Nutr. 37: 441-450 (1977).
53. Prentice, A.M., Whitehead, R.G., Roberts, S.B., Paul, A.A., Watkinson, M., Prentice, A. and Watkinson, A.A. Dietary supplementation of Gambian nursing mothers and lactational performance. Lancet ii: 886-888 (1980).
54. Prentice, A.M., Lunn, P.G., Watkinson, M. and Whitehead, R.G. Dietary supplementation of lactating Gambian women. II. Effect on maternal health, nutritional status and biochemistry. Hum. Nutr.: Clin. Nutr. 37C: 65-74 (1983).
55. Gopalan, C. Effect of protein supplementation and some so-called "galactogogues" on lactation of poor Indian women. Ind. J. Med. Res. 46: 31-37 (1958).
56. Chavez, A., Martinez, C. and Bourges, H. Role of lactation in the nutrition of low socio-economic groups. Ecol. Food Nutr. 4: 159-169 (1975).
57. Herrera, M.G., Mora, J.O., de Paredes, B. and Wagner, M. Maternal weight/height and the effect of food supplementation during pregnancy and lactation. In: Maternal Nutrition during Pregnancy and Lactation.

Aebi, H. and Whitehead, R.G., eds. Hans Huber Publishers: Bern, 252-263 (1980).

58. Lechtig, A. and Klein, R.E. Maternal food supplementation and infant health: results of a study in rural areas of Guatemala. In: Maternal Nutrition during Pregnancy and Lactation. Aebi, H. and Whitehead, R.G., eds. Hans Huber Publishers: Bern, 285-313 (1980).
59. Girija, A., Geervani, P. and Nageswara Rao, G. Influence of dietary supplementation during pregnancy on lactation performance. J. Trop. Pediatr. 30: 79-83 (1985).
60. Girija, A., Geervani, P. and Nageswara Rao, G. Influence of dietary supplementation during lactation on lactation performance. J. Trop. Pediatr. 30: 140-144 (1985).
61. Ashworth, A. and Feachem, R.G. Interventions for the control of diarrhoeal diseases among children: improving lactation. Bull. Wld. Hlth. Org. 64: (in press) (1986).
62. Prentice, A.M., Cole, T.J., Prentice, A. and Whitehead, R.G. Interventions to improve lactational performance. A practical proposition? Proc. XIII Int. Cong. Nutr. Brighton, England (in press) (1986).
63. Casey, C.E. and Hambridge, K.M. Nutritional aspects of human lactation. In: Lactation: Physiology, Nutrition and Breast-feeding. Neville, M.C. and Neifert, M.R., eds. Plenum Press: New York, 199-248 (1984).
64. Ashworth, A. and Feachem, R.G. Interventions for the control of diarrhoeal diseases among children: prevention of low birthweight. Bull. Wld. Hlth Org. 63: 165-186 (1985).
65. Rush, D. Effects of changes in protein and calorie intake during pregnancy on the growth of the human fetus. In: Effectiveness and Satisfaction in Antenatal Care, Clinics in Developmental Medicine. Chalmers, I. and Enkin, M., eds. Spastics International Medical Publications: London, 92-113 (1982).
66. Lunn, P.G., Austin, S., Prentice, A.M. and Whitehead, R.G. The effect of improved nutrition on plasma prolactin concentrations and post-partum infertility in lactating Gambian women. Am. J. Clin. Nutr. 39: 227-235 (1984).
67. Hartmann, P.E. and Prosser, C.G. Physiological basis of longitudinal changes in human milk yield and composition. Fed. Proc. 43: 2448-2453 (1984).
68. Orr-Ewing, A.K. A longitudinal study of infant growth in relation to breast-milk consumption, total food intake and morbidity. Ph.D. Thesis, University of London (1985).
69. Prentice, A. and Prentice, A.M. Unilateral breast dysfunction in lactating Gambian women. Ann. Trop. Paed. 4: 19-23 (1984).
70. Chen, X-C., Chang, Y., Wang, W-G., Bai, J-G. and Liu, D.S. Protein and energy intakes of lactating women and breast-milk production in urban and rural areas of Beijing. Proc. XIII Int. Cong. Nutr. Brighton, England (in press) and personal communication.
71. WHO Collaborative Study on Breast-Feeding. The quantity and quality of breast milk. World Health Organisation, Geneva (1985).
72. Devadas, R.P., Vijayalakshmi, P. and Vanitha, R. Impact of nutrition on pregnancy, lactation and growth performance of extero-gestate foetus. Ind. J. Nutr. Dietet. 15: 31-37 (1978).
73. Rattigan, S., Ghisalberti, A.V. and Hartmann, P.E. Breast-milk production in Australian women. Br. J. Nutr. 45: 243-249 (1981).
74. Dusdieker, L.B., Booth, B.M., Stumbo, P.J. and Eichenberger, J.M. Effect of supplemental fluids on human milk production. J. Paediatr. 106: 207-211 (1985).
75. Chandra, R.K. Breast-feeding, growth and morbidity. Nutr. Res. 1: 25-31 (1981).
76. Whitehead, R.G. and Paul, A.A. Diet and the pregnant and lactating woman. In: Nutrition and Health, a Perspective. Turner, M.R. ed. MTP Press: London, 159-168 (1982).

77. Hofvander, Y., Hagman, U., Hillervik, C. and Sjolin, S. The amount of milk consumed by 1-3 months old breast- or bottle-fed infants. Acta Paediatr. Scand. 71: 953-958 (1982).
78. McClelland, D.B.L., McGrath, J. and Sampson, R.R. Antimicrobial factors in human milk. Acta Paed. Scand. 271S: 1-20 (1978).
79. Lonnerdal, B., Forsum, E. and Hambreus, L. A longitudinal study of the protein, nitrogen and lactose contents of human milk from Swedish well-nourished mothers. Am. J. Clin. Nutr. 29: 1127-1133 (1977).
80. McKay, H., Rutishauser, I.H.E. and McKellar, W.J.D. A longitudinal study of breast-feeding. Proc. Nutr. Soc. Aust. 6: 111 (1981).
81. Strode, M.A., Dewey, K.G. and Lonnerdal, B. Effect of short-term maternal caloric restriction on breast milk volume and composition of well-nourished mothers. Fed. Proc. 43: 667 (1984).
82. Dewey, K.G. and Lonnerdal, B. Infant self-regulation of breast-milk intake. Fed. Proc. 53: 162 (1984).
83. Butte, N.F., Garza, C., Smith, E.O. and Nichols, B.L. Evaluation of the deuterium dilution technique against the test-weighing procedure for the determination of breast milk intake. Am. J. Clin. Nutr. 37: 996-1003 (1983).
84. Dewey, K.G., Strode, M.A. and Lonnerdal, B. Maternal vs infant factors related to breast milk volume. Fed. Proc. 44: 1675 (1985).
85. Bijerley, L.O. and Kirksey, A. Effects of different levels of vitamin C intake on the vitamin C concentration in human milk and the vitamin C intakes of breast-fed infants. Am. J. Clin. Nutr. 41: 665-671 (1985).
86. Picciano, M.F., Calkins, E.J., Garrick, J.R. and Deering, R.H. Milk and mineral intakes of breast-fed babies. Acta Paed. Scand. 70: 189-194 (1981).
87. Reinhardt, M.C. and Lauber, E. Prolonged lactation performance in a rural community of the Ivory Coast. J. Trop. Ped. 27: 74-77 (1981).
88. Coward, W.A., Cole, T.J., Sawyer, M.B., Prentice, A.M. and Orr-Ewing, A.K. Breast-milk intake measurement in mixed-fed infants by administration of deuterium oxide to their mothers. Hum. Nutr.: Clin. Nutr. 36C: 141-148 (1982).
89. Hennart, Ph., Ruchababisha, M. and Vis, H.L. Breast-feeding and post-partum amenorrhoea in Central Africa. 3. Milk production in an urban area. J. Trop. Pediatr. 29: 185-189 (1983).
90. Brown, K.H., Black, R.E., Robertson, A.D., Akhtor, N.A., Ahmed, G. and Becker, S. Clinical and field studies of human lactation: methodological considerations. Am. J. Clin. Nutr. 35: 745-756 (1982).
91. Linzell, J.L. Mammary blood flow and methods of identifying and measuring precursors in milk. In: Lactation: A comprehensive treatise. Vol. 1. The mammary gland/development and maintenance. Larson, B.L. and Smith, B.R., eds. Academic Press: New York, 143-225 (1974).
92. Neville, M.C., Allen, J.C. and Watters, C. The mechanisms of milk secretion. In: Lactation: Physiology, Nutrition and Breast-Feeding. Neville, M.C. and Neifert, M.R., eds. Plenum Press: New York, 49-102 (1984).
93. Prentice, A.M., Prentice, A., Lamb, W.H., Lunn, P.G. and Austin, S. Metabolic consequences of fasting during Ramadan in pregnant and lactating women. Hum. Nutr.: Clin. Nutr. 37C: 283-294 (1983).
94. Roberts, S.B., Cole, T.J. and Coward, W.A. Lactational performance in relation to energy intake in the baboon. Am. J. Clin. Nutr. 41: 1270-1276 (1985).
95. Ministry of Agriculture, Fisheries and Food. An introduction to cattle breeding. 1. Some theoretical aspects. MAFF Publications, Alnwick, U.K. (1982).
96. Sedgewick, J.P. A preliminary report of the study of breast-feeding in Minneapolis. Am. J. Dis. Child. 21: 455-464 (1921).

97. Davies, V. and Pratt, J.P. Stimulation and maintenance of lactation. Am. J. Nursing 46: 242-244 (1946).
98. Lunn, P.G. Maternal nutrition and lactational infertility: The baby in the driving seat. In: Maternal Nutrition and Lactational Infertility. Dobbing, J., ed. Nestle Nutrition. Vevey/Raven Press: New York, 41-64 (1985).
99. Prentice, A. The effect of maternal parity on lactational performance in a rural African community. (This volume).
100. Martin, J. and Monk, J. Infant feeding 1980. Office of Population Censuses and Surveys: London (1982).
101. Whitehead, R.G., Paul, A.A. and Rowland, M.G.M. Lactation in Cambridge and in The Gambia. In: Topics in Paediatrics 2. Nutrition. Pitman Medical: Tunbridge Wells, 22-33 (1980).

ETHNIC CULTURAL EFFECT UPON HUMAN LACTATION: INTRODUCTION TO WORKSHOP WITH SOME COMMENTS TO EXPERIENCE OBTAINED IN SCANDINAVIAN COUNTRIES DURING THE LAST TWO CENTURIES

Leif Hambraeus

Institute of Nutrition, University of
Uppsala, Uppsala, Sweden

> "The secretion of milk proceeds best in a tranquil state of mind and with a cheerful temper; then the milk is regularly abundant and agrees well with the child. On the contrary, a fretful temper lessens the quantity of milk."
> (Ashley Cooper, 1840) (1, 2)

INTRODUCTION

Successful breast-feeding in humans, as in all mammalian species, depends not only on what sometimes is called the biological instinct, but also on the interaction between the lactating mother and her infant. This interaction, described by Derrick Jelliffe as the "mother-child dyad" is also strongly influenced by the environment including socio-cultural factors, learned behaviour and emotional support.

Failure or success of breast-feeding is consequently related to many components which influence the physiology of lactation. These include physiological parameters such as the nutritional status of the mother during pregnancy and lactation as well as the physiological capacity of the mammary gland to produce milk. However, these physiological components are themselves influenced by socio-cultural factors, such as those that influence the maternal diet and the role of the mother in the society.

THE MOTHER-CHILD DYAD

In his lecture on "cultural traditions and nutritional practices related to pregnancy and lactation" during the Swedish Nutrition Foundation Symposium on "The Mother-Child Dyad - Nutritional Aspects" which was held in 1977, Jelliffe and Jelliffe (3) stressed that in order to assess the effects of cultural practices on breast feeding it was vital to recognize the reflexes that are operating between the lactating mother and her offspring. The maternal reflexes include the somatic prolactin reflex and the let-down (milk ejection) reflex, and the infant reflexes comprise the suckling and swallowing reflexes. The prolactin reflex seems to be related to sucking at the breast whilst the highly emotional and labile let-down reflex is much influenced by psychological factors.

It is quite obvious from above that all aspects of environmental factors, including the ethnic-cultural ones interact at various levels of the mother-child nursing dyad. In their review Jelliffe and Jelliffe (3) separated them into the following groups:

1. Attitudes towards the role of women in the society and the symbolism of breast and breastfeeding;

2. Techniques including not only cultural beliefs and traditions regarding breast-feeding but also the acceptance and availability of alternatives for infant feeding, i.e. anything from the use of wet nurses to artificial breast milk substitutes;

3. Maternal diet including cultural aspects and traditions regarding specific dietary regulations during pregnancy and lactation.

BREASTFEEDING PROMOTION

The Swedish physician and scientist Rosén von Rosenstein in his introduction to the first chapter "On nurses" in his famous textbook of Pediatrics (The Diseases of Children and Their Remedies) which was translated into English in 1776 (4) and thus seems to be the first textbook of pediatrics in the world, stated that.

> "A child ought to get a sufficient quantity of good nourishment, if it is to thrive well. The best food for it is, no doubt, the mother's milk. We therefore find, that children thrive well, suckled by their mother's milk, though that should not stand all the proofs which are required towards approving that of a nurse. Thus, if another child should suck the same milk, it would immediately grow sick. For this reason then, the mothers ought to suckle their own children; by this they gain a great deal: they will at least have easier deliveries, avoid several diseases, as milk-fever, purpura puerperarum, and inflammation of the womb, by a translation of milky matter....
>
> These motives ought to induce the mother to suckle the child herself, at least during those weeks she is obliged to stay within doors, especially as the mother's milk carries off the meconium better than anything, frees the child from many disorders, and makes it acquire her own temper and disposition. Therefore we see, that young lions, which have sucked a cow or a goat, have by this means been as it were tamed: and dogs on the contrary, who have sucked a she-wolf, have become beasts of prey."

The comments made by Rosén von Rosenstein, as cited above, illustrate the recognition of the very special physiological properties of human milk, which sometimes was referred to as the "white blood". This is of interest as, although Scandinavians domesticated and milked animals since long, milk from other species was rarely used in infant feeding before the 20th century.

SYMBOLISM OF BREAST FEEDING AND ITS INTERACTION WITH FERTILITY

Of special ethnic cultural interest is also the sexual symbolism associated with the female breasts and the effects of this symbolism on breastfeeding. There are reports from Scandinavian countries such as Sweden and Finland during the 19th century that husbands did not want their wives to breast-feed because they feared for their beauty (5). Also a mother was advised not to breast-feed during the middle of 18th century in Sweden if she had sexual relations with her husband as it was believed that the child could then be disturbed through the breastmilk and its life endangered (6).

In her studies on breastfeeding and reproduction Ulla Britt Lithell (7) reported that in some areas in Finland and Sweden during the 18th and 19th centuries children were breastfed for 2 years or even longer. In other areas breastfeeding for as long as 3-4 years has been reported. It has been assumed that one of the reasons that mothers continued to breastfeed was as a method of contraception.

The effects of attitudes and social norms such as "new knowledge" or "new dress fashion" on breastfeeding are illustrated by reports from Sweden by famous Swedish scientist and physician Carolus von Linné (8) that women belonging to the higher social classes did not breastfeed their infants during the 17th and 18th centuries but employed "wet nurses".

THE ROLE OF WET-NURSES

One factor of great impact on the prevalence of breast-feeding is the availability and acceptance of alternatives in infant feeding practices. The only alternative in ancient days was the use of wet nurses. Linné (8) in his article titled "Nutrix Noverca" (the wet nurse as a stepmother), like his contemporary collegue Rosén von Rosenstein, stressed the importance of choosing the right wet nurse in case one was needed. She should be "neither too young nor too old, neither too lean nor too fat and in good health".

> "But should it happen, that the mother has no milk, her nipples either being too small, or too large, too short, too hard, or too sharp pointed, that the child cannot hold them fast in its mouth to suck them: or if she should have fore ones, or herself be too sickly or weak, having the consumption, gravel, or any other disorder by which the milk thus affected might be propagated to the child: or if she is of a temper too easily moved by joy of sorrow, or in a situation where she cannot

avoid being often exasperated, then she ought not to suckle her child but procure a good nurse for it."

"Such a one (wet nurse) ought to be naturally of a serene, cheerful, sweet and virtuous disposition. She ought to be between 20 and 30 years of age, to have lain-in a little before the child's mother, and also to be used to the nursing of children; she ought to be of a strong constitution, and not afflicted with any hereditary disease, that might be transferred to the child; free also from the scurvy: therefore her gums ought to be well examined, whether they are hard and firm.... A fat nurse is preferable to a lean one, but if one can be found that nearly corresponds with the constitution of the child's mother, she will answer still better; she ought to be able to suckle the child at each breast..."

(Rosén von Rosenstein, 1776) (4)

OFFICIAL ENCOURAGEMENT OF BREASTFEEDING

From the socio-cultural and socio-economic point of view, it is interesting to note that the authorities took an interest in the discussion of breastfeeding practices in Sweden as early as during the 18th century. This might be because Rosén von Rosenstein was medical advisor to the King. Thus mothers were encouraged to treat their infants properly, as well as to breast-feed. In light of the discussion of the control of population growth and planned parenthood as well as of social benefits (governmental child allowance) of today, it is interesting to note the following statement which dates from 1801 and reads in translation as follows:

"quite equal to good care should be the encouragement ... that parents among peasantry should be freed of all personnal Taxes and Duties to the Crown, when they have in due form given evidence of having borne eight children, who survived the age of five years. The shortage which the common good would feel from such a freedom from taxation would in the future be replaced many times over when the crowd begins to increase."

From the nutritional and public health point of view it is interesting to note that the children should have survived the age of five years - an indicator as good as any about their knowledge of the need to take special care of children below 5 years of age!

Another illustration regarding the concern about breastfeeding is the proposal by the provincial Governor in one province of Finland during the 18th century that "a woman could be fined 10 silver coins if she refused to nurse her child". The proposal was, however, rejected by the local authorities, as it was impractical since the women often had to work in the field far from home (9).

THE ROLE OF INDUSTRIALIZATION

It is also of interest to analyze how any changes in the socio-economic situation in societies already the process of industrialization influence the breast-feeding pattern.

It is obvious that in all societies there seems to have been a slow change in infant care and breast-feeding habits in order to harmonize the wider aspects of community life, for good or for evil with the nutritional situation of the infant. This is perhaps best illustrated by the impact of the need of women as labor in heavy out-door work in rural districts or in fields far away from home or in industries in urban areas. In both cases the social situation is reported to have a detrimental effect on the breastfeeding and child care.

No doubt there have been fluctuations in the breast-feeding pattern in the Scandinavian societies throughout the last 2-3 centuries (7). The Scandinavian countries experienced a most remarkable socio-economic development during the last 100 years and we have been able to follow remarkable changes in the breast-feeding pattern (10).

It seems as the breastfeeding habits improved in Sweden as well as in Finland during the 19th century. Social and economic changes associated with industrialization which was very rapid during the end of the 19th and beginning of the 20th century, however, also had a negative impact on breastfeeding. Variations in social and economic factors which influenced nursing practices, as well as regional variations, may also have been considerable. Womens' liberation activities, as well as the need for female labor during the first and second world wars in addition to socio-cultural and ethnic factors also had a great impact on breastfeeding. Interestingly, an analysis of the infant mortality rate and mean duration of exclusive breastfeeding in Sweden 1911-1972 illustrates that there is no simple relationship (10). Fifty years ago the mortality and morbidity in Sweden were much higher in bottlefed than in breastfed babies but this is no longer the case in the 1960's. The reason for the great increase in breastfeeding during the 1970's and its high incidence today (52 per cent of the mothers more or less completely breastfeeding for at least 4 months and 29 per cent for 6 months in 1984) is thus a good illustration of the impact of fashion and socio-cultural components even in a modern, highly industrialized society.

CONCLUSION

Thus history reveals that the socio-economic, as well as socio-cultural, impact on breastfeeding in the past, as well as in the future, is substantial. This, in addition to the availability of more or less suitable human milk substitutes and their marketing, are certainly of great interest for further studies. The role of prolonged breast-feeding and its birth-spacing effect is another factor of socio-cultural and ethnic cultural interest. It is, however, still uncertain to what extent such knowledge exists and to what extent it is included in the ethnic-cultural rules.

In this workshop we will now have the opportunity to analyze more in detail some of the factors which I have tried to illustrate from a Scandinavian perspective. Thus we will discuss the problems and possibilities of performing biocultural studies as well as the specific relation between dietary, ethnical and anthropometric factors and human milk composition.

With reference to the local atmosphere of this meeting with Mexico's history and traditions all around us, what could be better to use as an illustration of or as a symbol for this workshop than the ancient Aztec heaven for children who died while nursing represented by the breast-tree from which succour is falling (2, 11).

REFERENCES

1. Cooper, A.P., 1840. The anatomy of the breast. Longmans, London. (cited by Jelliffe and Jelliffe, 1978).

2. Jelliffe, D.B. and Jelliffe, E.F.P., 1978. Human milk in the modern world. Oxford University Press, Oxford.

3. Jelliffe, D.B. and Jelliffe, E.F.P., 1979, Cultural traditions and nutritional practices related to pregnancy and lactation. , in "The Mother-Child Dyad - Nutritional Aspects. Symposia of the Swedish Nutrition Foundation XIV. L. Hambraeus and S. Sjölin, ed., Almqvist & Wiksell International, Stockholm.

4. Rosén von Rosenstein, N., 1977. A Nutrition Foundations' Reprint of The Diseases of children and their remedies. Translated into English by Anders Sparrman in 1776. Johnson Reprint Corporation, New York.

5. Aspelin, J.R., 1866. Kertomus Maalahden pitäjästä. (Reports from Malax). Helsingfors. (cited by Lithell, U.B. 1981).

6. Weiser-Aall, L. ,1976. Omkring lengden på dieperioden i folge nyere norske optegnelser. (On the length of breast-feeding period according to new Norwegian records). in Fataburen 1976. M. Vehere, B. af Klinteberg and R. Kvideland, eds. Lund.

7. Lithell, U.-B., 1981.Breast-feeding and reproduction. Studies in marital fertility and infant mortality in 19th century Finland and Sweden. Thesis. Acta Universitatis Upsaliensis. Studia Historica Upsaliensis No 120. Almqvist & Wiksell International, Stockholm.

8. von Linné, C., 1752. Amman som styvmoder (Nutrix Noverca). Uppsala.

9. Åkerblom, K. V., 1941. Korsholms historia. 1.(History of Korsholm 1.) Vasa. (cited by Lithell, 1981).

10. Vahlquist, B., 1975. Evolution of breast feeding in Europe. Env. Child Health 21, 11.

11. Bustamente, M.E., 1968. Commentario oficial al trabajo pediatria mexicana prehispanica. Gac. med. mex. 9, 1208. (cited by Jelliffe and Jelliffe, 1978)

MATERNAL FACTORS AFFECTING LACTATION

Lindsay H. Allen, Ann M. Ferris, and Gretel H. Pelto

Department of Nutritional Sciences*
University of Connecticut
Storrs, CT

INTRODUCTION

In the development of this paper, the topic "maternal factors affecting lactation" has been interpreted as encompassing not only biological characteristics but also social and psychological traits and the context within which they operate. Since the scope of the topic is very broad, this discussion is limited to aspects that are not covered by other participants in this workshop. In particular, the effects of diet and anthropometry on lactation outcome have not been reviewed, although they would obviously fit within the purview of the topic. The main purpose of this paper is to categorize the types of maternal factors that have been hypothesized, or are known, to affect lactation, and to explore the links between sociobehavioral factors and the biology of lactation.

The majority of research on factors that affect lactation outcome has focused on one of three areas: the initial selection of breast- vs bottle-feeding as the feeding mode; the duration of lactation; or breast milk volume and composition.

INITIAL FEEDING CHOICE

Table 1 provides a general outline of the factors that have been hypothesized or demonstrated to affect the decision to breast-feed or bottle-feed. These factors are primarily social and cultural, although lactation failure and medical conditions appear occasionally as reasons for selecting bottle-feeding. Women's roles apart from maternal responsibilities are an important reason for the wide-spread adoption of bottle-feeding. Butz[1] has developed an economic model of breast-feeding determinants based on the concept of scarce resources and competing demands, and Nerlove[2], with a large cross-cultural sample, demonstrated that infant feeding practices are strongly related to women's responsibilities in productive practices. Pelto[3] has reviewed some of the ways in which social roles affect decisions about breast-feeding.

Cultural beliefs have been significant factors affecting the choice

*Scientific Contribution No. 1160, Storrs Agricultural Experiment Station, University of Connecticut, Storrs, CT 06268.

Table 1. Factors in the Decision to Breastfeed

1. Maternal Roles	3. Social Pressure
Employment	Family
Productive Activities	Peers
Social Activities	Community
2. Cultural Beliefs	4. Lactation Failure
Health	5. Medical Problems
Prestige	
Sexual Mores	

of feeding mode. Until the advent of vigorous campaigns to promote breast-feeding, many women had come to see bottle-feeding as healthier for their infants[4] as well as representing a modern life-style and being more prestigious. Although the role of advertising in promoting such beliefs has been hotly debated, there is evidence that many cultures predispose women to believe that their own milk can become "spoiled" easily, and be unhealthy for the child.[5] Thus, there is often a cultural foundation to view bottle-feeding as a positive alternative to breast-feeding.[6]

Public health activities of recent years, and vigorous education campaigns during the last decade, are causing a significant increase in the proportion of women that choose to breast-feed their child, at least in industrialized countries,[7,8] and there may be a decline in the rate at which women in Third World countries are shifting to bottle-feeding.[9] While the issue of factors affecting feeding mode is still important on a worldwide basis, the issues of duration of lactation and volume of milk are assuming a more prominent position in lactation research.[10,11]

FACTORS AFFECTING MILK VOLUME

A summary of the most important factors that are known to affect milk volume, or that have been hypothesized to affect it, is provided in Table 2. Among these are maternal nutrition,[12] especially energy intake, and infant size. Whether the number of feeds per day, and/or the total time spent feeding per day, affect milk volume is somewhat controversial,[13-15] although it appears that a certain amount of suckling must occur on a daily basis if milk production is to be maintained. This is the rationale behind the frequently made statement that supplemental foods lead to a reduction in milk volume. While there is evidence that this sometimes occurs,[16] in many

Table 2. Factors Affecting Milk Volume

Maternal Nutrition	Frequency of Feeding?
Infant Size	Duration of Feeding?
Supplementation	Stress?
	Smoking?
	Activity?

studies it is not clear which came first; the need to supplement the infant because of insufficient milk production, or unnecessary supplementation followed by a subsequent decrease in milk volume.

Maternal stress or anxiety is often assumed to cause an overall decrease in milk volume, but evidence for this is lacking. It may, however impair milk let-down in a single feeding.[17] While the infants of breast-feeding mothers who smoke have slower growth rates,[18] a definite link to reduced milk secretion has not been confirmed. Finally, intensive material activity has been linked to lower milk volume in at least one study,[19] but whether this is due to higher maternal energy demands, or to less time spent feeding the infant, remains to be shown.

DURATION OF LACTATION

Factors affecting the duration of lactation have received the most attention in recent years, due to concern about the increasing frequency of early weaning.[10] In a recent publication[20] we categorized these factors as either biological, sociobehavioral, or biocultural. Examples of factors in each of these categories are provided in Table 3.

"Biological factors" refer to physically measurable characteristics of the mother and child that may relate to the ability of the dyad to produce an adequate and lasting milk supply, e.g., maternal and infant size, milk volume, and hormone levels. "Sociobehavioral factors" are primarily psychological or cultural in origin and are hypothesized to affect the mother's decisions about breast-feeding and her behavior during feeding. Finally, "biocultural" factors are those that _may_ involve an interaction between biological and sociobehavioral factors, one example being the hypothesis that feeding frequency affects milk production. However, an important conclusion of the present review is that we know almost nothing about the influence of sociobehavioral factors on maternal physiology or on milk production or composition.

In part, this situation has arisen because researchers tend to be experienced in _either_ biological or sociobehavioral research, so that biological and sociobehavioral factors are rarely studied simultaneously. Exploration of the biological links involves measurement of milk volume and composition, as well as relevant hormone levels, and such measurements are difficult especially in a field situation. Biologists are usually unaware of how to construct scales of sociobehavioral measures and have used such scales only rarely for the analysis of their data.

Table 3. Examples of Biological, Sociobehavioral and Biocultural Factors Affecting Lactation

Biological	Sociobehavioral	Biocultural
Anthropometry	Occupation	Hospital Practice
Infant Gender	Income	Feeding Frequency
Hormone Levels	Support	Perceived Adequacy
Time First Milk	Advice	Anxiety
Milk Volume	Desire to Breast-feed	Supplementary Food
Illness	Intended Duration	Time of First Feed
Parity	Experience	
Malnutrition	Desire to Lose Weight	

There is a clear need for studies in which both biological and sociobehavioral factors are examined simultaneously. The extent to which they are linked, and their relative importance, have tremendous policy implications, as will be explained below. From the very limited number of studies that have attempted simultaneously to study the effects of biological, sociobehavioral and biocultural factors on the duration of lactation, Allen and Pelto[20] reviewed four[21-24] in order to make a cross-cultural comparison of factors that predict outcome. The only biological factors associated with duration were maternal anthropometry and early first milk. In contrast, a substantial number of sociobehavioral factors predicted lactation duration, particularly external factors such as the advice and social support of the mother, and maternal attitudes and experience. In these studies, education, socioeconomic status and employment showed no associations, perhaps due to the homogeneity of the samples used. It appears that mothers will breastfeed longer if they have a strong desire to do so, if they feel confident about the process and comfortable feeding in public, and if they intend to feed for a long time. Analysis of the biocultural factors again points to the importance of maternal perceptions about the adequacy of her milk and of the growth of her infant, her previous experience, and the extent of supplementary feeding.

LINKS BETWEEN SOCIOBEHAVIORAL FACTORS AND LACTATION OUTCOME

The extent to which maternal behaviors and environmental factors affect the biological process of lactation is largely unknown. There are many such factors that can be hypothesized to affect milk volume or let-down, including: suckling frequency, time to first feed, stress, use of supplemental foods, alcohol consumption, smoking, and desire to lose weight. Some of these variables will be examined in terms of what is known about their effects on the secretion of oxytocin and milk let-down, and on the secretion of prolactin (HPL), since oxytocin and prolactin are the primary hormones that affect the physiology of lactation.

Situations that may affect milk let-down by changing oxytocin secretion are shown in Table 4. Oxytocin release is stimulated by the infant crying or suckling at the breast.[25,26] Interestingly, although the drinking of alcohol is often recommended in the belief that it will facilitate milk let-down, consuming more than 1-2 ounces of alcohol inhibits oxytocin release in a dose-related manner.[27] It is also often assumed that stress, pain and anxiety inhibit oxytocin and milk let-down, and there is considerable anecdotal evidence to this effect. There have, in fact, been very few studies in which oxytocin release or let-down have been measured quantitatively in a stressful situation. Perhaps the best attempt was that of Newton and Newton, who put the feet of a lactating woman in ice water, painfully pulled her toes, and asked her to solve mathematical problems. These tortures were

Table 4. Factors Affecting Oxytocin Secretion

Biocultural	Biological
Child Cry (+)	Suckling (+)
Alcohol (-)	
Pain (-)	
Anxiety (-)	

successful in inhibiting milk ejection! Milk was released when oxytocin was injected.[17]

Table 5 presents a summary of the biocultural and biological factors that may affect prolactin synthesis, and thereby reduce milk synthesis. The main biocultural influences on basal prolactin are suckling frequency, which increases blood levels of the hormone,[28] and supplemental feeding, which has the opposite effect.[29] Stress increases basal HPL in nonlactating adults, so that it is perhaps unlikely that maternal stress would decrease milk production. The effect of stress has not, however, been examined in relation to either basal or postsuckling levels of HPL in lactating women. The biological factors that affect basal HPL levels are associated with much more marked changes in the release of the hormone than are the biocultural factors. For example, for some time postpartum, both lactating and nonlactating women have elevated higher basal HPL levels, so that in one study these averaged 18 times the concentrations found in subjects who had not been recently pregnant or lactating.[31] Thus, breast-feeding is not necessary for basal HPL levels to be elevated in the early postpartum period. Basal levels are also much higher in the afternoon, and especially at night, than during the morning[32]. Malnutrition is also associated with large increases in basal HPL levels.[33] In contrast, basal levels fall dramatically with time regardless of the pattern and intensity of lactation, so that in many studies basal HPL has fallen to the levels found in nonpregnant, nonlactating women without any apparent effects on lactation capacity.[34]

It has been suggested that the magnitude and/or duration of postsuckling HPL response may be important for the maintenance of lactation,[35,36] although this is somewhat controversial. While suckling certainly induces prolactin release, the magnitude of this response appears to be more strongly affected by the time of day than by the extent and intensity of suckling.[32,34] Since the highest HPL response to suckling occurs at night, this might explain the delayed ovulation of women who breast-feed during the night.[34] The importance of night feeding to the maintenance of lactation remains to be determined. Finally, the postsuckling increase in HPL is substantially reduced after some months of lactation.[37]

From these data it appears that biocultural factors may exert some influence on the hormones involved in milk let-down and synthesis, but that their effects are small compared to those of biological influences. Thus, the relationship of let-down and production to duration remains problematic. The research directions that are required to resolve these issues involve

Table 5. Factors Affecting Prolactin Secretion

Biocultural	Biological
a) Basal Levels	
Smoking (-)	Malnutrition (+)
Suckling Frequency (+)	Parturition (+)
Stress? (+)	Time of Day, Later (+)
Supplements? (-)	Time Postpartum (-)
	Estrogens (+)
b) Postsuckling Response	
Supplements? (-)	Nipple Stimulation (+)
	Time of Day, Later (+)
	Time Postpartum (-)

studies of the effect of maternal behaviors on the biology of lactation.

MATERNAL PSYCHOLOGICAL CONDITION AND LACTATION OUTCOME

In a previous review of studies that had simultaneously examined socio-behavioral, biological and biocultural influences on breast-feeding, it was concluded that the mother's self-confidence and psychological attitude were among the strongest predictors of duration.[20] Figure 1 illustrates several paths by which the link between maternal anxiety and cessation of lactation might occur. The anxiety may be caused by a "perceived inadequacy" of milk, without real evidence of any failure of lactation. The anxious mother may suckle her infant less often, so that both oxytocin and HPL release are reduced, and the result is impaired milk volume. Alternatively, insecurity about the adequacy of her breast milk may cause a mother to wean her infant completely, or to introduce supplementary foods. Supplementation might

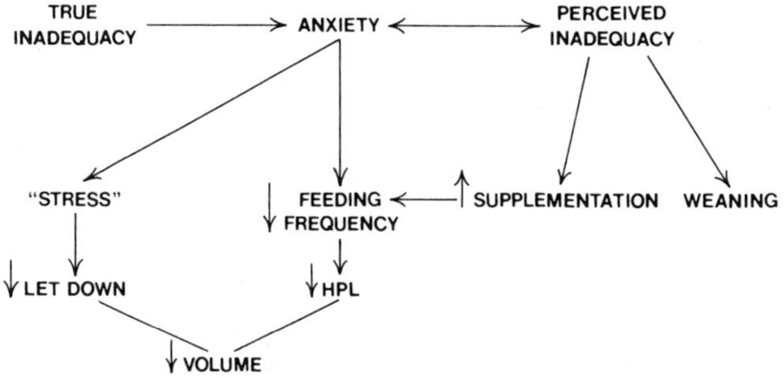

Figure 1. Pathways by which Maternal Psychological Condition may Affect Lactation.

reduce feeding frequency and impair milk synthesis as a consequence. Yet another possible pathway could be that a state of maternal anxiety might decrease milk volume via inhibition of oxytocin secretion,[17] or by vasoconstriction of the mammary gland and subsequent slow transport of oxytocin,[38] or by the stimulation of secretion of b-endorphins and their inhibition of oxytocin release.[39] Finally, anxiety about breast-feeding can be caused by a "true inadequacy," as evidenced by infant fussiness and crying or slow growth; this inadequacy may originate with psychological factors as described above, or, probably less frequently, with a biological insufficiency.

The relative importance of these pathways has not been tested. Given the apparent importance of maternal anxiety as a determinant of early weaning, it is important to clarify the processes involved and the reasons for resulting changes in feeding practices. When questioned about the reason for early weaning, many women respond that their milk supply was inadequate. It is rare, however, that frequently available data such as infant growth are collected in order to substantiate this belief. It is important to know whether western feeding practices such as a reduced frequency of feeding, and cultural influences that lead a mother to doubt her lactational adequacy, do lead to an impairment of milk production. The strategy which could be taken to solve the problem would be quite different depending on which of the above pathways occurred.

TIME OF FIRST FEED AND LACTATION OUTCOME

A similar model might be used to explore the relationship between the time of the infant's first feed and lactation outcome. An infant can start to feed anytime from immediately after birth up to two or three days later. In many cultures there is a belief that colostrum is harmful, so that the infant is not suckled for several days.[40] In spite of this delayed onset of feeding, it is rare for such women to experience difficulties in either the initiation or the maintenance of lactation. There are many natural examples of situations in which the time of first breast-feeding is substantially delayed, without apparent prejudice to a good lactation outcome. In spite of such examples, there is a growing belief among professionals, and mothers themselves, that the baby must be put to the breast as soon as possible after birth, even in the delivery room.

A review of the available literature on this question shows that the importance of an early first feed is still controversial. For example, an "early" first feed was a predictor of the eventual duration of lactation in the studies of McCabe[22] and Wright and Walker[24] but not in that of Salariya et al. in Scotland.[41] Much of the inconsistency in these studies is probably caused by different methods of analysis, and lack of standardization among studies in the construction of the variable "early first feed"; this was defined variously as in the first 10 minutes, the first 6 hours, the first 12 hours, etc., and as a bivariate or continuous variable. Thus, methodologies and units must be standardized across studies when attempting to make cross-cultural comparisons of factors affecting lactation outcome. Sociobehavioral factors are most usefully measured as continuous variables, if they are to be used in analyses of the association between factors that affect lactation outcome.

If an early first feed does affect either the initiation of lactation or its duration, it is important to understand whether it does so through a biological/physiological link or through an effect on the mother's attitude or behavior. We lack sufficient information to determine which pathway is most likely. Potential biological effects of a late first feed include: breast engorgement and infant sucking problems,[17] or a permanent reduction in milk volume.[42] On the other hand, early mother-infant interaction has been shown to have effects on mother-infant bonding.[43] If an early first feed improves this bonding, or changes the mother's perception of the importance of lactation, then the initiation and duration of lactation may be largely determined by the mother's attitude and behavior.

The importance of knowing which of these situations is correct lies in its policy implications. Delayed first feeding is often the situation, especially in cases of medical complications of the mother or infant. An adverse biological impact of late first feeding should be addressed by changes in hospital practices where possible to permit earlier feeding and stimulate maternal milk production, and/or to monitor the infant's growth adequacy. In contrast, if mother-infant bonding is adversely affected, then education and motivation may be more beneficial. In the mother who is highly motivated to breast-feed in any case, a delayed time of first feeding may not be important.

FREQUENCY OF FEEDING AND LACTATION OUTCOME

In Third World countries, infants are usually fed on demand, which may result in about 20 suckling episodes per day. In contrast, the relatively low frequency of suckling in industrialized nations has been hypothesized by some to lead to a diminution of milk volume and subsequently to a reduced duration of lactation. Thus, a maternal behavior, "feeding frequency," may have an adverse effect on the biological process of lactation. The hypothesized mechanism would be a reduced secretion of prolactin in the women who suckle less frequently.[44] An alternative explanation might be that the infant who has to wait a long time between feeds becomes fretful, and subsequently has a problem suckling at feeding time. To date, the evidence for a biological linkage is controversial, and in our own studies, successful lactation has been observed in women who suckle as few as four times per day.[21]

SUMMARY

It is apparent from this review that maternal sociobehavioral and biocultural factors may have a very important influence on the initiation of lactation, on infant feeding patterns, on the introduction of supplements, and on the adequacy and duration of lactation. Sociobehavioral, biocultural and biological factors rarely have been studied concurrently, so that it is difficult to interpret their relative importance. In particular, the links between maternal behaviors and psychological state, and the physiological process of lactation, are poorly understood. There is a need to develop standardized scales to measure appropriate sociobehavioral factors such as: level of maternal stress, perception of lactation adequacy, desire to breast-feed, and so on. For example, we have constructed a scale to estimate the degree of maternal stress during pregnancy, that is a strong predictor of pregnancy weight gain.[45] This scale could be modified to measure relevant stressful influences in lactation. An additional concern is that both biological and sociobehavioral data need to be recorded as continuous variables whenever possible.

There are several reasons why it is important to understand the links between maternal behaviors and the physiological process of lactation. Sociobehavioral factors may confound the interpretation of purely "biological" studies: for example, maternal anxiety may affect the relationship between suckling frequency and milk volume, or energy intake and milk volume, or time of first feed and lactation outcome. Maternal activity levels and behavior may often explain changes in milk volume and lactation duration.

The extent to which maternal behavior affects lactation biology also has considerable policy implications. For example, if the time of first feed simply affects lactation outcome by improving mother-infant bonding, or the mother's perception of the importance of breast-feeding, then feeding problems might be resolved by improved maternal education and motivation. In women who are already highly motivated, the elapsed time to first feed may be relatively unimportant. On the other hand, time to first feed may influence the physiological process of lactation initiation through an effect on prolactin levels, or through breast engorgement and infant sucking problems. In this case, every effort should be made to allow breast-feeding to start as soon as possible after delivery.

REFERENCES

1. W. Butz, Economic aspects of breast feeding, *in*: "Nutrition and Human Reproduction,"W. H. Mosley, ed., Plenum, New York (1977).
2. S. B. Nerlove, Women's workload and infant feeding practices: a relationship with demographic implications, *Ethnology* 13:114 (1974).
3. G. H. Pelto, Perspectives on infant feeding: decision-making and ecology, *Food Nutr. Bull.* 3:16 (1981).
4. J. Prince, Infant feeding through the ages, *Midwives Chron. & Nurs. Notes* 7:283 (1976).
5. C. A. Bryant, Impact of kin, friend and neighbor networks on infant feeding practices, *Soc. Sci. Med.* 16:1757 (1982).
6. G. H. Pelto, Infant feeding practices in the Third World: beliefs and motivations, *in*: "Infant and Young Child Feeding," J. Bond et al., eds., Academic Press, New York.
7. G. S. Martinez and P. A. Dodd, Milk feeding practices in the U.S. during the first twelve months of life, *Pediatrics* 74:591 (1983).
8. G. E. Hendershot, Trends in breast feeding, *Pediatrics* 74:591 (1984).
9. F. Notzon, Trends in infant feeding in developing countries, *Pediatrics* 74:648 (1984).
10. A. P. Simopoulos and G. D. Grave, Factors associated with the choice and duration of infant-feeding practice, *Pediatrics* 74:603 (1984).
11. M. R. Forman, Review of research on the factors associated with choice and duration of infant feeding in less-developed countries, *Pediatrics* 74:667 (1984).
12. A. Chavez, C. Martinez, and H. Bourges, Role of lactation in the nutrition of low socio-economic groups, *Ecol. Food Nutr.* 4:159 (1975).
13. M. de Carvalho, S. Robertson, R. Merkatz, and M. Klaus, Milk intake and frequency of feeding in breast-fed infants, *Early Hum. Dev.* 7:155 (1982).
14. G. E. Egli, N.S. Egli, and M. Newton, The influence of the number of breast feedings on milk production, *Pediatrics* 27:314 (1961).
15. M. de Carvalho, S. Robertson, A. Friedman, and M. Klaus, Effect of frequent breast-feeding on early milk production and infant weight gain, *Pediatrics* 72:307 (1983).
16. A. Glasier, A. S. McNeilly, and P. W. Howie, The prolactin response to suckling, *Clin. Endocrinol.* 21:109 (1984).
17. N. Newton and M. Newton, Relation of the let-down reflex to ability to breast-feed, *Pediatrics* 5:726 (1950).
18. A. N. Andersen, C. Lund-Andersen, J. F. Larsen, N. J. Christensen, J. J. Legros, F. Louis, H. Angelo, and J. Molin, Suppressed prolactin but normal neurophysin levels in cigarette smoking breastfeeding women, *Clin. Endocrinol.* 17:363 (1982).
19. A. M. Prentice, R. G. Whitehead, A. Paul, A. Prentice, S. B. Roberts, M. Watkinson, and A. A. Watkinson, Dietary supplementation of Gambian nursing mothers and lactational performance, *Lancet* (ii): 886 (1980).
20. L. H. Allen and G. H. Pelto, Research on determinants of breastfeeding duration: suggestions for biocultural studies, *Med. Anthro.* 9:97 (1986).
21. A. M. Duthie, Biological and sociocultural predictors of the extent and duration of breastfeeding, Ph.D. Dissertation, Univ. of Conn. (1983).
22. T. L. McCabe, The assessment of factors that affect the duration of lactation of women residing in Eastern Connecticut: a predictive model, M.S. Thesis, Univ. of Conn. (1982).
23. S. Sjolin, Y. Hofvander, and C. Hillervik, Factors relating to early termination of breastfeeding, *Acta Paediat. Scand.* 66:505 (1977).
24. H. J. Wright and P. C. Walker, Prediction of duration of breastfeeding in primiparas, *J. Epidemiol. Comm. Health* 37:89 (1983).

25. A. S. McNeilly, I. C. A. F. Robinson, M. J. Houston, and P. W. Howie, Release of oxytocin and prolactin in response to suckling, Br. Med. J. 286:255 (1983)
26. R. F. Drewett, A. Bowen-Jones, and J. Dogterom, Oxytocin levels during breast-feeding in established lactation, Horm. Behav. 16:245 (1982).
27. E. Cobo, Effect of different doses of ethanol on the milk-ejecting reflex in lactating women, Am. J. Obstet. Gynecol. 115:817 (1973).
28. P. W. Howie, A. S. McNeilly, M. J. Houston, A. Cook, and H. Boyle, Fertility after childbirth: infant feeding patterns, basal PRL levels and post-partum ovulation, Clin. Endocrinol. 17:315 (1982).
29. P. W. Howie, A. S. McNeilly, M. J. Houston, A. Cook, and H. Boyle, Effect of supplementary food on weaning patterns and ovarian activity during lactation, Br. Med. J. 283:757 (1981).
30. G. L. Noel, H. K. Suh, J. G. Stone, and A. G. Frantz, Human prolactin and growth hormone release during surgery and other conditions of stress, J. Clin. Endocrinol. Metab. 35:840 (1972).
31. R. E. Weitzman, R. D. Leake, R. T. Rubin, and D. A. Fisher, The effect of nursing on neurohypophyseal hormone and prolactin secretion in human subjects, J. Clin. Endocrinol. Metab. 51:836 (1980).
32. A. Glasier, A. S. McNeilly, and P. W. Howie, The prolactin response to suckling, Clin. Endocrinol. 21:109 (1984).
33. P. G. Lunn, S. Austin, A. M. Prentice, and R. G. Whitehead, The effect of improved nutrition on plasma prolactin concentrations and post-partum infertility in lactating Gambian women, Am. J. Clin. Nutr. 39:227 (1984).
34. D. L. Bunner, E. F. VanderLaan, and W. P. VanderLaan, Prolactin levels in nursing mothers, Am. J. Obstet. Gynecol. 131:250 (1978).
35. A. N. Andersen and V. Schioler, Influence of breast-feeding pattern on pituitary-ovarian axis of women in an industrialized community, Am. J. Obstet. Gynecol. 143:673 (1982).
36. P. Delvoye, M. Demaegd, J. Delogne-Desnoeck, and C. Robyn, The influence of the frequency of nursing and of previous lactation experience on serum prolactin in nursing mothers, Biosoc. Sci. 9:447 (1977).
37. R. D. Leake, C. B. Waters, R. T. Rubin, J. E. Buster, and D. A. Fisher, Oxytocin and prolactin releases in long-term breast-feeding, Obstet. Gynecol. 62:565 (1983).
38. B. A. Cross, Neurohormonal mechanisms involved in emotional inhibition of milk ejection, J. Endocrinol. 12:29 (1955).
39. G. Clarke, P. Wood, L. P. Merrick, D. W. Lincoln, Opiate inhibition of peptide release from the neurohormonal terminals of hypothalamic neurons, Nature 282:746 (1979).
40. A. Niehoff and N. Meister, The cultural characteristics of breast-feeding: a survey, Environ. Child Health March:16 (1972).
41. E. M. Salariya, P. M. Easton, and J. I. Cater, Duration of breast-feeding after early initiation and frequent feeding, Lancet 2:1141 (1978).
42. T. Aono, T. Shioli, T. Shoda, and K. Kurachi, The initiation of human lactation and prolactin response to suckling, J. Clin. Endocrinol. Metab. 44:1101 (1977).
43. M. E. Lamb, Early contact and maternal-infant bonding: one decade later, Pediatrics 70:763 (1982).
44. J. D. Gussler and L. H. Briesemeister, The insufficient milk syndrome: a biocultural explanation, Med. Anthro. 4:1 (1980).
45. T. A. Picone, L. H. Allen, M. M. Schramm, and P. N. Olsen, Pregnancy outcome in North American women. I: effects of diet, cigarette smoking and psychological stress on maternal weight gain, Am. J. Clin. Nutr. 3:1205 (1982).

ANTHROPOMETRY IN THE APPRAISAL OF LACTATION PERFORMANCE AMONG WELL-NOURISHED WOMEN

Nancy F. Butte and Cutberto Garza

USDA/ARS Children's Nutrition Research Center
Department of Pediatrics, Baylor College of
Medicine and Texas Children's Hospital, Houston, Texas

The energy needed for milk production is provided by the maternal diet and the mobilization of tissue reserves. Anthropometric indices may be useful to identify women who are at risk of lactation insufficiency. In a study to evaluate milk production and milk composition, anthropometric indices of lactating women were monitored and related to lactation performance.

METHODS

Forty-five well-nourished women were recruited from the middle-upper socioeconomic stratum of Houston, Texas. Adequate weight gains during pregnancy [14.4 (3.3) kg] [mean (SD)] indicated satisfactory nutrition status during pregnancy. Maternal tissue reserves were ample at the onset of lactation. The mothers were exclusively breastfeeding their infants. Mean maternal age was 28.0 (3.1) years and parity was restricted to one or two.

Measurements of maternal weight, height, and skinfold thicknesses were made postpartum and at 4 monthly intervals thereafter. Skinfold thicknesses were measured using Lange calipers at the following sites: triceps, biceps, suprailiac, and subscapular. Maternal body fat was predicted from skinfold thicknesses based on the equation derived by Durnin and Womersley (1). Maternal body fat also was calculated according to Siri (2) from water displacement measurements in a Whitmore volumeter. The amount of milk produced over a 24-hr period was determined by the test-weighing procedure in which the infant was weighed before and after each feeding on an automatic, electronic balance (Sartorius 3804 MP). Milk was expressed with an electrical pump (Egnell, Inc., Cary, IL) over a 24-hr period for routine analysis of total nitrogen, protein nitrogen, lactose, fat, and caloric content. Maternal dietary intake was estimated from a 3-day written dietary record. Statistical analyses included Pearson correlation coefficient, analysis of variance, and independent t-tests.

RESULTS

A wide range of maternal body sizes was represented in this study.

Table 1. Maternal Body Weight During Lactation

Index	Postpartum	Mo 1	Mo 2	Mo 3	Mo 4
Wt (kg)	64.6(9.1)[a]	61.3(9.5)	60.7(10.0)	60.2(10.4)	59.3(10.5)
Wt/ht[b] (kg/cm)	0.40(0.04)	0.37(0.05)	0.37(0.05)	0.37(0.05)	0.36(0.06)
Wt/ht (kg/cm^2 x 1000)	2.43(0.25)	2.30(0.26)	2.28(0.28)	2.25(0.30)	2.22(0.30)
Wt/prepregnancy[c] wt	1.16(0.06)	1.08(0.05)	1.07(0.05)	1.06(0.05)	1.05(0.07)
Wt change (kg/mo)		-3.83(2.26)	-0.59(1.20)	-0.62(1.12)	-0.80(1.86)

[a] Mean (SD)
[b] Maternal height = 163.0(6.3)cm
[c] Weight gain during pregnancy = 14.4(3.3)kg

Maternal body weight ranged from 43.6 to 85.0 kg at the onset of lactation (Table 1). There was considerable variability in the rate of weight change among the women; the average change varied from -10.7 to 5.5 kg/month. The Quetelet index (wt in kg relative to ht^2 in cm x 1000) declined from 2.43 (.25) postpartum to 2.22 (.30) at 4 months postpartum. The 50th percentile value of the Quetelet index for nonpregnant, nonlactating white females, ages 27 to 29 yr in the First Health and Nutrition Examination Survey (3) was 2.21 (kg/cm^2 x 1000). As lactation progressed, the Quetelet index approached the expected normal distribution: immediately postpartum, 85% of the women were above the 50th percentile and 43% remained above after 4 months of lactation. Another indication of ample postnatal tissue stores was that the mothers were 16(6)% above their prepregnancy weight after delivery and 5 (7)% at 4 months postpartum.

Lactation performance evaluated by the quantity and quality of milk produced and by the growth of the recipient infant was considered adequate (4). The mean milk production of 733(89) g/day was in accord with other reports in the literature and milk composition was within expected norms (5-7).

The skinfold measurements are presented in Table 2. There were no significant changes over time in the triceps and biceps skinfold thicknesses. Measurements of the suprailiac and subscapular skinfolds ($p < .001$) and the sum of all sites ($p < 0.002$) decreased significantly over the four months of lactation.

Maternal body fat predicted from skinfold thicknesses decreased significantly over the four months of lactation ($p < .001$) (Table 3). Measured by the water displacement method, maternal body fat decreased significantly from 28.0 (7.4)% at one month postpartum to 26.3 (7.6)% at 4 months postpartum ($p < 0.001$). The estimations of maternal body fat by these two methods did not differ significantly.

There were no significant correlations between milk production or milk composition and the battery of anthropometric indices. The variables explored were maternal weight, height, metabolic size (weight 3/4), weight/height, weight/height^2, prepregnancy weight, weight gain during pregnancy, weight/prepregnancy weight, triceps, biceps, subscapular, and suprailiac skinfolds, and the sum of skinfold thicknesses. The percentage body fat predicted from skinfolds or water displacement was not related to milk production or composition, nor was the rate of change of body weight, body fat, or skinfold thicknesses significantly correlated to lactation outcome.

Table 2. Skinfold Thicknesses of Lactating Women During the First Four Months Postpartum

Parameter	Postpartum	Mo 1	Mo 2	Mo 3	Mo 4
Triceps (mm)	16.3(5.1)[a]	16.9(4.6)	17.0(4.7)	17.3(5.3)	17.2(5.2)
Subscapular (mm)	18.2(7.1)	16.8(6.4)	16.4(7.4)	15.7(7.2)	15.1(7.3)
Biceps (mm)	7.8(3.9)	6.9(3.2)	6.9(3.3)	7.3(4.6)	6.8(3.4)
Suprailiac (mm)	26.1(8.5)	25.7(6.9)	25.2(7.6)	23.1(8.1)	22.2(8.0)
Sum Skinfolds (mm)	68.4(20.2)	66.3(18.9)	65.5(20.6)	63.4(22.9)	61.7(21.8)

[a] Mean (SD)

Table 3. Maternal Body Fat During Lactation Predicted From Measurements of Skinfold Thicknesses and Water Displacement

Month	Skinfold thickness[a]		Water displacement	
Postpartum	Body density	Body fat %	Body density	Body fat %
0	1.036(0.011)[b]	28.1(5.0)		
1	1.036(0.010)	27.6(4.6)	1.036(0.016)	28.0(7.4)
2	1.037(0.011)	27.3(5.0)	1.038(0.014)	27.2(6.3)
3	1.037(0.011)	27.2(5.3)	1.039(0.016)	26.3(6.8)
4	1.038(0.011)	27.0(5.1)	1.040(0.016)	26.3(7.6)

[a] Body fat (%) calculation based on triceps, biceps, and subscapular skinfold thicknesses
[b] Mean (SD)

Table 4. Energy Availability During Lactation Predicted from Changes in Maternal Weight and Body Fat

Month postpartum	Energy intake	Energy Equiv.[a] wt change	Energy Equiv. skinfolds	Body fat changes[b] water displacement
1-2	2098(536)	-141(275)	-82(335)	-268(691)
2-3	2232(594)	-147(287)	-22(423)	-119(738)
3-4	2089(496)	-251(432)	-193(322)	-126(801)
1-4	2182(453)	-154(243)	-110(216)	-137(316)

[a] Assumption: energy equivalent of wt changes = 6500 kcal/kg
[b] Assumption: energy equivalent of body fat change = 9100 kcal/kg

The energy mobilized from tissue stores during lactation may be estimated from anthropometric measurements (8). Calculations based on the energy equivalence of changes in weight (6500 kcal/kg) indicated that 154(243) kcal/d were mobilized from tissue reserves during months 1 to 4 (Table 4). Computed values of the energy provided from fat mobilization averaged 110(216) kcal/day and 137(316) kcal/day based on skinfold thicknesses and the water displacement method, respectively. By difference, the energy derived from losses of lean body mass was determined to be -18(28) kcal/day and -6(39) kcal/day, based on the two respective techniques. The amount of energy mobilized from tissue reserves was not predictive of the lactation performance, nor was milk production significantly correlated to the combined amount of energy available from the diet and tissues.

Lactation performance of women classified in the highest and lowest deciles for body weight and percentage body fat was compared (Table 5). Milk production tended to be greater among women with high body weights compared with that of leaner women [818(211) vs 643(115) g/day; $p = 0.06$]. The protein nitrogen content of the milk was significantly higher in the heavier women than that in lighter women [1.57(0.16) vs 1.34(0.13) mg/g; $p = 0.003$]. No significant differences were seen in lactose, fat, or energy content. The women in the upper decile were heavier even when adjustments were made for body height. The mean Quetelet index (wt/ht^2) of the upper decile was 2.72(0.28) vs 2.00 (0.06) $kg/cm^2 \times 1000$ for the lower decile. Infant weights at birth and at 4 months were not significantly different between the two groups. Classification according to percentage body fat revealed no statistically significant findings, although the leaner women tended to produce less milk [736(110) g/day vs 842(185) g/day; $p = 0.29$] of lower caloric value [0.62(0.05) vs 0.69(0.08) kcal/g; $p = 0.22$]. The small sample size ($r = 4$) in the lower and upper deciles was a limiting factor in detecting stronger relationships.

For a further examination of the relationship between lactation performance and body composition, the study population was divided into two groups; those who lost body fat during lactation and those who gained body fat or whose weight remained stationary based on the water displacement technique. The women who lost body fat tended to consume fewer calories than those who gained body fat or whose weight remained stationary [2045(474) vs 2283(497) kcal/day; $p = 0.07$]. Milk production and protein nitrogen and lactose contents were not different between the two groups, however, the fat concentration of the milk tended to be lower among the women in negative fat balance [33.1(7.1) vs 36.8(9.7) mg/g; $p = 0.10$]. There were no significant differences between groups with respect to feeding frequency or length of feeding.

DISCUSSION

Several investigators have monitored the anthropometric changes of well-nourished (9-11) and marginally-nourished women (12,13) during lactation, but few (14-16) have related these changes to lactation performance. Reproductive women in rural Gambia appeared to maintain long-term energy balance despite seasonal fluctuations in food availability. Marked seasonal changes seen in body weight and skinfold thicknesses were related to changes in energy intake and milk output (14). The fat concentration of the human milk paralleled seasonal variations in maternal subcutaneous fat reserves estimated by triceps skinfolds (15). There was a positive correlation ($r = 0.27$) between the relative triceps skinfold and the fat concentration. In another study (16) conducted in rural Kenya, lactating women were categorized according to international weight-for-height standards. The women who fell between 70 to 80% of the reference standard (Quetelet index = 1.83) produced significantly less milk ($p < 0.028$) than those classified between 90 to 115% of the standard (Quetelet index = 2.36). The milk of the underweight women had significantly higher concentrations of fat and lactose.

In contrast, we detected no significant associations between anthropometric indicators and lactation performance. Several explanations are possible. First, the study population was relatively homogeneous. Although a wide range of maternal body sizes was examined, the sample was representative of well-nourished women with normal to excessive body weights. Had the population sample extended to undernourished women with suboptimal levels of milk production, significant relationships may have been detected. Second, in the energy balance of lactation, mobilization of tissue reserves indicated by anthropometric indices is a relatively minor component when compared with dietary sources of energy. The compensatory interaction between dietary energy and energy mobilized from tissue reserves may preclude any direct relationship between lactation and anthropometric variables. Third, variable energy needs for maintenance and activity will affect the availability of energy for lactation. Strenuous work demands and associated stress may interfere with milk production. These confounding factors may have obscured detection of significant relationships between maternal anthropometry and lactation outcomes. Finally, the imprecision and inaccuracy of the anthropometric measurements may have obscured significant differences. The ability to predict body composition of an individual from measurements of skinfold thicknesses is poor (18). Alternative methodologies, e.g., isotope dilution techniques and total body electrical conductivity, may be more discriminating.

Our findings are in contrast with those of Quandt (17) who reported that declining maternal adiposity was associated with a breast-feeding pattern of short, frequent feeds. She hypothesized that fat mobilization during lactation was caused by prolactin-mediated suppression of lipoprotein lipase in the peripheral adipose tissue and augmentation of activity in the mammary gland. Frequent feeds promote elevated levels of prolactin and thus would facilitate fat uptake by the mammary gland at the expense of adipose tissue.

Table 5. Milk Production and Composition of Women Classified into the Lowest and Highest Deciles for Body Weight

	Milk Production (g/d)				
Decile	Mo 1	Mo 2	Mo 3	Mo 4	ANOVA
> 90	819	801(268)	833(186)	822(164)	F = 5.2
< 10	662(85)	625(165)	673(68)	630(89)	p = .06
	Protein Nitrogen (mg/d)				
< 90	1.80(.26)	1.62(.18)	1.39(.08)	1.50(.04)	F = 19.2
> 10	1.53(.12)	1.33(.12)	1.29(.14)	1.20(.14)	p = .003
	Fat (mg/g)				
< 90	32.5(4.9)	33.2(3.5)	33.3(5.6)	35.2(9.3)	F = 0
> 10	36.0(7.8)	34.9(10.0)	32.2(8.1)	31.5(6.0)	p = .98
	Energy (kcal/g)				
> 90	.69(.03)	.65(.05)	.65(.04)	.64(.05)	F = .72
< 10	.67(.07)	.65(.10)	.58(.06)	.61(.05)	p = .42

[a] Mean maternal weights of highest decile = 81.7(3.9) kg postpartum and 78.5(7.7) kg at 4 mo and of lowest decile = 51.7(4.6) kg postpartum and 44.4(3.2) kg at 4 mo.

CONCLUSION

The changes in anthropometric measurements of a population of well-nourished, lactating women have been described. A gradual, moderate weight reduction over the first 4 months postpartum was observed in most women. Significant decreases in triceps and suprailiac skinfolds were seen along with a slight, but significant decline in body fat. These changes were not significantly correlated to the rates of milk production or milk composition. Women classified into the highest decile for body weight, however, produced more milk of higher protein content than those in the lowest decile. Also, the women who were losing body fat tended to have lower concentrations of fat in their milk. Overall, anthropometric indices were not predictive of lactation performance of these women, with the possible exception of those at the extremes of the study population.

ACKNOWLEDGMENTS

This work is a publication of the USDA/ARS Children's Nutrition Research Center, Department of Pediatrics, Baylor College of Medicine and Texas Children's Hospital, Houston, TX. This project has been funded in part with Federal funds from the U.S. Department of Agriculture, Agriculture Research Service under Cooperative Agreement number 58-7MNI-6-100. The contents of this publication do not necessarily reflect the views or policies of the U.S. Department of Agriculture, nor does mention of trade names, commercial products, or organizations imply endorsement by the U.S. Government.

REFERENCES

1. J.V.G.A. Durnin and J. Womersley, Body fat assessed from total body density and its estimation from skinfold thickness: measurements on 481 men and women aged from 16 to 72 years, Br. J. Nutr. 32:77 (1974).
2. W.E. Siri, Body composition from fluid spaces and density, University of Colorado Donner Laboratory Medical Physics Report, March 19, no. 3349 (1956).
3. C.E. Cronk and A.F. Roche, Race- and sex-specific reference data for triceps and subscapular skinfolds and weight/stature^2, Am. J. Clin. Nutr. 35:347 (1982).
4. N.F. Butte, C. Garza, E.O. Smith, and B.L. Nichols, Human milk intake and growth performance of exclusively breast-fed infants, J. Pediatr. 104:187 (1984).
5. A. Wallgren, Breast milk consumption of healthy full-term infants, Acta Pediatr. Scand. 32:778 (1945).
6. R.G. Whitehead and A.A. Paul, Infant growth and human milk requirements, Lancet 2:161 (1981).
7. K.G. Dewey, D.A. Finley, and B. Lonnerdal, Breast milk volume and composition during late lactation (7-20 months), J. Pediatr Gastroenterol. Nutr. 3:713 (1984).
8. N.F. Butte, C. Garza, J.E. Stuff, E.O. Smith, and B.L. Nichols, Effect of maternal diet and body composition on lactational performance, Am. J. Clin. Nutr. 34:296 (1984).
9. D.J. Naismith and C.D. Ritchie, The effect of breast-feeding and artificial feeding on body weights and skinfold measurements and food intakes of forty-two primiparous women, Proc. Nutr. Soc. 34:116A (1975).

10. C. Manning-Dalton and L.H. Allen, The effects of lactation on energy and protein consumption, postpartum weight change and body composition of well-nourished North American women, Nutr. Res. 3:293 (1983).
11. E.H. Morse, R.P. Clarke, S.B. Merrow, and B.E. Thibault, Comparison of the nutritional status of pregnant adolescents with adult pregnant women II. Anthropometric and dietary findings, Am. J. Clin. Nutr. 28:1422 (1975).
12. G.A. Harrison, A.J. Boyce, and C.M. Platt, Body composition changes during lactation in a New Guinea population, Ann. Hum. Biol. 2:395 (1975).
13. L.S. Adair, E. Pollitt, and W.H. Mueller, Maternal anthropometric changes during pregnancy and lactation in a rural Taiwanese population, Hum. Biol. 55:771 (1984).
14. E.M. Mueller and R.G. Whitehead, Seasonal variations in energy intake, body-weight and skinfold thickness in pregnant and lactating women in rural Gambia, Proc. Nutr. Soc. 38:28A (1979).
15. A. Prentice, A.M. Prentice, and R.G. Whitehead, Breast-milk fat concentrations of rural African women 2. Long-term variations within a community, Br. J. Nutr. 45:495 (1981).
16. W.M. Van Steenbergen, J.A. Kusin, C. DeWith, E. Lacko, and A.A.J. Jansen, Lactational performance of mothers with contrasting nutritional status in rural Kenya, Acta Pediatr. Scand. 72:805 (1983).
17. S.A. Quandt, Changes in maternal postpartum adiposity and infant feeding patterns, Am. J. Phys. Anthropol. 60:455 (1983)
18. N.F. Butte, C. Wills, E.O. Smith, and C. Garza, Prediction of body density from skinfold measurements in lactating women, Br. J. Nutr. 53:485 (1985).

ETHNIC DETERMINANTS OF LACTATION IN A POPULATION OF MOTHERS IN THE UNITED STATES

David K. Rassin[1], C. Joan Richardson[1] and Tom Baranowski[2]

[1]Division of Perinatal Pediatrics
Department of Pediatrics, and
[2]Department of Preventive Medicine and Community Health
University of Texas Medical Branch at Galveston
Galveston, Texas 77550

INTRODUCTION

The American Academy of Pediatrics (1), as well as other professional organizations (2), has strongly endorsed breastfeeding as the nutrition of choice for the healthy term infant during the first four to six months of life. These endorsements reflect an impetus to increase the incidence of breastfeeding in the United States after many years of decline, the low point of which occurred in the 1960's (3). There has been an apparent increase in the incidence of breastfeeding with approximately 50% of the mothers nourishing their infants in this fashion at the time of discharge from the hospital in 1980 compared to approximately 26.5% in 1965 (3,4). However, this increase in the incidence of breastfeeding has not been as apparent in the lower socioeconomic groups: for example only 37.3% of mothers from families earning less than $7000 per year were breastfeeding in the week after delivery in 1979 versus 55.2% of mothers earning more than $15,000 per year (4). The gradual increase in breastfeeding has continued (61% in 1984) as has the low incidence among families earning less than $7000 per year (36.6% in 1984) (5).

This relatively low incidence of breastfeeding in the United States continues despite evidence that there are both physiological and psychological benefits to the neonate. Immunologic, biochemical, allergenic, nutritional, psychological and economic advantages have been documented and extensively reviewed (6-8). More recently, a task force appointed by the Assistant Secretary of Health and Human Services has reviewed the data and suggested that, while not conclusive, the evidence is persuasive that breastfed infants are healthier long-term than formula fed infants (9). In addition, a workshop convened by the Surgeon General of the United States has issued a report encouraging greater efforts to increase the incidence of breastfeeding, especially among lower socioeconomic groups and targeted ethnic groups (10).

If it is accepted that breastfeeding is the preferred method of infant nutrition several aspects must then be addressed. One, which is the topic of most of the rest of this volume, is to arrive at an understanding of what factors influence the composition of human milk and how does one evaluate the quality of human milk. A second important aspect is to understand which mothers elect to, or not to, breastfeed and what factors play a role in that decision. If a major public health goal is to increase the incidence of breastfeeding, an understanding of the maternal decision making process is important to the design of appropriate intervention programs. One area in particular that has been largely neglected has been the influence and/or association of ethnicity on the breastfeeding decision. It is the intent of this presentation to briefly review some of what is known regarding infant feeding practices amongst different ethnic groups in the United States and then to examine some of the differences in social support and attitudes that we have detected among ethnic groups in a low socioeconomic group of mothers.

The available data regarding the incidence of breastfeeding among various ethnic groups is sparse. The longest series of national data regarding the incidence of breastfeeding has been collected in a continuing mail-in survey of new mothers by Ross Laboratories, some of the data has been mentioned above (3,4). Only recently has this survey presented data related to ethnicity (5, reported in 10). As of 1984 the percent of black mothers who indicated that they intended to breastfeed was 33%, in contrast 65% of white mothers indicated that they would breastfeed. These data reflect several problems that may have resulted in overestimations. The study population was different from the census population (generally being from a higher socioeconomic group) resulting in the necessity for the application of various weighting factors to "normalize" the data (3). For example, unweighted data indicated that 49.7% of the population had educational levels of high school or less while other data indicates the population in this category ought to be 71.1%, thus a fairly large weighting factor is needed (3). These weighting factors have changed with time and available information, but are still used, especially with respect to ethnicity (5). The lower socioeconomic group that is under represented in this data would appear to be both those least likely to breastfeed and those least likely to be respondents to a mail or telephone questionnaire.

Other national data regarding the incidence of breastfeeding among black and white mothers has come from the National Surveys of Family Growth. Analyses of these data have shown a decline amongst black mothers breastfeeding from about 59% (versus 49% in white mothers) in 1951 to 1959 to 14% (versus 29%) in the period 1966 to 1970 (11). Similar data were observed in analyses of a second cycle of this study, 38% breastfeeding black mothers in 1955 to 1959 (versus 30%) to 19% (versus 26%) from 1965 to 1969 (12). A decline in the incidence of breastfeeding has also been observed in mothers of hispanic origin over this time period from 58% to 35% (11). The surveys of family growth are also not completely representative of the population because of changes in the eligibility criteria of mothers at the time of their interviews over the course of the data collections (discussed in 13). Also, National Natality Surveys of 1969 and 1980 indicate that Black women breastfeed much less frequently than white women (9% versus 19% in 1969, 25% versus 51% in 1980 - Black versus white respectively (14)). Those studies were also based on mail-in questionnaires and exclude unwed mothers who would be expected to be primarily from a low socioeconomic group.

Thus, available national data has indicated that black mothers may breastfeed at a reduced incidence compared to white mothers. However, these differences are probably underestimates as the design of the data collections has been such as to make it least likely that these mothers would be included.

In an effort to further understand the ethnic influences on or associations with breastfeeding behavior we have performed a series of investigations in the patient population of the obstetric service at the University of Texas Medical Branch at Galveston. This service provides health care to a predominantly lower socioeconomic population. The population offers the advantages of being triethnic (significant representation from white-Black-and Mexican-American groups); relatively large (approximately 400 admissions per month); representative of a fairly broad geographic area (the only state supported hospital medical facility available to patients from anywhere in Texas); and available for confirmation of reported intentions (identification of actual practices in the nursery to insure that self-report data is correct). In our first and most completely analyzed investigation we examined the demographics of our population as well as the available social support systems and the attitudes of respondents towards breastfeeding (15-17). We have collected subsequent data to further confirm the rates of breastfeeding in the various ethnic groups and to do more in depth analysis of some of the reported maternal attitudes. Some follow-up investigations of identified breastfeeding mothers have also been conducted to examine the factors that influence their continuation or discontinuation of breastfeeding.

DEMOGRAPHICS

We have been able to collect almost complete population data on one month samples of our patient population. For example, in July of 1981, 379 women gave birth at UTMB. Completed questionnaires checked with nursery personnel for actual feeding practices were collected from 358 or 94.5% of these mothers. Of the remaining 21 mothers, 9 delivered stillborn infants and were not interviewed and the remaining 12 were lost due to early discharge - 7, declined to participate - 4, or lost questionnaire - 1. Thus, data was not available from only 3% of the 370 mothers available to breastfeed. The population was young (49% less than 21 years of age), with a large number of unmarried mothers (39%), relatively undereducated (52% some high school or less), low income (35% less than $5000 per year), and with a high degree of head of household unemployment (25%) (Table 1).

Table 1. Characteristics of the Study Population

Characteristic	No.	%BF	Characteristic	No	%BF
Age (yr)			**Maternal Ethnicity		
13-17	58	25.9	Anglo-American	145	43.5
18-21	116	23.3	Black-American	131	9.2
22-25	110	28.2	Mexican-American	62	22.6
26-40	71	32.4	Other	19	42.1
**Marital Status			**Paternal Ethnicity		
Married	218	35.8	Anglo-American	133	44.4
Single	93	14.0	Black-American	138	9.4
Other	45	13.3	Mexican-American	63	19.1
			Other	21	57.1
**Head of Household			*Maternal Ethnicity		
Husband	200	36.0	Grade 8 or less	68	29.4
Self	56	19.6	Some High School	117	18.0
Other	101	13.9	Grad. High School	102	28.4
*Annual Family Income					
$5000	61	18.0			
$5000-15000	75	33.3	Employment Status		
$15000	38	47.4	Head of Household		
Don't know/no response	184	23.9	Employed	267	28.5
			Unemployed	89	23.6

*$p < 0.5$ or ** $p < 0.0001$ by x^2 test for equality of proportions for breastfeeding behavior. BF = breastfeeding.

Table 2: Breastfeeding Proportions by Ethnicity Controlling for Marital Status, Head of Household and Maternal Education.

Maternal Ethnicity	Marital Status			Head of Household		
	**Married	Single	Other	**Husband	Self	Other
	% Breastfeeding					
Anglo-American	48.6	26.3	29.4	48.5	35.7	28.6
Black-American	9.1	12.3	0	9.8	8.8	8.9
Mexican-American	27.1	0	16.7	26.2	40.0	6.7
Other	47.1	0	0	50.0	33.3	0
Total	35.8	14.0	13.3	36.0	19.6	13.9

	Maternal Education			
	Grade 8* or Less	Some High	**Grad High	*Some College
Anglo-American	40.0	24.5	52.4	66.7
Black-American	0	9.3	8.0	12.9
Mexican-American	25.9	15.0	22.2	40.0
Other	33.3	100	100	50
Total	29.4	17.9	28.4	39.7

Significant ethnic difference for mothers who breast-fed within this category, *$p < 0.05$ or **$p < 0.0001$.

It should be noted that a large population (51%) did not know (or did not wish to report, although when given the option of indicating these two choices they usually selected "did not know") their annual income. The population was tri-ethnic (40% Anglo-, 37% Black- and 17% Mexican-American). Only 27.2% (98 mothers) of the population indicated that they intended to breastfeed their infant. The demographic characteristics that exhibited disparity among breastfeeding proportions by X^2 analysis were marital status, head of household, maternal education, annual family income, and maternal ethnicity (paternal ethnicity had a like pattern). The difference in proportion of mothers breastfeeding among the ethnic groups appeared to be the most dramatic of all the demographic characteristics that showed significant disparity (Table 2). Further follow-up studies in 1983 and 1984 indicated that while there were some increases in overall incidence of breastfeeding, the disparity among the ethnic groups remained (Table 3).

When the data were examined to see whether or not the relationship of some of these variables to breastfeeding persisted when other variables also related to breastfeeding are controlled, we found persistent significance with respect to ethnic differences within: the groups of married mothers; families in which the husband was the head of the household; and mothers who had at least a high school education. The relationship of maternal ethnicity to breastfeeding appears to be the strongest of all of the demographic variables examined.

Table 3: Distribution of Breastfeeding Mothers by Ethnicity With Time.

	1981	1983	1984	1984*
Maternal Ethnicity		% Breastfeeding		
Anglo-American	44	45	43	73
Black-American	9	20	10	50
Mexican-American	23	29	33	33
Other	42	37	—	—
Total n	357	411	116	103
Total %BF	27	34	32	70

* A population of middle class mothers from a private practice setting (note only two Black-Americans and 6 Mexican-American mothers are in this group).

Social class might be an underlying factor to ethnicity. However, in this type of population there is little difference between the Anglo- and Black-American groups with respect to social class if education is taken as an indicator. Indeed, 65% of the Black-Americans had completed high school and/or had some college versus 58% of the Anglo-Americans. The difficulty in evaluating this type of population is further illustrated by the problems encountered in attempting to do a six month follow-up study of the mothers who were breastfeeding their infants in the hospital. Of the original 98 mothers only 63 (64.3%) could be contacted despite extensive searches of hospital and telephone records. No differences were noted between those who could be contacted and those who could not be contacted with respect to ethnicity, income, maternal education or marital status. Only 13 (20.1%) of the mothers who could be contacted were still breastfeeding their infants six months after delivery.

SOCIAL SUPPORT

Professional support (18) and psychosocial factors (19) have been implicated as influences in the decision to breastfeed. In addition, support from the husband (20-22), mother of the index mother (23,24) and health care providers (18,25,26) have been identified as being important in influencing the decision of the mother. We have examined the influence and level of support from a preidentified set of social sources and examined their relationship to the breastfeeding decision within the various ethnic groups in our subject population.

Social support was assessed by asking the respondents to evaluate the degree of supportiveness to breastfeeding of the mother's male partner, mother, grandmother, best friend, favorite aunt and children. The question was answered whether or not the mother intended to breastfeed. Social influence was assessed by asking the mother to indicate any two of a list of people and things (husband, mother, grandmother, newspaper article, magazine article, etc.) that were most important in influencing her in her decision to breastfeed.

Table 4. Distributions by Ethnicity for Maternal Perceptions of Social Support for Breastfeeding

	Non Supportive		Unsure		Supportive	
	Total	BF	Total	BF	Total	BF
Anglo-Americans (n=145, BF=63)						
** Male Partner	13	1	35	6	81	52
** Mother	14	4	31	5	90	50
** Grandmother	12	2	33	6	61	35
** Best Friend	13	3	37	7	81	49
** Children	8	1	51	14	24	18
Black-American (n=131, BF=12)						
Male Partner	16	1	53	4	46	6
Mother	17	1	47	1	50	7
Grandmother	10	0	44	3	40	4
Best Friend	24	0	57	4	32	5
Children	9	0	57	6	14	1
Mexican-American (n=62, BF=14)						
*Male Partner	6	1	14	0	38	12
Mother	5	1	14	1	35	10
Grandmother	2	0	15	1	23	8
Best Friend	4	0	21	5	19	6
Children	2	0	16	2	5	2

Significance level of * $p < 0.05$ or ** $p < 0.001$ when testing for independence of the decision to breastfeed and social support.

The degree of social support was rated as non-supportive, unsure or supportive. Each social support variable was significantly different across breastfeeding groups within the Anglo-American group. Thus, the intention to breastfeed is dependent upon social support. In contrast, no such significant differences were seen in the Black-American population and only the male partner was related to breastfeeding in the Mexican-American population (Table 4).

Social influence variables were different among the ethnic groups within the married but not the unmarried mothers. Among the married mothers Anglo- and Black-Americans saw the husband as most influential while the Mexican-Americans saw their mother and husband as the most influential in their decision to breastfeed. Among the not-married group, mother was the most important social influence regardless of the ethnic group (Table 5). The perception of influence was independent of the decision to breastfeed with only a few exceptions: married Anglo-Americans and unmarried Black-Americans with previous breastfeeding experience; and both married and unmarried Mexican-Americans who perceived that the doctor influences their decision to breastfeed.

Table 5. Distribution by Ethnic Group and Marital Status for Two Maternally Perceived Social Influences on the Decision to Breastfeed.

	Married Perceived Influence				Not Married Perceived Influence			
	Yes		No		Yes		No	
	Total n	BF n	Total n	BF n	Total n	BF n	Total n	BF n
Anglo-American								
Husband	48	25	61	28	-	-	-	-
Mother*	21	6	88	47	16	4	20	6
Doctor	11	6	98	47	1	1	35	9
Friend	22	12	87	41	6	2	30	8
Previous BF *	16	13	93	40	7	4	29	6
Black-American								
Husband	19	1	25	3	-	-	-	-
Mother	12	2	32	2	36	3	50	5
Doctor	5	1	39	3	7	1	70	7
Friend	4	1	40	3	16	1	70	7
Previous BF**	0	0	44	4	1	1	85	
Mexican-American								
Husband	16	5	32	8	-	-	-	-
Mother	18	7	30	6	4	0	10	1
Doctor**	7	4	41	9	2	1	12	0
Friend	3	2	45	11	3	1	11	0
Previous BF	0	0	48	13	0	0	14	1

Significance level of $p < 0.05$ when testing for independence of decision to breastfeed and perceived influence in the married * or not married** group.

Interpretation of these data is complicated by the small number of Black and Mexican-Americans who indicated an intent to breastfeed. Also, there is quite a disparity in the marital status of the Anglo-Americans (75% married) versus the Black-Americans (37%). It should also be noted that although the variables of social support and social influence are similar in some cases, further analysis of various combinations showed that only the Anglo-Americans had an apparent dependence in their responses regarding the influence of their husband versus the supportiveness of their male partner. Thus, the lack of strong correlations between the responses to the social influence items and the social support items would imply that there is a difference between perceived social support and social influence.

A logistic model analysis of social support again delineated differences among the ethnic groups. For Anglo-Americans, the male partner's support provides the best explanatory variable with some mild improvement if Best Friend is added to the model. For Black-Americans, Best Friend is most significant in estimating probability of breastfeeding. For the Mexican-Americans, the mother is the most important variable with an independent but secondary contribution from the male partner.

A similar analysis for the social influence variables resulted in no reasonable model for the Black-Americans. Influence variables do not appear to be predictive of breastfeeding in this group. Among the Anglo-Americans, previous breastfeeding experience appears to be the best explanatory variable while for the Mexican-Americans a combination of doctor (most important) mother and best-friend results in the best model for estimating probability of breastfeeding. It was interesting to note that among Anglo-Americans the mother's mother had a consistently negative effect, implying that this individual's influence was usually in a direction away from breastfeeding.

These data imply that in order to increase support for breastfeeding programs should be developed that include the male partner of Anglo-Americans and avoid the mother of the index mother. Friends would appear to be much more important to Black-American women. Mexican-Americans should first be supported via their doctors and then mother of the mother and friends.

ATTITUDES

These mothers also responded to 26 statements about their attitudes to or beliefs about breastfeeding. Their responses were submitted to a factor analysis, such an analysis is a mathematical approach used to reduce the complexity in a common set of items by identifying groups of items which are highly interrelated. These groups of items are called factors and may then be treated as variables in their own right. The name of each factor is generated to reflect the common theme in the items composing that factor. The success of the factor analysis may be assessed by the ease with which such a common theme may be identified. Four factors were found among these 26 items, and we named them as follows: 1. Benefits for infant; 2. Social inconvenience; 3. Personal inconvenience; 4. Physical inconvenience (Table 6). Each factor is important to the extent that it gives us insight into the thinking of the respondents about breastfeeding.

It is important to note from this study that the first factors had the highest item loadings for "benefits for infant", but benefits for other actors were also included. This fact indicates either that mothers have an undifferentiated picture of the benefits of breastfeeding, or that we did a poor job of specifying the many possible benefits. The mothers obviously had a more differentiated picture of the inconveniences in that three factors were necessary to define these items. These factors had a differential importance among the three ethnic groups. The "benefits for infant" factor was proportionately highest among Anglo-American and married mothers. The "social" inconvenience" factor was highest among Black-American and unmarried mothers. The "physical inconvenience" factor was proportionally highest among Mexican-American mothers, adolescents and first pregnancies. In all cases as perceived benefits to the baby increased so did the incidence of intended breastfeeding. The appropriate direction held for the three inconvenience factors, as well.

The initial study of attitudes was limited in that the 26 statements used were taken from items or comments included in the literature and from comments made by mothers during pretesting of the original form. Thus, no theoretical rationale guided the selection of items. As a result, the resulting factor structures might misrepresent the true beliefs/attitudes because not all the domains of these attitudes/beliefs were adequately sampled in the original set of items. Review of the items included in the obtained factors indicated that there may be up to eight factors. We, therefore, generated 98 statements of attitudes/beliefs about breastfeeding. These 98 statements were generated to reflect the eight anticipated factors, including: 1) benefits to the mother, 2) benefits to the child, 3) benefits

Table 6. Four Factors Derived from Maternal Statements Regarding Their Attitudes Towards Infant Feeding Practices

Item	Loading
Factor 1 (27.5% Variance) Benefits for Infant	
Breastfeeding	
...is best for the baby	0.86
...is best for the health of my baby	0.79
...is more natural	0.79
...is more nutritional	0.75
...brings mother and child close together	0.66
...is more personally satisfying	0.60
...for even a short time is important	0.57
...gives my baby special immunities	0.55
...is more convenient	0.52
Factor 2 (9.2% Variance) Social Inconvenience	
Breastfeeding	
...causes people to have sex less often	0.75
...would make it difficult for me to see my friends	0.74
...would come between me and my husband or boyfriend	0.68
...would make it difficult for me to go to meetings	0.58
...in public is embarrassing	0.43
Factor 3 (6.1% Variance) Personal Inconvenience	
Breastfeeding can be very annoying	0.69
Breastfeeding does not appeal to me	0.65
Bottle feeding is more convenient	0.61
Breastfeeding ties me down	0.60
I am too nervous to breastfeed	0.48
Breastfeeding would make it difficult for me to go to meetings	0.44
Breastfeeding is more convenient	-0.55
Factor 4 (4.9%) Variance) Physical Inconvenience	
Breastfeeding may hurt	0.72
Breastfeeding makes the breast too big	0.52
There is no medical proof that breastmilk is best for my baby	-0.40
Breastfeeding prevents allergies	-0.43
Breastfeeding gives my baby special immunities	0.47

to the mother-child relationship, 4) physical convenience - inconvenience, 5) personal convenience - inconvenience, 6) social convenience - inconvenience, 7) attitudes toward the nursing act, and 8) work-school related attitudes. Items were written in roughly equal proportions about these potential factors in regard to breast and formula feeding separately. Within each factor/type of feeding item group, items were written in roughly equal numbers to be positive or negative to the factor/type of feeding concept. All these items were included in a questionnaire completed by a sample of all mothers.

Items from each of the proposed benefits scales loaded on the first factor. This finding indicates that the mothers have a general perception of undifferentiated benefits of breastfeeding. In addition, this factor taps only breastfeeding items, and not formula feeding items. indicating that the beliefs of the benefits of one form of infant feeding are not related to the beliefs about the benefits of the other form of feeding.

The second factor included items on the social inconveniences of breastfeeding and conveniences of formula feeding, including both breastfeeding and formula feeding items. The third factor concerned the inconveniences of formula feeding, including virtually no breastfeeding items. The fourth factor generally included statements relating to health concerns about either breast- or formula-feeding.

Several things are important to note from these analyses. Beliefs about the benefits of breastfeeding are independent of beliefs about formula feeding. This finding would indicate that mothers who believe that breastfeeding is beneficial do not necessarily believe that formula feeding is not beneficial. In addition, the perception of the benefits of breastfeeding in this sample are broadly undifferentiated. This data tends to indicate that if a mother perceives one kind of benefit she sees many others as well.

Breastfeeding and formula feeding beliefs are interrelated, however, in the areas of social convenience/inconvenience and health concerns. In particular, if a mother perceives social inconveniences from breastfeeding, she is likely to see a variety of conveniences from formula feeding. In the same way, if a mother perceives health concerns from breastfeeding, the mother is likely to see some health benefits from formula feeding.

The generally perceived inconveniences of formula feeding are not tied to inconveniences of breastfeeding. Why the benefits of breastfeeding constitute one factor, while the inconveniences of formula feeding constitute a separate independent factor is worth further exploration.

When these same items were given to a middle class population of mothers in a private pediatric practice the factors were similar, with some notable differences. The factors among these middle class mothers more closely interrelated the breast and formula feeding beliefs. The first factor provided a clear picture of positive attitudes toward the general benefits of breastfeeding, which were negatively correlated with attitudes toward formula feeding. It is also important to note that there is no differentiation in the first factor among the various categories of benefits to breastfeeding.

Social factors were contained in the second factor, emphasizing, however, the social inconveniences of breastfeeding without emphasizing the benefits of formula feeding. The health concerns of both formula and breastfeeding were identified in factor 3, without an expected inverse relationship between the value of formula versus breastfeeding items in the factor. The determination of the relationship of these items to the act of breastfeeding remains to be completed. Reflecting our earlier analyses, we expect these relationships to be significant and in the expected directions.

Several general points can be made about these analyses. There seem to be similar structures in the two samples, including three factors: general benefits of breastfeeding, social inconveniences of breastfeeding, and health concerns. Four differences in structure exist between the two populations, especially in the extent to which attitudes toward breastfeeding and formula feeding are integrated. The lack of differentiation among perceived benefits, or perceived inconveniences, probably reveals a lack of intense thought and discussion about these issues. We obviously know little about the beliefs of mothers toward infant feeding. Further exploration of these relationships are clearly warranted to provide a sounder basis for intervention programs to promote breastfeeding.

These latter investigations have not yet been fully investigated with respect to the ethnic influences on attitudes. However, the initial investigation showed that this would appear to be a fruitful avenue of investigation in further understanding the factors involved in deciding to initiate and maintain breastfeeding.

CONCLUSIONS

Ethnicity appears to be an important factor in breastfeeding behavior in the United States. We have identified and characterized a population of predominantly disadvantaged mothers who are more likely to formula-feed than breastfeed. Ethnicity appears to be the overriding influence on the breastfeeding decision in this population. The key supportive individuals vary by ethnic background. Maternal attitudes; such as regards benefits to baby, and personal inconvenience, are strongly related to the breastfeeding decision, but these also vary by ethnic group. Our overall conclusions are that:

- The incidence of breastfeeding is low in a low socioeconomic group of U.S. mothers.
- The incidence of breastfeeding is especially low among Black-American mothers.
- Prenatal care does not appear to influence breastfeeding.
- Education and social class influence breastfeeding.
- Maternal or neonatal medical problems decrease breastfeeding.
- Previous breastfeeding behavior increases breastfeeding.
- Women with greater self-efficacy are more likely to breastfeed.
- Social support is important to the decision to breastfeed but varies by ethnic group and marital status.
- Maternal attitudes are important to the decision to breastfeed and vary by ethnic background.
- Personal inconvenience is a significant detractor to breastfeeding behavior.
- Maternal concern for the infant's welfare tended to be a better predictor of breastfeeding as opposed to her concerns for her own welfare.

Thus, a number of important features to the decision to breastfeed may be observed in examining this triethnic population. It must especially be kept in mind that programs to encourage breastfeeding behavior must address these ethnic differences that exist among U.S. mothers. In addition, our data regarding distribution of breastfeeding mothers among ethnic groups compares well with national data (5,10,14), implying that extrapolation to the national situation may be valid. Previous comparisons of cultural influences on lactation performance have primarily examined such disparate, but homogeneous, areas as Kenaba in The Gambia versus Cambridge, England or Swedish mothers versus Ethiopian mothers (see elsewhere in this volume). It may be of more importance in understanding cultural influences to examine variations within a single heterogenous population, such as in the urban areas of the United States or the United Kingdom, where similar environmental or geographic influences still breed very different behaviors with respect to breastfeeding as a result of varying cultural beliefs.

REFERENCES

1. Committee on Nutrition of the American Academy of Pediatrics, Breast-feeding: A commentary in celebration of the international year of the child, 1979, Pediatrics 62:591 (1978).
2. ESPGAN Committee on Nutrition, Guidelines on infant nutrition: I. Recommendations for the composition of an adapted formula, Acta Paediatr. Scand. (Suppl.) 262:3 (1977).
3. G.A. Martinez, D.A. Dodd, and J.A. Samartgedes. Milk feeding patterns in the United States during the first 12 months of life, Pediatrics 68:863 (1981).
4. G.A. Martinez and J.P. Nalezienski. 1980 Update: The recent trend in breastfeeding, Pediatrics 67:260 (1981).
5. G.A. Martinez and F.W. Krieger, 1984 Milk-feeding patterns in the United States, Pediatrics 76:1004 (1985).
6. D.B. Jelliffe and E.F.P. Jelliffe, "Human Milk in the Modern World", Oxford University Press, Oxford (1978).
7. "Breastfeeding and the Mother", Ciba Foundation Symposium 45 (new series), Elsevier, North Holland (1976).
8. G.E. Gaull, R.G. Jensen, D.K. Rassin, and M.H. Malloy. Human milk as food, Advances in Perinatal Med. 2:47(1982).
9. Report of the task force on the assessment of the scientfic evidence relating to infant-feeding practices and infant health, Pediatrics 74:579 (1984).
10. Report of the surgeon general's workshop on breastfeeding and human lactation, DHHS Publication No. HRS-D-MC 84-2, (1984).
11. C. Hirschman and G.E. Hendershot. Trends in breastfeeding among American mothers, USDHEW Pub. No. PHS 79-1979 (1979).
12. G.E. Hendershot. Trends in breastfeeding, USDHEW Pub. No. 80-1250 (1980).
13. A.P. Simopoulos and G.D. Grove. Factors associted with the choice and duration of infant-feeding practice. Pediatrics 74:603 (1984).
14. M.R. Forman, K. Fetterly, B.I. Graubard, and K.G. Wooten. Exclusive breastfeeding of newborns among married women in the United States: The National Natality Surveys of 1969 and 1980, Am. J. Clin. Nutr. 42:864 (1985).
15. D.K. Rassin, C.J. Richardson, T. Baranowski, P.R. Nader, N. Guenther, D.E. Bee, and J.P. Brown. Incidence of breastfeeding in a low socioeconomic group of mothers in the United States: Ethnic patterns, Pediatrics 73:132 (1984).
16. T. Baranowski, D.E. Bee, D.K. Rassin, C.J. Richardson, J.P. Brown, N. Guenther, and P.R. Nader. Social support, social influence, ethnicity and the breastfeeding decision, Soc. Sci. Med. 17:1599 (1983).

17. T. Baranowski, D.K. Rassin, C.J. Richardson, J.P. Brown, D.E. Bee, and N. Guenther. Attitudes toward breastfeeding (submitted).
18. B. Winikoff and E.C. Baer. The obstetrician's opportunity: Translating "Breast is best" from theory to practice. Am. J. Obstet. Gynecol. 138:105 (1980).
19. A. Bentovim. Shame and other anxieties associated with breastfeeding: A systems theory and psychodynamic approach, in: "Breastfeeding and the Mother". Ciba Foundation Symposium 45 (new series), Elsevier, North-Holland (1976).
20. C.J. Bacon and J.M. Wylie. Mother's attitudes to infant feeding at Newcastle General Hospital in Summer, 1975. Br. Med J. 1: 308 (1976).
21. E. Eastham, D. Smith, D. Poole, and G. Neligan. Further decline of breastfeeding, Br. Med. J. 1:305 (1976).
22. E.H. Rousseau, J.N. Lescop, S. Fontaine, J. Lambert and C.C. Roy. Influence of culture and environmental factors on breast-feeding, Can. Med. Assoc. J. 127:701(1982).
23. S. Mackey and P.A. Fried. Infant breast bottle feeding practices: Some related factor and attitudes, Can. J. Publ. Hlth. 72:312 (1981).
24. B. Oseid, J.P. Carter, J. Brown, J. Sullivan, C. Chang, and P. Gendel. Characteristics and outcome of low-income urban women who choose to breastfeed, APA Abstract, Washington, D.C., 1982.
25. R.A.K. Jones and E.M. Belsey. Breastfeeding in an inner London borough - A study of cultural factors, Soc. Sci. Med. 11:175 (1977).
26. D.L. Yeung, M.D. Pennell, M. Leung, and J. Hall. Breastfeeding: Prevalence and influencing factors, Can. J. Publ. Hlth. 72:323 (1981).

EFFECTS OF VEGETARIAN DIETS UPON THE COMPOSITION OF HUMAN MILK

Dorothy Ann Finley

Department of Nutrition
University of California
Davis, CA

INTRODUCTION

Nutrients of concern when vegetarian diets are analyzed for adequacy include: protein, iron, calcium, zinc, iodine, riboflavin, vitamin B-12 and vitamin D. With careful planning it is possible for a lacto-ovo-vegetarian to meet or exceed the dietary requirement for all nutrients. Since vitamin B-12 is found only in animal products, very strict vegetarians cannot meet their vitamin B-12 requirement through diet. In this review, the effect of diet on breast milk composition will be examined with particular emphasis on those nutrients likely to be inadequate in vegetarian diets. In addition, the effect of dietary fat on the composition of breast milk will be considered.

PROTEIN

Early research on the effect of maternal diet on the protein concentration of milk suffered from methological inadequacies.[1] Many recent studies have reported that protein concentration of milk from poor malnourished women is not different from that of relatively affluent, well-nourished women.[2-5] Exceptions have been noted, however.[6,7]

One recent study examined the protein concentration of milk from well-nourished lacto-ovo-vegetarian and non-vegetarian American women.[8] The protein concentration of the milk decreased rapidly during the first month of lactation, but there was no significant correlation between month of lactation and protein concentration for the period 2-15 months of lactation. The level of protein in milk from the two groups of women was not significantly different during the first 6 months of lactation, however, during months 7-15 of lactation, the milk from vegetarians contained a significantly lower percentage of protein (1.44 ± 0.46%, mean ± SD, n=52 samples from 11 women) than milk from non-vegetarians (1.83 ± 0.48%, n=21 samples from 16 women). There was no significant difference in total energy intake between the two groups of women. Although mean protein intake of both groups of women was over 100% of the RDA for protein, the protein intake of the vegetarian women (79 ± 26 g/day, n=99 records from 11 women) was significantly less than that of the non-vegetarian women (95 ± 30 g/day, n=73 records from 16 women). Vegetarians consumed 31% of their protein as animal protein and non-vegetarians consumed 64% as animal protein. Unfortunately, in this research the effect of total protein intake cannot be separated from that of protein source.

The results of protein supplementation on human milk protein levels have been inconsistent. Of six studies identified, three reported an increase in protein concentration following supplementation;[9-11] two showed no change in protein concentration;[12,13] and a sixth study reported that milk protein concentration decreased and milk volume increased following protein supplementation with the result that 24-hour total protein output did not change.[14,15] Edozien et al.[13] have also found an increase in milk volume with protein supplementation, but Karmarkar et al.[9] and Deb and Cama[12] found no increase in milk yield with supplementation. Most of these studies were confounded in that the supplementation not only increased maternal protein intake, but also total energy intake. Although Deb and Cama[12] did not find any change in protein concentration in milk with supplementation, they reported that the protein supplementation had an effect on protein composition of the milk.

Forsum and Lonnerdal[11] studied three healthy, well-nourished Swedish women who consumed between 40 and 52 grams protein/day (8% energy from protein) followed by between 100 and 165 grams protein/day (20% energy from protein) and found significantly higher total nitrogen, true protein, non-protein-nitrogen concentrations and total output of milk during the period of higher protein intake. For each woman, total energy intake was similar in the two dietary periods.

It appears therefore that at least under certain conditions, the protein fraction of milk can be affected by maternal dietary intake of protein and/or of total energy. Further work should attempt to separate the effects of source and amount of protein from those of total energy.

MINERALS

Most recent studies have concluded that there is little, if any, change in milk calcium with changes in calcium intake,[7,16,17] with milk from malnourished women having concentrations in the lower region of the normal range. However, a study from Brazil reported that milk from women in the low socioeconomic group showed a tendency to have higher mean values than that from women in the higher socioeconomic group.[2] Similar results were found when milk from Ethiopian women was compared with that from Swedish women: higher mean calcium concentration was found in milk samples from the Ethiopian women than in those from the Swedish women, the highest mean concentration being noted in the non-privileged Ethiopian group.[18] On the other hand, Bailey[19] and Jansen et al.[20] reported low milk calcium levels in women from New Guinea compared to published normal values. This finding may be explained by exceptionally low intakes of calcium in this region and agree with findings of poor skeletal calcification of infants in this area. Greer et al.[21] reported a correlation between maternal calcium intake and milk calcium in American women; however, others have not found a correlation between them.[8,22] In a study of American lactating lacto-ovo-vegetarian women,[8,23] there was no difference in calcium intake between the vegetarians and non-vegetarians and no difference in the calcium concentration of their milk.

Most recent work has found no relationship between the iron status of the mother and the iron content of her milk.[15,26-28] However, Fransson et al.[29] found milk iron levels were significantly higher in severely anemic Indian mothers (Hb ≤ 8 g/dl) than in mothers having higher or normal hemoglobin values. Concentration of the major iron-binding protein of human milk, lactoferrin, was also higher in anemic mothers. No effect of dietary iron has been found on the level of iron in the milk.[7,8,17,18,22,25,27,30] Supplemental iron did not increase milk iron in humans,[25] cows[31] or sows,[32] although iron level in milk of rats can be increased by iron supplementation.[33-35]

In well-nourished women, no relationship has been found between maternal dietary zinc intake and the zinc concentration in her milk.[8,17,22,30] In addition, supplemental zinc did not increase milk zinc levels.[17,36,37] In one study, however, milk zinc was slightly higher in late lactation (months 9-12) in women supplemented with 13 mg zinc/day during lactation than in unsupplemented women.[38] There is one report in which low levels of breast milk zinc might have been related to zinc deficiency.[39] However, dietary supplementation of the mothers did not increase the zinc content of their milk. It has been pointed out, however, that the concentration of zinc in milk from mothers living in parts of the world where populations show chronic zinc deficiency has not been determined.[24] There is evidence from work with sows,[40] cows[41] and rats[35,42] that zinc intake can affect milk zinc levels.

Recent reports on the effect of maternal dietary iodine intake on breast milk iodine are inconsistent.[44,45] Iodine which is concentrated in breast milk (higher levels than in serum) can be absorbed from medical preparations of iodine.[43] It appears that milk iodine concentrations are higher today than in the 1930's.[44]

In summary, it appears that the concentrations of calcium, iron, zinc and iodine in milk are relatively independent of maternal mineral intake. Since vegetarian women are more likely to consume lower levels of these nutrients in readily available forms than non-vegetarians, a major concern is whether maternal mineral status is being compromised if intake does not provide sufficient mineral to meet the increased demands of lactation.

VITAMINS

The concentrations of water soluble vitamins appear to be dependent upon maternal dietary intake, particularly when maternal intake is low. The milk of malnourished women with low riboflavin intakes contains low levels of these vitamins, and the levels can be increased by vitamin supplementation.[10,46,47] In well-nourished American women milk riboflavin levels were increased by increasing maternal intake.[48]

The level of vitamin B-12 in milk usually reflects maternal dietary intake,[46,49-52] although Sandberg et al.[53] reported that the vitamin B-12 content of milk from 10 American mothers taking between 5 and 100 μg of supplemental cyanocobalamin daily was not significantly different from that of unsupplemented mothers. Jathar et al.[54] reported mean serum and milk vitamin B-12 levels in lacto-vegetarian women and non-vegetarian women. The vegetarians had lower serum values but milk levels were not different between the groups, and there was no significant correlation between the vitamin B-12 content of serum and that of milk. The authors point out that the values for milk vitamin B-12 were very low compared to those reported for milk from women in developed countries using similar methods. There is clinical evidence that milk vitamin B-12 levels are related to maternal intake. Solely breast-fed Indian infants have developed a syndrome of tremors ascribed to a deficiency of vitamin B-12 in their mother's milk.[55] There is also a report of a vitamin B-12 deficient American child who was nursed by a strict vegetarian.[56] Other workers have reported low vitamin B-12 concentrations in milk of women consuming a largely vegetarian diet.[46] Supplementation of such women with vitamin B-12 increased milk vitamin B-12 levels.[46]

Low maternal vitamin D status results in a low level of vitamin D in milk,[57] while supplemental vitamin D given to mothers with adequate vitamin D status results in significantly higher levels of milk vitamin D.[57,58] Vitamin D deficiency has been reported in breast fed black American children who were not receiving vitamin D supplements.[59,60]

In summary, the levels of riboflavin, vitamin B-12 and vitamin D in breast milk are related to maternal intake. If the mother is a vegetarian, particularly a very strict one, maternal intake of these vitamins is likely to be low, and this would be reflected in her breast milk.

FAT

Karmarkar and Ramakrishnan[7,61] reported that the concentration of fat in the milk of Indian women was correlated with the level of dietary fat during lactation when a woman's dietary fat level was 70 g/day or lower, but that when women consumed between 70 and 115 g/day the fat level in their milk was not higher than that in women consuming between 50 and 70 g fat/day. Milk fat concentration increased with supplementary dietary fat up to a total fat intake of 50-55 g/day but did not increase further when total fat intake was increased to 60-65 g/day.[9] (Lactating American women consume approximately 90 grams fat per day.) Crawford et al.[62] reported that samples obtained when one breast was completely emptied by undernourished East African mothers often contained less than 1-2% fat.

Deb and Cama[12] studied one Indian woman whose habitual protein intake was 46 g protein/day. Her dietary protein intake was controlled from day 48 to day 240 of lactation: first she consumed 46 g protein/day for 40 days, this was followed by four 40 day periods in which she consumed 60, 46, 70 and 46 g/day, respectively. With each cycle the fat concentration of her milk increased or decreased according to the dietary protein level. Similar results were seen when 9 other women were supplemented in a like manner.

It may be that the effects of supplementary fat or protein on milk fat are because the supplements increase maternal total energy intake rather than an effect of the particular nutrient per se. A recent study of rural African women by Prentice et al.[63] found that mean breast milk fat concentrations were affected by season of the year in a manner that correlated with seasonal changes in maternal subcutaneous fat stores but not with seasonal variations in maternal energy intake.

Maternal nutritional status can therefore affect milk fat concentration: milk fat concentration may be related to low energy intakes, extremely low dietary fat intake and subcutaneous fat stores (produced by a balance of energy intake and energy expenditure) when nutritional status is low.

The fatty acid pattern of milk can be changed without affecting the milk volume or milk fat output by changes in the type of dietary fat,[64-70] by changes in energy intake,[64] and by changes in dietary carbohydrate level.[64,70-74] During energy equilibrium and low to moderate carbohydrate intake, milk fat resembles dietary fatty acid pattern; when there is inadequate energy consumption, milk fat reflects the composition of subcutaneous depot fat.[64] High dietary carbohydrate levels, either a high percentage of carbohydrate in the diet[72,73] or excess dietary energy due to excess carbohydrate,[64] result in breast milk with high levels of lauric (C12:0) and myristic (C14:0) acids and low levels of linoleic acid (C18:2n-6).

Two papers have studied the specific effects of vegetarian diets on the fatty acid composition of breast milk. In one study milk from 4 vegans was analyzed;[75] in the other, milk from 27 lacto-ovo-vegetarians was analyzed.[76] Among vegetarians in both studies milk levels of C16:0, C16:1, C18:0 and C18:1, all fatty acids high in animal fat, were either significantly lower or showed strong downward trends compared to non-vegetarians.

Milk from women supplemented with fish oil[77] or who frequently consume fish,[76,78] the only food containing C22:6n-3 in significant quantities, contains more of this fatty acid than milk from women who do not consume fish oil or fish. The fatty acid C22:6n-3 is abundant in the brain's structural lipids[79] and therefore its level in human milk is of particular interest.

In a like manner, maternal intake of trans fatty acids is reflected in milk.[76,80-82] Vegetarian women who choose solid vegetable oil over butter as a spread and for cooking would, therefore, likely produce milk with a higher proportion of trans-fatty acids than women who consume butter and oils. On the other hand, Akesson and coworkers[83] reported that the trans-fatty acid content of commonly consumed vegetarian diets in Sweden is lower than that of non-vegetarian diets. Intake of trans-fatty acids by rapidly growing children is a particular concern since these unsaturated fatty acids behave like saturated fatty acids.[84]

SUMMARY AND CONCLUSION

There is considerable evidence that maternal diet has an effect on the composition of her milk. Milk from well-nourished vegetarians would be expected to be similar to that of well-nourished non-vegetarian women except that the fatty acid pattern would reflect the lower intake of saturated fatty acids and higher intake of unsaturated fatty acids by the vegetarians.

The situation among poorly-nourished vegetarians is more complicated. There are several reasons for malnutrition among vegetarian women: poverty and the subsequent inability to obtain an adequate diet, inattention to diet planning or participation in a cult that not only severely restricts intake of animal products, but also other foods. It appears that supplementation with either protein or fat can have an effect on milk composition and perhaps milk yield if the woman is eating insufficient energy. In addition, breast milk will reflect low dietary intake of vitamins. More work is needed to determine specific effects of malnutrition on the composition of milk from vegetarian women particularly the effects of low mineral intake on maternal mineral status.

REFERENCES

1. S. D. Morrison, Human Milk: Yield, Proximate Principles and Inorganic Constituents, Technical Communications No. 18, Commonwealth Agricultural Bureau, Slough, England (1952).
2. T. A. Carneiro and J. E. Dutra de Oliveira, Nutritional studies in human lactation in Brazil. 1. Chemical composition of breast milk. J. Trop. Pediatr. Environ. Child Health 19:284 (1973).
3. B. S. Lindbald and R. J. Rahimtolla, A pilot study of the quality of human milk in a lower socio-economic group in Karachi, Pakistan. Acta Paediatr. Sand. 63:125 (1974).
4. B. Lonnerdal, E. Forsum, M. Gebre-Medhin, and L. Hambraeus, Breast milk composition in Ethiopian and Swedish mothers. II. Lactose, nitrogen, and protein contents. Am. J. Clin. Nutr. 29:1134 (1976).
5. W. M. Van Steenbergen, J. A. Kusin, C. De With, E. Lacko, and A. J. Jansen, Lactating performance of mothers with contrasting nutritional studies in rural Kenya, Acta Paediatr. Scand. 72:805 (1983).
6. M. M. Hanafy, M. R. A. Morsey, Y. Seddick, Y. A. Habib, and E. el Lozy, Maternal nutrition and lactation performance, J. Trop. Pediatr. Environ. Child Health 18:187 (1972).
7. M. G. Karmarkar and C. V. Ramakrishnan, Studies on human lactation. Relation between the dietary intake of lactating women and the chemical composition of milk with regard to principal and certain inorganic constituents. Acta Paediatr. 49:599 (1960).
8. D. A. Finley, B. Lonnerdal, K. G. Dewey, and L. E. Grivetti, Inorganic constituents of breast milk from vegetarian and non-vegetarian women: Relationships with each other and with organic constituents, J. Nutr. 115:772 (1985).
9. M. G. Karmarkar, R. Rajalakshmi, and C. V. Ramakrishnan, Studies on human lactation. I. Effect of dietary protein and fat supplementation of protein, fat and essential amino acid contents of breast milk. Acta Paediatr. 52:473 (1963).
10. A. M. Prentice, S. B. Roberts, A. Prentice, A. A. Paul, M. Watkinson, A. A. Watkinson, and R. G. Whitehead, Dietary supplementation of lactating Gambian women. I. Effect on breast-milk volume and quality. Human Nutr.: Clin. Nutr. 37C:53 (1983).
11. E. Forsum and B. Lonnerdal, Effect of protein intake on protein and nitrogen composition of breast milk, Am. J. Clin. Nutr. 33:1809 (1980).
12. A. K. Deb and H. R. Cama, Studies on human lactation. Dietary nitrogen utilization during lactation, and distribution of nitrogen in mother's milk. Brit. J. Nutr. 16:65 (1962).
13. J. C. Edozien, M. A. Rahim Khan, and C. I. Waslien, Human protein deficiency: Results of a Nigerian village study. J. Nutr. 106:312 (1976).
14. C. Gopalan, Studies on lactation in poor Indian communities. J Trop. Pediatr. 4:87 (1958).
15. C. Gopalan and B. Belavady, Nutrition and lactation. Fed. Proc. 20(suppl. 7):177 (1961).
16. L. J. Filer, Maternal nutrition in lactation, in: "Clinics in Perinatology," L. A. Barness and R. M. Pitkin, eds., W. B. Saunders Co., Philadelphia (1975).
17. A. Kirksey, J. A. Ernst, J. L. Roepke, and T.-L. Tsai, Influence of mineral intake and use of oral contraceptives before pregnancy on the mineral content of human colostrum and of more mature milk. Am. J. Clin. Nutr. 32:30 (1979).

18. G.-B. Frannson, M. Gebre-Medhin, and L. Hambraeus, The human milk contents of iron, copper, zinc, calcium and magnesium in a population with a habitually high intake of iron, Acta Paediatr. Scand. 73:471 (1984).
19. K. V. Bailey, Quantity and composition of breastmilk in some New Guinean populations, J. Trop. Pediatr. 11:35 (1965).
20. A. A. Jansen, R. Luyken, S. H. Malcolm, and J. J. L. Willems, Quantity and composition of breast milk in Biak Island (Net. New Guinea), Trop Geog. Med. 2:138 (1960).
21. F. R. Greer, R. C. Tsang, J. E. Saercy, R. S. Levin, and J. J. Steichen, Mineral homeostasis during lactation-relationship to serum 1,25-dihydroxyvitamin D, 25-hydroxyvitamin D, parathyroid hormone, and calcitonin, Am. J. Clin. Nutr. 36:431 (1982).
22. L. A. Vaughn, C. W. Weber, and S. R. Kemberling, Longitudinal changes in the mineral content of human milk, Am. J. Clin. Nutr. 32:2301 (1979).
23. D. A. Finley, K. G. Dewey, B. Lonnerdal, and L. E. Grivetti, Food choices of vegetarians and nonvegetarians during pregnancy and lactation, J Am. Diet. Assn. 85:678 (1985).
24. E. C. Casey and K. M. Hambidge, Nutritional aspects of human lactation, in: "Lactation. Physiology, Nutrition and Breast-Feeding," M. E. Neville and M. R. Neifert, eds., Plenum Press, New York (1983).
25. M. F. Picciano and H. A. Guthrie, Copper, iron, and zinc contents of mature human milk, Am. J. Clin. Nutr. 29:242 (1976).
26. T. T. Loh and T. A. Sinnathury, Haematological data and milk iron in Malaysian women, Aust. N.Z. J. Obstet. Gynaecol. 11:254 (1971).
27. M. J. Murray, A. B. Murray, N. J. Murray, and M. B. Murray, The effect of iron status of Nigerien mothers on that of their infants at birth and 6 months, and on the concentration of Fe in breast milk, Brit. J. Nutr. 39:627 (1978).
28. A. Celada, R. Brusset, J. Gutierrez, and V. Herreros, No correlation between iron concentration in breast milk and maternal iron stores, Helv. Paediatr. Acta 37:11 (1982).
29. G.-B. Fransson, K. N. Agarwal, M. Gebre-Medhin, and L. Hambraeus, Increased breast milk iron in severe maternal anemia. Physiological trapping or leakage? Acta Paediatr. Scand. 74:290 (1985).
30. E. Vuori, S. M. Makinen, R. Kara, and P. Kuitunen, The effects of the dietary intakes of copper, iron, manganese, and zinc on the trace element content of human milk, Am. J. Clin. Nutr. 33:227 (1980).
31. E. J. Underwood, "Trace Elements in Human and Animal Nutrition," Academic Press, New York (1971).
32. W. G. Pond, T. L. Veum, and V. A. Lazar, Zinc and iron concentrations of sows' milk, J. An. Sci. 24:668 (1965).
33. E. Ezekiel and E. H. Morgan, Milk iron and its metabolism in the lactating rat, J. Physiol. 165:336 (1963).
34. D. Carmichael, J. Hegenauer, M. Lem, L. Ripley, P. Saltman, and L. Hatlen, Iron supplementation of the lactating mouse and suckling neonates, J. Nutr. 107:1377 (1977).
35. C. L. Keen, B. Lonnerdal, M. V. Sloan, and L. S. Hurley, Effect of dietary iron, copper and zinc chelates of nitrilotriacetic acid (NTA) on trace metal concentrations in rat milk and maternal and pup tissues, J. Nutr. 110:897 (1980).
36. R. M. Freeley, R. R. Eitenmiller, J. B. Jones, Jr., and H. Barnhart, Copper, iron and zinc contents of human milk at early stages of lactation, Am. J. Clin. Nutr. 37:443 (1983).
37. P. B. Moser, D. Allen, and R. Reynolds, Analyzed zinc intakes of postpartum women and zinc concentration of breast milk, Fed. Proc. 41:351 (1982).

38. N. F. Krebs, K. M. Hambidge, M. A. Jacobs, and J. D. Rasbach, The effects of a dietary zinc supplement during lactation on longitudinal changes in maternal zinc status and milk zinc concentrations, Am. J. Clin. Nutr. 41:560 (1985).
39. A. W. Zimmerman and K. M. Hambidge, Low zinc in mothers' milk and zinc deficiency syndrome in breast-fed premature infants, Am. J. Clin. Nutr. 33:951 (1980).
40. I. P. Earle and J. W. Stevenson, Relation of dietary zinc to composition of sow colostrum and milk, J. An. Sci. 24:325 (1965).
41. W. J. Miller, C. M. Clifton, and P. R. Fowler, High levels of dietary zinc on content in milk, J. An. Sci. 23:885 (1964).
42. P. B. Mutch and L. S. Hurley, Effect of zinc deficiency during lactation on postnatal growth and development of rats, J. Nutr. 104:828 (1974).
43. D. C. Postellon and R. Aronow, Iodine in mother's milk, JAMA 247:463 (1982).
44. C. A. Gushurst, J. A. Mueller, J. A. Green, and F. Sedor, Breast milk iodide: Reassessment in the 1980's, Pediatr. 73:354 (1984).
45. J. C. Bruhn and A. A. Franke, Iodine in human milk, J. Dairy Sci. 66:1396 (1983).
46. A. D. Deodhar, R. Rajalakshmi, and C. V. Ramakrishnan, Studies on human lactation. Part III. Effect of dietary vitamin supplementation on vitamin contents of breast milk. Acta Paediatr. Scand. 53:42 (1964).
47. C. J. Bates, D. Phil, A. M. Prentice, M. Watkinson, P. Morrell, B. A. Sutcliffe, F. A. Foord, and R. G. Whitehead, Riboflavin requirements of lactating Gambian women: A controlled supplementation trial, Am. J. Clin. Nutr. 135:701 (1982).
48. P. A. Nail, M. R. Thomas, and R. Eakin, The effect of thiamin and riboflavin supplementation on the level of those vitamins in human breast milk and urine, Am. J. Clin. Nutr. 33:198 (1980).
49. A. M. Prentice, Variations in maternal dietary intake, birthweight and breast-milk output in The Gambia, in: "Maternal Nutrition During Pregnancy and Lactation," H. Aebi and R. Whitehead, eds., Hans Huber Publishing (1979).
50. M. R. Thomas, J. Kawamoto, S. M. Sneed, and R. Eakin, The effects of vitamin C, vitamin B-6 and vitamin B-12 supplementation on the breast milk and maternal status of well-nourished women, Am. J. Clin. Nutr. 32:1679 (1979).
51. M. R. Thomas, S. M. Sneed, C. Wei, P. A. Nail, M. J. Wilson, and E. E. Sprinkle III, The effects of vitamin C, vitamin B-6, vitamin B-12, folic acid, riboflavin and thiamin on the breast milk and maternal status of well-nourished women at 6 months postpartum, Am. J. Clin. Nutr. 33:2151 (1980).
52. S. M. Sneed, C. Zane, and M. R. Thomas, The effects of ascorbic acid, vitamin B-6, vitamin B-12 and folic acid supplementation on the breast milk and maternal nutritional status of low socioeconomic lactating women, Am. J. Clin. Nutr. 34:1338 (1981).
53. D. P. Sandberg, J. A. Begley, and C. A. Hall, The content, binding and forms of vitamin B-12 in milk, Am. J. Clin. Nutr. 34:1717 (1981).
54. V. S. Jathar, S. A. Kamath, M. N. Parikh, D. V. Rege, and R. S. Satoskar, Maternal milk and serum vitamin B-12, folic acid, and protein levels in Indian subjects, Arch. Dis. Child. 45:236 (1970).
55. M. Jadhav, J. K. G. Webb, S. Vaishnava, and S. J. Baker, Vitamin B-12 deficiency in Indian infants, Lancet 2:903 (1962).
56. M. C. Higginbottom, L. Sweetman, and W. L. Nyhan, A syndrome of methylmalonic aciduria, homocystinuria, megaloblastic anemia and neurological abnormalities in a vitamin B-12 deficient breast-fed infant of a strict vegetarian, N. Engl. J. Med. 299:317 (1978).

57. B. W. Hollis, P. W. Lambert, and R. L. Horst, Factors affecting the antirachitic sterol content of native milk, in: "Perinatal Calcium and Phosphorus Metabolism," M. F. Holick, T. K. Gray, and C. S. Anast, eds., Elsevier, Amsterdam (1983).
58. L. J. Polskin, B. Kramer, and A. E. Sobel, Secretion of vitamin D in milks of women fed fish liver oil, J. Nutr. 30:451 (1945).
59. P. O'Connor, Vitamin D-deficiency rickets in two breast-fed infants who were not receiving vitamin D supplementation, Clin. Pediatr. 16:361 (1977).
60. J. T. Dwyer, W. H. Dietz, G. Hass, and R. Suskind, Risk of nutritional rickets among vegetarian children, Am. J. Dis. Child. 133:134 (1979).
61. M. G. Karmarkar and C. V. Ramakrishnan, Relation between dietary fat, fat content of milk and concentration of certain enzymes in human milk, J. Nutr. 69:274 (1959).
62. M. Crawford, B. Hall, B. M. Laurance, and A. Munhambo, Milk lipids and their variability, Current Med. Res. Opinion 4:33 (1976).
63. A. Prentice, A. M. Prentice, and R. G. Whitehead, Breast-milk fat concentrations of rural African women. 2. Long-term variations within a community, Brit. J. Nutr. 45:495 (1981).
64. W. Insull, Jr., J. Hirsch, T. James, and E. H. Ahrens, Jr., The fatty acids of human milk. II. Alternations produced by manipulation of calorie balance and exchange of dietary fats, J. Clin. Invest. 33:442 (1959).
65. M. Kramer, K. Szoke, K. Linder, and R. Tarjan, The effect of different factors on the composition of human milk and its variation. III. Effect of dietary fats on the lipid composition of human milk, Nutr. Dieta. 7:71 (1965).
66. J. A. F. Rook and R. C. Witter, Diet and milk secretion in the sow, Proc. Nutr. Soc. 27:71 (1968).
67. G. M. Miller, J. H. Conrad, and R. B. Harrington, Effect of dietary unsaturated fatty acids and stage of lactation on milk composition and adipose tissue in swine, J. An. Sci. 32:79 (1971).
68. M. Wellby, M. W. O'Halloran, and M. L. Wellby, Maternal diet and lipid composition of breast milk, Lancet 2:458 (1973).
69. M. J. Mellies, T. T. Ishikawa, P. S. Gartside, K. Burton, J. MacGee, K. Allen, P. M. Steiner, D. Brady, and C. J. Glueck, Effects of varying maternal dietary fatty acids in lactating women and their infants, Am. J. Clin. Nutr. 32:229 (1979).
70. E. Vuori, K. Kiuru, S. M. Makinen, P. Vayrynen, R. Kara, and P. Kuitunen, Maternal diet and fatty acid pattern of breast milk, Acta Paediatr. Scand. 71:959 (1982).
71. W. Insull, Jr. and E. H. Ahrens, Jr., The fatty acids of human milk from mothers on diets taken ad libitum, Biochem. J. 72:27 (1959).
72. W. W. C. Read, P. G. Lutz, and A. Tashjian, Human milk lipids. II. The influence of dietary carbohydrates and fat on the fatty acids of mature milk, A study in four ethnic groups, Am. J. Clin. Nutr. 17:180 (1965).
73. W. W. C. Read, P. G. Lutz, and A. Tashjian, Human milk lipids. III. Short-term effects of dietary carbohydrate and fat, Am. J. Clin. Nutr. 17:184 (1965).
74. R. W. Seerly, F. M. Griffin, and H. C. McCampbell, Effect of sow's dietary energy source on sow's milk and piglet carcass composition, J. An. Sci. 46:1009 (1978).
75. T. A. B. Sanders, F. R. Ellis, and J. W. T. Dickerson, Studies of vegans; the fatty acid composition of plasma choline phosphoglycerides, erythrocytes, adipose tissue, and breast milk, and some indicators of susceptibility to ischemic heart disease in vegans and omnivore controls, Am. J. Clin. Nutr. 31:805 (1978).

76. D. A. Finley, B. Lonnerdal, K. G. Dewey, and L. E. Grivetti, Breast milk composition: fat content and fatty acid composition in vegetarians and non-vegetarians, Am. J. Clin. Nutr. 41:787 (1985).
77. W. S. Harris, W. E. Conner, and S. Lindsey, Will dietary ω-3 fatty acids change the composition of human milk?, Am. J. Clin. Nutr. 40:780 (1984).
78. B. Hall, Uniformity of human milk, Am. J. Clin. Nutr. 32:304 (1979).
79. A. J. Sinclair, Long-chain polyunsaturated fatty acids in the mammalian brain, Proc. Nutr. Soc. 29:54 (1975).
80. J. M. Aitchison, W. L. Dunkley, N. L. Canolty, and L. M. Smith, Influence of diet on trans fatty acids in human milk, Am. J. Clin. Nutr. 30:2006 (1977).
81. M. C. Craig-Schmidt, J. D. Weete, and S. A. Faircloth, The effect of hydrogenated fat in the diet of nursing mothers on lipid composition and prostaglandin content of human milk, Am. J. Clin. Nutr. 39:778 (1984).
82. J. E. Chappell, M. T. Clandinin, C. Kearney-Volpe, Trans fatty acids in human milk lipids: Influence of maternal diet and weight loss, Am. J. Clin. Nutr. 42:49 (1985).
83. B. Akesson, B.-M. Johansson, M. Svensson, P.-A. Ockerman, Content of trans-octadecenoic acid in vegetarian and normal diets in Sweden, analyzed by the duplicate portion technique, Am. J. Clin. Nutr. 34:2517 (1981).
84. G. J. Brisson, "Lipids in Human Nutrition. An Appraisal of Some Dietary Concepts," JK Burgess, New Jersey (1981).

CULTURAL AND ENVIRONMENTAL INFLUENCES ON THE NUTRITIONAL STATUS OF LACTATING WOMEN AND THEIR INFANTS IN NEPAL

Philip Burbrink Moser, Suniti Archarya,
and Robert D. Reynolds

Department of Food, Nutrition and Institution Administration
University of Maryland, College Park, Maryland 20742

Department of Family Planning, Ministry of Health
Kathmandu, Nepal

Human Nutrition Research Center, U.S. Department
of Agriculture, Beltsville, Maryland 20705

ABSTRACT

The culture and environment of lactating women not only affects the nutritional status of the mother through their effects in the selection of the diet and utilization of that diet, but also the nutritional status of the infant through their effects on the mother. Culture and environment can also have a more direct effect on the nutritional status of the infant, such as feeding practices. An intensive health and nutrition study was conducted on 26 lactating women and their infants in six villages in the Kathmandu Valley of Nepal which considered how the culture and environment influenced the nutritional status of this population. A detailed socioeconomic profile, health history and dietary history were obtained from the mothers by Nepalese public health workers. Anthropometric measurements and a physical examination by the team physician were performed on both the mothers and infants. During the three day study period, a 24-hour duplicate food composite was collected and subsequently analyzed for various nutrients. Analysis of the dietary composites indicated that the mothers consumed a low fat high carbohydrate diet. These diets were also higher than American Diets in neutral detergent fiber and phytate, which may exascerbate problems with minerals consumed in low amounts such as calcium (482 mg/day) and may even compromise minerals such as iron (33 mg/day) which was consumed in large amounts. Two special foods, jwano and gundruk, consumed by Nepalese women were examined for nutrient content and found to contain significant amounts of calcium, iron and magnesium. Fifty percent of the women studied supplemented their infants with lido, a rice water paste, because they felt their milk supply was inadequate. Anthropometric measurements and physical examination of the infants indicated adequate infant growth. The mothers physical exam revealed a 100% incidence of hepatitis A, a high apparent intestinal parasitic infestation and a stunting of growth.

INTRODUCTION

The culture and environment of lactating women not only affects the nutritional status of the mother through their effect on the selection of diet and the utilization of that diet, but also the nutritional status of the infant through their effects on breast milk. Culture and environment can also have a direct effect on the nutritional status of the infant, such as on feeding practices. The purpose of the present report is to describe the nutritional status of mother and infant pairs living in the Kathmandu Valley of Nepal and how the culture and environment of this population influenced nutritional status.

An in-depth nutrition survey was conducted of lactating women and their infants in the Kathmandu Valley of Nepal. The country of Nepal is located between India and China and is the home of the Himalayan Mountains. This kingdom has been open to Western influence for only the past 30 years and much of the population can be reached only by foot due to the rugged terrain.

MATERIALS AND METHODS

This survey was conducted during October and November of 1983, the harvest season, when there is the greatest availability and variety of food. This must be considered when interpreting the data collected.

Twenty-six lactating mothers and their infants living in six villages outside of the capital city of Nepal took part in a comprehensive nutritional status study. All women were two to six months postpartum and had given birth to a single child. Informed verbal consent was obtained from all women prior to their participation in the study. Public health workers in the Family Planning Division of the Ministry of Health acted as translaters and assisted in the collection of the samples and the data. Following the selection of the six villages surrounding Kathmandu, our research team spent three days in each of the villages. Following recruitment of the mothers on the first day, a detailed socioeconomic profile, health history and dietary history were obtained by the Nepalese public health workers. Anthropometric measurements were also obtained on the first day on both the mothers and infants. A physical examination by the team physician with an emphasis on nutrient related parameters was performed on both the mothers and infants.

On the second day in each village, the subjects went through a normal day of activity. One public health worker stayed with each subject from the first light in the morning, which would be when our subjects were waking up, until after the evening meal. During this time the public health worker recorded everything that was consumed by the subject and helped the subject prepare a duplicate composite of everything that she had consumed during that period of time. The composites were taken to our makeshift lab in Kathmandu, homogenized and aliquots were frozen for shipment back to the United States where they were analyzed.

Early on the morning of the third day, a breastmilk and urine sample was collected from the mothers and a blood sample was obtained from both the mother and the infant. These samples were also transported back to our makeshift lab where aliquots were frozen in liquid nitrogen for shipment back to the United States for analysis. Details of methods and procedures are published elsewhere.[1-4]

RESULTS AND DISCUSSION

Table 1 describes the subjects who participated in this survey. The mothers were an average age of 27.5 years with a range of 16-45 years. The infants were between 2 and 6 months of age with an average age of 3.8 months. Half of these infants were girls and half were boys. The mean total pregnancies for this group of women was 3.5 with a range of 1-10. The mean number of live births was 3.1 with a range

Table 1. Description of Subjects
Means and Ranges

Age	27.5 years (16-45)
Total Pregnancies	3.5 (1-10)
Live Births	3.1 (1-9)
Children Living	2.5 (1-5)
Childhood Mortality	25%

of 1-9. The mean number of living children was 2.5 with a range of 1-5. Thus, the mean childhood mortality rate for our group of mothers was approximately 25%. Half of the mothers who participated in this study delivered their infants at home with the other half delivering their infants in health care facilities. Although the infants examined by our physician were healthy with no unusual physical findings, several other children in the study villages between the ages of 2-5 were found to be suffering from protein calorie malnutrition.

Table 2 shows the results of the proximate analysis of the maternal food composites and compares those values to values calculated from 3-day dietary records of lactating women we previously studied in the United States.

Table 2. Comparison of Dietary Intake of Lactating Women From Nepal and Annapolis Maryland

	Nepal	Annapolis, MD
KILOCALORIES	2,150	1,901*
PROTEIN	62g	80g*
(% Kilocalories)	11.6%	16 8%
FAT	21g	81g*
(% Kilocalories)	8.6%	38 4%
CARBOHYDRATE	392g	221g*
(% Kilocalories)	73.3%	46.5%
NEUTRAL DETERGENT FIBER	24.0g	7.7g**
PHYTATE	2.15g	0 61-1.26g**

* Calculated from diet records rather than analyzed from diet composites.
**Calculated for women in the USA.

The kilocalorie intake of the Nepalese women is higher than women in the United States, yet the Nepalese women are smaller. This difference probably relates to the heavy manual labor carried out by the Nepalese mothers and the higher rates of disease and infections in Nepal The diet of the Nepalese women is lower in protein and dramatically lower in fat. The Nepalese women also consumed more of their kilocalories as carbohydrates than the U.S women. The high carbohydrate diet of these women was predominantly complex carbohydrates from rice and vegetables. The percent of kilocalories in the Nepalese do not add up to 100%. Alcohol that was consumed by several subjects could have led to an underestimation of the calories coming from carbohydrates.

Table 2 also shows the neutral detergent fiber and phytate content of the Nepalese women diets in comparison to the diets of American women. The neutral detergent fiber and phytate are two and three times that reported for U.S women. These high phytate and fiber intakes may exascerbate problems with minerals consumed in low amounts such as calcium (482 mg/day), and may even compromise minerals such as iron (33 mg/day) which was consumed in large amounts relative to its recommended intake.[5]

Often isolated people adopt certain foods as conferring special benefits to them. Lactating women will consume food that they believe will increase their milk supply. Two foods that Nepalese women consume to enhance lactation are locally referred to as jwano and gundruk. Jwano, a locally grown seed is a member of the same family as fennel, dill, cumin, corriander and caraway. This seed is reported to be a lactogen by both the Nepalese and Westerners who work with the Nepalese women. However, the action has not been documented scientifically. New mothers who appear to have difficulty in establishing adequate lactation are given a thin soup prepared from the jwano seeds, which are first fried in a bit of oil and then boiled in water The average daily intake of the seeds is estimated to be about 50 grams. The women may also occasionally consume the jwano soup to sustain or enhance established lactational performance.

Gundruk is prepared from dried greens, predominantly from mustard or radish. The greens are picked, air-dried and then fermented in a covered clay pot with a bit of water. This fermentation process takes a few days to a week. At the end of this time, the gundruk can be consumed as a boiled side vegetable or redried for later consumption. Table 3 shows the nutrient content of these two foods. Both the jwano

Table 3. Nutrient Content of Selected Food Items

	Jwano	Gundruk	Short Grain Rice	Dry Whole Milk Powder	Raw Beef Liver
	μg/g Food*				
Calcium	17,400	18,840	81	9,120	80
Iron	1,721	1,430	18.4	4.7	65
Magnesium	3,121	2,720	507	850	200

*Nutrient content listed on dry weight basis, except for beef liver.

and gundruk are high in calcium, iron and magnesium compared to dry whole milk or raw beef liver. Table 4 shows the nutrient contribution of jwano and gundruk, compared to rice if they were consumed in normal amounts on a daily basis. Even though rice provides the bulk of the Nepalese diet, a small serving of either jwano soup or gundruk would provide substantial amounts of calcium, iron and magnesium to the daily diet of lactating women

The results of the diet history showed that 23% of the women in our study consumed jwano as a special food during lactation and 7% reported consuming radish or mustard greens as a special food but not gundruk. However, during the 24-hour diet composite collection, none of the women consumed jwano but 19% consumed gundruk. Since jwano is viewed primarily as a lactogen to initiate lactation, and all of our subjects were already lactating, this may explain why none of the women consumed jwano during the 24-hour food collection period.

Table 4. Contribution To Daily Diet

	Jwano	Gundruk	Rice
Daily Intake (g)*	50	10	238
Calcium (mg/day)	850	188	19.3
Iron (mg/day)	86.0	14.0	4.4
Magnesium (mg/day)	156	27	121

*Intake listed as g dry weight of food item.

Sixty-two percent of the women in the study reported consuming one or more "special foods" at some point in their lactation. These foods included jwano soup, fresh radish or mustard greens, meat soup, and/or brown sugar.

Although the anthropometric measurements and physical examination indicate adequate infant growth, 54% of our subjects stated that they felt their milk supply was inadequate for the needs of their infants. As a result, 50% of the supposedly exclusively breastfed infants[6] were supplemented with lido, which is a pablum-like rice and water paste. This high percentage of supplemental feeding is in contrast to the 93% exclusive breast feeding of Nepalese as reported by the World Fertility Study of 1976.[6] It is difficult, however, to extrapolate our small sample size to all of Nepal.

In addition 65% of the women reported taking traditional ayurvedic herbs and medicines during lactation, which was down from the 88% of the women taking ayurvedic medicine during their pregnancy. These ayurvedic medicines have not been analyzed for their nutrient content.

Table 5 shows the major physical findings for both the mothers and infants Nineteen percent of the mothers examined had palpable hepatomegaly which is probably related to the 100% incidence of hepatitis A in the women. Sixteen percent were observed to have cheilosis and angular stomatitis, characteristic of impaired B vitamin status. The dry blood smears showed 92% of the women had eosinophilia which was most probably tropical eosinophilia due to the presence of intestinal parasites. As stated above, 100% of the mothers in our study had antibodies to hepatitis A. Viral hepatitis A is primarily spread by fecal-oral contact. Water and food-borne epidemics are common especially in underdeveloped countries like Nepal. This high percentage of incidence of eosinophilia and hepatitis A is probably related to the lack of a sanitary water supply in Nepal. Eight percent of the mothers had antibodies to hepatitis B. Virus B is mainly transmitted parenterally. Transfusions of contaminated blood or blood products is the usual source, along with using contaminated needles. As stated previously, on physical examination, the infants appeared healthy with no unusual findings.

Table 5. Major Physical Findings

Mothers	
Hepatomegaly	19%
Cheilosis & Angular Stomatitis	16%
Blood Smears Eosinophilia	92%
100% of mothers had antibodies to Hepatitis A	
8% of mothers had antibodies to Hepatitis B	
Infants	
No unusual physical findings	

Table 6 shows the results of the maternal anthropometric measurements. The women averaged 151 cm or 4'10" in height and 46.5 kg or 102 lbs. in weight. Using Jelliffe's standards of weight for height, these women would be 92% of standard.[7] Using data from the 1971-1974 HANES study, these women would be in the 10-25 percentile, indicating they are small.[8] Mid-arm circumferences which are used as a field measure to evaluate protein reserves indicate the women in this survey to be 80% of Jelliffe's standard which would indicate mild protein malnutrition[7]. If U.S. standards from Frisancho are applied, the protein malnutrition would appear more severe.[9] Triceps skinfolds are used to evaluate kilocalorie reserves by measuring fat in a precise location of the arm. Our women were 82% of Jelliffe's standard indicating a mild deficit in kilocalorie reserves.[7] If the Frisancho standards are applied, the kilocalorie reserves would be considered moderately depleted.[9]

Table 6. Maternal Anthropometrics

Height	151±1.5 cm
Weight	46.5±1.65 kg
Weight for Height	
Jelliffe	92% STD
NCHS	10-25% TILE
Mid-Arm Circumference	22.8±0.51 cm
Jelliffe	80% STD
NCHS	<5% TILE
Triceps Skinfold	13.5±1.04 mm
Jelliffe	82% STD
NCHS	10% TILE

In order to summarize the data from infants 2 to 6 months of age and both sexes, the different centiles for growth were examined. The standards used were those suggested by WHO[10] which are based on National Center for Health Statistics data from the U.S. Table 7 shows the weight for age distribution. The one category that is substantially greater than expected is the 10-25 percentile. Only two infants are below the 10th percentile and would be considered to be at risk for nutritional problems. Table 7 also shows the length data. As with the weight data most of the infants length for age fell in the 25-75 percentile. However, the length data indicate that four infants are below the 10th percentile and would be thought to be at possible risk for nutritional problems. In general from these data most of the breastfed infants in this study are demonstrating what would be considered normal weight and length for age. These observations are consistent with no unusual findings from the physical examinations of the infants.

To summarize, the maternal diets were high in carbohydrates and low in fat compared to diets consumed by lactating women in the United States. The maternal diets were also high in fiber and phytates which may compromise the mineral status of these women. The consumption of several locally grown foods considered to be special for lactating women in Nepal could

Table 7. Comparison of Expected and Actual Centiles for Weight for Age and Length for Age of Nepalese Breast Fed Infants

Centile	Expected	Actual Weight For Age	Actual Length For Age
	%		
< 3	3	4	4
3-10	7	4	12
10-25	15	35	35
25-75	50	54	50
>75	25	4	0

add substantially to the mineral intake of these women, if they are consumed on a frequent basis. The lactating women in this study had a 100% incidence of hepatitis A, and a high apparent intestinal parasitic infection which could put these women at risk for problems with iron nutriture. And, although the mother's anthropometric measurements indicated a stunted growth, the breastfed infants appear to be growing adequately.

REFERENCES

1. R. D. Reynolds, S. Acharya, W. McConnell, M. B. Andon, M.P. Howard and P.B. Moser. Nutritional and medical status of lactating women and their infants in the Kathmandu Valley of Nepal. Am. J. Clin. Nutr. (submitted)
2. P. B. Moser, S. Acharya, M. B. Andon, M. P. Howard and R. D. Reynolds. Nutritional intakes and status of calcium and magnesium in Nepalese lactating women and their breast-fed infants. Am. J. Clin. Nutr. (submitted)
3. P. B. Moser, S. Acharya, M. P. Howard, M. B. Andon, S. Lewis and R. D. Reynolds. Nutritional intake and status of selected trace elements in Nepalese lactating women and their breast-fed infants. Am. J. Clin. Nutr. (submitted)
4. R. D. Reynolds, S. Acharya, M. B. Andon, M. P. Howard, J. E Leklem and P. B. Moser. Nutritional intake and status of vitamin B-6 in Nepalese lactating women and their breast-fed infants. Am. J. Clin. Nutr. (submitted)

5. Food and Nutrition Board. Recommended dietary allowances, 8th ed. Washington, D.C.: National Academy of Sciences, National Research Council, 1980.
6. The World Fertility Survey: January 1978 - December 1980 Annual Report. International Statistical Institute. The Hague, 1981.
7. D. B. Jelliffe. The assessment of the nutritional status of the community Geneva, Switzerland, World Health Organization, 1966.
8. National Center for Health Statistics. Weight by height and age for adults 18-74 years: United States, 1971-74. Series 11, Number 208, DHEW Publication No. (PHS) 79, 1656, 1979.
9. A. R. Frisancho. New norms of upper limb fat and muscle areas for assessment of nutritional status. Am. J. Clin. Nutr. 1981; 34:2540-2545.
10. World Health Organization. Measuring change in nutritional status. Geneva, Switzerland, 1983.

LACTATIONAL PERFORMANCE AND MILK COMPOSITION IN RELATION TO DURATION OF PREGNANCY AND LACTATION

Stephanie A. Atkinson and
Karyn J. Kaufman

Faculty of Health Sciences
McMaster University
Hamilton, Ontario, Canada

INTRODUCTION

The dynamic changes that occur in milk composition associated with duration of lactation have been recognized for over a century as documented in several early publications some dating back to 1874 (1-3). In the mid 1900s Macy (4) reviewed 1500 publications on milk composition from many countries and selected 268 papers based on "the characteristics of subjects, methods of collecting samples, analytical techniques, diet and environmental factors". From the data surveyed, they compiled a table of composite values for more than 50 components in human milk at three lactational stages: colostrum, representing one to five days postpartum; transitional milk, representing days six to ten postpartum; and mature milk, representing day 15 to 15 months postpartum. Since that time and particularly since the mid 1970s, a plethora of information on milk composition has emerged providing further characterization of important biological components in human milk and knowledge of those factors which are associated with alterations in the composition and volume of human milk produced by the average healthy lactating woman (Table 1).

The objective of the present review of lactational performance and milk composition is two-fold. Firstly, is to briefly summarize the state of recent information on a selection of components of human milk in relation to longitudinal changes in composition during lactation. Secondly, the concept of a "preterm" milk will be explored based on information stemming from the early studies of Atkinson and colleagues (5-8) and subsequently others (9-18) on the production and composition of milk from mothers giving birth prematurely. As well as highlighting the descriptive data, it is important to address the interpretation and biological implications of accumulated information on the characterization and patterning of components in human milk. Such information is impotant for the expansion of our understanding of the physiological mechanisms of lactation. For instance, do changes in milk composition with duration of lactation occur in response to a "biological clock" or do they simply represent a response to maternal endocrine events elicited by the suckling process? The other application of knowledge of milk composition is in relation to estimating the needs of the developing infant for the nutritional and immunological components of human milk, but this falls outside the theme of this conference. The information provided in this chapter is intended to set the stage for the new

Characterization of changes in various components of milk is useful, particularly if the data represent longitudinal rather than cross-sectional milk samples so that between mother biological variability is minimized. Hartman and co-workers from Australia have produced some excellent data on changes in composition of several nutrients in human milk in the prepartum period (60 days prior to term); during the initiation of lactation (through the first 50 hours) (32); during early lactation (1 to 10 postpartum days) (32) and longitudinally through the first 12 months of lactation (33). Although they tracked milk from left and right breasts, no significant differences could be found.

As demonstrated by many investigators since the early 1900s, total nitrogen and the major proteins (lactalbumin, immunoglobulins and lactoferrin) (4,5,33,34,35) decrease in concentration precipitously over the first days and weeks of lactation and then remain relatively constant. Changes in the non-protein nitrogen fraction are not so marked (6,34). More recently, Donovan and Lonnerdal (36) have shown that the relative proportion of components within the acid-soluble fraction (non-protein nitrogen) change from colostrum to mature milk with increases in the proportion of urea N being particularly notable. Milk minerals and lactose also undergo their most significant changes during the very early stages of lactation. Sodium and chloride in milk decrease most precipitously in the first 3 to 5 days of lactation and potassium and lactose increase reaching a plateau by day 2 and day 4 to 6, respectively (8,32,33). The dramatic changes in ionic and protein composition in the early post parturient stage are thought to be a consequence of the closure of the junctional complexes between the alveolar cells thus preventing paracellular transport of plasma constituents directly into milk and the reverse movement of potassium and lactose to maintain isotonicity (37).

The other major cations in milk, calcium, phosphorus and magnesium, demonstrate variable patterns of change during early lactation but remain relatively constant in concentration thereafter. In one study, calcium decreased significantly from 8 to 7 mmol/L while phosphorus rose from about 3.5 to 5 mmol/L over the first week of lactation (7). The Ca:P molar ratio thus declined from 2.1 (2.9 mg/mg) to 1.5 (2.0) over this time period. Frequency distributions of data on calcium, phosphorus and magnesium in milk over 45 days of lactation found the values to be normally distributed with similar median and mean values observed at each lactational stage (27). Magnesium tends to remain relatively constant throughout lactation although inter-subject variability is usually quite considerable (7,10,27).

Knowledge of the characteristic changes of milk during normal suckling has allowed investigators to more easily investigate and recognize aberrations in milk composition in association with abrupt and gradual weaning, maternal disease states such as diabetes, cystic fibrosis or Cushing's Syndrome; induced lactation of non-biological mothers; or in association with preterm birth. Most of these topics are highlighted in other sections of the Workshop proceedings and preterm milk composition will be reviewed later in this chapter.

The total lipid and lipid fractions in human milk have been shown to also follow distinctive patterns in concentration with progressing lactation. Total lipids rise dramatically over the first week of lactation (8,11,25,38) to values in human milk which are highly variable between women and range from 2.6 to greater than 4.3 g/100 ml (39,40). The total triglycerides of milk parallel changes in total lipid since they represent 98% or more of milk lipid (40). While phospholipid content does not appear to change over the first four weeks in one study (38) others have described an exponential decline over the first three months of lactation (11). Milk cholesterol content decreases initially reaching a nadir at about two weeks of lactation (38,11). Teleologically, one could postulate that milk lipid is initially low and increases postnatally to parallel the developmental increases in the infant's capacity to produce pancreatic lipase and bile salts for the digestion of fat. It is more likely, however, that the dramatic early rise in milk lipid reflects induction of the suckling induced hormonal regulators of de novo lipid synthesis and transport of long chain fatty acids into mammary secretions from plasma sources. In contrast to total lipid, the relative pattern of fatty acids does not appear to be altered by duration of lactation but rather by maternal dietary fatty acids (11,38,40-45).

Longitudinal analysis of the lipid content of milk has been useful to establish reference levels of fat for infant formulas and to assess aberrations in fat content of human milk in association with undernutrition and low fat diets (42) or type 1 hyperlipoproteinemia (43). The cholesterol content of 'normal' milk has served as a reference point in assessing composition of milk of mothers receiving diets with varying ratios of dietary polyunsaturated fatty acids (44,45) and plant sterols (44).

Patterns of change in vitamin content of human milk have been less well defined compared to the macronutrients and minerals, possibly because vitamin levels in milk are so vulnerable to the vitamin nutriture of the mother. Vitamin A (retinol) and B-carotene and vitamin E are higher in colostrum and fall with time (46-48). Despite being lipid soluble, these vitamins do not appear to reflect changes in total lipid content of the milk (48). An extensive summary of vitamin D in milk is provided in the chapter by Hollis.

For the water soluble vitamins, some recent studies in which maternal dietary intake was controlled have aided in the elucidation of longitudinal changes in milk vitamin content. Vitamin C has been shown to decline gradually over the first four to five months of lactation by one group (49) while others have shown either an initially low concentration in the first compared to the second and fourth weeks of lactation (17) or a constant concentration over the first seven weeks of lactation (26). Both free and total folate increased significantly from early (4-7 days postpartum) to mature (35-90 days postpartum) milk by 100% or more (17,50,51). Levels of thiamin (52), riboflavin (53) and vitamin B_6 (54) tend to increase with duration of lactation although the time frames are very variable between vitamins.

Longitudinal changes in trace elements in human milk have been demonstrated in several recent studies from both North America and Scandinavia. Compared to changes in protein and electrolytes in milk, the decreases in copper and zinc over time are more gradual taking 8 to 12 weeks postpartum before a nadir is reached (55-57). Recently, Casey and co-workers (58) reported a careful tracking of changes in copper, zinc, manganese and chromium over the first 30 days postpartum. The pattern of change for manganese parallels that described for zinc while that of chromium displays an initial rise over the first postpartum week followed by a plateau (58). Information on the trace element content of human milk has been particularly helpful in the diagnosis of nutritional zinc deficiency in solely breastfed infants. For example in a recent patient case, a premature infant (33 weeks gestation at birth) presented at four and one-half months postnatally at McMaster University Medical Centre (Atkinson, unpublished data) with clinical and biochemical evidence of zinc deficiency that could be attributed to abnormally low zinc in the mother's milk. In similar case reports in the literature (59-61), fulminant nutritional zinc

Table 1. Factors Associated with Alterations in the Composition and Volume of Human Milk

I Stage of Lactation
"Early" vs "Late or Mature" Milk
Factors: Maturation of mammary structure and milk synthesis mechanisms
: Endocrine regulation of milk synthesis
: Physiological to meet infants needs

II Stage of Gestation at Parturition
"Very Preterm" vs "Preterm" vs "Full-Term" Milk
Factors: Maturation of mammary gland
: Endocrine regulation of milk synthesis
: Nipple stimulation - initiation, frequency, duration
: Anxiety state
: Return of ovulation/menses

III Environmental Influences
Acute and gradual weaning
Tandem nursing
Non-biologic induced lactation
Smoking
Maternal drug ingestion and diet
Anxiety/stress/problems
Help and support

information which will evolve from the Workshop on, "The Effect of Duration of Pregnancy and Lactation upon Composition of Human Milk" (Pages 103 through 205).

DEFINITION OF STAGES OF LACTATION

Throughout the years comparison of published values for specific components of milk have often been hampered by a lack of agreement amongst investigators on the definition of the stages of lactation often referred to as 'colostrum', 'transitional milk' and 'mature milk'. Generally, there is agreement that lactational days are counted as postpartum days with day one being the day following delivery. However, in some studies, day one of lactation may be considered as day of delivery (19) while others have determined the first day of lactation as the first day of production of transitional milk which was usually day two or three postpartum (20). For colostrum, the time interval has been determined as postpartum days 1 to 3 (21,22,23), 1 to 4 (11), 0 to 5 (24), 1 to 5 (4), or 3 to 5 (25). Transitional milk has been ascribed a similar variable time interval ranging from postpartum days 6 to 10 (4,21,26) to 5 or 6 to 15 (23) or 10 to 14 (27). The term mature then refers to milk produced anytime after the transitional stage (after 10 to 15 days postpartum), although some investigators have defined milk to be 'mature' as early as postpartum day 7 (11) and as late as day 40 (26). Definition of the final stage of mature milk has not, to my knowledge, ever been attempted. However, since changes in milk composition occur during gradual (28-30) and abrupt weaning (31), this interval of lactation is not truly representative of the composition of mature milk produced during full lactation. Clearly, an important challenge for this meeting would be to achieve a consensus as to the preferred designation for stages of lactation represented by common characteristics of milk composition.

deficiency presenting with severe perioral dermatitis, delayed wound healing, low serum zinc and delayed growth have been attributed to ingestion of mothers' milk with zinc concentrations below the range for lactational stage-adjusted values of normal mothers' milk. In our case, milk zinc was 230 ug/dl at a lactational stage of 4.5 months (normal median value - 780 ug/dl (55).

Identification of new components in human milk has included analysis of non-nutritional substances with as yet undetermined physiological function. Two such components are the cyclic nucleotides and N-acetylneuraminic acid. Changes in cyclic adenosine monophosphate (cAMP) and cyclic guanosinemonophosphate (cGMP) over the first 40 days of lactation have been reported (62). Because of the great degree of individual variability, distinct patterns of change with time could not be determined. In contrast, both glycoprotein and oligosaccharide derived N-acetylneuraminic acid demonstrated precipitous decreases in concentration over the first nine weeks of lactation, thereafter levelling off up to 28 weeks postpartum at levels of one-third and one-seventh of the initial values, respectively (63). Growth-promoting activity of human milk during lactation has also been described (64). Insulin and epidermal growth factor were found in very high concentrations in day 1 colostrum falling dramatically over the first 3 days postpartum. In mature milk, concentratins of these components represented only 10% of those in colostrum. Definition of growth-promoting components in human milk may be important to our understanding of their role in the proliferation and differentiation of infant tissues.

"PRETERM" MILK: FACT OR ARTIFACT?

1. Preterm Milk Composition

Since 1978, more than 40 published studies have reported on the comparative analysis of milk produced by mothers delivering prematurely or at term, often referred to as preterm milk and term milk, respectively (5-18,22,25,41,48,50). Observations from many of these studies suggest that preterm milk is unique in nutrient composition compared to term milk but agreement on these observations is not universal. A summary of some of the comparative analyses of preterm and term milk for selected nutrients is found in Table 2.

In general, the pattern of changes in milk composition in term milk is also observed in preterm milk. What then could be the possible physiological basis for the reported differences in nutrient density between the two sources of milk? There is little evidence to suggest that this milk secretion has a teleological basis making it uniquely suited to meet the nutritional needs of the premature infant. However, there is indirect evidence from lactating animals to support the hypothesis that differences in milk composition may be secondary to an altered or an interrupted hormonal status at parturition, altered development of hormone receptors within the mammary gland and/or simply a lack of cellular differentiation and maturation. A discussion of these hypotheses may be found in the chapter by Atkinson in this book.

The concept that preterm mothers have an immature mammary system which permits paracellular leakage of serum proteins and ions through incompletely matured tight junctions is based on the concept of "leaky junctions" between apical membranes as found in the goat where prepartum paracellular transport causes elevated concentrations of serum proteins (IgG), sodium and chloride and lowered lactose and potassium content compared to milk obtained post parturition (65,66). Based on recent studies in the author's (SAA)

Table 2. Composition of Selected Components in Preterm Milk as Compared to Term Milk

Stage of Lactation (days)	Protein Nitrogen	NPN[1]	IgA	Total Lipids	MCFA[2]	Sodium	Reference
3–28	P>F[3]	P>F	–	P>F	–	P=F	5–8
3–28	P>F	–	–	P=F	–	P>F	9
7–28	P>F	P=F	–	P=F	–	P>F	10
6–≥15	P=F	–	–	P=F	–	P=F	15
3–14	P>F	–	P>F	–	–	–	16
5–30	VP>F[3] P=F	VP>F	–	VP>F P=F	VP>F P=F	–	14
14–84	P>F	P=F	–	–			12
4–37	–	–	–	P>F	P>F	–	13
3–14	P=F	–	–	P=F	–	–	22
	–	–	–	P>F	–	–	18

1 NPN – non-protein nitrogen
2 MCFA – medium chain fatty acids
3 P = preterm milk; F = full-term milk; VP = very preterm milk

laboratory (described elsewhere in this publication) the concept of paracellular leakage of minerals into milk would not appear valid in relation to the "premature" mammary gland.

Unfortunately, variability in design methodology limits the comparison of results between many of the reported studies on preterm milk composition. Some of the major important variables which have not been controlled between studies include: inclusion of wide ranges of gestational stage in preterm groups; collapsed time intervals for stage of lactation; milk sampling methodology which may represent a random sample, a pool of fore and hind milk, a single breast expression, a complete feeding expression (both breasts) or a complete 24-hour expression of milk. Unless one of the two latter collection methods are employed assessment of the lactational capacity by measurement of milk volume cannot be achieved. In some but not all studies milk volume has been measured. When milk volume produced by a mother is less than that which meets her infant's needs, one should consider whether indeed this is representative of "normal" lactation. For example, in studies by Anderson et al (22) and Gross et al (9), reported 24-hour milk volumes are interpolated to be as low as 16 and less than 50 ml – values that are difficult to accept as being reflective of "full" or normal lactation. At such abnormally low volumes, volume may become a primary determinant of composition and negate a clear perspective on the nutrient composition of preterm milk. Anderson (22) noted that protein content of milk was negatively correlated with milk volume but this would be predicted since milk volume increases and protein decreases with progressive stage of lactation. Statistical analysis of differences in preterm and term milk composition adjusted for milk volume as a cofactor has not found milk volume

Table 3. Perinatal Events Related to Preterm Birth which may Affect the Lactational Process and Milk Composition

Delay in initiating pumping
- Mother too ill/anxious
- Lack of nursing support for teaching
- Unavailability of appropriate pumps

Pattern of nipple stimulation --- milk volume
- Time of initiation of breast expression
- Pumping frequency (1-6 times/day) and duration
- Type of breast pump
- Amount of suckling

Anxiety related to babe's medical condition
- Poor milk letdown --- low milk volumes
  --- ? affect on composition

Perinatal drugs - e.g. glucocorticoids, oxytocin

Early return of menses

Degree of prematurity

to be a significantly associated variable when the milk produced is a reasonable amount (1).

Finally, many investigators have demonstrated a greater degree of inter-individual variability in milk composition in preterm as compared to term milk. Whether such exaggerated variability in milk composition between prematurely delivered mothers reflects true biological variability or is an artifact of the lactational process and milk sampling methodology indigenous to this population has not been examined in detail. We propose that there are a number of perinatal events associated with preterm birth (Table 3) which may indeed influence the lactational process and the endocrine events which regulate milk synthesis and secretion. Further studies are needed to properly evaluate the impact of such perinatal events on the lactational capacity of mothers giving birth prematurely.

2. Lactation Performance of Mothers Delivering Prematurely

Success in initiating and maintaining lactation in prematurely delivered women may be related to perinatal events either similar to or different from those affecting mothers delivering at term. The observed differences in composition and volume of milk produced by mothers giving birth prematurely may indeed be influenced by the mother's lactation experience. A small body of literature suggests that mothers of preterm infants have a qualitatively different experience than term mothers. Auerbach and Avery (67) surveyed 117 mothers who provided breast milk for preterm infants. Ninety percent of mothers reported difficulties including fatigue, maintaining a milk supply and getting the baby to nurse at the breast. Verronen (68) commented on the difficulty of promoting breast feeding in small infants because the methods used to encourage lactation such as early nursing, rooming-in, and demand feeding are not usually possible in the care of preterm infants. Average duration of lactation was noted to be significantly shorter in preterm mothers: their mean duration was 5.6 months compared to 7.0 months in term mothers (69). In a prospective study of the course of lactation in mothers of very low birth weight infants, early termination of lactation was attributed to the difficulties mothers had in supplying expressed breast milk to the nursery, the frequent report of milk insufficiency and the anxiety and inadequacy mothers felt about losing their milk supply (70).

In the tertiary neonatal intensive care unit at McMaster University, a study of the influences on breast feeding of preterm infants was conducted during 1984-85 by one of us (KK). The purposes of the study included an examination of influences on the duration of lactation in mothers choosing to provide breast milk. Of 125 consecutively admitted singleton birth infants who were <2500 g and <36 weeks gestation, 88 of the mothers (70.4%) chose to breast feed and all but eight found it necessary to initiate milk expression. The 88 infants had a mean birthweight of 1699 g, and mean gestation of 31.5 weeks; 57 (64.8%) were males and 37 (29.6%) were categorized as critically ill on the first day of life.

The course of lactation was studied prospectively and data were obtained by telephone interviews at two week intervals. During the 43 weeks of the study, 62 of 88 (70.5%) mothers were observed to completely stop breast expression/feeding, 24 (27.3%) were continuing to breast feed at the study's end and two were lost to follow up. Sixty-one mothers initiated infant suckling at the breast; the infant's postnatal age at first suckling varied from 1 to 91 days (mean $\pm$ S.D. was 17 $\pm$ 17 days). The remaining 27 mothers discontinued milk expression before the infant could be put to the breast. Sixteen of the mothers who were able to initiate breast feeding stopped when they were combining some nursing with milk expression. In all, then, nearly 50 percent of mothers failed to establish effective infant suckling.

The observed duration of <u>any</u> breast expression/feeding varied from 5 to 195 days (mean $\pm$ SD = 74 $\pm$ 71 days). A rapid drop was observed in the early weeks: at 30 postnatal days 67% of mothers were maintaining partial or full lactation, 46% at 60 days, and 30% at 120 days. The median duration was 54 days or approximately 8 weeks. This compares with 1982 national Canadian data of 83% and 59%of breast feeding mothers persisting at 2 and 4 months respectively (71).

Table 4 shows the reasons given by mothers for stopping lactation and it is evident that the perception of insufficient milk was a frequent concern (44%). There were other stated reasons for stopping lactation, with difficulty establishing infant suckling at the breast being the second most frequent reason. Based on the mothers' descriptions of experiences leading to the decision to stop lactation, it was apparent that the stated reason was often the most proximal reason or event in a chain of events.

Table 4. Frequency of Cited Reasons for Stopping Breast Expression/Feeding

Stated Reason	f	%
Insufficient milk	27	43.6
Infant did not nurse well	11	17.7
Mother returned to work	6	9.7
Difficulty with breast pump	5	8.1
Mother ill; advised to stop	4	6.5
Infant illness	4	6.5
Other	5	8.1
	62	100.2

Table 5. Comparison of Duration of Lactation in Subgroups of Mothers

Subgroup	n	Cumulative proportion continuing at 30 days	Cumulative proportion continuing at 60 days	Median days of lactation	Mean * U score	Lee-Desu statistic D **	df	P
Cited Supports								
None	18	0.111	0.000	16.9	-61.33			
1	12	0.750	0.333	48.0	- 1.67			
2	17	0.765	0.529	64.7	6.47			
3 or 4	30	0.797	0.543	58.0	13.27			
5 or 6	11	1.000	1.000	270.0	56.00	44.744	4	<0.0001
	88							
Problems Per Contact								
> 2.66	42	0.518	0.265	32.2	-21.33			
≤ 2.66	46	0.804	0.628	106.9	19.48	15.117	1	<0.0001
	88							
Infant Condition								
Not recovered	26	0.308	0.039	21.7	-42.27			
Fully recovered	60	0.814	0.642	93.5	18.63	28.982	1	<0.0001
	86							
Planned Duration								
< 6 months	47	0.617	0.336	42.5	-13.30			
≥ 6 months	37	0.781	0.667	144.6	16.89	8.653	1	<0.0033
	84							
Maternal Age								
< 27	44	0.564	0.228	35.7	-17.91			
≥ 27	44	0.773	0.681	108.8	17.91	11.668	1	0.0006
	88							
Education								
≤ High school	46	0.582	0.381	42.3	-10.63			
> College/university	42	0.762	0.541	73.9	11.64	4.503	1	0.0338
	88							
Previous Breast-feeding								
No	57	0.611	0.359	43.2	-8.25			
Yes	31	0.774	0.640	103.8	15.16	4.548	1	0.0330
	88							
Current Smoking								
Yes	22	0.581	0.278	38.1	-16.86			
No	66	0.697	0.513	65.8	5.62	3.449	1	0.0633
	88							

Note: Missing data causes some totals of subgroup n's ≠ 88.

* U compares an individual's duration time with all others. U is initially 0 and is incremented by one for each case whose duration is less and decremented by one for each case whose time is greater (72).

** D describes the probability that the subgroups have different survival distributions. D is based on the U scores of all subjects in the subgroup and is distributed as chi square (degrees of freedom equal to subgroups minus one) (72).

Multiproblem situations often involved a concern about insufficient volume. For example, the anxiety associated with the variable course of recovery for some infants was reported by mothers to influence their milk production. Other mothers experienced health problems themselves that adversely affected their milk production. Often, then, the concern about milk volume was an underlying feature of the events leading to a decision to stop either breast expression or feeding.

Several variables were examined for their potential prognostic relationship with duration of lactation. Table 5 shows that socio-demographic variables like age and education were significantly related to duration but that several other influences were present as well. Variables like the number of supportive persons, the infant's condition and the number of problems experienced by mothers reflected the complexity of maintaining lactation with a preterm infant. A more detailed description of these variables follows.

The sources of help and support for breastfeeding which mothers reported receiving in the perinatal period are shown in Table 6. The prominence of husband/partner support is consistent with findings from the literature (73-77). Mothers described the value of their partner's general encouragement and his tangible help with other children or household tasks. Nurses were the second most frequently cited source of support; likely reflecting the longer period of specialized hospital care needed by these infants. The number of cited sources of support showed considerable variation with nearly a quarter of the group reporting no source of support. It was shown in Table 6 that number of supports was highly significantly related to length of lactation.

Mothers' descriptions of problems they encountered related to their breastfeeding experience were recorded throughout the follow up time and summarized under problem areas. Undue fatigue was the most frequently mentioned problem (63% of mothers), followed by milk insufficiency (55%), painful nipples/breast (40%), difficulty getting the baby to nurse well (18%), and problems using or getting access to a breast pump (16%). More than one problem area was frequently reported with 51 mothers (58%) citing two or more kinds of difficulties. Mothers who reported an equal or greater number of problems per contact than the mean of 2.7 had a significantly shorter median duration of lactation.

Table 6. Sources of Help/Support for Breast-feeding

Source	Number citing source according to amount of help provided			Total number citing source	% of mothers
	Some	Moderate	Very much		
Husband/partner	4	9	53	66	75.0
Own mother	2	3	16	21	24.0
Mother-in-law	2	6	6	14	16.0
Friend	2	5	8	15	17.0
Organized group (LLL)[1]	-	4	2	6	0.8
Doctors	-	13	7	20	23.0
Nurses	3	15	11	29	33.0
Other family members	6	11	6	23	26.0

[1] La Leche League

The infant's condition was often an underlying feature of lactation problems. The illness state dictated to a large extent the length of time milk expression was needed, when the infant could be introduced to suckling, the need for continued visits to the hospital, and the overall level of parent stress. The mother's perception of whether her infant was recovered by the end of the follow up time was significantly related to duration.

Mothers were asked at the time of enrollment their planned length of time to breast feed. Over 40% indicated they wanted to breast feed for more than six months (Table 7). The planned duration was assumed to reflect in part a motivational influence and there is some evidence for this assumption. Mothers who knew they wanted to breast feed, even before becoming pregnant, were more likely to plan to breast feed for more than 6 months ($p = 0.02$).

The significant association of higher maternal age, more education, and previous breast feeding with longer duration seen in Table 5 is consistent with other investigators' reports (78). The relationship of smoking to duration was just beyond the conventional significance level (Table 6), but the observed difference in median duration between smokers and nonsmokers (38 days vs. 65 days) is consistent with others' observations (77,79,80) and with the potential effects of nicotine on milk production.

The relative importance of the variables that were significant in Table 5 was investigated with Cox's regression model for survival data (81). This model defines a prognostic index from a linear combination of variables. A stepwise procedure ranks the variables and provides a significance level at each step based on a likelihood ratio test distributed as chi square with one degree of freedom (81). Results of the regression analysis are shown in Table 8 and indicate that number of social supports was the most important influence on duration in this study sample. In order of their selection, viewing the infant as recovered, planning a longer breast feeding time, being older and experiencing fewer problems were the other significant influences on longer duration.

The findings from this study support the earlier mentioned observations that mothers of preterm infants experience considerable difficulty with lactation and do not persist as long as mothers of term infants. The several variables that were related to duration of lactation suggest that a complex multicausal set of events determines when a decision will be made to stop lactation. One implication of this view is that it may be difficult to identify strategies that are uniformly effective in assisting mothers of

Table 7. Distribution of Responses to Planned Length of Breast-feeding

	f	% of valid responses	% of breast-feeding mothers (n = 88)
Less than 1 month	2	2.4	2.3
1 to 2 months	4	4.8	4.6
3 to 4 months	25	29.8	28.4
5 to 6 months	16	19.0	18.2
More than 6 months	37	44.0	42.0
Total	84	100.0	95.5

preterm infants. The finding from this study about the relative importance of social support lends credence to interventions that provide a support person(s) to assist with problem solving. The significant association of maternal education, age and infant condition may help define mothers most likely to benefit from interventions, e.g. those whose infants are slowest to recover, the younger and less well educated mothers. The finding that planned length of breast feeding was a significant influence is a reminder that mothers have their own perceptions about an appropriate duration of lactation. This information is important to obtain from mothers so that efforts can be directed to helping women achieve their goals. Strategies that can help women breast feed more easily may then make it possible for more women to want to breast feed for a longer time.

SUMMARY

The composition of human milk is influenced by biological and environmental factors many of which are well understood and predictable, e.g. stage of lactation and maternal dietary factors, but many for which our understanding is much more limited. 'Preterm' milk is a more recently described phenomenon which may be attributed to one or a combination of altered hormonal milieu, 'immature' mammary gland morphology or artifact of perinatal events associated with premature birth. Future studies must be directed towards elucidating those single and interactive factors responsible for the synthesis and secretion of human milk. From this knowledge one can develop a more comprehensive understanding of the basic physiology of lactation and the environmental modulators which must be controlled in order for a mother to achieve maximal lactational performance with optimal milk composition to meet the needs of her developing suckled infant.

Table 8. Cox's Regression Model of Variables Related to Hazard Function

Variable	Regression coefficient	df	Improvement in X^2	P2	Global X^2	Global P
Number of supports	-0.310	1	11.313	0.001	33.499	<0.001
Condition of infant	-0.393	2	11.313	0.001	58.423	<0.001
Planned length of breast-feeding	-0.651	3	9.048	0.003	68.771	<0.001
Maternal age	-0.103	4	8.475	0.004	74.007	<0.001
Problems per contact	0.262	5	6.485	0.011	78.527	<0.001

ACKNOWLEDGMENT

The authors gratefully acknowledge all the nursing mothers who so generously gave of their time and milk samples for the conduct of the studies described. Dr. Atkinson is supported by a Career Scientist Award from the Ministry of Health of Ontario. Dr. Kaufmán was supported by a doctoral fellowship and research award from the National Health Research and Development Program, Health and Welfare Canada, for the research reported herein.

REFERENCES

1. E. F. von Gorup-Besaneg, Lehrbuch der physiologischeu Chemie, Braunschweig 421 (1874).
2. F. S. Hammett, Variations in the composition of human milk during the first eleven days after parturition, J. Biol. Chem. 29(3):381 (1917).
3. M. Bell, Studies on the composition of human milk, J. Biol. Chem. 80:239 (1928).
4. I. G. Macy, Composition of human colostrum and milk, Am. J. Dis. Child 78:589 (1949).
5. S. A. Atkinson, M. H. Bryan, and G. H. Anderson, Human milk: difference in nitrogen concentration in milk from mothers of term and premature infants, J. Pediatr. 93:67 (1978).
6. S. A. Atkinson, G. H. Anderson, and M. H. Bryan, Human milk: comparison of the nitrogen composition in milk from mothers of premature and full-term infants, Am. J. Clin. Nutr. 33:811 (1980).
7. S. A. Atkinson, I. C. Radde, G. W. Chance, M. H. Bryan, and G. H. Anderson, Macromineral content of milk obtained during early lactation from mothers of premature infants, Early Hum. Dev. 4:5 (1980).
8. G. H. Anderson, S. A. Atkinson, and M. H. Bryan, Energy and macronutrient content of human milk during early lactation from mothers giving birth prematurely and at term, Am. J. Clin. Nutr. 34:258 (1981).
9. S. J. Gross, R. J. David, L. Bauman, and R. M. Tomarelli, Nutritional composition of milk produced by mothers delivering preterm, J. Pediatr. 96:641 (1980).
10. J. A. Lemons, L. Moye, D. Hall, and M. Simmons, Differences in the composition of preterm and term milk during early lactation, Pediatr. Res. 16:113 (1982).
11. J. Bitman, D. L. Wood, N. R. Mehta, P. Hamosh, and M. Hamosh, Comparison of the lipid composition of breast milk from mothers of term and preterm infants, Am. J. Clin. Nutr. 38:300 (1983).
12. N. F. Butte, C. Garza, C. A. Johnson, E. O'Brian-Smith, and B. L. Nichols, Longitudinal changes in milk composition of mothers delivering preterm and term infants, Early Hum. Devel. 9:153 (1984).
13. J. E. Chappell, M. T. Clandinin, G. J. Barbe, and D. T. Armstrong, Prostanoid content of human milk: relationships to milk fatty acid content, Endocrinol. Exp. 17:351 (1983).
14. G. LePage, S. Collet, D. Bougle, L. C. Kien, D. LePage, L. Dallaire, P. Darling, and C. Roy, The composition of preterm milk in relation to the degree of prematurity, Amer. J. Clin. Nutr. 40:1042 (1984).
15. L. Sann, F. Bienvenu, C. Lahet, J. Bienvenu, and M. Bethenod, Comparison of the composition of breast milk from mothers of term and preterm infants, Acta Paediatr. Scand. 70:115 (1981).
16. R. K. Chandra, Immunoglobulin and protein levels in breast milk produced by mothers of preterm infants, Nutr. Res. 2:27 (1982).

17. S. A. Udipi, A. Kirksey, K. West, and G. Giacoia, Vitamin B_6, Vitamin C and folacin levels in milk from mothers of term and preterm infants during the neonatal period, Am. J. Clin. Nutr. 42:522 (1985).
18. P. Guerrini, G. Bosi, R. Chierici, and A. Fabbri, Human milk: relationship of fat content with gestational age, Early Hum. Dev. 5:187 (1981).
19. K. J. Kaufman, Social-psychological influences on breast-feeding of of preterm infants, Doctoral Dissertation, The University of North Carolina at Chapel Hill (1986).
20. C. M. Hibberd, O. G. Brooke, N. D. Carter, M. Haug, and G. Harzer, Variation in the composition of breast milk during the first 5 weeks of lactation: implications for the feeding of preterm infants, Archives of Dis. in Childhood 57:658 (1982).
21. C. Conde, E. Casado des Frias, and M. Moro, Essential fatty acids in phosphoglycerides in human milk. Milk from mothers of term and preterm infants, Acta Pediatr. Scand. 72:255 (1983).
22. D. M. Anderson, F. H. Williams, R. B. Merkatz, P. K. Schulman, D. S. Kerr, and W. B. Pittard, Length of gestation and nutritional composition of human milk, Am. J. Clin. Nutr. 37:810 (1983).
23. G. Harzer, V. Franzke, and J. G. Bindels, Human milk nonprotein nitrogen components: changing patterns of free amino acids and urea in the course of early lactation, Am. J. Clin. Nutr. 40:303 (1984).
24. R. A. Ehrenkranz, B. A. Ackerman, and C. M. Nelli, Total lipid content and fatty acid composition of preterm human milk, J. Ped. Gastro. Nutr. 3:755 (1984).
25. R. A. Gibson, and G. M. Kneebone, Fatty acid composition of human colostrum and mature breast milk, Am. J. Clin. Nutr. 34:252 (1981).
26. J. R. Moran, R. Vaughan, S. Stroop, S. Coy, H. Johnston, and H. L. Greene, Concentrations and total daily output of micro nutrients in breast milk of mothers delivering preterm: A longitudinal study, J. Pediatr. Gastro. Nutr. 2:629 (1983).
27. R. Feeley, R. Eitenmiller, J. Jones, and H. Barnhart, Calcium, phosphorus and magnesium contents of human milk during early lactation, J. Ped. Gastro. Nutr. 2:262 (1983).
28. C. Garza, C. A. Johnson, E. O. Smith, and B. L. Nichols, Changes in the nutrient composition of human milk during gradual weaning, Am. J. Clin. Nutr. 37:61 (1983).
29. K. G. Dewey, D. A. Finley, and B. Lonnerdal, Breast milk volume and composition during late lactation (7-20 months), J. Pediatr. Gastro. and Nutr. 3:713 (1984).
30. E. Lauber, and M. Reinhardt, Studies on the quality of breast milk during 23 months of lactation in a rural community of the Ivory Coast, Am. J. Clin. Nutr. 32:1159 (1979).
31. P. E. Hartman, and J. K. Kulski, Changes in the composition of the mammary secretion of women after abrupt termination of breast-feeding, J. Physiol. 275:1 (1978).
32. J. K. Kulski, and P. E. Hartman, Changes in human milk composition during the initiation of lactation, Aust. J. Exp. Biol. Med. Sci. 59:101 (1981).
33. J. K. Kulski, P. E. Hartman, and W. J. Saint, Changes in the milk composition of nonpuerperal women, Am. J. Obstet. Gynecol. 139:597 (1981).
34. B. Lonnerdal, E. Forsum, and L. Hambraeus, A longitudinal study of the protein, nitrogen, and lactose contents of human milk from Swedish well-nourished mothers, Am. J. Clin. Nutr. 29:1127 (1976).
35. K. N. P. Mickleson, and K. M. Moriarty, Immunoglobulin levels in human colostrum and milk, J. Pediatr. Gastro. and Nutr. 1:381 (1982).
36. S. M. Donovan, and B. Lonnerdal, Non-protein nitrogen constituents in mature human milk and colostrum, Fed. Proc. 44(4):A7399 (1985).

37. M. C. Neville, J. C. Allen, and C. Watters, The mechanisms of milk secretion, in: "Lactation - Physiology, Nutrition and Breast-feeding," M. C. Neville and M. R. Niefert, eds. (1983).
38. G. Harzer, M. Haug, I. Dieterich, and P. R. Gentner, Changing patterns of human milk lipids in the course of the lactation and during the day, Am. J. Clin. Nutr. 37:612 (1983).
39. Department of Health and Social Security, The composition of mature human milk, Her Majesty's Stationery, U.K. office (1977).
40. R. G. Jensen, M. M. Hagerty, and K. E. McMahon, Lipids of human milk and infant formulas: a review, Am. J. Clin. Nutr. 31:990 (1978).
41. J. E. Chappell, M. T. Clandinin, and C. Kearney-Volpe, Trans fatty acids in human milk lipids: influence of maternal diet and weight loss, Am. J. Clin. Nutr. 42:49 (1985).
42. D. B. Jeliffe, and E. F. P. Jeliffe, The volume and composition of human milk in poorly nourished communities: a review, Am. J. Clin. Nutr. 31:492 (1978).
43. G. Steiner, J. J. Myher, and A. Kuksis, Milk and plasma lipid composition in a lactating patient with type I hyperlipo proteinemia, Amer. J. Clin. Nutr. 41:121 (1985).
44. M. J. Mellies, T. T. Ishikawa, P. Gartside, K. Burton, J. MacGee, K. Allen, P. M. Steiner, D. Brady, and C. J. Glueck, Effects of varying maternal dietary cholesterol and phytosterol in lactating women and their infants, Am. J. Clin. Nutr. 31:1354 (1978).
45. J. M. Potter, and P. J. Nestel, The effects of dietary fatty acids and cholesterol on the milk lipids of lactating women and the plasma cholesterol of breast-fed infants, Am. J. Clin. Nutr. 29:54 (1976).
46. I. G. Macy, and H. J. Kelly, Human milk and cows' milk in infant nutrition, in: "Milk: The Mammary Gland and its Secretion," Vol. II, B.K. Kon and A.T. Cowie, eds., Academic Press, N.Y. (1961).
47. H. Koboyashi, C. Kanno, K. Yanauchi, and J. Tsugo, Identification of α, β, γ and δ tocopherols and their contents in human milk, Am. J. Clin. Nutr. 33:198 (1980).
48. J. E. Chappell, T. Francis, and M. T. Clandinin, Vitamin A and E content of human milk at early stages of lactation, Early Human Develop. 11:157 (1985).
49. M. D. Salmenpera, Vitamin C nutrition during prolonged lactation: optimal in infants while marginal in some mothers, Am. J. Clin. Nutr. 40:1050 (1984).
50. J. Ek, Plasma, red cells, and breast milk folacin concentrations in lactating women, Am. J. Clin. Nutr. 38:929 (1983).
51. R. R. Eitenmiller, W. D. Bryan, I. K. Khalsa, R. M. Feeley, and H. M. Barnhart, Folate content of human milk during early lactational stages, Nut. Res. 4:391 (1984).
52. P. A. Nail, M. R. Thomas, and R. Eakin, The effect of thiamin and riboflavin supplementation on the level of those vitamins in human breast milk and urine, Am. J. Clin. Nutr. 33:198 (1980).
53. C. Roderuck, M. N. Coryell, H. H. Williams, and I. G. Macy, Metabolism of women during the reproductive cycle. IX. The utilization of riboflavin during lactation, J. Nutr. 32:267 (1946).
54. J. L. B. Roepke, and A. Kirksey, B_6 nutriture during pregnancy and lactation. II. The effect of long-term use of oral contraceptives, Am. J. Clin. Nutr. 32:2249 (1979).
55. E. Vuori, and P. Kuitunen, The concentrations of copper and zinc in human milk. A longitudinal study, Acta Paediatr. Scand. 68:33 (1979).
56. L. A. Vaughan, C. W. Weber, and S. R. Kemberling, Longitudinal changes in the mineral content of human milk, Am. J. Clin. Nutr. 32:2301 (1979).

57. N. F. Krebs, K. M. Hambidge, M. A. Jacobs, and S. Mylet, Zinc in human milk: diurnal and within-feed patterns, J. Pediatr. Gastro. and Nutr. 4:227 (1985).
58. C. E. Casey, K. M. Hambidge, and M. C. Neville, Studies in human lactation: zinc, copper, manganese and chromium in human milk in the first month of lactation, Am. J. Clin. Nutr. 41:1193 (1985).
59. A. W. Zimmerman, K. M. Hambidge, M. L. Lepow, D. Greenberg, M. L. Stover, and C. E. Casey, Acrodermatitis in breast fed premature infants: evidence for a defect of mammary zinc secretion, Pediatrics 69:176 (1982).
60. P. S. Aggett, D. J. Atherton, J. More, J. Davey, H. T. Delves, and J. T. Harries, zinc deficiency in a breast-fed pre-term infant, Arch. Dis. Child 55:547 (1980).
61. P. H. Parker, G. L. Helinek, R. Meneely, S. Stroop, F. K. Ghishan, and H. L. Greene, Zinc deficiency in a premature infant fed exclusively human milk, Am. J. Dis. Child 136:77 (1982).
62. J. P. Skala, O. Koldovsky, and P. Hahn, Cyclic nucleotides in breast milk, Am. J. Clin. Nutr. 34:343 (1981).
63. S. E. Carlson, N-Acetylneuraminic acid concentrations in human milk oligosaccharides and glycoproteins during lactation, Am. J. Clin. Nutr. 41:720 (1985).
64. L. C. Read, F. M. Upton, G. L. Francis, J. C. Wallace, G. W. Dahlenberg, and F. J. Ballard, Changes in the growth-promoting activity of human milk during lactation, Pediatr. Res. 18(2):133 (1984).
65. J. L. Linzell, and M. Peaker, Changes in colostrum composition and in the permeability of the mammary epithelium at about the time of parturition in the goat, J. Physiol. 243:129 (1974).
66. M. Peaker, Secretions of ions and water, in: "Biochemistry of Lactation," R. B. Mepham, ed., Elsevier Science Pub., N.Y. (1983).
67. K. G. Auerbach, and J. L. Avery, Relactation and the premature infant: report from a survey, RHNI Monograph #3, Resources in Human Nuturing, Denver (1979).
68. P. Verronen, Breast feeding of low birthweight infants, Acta Paediatr. Scand. 74:495 (1985).
69. A. Meberg, S. Willgraff, and H. A. Sande, High potential for breast feeding among mothers giving birth to preterm infants, Acta Paediat. Scand. 71:661 (1982).
70. V. Yu, J. Jamieson, and B. Bajuk, Feeding fresh breast milk to extremely preterm infants, Aust. Pediat. J. 17:186 (1981).
71. E. McNally, S. Hendricks, and I. Horowitz, A look at breast-feeding trends in Canada (1963-1982), Can. J. Pub. Health 76:101 (1985).
72. C. H. Hull, and N. H. Nie, SPSS Update 7-9, McGraw-Hill Book Company, N.Y. (1981).
73. J. P. Cole, Breastfeeding in the Boston suburbs in relation to personal-social factors, Clin. Pediatr. 16:352 (1977).
74. D. R. Entwisle, S. G. Doering, and T. W. Reilly, Sociopsychological determinants of women's breast feeding behaviour: A replication and extension, Amer. J. Orthopsychiatry 244 (1982).
75. M. L. Lyon, G. Chilver, D. G. White, and A. Woolett, Current maternal attitudes to infant feeding methods, Child Care, Health and Development 7:145 (1981).
76. L. T. Switzky, P. Vietze, and H. M. Switzky, Attitudinal and demographic predictors of breast feeding and bottle feeding behavior by mothers of six-week old infants, Psychological Reports 45:3 (1979).
77. D. L. Yeung, M. D. Pennell, M. Leung, and J. Hall, Breastfeeding: Prevalence and influencing factors, Can. J. Pub. Health 72:323 (1981).
78. A. P. Simopoulos, and G. D. Grave, Factors associated with the choice and duration of infant-feeding practice, Pediatrics (Suppl) 603 (1984).

79. A. J. Lyon, Effects of smoking on breast feeding, Arch. Dis. Childhood 58:378 (1983).
80. M. Wichelow, Breast-feeding in Cambridge, England: Factors affecting the mother's milk supply, J. Adv. Nursing 4:253 (1979).
81. E. T. Lee, Statistical methods for survival data analysis, "Lifetime Learning," Belmont, CA. (1980).

PATTERN OF CHANGE IN MILK COMPOSITION DURING LACTOGENESIS IN TERM AND PRETERM MOTHERS

Stephanie A. Atkinson,
Carol L. Wade,
Ruthann Stanhope and
Debra Fraser

Department of Pediatrics
McMaster University
Hamilton, Ontario, Canada L8N 3Z5

INTRODUCTION

Determination of the biochemical composition of milk from mothers giving birth prematurely (preterm milk) by Atkinson *et al*, (1-3) and subsequently by others (4-9) demonstrated that preterm milk had greater concentrations of nitrogen, lipid, medium chain fatty acids, energy and some minerals when compared to term milk at similar lactational stages. Evidence for these compositional differences is not universal and such lack of agreement amongst investigators may be attributed to differences in sample collection methodology, the inclusion of wide ranges of gestational stage and the greater degree of inter-individual variability in milk composition in preterm compared to term milk. For a more complete discussion of these areas, see chapter by Atkinson and Kaufman in this book.

In general, the patterns of change in milk composition in term milk have also been observed in preterm milk. What then could be the possible physiological basis for the reported differences in nutrient density between the two sources of milk? There is little evidence to suggest that this milk secretion has a teleological basis making it uniquely suited to meet the nutritional needs of the premature infant. A number of possible alterations in physiological mechanisms related to the lactational process can be proposed as explanations for the production of preterm milk of different nutrient composition. Milk composition might be affected by variations in breast stimulation due to incomplete emptying of the breast because of weak sucking of the small premature infant or use of a breast pump versus suckling. Alternatively, there is indirect evidence from lactating animals to support the hypothesis that differences in milk composition may be secondary to an altered or an interrupted hormonal status at parturition and/or altered development of hormone receptors within the mammary gland. Prepartum lactation is thought to be repressed by high placental-luteal hormone levels which serve to inhibit proliferation of mammary PRL receptors (10). Since women at 30 weeks of gestation have relatively lower circulating progesterone/estrogen levels compared to 38 to 40 weeks of gestation (11-13), proliferation of PRL receptors and magnitude of PRL release may be greater at preterm parturition. This hormonal milieu would be conducive to higher rates of mammary synthesis of lipid (4,9,14), protein

(1,2,5,6,8) or medium chain fatty acids (7,9) as has been reported. Hypothetically, rate of milk production may also be affected by the interference of high maternal anxiety states with oxytocin secretion and "let down" of milk. As well, decreased blood flow to the mammary gland could alter substrate availability or the hormonal milieu with subsequent alterations in milk composition. Neither of the latter explanations have been systematically investigated.

A further possible explanation for altered composition of preterm milk is based on the hypothesis that preterm mothers have an immature mammary system which permits paracellular leakage of serum proteins and ions through incompletely matured tight junctions or "leaky junctions" between apical membranes as has been described in the goat. During the prepartum period paracellular transport is thought to allow direct diffusion between the extracellular fluid and milk thus causing elevated concentrations of serum proteins (IgG), sodium and chloride and lowered lactose and potassium content compared to milk obtained post parturition in the animal (15). In women, indirect evidence does exist for the presence of paracellular transport of ions in pregnancy (16), in the mastitic breast (17) and during mammary gland involution (18,19). In these situations mammary secretions comprise elevated concentrations of sodium and chloride and lower lactose and potassium than mature milk but not altered protein content. The factors which regulate alveolar tight junction structure and thereby permeability via paracellular transport are not well defined. Among the possibilities suggested are frequent breast stimulation which may alter integrity of the mammary epithelium (15); local chemical mediators such as prostaglandins (20) or ionic calcium concentration (21); or a physical defect in epithelial cells (22).

To date, comparative studies of milk composition in mothers delivering prematurely and at term have been descriptive in nature and have not attempted to examine possible physiological mechanisms that may account for the observed differences in milk composition. Furthermore, the multitude of perinatal events associated with preterm birth that may affect the lactational process (see preceding Chapter) have not been controlled for. Two such important variables - postpartum timing of the initiation of lactation and the frequency of suckling or breast expression - have been addressed in the present study.

The objective of this study was to track changes in the concentrations of specific ions, lactose and urea from the first suckling/pumping through the initial days of lactation to determine if patterns of change in these milk components during lactogenesis might provide indirect evidence of differences in secretory mechanisms for specific components which may reflect altered mammary gland morphology.

METHODS

Subjects

Mothers delivering at Chedoke-McMaster Hospital who indicated a desire to breast feed were asked to participate in the study protocol as approved by the Research Advisory Group, Faculty of Health Sciences, McMaster University either during a visit to the prenatal clinic for full term mothers (FT) or shortly after birth for FT and preterm mothers (PT). The purpose and procedures of the study were explained by one of the research team (CLW or RS) and informed written consent obtained. Information on perinatal events, parity, previous breastfeeding experience, age, and drug use were obtained from the hospital chart and personal interview of the mother.

Collection of Milk Samples

Milk samples were obtained serially at each pumping or suckling beginning with the first time postpartum. Milk was collected using an electric pump (Egnell Ltd. or Medella Inc.) and stored in 5 ml polyethylene screw-top vials at -20°C until analysis. For mothers suckling their infants samples were obtained at the end of the feeding. In the case of manually pumped milk, the entire pumpings of milk from both breasts were measured for volume and then an aliquot removed for future analysis. These two methods of collection were presumed comparable as within feed variations of the components being analyzed have not been demonstrated (23). Milk samples were collected serially for the first 20 pumpings/sucklings. The time of day the milk was pumped and the volume of milk pumped were recorded for each sample.

Milk Analyses

For quantitation of sodium and potassium in milk, whole milk samples were warmed to 37°C and mixed by multiple manual inversions and diluted 2:1 with deionized water. Ion concentration was measured using potentiometric analysis with Na/K ion selective electrodes (KNa 1, Radiometer, Copenhagen, Denmark) run in the urine mode (24). Chloride ions were measured directly on whole milk using potentiometric titration with silver (25). Lactose was measured using the enzymatic method of the Boehringer-Mannheim lactose-galactose kit as previously described (4). Urea nitrogen was measured in defatted milk samples by the Sigma Urea nitrogen kit (Sigma No. 640, Sigma Chemical Co., St. Louis, MO.). Non-protein nitrogen was measured in defatted milks as previously described (26).

Statistical Analysis

Changes in individual milk components with progressing lactation underwent regression analysis. Differences between PT and FT groups were tested by employing analysis of variance (27). Patterns of change in milk components with progressing lactation were analyzed using both pumping number and postpartum day as the x variable.

RESULTS AND DISCUSSION

Ten mothers giving birth prematurely (<33 weeks gestation) and 10 mothers giving birth at term (>37 weeks gestation) were enrolled in the study. Characteristics of the two groups of mothers are summarized in Table 1. Neither the number of pregnancies nor the number of live born children differed between the groups. The major variable between the two groups was that 50% of the FT mothers were suckling their infants whereas all PT mothers were pumping milk. With respect to perinatal drug use, most mothers received intravenous Syntocinon (synthetic oxytocin, Sandoz Pharmaceuticals). Celestone (betamethasone, Schering Canada Inc.) was given predelivery to 6 of the PT mothers for the therapeutic purpose of inducing synthesis of fetal lung maturation when premture delivery was pending. Of course, no FT mothers received this drug.

Analysis of the frequency and timing of the milk samples obtained revealed striking differences between PT and FT groups in the cumulative number of pumpings/sucklings that had occurred at each postpartum day from one to seven. By postpartum day 3 the PT group had only 4.9 ± 1.2

Table 1. Characteristics of study population

	Preterm Mothers	Fullterm Mothers
n	10	10
Age, yr	26.5 ± 1.0[1]	28.7 ± 1.2
Gestational stage at delivery, wk	28.7 ± 1.1[2]	39.3 ± 0.5
Birthweight of infant, g	1235 ± 194[2]	3550 ± 190
Parity		
Primiparous	7/10	9/12
Mode of delivery		
Vaginal	6	6
Caesarian section	4	4
Previous breastfeeding experience	5/10	5/10
Mode of breastfeeding		
Suckling	0	5
Pumping	10	5

[1] X ± SEM

[2] ANOVA, $p<0.01$

cumulative milk pumpings versus 14.0 ± 2.5 in the FT group, $F = 9.807$, $p<0.01$. For the remaining days PT mothers had cumulative pumpings of <50% those of the FT mothers. If one looks at this another way, the postpartum days represented over the interval of the first 20 pumpings was different between groups (PT = 4.6 ± 0.1, FT = 3.5 ± 0.1, $F = 27.2$, $p<0.01$) owing to the initial delay in initiating pumping by PT mothers and the fact that they pump less frequently. This emphasizes the importance when undertaking comparative analysis of milk composition to consider whether matching of mother groups should be done by postpartum day or pumping/suckling interval, since the pumping patterns, i.e. initiation and frequency, of PT mothers is likely to differ dramatically from FT mothers suckling their infants. Presumably, the greater stimulation of the breasts with more frequent pumping will induce the final differentiation in mammary morphology and establish full milk synthesis at a faster rate. Accordingly, it was determined that a more appropriate comparison of milk composition would be by pumping number rather than postpartum or lactational day as is conventionally done.

The volume of milk produced by PT and FT mothers who were exclusively expressing milk was not different over the time period studied. Mean volumes of single pumpings were 73 ± 8 ml and 91 ± 11 ml for PT and FT milks, respectively. Volume of milk has no apparent relationship to ion concentration. Multiple regression analysis of ion concentrations over time, with volume of a single pumping as a covariable, showed no effect of milk volume on the changes in ion concentration with time.

Over the first twenty pumping/sucklings, milk Na^+ and Cl^- decreased significantly (Figure 1a & b) and were highly correlated (PT, r=0.890, FT, r=0.933, p<0.05) in both groups. In contrast, milk K^+ demonstrated a significant rise in FT milk and no change in PT milk over the same lactational interval (Figure 1c). Milk Na and K were inversely related: PT, $y = 21.8 - 0.140x$, $r = -0.500$, $p<0.01$; FT, $y = 19.2 - 0.065x$, $r = -0.214$, $p<0.05$).

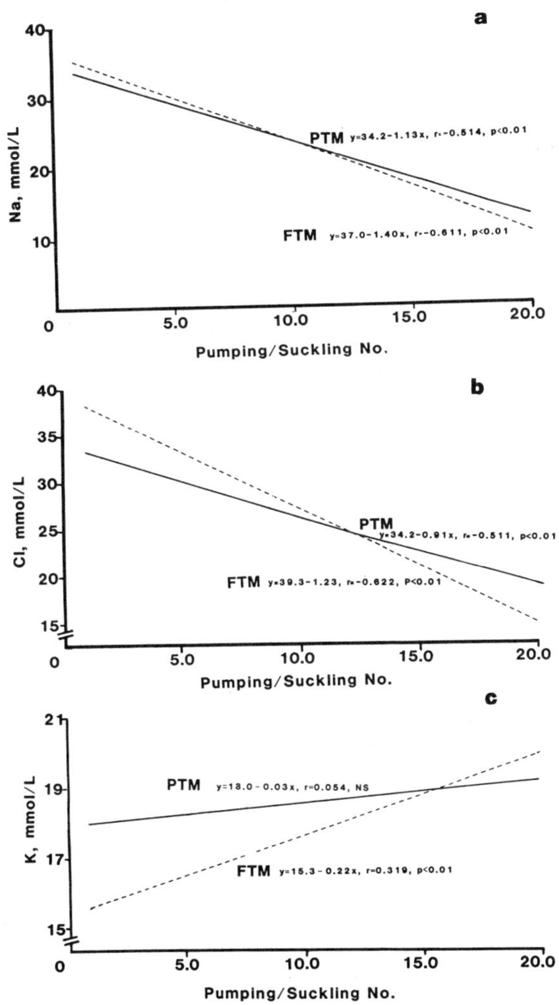

Figure 1. Regression equations describing the relationship between sequential pumpings/sucklings and concentration of Na (a), Cl (b) and K (c) in preterm milk (PTM, ——) and term milk (FTM, ---) during lactogenesis.

In this study, in contrast to the findings of some previous studies (5,6), no significant differences in ion content was observed between PT and FT milk during early lactation. However, this is the first study to control for the number of pumpings or breast stimulations that had taken place in each population in relation to milk content. We analyzed the milk composition data using postpartum day as the x variable rather than pumping number and obtained, not surprisingly, very different regression equations. The data employing postpartum day as the dependent variable have not been included as this approach has been deemed inappropriate for the comparison of milk composition between PT and FT mothers for reasons previously stated.

In a subgroup of 60 PT milks (n=3 PT mothers) and 60 FT milks (n=3 FT mothers) further analysis were completed on the first 10 pumpings/sucklings, including measurements of lactose, urea and non-protein nitrogen (NPN) composition. The regression equations describing the changes in concentration of Na, Cl, K and lactose over the first 10 pumpings/sucklings are summarized in Table 2. Sodium and Cl declined significantly and in parallel in both PT and FT milk although the rate of decline as indicated by the slope was greater than that determined by data from the first 20 pumpings/sucklings (Figure 1). Neither K nor lactose content changed significantly in either PT or FT milk. In FT milk, lactose is inversely correlated with Na and Cl ($p<0.01$) and positively correlated with K ($p<0.05$) but none of these relationships hold for PT milk.

The pattern of change with lactational stage in FT milk follows that demonstrated by Linzell and Peaker (15) in the goat during the stage of lactation around parturition when paracellular transport of ions and lactose is thought to occur. For PT mothers, the interrelationships of ions and lactose were not significant suggesting that transport mechanisms of ions are different from that of FT mothers. Certainly, in PT milk the patterns of change in ions observed do not reflect the "leaky junction" concept as described for the parturient goat and purported as an explanation of preterm milk composition (28). In general, the increase in the concentrations of

Table 2. Relationships between ions and lactose over the first 10 pumping/sucklings in PT and FT milk

Variable	Regression Equation	r	P
Milk Na (mmol/L)/PSNo[1]	PTM[2] - y = 40.6 - 2.87x	-0.619	<0.01
	FTM[3] - y = 35.8 - 1.60x	-0.370	<0.05
Milk Cl (mmol/L)/PSNo	PTM - y = 40.6 - 2.33x	-0.590	<0.01
	FTM - y = 35.4 - 0.96	-0.230	<0.05
Milk K (mmol/L)/PSNo	PTM - y = 18.4 + 0.24x	0.225	NS
	FTM - y = 15.2 + 0.13x	0.197	NS
Milk lactose/milk Na	PTM - y = 6.69 - 0.02x	-0.330	NS
	FTM - y = 7.85 - 0.06x	-0.791	<0.01
Milk lactose/milk Cl	PTM - y = 6.48 - 0.01x	-0.130	NS
	FTM - y = 7.82 - 0.05x	-0.673	<0.01
Milk lactose/milk K	PTM - y = 5.10 + 0.05x	0.164	NS
	FTM - y = 2.98 + 0.20x	0.390	<0.05

[1]PSNO = Pumping Suckling Number
[2]PTM = Preterm milk
[3]FTM = Full-term milk

lactose and K and the decrease in the concentrations of Na and Cl in mammary secretions during lactogenesis are consistent with the existence of a paracellular pathway across the mammary gland just prior to parturition (16). Why there would be differences in the transport pathways between PT and FT milk during lactogenesis requires further study. The concept of "paracellular" transport in mammary glands has not been well explored in humans. In fact, the observation that milk glucose was not increased in association with other changes indicative of mammary epithelium permeability, during the colostral phase in women (16,29) casts some doubt as to whether the observations of mammary permeability in the goat (15) should be directly extrapolated to women (18).

For those components which did not change significantly over the first 10 pumpings, only NPN was significantly different between groups being higher in PT milk (Table 3) as previously demonstrated by Atkinson et al (2). Again, it is surprising that if paracellular transport occurs in early lactation why would a small molecule such as urea not be subject to alterations in transport into mammary secretions via this route.

CONCLUSION

In the population studied, mothers giving birth prematurely demonstrated a different timing pattern than mothers delivering at term in the initiation of lactation and frequency of pumping during early lactation. Accordingly, comparison of milk composition between PT and FT milk using postpartum day as the dependent variable will misrepresent the cumulative lactational experience of these two groups of mothers. Because of this, the current study employed sequential pumping/suckling numbers as the dependent variable.

The pattern of breast or nipple stimulation during lactogenesis may impact an important effect on the post-parturient differentiation of the mammary gland which in turn effects transport of components into early milk. Certainly in the goat, pre-parturient milking of one mammary gland evoked changes in milk composition which were not evident in the contralateral non-milked gland (15). The change in composition in the milked gland was matched by decreases in the permeability to labelled sucrose, sodium and chloride passing from blood to milk (15). Maule and colleagues (20) have suggested that a local factor such as a prostaglandin operates in late pregnancy to keep open the paracellular pathway and that this factor can be removed by milking. Future studies designed to examine preterm milk composition and the physiology of lactation in mothers giving birth prematurely should consider the breast stimulation and pumping pattern of the mothers since these activities may impact considerably on the composition of the milk produced.

Table 3. Comparison of Components in Term and Preterm Milk During Early Lactation[1]

Component	Preterm	Term	F	P
Lactose, g/dl	6.12 $\pm$ 0.20[2]	6.19 $\pm$ 0.20	0.06	NS
NPN, mg/dl	85.0 $\pm$ 7.5	66.5 $\pm$ 5.1	4.33	$p<0.05$
Urea N, mg/dl	14.7 $\pm$ 0.7	12.6 $\pm$ 0.9	3.31	NS
Urea N/NPN, %	19.1 $\pm$ 1.7	21.5 $\pm$ 2.2	0.68	NS

[1] averaged over pumpings 1 to 10, n=30 samples per group
[2] $\bar{X} \pm SEM$

ACKNOWLEDGEMENT

The authors are very grateful to all the mothers who so willingly followed the study protocol and to Karen Distefano, R.N. and Kerri Timoffee who assisted in data collection and analysis. Dr. Atkinson is a Career Scientist of the Ministry of Health of Ontario. Ms. Wade was recipient of a Medical Research Council summer studentship in support of this research project.

REFERENCES

1. S. A. Atkinson, M. H. Bryan, and G. H. Anderson, Human milk: difference in nitrogen concentration in milk from mothers of term and premature infants, J. Pediatr. 93:67 (1978).
2. S. A. Atkinson, G. H. Anderson, and M. H. Bryan, Human milk: comparison of the nitrogen composition in milk from mothers of premature and full-term infants, Am. J. Clin. Nutr. 33:811 (1980).
3. S. A. Atkinson, I. C. Radde, G. W. Chance, M. H. Bryan, and G. H. Anderson, Macromineral content of milk obtained during early lactation from mothers of premature infants, Early Hum. Dev. 4:5 (1980).
4. G. H. Anderson, S. A. Atkinson, and M. H. Bryan, Energy and macronutrient content of human milk during early lactation from mothers giving birth prematurely and at term, Am. J. Clin. Nutr. 34:258 (1981).
5. S. J. Gross, R. J. David, L. Bauman, and R. M. Tomarelli, Nutritional composition of milk produced by mothers delivering preterm, J. Pediatr. 96:641 (1980).
6. J. A. Lemons, L. Moye, D. Hall, and M. Simmons, Differences in the composition of preterm and term milk during early lactation, Pediatr. Res. 16:113 (1982).
7. J. Bitman, D. L. Wood, N. R. Mehta, P. Hamosh, and M. Hamosh, Comparison of the lipid composition of breast milk from mothers of term and preterm infants, Am. J. Clin. Nutr. 38:300 (1983).
8. N. F. Butte, C. Garza, C. A. Johnson, E. O'Brian-Smith, and B. L. Nichols, Longitudinal changes in milk composition of mothers delivering preterm and term infants, Early Hum. Devel. 9:153 (1984).
9. J. E. Chappell, M. T. Clandinin, G. J. Barke, and D. T. Armstrong, Prostanoid content of human milk: Relationship to milk fatty acid content, Endocrinol Exp. 17:351 (1983).
10. J. Djiane, and P. Durand, Prolactin-progesterone antagonism in self regulation of prolactin receptors in the mammary gland during pregnancy and lactation, Nature 266:641 (1977).
11. C. R. Parker, R. B. Everett, J. G. Querk, P. J. Whalley, and N. F. Gant, Hormone production during pregnancy in the primigravida patient I plasma levels of progesterone and 5-alpha-pregnone - β 3,20 dione throughout pregnancy of normal women and women who developed pregnancy-induced hypertension, Am. J. Obstet. Gynecol. 135:778 (1979).
12. J. E. Buster, R. J. Chang, D. L. Preston, B. M. Slashaff, L. M. Cousins, G. E. Abraham, C. S. Hobel, and J. R. Marshall, Interrelationships of circulating maternal steroid concentrations in third trimester pregnancies, J. Clin. Endocrinol. Metab. 48:133 (1979).
13. H. H. Goh, L. S. Lim, P. C. Wong, and S. S. Ratnam, Plasma oestriol in pregnancies complicated by diabetes mellitus, Aust. J. Exp. Biol. Med. Sci. 60:529 (1982).
14. G. Lepage, S. Collet, D. Bougle, L. C. Kien, D. Lepage, L. Daillaire, P.

Darling, and C. Roy, The composition of preterm milk in relation to the degree of prematurity, Amer. J. Clin. Nutr. 40:1042 (1984).

15. J. L. Linzell, and M. Peaker, Changes in colostrum composition and in permeability of mammary epithelium at about the time of parturition in the goat, J. Physiol. (London) 243:129 (1974).

16. J. K. Kulski, and P. E. Hartman, Changes in milk composition during the initiation of lactation, Aust. J. Exp. Biol. Med. Sci. 59:101 (1981).

17. A. E. Conner, Elevated levels of sodium and chloride in milk from mastitic breast, Pediatrics 63:910 (1979).

18. P. E. Hartman, and C. G. Prosser, Physiological basis of longitudinal changes in human milk yield and composition, Fed. Proc. 43:2448 (1984).

19. C. Garza, C. A. Johnson, E. O'Brian Smith, and B. L. Nichols, Changes in the nutrient compositon of human milk during gradual weaning, Am. J. Clin. Nutr. 37:61 (1983).

20. F. M. Maule-Walker, and M. Peaker, Local production of prostaglandins in relation to mammary function at the onset of lactation in the goat, J. Physiol. 309:65 (1980).

21. M. C. Neville, and M. Peaker, Ionized calcium in milk and integrity of the mammary epithelium in the goat, J. Physiol. 313:561 (1981).

22. O. M. Shannon, and D. R. Pitelka, Influence of cell shape on the induction of functional differentiation in mouse mammary cells in vitro, In Vitro 17:1016 (1981).

23. M. C. Neville, R. P. Keller, J. Seacat, C. E. Casey, J. C. Allen, and P. Archer, Studies on human lactation: Within-feed and between breast variation in selected components of human milk, Am. J. Clin. Nutr. 40:635 (1984).

24. M. C. Neville, R. P. Keller, B. Lonnderdal, S. Atkinson, C. L. Wade, N. Butte, and P. B. Moser, Measurement of electrolyte and macromineral concentrations in human milk, in: "Human Lactation: Milk Components and Methodologies," R. G. Jensen and M.C. Neville, Eds., Plenum, N.Y. (1985).

25. E. Cotlove, Determination of chloride in biological materials, Meth. Biochem. Anal. 12:277 (1964).

26. S. A. Atkinson, Characterization of the non-protein nitrogen fraction of human milk: methodological considerations, in: "Human Lactation: Milk Components and Methodologies," R.G. Jensen and M.C. Neville, Eds., Plenum, N.Y. (1985).

27. G. W. Snedecor, and W. G. Cochrane, Statistical Methods, 6th Edition, Iowa State Uniersity Press, Iowa (1967).

28. G. H. Anderson, The effect of prematurity on milk composition and its physiological basis, Fed. Proc. 43:2438 (1984).

29. C. G. Prosser, and P. E. Hartman, Saliva and milk composition during the menstrual cycle of women, Aust. J. Exp. Biol. Med. Sci. 61:265 (1983).

LIPID COMPOSITION OF PREPARTUM, PRETERM AND TERM MILK

Joel Bitman, D.L. Wood, Margaret C. Neville, L.M. Freed, N.R. Mehta, P. Hamosh and Margit Hamosh

USDA-Agricultural Research Service, Beltsville, MD
University of Colorado School of Medicine, Denver, CO and
Georgetown University Medical Center, Washington, D.C.

INTRODUCTION

The mammary gland undergoes a gradual development in preparation for lactation throughout the 40-week pregnancy period. During this period, the mammary gland is subjected to both maternal and placental hormonal influences. It would be expected that a mother giving birth prematurely would have less developed mammary glandular tissue than a term mother. The mammary glands of preterm mothers might be considered to be immature and this might be of significance for nutrition of the premature infant.

We had several objectives:

1) do different gestation lengths result in differences in milk lipids?

   We compared milk lipid composition of mothers who gave birth prematurely at 26-30 and at 31-36 weeks with that of term mothers.

2) do changes occur in milk lipids during the course of lactation?

   We studied milk lipid composition of all groups at day 3 for colostrum, day 7 for transitional milk and days 21, 42 and 84 for mature milk.

3) are the lipids of mammary secretions before parturition different from those present in milk?

   Small amounts of a milky secretion can be expressed from the breast from early pregnancy onwards. This secretion has been termed precolostrum. We studied lipid composition of mammary secretions at 42 and 10 days before parturition and at 3, 7 and 56 days postpartum in a group of term mothers.

TABLE 1. LIPID CONTENT OF PREPARTUM SECRETION AND OF HUMAN MILK

	---Prepartum--		------------Postpartum---------		
	Early	Late	Colostrum	Transitional	Mature
Lipid g/dl	1.15[a]	1.28[a]	3.16[b]	3.49[b]	4.14[b]
SE	0.16	0.42	0.17	0.40	0.44
Days	-42.00	-9.50	3.00	7.20	56.20
N	6	6	6	6	6

[a,b]Means in the same row with different superscripts differ ($p < 0.05$)

EXPERIMENTAL

Milk was collected on postpartum days 3 (colostrum), 7, 21, 42 and 84 from 18 preterm mothers who delivered infants between 26-30 weeks of gestation, from 28 preterm mothers who delivered infants between 31-36 weeks of gestation, and from six term mothers who delivered infants at 37-40 weeks of gestation. Samples were stored frozen at -20°C until lipid analysis (1,2). A group of 5 subjects who delivered at term provided samples of mammary secretions at times designated as Early Prepartum (-42.0 days) and Late Prepartum (-9.5 days). Mammary secretions before parturition are termed precolostrum; secretions during days 0-4 are defined as colostrum. Milk secreted from postpartum days 7-14 is termed transitional milk and milk secreted after day 14 postpartum is termed mature milk.

Lipids were extracted by the method of Folch et al (3). Total lipids were determined gravimetrically on aliquots of the chloroform extract. Fatty acids (FA) were determined by temperature-programmed gas liquid chromatography of fatty acid methyl esters (1,2). Neutral lipid (NL) classes were determined by quantitative densitometry in situ after separation by two-stage thin layer chromatography (TLC) as described earlier (1). Phospholipids (PL) were separated from NL using commercially available, pre-packed disposable silica gel Sep-Pak cartridges and PL classes separated by TLC (2). The NL and PL were quantitatively determined by spectrophotodensitometry in situ using the Shimadzu CS-910 Dual Wavelength TLC Scanner (1,2).

RESULTS

Fat Concentration and Neutral Lipid Classes

Fat, contained mainly in the core of the milk globules, increases gradually from 2% in colostrum to 2.9% in transitional and to 3.6% in mature milk (1). Fat concentrations increased significantly in all maternal groups during the first 21 days of lactation and were not different among mothers of preterm or term infants. Fat concentrations were relatively constant in mature milk at 21, 42 and 84 days.

The concentration of lipid in the mammary secretions during the prepartum period was relatively constant, being about 1 g/dl (Table 1). Postpartum, fat concentrations increased so that colostrum contained 3 times the prepartum level ($p < 0.05$). Fat concentration in colostrum in this group of mothers, 3.16%, was higher than that observed in colostrum from preterm and term mothers, 2.04% (1). This may represent the influence of physical stimulation of the mammary gland since these mothers had been taking prepartrum mammary secretion samples from their

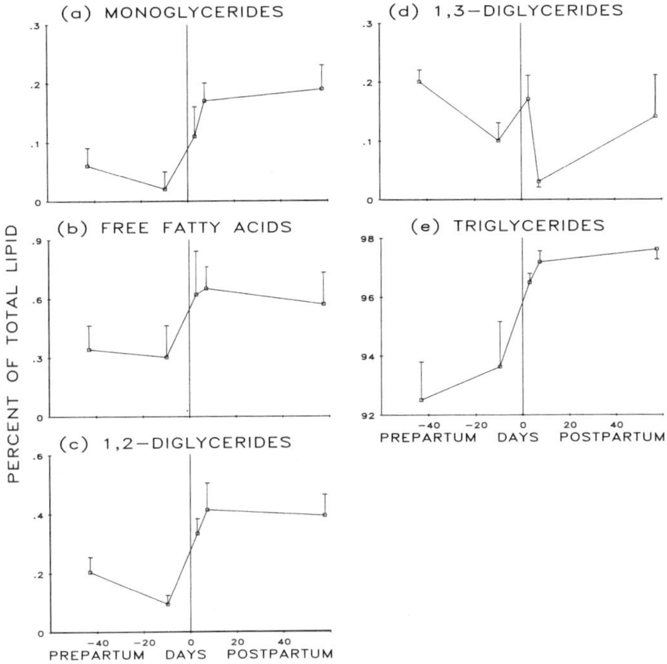

Fig. 1. Changes in distribution of neutral lipid classes in the mammary secretion of women pre- and postpartum.

breasts by manual expression or may represent individual or nutritional differences present in these 5 mothers.

The fat in milk is present in the form of globules composed of an outer membrane of polar lipids and protein and an inner core of neutral fat. The core of the globules consist primarily of triglycerides containing almost all of the milk fat, 98-99%. The milk fat globule membrane, in contrast, is composed mainly of PL and cholesterol.

Prepartum secretions were clearly different from postpartum secretions in distribution of the lipids among the various classes (Fig. 1). Almost all of the lipid present in either pre- or postpartum secretion was triglyceride (TG) (Fig. 1e). Early prepartum secretion contained 93% TG but this increased to 97% in postpartum secretions ($p < 0.05$). 1,2-diglycerides, monoglycerides and free fatty acids all exhibited increases from prepartum to postpartum levels.

Cholesterol exhibited a decline during lactation. Cholesterol was high in colostrum and decreased to lower levels in transitional and mature milk (Fig. 2). The concentration in mature milk was 13.5 mg/dl distributed as 87% free cholesterol and 13% cholesteryl ester (CE). Two interesting trends were apparent:

1) as previously observed (1,2), cholesterol was high in colostrum and declined during lactation,

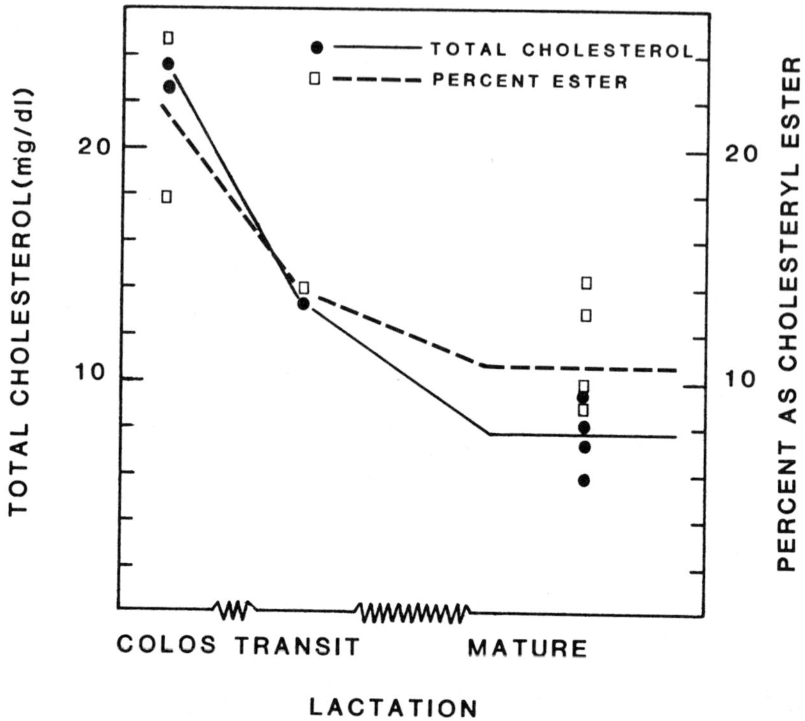

Fig. 2. Proportion of cholesteryl ester in human milk during lactation.

2) the percentage of cholesteryl ester was about two times higher in colostrum (20%) than in mature milk. Thus, the amount of cholesteryl ester was about 5 mg per dl in colostrum but was only 1 mg per dl in mature milk.

The lipid of prepartum secretions contained a higher proportion of cholesterol and cholesteryl esters than colostrum and milk (Fig.3). In early prepartum secretions, cholesterol and cholesteryl ester concentrations totaled 39 mg/dl which comprised 3.4% of total lipid. Shifts in lipid class distribution occurred postpartum, and cholesterol showed a progressive decrease to the 10-15 mg/dl usually found in colostrum, transitional and mature milk. Cholesteryl esters also decreased to the small percentages usually found in milk. The relative proportion of cholesterol present as ester was considerably higher in precolostrum and colostrum (27-40%) than in mature milk (20%).

Phospholipids

Several differences were observed in the PL from preterm and term milks: 1) PL from preterm mothers were higher than term; 2) PL from preterm mothers exhibited a continuous curvilinear decline; 3) term PL showed a smaller linear decline (2). PL were present at a concentration of 0.5% of total lipids, or 15-20 mg per deciliter. Our results are in agreement with the level of 0.26% reported by Bracco et al (4). Many reports gave values 2 to 10 times higher than the amounts we found by

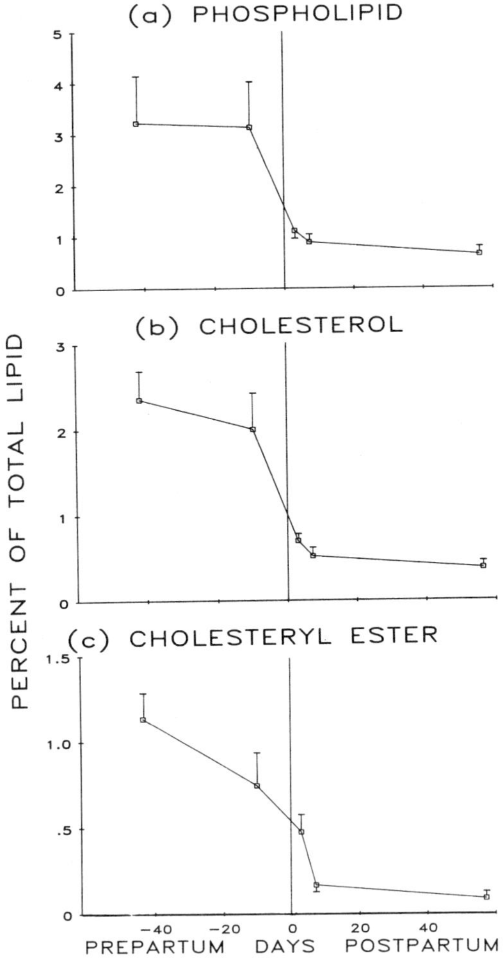

Fig. 3. Changes in distribution of phospholipid, cholesterol and cholesteryl ester in the mammary secretion of women pre- and postpartum.

direct quantitation of the separated phospholipids. Almost all of these results were obtained by non-specific colorimetric procedures to determine lipid phosphorus. Relative comparisons are difficult because of differences in sampling, analytical methodology and handling as well as possible biological differences.

Phospholipid concentrations in pre- and postpartum mammary secretions of the 5 women are shown in Table 2. Total PL remained relatively constant in the prepartum period, being about 40 mg/dl, and decreased after parturition to about 27 mg/dl. As a perccent of total lipid, PL showed progressive declines, decreasing from 1.12% in colostrum to half of that in mature milk.

TABLE 2. Phospholipid class composition of prepartum secretion and of human milk during lactation

Group	mg/dl	% of total lipid	Percentage in phospholipid class: S	PC	PS	PI	PE
Early PP*	37 ±6	3.23[a]	51.6[a]	24.8	8.6	6.2[a]	8.9[a]
Late PP	40 ±4	3.14[a]	47.7[b]	27.3	9.0	6.0[a]	10.0[a]
Colost	35 ±3	1.12[b]	33.2[c]	28.8	10.2	9.5[c]	18.2[b]
Transit	31 ±3	0.90[b]	36.3[c]	30.2	8.2	7.2[ab]	18.1[b]
Mature	27 ±3	0.65[b]	35.0[c]	28.8	7.5	8.2[bc]	20.5[b]

*PP = Prepartum Values represent means ± standard errors
S = sphingomyelin, PC = phosphatidyl choline, PS = phosphatidylserine, PI = phosphatidylinositol, PE = phosphatidylethanolamine

[a,b,c]Means in the same column with different superscripts differ ($p < 0.05$)

The distribution of the PL of preterm and term milk into their 5 major constituent classes revealed that changes occurred primarily in early lactation as secretion changed from colostrum to transitional to mature milk (2). Milk PL did not exhibit any marked differences attributable to length of gestation after day 21. The constancy of the phospholipid distribution indicated that the composition of the membrane of the milk fat globule was identical at all stages of lactation. This is not surprising since the PL probably fulfill similar structural functions in these milks.

Prepartum mammary secretion was clearly different from postpartum in distribution of PL among classes (Table 2). The largest differences were noted in content of sphingomyelin (S) and phosphatidyl ethanolamine (PE). In prepartum secretions, S was 50% of total PL, about 15% higher than the amount present postpartum ($p < 0.05$). Prepartum PE was only half the postpartum level ($p < 0.05$). As lactation progressed, PL class composition was relatively constant in colostrum, transitional and mature milk (Table 2). Mean values for PL class composition for postpartum samples of these 5 women for sphingomyelin (S), phosphatidyl choline (PC), phosphatidyl serine (PS), phosphatidyl inositol (PI), and phosphatidyl ethanolamine (PE), were 35, 29, 9, 8 and 19% respectively. These values were very similar to those of preterm and term milks (2), 38, 28, 9, 6 and 19% for S, PC, PS, PI, and PE respectively.

Fatty Acids

Composition of milk lipids changed as lactation progressed from secretion of colostrum to transitional and mature milk (1). In milk from preterm mothers, medium-chain saturated fatty acids, 10:0, 12:0 and 14:0, which comprise 15% of total fatty acids, increased about 100% over concentrations in colostrum. The 2-fold increase in shorter-chain fatty acids in VPT and PT milk means that for 2 to 3 months of lactation, the preterm infant ingesting its' own mother's milk is receiving about 17% of total lipid in fatty acid of medium length whereas term infants receive about 10%. Few differences were observed among gestational groups in concentrations of palmitic, stearic and linoleic acids. Oleic acid, 18:1, was the major fatty acid which compensated in a reciprocal manner for the differences observed with the medium-chain fatty acids.

There has been considerable interest in levels of polyunsaturated fatty acids in breast milk with regard to providing adequate amounts of essential fatty acids for growth of the newborn. Crawford et al (5,6) emphasized the importance of C20-C22 polyunsaturated fatty acids as essential nutrients because they are structural lipids for growth of the brain and nervous tissue. Early high levels of 20:4 serve for brain cell proliferation, then decrease as myelination increases and that increasing amounts of 24:1 are used. Crawford et al (5) found that these changes occurred in the milk over a 9-month lactation period.

We found few if any differences in levels of long-chain polyunsaturated (LCP) fatty acids, C20 to C22, in mature milk after 21 days of lactation (1,2). We observed a definite trend in all three gestational groups. Colostrum contained higher amounts of these LCP fatty acids, derived from both linoleic acid (20:2w6, 20:3, 20:4, 22:4, 22:5w6) and from linolenic acid (20:5, 22:5w3, 22:6), than transitional milk and these levels were further reduced in mature milk. Moreover, those mothers who delivered at the earliest times had higher amounts of LCP in their milk than those who delivered closer to term.

A comparison of the fatty acid composition of pre- and postpartum secretions with preterm and term milk is shown in Table 3. In contrast to large differences observed in lipid class distribution (Fig. 1 and 3) and in PL class composition (Table 2) between pre- and postpartum secretions, only small differences were seen in fatty acid composition (Table 3). In prepartum secretions, the medium-chain fatty acids (8:0 to 14:0), which are synthesized in the mammary gland, showed a small increase of about 3% ($p < 0.05$). This was compensated for by decreases in 16:0, 18:0, 18:1 and by a decrease ($p < 0.05$) in nine minor long-chain polyunsaturated fatty acids.

DISCUSSION

The similarity of the FA composition of prepartum secretions to that of postpartum secretions indicated that the enzymatic systems involved in generation of the core lipid components were in place and functioning adequately throughout the prepartum period, long before the birth of the infant. Since FA composition changed only slightly but fat content increased from 1% to 3%, the same systems apparently were operating after initiation of lactogenesis but at a higher synthetic rate. Thus, in term mothers, a fatty acid composition was produced in milk postpartum that was very similar to the FA composition of prepartum mammary secretions.

In mothers delivering prematurely, however, milk FA composition exhibited larger differences (1). Concentrations of 12:0 and 14:0 were about 2X the concentrations found in prepartum secretions or in term milk. Preterm LCP in colostrum and transitional milk were about 2X LCP concentrations in term mothers (1), suggesting that the synthetic systems in preterm mothers were operating differently to generate these medium-chain and long-chain polyunsaturated fatty acids.

Smith (7) has examined the time course of development of lipogenic enzymes in the rat and showed that the enzymes involved in synthesis of medium-chain and long-chain fatty acids are regulated independently.

TABLE 3. Fatty acid composition of pre- and postpartum mammary secretions and of mature preterm and term milk (weight percent)

Fatty acid	Prepartum*	Postpartum+	Term Milk**	Preterm Milk**
10:0+	0.1[a]	0.7[b]	1.0	1.3
12:0	1.7[a]	3.9[b]	4.5	7.0
14:0	4.9	5.3	5.7	8.0
14:1	0.3	0.3	-	-
15:0	0.4	0.4	0.3	0.2
16:0	21.4	20.6	22.2	21.6
16:1	2.8	3.0	3.8	2.7
17:0	0.7	0.9	0.5	0.5
18:0	8.1	6.9	7.7	7.2
18:1	34.9	33.7	35.5	33.6
18:2	15.0	16.7	15.6	14.8
18:3	2.4	2.4	1.0	0.8
20.0	0.6	0.5	0.3	0.1
21.0	0.3	0.4	0.2	0.1
LCPo	6.3[a]	4.1[b]	1.8	2.2

* Mean of Early Prepartum and Late Prepartum samples
+ Mean of colostral, transitional and mature milk samples
**Term and preterm milk data from mature milk of mothers (1)
+ 8:0, 10:1, 12:1 (not shown) all increased from 0.0 wt% prepartum to trace concentrations postpartum
o Long-chain polyunsaturated fatty acids + sum of 20:2, 20:3, 20:4, 20:5, 22:2, 22:4, 22:5w6, 22:5w3, 22:6

[a,b]Means with different superscripts in pre- and postpartum rows differ ($p < 0.05$)

During pregnancy the enzyme responsible for medium-chain fatty acid synthesis increased and reached a maximum before parturition. This would provide a high proportion of medium-chain fatty acids on initiation of lactation, supplying a readily digestible energy source at early lactation times, when the neonate's digestive system is immature.

In the study reported here in women, after initiation of lactogenesis, fatty acid composition changed only slightly but fat content increased from 1% in the prepartum mammary secretions to 3%. In both rats and cows, in vitro metabolic studies by Smith (7) and Mellenberger et al (8) demonstrated that the ability of mammary gland tissue to synthesize fat increased greatly after parturition. Before birth, synthetic capacity was relatively low and the pattern of fatty acids synthesized was predominantly long-chain acids with low amounts of medium-chain fatty acids. After parturition, the rate of lipogenesis increased and the pattern shifted towards increased short and medium-chain fatty acids, typical of functional secretory lactating mammary tissue. This would serve to supply increased energy for nutrition of the young.

There is almost no information in the literature concerning the lipid composition of prepartum mammary secretions in the human. In a recent report, Parodi (9) found that prepartum mammary secretion in the cow differed greatly from normal milk. As lactation progressed, concentrations of the small and medium-chain length fatty acids (4:0, 6:0, 8:0, 10:0) increased. Large increases were also observed in 18:0 and 18:1.

The decline that we observed in the concentration of cholesterol, phospholipids and cholesteryl esters from the prepartum period may be related to abrupt permeability changes which occur in the mammary gland at about the time of parturition. The abrupt shifts that occur in lipid components parallel abrupt shifts observed in a number of other mammary constituents in women (10) and in ruminants (11). Several investigators (23-26) demonstrated that immunoglobulins, lactoferrin, c-lactalbumin, albumin, Na and Cl were high in prepartum secretions in women, goats and cows and by day 3 postpartum, concentrations approached those of normal milk. Linzell and Peaker (11,12) concluded that these changes in composition were brought about by transport through the spaces between the mammary epithelial cells. This paracellular pathway involves an alteration in the permeability of the junctions between adjacent cells from leaky in pregnancy to tight near term.

The larger amounts of PL, cholesterol and cholesteryl esters might be present in prepartum secretions as residual fragments of epithelial cells, leukocytes, red blood cells, or might represent contamination with small amounts of plasma. Indeed, almost all plasma lipids are transported primarily in equal amounts in PL and in cholesteryl esters (13-15). Leaky junctions between mammary gland cells, permitting a small contamination with blood plasma, could explain the presence of high amounts of cholesterol, phospholipids and cholesteryl esters. Thus, the permeability changes documented in women (10) and in ruminants (11, 12) which result in abrupt changes in carbohydrates, proteins and electrolytes, could also be responsible for the dramatic changes in lipids that were observed between prepartum and postpartum mammary secretions. Alternatively, the presence of higher amounts of cholesterol and phospholipids prepartum might represent either greater synthesis by the mammary gland or different lipid transport mechanisms.

SUMMARY

Changes in the lipid composition of mammary secretions of 5 women were studied at two prepartum periods and compared to the composition of colostrum, transitional and mature breast milk. Fat content was about 1 g/dl prepartum and increased to 3-4 g/dl postpartum. Triglycerides were 93% of total lipids prepartum and increased to 97% postpartum. All fat globule core lipids, with the exception of 1,3-diglycerides, increased postpartum. Prepartum secretions contained higher amounts of the membrane components, phospholipids, cholesterol and cholesteryl esters, which declined postpartum. Comparisons were also made with the lipid composition of milk from 46 mothers delivering prematurely and with milk from 6 term mothers. Fat content of preterm and term milks increased during lactation, whereas phospholipids and cholesterol declined. Concentrations of medium-chain fatty acids increased from colostrum to mature milk and were highest in preterm milk.

REFERENCES

1. Bitman J, Wood DL, Hamosh M, Hamosh P, Mehta NR. Comparison of the lipid composition of breast milk from mothers of term and preterm infants. Am J Clin Nutr 1983;38:300-12.
2. Bitman J, Wood DL, Mehta NR, Hamosh P, Hamosh M. Comparison of the phospholipid composition of breast milk from mothers of term and preterm infants during lactation. Am J Clin Nutr 1984;40:1103-19.

3. Folch J, Lees M, Sloane-Stanley GH. A simple method for the isolation and purification of total lipids from animal tissues. J Biol Chem 1957;226:497-509.
4. Bracco U, Hidalgo J, Bohren H. Lipid composition of the fat globule membrane of human and bovine milk. J Dairy Sci 1972;55:165-72.
5. Crawford MA, Hall B, Laurance BM, Munhambo A. Milk lipids and their variability. Curr Med Res Opinion 1976; 4 (Suppl 1):33-43.
6. Crawford MA, Hassan AG, Rivers JPW. Essential fatty acid requirements in infancy. Am J Clin Nutr 1978;31:2181-5.
7. Smith S. Mechanism of chain length determination in biosynthesis of milk fatty acids. J Dairy Sci 1980;63:337-52.
8. Mellenberger RW, Bauman DE, Nelson DR. Metabolic adaptations during lactogenesis. Fatty acid and lactose synthesis in cow mammary tissue. Biochem J 1973;136:741-8.
9. Parodi PW. Positional distribution of fatty acids in triglycerides from prepartum mammary gland secretion and early postpartum milk. J Dairy Sci 1983;66:912-9.
10. Kulski JK, Hartmann PE. Changes in human milk composition during the initiation of lactation. Aust J Exp Biol Med Sci 1981;59:101-14.
11. Linzell JL, Peaker M. Changes in colostrum composition and in permeability of the mammary epithelium at about the time of parturition in the goat. J Physiol 1974;243:129-51.
12. Peaker M. Secretion of ions and water. In Mepham TB, ed, Biochemistry of Lactation. Elsevier, Amsterdam-New York. 1983:285-305.
13. Patton S, Jensen RG. Biomedical aspects of lactation. Elmsford, NY: Pergamon Press, 1976.
14. Margolis S, Capuzzi D. Serum-lipoprotein synthesis and metabolism. Chap. 16. In Nelson GJ, ed. Blood lipids and lipoproteins: Quantitation, composition and metabolism. Wiley-Interscience, New York, NY. 1972:825-80.
15. Bitman J, Wood DL, Tyrrell HF, Bauman DE, Peel CJ, Brown ACG, Reynolds PJ. Blood and milk lipid responses induced by growth hormone administration in lactating cows. J Dairy Sci 1984;67:2873-80.

CHANGES IN MILK COMPOSITION AFTER SIX MONTHS OF LACTATION: THE EFFECTS OF DURATION OF LACTATION AND GRADUAL WEANING

Margaret C. Neville, Clare E. Casey, Ronald P. Keller, and Philip Archer

Departments of Physiology, Pediatrics, and Preventive Medicine and Biometrics
University of Colorado School of Medicine
Denver, Colorado 80262

SUMMARY

We followed lactation to one year or more in 8 women measuring both milk yield and composition. During the period from six months to one year four women showed milk yields which declined significantly while four women had yields which remained above 450 g per day. In order to determine whether changes in composition were due to changes in duration of lactation, declining milk yield, or both, the time-dependance of the concentration of several milk components was compared with the time-dependance of the milk yield. The following conclusions were drawn: (i) Within the accuracy of the analysis lactose, potassium and copper concentrations depended neither on milk yield nor duration of lactation. (ii) Lipid increased with duration of lactation and citrate and zinc decreased with duration of lactation. Changes in milk yield did not affect these components. (ii) Sodium, chloride, total protein, and magnesium increased and glucose decreased with decreasing milk yield. Duration of lactation did not affect these components. (iv) Calcium decreased with duration of lactation and increased with declining milk yield. These conclusions are compared with conclusions derived from multiple regression analysis of the same data. It is concluded that both types of analysis used in conjunction with inspection of graphical data are useful in the analysis of longitudinal data.

INTRODUCTION

Changes in milk composition after six months of lactation have been measured by a number of authors (1-8) while others (9,10) have documented changes that occur with gradual weaning. A problem, when studying lactation during this period, is to separate changes in milk composition associated with duration of lactation from changes associated with decreases in milk volume production. This separation is only possible if composition and yield are measured in the same individual. Some data of this sort are available. Macy (1), Ferris and Jensen (7) and Dewey et al. (6) measured milk yields on at least some of their subjects. However, no systematic study has appeared in which both volume and composition were measured regularly in the same women over a substantial period of time. Further no standard statistical method is currently available for analysis of longitudinal data of this sort.

In a recent study we followed the course of lactation to one year or more in 12 women, measuring both milk yields and composition at monthly intervals. After six months all women showed declining milk yields. However, some declined to zero in the course of the study; others remained above 450 ml/day. In this paper we examine the relation between duration of lactation, milk yield and milk composition in eight women for whom we have relatively complete monthly data for milk composition and volume between five and twelve months of lactation. We use a new statistical technique called three-step regression (TSR), comparing the results of this analysis with the results of multiple linear regression (MLR).

METHODS

Subjects

Each subject volunteered for this study during pregnancy and was chosen on the basis of her stated intention to breast-feed her infant exclusively for six months and to continue breast-feeding without supplementation with formula for at least one year. All had breast-fed at least one previous infant for a year or more. They were all healthy middle-class Caucasian women between the ages of 26 and 39 who bore a normal infant in an uncomplicated vaginal delivery at term. The protocol of the study was approved by the Human Subjects Committee of the University of Colorado Health Sciences Center and all subjects gave their informed consent based on a complete description of the study by a health service worker.

Measurement of Milk Yield

Subjects were asked to test-weigh their infants before and after every feed for a 24 hour period plus at least two feeds into the next 24 hour period. This protocol was performed once a month in the subject's home. Because all subjects had weighed their infants from birth they had had considerable experience in the operation of the equipment. An electronic balance, usually a Mettler model PE24 but occasionally a Sartorius model 3862 MP was used. The balance was mounted on a platform above an infant swing and interfaced with a computer programmed to collect multiple weighings in a way which minimized the effect of infant movement (Keller, unpublished), making it possible for our subjects to obtain data on active infants over six months old. The mothers recorded all weights and times; a computer printout of the data was also obtained.

Collection and Storage of Milk Samples

Milk samples were obtained by manual expression into an acid-washed plastic vial after washing the breast with distilled water. Five ml samples were taken from each breast in the middle (2-3 minutes after let-down) of a mid-morning feed either on the day of test-weighing or the day after. Triplicate tubes for fat analysis by creamatocrit (11) were immediately drawn up from each vial by the subject and sealed on both ends with Critoseal®. The vial was capped and refrigerated along with the fat tubes until picked up by the health service worker within 24 hours (usually within 4 hours) of expression. The sample was returned to the laboratory on ice where it was aliquoted into 0.5 and 1 ml aliquots in a laminar flow hood to prevent trace element contamination. Aliquots for trace element analysis were stored in trace element free tubes. All aliquots were immediately frozen and stored at -70°C.

Milk Composition: Analytical Techniques

Total lipid. Total lipid content was estimated by creamatocrit as described by Lucas et al. (11). A new standard curve was compared with the Folch extraction for each technician reading the creamatocrit tube.

Lactose and Glucose. Lactose and glucose were analyzed by enzyme-linked electrometry (Yellow Springs Instrument Company).

Protein. Protein was analyzed by the BCA assay (Pierce Chemical Company). A 1:60 dilution of milk was defatted by centrifugation and incubated 15 minutes prior to reading on the spectrophotometer (12). Human milk samples the nitrogen content of which was determined by Kjehldal were used as standards. The non-protein nitrogen content of these standards had been determined by Kjehldal analysis of the supernatants resulting from tri-chloroacetic acid precipitates and subtracted from the total.

Sodium and potassium. Sodium and potassium were determined by ion-selective electrode using a Beckman E2A analyzer and urine standards.

Chloride. Chloride was analyzed colorimetrically on defatted milk samples.

Calcium and magnesium. Calcium and magnesium were measured colorimetrically on defatted milk samples (13).

Citrate. Citrate was measured with the Boehringer-Mannheim test kit which uses the reactions of citrate lyase and malate dehydrogenase to reduce NADH to NAD. The reduction in NADH is read spectrophotometrically.

Zinc. Zinc was analyzed in whole milk by flame atomic absorption spectrophotometry, after low temperature ashing (14).

Copper. Copper was analyzed in liquid whole milk samples by graphite furnace atomic absorption (Perkin-Elmer 5000 with HGA500; Perkin-Elmer Corp. Norwalk CT 06856), using the method of standard additions (14).

Data Analysis

The milk yield was calculated in three ways in order to assure that the most representative value was obtained for that time period. The sums of the volumes obtained during the first and last 24 hours of the weighing period were calculated as well as a weighted average obtained by summing the volumes of all the feeds except the first, dividing by the time in hours elapsed between the first and last feeds and multiplying by 24 hours. The three values were compared and unless there was an obvious reason to do otherwise, the median value was considered to be the most representative. This was usually, but not always, the weighted average. The milk yields given in this publication represent the sum of the values obtained from test-weighing the infant plus any milk obtained by breast pump during the observation interval. They are uncorrected for specific gravity or insensible weight loss.

All compositional data represent the mean of two milk samples, one from each breast. Methods of statistical analysis are described in the results section. The program ABSTAT (Anderson-Bell) was used with an IBMPC-XT to make the relevant calculations.

RESULTS

Milk yields

The milk yields for each subject from four months until the end of the study are depicted in Fig. 1. All subjects were producing between 700 and 1000 g of milk at four months of lactation and the yield from all subjects declined after that time, but at varying rates. Four of the eight subjects (Numbers 4,6,7,11) made an active effort to wean their infants by decreasing the number of feeds and increasing the amount of supplementary food between six months and one year. Although the other subjects also introduced supplementary foods, there was no effort to supplant breast feeding. Because the data were reasonably complete between 5 and 13 months and each individual's data were reasonably linear over time, the mean rate of decline in milk yield was calculated using linear regression analysis. The slopes obtained from this analysis are given in Table 1 along with the slopes obtained from a similar analysis of the number of feeds per day. Thus, over this period the decline in milk yield varied between 100 ml/month and 15 ml/month. In all but one subject the decline was accompanied by a decrease in feed frequency which tended to be greater in those subjects with a greater decline in milk yield (Table 1).

Changes in Milk Composition

During the second six months of lactation there were changes in the concentration of a number of milk components. Fig. 2 shows two examples of milk components plotted as a function of duration of lactation for each

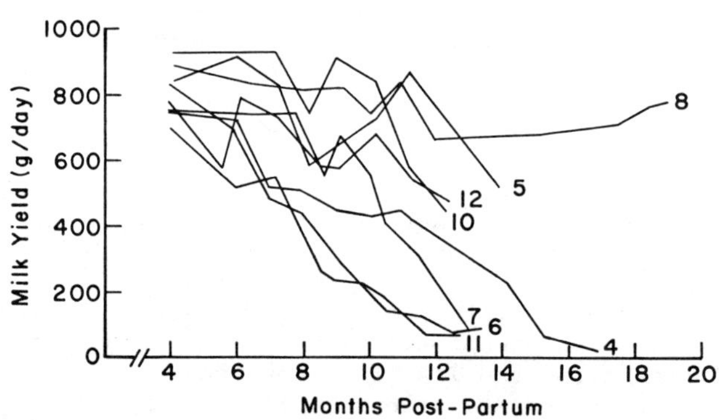

Fig. 1. **Daily milk yield in 8 breast feeding women after 4 months lactation.** Milk yields were measured by test-weighing as described and any milk pumped from the breasts was added to infant intake. The numbers are the subject codes for the individuals in the study.

individual. Fig. 2A shows the concentration of milk glucose. The patterns appear to be similar to the yield patterns shown in Figure 1. Fig. 2B shows the changes in zinc concentration. Here all subjects show a consistent downward trend with duration of lactation, one subject being more pronounced than the others.

Table 1

Monthly Change in Milk Yield and Feeding Frequency*

Subject Number	Change in Milk Yield (g/month)[a]	r[b]	Change in Feed Frequency (Feeds/day/month)	r[b]
11	-101	0.98	-0.75	0.96
6	- 93	0.97	-0.72	0.97
7	- 85.6	0.89	-0.33	0.64
10	- 60.8	0.81	-0.30	0.61
4	- 43.2	0.84	-0.54	0.68
12	- 30.6	0.32	-0.21	0.68
8	- 21.6	0.73	-0.57	0.59
5	- 14.9	0.28	0.005	0.28

*Values obtained from linear regression analysis of yield and feed frequency data from 5 through 13 months of lactation. The mean feed frequency was 7.4 ± 2.5 (S.D.) at 6 months and 4.7 ± 2.6 at 12 months. [a]Equivalent to β_2, Eq. 2. [b]Correlation coefficient

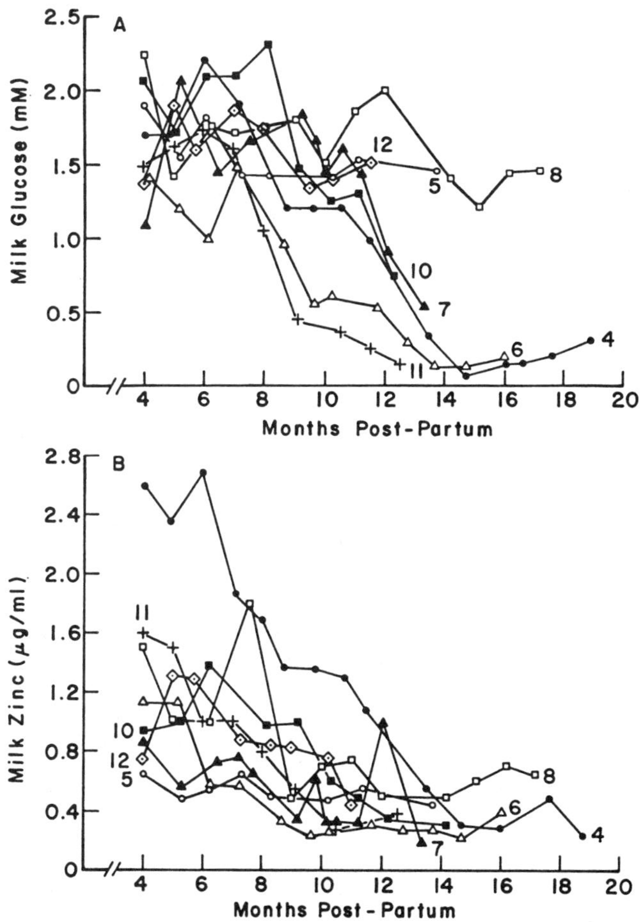

Fig. 2. **The relation between duration of lactation and milk composition for 8 lactating women.** Individual values for milk glucose concentration (A) and milk zinc concentration (B) are shown as a function of the duration of lactation.

The question we asked was: "Are the changes in these and the other compositional variables related to duration of lactation, declining milk yield, or both?" To answer this question we undertook a preliminary statistical analysis which involved fitting two regression lines *for each subject* for each milk constituent analyzed. One line describes the change in concentration over time:

$$C = \alpha_1 + \beta_1 t, \tag{1}$$

where C is concentration, t, time and α_1 and β_1 are constants. The second describes the change in milk volume over time:

$$V = \alpha_2 + \beta_2 t, \tag{2}$$

where V is volume.

The relation of these lines *across subjects* was examined by fitting a third regression line to the slopes, β_1 and β_2, of the above regressions for each milk constituent across all individuals:

$$\beta_1 = \alpha_3 + \beta_3 \beta_2. \tag{3}$$

In these relationships the slopes of the first two lines represent changes with time for individuals:

$$\frac{dC}{dt} = \beta_1 , \quad \frac{dV}{dt} = \beta_2. \tag{4}$$

If the change in concentration is related to the change in volume, this would be indicated by a significant slope, β_3, of the regression across individuals. If the concentration change is independent of volume change (i.e., $\beta_3 = 0$), a significant intercept, α_3, would reflect non-zero slopes in most, if not all of the individual regressions versus time.

The slopes, β_1, for the first step of this analysis, from the regressions of each of the compositional variables versus time for each individual, are given in Table 2. Because of the sample size any correlation greater than 0.3 was considered significant. A majority of the correlation coefficients are significant for sodium, potassium, chloride, lipid, calcium, magnesium, glucose, citrate, and zinc. However, since the volume is also decreasing in most subjects during this period, this observation alone does not give us information about the effect of duration of lactation on composition.

The second step is to calculate the change in milk yield for each individual. This has already been done in Table 1. In most cases the slope, β_2, is highly significant suggesting that a linear regression is appropriate and that there is a change in volume with time as noted previously.

The final step is to perform a regression of the rates of change in milk composition (i.e., β_1) for each of the 12 components against the rate of change of milk volume (i.e., β_2). The results of this analysis break down into four cases:

Case 1: There is no significant concentration change with either volume change or duration of lactation. Figure 3 shows a plot of β_1 *vs.* β_2 for potassium, lactose and copper. Neither the slope, β_3, nor the intercept, α_3, is significant for these three milk components. This is consistent with the relatively low correlation coefficients and the inconsistent signs for the slopes β_1 in Table 2.

Table 2

Slopes (β_1) from Regression Analysis of Changes in Milk Composition between 150 and 390 Days Postpartum

Subject	Sodium mM/mo	r	Potassium mM/mo	r	Chloride mM/mo	r	Protein mM/mo	r
11	1.74	0.87	0.08	0.10	3.10	0.86	0.09	0.74
6	2.33	0.78	-0.20	0.20	2.31	0.85	0.12	0.89
7	0.24	0.32	0.42	0.52	1.08	0.74	0.03	0.28
10	-0.38	0.67	0.33	0.32	0.54	0.51	0.01	0.28
4	0.21	0.35	0.21	0.44	0.63	0.39	-0.02	0.27
12	0.59	0.29	0.57	0.35	-0.09	0.04	-0.01	0.12
8	-0.60	0.43	0.57	0.57	-0.06	0.05	0.03	0.59
5	0.02	0.03	-0.27	0.54	0.87	0.50	0.01	0.15

Subject	Lipid %/mo	r	Calcium mM/mo	r	Magnesium mM/mo	r	Glucose mM/mo	r
11	0.04	0.09	-.015	0.06	0.075	0.54	-0.24	0.95
6	0.30	0.36	0.12	0.44	0.088	0.79	-0.13	0.74
7	0.27	0.29	-0.11	0.48	0.025	0.38	-0.09	0.49
10	0.54	0.56	-0.27	0.66	-0.025	0.30	-0.16	0.72
4	0.24	0.24	-0.09	0.24	0.039	0.55	-0.18	0.79
12	0.64	0.63	-0.37	0.81	-0.022	0.38	-0.04	0.36
8	0.21	0.45	-0.09	0.46	-0.025	0.61	0.06	0.64
5	0.48	0.43	-0.30	0.76	0.001	0.02	-0.02	0.14

Subject	Lactose mM/mo	r	Citrate mM/mo	r	Zinc ug/ml/mo	r	Copper ug/ml/mo	r
11	-3.9	0.61	-0.06	0.66	-0.15	0.93	-0.0006	0.38
6	0.57	0.09	-0.06	0.32	-0.09	0.78	0.0042	0.36
7	2.77	0.30	-0.09	0.69	-0.01	0.08	-0.018	0.56
10	-3.54	0.59	-0.12	0.53	-0.12	0.70	-0.018	0.69
4	6.0	0.50	-0.06	0.32	-0.27	0.90	-0.003	0.27
12	-2.7	0.41	-0.24	0.99	-0.09	0.78	0.0021	0.12
8	0.87	0.23	-0.06	0.33	-0.09	0.53	-0.005	0.03
5	1.73	0.28	-0.27	0.77	-0.01	0.14	0.005	0.26

r: correlation coefficient (Pearson Product Moment)

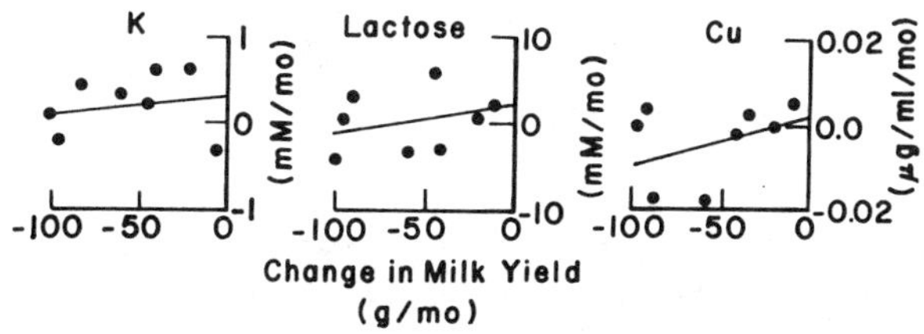

Fig. 3. **Rate of change of milk composition as a function of rate of change of milk yield for Case 1.** Ordinate is β_1; abscissa is β_2. See text for further explanation.

Case 2: There is a significant relation between composition change and volume change but not duration of lactation. In this case β_3 is significant but α_3 is not. Fig. 4 shows a plot of β_1 *vs.* $\beta 2$ for sodium, chloride, glucose, magnesium and protein. Because we used this treatment of the data as a preliminary screening method, the probability level for significance was tentatively set at $P < 0.1$ and the relation further investigated by other means (see below).

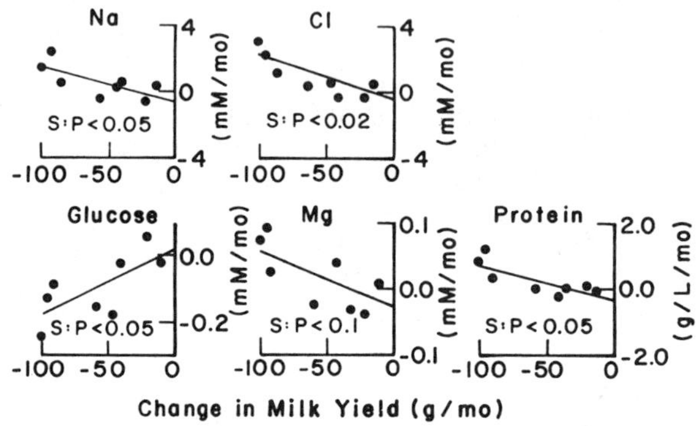

Fig. 4. Rate of change of milk composition as a function of rate of change of milk yield for Case 2. S: is the probability that the slope is different from zero.

Case 3: There is a significant relation between composition change and duration of lactation but not between composition change and milk volume (Fig. 5). In this case, which applies to citrate, lipid and zinc, β_3 is not significantly different from zero allowing the β_1's to be pooled across women. (This procedure is equivalent to collapsing the points shown in Fig. 5 on the ordinate and taking the mean). When this is done the results become highly significant.

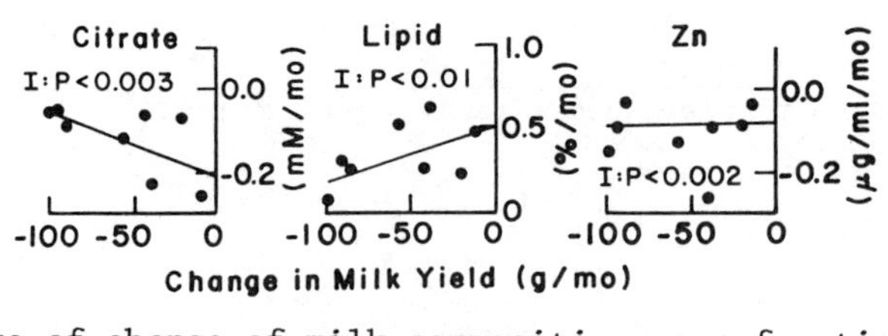

Fig. 5. Rate of change of milk composition as a function of rate of change of milk yield for Case 3. I is the probability that the intercept differs from zero.

Case 4: There is a significant relation between both composition change and duration of lactation and between composition change and milk volume change (Fig. 6). In this case, which applies only to calcium in this study, both β_3 and α_3 are significant.

Fig. 6. Rate of change of milk composition as a function of rate of change of milk yield for Case 4. See Figs 4 and 5 for meaning of S and I.

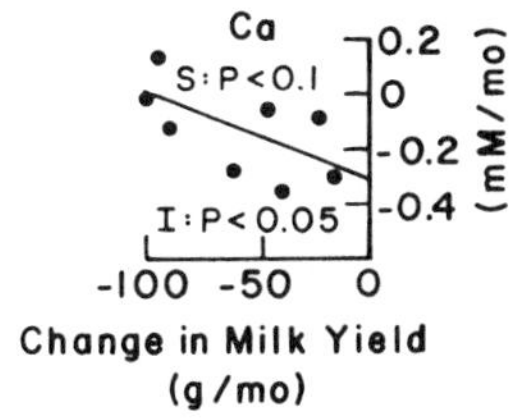

In order to check the pertinence of this analysis we further examined the changes in lipid, citrate and zinc as a function of duration of lactation. The mean concentrations of these constituents in the eight subjects are shown in Figure 7. The changes with time are clear.

Because calcium apparently decreased with duration of lactation only when weaning did not occur the mean calcium concentration has been plotted only for those four subjects in which the decline in milk volume was less than 50 ml per month (Fig. 7). Again there appeared to be a fairly linear decline in concentration suggesting that the use of the intercept α_3 to predict changes with duration of lactation is valid.

A lack of effect of duration of lactation on sodium, chloride, protein, magnesium and glucose is consistent with the generally lower correlation coefficients in Table 2 for the subjects with smaller decreases in volume. The effect of milk yield on these components is more complex and will be discussed in the next section.

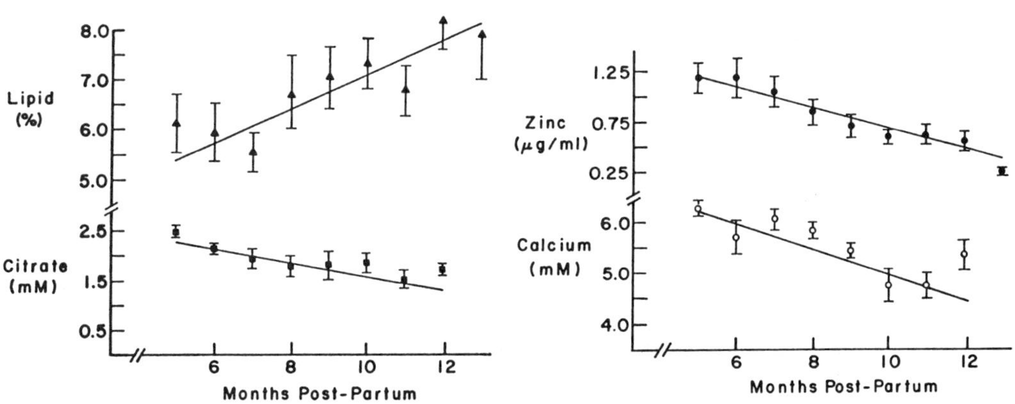

Fig. 7. **Change in concentration with duration of lactation for certain milk components.** Mean values by month of lactation for eight subjects for lipid, citrate and zinc and for four subjects who showed relatively less decline in milk volume for calcium. Distance between bars represents two standard errors of the mean. The lines are based on the mean slopes and intercepts obtained by regression analysis of the data from each individual.

Changes in Milk Composition with Decreasing Milk Yield

In the analysis above (Case 2) we made the assumption that a linear regression produced a reasonable fit to the data. In order to further investigate the validity of this assumption we have graphed the sodium and chloride as a function of duration of lactation for each of the four subjects who showed a marked decline in milk yield during the period of this study (Fig. 8). It can be seen that the pattern of change in these two ions shows marked individual variation. In subjects 11 and 6 there is indeed a fairly linear rise with declining milk yield. In subjects 4 and 7, on the other hand, there is little change in these substances until milk yield has fallen below 200 ml per day. At that point there is a decisive rise, with both ions going above 80 mM in the case of subject 4. The changes in these two ions are parallel in all four cases and generally proportional to changes in protein concentration (not shown). This is to be expected if the increased concentration results from a loosening of the tight junctions between the mammary alveolar cells. The variability of the results suggests that the conditions under which these junctions open vary from woman to woman. The changes in calcium and magnesium with volume were less significant and will not be further discussed here.

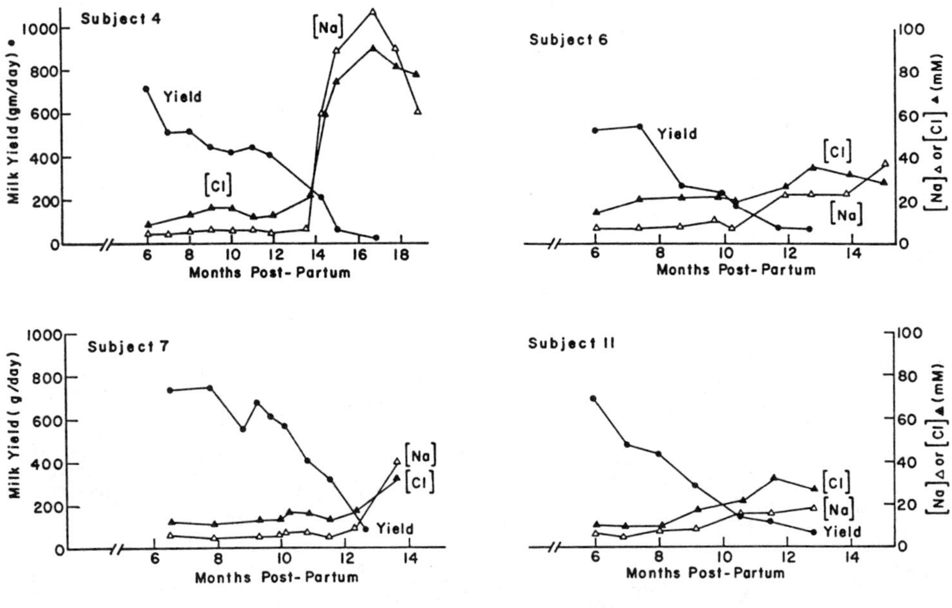

Fig. 8. **Changes in milk sodium and chloride concentrations and milk yield as a function of duration of lactation.** Data are plotted for four subjects who weaned their infants during the study.

From the data shown in Fig. 4 as well as Table 2, it can be seen that glucose shows a strong tendency to decrease with a decrease in milk volume. This phenomenon has been previously observed by Hartmann and coworkers (10) and is further discussed in another paper in this meeting (15).

DISCUSSION

Statistical techniques

The three-step regression (TSR) technique for the analysis of longitudinal data used in this paper has several advantages. TSR is straightforward and can be used, at least in a preliminary way, to sort through large amounts of data utilizing available statistical packages. Relationships between trends in the data are revealed by taking full advantage of the multiple data points obtained from the same individual over time. One limitation is that use of linear regression analysis implies that the data trends are linear with respect to time. We plotted all the data before commencing the analysis and in general this assumption appeared to be valid. There were some problems with components which vary with milk volume. Thus there is a major increase in sodium, chloride and protein which occurs only after the milk volume has fallen to a very low level. These changes are not modelled satisfactorily by a linear regression. A change in copper at very low milk volumes was not significant using this technique (see below).

It can be shown that Eqns 1,2, and 3 can be combined to give:

$$C = \alpha' + \alpha_3 t + \beta_3 V, \qquad (5)$$

where α' is a constant. This equation can be fit to the individual data points using the technique of multiple linear regression (MLR). Trends in the data for the individuals are lost when this method, often applied to cross sectional studies, is used. It is instructive to compare the results obtained MLR with those obtained with TSR. Table 3 shows the results of this comparison.

Potassium, lactose and copper are predicted by TSR not to change with volume or time. MLR on the other hand predicts that lactose increases with duration and decreases with decreased volume illustrating a tendency of MLR to predict offsetting changes with duration and volume that are not borne out by individual trends. However MLR also predicts a small decrease in copper with decreasing volume. This change can be observed graphically at very low volumes in some individuals but was not significant by TSR which has only 7 degrees of freedom in the third regression compared with about 100 degrees of freedom for MLR. The small number of degrees of freedom in the final step of TSR means that some significant changes can be overlooked.

For those variables predicted by TSR to change with duration of lactation, lipid, calcium, citrate, and zinc, MLR made correct predictions only for calcium and zinc. Again the failure to predict the correct conclusion for lipid and citrate was again due to prediction of offsetting changes in the effects of duration and volume. Those variables predicted by TSR to change with milk yield were also predicted by MLR linear regression to change with yield. In some cases (i.e., sodium, chloride, and protein) the values of α_3 obtained by the two methods differed. This is not surprising since the graphs in Fig. 8 indicate that a linear model does not fit these data very well in any case.

The choice of statistical methods for the analysis of longitudinal data should be made only after all data are plotted as a function of time and inspected by the investigator. The above analysis suggests that a combination of TSR with MLR and judicious curve inspection provides the least chance of erroneous conclusions. Because the number of subjects in the reported study was small, any conclusions derived here should also be replicated in other studies.

Table 3

Comparison of Coefficients Obtained by Two Statistical Methods

Component	Units	α_3: Change with duration per month		β_3: Change with volume per 100 g increase	
		MLR	TSR	MLR	TSR
Sodium	mM	n.s.	n.s.	-0.93 ± 0.17*[a]	-2.20 ± 0.8 *
Potassium	mM	n.s.	n.s.	n.s.	n.s.
Chloride	mM	n.s.	n.s.	-1.2 ± 0.20*[a]	-2.7 ± 0.8 *
Lipid	%	-0.54 ± 0.12[b]	0.34 ± 0.06*	-0.52 ± 0.09*[b]	n.s.
Calcium	mM	-0.017± 0.006*	-0.032± 0.014*	-0.015± 0.005*	-0.032± 0.015*
Magnesium	mM	n.s.	n.s.	-0.19 ± 0.02*	-0.19 ± 0.09*
Protein	g/dl	n.s.	n.s.	-0.06 ± 0.01*	-0.11 ± 0.04*
Glucose	mM	n.s.	n.s.	0.17 ± 0.02*	0.20 ± 0.08*
Lactose	mM	3.12 ± 0.99*[b]	n.s.	4.1 ± 0.79*[b]	n.s.
Citrate	mM	n.s.	-0.12 ± 0.03*	0.07 ± 0.03*[b]	n.s.
Zinc	ug/ml	-0.11 ± 0.03*	-0.11 ± 0.03*	n.s.	n.s.
Copper	ng/ml	n.s.	n.s.	8.0 ± 3.0 *[b]	n.s.

*P < 0.1
[a] Value obtained by MLR significantly (P<0.05) different from value obtained by TSR.
[b] Conclusion drawn from MLR different from conclusion drawn from TSR

Changes in milk composition with duration of lactation

Four of the twelve milk components examined here were found to change significantly with duration of lactation in the second six months postpartum. A marked longitudinal decrease in zinc concentration starting soon after lactogenesis has been observed by many investigators (5,14,16). Our values from six to 12 months are similar to those of Vaughn et al. (14). A decrease in calcium content during this period has also been widely documented (1-3, 14). The decrease is larger than can be accounted for by the concomitant decrease in citrate, a major calcium binding ligand. To our knowledge the decrease in citrate has not been previously reported. The marked increase in lipid has not been observed by other investigators although Macy (1), Abdel Kader et al. (4) and Ferris and Jensen (7) reported smaller increases in lipid between six and twelve months lactation. Our data on lipid composition must be viewed with caution because we analyzed only small mid-morning mid-feed samples which may not provide a representative sample for this milk constituent (7).

Changes in milk composition on weaning

Fewer studies of milk composition during weaning exist. The earliest report was that by Hartmann and Kulski (17) in which they showed that abrupt weaning was accompanied by a rapid decrease in milk volume with marked increases in sodium and chloride and decreases in glucose, lactose and potassium. With gradual weaning the same changes take place only much more slowly (9-10). The changes we observed in sodium, chloride and total protein are entirely consistent with those observed by the previous authors. Although not shown in our statistical analysis, when sodium and chloride go to very high levels in the milk, we observed a decrease in lactose similar to that observed by other authors. These changes are thought to represent changes in the permeability of the paracellular pathway between the mammary alveolar cells which increases the ability of extracellular fluid components to enter the milk spaces. The activity of the mammary alveolar cells must also change in character at this time to produce the high concentrations of lactoferrin and IgA observed in post-weaning milk (17). Other changes with weaning are more gradual, particularly the tendency for calcium and magnesium to increase. The physiological basis for these observations is unknown. There are striking and consistent changes in milk glucose on weaning. These are discussed in another paper in this volume (15).

ACKNOWLEDGEMENT

The research described in this study was supported by contract number HD 2-2801 from NIHCD and by NIH grants HD 19547 and AM 12432. The investigators are profoundly grateful to the subjects of these experiments who selflessly provided milk samples and volume data through the course of a long and difficult experiment.

REFERENCES

1. I. G. Macy, Human Milk Studies. X. Daily and monthly variations in milk components as observed in two successive lactation periods. Am J. Dis. Child. 43:1062-1067 (1944).
2. D. Winikoff, 1944, Calcium, magnesium and phosphorus in the milk of Australian women. Med. J. Australia 660-665 (1944).

3. S.D. Morrison, "Human Milk: Yield, Proximate Principles and Inorganic Constituents". Commonwealth Agricultural Bureaux, Farnham Royal, Slough, Bucks, U.K. (1952).
4. M.M. Abdel Kader, R. Bahgat, M.T. Aziz, F. Hefnawi, M.H.H. Badraoul, N. Younis, and F. Hassib, Lactation patterns in Egyptian women. II. Chemical composition of milk during the first year of lactation. J. Biosoc. Sci. 4:403-409 (1972).
5. L.A. Vaughan, C.W. Weber, and S.R. Kemberling, Longitudinal changes in the mineral content of human milk. Am. J. Clin. Nutr. 32: 2301-2306 (1979).
6. K.J.G. Dewey, D.A. Finley, and B. Lönnerdal, Breast milk volume and composition during late lactation (7-20 months). J. Ped. Gastroent. Nutr. 3:713-720 (1984).
7. A.M. Ferris, and R.G. Jensen, Lipids in human milk: A review. 1. Sampling, determination and content. J. Ped. Gastroent. Nutr. 3:108-122 (1984).
8. WHO Collaborative Study on Breast-feeding: The Quantity and Quality of Breast Milk. WHO, Geneva, (1985).
9. C. Garza, C.A. Johnson, E. O'Brian-Smith, and B.L. Nichols, Changes in the nutrient composition of human milk during gradual weaning. Am.J.Clin.Nutr. 37:61-65 (1983).
10. C.G. Prosser, L. Saint, and P.E. Hartmann, Mammary gland function during gradual weaning and early gestation in women. Aust.J.Exp.Biol.Med.Sci. 62:215-228 (1984).
11. A. Lucas, J.A.H. Gibbs, R.L.J. Lyster, J.P. Baum, Creamatocrit:simple clinical technique for estimating fat concentration and energy value of human milk. Brit. Med. J. 1:1018-1020 (1978).
12. R.P. Keller and M.C. Neville, Determination of total protein in human milk: comparison of methods. Clin.Chem. 32:120-123 (1986).
13. M.C. Neville, R.P. Keller, B. Lonnerdal, S.A. Atkinson, C.L. Wade, N. Butte, and P.B. Moser, Measurement of electrolyte and macromineral concentrations in human milk. in Human Lactation: I. Milk Components and Methodologies. Plenum Press, N.Y. pp 129 - 140 (1985).
14. C.E. Casey, K.M. Hambidge, and M.C. Neville, M.C., Studies in Human Lactation. Zinc, Copper, Manganese and Chromium in Human milk in the first eight weeks of lactation. Am. J. Clin Nutr. 41:1193-1200 (1985).
15. M.C. Neville, J.C. Allen and C.E. Casey, Regulation of the rate of lactose production. These proceedings.
16. E. Vuori, and P. Kuitunen, The concentrations of copper and zinc in human milk: A longitudinal study. Acta Paed. Scand 68:33-37 (1979).
17. P.E. Hartmann and J.K. Kulski, Changes in the composition of the mammary secretion of women after abrupt termination of breast feeding. J. Physiol 275: 1-11.

COMPLEMENTATION AND WEANING PHASES OF LACTATION

Cutberto Garza, Janice Stuff, Nancy Butte,
and Corinne Montandon

USDA/ARS Children's Nutrition Research Center
Department of Pediatrics, Baylor College of
Medicine and Texas Children's Hospital, Houston, Texas

INTRODUCTION

Breastfeeding is recommended as the best feeding choice by most major national and international agencies concerned with maternal-infant health. However, a clear consensus regarding the implementation of this recommendation is not possible because of unresolved issues concerned with the nutrient needs of infancy, maternal physiology, the use of human milk substitutes, the impact of environmental contaminants on milk consumption, and economic and social factors that affect the infant feeding choice made by the mother. There is no agreement, therefore, on the optimal duration of exclusive breastfeeding (1,2). Such guidelines, however, should be an implicit component of current feeding recommendations. The development of guidelines that best meet the needs of the weanling poses a dilemma: the premature introduction of solid foods increases the risk of infectious illnesses and the inappropriately delayed introduction of solid foods may result in stunting and wasting (3,4).

Specific issues that have emerged from this dilemma have been addressed in our laboratory: 1) the quantification of nutrient intake during the periods of exclusive breastfeeding and the introduction of solid foods in infants of women at minimal risk of malnutrition with available lactation support services, 2) the estimation of human milk composition during these periods, and 3) maternal adaptations to the decreased production of milk. This discussion will focus on the first two issues.

INTAKES OF EXCLUSIVELY BREAST-FED INFANTS

Interest has grown in the quantification of intakes of exclusively breast-fed infants because studies have shown discrepancies between the amounts of milk required to meet estimated nutrient allowances and usual rates of milk production (5-9), with one possible exception (10). We documented milk intake and growth in a prospective, longitudinal study of 45 exclusively breast-fed infants during the first 4 months of life (2). Infants were required to be healthy, term, and appropriate size for gestational age. Measurements of milk intake, sampling of milk for compositional studies, and monitoring of infant growth were performed at monthly intervals. The amount of milk ingested daily was determined by the test-weighing method (11) during a 24-hour period. Milk also was obtained for compositional studies; feeding and pumping were alternated between breasts with successive feeds during a 24-hour period. Compositional analyses were performed on a monthly 24-hour milk sample for each subject.

Energy and protein intakes were found to be substantially less than current estimates of requirements derived by the factorial approach (12). Requirements for protein are based on the sum of obligatory N losses, N needed for growth, and N needed to adjust for the inverse relationship between N intake and efficiency of N utilization. Energy requirements are based on the sum of energy needed for basal metabolism, thermic response to food, caloric content and cost of synthesis of tissues gained as the infant grows, and activity. Energy intakes declined significantly from 110 $\pm$ 24 kcal/kg/day at month 1 to 71 $\pm$ 17 kcal/kg/day at month 4. Protein intake decreased from 1.6 $\pm$ 0.3 g/kg/day at month 1 to 0.9 $\pm$ 0.2 g/kg/day at month 4. Although the mean weights of these infants were consistently greater than the mean weights of NCHS reference population, weight-for-age percentiles decreased after the first month at a rate of 2.6 percentiles per month. Excluding birth measurements, length-for-age percentiles did not vary significantly throughout the study, and weight-for-length percentiles declined at a rate of 3.9 percentiles per month. Length-for-age percentiles were correlated positively with those for weight-for-age and negatively with those for weight-for-height.

The results of our studies of exclusively breast-fed infants may be interpreted to support several views: protein and energy requirements have been overestimated, falling weight-for-age and weight-for-length percentiles indicate that exclusive human milk feeding cannot support "normal" growth after the third month of life, or alternatively, this growth pattern represented the regression of the group toward the mean. The first view assumes that ad libitum intakes of exclusively breast-fed infants generally meet nutrient requirements in early life if there is reasonable assurance that maternal lactation performance is not impeded significantly by physiologic or environmental factors. The second view assumes that NCHS standards represent "normal" growth, although this assumption has been questioned recently (13). An evaluation of the validity of the third view requires the study of infants with birth characteristics distinct from those of our study population.

INTAKE DURING THE PERIOD OF COMPLEMENTATION

We planned and initiated a pilot study to address these issues (14). Intakes of infants were measured during the transition from an exclusive human milk diet to one that included solid foods. If human milk were indeed limiting by the third month of lactation, we proposed that energy intakes would increase with the ad libitum introduction of solid foods, and furthermore that we would observe an accelerated growth rate. Seventeen infants were studied; 9 were studied at months 5 and 6, and 8 at months 6 and 7. All were exclusively breast-fed for 5 full months after which solid foods were added to the diet. Each infant was studied for 5 consecutive 24-hour periods. Serial measurements were made of milk intake (test-weighing) and solid food intake (pre- and post-feeding jar weighing). Intakes are summarized in Fig 1. Growth data for the observation period are summarized in Fig 2. Our observations of the infants' growth and total energy intakes after the introduction of solid foods, approximately 70 kcal/kg/day, showed that energy intakes remained below levels recommended by the RDA (15) and WHO/FAO (12). Intakes at 5 months coincided with estimates made in our previous study (2).

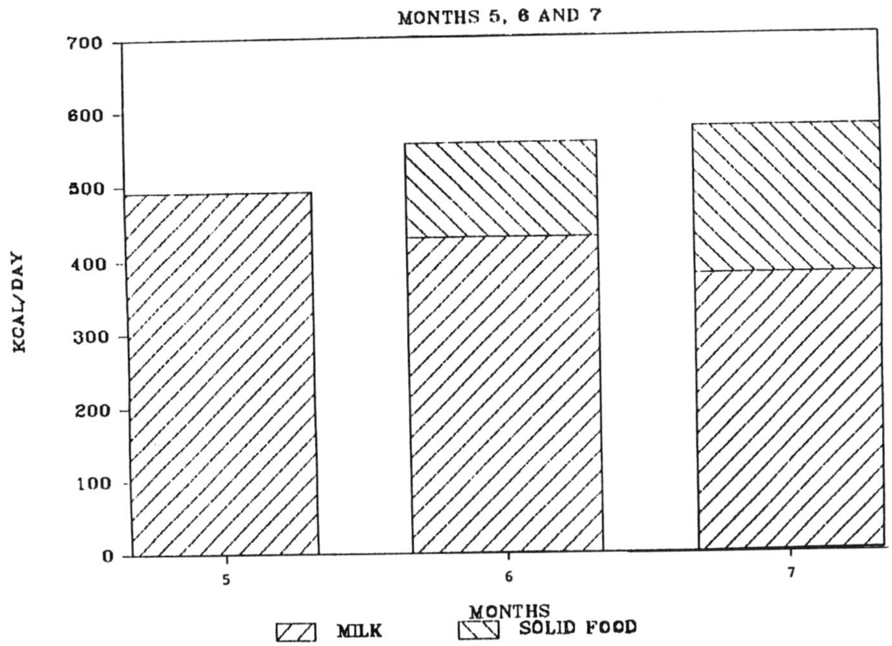

Fig. 1. Total caloric intake subdivided into calories from human milk (▨) and solid food (▧) in 5-, 6-, and 7-month-old infants.

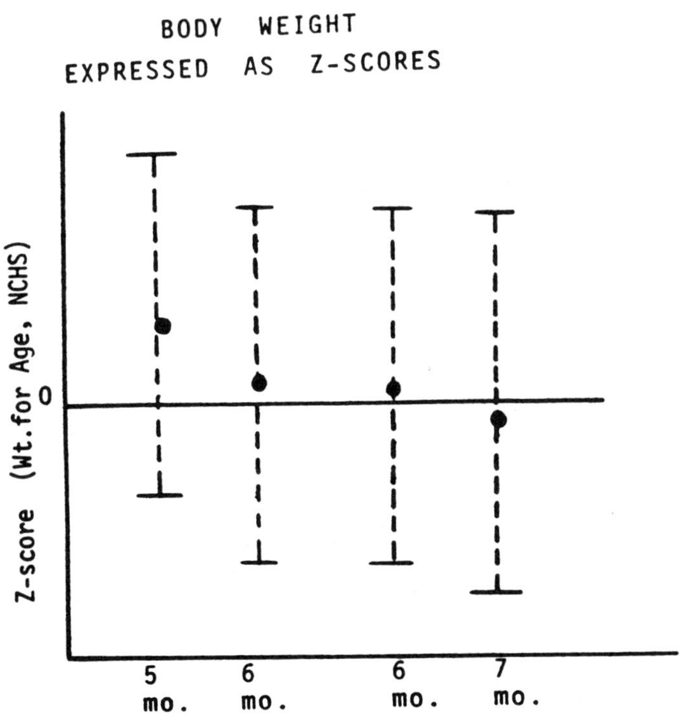

Fig. 2. Z scores for weight/age of infants followed at months 5 and 6 and months 7 and 8. Infants were breastfed exclusively during month 5 and fed a mixture of human milk and solid foods during months 6, 7, and 8.

As a follow-up to these observations, we have begun a longitudinal study in which we will evaluate maternal lactation performance by measuring the intake and growth of the infant before and immediately after the transition from an exclusive human milk diet to one including solid foods (16). Fifty women will be recruited during the last trimester of pregnancy from potential subjects who plan to breastfeed their infants exclusively from 4 to 6 months. Only women who have no children or one child are recruited. Those enrolled must have given birth to full-term, appropriate for gestational age, healthy infants. The infants will be studied from birth until at least three months after solid foods are added to their diets. The timing of the introduction of solid foods is made by each mother in consultation with the infant's pediatrician. Other than the initial introduction of rice cereal, the sequence of solid foods added to the infant's diet is made by the mother and infant's pediatrician. Mothers are asked to offer solid foods only after the infant has nursed. Each infant's weight, length, and selected skinfold thicknesses and body circumferences are measured weekly for the first 2 months of life, biweekly during months 3 and 4, and weekly thereafter until 3 months after solid foods have been added. Nutrient intakes are measured monthly from 16 weeks of life until 3 months after the introduction of solid foods. The volume of daily milk intake is measured by the test-weighing technique for 5 consecutive days. The composition of each mother's milk is determined monthly from laboratory analyses of a 24-hour milk sample. Nutrient intake from solid foods also is determined for 5 consecutive days. Mothers are supplied with preweighed jars of food and detailed instructions for their storage after their use. Nutrient analyses are performed by our laboratory on each lot of the 12 types of solid foods used in the study.

Preliminary results are based on the first 7 males and 6 females who have completed the study protocol. Intake data for these 13 infants are summarized in Table 1. Because analyses of each subject's milk are not completed, a caloric concentration of 67 kcal/dl has been assumed. Preliminary data support this assumption. Milk intake appears to have dropped after the introduction of solid foods and caloric intakes from solid foods appear to have increased gradually. Although the number of nursings decreased by 20 to 30% after solid foods were added to the infants' diets, the amount of milk consumed dropped approximately 40%. Estimated total caloric intakes from both human milk and solid foods did not appear to rise during this period. Weight/age percentiles remained relatively stable at approximately 65 before and after the ad libitum availability of solid foods.

Because dietary energy intakes did not increase, these data support the view that energy requirements of infants may have been overestimated. The stability of energy intakes during this period does not support the premise that the low energy intakes of breast-fed infants at 4 months and beyond are the necessary outcome of inadequate maternal lactation capacity. However, it is not possible to determine if maternal behavior is responsible for the low intakes. The number of nursings did fall, but there is no apparent reason to explain why a possible shortfall in energy would not be compensated by an increase in the amount of solid foods ingested. Also noteworthy is our observation that infants fed artificial formulas have intakes higher than those of breast-fed infants (17). The basis for this difference requires exploration. Attention should be given to potential physiologic factors and methodological approaches to estimate intakes in both populations.

Table 1. Energy Intakes of Infants Before and After the Addition of Solid Foods to an Exclusive Human Milk Diet

Age (wk)	Food Source: Milk[a] (kcal/d)	Food Source: Solid Foods (kcal/d)	Total (kcal/d)	Total (kcal/kg)
16				
-SF[b]	504 ± 93[c]	0	504 ± 93	77 ± 14
20				
-SF[b]	513 ± 130	0	513 ± 130	70 ± 18
+SF	371 ± 112	82 ± 160	453 ± 119	64 ± 19
24				
-SF	580 ± 117	0	580 ± 117	76 ± 18
+SF	294 ± 127	161 ± 105	456 ± 142	61 ± 21
28				
+SF	405 ± 127	135 ± 96	553 ± 133	67 ± 18
32				
+SF	376 ± 150	196 ± 66	573 ± 166	67 ± 20

[a] Assumed caloric concentration = 67 kcal/dl
[b] -SF = exclusive human milk diet; +SF = solid foods plus human milk
[c] Mean ± SD

MILK COMPOSITION

We have measured the concentrations of selected nutrients (2) and immunologic factors (18-19) during the phases of exclusive breastfeeding and decreasing milk production (20-21). Analyses of 24-hour milk samples obtained in our study of exclusively breast-fed infants during the first four months of life demonstrated a general stability in the nutrient concentrations of milk collected during months 3 and 4.

Values for nutrient concentrations obtained for milk collected during months 3 and 4 postpartum are similar to those measured in single samples of milk collected from 6 women at approximately 6 months postpartum before they began to wean their infants gradually from an exclusively human milk diet (Figs. 3 and 4). These 6 subjects were asked to reduce the frequency or duration of nursings by approximately one-third each month for a period of 3 months. All subjects elected to reduce the frequency of feedings. The contents of a single breast were collected for analysis between 8:00 AM and 12:00 noon before weaning began and at 2-week intervals for 12 weeks after weaning began. Although mean protein N concentrations appeared to rise minimally (133 ± 15 mg N/100 ml to 142 ± 24 mg N/100 ml) from the preweaning period to the half-way point of the study (week 6), caloric concentrations were much more erratic. The higher caloric concentrations observed at week 6 corresponded to high concentrations of fat measured in these samples. The collection of only single samples and the relatively small number of subjects studied complicate the interpretation of these data. Moreover, we have found that the concentration of energy in single milk samples may depend on individual feeding patterns. The energy content of single milk samples was related negatively to the volume expressed and to the sampling time preceding the index sample. A positive relationship was observed between milk volume and the time elapsed prior to sampling (unpublished results). If milk samples in the ongoing longitudinal study demonstrate similar fluctuations

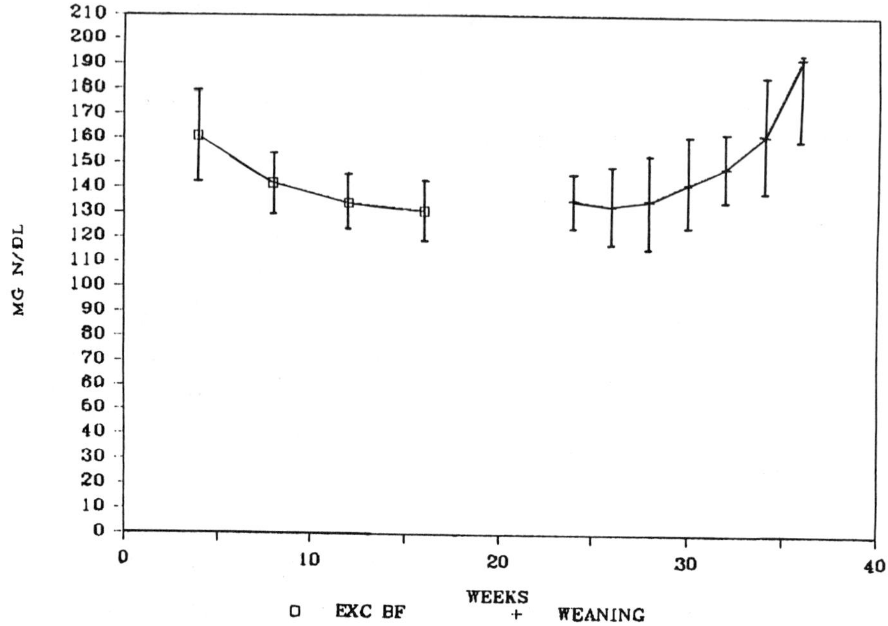

Fig. 3. Milk protein nitrogen concentrations during the period of exclusive breastfeeding and gradual weaning. 24-hour samples were obtained during the exclusive breastfeeding phase; only single samples were available during the gradual weaning phase.

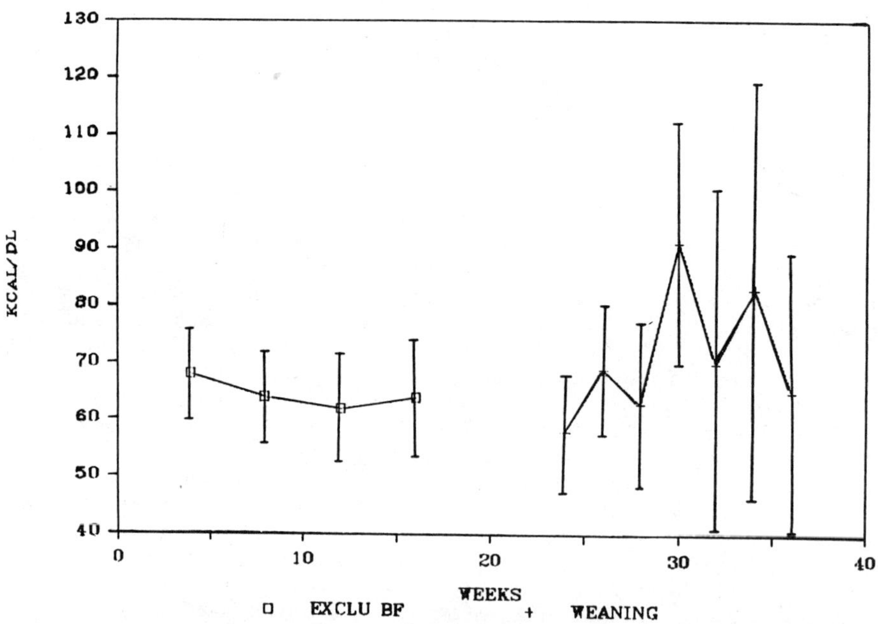

Fig. 4. Energy concentrations in milk during the period of exclusive breastfeeding and gradual weaning. 24-hour samples were obtained during the exclusive breastfeeding phase; only single samples were available during the gradual weaning phase.

in energy content as the weaning process progresses, the estimates of the caloric intakes of infants would be affected significantly. These observations and the results of our pilot study underscore the importance of care when nutrient concentrations are extrapolated during phases of lactation in which milk volumes change. The preliminary estimates of intakes in Table 1, therefore, must be considered cautiously.

In collaboration with Drs. A.S. Goldman and R.M. Goldblum, we also measured the concentrations of SIgA, lactoferrin, lyzozyme and SIgA antibodies to a pool of E. coli somatic O antigens during gradual weaning in 6 subjects (21). The preweaning levels of these factors were similar to levels found in human milk obtained at 6 months in a separate group of lactating subjects. SIgA was observed to increase steadily as weaning progressed. SIgA antibody titers to E. coli somatic antigens rose more than fourfold in 4 subjects. Lysozyme levels rose in 4 and lactoferrin increased in 5 of the 6 individuals studied. Correlations were found between the slopes relating concentrations of lysozyme and lactoferrin to time, and between lysozyme and total IgA. These studies also demonstrate the difficulties that may be encountered if one attempts to extrapolate values from the literature in studies of lactational periods characterized by changing milk volumes. Although the increased concentrations of IgA, lysozyme, and lactoferrin may be explained in part by decreases in milk volume, the changes in antibody levels were too marked to have resulted from this variable. Our observations based on results thus far suggest that the enteromammary pathway continues to function during periods of decreased breast stimulation, and that increases in concentration partially compensate or overcompensate for the decreases in milk production that accompany weaning. Therefore, the potential protection provided by human milk feedings during this high-risk period is sustained. The longitudinal study in progress should contribute to the understanding of the regulation of the immunologic system of human milk during the weaning phase of infant feeding.

SUMMARY

Studies during the complementation and weaning phases of lactation indicate that the low energy intakes of breast-fed infants likely are not due to limitations in maternal lactation capacities, but represent physiologically regulated intakes. Preliminary studies of nutrient and immunologic composition of human milk during gradual weaning support the need for detailed compositional analyses of milks during this period. Such descriptive studies should provide insights for future investigations that focus on the regulation of milk composition during weaning.

ACKNOWLEDGMENTS

This research is supported by a contract (NO 1-HD-2-2814) from the National Institutes of Health and by the USDA/ARS Children's Nutrition Research Center, Department of Pediatrics, Baylor College of Medicine and Texas Children's Hospital, Houston, TX. This project has been funded in part with Federal funds from the U.S. Department of Agriculture, Agriculture Research Service under Cooperative Agreement number 58-7MNI-6-100. The contents of this publication do not necessarily reflect the views or policies of the U.S. Department of Agriculture, nor does mention of trade names, commercial products, or organizations imply endorsement by the U.S. Government.

REFERENCES

1. J.C. Waterlow and A.M. Thomson, Observations on the adequacy of breastfeeding, Lancet 2:238 (1979).
2. N.F. Butte, C. Garza, E.O. Smith, and B.L. Nichols, Human milk intake and growth performance of exclusively breast-fed infants, J. Pediatr. 104:187 (1984).
3. S.A. Sarker, A.M. Molla, and M.M. Rahaman, Impact of supplementary food on intake of breast milk in diarrhoea, Lancet Dec 10:1349 (1983).
4. M. Watkinson, Delayed onset of weanling diarrhoea associated with high breast milk intake, Transactions of the Royal Soc. Trop. Med. Hyg. 75:432 (1981).
5. A. Wallgren, Breast milk consumption of healthy, full-term infants, Acta Paediatr. Scand. 32:778 (1945).
6. M.F. Picciano, E.J. Calkins, J.R. Garrick, and R.H. Deering, Milk and mineral intake of breast-fed infants, Acta Paediatr. Scand. 70:189 (1981).
7. K.G. Dewey and B. Lonnerdal, Milk and nutrient intake of breast-fed infants from 1 to 6 months: relation to growth and fatness, J. Pediatr. Gastroenterol. Nutr. 2:497 (1983).
8. L. Kohler, G. Meeuwisse, and W. Morttensson, Food intake and growth of infants between six and twenty-six weeks of age on breast milk, cow's milk formula, or soy formula, Acta Paediatr. Scand. 73:40 (1984).
9. R.K. Chandra, Breast-feeding, growth, and morbidity, Nutr. Res. 1:25 (1981).
10. S. Rattigan, A.V. Ghisalberti, and P.E. Hartmann, Breast milk production in Australian women, Br. J. Med. 45:243 (1981).
11. M.W. Woolridge, N.F. Butte, K.G. Dewey, A.M. Ferris, C. Garza, and R.P. Keller, Methods for the measurement of milk volume intake of the breast-fed infant, in: "Human Lactation: Milk Components and Methodologies," R. Jensen and M. Neville, eds., Plenum Press, New York (1985).
12. FAO/WHO Energy and Protein Requirements, WHO Technical Report Series, No. 522. FAO Nutrition Meeting, Report Series, No. 52, Geneva (1973).
13. R.G. Whitehead and A.A. Paul, Infant growth and human milk requirements. A fresh approach, Lancet July 25:161 (1981).
14. J. Stuff, C. Garza, C. Boutte, J.K. Fraley, E.O. Smith, E.R. Klein, and B.L. Nichols, Sources of variation in milk and caloric intakes in breast-fed infants: implications for lactation study design and interpretation, Am. J. Clin. Nutr. 43:361 (1986).
15. Committee on Dietary Allowances, Food and Nutrition Board: Recommended dietary allowances, Washington, D.C., National Academy of Sciences (1980).
16. J.E. Stuff, C. Garza, C. Boutte, and B.L. Nichols, Caloric intakes of older breast-fed infants: human milk and solid food (abstr), Am. J. Clin. Nutr. 43:679 (1986).
17. C.M. Montandon, C.A. Wills, C. Garza, E.O. Smith, and B.L. Nichols, Formula intake of one- and four-month old infants, J. Pediatr. Gastroenterol. Nutr. 5:434 (1986).
18. A.S. Goldman, C. Garza, B.L. Nichols, and R. Goldblum, Immunologic factors in human milk during the first year of lactation, J. Pediatr. 100:563 (1982).
19. N.F. Butte, R.M. Goldblum, L.M. Fehl, K. Loftin, E.O. Smith, C. Garza, and A.S. Goldman, Daily ingestion of immunologic components in human milk during the first four months of life, Acta Paediatr. Scand. 73:296 (1984).

20. C. Garza, C.A. Johnson, E.O. Smith, and B.L. Nichols, Changes in the nutrient composition of milk during gradual weaning, Am. J. Clin. Nutr. 37:61 (1983).
21. A.S. Goldman, C. Garza, B.L. Nichols, E.O. Smith, and R.M. Goldblum, Immunologic components in human milk during gradual weaning, Acta Paediatr. Scand. 72:133 (1983).

THE EFFECT OF MATERNAL PARITY ON LACTATIONAL PERFORMANCE IN A RURAL AFRICAN COMMUNITY

Ann Prentice

MRC Dunn Nutrition Unit
Cambridge U.K. and
Keneba, The Gambia

INTRODUCTION

In the developing world, particularly in areas of high infant mortality, many mothers produce their first child soon after menarche and continue with repeated cycles of pregnancy and lactation throughout their reproductive life. The children of mothers living in such circumstances generally rely heavily on breast-milk as their major source of nutrients during infancy and early childhood. Breast-milk also provides these children with non-nutritive factors, such as antimicrobial agents and growth modulators, which may be crucial assets in their fight for survival. Consequently, any alteration in the lactational performance of a mother, in terms of breast-milk quality and volume, is likely to be reflected in the health of her child.

The Dunn Nutrition Unit has been studying the lactational performance of rural West African mothers living in Keneba, The Gambia, for many years.[1] Mothers in this community breast-feed each child for at least 18 months, continuing in many cases into a third year of lactation, and may have 10 or more children. Complementary food is given to the infants after 3 months of age but even at 18 months, breast-milk provides over 40% of the children's daily protein and energy intakes. Breast-milk quality and volume of Keneba mothers were shown to vary with both stage of lactation and season of the year.[2-5] Breast-milk quality was altered slightly by the introduction of a nutritionally balanced dietary supplement designed to raise the energy intakes of the mothers to recommended levels but milk volume was not affected.[6] In addition it was demonstrated that each mother in Keneba had a lactational performance which, despite the variations due to stage of lactation, season of the year and supplementation, was characteristic of the individual not only within one lactational period but also during successive lactations.[3,7,8] The difference noted in characteristic lactational performance between individuals were substantial. For example, a five-fold variation in relative daily fat production was observed between different mothers. The data presented in this report establish that one of the major determinants of an individual's characteristic lactational performance is maternal parity.

MATERIALS AND METHODS

All lactating mothers living in Keneba between 1978-1981 (n=180) took part in this study which had the approval of the Ethical Committees of the Dunn Nutrition Unit, Cambridge and MRC Laboratories, The Gambia. After 1979 all subjects received an energy-rich dietary supplement which was extended to pregnant mothers in 1980.[6] Measurements were only made on mothers between 14 days and 18 months of lactation to avoid the periods of lactogenesis and involution. The results from subjects with clinical mastitis or chronic breast dysfunction have been removed from the analysis.

The obstetric histories of the mothers were obtained at routine antenatal clinics and were checked against a twice-yearly census which had been carried out in the area since 1952. The parity of a woman was taken as the number of live births achieved plus any stillbirths in the last trimester of pregnancy. Twins increased the parity score by 2. The highest parity score in the study was 13. All the mothers in the study had had their first child in their late teenage, no primiparous mother being older than 20 at parturition. As a consequence, maternal age and parity were inextricably linked in these subjects and no differentiation between their separate effects on lactational performance could be made.

Breast-milk volumes

Breast-milk intakes of infants were measured by test-weighing over a 12 h period from 07.00-19.00 hours. The measurements were made at routine sessions designed to be as close to everyday life as possible with the minimum of interference with the normal pattern of lactation.[2] The frequency of feeding was also carefully noted during these sessions. Volumes obtained over this 12 h period were closely correlated with 24 h intakes measured in a series of 95 determinations conducted at different seasons of the year. Volume measurements were made on 100 of the subjects every month during their lactation. The results of this study were compared with a larger set of volume determinations on Keneba mothers from 1976-1982 (number of lactations = 387, number of subjects = 184, number of data points = 4430).[8]

Breast-milk composition

The breast-milk concentrations of fat, nitrogen, lactose and 7 antimicrobial proteins (IgA, IgG, IgM, C3, C4, lactoferrin and lysozyme) were measured for each mother (n=180) every month during a single lactational period (up to 18 determinations per subject).

Milk samples for fat analysis were collected using a protocol designed to minimise within-feed and diurnal variations in fat concentration.[9] Small volumes of milk (0.5 ml) were expressed manually from both breasts, before and after a mid-afternoon feed and aliquots pooled. The mean fat content at this specific feed was related to the daily mean fat concentration in these mothers.[9]

No consistent within-feed or diurnal variations in the concentrations of any other breast-milk component assayed were found in Keneba milks. Consequently the samples collected for fat measurements were also assayed for nitrogen and lactose while samples for antimicrobial factor determinations (up to 6 per subject) were collected at 08.00-10.00 h.

Breast-milk analysis

All samples were stored in polystyrene tubes at -20°C. Milks were defatted by centrifugation where necessary prior to analysis.

Fat was measured by the creamatocrit method with calibration against the British Standard Method (1968).[9] Lactose was measured by the p-hydroxybenzoic acid hydrazide method,[10] nitrogen by the micro-Kheldahl technique. Total energy was calculated from modified Atwater factors,[11] with no corrections for unavailable nitrogen or growth requirements. The antimicrobial proteins were determined by single radial diffusion as described in detail elsewhere.[4] Secretory component (free + bound) was quantitated in order to differentiate changes in the proportion of secretory-IgA and serum-IgA in milk.

Daily intakes of each breast-milk constituent were estimated by combining the concentration data with measurements of milk volume made for the same mother on or close to the day of milk sampling.

Data Analysis

Standardisation of the data for stage of lactation, season of the year and supplementation was achieved by expressing each measurement as a percentage of the mean value recorded for all mothers in the same trimester of lactation during the month in which the particular sample was collected. These adjusted figures gave a measure of the breast-milk quality and volume of the individual relative to other mothers in the community at that time. All immunoprotein results were transformed to logarithms before data processing to correct a marked positive skew in the distribution of values.

The effects of parity on breast-milk volume and feed frequency were confirmed by step-wise multiple regression analysis on the larger data set using the GENSTAT statistical language. Each lactational period of a mother was treated as a separate entity.

Characteristic lactational performance

One-way analysis of variance demonstrated that the quality and quantity of milk produced by a mother, once adjusted for season, stage of lactation and plane of nutrition, were characteristic of the individual during successive months of the same lactational period ($p<0.001$ for all instances, e.g. volume $F = 8.7$, df = 349,4052; fat $F = 3.7$, dfs = 100,633; lysozyme $F = 5.8$, dfs = 70,144).[3,8] An individual's characteristic concentration and daily production of each milk component during a particular lactation was represented by the mean of all the data, after standardisation, obtained for the mother over the entire lactational period. Only one value per subject was therefore used in determining the effect of parity on each of the milk components studied and on milk production. The variation in these relative mean values between different subjects was high. For example the range of fat production varied between 37% and 195% of the mean and lactoferrin production varied from 49% to 228% of the mean.

Analysis of variance also demonstrated that there was a significantly greater between-mother than within-mother variation in mean relative milk volumes measured in successive lactations after allowing for the sex and parity of each child ($F = 4.0$, dfs = 172,148) showing that the volume produced by a mother is characteristic of the individual throughout life.[8]

RESULTS

Breast-milk volume

Increasing maternal parity had little effect on breast-milk volume up to parity 9 (Fig. 1). There was a marked decrease in volume produced by mothers of parity 10 and above such that primiparous mothers produced 30% more milk ($p<0.02$) relative to mothers of very high parity. The decline in daily output was caused by a reduction in the volume of milk produced per feed as feed frequency was not affected by maternal parity. This pattern of variation in milk volumes with parity noted in the study mothers was confirmed by a step-wise multiple regression analysis of the larger data set for whom parity values were available (n=341). This analysis also established that the daily volumes produced by mothers of parity 1 and 2 were slightly, but significantly, higher than those of mothers of parity 3-9 (Fig. 1).

Breast-milk nutritional factors

Maternal parity was found to have a marked influence on the concentrations and daily production of breast-milk fat, nitrogen, lactose and total energy (Table 1).

Milk fat concentrations decreased substantially after parity 1 until a steady level was reached after parities 3-4. Primiparous mothers produced milk with a fat concentration 23% above that produced by mothers of parity greater than 3. When combined with the variation in milk volume, this led to a pronounced decrease in daily fat production with increasing parity: infants of primiparous mothers consumed 40% more fat per day than infants of mothers of parity 4-9 and 80% more than infants of mothers of parity 10 and higher.

The influence of maternal parity on milk nitrogen concentrations and daily production was similar to the pattern seen for fat, but the size of the effect was smaller. First-born infants consumed 19% more nitrogen per day than children of mothers of parity 4-9 and 51% more than mothers of higher parity.

Lactose concentrations were unaffected by parity. Consequently the variation in daily lactose production followed that observed for milk volume, with 30% higher intakes by first-born infants compared with children of mothers of parity 10 and above.

As a result of the combined effects on fat, nitrogen and volume, the calculated energy content and daily energy production of breast-milk were also influenced by maternal parity. Infants of primiparous mothers consumed 13% more energy than infants of mothers of parity 4-9 and 41% more than those of mothers of very high parity.

Breast-milk antimicrobial proteins

The variations in the concentrations and daily production of IgA, IgG, IgM, C3, C4, lactoferrin, lysozyme and secretory component with maternal parity are given in Table 2. The pattern of change was similar for all the proteins although the magnitude of the effect varied between them.

The milk of primiparous mothers was richer in all the antimicrobial proteins than that of mothers of parity 3-9. Unlike the nutritional components, however, the concentrations of the immunoproteins tended to increase again in the milks of mothers of very high parity. As a result

Table 1. Effect of maternal parity on breast-milk nutrient concentrations and daily intakes

		Maternal Parity				
		1	2	3-8	9	10+
Fat	Conc[a]	116.2 (±3.5)[b]	104.2 (±3.6)[c]	95.1 (±1.4)	88.8 (±2.7)	94.9 (±3.8)
	Intake[a]	128.2 (±8.6)[b]	111.7 (±9.9)[c]	93.9 (±2.7)	89.8 (±9.5)	71.3 (±6.7)[c]
Nitrogen	Conc	106.4 (±3.8)[b]	106.4 (±4.5)[d]	98.7 (±1.5)	96.8 (±4.3)	94.2 (±4.6)
	Intake	115.7 (±8.4)[d]	109.6 (±9.7)	97.1 (±3.0)	94.8 (±7.3)	76.5 (±8.8)[d]
Lactose	Conc	98.5 (±1.0)[b]	99.7 (±1.1)[d]	99.8 (±0.6)	103.6 (±1.3)	101.4 (±0.5)
	Intake	105.6 (±7.5)[d]	105.3 (±7.0)	100.2 (±2.9)	94.4 (±5.5)	87.0 (±8.8)[d]
Calculated Energy	Conc	105.4 (±1.7)[b]	102.5 (±1.9)[d]	98.8 (±0.9)	97.0 (±1.8)	97.6 (±1.8)
	Intake	111.4 (±7.1)[d]	108.1 (±8.6)	99.8 (±2.9)	96.6 (±8.7)	79.0 (±7.6)[d]
Numbers	Conc	30	19	99	13	19
	Intake	14	11	62	5	8

[a]Values are arithmetic mean ± standard error after standardisation for season, stage of lactation and supplementation (percentage of mean)
Significance of differences from parities 3-9: b $p<0.001$; c $p<0.01$; d $p<0.05$

Table 2. Effect of maternal parity on breast-milk immunoprotein concentrations and daily intakes

		Maternal Parity				
		1	2	3-8	9	10+
Lactoferrin	Conc[a]	123.6 (+10.2)[b]	110.7 (+ 9.7)[d]	94.7 (+2.6)	82.6 (+ 7.0)	108.5 (+ 7.5)
	Intake[a]	134.1 (+ 9.3)[b]	105.8 (+10.4)	94.5 (+3.3)	72.0 (+12.7)	79.5 (+10.9)
Lysozyme	Conc	136.7 (+13.5)[b]	117.8 (+14.7)[c]	89.8 (+3.6)	95.9 (+ 8.4)	110.4 (+10.5)
	Intake	155.7 (+15.1)[b]	116.1 (+22.5)[d]	85.1 (+4.4)	93.7 (+13.4)	97.6 (+10.3)
IgA	Conc	102.7 (+ 8.8)	114.3 (+11.6)[d]	95.7 (+3.0)	86.4 (+ 8.8)	125.2 (+ 7.3)[c]
	Intake	110.1 (+10.0)	111.2 (+13.2)	95.8 (+3.8)	76.9 (+17.5)	95.5 (+10.8)
Secretory Component	Conc	115.3 (+ 6.6)[b]	108.7 (+ 8.2)[d]	96.5 (+2.2)	91.9 (+ 7.7)	107.8 (+ 4.8)
	Intake	119.6 (+ 6.8)[c]	104.2 (+12.0)	94.7 (+3.3)	79.8 (+10.7)	88.9 (+10.1)
IgG	Conc	114.2 (+11.0)[d]	118.1 (+ 9.0)[c]	94.3 (+2.8)	86.7 (+10.3)	106.2 (+ 6.2)
	Intake	120.4 (+14.4)[d]	120.5 (+10.7)[d]	93.3 (+4.0)	81.3 (+11.1)	82.4 (+12.1)
IgM	Conc	125.5 (+10.6)[c]	128.1 (+18.8)[c]	93.4 (+3.7)	71.8 (+13.0)	122.0 (+13.9)[d]
	Intake	134.9 (+15.7)[c]	119.0 (+24.6)	94.1 (+5.5)	79.9 (+22.6)	86.7 (+10.4)
C3	Conc	127.1 (+15.5)[c]	113.5 (+14.5)	94.3 (+3.9)	81.4 (+ 9.5)	107.3 (+11.0)
	Intake	145.9 (+20.8)[b]	103.7 (+18.9)	93.7 (+4.7)	68.7 (+11.2)	87.4 (+10.4)
C4	Conc	144.8 (+25.8)[c]	136.2 (+30.7)[c]	90.3 (+5.8)	65.4 (+21.2)	107.6 (+13.2)
	Intake	179.4 (+31.1)	107.4 (+29.9)	90.2 (+5.9)	45.4 (+23.0)	91.8 (+15.8)
Numbers	Conc	20	19	93	8	12
	Intake	14	11	62	5	8

[a]Values are geometric mean (+1 geometric standard error) after standardisation for season, stage of lactation and supplementation (percentage of mean)
Significance of difference from parities 3-9: b $p<0.001$; c $p<0.01$; d $p<0.05$

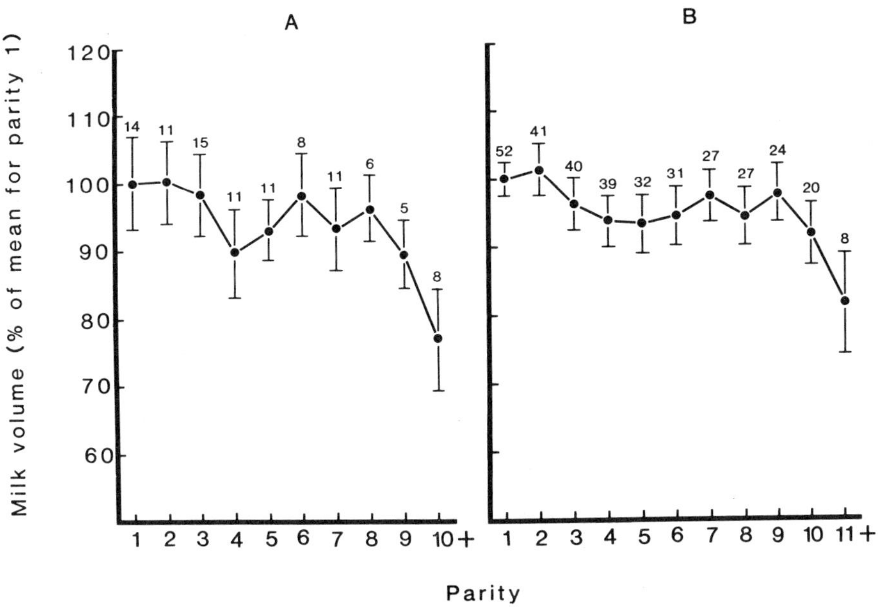

Fig. 1. Effect of parity on breast-milk volume. Values are expressed relative to parity 1 after standardisation for season and stage of lactation. A = subjects in milk composition study B = full data set.

the daily intake of immunoproteins by first-born infants was substantially higher than for infants of mothers of parity 3-9 but there was no further decline in consumption by the children of mothers of parities 10 and above. The increases in the daily consumption of immunoproteins by the infants of primiparous mothers compared with those of mothers of parity 3 and higher are as follows: Lactoferrin 47%, lysozyme 79%, IgA 17%, IgG 31%, IgM 47%, C3 60% and C4 108%.

DISCUSSION

The mothers of Keneba are representative of many thousands of women living in underprivileged circumstances throughout the developing world. These mothers live and produce a succession of children in conditions of severe hardship including chronic undernutrition, high prevalence of infection, strenuous physical activity and poor living conditions. The results of this study clearly demonstrate that the lactational performance of underprivileged mothers deteriorates with increasing maternal parity and this finding is particularly striking when the daily production of milk components is considered.

A number of mechanisms can be suggested to explain the effect of parity on lactational performance. It is possible, for example, that infants of mothers with poor milk production have a higher risk of dying during the period of breast-feeding. These mothers would have smaller intervals between births and would ultimately reach higher parity scores. The decrease in milk volume observed at very high parities in this cross-sectional analysis could then be attributed to a selection effect. This suggestion, however, seems unlikely as most deaths in early childhood in Keneba occur in the perinatal period or after the cessation of breast-feeding.

A second explanation is that there is a reduction in the availability of essential nutrients which might limit lactation in mothers of high parity. However in Keneba no evidence for the maternal depletion syndrome has yet been found as maternal weight-for-height, subcutaneous fat stores and food intakes do not decrease with increasing parity.[3,12] A third hypothesis is that a progressive deterioration in secretory function of the mammary gland occurs with increasing parity. Such a mechanism would not be surprising when it is considered that by the time a Keneba mother starts her tenth lactation she will have already secreted 3000-4000 litres of milk.

The close relationship between parity and maternal age in Keneba makes it impossible to draw any conclusions about whether the high relative lactational performance of primiparous mothers in Keneba is also a feature of the older primiparous mother typical of Western and Chinese societies. It can be appreciated, however, that any cross-cultural comparison of breast-milk quality and quantity must include careful matching of subjects for age and parity. Failure to do so in the past may have contributed to the false impression that mothers living in underprivileged communities necessarily have inferior breast-milk quality and volumes to mothers in more affluent societies.[8]

A recent analysis of the growth of Keneba infants[13] has shown that first-born children, who have smaller birth-weights than other infants, have high growth velocities during the first few months of life so that by 3 months their weights are indistinguishable from those of children of mothers of medium parity. By contrast the growth of children born to mothers of very high parity during this period is poor. After 3 months of age the growth patterns of all children are similar with the result that the differential in anthropometric status that was evident at 3 months between children of mothers of low and high parity is maintained throughout infancy. The influence of maternal parity on child growth, therefore, paralleled the variations in lactational performance of Keneba mothers observed with increasing parity. In addition, the impact of parity on child growth was most apparent between birth and 3 months of age, the period of exclusive breast-feeding in this community. The results of this study, therefore, strongly suggest that the long-term differences in breast-milk composition and volume between mothers of different parity are a major contributory factor in determining the relative growth and well-being of their infants.

SUMMARY

High concentrations of fat, nitrogen and immunoproteins in the breast-milk of Gambian mothers nursing their first baby led to substantially greater daily intakes of these factors by their infants compared with other children in the community. The daily consumption of breast-milk fat, nitrogen and lactose was further reduced in the children of mothers of very high parity (10 and above) owing to a decline in daily milk volume. A compensatory increase in milk immunoprotein concentrations prevented a similar decrease in immunoprotein intakes by these infants.

ACKNOWLEDGEMENTS

I would like to thank all members of the Keneba team, especially Drs. A.M. Prentice (project leader), T.J. Cole (statistician) and R.G. Whitehead (director). The study would not have been possible without the cheerful co-operation of the Keneba villagers. A.P. is currently supported by an award from the Bristol-Myers Fund to the Dunn Nutrition Unit.

REFERENCES

1. Dunn Nutrition Unit, "Maternal and child nutrition publications 1974-1984", A. M. Prentice, ed., Dunn Nutrition Unit, Cambridge (1985).
2. A. M. Prentice, Variations in maternal dietary intake, birthweight and breast-milk output in The Gambia, in: "Maternal nutrition during pregnancy and lactation", H. Aebi and R. G. Whitehead, eds., Hans Huber Publishers, Bern (1980).
3. A. Prentice, A. M. Prentice and R. G. Whitehead, Breast-milk fat concentrations of rural African women. II. Long-term variations within a community, Brit. J. Nutr. 45:495 (1981).
4. A. Prentice, A. M. Prentice, T. J. Cole and R. G. Whitehead, Breast-milk antimicrobial factors of rural Gambian mothers. I. Influence of stage of lactation and maternal plane of nutrition, Acta Paediatr. Scand. 73:796 (1984).
5. A. Prentice, M. Watkinson, A. M. Prentice, T. J. Cole and R. G. Whitehead, Breast-milk antimicrobial factors of rural Gambian mothers. II. Influence of season and prevalence of infection, Acta Paediatr. Scand. 73:803 (1984).
6. A. M. Prentice, S. B. Roberts, A. Prentice, A. A. Paul, M. Watkinson, A. A. Watkinson and R. G. Whitehead, Dietary supplementation of lactating Gambian women. I. Effect on breast-milk volumes and quality, Human Nutr.: Clin. Nutr. 37C:53 (1983).
7. A. Prentice, A. M. Prentice, T. J. Cole and R. G. Whitehead, Determinants of variations in breast-milk protective factor concentrations of rural Gambian mothers, Arch. Dis. Chld. 58:518 (1983).
8. A. M. Prentice, A. A. Paul, A. Prentice, A. E. Black, T. J. Cole and R. G. Whitehead, Cross-cultural differences in lactational performance, in: "Human lactation - Effect of maternal environmental factors", Plenum Press, New York (1986).
9. A. Prentice, A. M. Prentice and R. G. Whitehead, Breast-milk fat concentrations of rural African mothers. I. Short-term variations within individuals, Brit. J. Nutr. 45:483 (1981).
10. G. J. Hudson, P. M. V. John, B. S. Bailey and D. A. T. Southgate, The automated determination of carbohydrate, J. Sci. Food Agric. 27:681 (1976).
11. Department of Health and Social Security, "The composition of mature human milk", Report on Health and Social Subjects no. 12 (1977).
12. A. M. Prentice, R. G. Whitehead, S. B. Roberts, A. A. Paul, Long-term energy balance in child-bearing Gambian women, Am. J. Clin. Nutr. 34:2790 (1981).
13. A. Prentice, T. J. Cole, A. M. Prentice and R. G. Whitehead, The effect of maternal parity on child growth in rural West Africa, (in preparation).

COMPARATIVE PROSTAGLANDIN CONTENT IN HUMAN MILK

Janet E. Chappell,
David T. Armstrong and
M. Thomas Clandinin

Medical Department
Bristol-Myers Pharmaceutical Group
Ottawa, Canada
Department of Obstetrics and Gynaecology
The University of Western Ontario
London, Canada
Department of Foods and Nutrition
University of Alberta
Edmonton, Canada

INTRODUCTION

Current understanding of the physiology of human lactation is derived largely from principles drawn from animal experiments, tissue explant data and acute human studies of varying physiological states. Extrapolation of controlling mechanisms from these sources must be viewed with some caution. As plasma profiles of hormones and other appropriate compounds can be artificially influenced by factors unrelated to mammary gland lactogenesis, analysis of breast fluid[1] and milk might serve to identify prior synthetic events.

LACTOGENESIS: PROLACTIN EFFECT

In the human, numerous hormones have been linked to the lactational process, although it has been impossible to associate individual hormones with each point in the cascade of events[2]. Prolactin, however, continues to be identified as a major initiating lactogenic factor[3,4]. Indeed, inhibition of prolactin secretion by pharmacological means at any stage in the postpartum period causes prompt cessation of lactation. Prolactin seems to initiate its action by interacting with a specific receptor on the cell surface of the mammary epithelial cell. Incomplete information is available regarding the cellular events involved subsequent to binding and prior to milk synthesis. Whether by internalization after binding or by paracellular transport, prolactin is present within the secretory cell and is lysosomally degraded. An unknown percentage of cellular prolactin is released into human milk[5,6]. Healey and coworkers[6] suggest that the lactational stage profile of milk prolactin levels correlates with at least two known compositional changes. Clinically it is suggested that the physiology associated with lactation failure, galactorrhea or relactation may be chronicled by milk hormonal patterns.

Recent observations by some laboratories[7-11] indicate that the milk lactated by mothers delivering prematurely differs in macronutrient content when compared with milk from mothers delivering at term. As there is little evidence to suggest that this milk secretion has a teleologic origin, it does raise the possibility of an underlying hormonal relationship responsible for these differences in milk composition. Reported variance and inconsistancies[12,13] may be better understood if 'preterm milk' is examined in terms of subgroups and as an event secondary to an altered or interrupted hormonal status.

In this regard, during late gestation high progesterone levels are thought to inhibit the proliferation of mammary prolactin receptors and thus prepartum lactation. Since circulating progesterone levels are lower at 30 weeks of gestation than at 38-41 weeks of gestation[14,15], it may be that women who deliver premature infants initiate lactation with lower circulating progesterone levels and therefore with relatively greater levels of prolactin and/or potentially increased number of mammary prolactin receptors. Furthermore, there are reports that progesterone levels are lower in some women prior to and during premature labour when compared to women of similar gestational stage who carry their fetus to term[16,17].

Difficulties in milk prolactin analysis - such as resistant protein-prolactin complexes[18], uncertain solubility[19] and location of receptors[20] - may obscure subsequent prolactin measurements. In recent years prostaglandins have been shown to possess a multitude of physiologic effects. These ubiquitous 20-carbon carboxylic fatty acids are synthesized and released in response to cell stimulation. The subsequent rapid metabolism of prostaglandins has meant that the specifics regarding function remain illusive. One concept is that prostaglandins are constantly turning on or off adenosine 3',5'-cyclic monophosphate (cAMP), a key intracellular mediator of tissue response to hormones (Scheme 1).

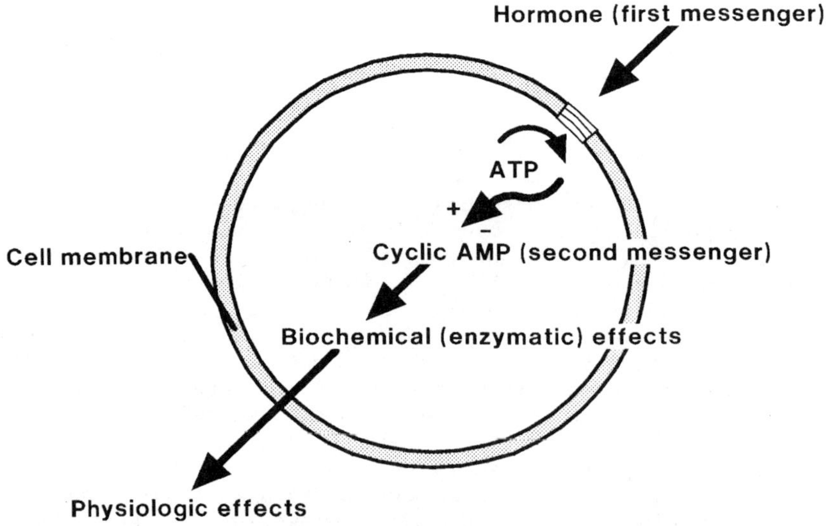

Scheme 1. Mediator hypothesis. The Yin-Yang theory postulates that the cAMP to cGMP ratio controls cell function. (Adapted from 'The Prostaglandins', The Upjohn Co., 1973.)

From animal and cell culture data, it has been proposed that prostaglandins mediate critical lactogenic processes[21]. This observation has not, however, been reported by Matusik and Rosen[22]. Shiu and Friesen[23] suggest that the action of prolactin, unlike most hormones, may be mediated by an elevated level of guanosine 3',5'-cyclic monophosphate (cGMP) coupled with a reduced intracellular concentration of cAMP. Prostaglandins from series 1 have been shown to stimulate adenylate cyclase activity and thus to increase cAMP concentration in rabbit and mouse mammary glands[24]. Series 2 prostaglandins have the opposite effect and therefore have been labeled as lactogenic. The action of series 3 prostaglandins regarding mediated prolactin effects is currently unknown. If prostaglandins do mediate the prolactin effect within the mammary gland, milk prostaglandin content may indirectly reflect a stage of lactogenic function. Prostaglandins have been reported to be present in human milk[25-28], although discussion has been limited to their potential gastrointestinal effect in the breastfed infant.

PERIPARTURIENT PROSTAGLANDINS

The role of prostaglandins during the peripartum period of women has not been well established. Prostaglandins, particularly those of the E series, play an important part in the control of fetal and placental haemodynamics[29]. While they are released into the maternal circulation and amniotic fluid during labor, there is conflicting evidence as to their involvement in the initiation of labor[30]. Smith and Abraham[31] have reported that lactation occurs in many women following therapeutic abortion with prostaglandin $F_{2\alpha}$. Maternal plasma prostaglandin levels appear to be elevated during lactation and have been observed to respond to suckling[32]; yet the significance is also unknown. Finally, prostaglandins have been found to be both synergistic and antagonistic to the milk ejection process in women[33].

This pattern of opposing actions is not limited to pregnancy and lactation. Indeed it has been suggested that in tissues where different prostaglandins have opposing actions, the ability to alter the amount of individual prostaglandins produced provides a mechanism for controlling physiologic processes[34]. Maule and Peaker[35], working with goats, have perhaps best described and speculated as to the role of prostaglandins in mammary gland function. They have proposed that prostaglandin $F_{2\alpha}$ serves as a prepartum inhibitor of milk secretion. After parturition, increases in prostaglandin synthesis with subsequent rapid metabolism and excretion into milk appears to facilitate milk release. Spooner and coworkers[36] have speculated that F prostaglandins are indirectly involved in milk lipid synthesis via their removal of the inhibitory progesterone effect on rat mammary gland lipoprotein lipase activity during parturition.

HUMAN MILK PROSTAGLANDINS

Prostaglandins are not stored preformed but rather are synthesized and released as required. Therefore, their presence is thought to be indicative of prior stimuli. Two laboratories demonstrated in 1980 that human milk contains large quantities of prostaglandins of the E and F series, which are present in over 100 times the amounts found in control adult plasma[25,26] (Figure 1). Unlike observations in the goat[35], Lucas and Mitchell[25] found low metabolite to parent prostaglandin ratios in milk, when compared with plasma ratios. Since fore- and hindmilk collection procedures were followed by these investigators, interpretation from averaged values must be made with some reservation (Table 1).

TABLE 1

PROSTANOID CONTENT OF COLOSTRUM AND HUMAN MILK[1]
(ng/100 mL)

		PGE[2]	PGF	6-Keto $PGF_{1\alpha}$
Craig-Schmidt et al[28] [8]	C[3]	-	-	-
	HM	14 ± 1	11 ± 2	-
Reid et al[26] [6]	C	8 ± 6	61 ± 23	-
	HM	11 ± 5	38 ± 21	-
Lucas & Mitchell[25] [10]	C	19 ± 5	55 ± 24	22 ± 6
	HM	-	-	-
Chappell et al[27] [13]	C	140 ± 21	97 ± 24[4]	24 ± 2
	HM	692 ± 69	68 ± 18	133 + 15

[1]Values are means ±SEM; [] represents number of fullterm samples. [2]Due to small but measurable cross reactivities between the series 1 and 2 prostaglandins, PGE_2 and $PGF_{2\alpha}$ are described only as PGE and PGF. [3]C=Colostrum, HM=Human milk. [4]Representative of 5 samples only.

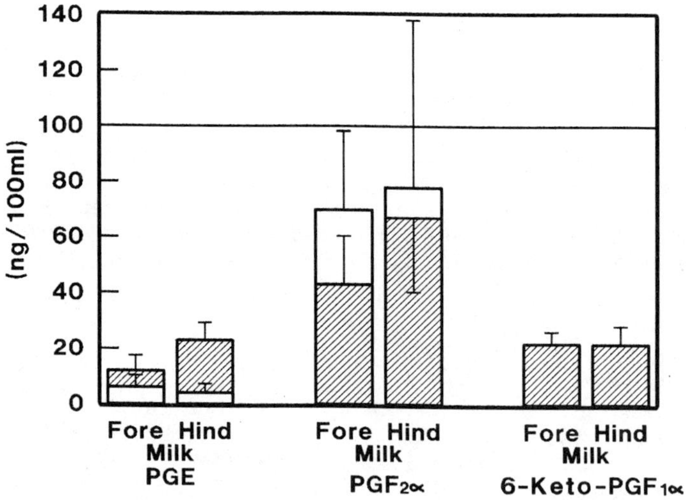

Fig. 1. Reported prostanoid levels in fore- and hindmilk at days 5-9 postpartum. ▨ Lucas and Mitchell[25], ▯ Reid et al[36], mean ±SEM.

Given the reported increased levels of measured prostaglandins in hindmilk and theoretical lipid solubility, we attempted to examine serial milk samples representative of complete expression, also known to be different in total lipid content (Figure 2). Since the dynamics of human mammary gland lipogenesis are not well understood, analysis of human milk was conducted to determine if known transitions in milk lipid and fatty acid composition are related to levels of specific milk prostanoids. Since it is conceivable that a difference in 'hormonal milieux' may result in the higher rates of mammary lactogenesis reported for some mothers of preterm infants[11,37,38], milk from mothers who delivered infants at term and from women who delivered prematurely (28-33wks) was compared to examine potential relationships between prostanoid concentration and gestational age effects on milk lipid content. Findings of increased preterm milk 'de novo' fatty acid synthesis[11,38,39] and the work of Borst[40] (which associated increased medium chain fatty acid synthesis in mouse mammary gland explants with prolactin regulation) was considered further support for this comparative approach.

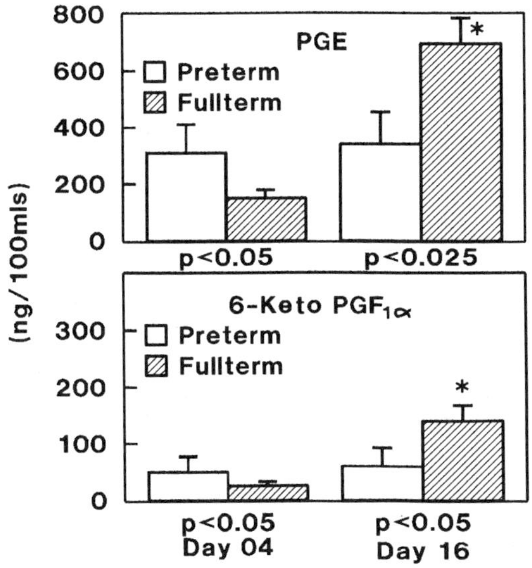

Fig. 2. Effect of gestational age and lactational stage on milk prostaglandin E and 6-keto prostaglandin $F_{1\alpha}$ content. The mean ±SEM for prostaglandin E in PT and FT ml on days 4 and 16 was 320±73 and 140±21 ng/dl, and 331±66 and 692±69 ng/dl, respectively. The mean ±SEM for 6-keto-prostaglandin $F_{1\alpha}$ in PT and FT milk on day 4 of lactation was 53.5±10 and 24±2 ng/dl and on day 16 of lactation was 64.0±16 and 133.2±15 ng/dl, respectively. *p<0.01 representative of lactational stage influence[27].

Prostaglandin E, F, and the metabolite of prostacyclin (6-keto-prostaglandin $F_{1\alpha}$) were determined by radioimmunoassays[41], and fatty acids were analyzed quantitatively by capillary gas liquid chromatography[42]. The instability of prostacyclin necessitates the analysis of its metabolite 6-keto-prostaglandin $F_{1\alpha}$ with no examination of time course possible. 6-keto-prostaglandin $F_{1\alpha}$ may, however, be further metabolized to an active form 6-keto-prostaglandin E_1[43]. It was again apparent that prostanoids are present in human milk at all stages of lactation (Figure 2). Prostaglandin values for day 37 were not significantly different from day 16 within each group and therefore are not illustrated (Figure 2). As no apparent gestational age influence was observed for prostaglandin F, these results are only summarized in Table 1. Milk content of prostaglandin E was highly correlated with the concentration of 6-keto-prostaglandin $F_{1\alpha}$ for all days of lactation studied and for both groups of mothers (Figure 3).

Fullterm Milk

Although drawn from a limited number of milk samples, milk prostaglandin F content appears to decrease with maturation of lactation (Table 1). This observation, however, was not statistically significant due to marked inter-individual variation. This trend is perhaps consistent with Maule and Peaker's findings in goats[35] and may therefore indicate a decreased inhibition of milk secretion. Early serial colostrum analysis of prostaglandin F is, however, required to support this hypothesis.

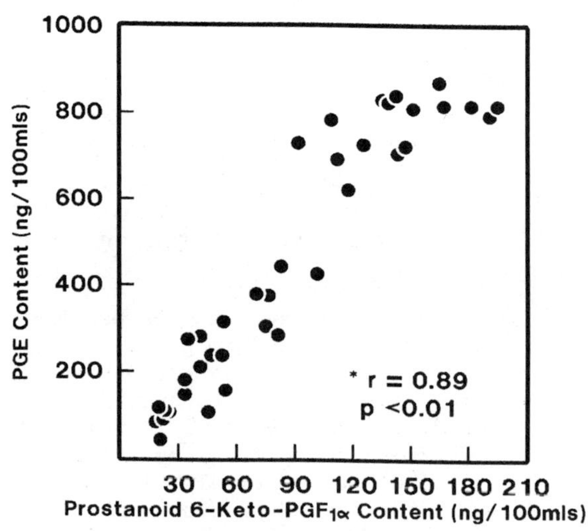

Fig. 3. Relationship between milk content of prostaglandin E and 6-keto-prostaglandin $F_{1\alpha}$.[27]

A reverse longitudinal pattern was observed by us for 6-keto-prostaglandin $F_{1\alpha}$ and prostaglandin E. It would appear that for this group of mothers who delivered at term, a relationship exists between the prostaglandin levels and milk total fatty acid levels reported (Figures 2 and 4). These compositional correlations cannot yet be directly interpreted as a cause and effect relationship but we believe that the presence of prostanoids in full term human milk may reflect the balance of hormonal subcellular controls over lactation. This is further supported by the positive correlation between fullterm milk prostaglandin (PGE and 6-keto-$PGF_{1\alpha}$) and C8:0, C10:0, C12:0, C14:0 fatty acid levels which are present in milk as a consequence of mammary gland 'de novo' synthesis ($p<0.05$).

The obvious differences in reported human milk prostaglandin E content are not easily explained (Table 1). Critical analytical differences are not apparent. Nonetheless, existing methodology developed for 'non milk' systems perhaps should be re-examined to ensure appropriateness for direct transfer for milk analysis. These might include column conditions for the removal of interfering substances, pH target for optimal recovery and 'boundfree' separation techniques which minimize dissociation of the antigen-antibody complex. The freezing of samples prior to prostaglandin analysis when compared to immediate post collection analysis does not explain the between-study prostaglandin E differences.

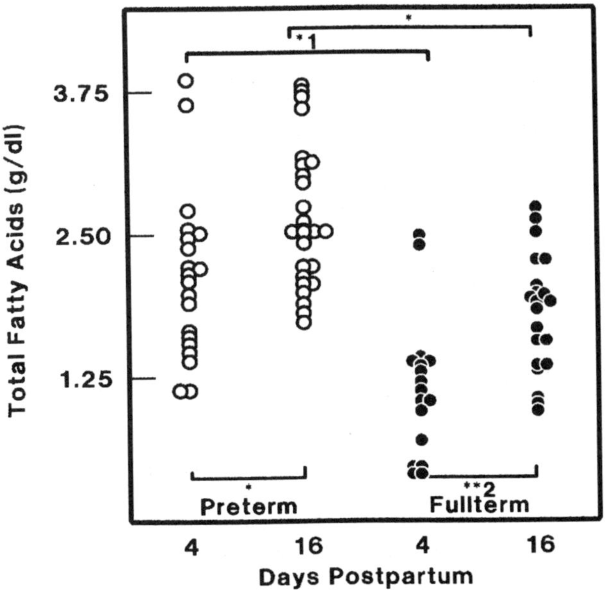

Fig. 4. Effect of lactational and gestational age on milk total fatty acid concentration. The mean ±SEM for the PT and FT milk was 2.1±0.2 and 1.3±0.2 g/dl for day 4 of lactation ($p<0.05$) and 2.5±0.3 and 1.9±0.12 g/dl on day 16 of lactation[1] *$p<0.05$, [2]**$p<0.01$[27].

The major collection difference is that while Reid and coworkers[26] and Lucas and Mitchell[25] manually collected small fore- and hindmilk samples (Craig-Schmidt and colleagues[28] manually collected 10 - 15 mls of hindmilk only), we collected a complete breast expression using a mechanical or electric pump. It is perhaps feasible that the time interval required for a complete expression is such that enzymes capable of transforming one active prostaglandin to another[44] or prostaglandin releasing macrophages[45] may be stimulated. Factors such as length of time at body temperature or at room temperature and/or degree of milk contact with the collection container material may be involved. It is, however, unlikely that only prostaglandin E would be sensitive to these collection procedures. Milk collection and sampling with known prostaglandin synthetase inhibitors (indomethacin) may serve to indirectly identify the source of milk prostaglandin release.

Dietary Influences

The literature indicates that precursor fatty acid availability and therefore dietary fat intake, influence the synthesis and release of prostaglandins[46-48]. Craig-Schmidt and coworkers[28], however, did not find significant differences in milk prostaglandin E or $F_{2\alpha}$ content following maternal dietary cross-over trials. Milk levels of elaidic acid (C18:1(9)t) were significantly higher following consumption of hydrogenated fat (6.5% of total fatty acid intake) when compared with lower intakes (1.8% of total). The investigators concluded that the currently consumed range of hydrogenated fat intakes does not contain sufficient C18:2(6)tt and C18:2(6)ct to affect precursor fatty acid availability for prostaglandin synthesis.

Similarly, for women consuming ad libitum diets, we did not find a correlation between milk prostanoid content and C18:2(6) or the immediate precursor fatty acids C20:3(6)/C20:4(6) from milk neutral lipids or phospholipids. The Bargmann-Knoop model of milk secretion suggests that the milk fat globule is enveloped by the plasma membrane prior to expulsion into the alveolar lumen. The phospholipid fatty acid profile of milk and alveolar cell should therefore be similar. While a relationship between precursor fatty acids and prostaglandin content might have been expected, the competition for elongation, desaturation and synthesis is a complex process. Furthermore, the physiologic range may not be sufficiently extensive to provide a means of comparison.

Preterm Milk

Although a full spectrum of nutrient profiles has been reported for preterm milk, colostrum (early lactation) observations have tended to be less variable between laboratories. It is perhaps these initial marked differences in preterm as compared to fullterm milk which might serve to identify the events or factors involved in this altered lactation state. We found the total fatty acid, 'de novo' synthesized fatty acid and prostaglandin levels to be significantly higher in preterm colostrum than in similarly collected fullterm samples (Figures 2, 4, 5). Between-mother variability was greater in preterm milk when compared to fullterm milk for all measured milk components. A linear relationship was not observed between milk prostaglandin levels and milk lipid components in preterm milk. Furthermore, a parallel increase in prostaglandin levels relative to lipogenesis was not observed with the maturation of lactation. The significance of the observed preterm prostaglandin lactational stage profile relative to the fullterm milk pattern is unknown.

Although total fatty acid and 'de novo' synthesized fatty acid levels increased over time for both preterm and fullterm milk, the magnitude of the increase was relatively greater in fullterm milk. From the serial prostaglandin profile, it may be suggested that the preterm mammary gland lipogenic set point is acutely operative whereas the term gland physiologic

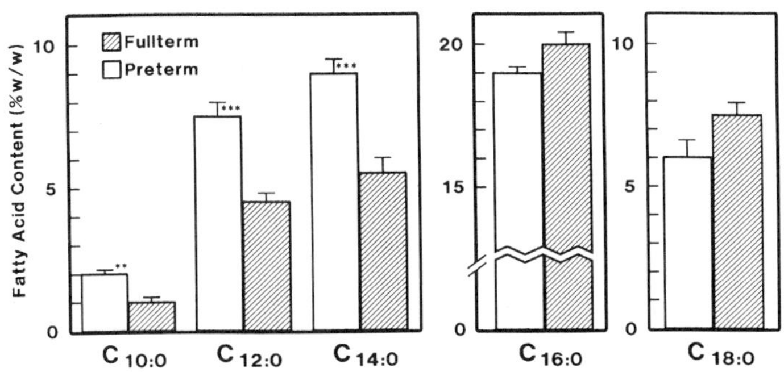

Fig. 5. Effect of gestational period on major saturated fatty acid profile of early human milk. $C_{8:0}$ (not illustrated) and $C_{10:0}$ **p<0.01; ***p<0.005[38].

activity is more transitional. Subsequent studies using a larger data set might find that subgroup analysis would allow for stratification of the observed variance into high and low responders. Novel analytic approaches as outlined by Atkinson and colleagues and by Neville in other chapters in this book will also serve to expand our understanding of the preterm milk phenomenon.

FUTURE INVESTIGATION

Human milk prostaglandin data is limited. Therefore, additional analysis of human milk throughout the lactation cycle is required to better characterize the pattern of prostaglandin secretion. Prostaglandin analysis in milks of known compositional differences and determination of the milk prostanoid metabolite to prostaglandin ratio may be best examined by adapting mammary epithelial cell absorption procedures[49]. In addition, comparative maternal plasma and milk prostaglandin analysis during lactation may identify a possible sequencing of events.

Fatty acid intake has been reported to influence prostaglandin synthesis in humans. Therefore, 'significantly' altered maternal fatty acid diets and subsequent prostaglandin milk content might be investigated to determine the degree to which mammary gland prostaglandin synthesis operates independent of external influences. Acute and chronic acetylsalicylic acid ingestion might be expected to reduce milk prostaglandin content. If synthetic milk constituents were also influenced, a direct relationship between milk prostaglandin levels and lactogenic control might be proposed.

SUMMARY

Although prostaglandins have been reported to be produced in significant quantities by the mammary gland of many species, they have received relatively little attention as possible regulators of mammary function. Prostaglandins (PGE and PGF) and prostaglandin metabolites (PGFM, TXB_2 and 6-keto-$PGF_{1\alpha}$) are present in human milk at all stages of lactation. However, standardized sampling criteria, storage conditions and analytical procedures have not been established. Although this inference is drawn from a limited number of observations, it would appear that specific postpartum patterns of prostaglandin release are evident. A significantly different prostaglandin profile has been reported in preterm milk. The influence of precursor fatty acid availability from milk neutral lipid or phospholipid or the maternal diet on subsequent milk prostaglandin levels has not been observed. The lactogenic significance of human milk prostaglandins remains unknown. Given the observed postpartum prostaglandin pattern which parallels many known compositional changes, milk prostaglandin levels may indicate the degree of mammary gland synthetic activity.

REFERENCES

1. J. K. Kulski, P. E. Hartmann, W. J. Saint, P. F. Giles, and D. H. Gutteridge, Changes in the milk composition of nonpuerperal women, Am. J. Obstet. Gynecol. 139:597 (1981).
2. H. A. Tucker, Endocrinology of lactation, Semin. Perinatol. 3:199 (1979).
3. S. J. Nillius, Prolactin, Acta Endocrinol. (Suppl. 216) 88:99 (1978).
4. J. Skarda, E. Urbanova, L.-M. Houdebine, C. Delouis, and J. Bilek, Effects of insulin, cortisol and prolactin on lipid, protein and casein synthesis in goat mammary tissue in organ culture, Reprod. Nutr. Develop. 22:379 (1982).
5. R. R. Gala, I. A. Forsyth, and A. Turvey, Milk prolactin is biologically active, Life Sc. 26:987 (1980).
6. D. L. Healey, S. Rattigan, P. E. Hartmann, A. C. Herington, and H. G. Burger, Prolactin in human milk: Correlation with lactose, total protein, and α-lactalbumin levels, Am. J. Physiol. 238:E83 (1980).
7. S. A. Atkinson, M. H. Bryan, and G. H. Anderson, Human milk: difference in nitrogen concentration in milk from mothers of term and preterm infants, J. Pediatr. 93:67 (1978).
8. S. J. Gross, R. J. David, L. Bauman, and R. M. Tomarelli, Nutritional composition of milk produced by mothers delivering preterm, J. Pediatr. 96:641 (1980).
9. J. A. Lemons, L. Moye, D. Hall, and M. Simmons, Differences in the composition of preterm and term human milk during early lactation, Pediatr. Res. 16:113 (1982).
10. R. K. Chandra, Immunoglobulin and protein levels in breast milk produced by mothers of preterm infants, Nutr. Res. 2:27 (1982).
11. J. Bitman, D. L. Wood, M. Hamosh, P. Hamosh, and N. R. Mehta, Comparison of the lipid composition of breast milk from mothers of term and preterm infants, Am. J. Clin. Nutr. 38:300 (1983).
12. L. Sann, F. Bienvenu, C. Lahet, J. Bienvenu, and M. Bethenod, Comparison of the composition of breast milk from mothers of term and preterm infants, Acta Paediatr. Scand. 70:115 (1981).

13. D. M. Anderson, F. H. Williams, R. B. Merkatz, P. K. Schulman, D.S. Kerr, and W. B. Pittard, Length of gestation and nutritional composition of human milk, Am. J. Clin. Nutr. 37:810 (1983).
14. J. E. Buster, R. J. Chang, D. L. Preston, R. M. Elashoff, L. M. cousins, G. E. Abraham, C. J. Hobel, and J. R. Marshall, Interrelationships of circulating maternal steroid concentrations in third trimester pregnancies. I. C_{21} steroids: Progesterone, 16α-hydroxyprogesterone, 17α-hydroxyprogesterone, 20α-dehydroprogesterone, delta^5-pregnenolone sulfate, and 17-hydroxy delta^5-pregnenolone, J. Clin. Endocrinol. Metab. 48:133 (1979).
15. C. R. Parker, R. B. Everett, J. G. Quirk, P. J. Whalley, and N. F. Gant, Hormone production during pregnancy in the primigravid patient: I. Plasma levels of progesterone and 5α-pregnane-3,20-dione throughout pregnancy of normal women and women who developed pregnancy induced hypertension, Am. J. Obstet. Gynecol. 135:778 (1979).
16. A. I. Csapo, O. Pohanka, and H. L. Kaihola, Progesterone deficiency and premature labor, Br. Med. J. 1:137 (1974).
17. L. M. Cousins, C. J. Hobel, R. J. Chang, D. M. Okada, and J. R. Marshall, Serum progesterone and estradiol - 17β levels in premature and term labor, Am. J. Obstet. Gynecol. 127:612 (1977).
18. A. A. van der Gugten, M. J. Waters, G. S. Murthy, and H. G. Friesen, Studies on the irreversible nature of prolactin binding to receptors, Endocrinology 106:402 (1980).
19. R. P. C. Shiu and H. G. Friesen, Solubilization and purification of a prolactin receptor from the rabbit mammary gland, J. Biol. Chem. 249:7902 (1974).
20. M. J. Waters, A. S. McNeilly, S. Ohgo, and H. G. Friesen, Prolactin receptor content of rabbit milk, Endocrinology 107:816 (1980).
21. J. A. Rillema, Possible role of prostaglandin $F_{2\alpha}$ in mediating effect of prolactin on RNA synthesis in mammary gland explants of mice, Nature 253:466 (1975).
22. R. J. Matusik and J. M. Rosin, Prolactin regulation of casein gene expression: Possible mediators, Endocrinology 106:252 (1980).
23. R. P. C. Shiu and H. G. Friesen, Mechanism of action of prolactin in the control of mammary gland function, Ann. Rev. Physiol. 42:83 (1980).
24. J. A. Rillema and E. A. Wild, Prolactin activation of phospholipase A activity in membrane preparations from mammary glands, Endocrinology 100:1219 (1977).
25. A. Lucas and M. D. Mitchell, Prostaglandins in human milk, Arch. Dis. Child. 55:950 (1980).
26. B. Reid, H. Smith, and Z. Friedman, Prostaglandins in human milk, Pediatrics 66:870 (1980).
27. J. E. Chappell, M. T. Clandinin, G. J. Barbe, and D. T. Armstrong, Prostanoid content of human milk: relationships to milk fatty acid content, Endocrinol. Exper. 17:351 (1983).
28. M. C. Craig-Schmidt, J. D. Weete, S. A. Faircloth, M. A. Wickwire, and E. J. Livant, The effect of hydrogenated fat in the diet of nursing mothers on lipid composition and prostaglandin content of human milk, Am. J. Clin. Nutr. 39:778 (1984).
29. I. Z. MacKenzie, D. A. MacLean, and M. D. Mitchell, Prostaglandins in the human fetal circulation in mid-trimester and term pregnancy, Prostaglandins 20:649 (1980).
30. G. C. Liggins, C. S. Forster, S. A. Grieves, and A. L. Schwartz, Control of parturition in man, Biol. Reprod. 16:39 (1977).

31. S. Smith and S. Abraham, Lactation following therapeutic abortion with prostaglandin $F_{2\alpha}$, Nature 240:411 (1972).
32. O. Ylikorkala and L. Viinikka, Prostacyclin, thromboxane, and prostaglandin $F_{2\alpha}$ in maternal plasma during breast feeding, Am. J. Obstet. Gynecol. 139:690 (1981).
33. H. Vorherr, Effect of prostaglandins on milk ejection, Endokrinologie 74:257 (1979).
34. P. M. Olley and F. Coceani, The prostaglandins, Am. J. Dis. Child. 134:688 (1980).
35. F. M. Maule Walker and M. Peaker, Local production of prostaglandins in relation to mammary function at the onset of lactation in the goat, J. Physiol. 309:65 (1980).
36. P. M. Spooner, M. M. Garrison, and R. O. Scow, Regulation of mammary and adipose tissue lipoprotein lipase and blood triacylglycerol in rats during late pregnancy, J. Clin. Invest. 60:702 (1977).
37. G. H. Anderson, S. A. Atkinson, and M. H. Bryan, Energy and macronutrient content of human milk during early lacation from mothers giving birth prematurely and at term, Am. J. Clin. Nutr. 34:258 (1981).
38. J. E. Chappell, and M. T. Clandinin, Comparative fatty acid content of human milk, Feder. Proc. 41:473A (1982).
39. G. Lepage, S. Collet, D. Bougle, L. C. Kien, D. Lepage, L. Dallaire, P. Darling, and C. C. Roy, The composition of preterm milk in relation to the degree of prematurity, Am. J. Clin. Nutr. 40:1042 (1984).
40. D. W. Borst, Hormonal regulation of medium chain fatty acid synthesis by mouse mammary gland explants, Lipids 15:913 (1980).
41. C. A. Evans, T. G. Kennedy, J. E. Patrick, and J. R. G. Challis, Uterine prostaglandin concentrations in sheep during late pregnancy and adrenocorticotropin-induced labor, Endocrinology 109:1533 (1981).
42. J. E. Chappell, M. T. Clandinin, and C. Kearney-Volpe, Trans fatty acids in human milk lipids: Influence of maternal diet and weight loss, Am. J. Clin. Nutr. 42:49 (1985).
43. P. Y-K. Wong, W. H. Lee, C. P. Quilley, and J. C. McGiff, Metabolism of prostacyclin: formation of an active metabolite in the liver, Federation Proc. 40:2001 (1981).
44. W. E. M. Lands, The biosynthesis and metabolism of prostaglandins, Ann. Rev. Physiol. 41:633 (1979).
45. H. Blau, J. H. Passwell, J. Levanon, J. Davidson, F. Kohen, and B. Ramot, Studies on human milk macrophages: effect of activation of phagocytosis and secretion of prostaglandin E_2 and lysozyme, Pediatr. Res. 17:241 (1983).
46. B. R. Culp, B. G. Titus, and W. E. M. Lands, Inhibition of prostaglandin biosynthesis by eicosapentaenoic acid, Prostaglandins and Medicine 3:269 (1979).
47. M. G. Lewis, T. L. Kaduce, and A. A. Spector, Effect of essential polyunsaturated fatty acid modifications on prostaglandin production by MDCK canine kidney cells, Prostaglandins 22:747 (1981).
48. O. Adam and G. Wolfram, Effect of different linoleic acid intakes on prostaglandin biosynthesis and kidney function in man, Am. J. Clin. Nutr. 40:763 (1984).
49. B. J. Thompson and S. Smith, Biosynthesis of fatty acids by lactating human breast epithelial cells: an evaluation of the contribution to the overall composition of human milk fat, Pediatr. Res. 19:139 (1985).

THE RELATIONSHIP OF MATERNAL FACTORS TO COMPOSITION AND STRUCTURE OF CASEINS

Rae Greenberg

P.O. Box 46454
Philadelphia, PA 19160

INTRODUCTION

The phosphoproteins of human milk occur as colloidal particles referred to as casein micelles. Recent reports on the size distribution, morphology, and composition of this micellar system (1,2) indicate that human casein micelles are smaller than the bovine equivalents but are probably also formed from spherical submicellar units. The isolation and characterization of human β- and κ-caseins (3,4), probable lack of α_s-casein (5), and extrapolation from bovine micelle structure would suggest that these small, somewhat fragile human casein particles are composed of mainly β-casein with a much smaller amount of κ-casein. Investigators have begun to characterize the protein interactions in this system (6) but no definitive model for the human milk micelle has emerged.

COMPOSITION AND STRUCTURE OF β-CASEIN

Beta-casein was isolated from mature human milk (7) and its primary structure elucidated by classical sequencing strategy (3). The basis for this sequence was provided by the arrangement of cyanogen bromide cleaved and trifluoroacetyl blocked trypsin cleaved peptides to provide unambiguous overlapping data. Sequencing was carried out on a liquid phase sequencer with a variety of procedures to accomplish Edman degradation. Human β-casein (H-β-Cn) is a single chain molecule of 212 amino acids as shown in Fig. 1 and is comparable in size to the bovine homologue. During the course of sequencing, two amino acids in equal amounts were identified at positions 142 (ile/pro) and 169 (leu/gln). This suggests genetic polymorphism at these sites involving no change of charge - a so called "silent" genetic variant. Seven genetic variants of bovine β-casein have been reported (8), all demonstrable by acid or alkaline polyacrylamide gel electrophoresis. These variants, containing one or more charged residue differences, have been confirmed as truly genetic by gel pattern analysis of dam, sire, daughter relationships. For substitutions of uncharged residues, the case in H-β-Cn, there is no easy way to demonstrate this phenomenon. Careful sequence analysis with good quantitation should suffice to confirm the existence of heterozygosity in the

1 5 10 15 20 25
Arg-Glu-Thr-Ile-Glu-Ser-Leu-Ser-Ser-Ser-Glu-Glu-Ser-Ile-Pro-Glu-Tyr-Lys-Gln-Lys-Val-Glu-Lys-Val-Lys-

30 40 50
His-Glu-Asp-Gln-Gln-Gln-Gly-Thr-Asp-Gln-His-Gln-Asp-Lys-Ile-Tyr-Pro-Ser-Phe-Gln-Pro-Gln-Pro-Leu-Ile-

55 65 75
Tyr-Pro-Phe-Val-Glu-Pro-Ile-Pro-Tyr-Gly-Phe-Leu-Pro-Gln-Asn-Ile-Leu-Pro-Leu-Ala-Gln-Pro-Ala-Val-Val-

80 90 ↓γ_2 ↓γ_3 100
Leu-Pro-Val-Pro-Gln-Pro-Glu-Ile-Met-Glu-Val-Pro-Lys-Ala-Lys-Asp-Thr-Val-Tyr-Thr-Lys-Gly-Arg-Val-Met-

105 115 125
Pro-Val-Leu-Lys-Gln-Pro-Thr-Ile-Pro-Phe-Phe-Asp-Pro-Gln-Ile-Pro-Lys-Leu-Thr-Asp-Leu-Glu-Asn-Leu-His-

130 140 150
Leu-Pro-Leu-Pro-Leu-Leu-Gln-Pro-Ser-Met-Gln-Gln-Val-Pro-Gln-Pro-Ile-Pro-Gln-Thr-Leu-Ala-Leu-Pro-Pro-

155 165 175
Gln-Pro-Leu-Trp-Ser-Val-Pro-Glu-Pro-Lys-Val-Leu-Pro-Ile-Pro-Gln-Glu-Val-Leu-Pro-Tyr-Pro-Val-Arg-Ala-

180 190 200
Val-Pro-Val-Gln-Ala-Leu-Leu-Leu-Asn-Gln-Glu-Leu-Leu-Leu-Asn-Pro-Pro-His-Gln-Ile-Tyr-Pro-Val-Pro-Glu-

205 212
Pro-Ser-Thr-Thr-Glx-Ala-Asx-His-Pro-Ile-Ser-Val

Figure 1. Amino acid sequence of human β-casein with plasmin cleavage points indicated. Phosphorylation sites are residues 3,6,8,9,10.

human protein. Screening for genetic polymorphism using such a technique is of course an unthinkable task but alternative possibilities will be addressed later in this report.

Human β-casein occurs in multiphosphorylated forms having 0 to 5 phosphate groups/molecule; the bovine homologue differs in that it is usually found as a fully phosphorylated molecule. It was determined that each of the multiphosphorylated forms of H-β-Cn contained phosphate groups on specific seryl or threonyl residues and were not mixtures of species having a certain number of phosphate groups randomly distributed (9). The phosphorous containing sequence cluster, located within the first 12 residues of the H-β-Cn molecule is also found at varying locations in bovine β-, α_{s1}-, and α_{s2}-caseins (10). According to Mercier the configuration Thr/Ser-X-A, were X represents any amino acid, and A, an acidic residue, is required for casein phosphorylation. Sites where A is a dicarboxylic amino acid are termed primary sites (cf. positions 3,9,10, Fig 1); and those with phosphoserine in that position, secondary sites (positions 6 and 8). For a more detailed discussion on this subject see Greenberg et al (3). Monti and Jolles (36) reported on the isolation of a human whey protein which they concluded was intact O-P β-casein. Increased solubility of this form during casein precipitation at pH 4.6 allows its distribution between the whey and casein fractions. The reason for the existence of multiphosphorylated forms in H-β-Cn as compared with the fully phosphorylated cow equivalent remains unclear. Possible explanations involve single or multiple kinase or phosphatase activity during biosynthesis or a variability in transport mechanism between the two species.

The appearance of quantitative variation among the six H-β-Cn forms is an additional point to be considered. On the aforementioned gel pattern the 2-P and 4-P forms usually show greater intensities than the other bands for many individual and pooled milk samples. However, during our limited screening studies of individual samples, variations in band intensity patterns have been encountered. In addition to genetic control other factors such as stage of lactation, maternal health, or altered chemistry of calcium and phosphate, may also play a role in governing the quantitative variation.

In the comparison of the human β-casein sequence with the ruminant homologues, bovine (11) and ovine (12), the only other β-caseins for which such data are available, it is necessary to place the amino terminus of the human molecule at position 10 of the other two sequences to align the structures. A compensating carboxyl-terminal extension of the human protein provides for the approximate size equivalency. This "frame shift" relationship is rather unusual, and considering that several residues at the amino and carboxyl termini of the three proteins are identical, the mutation may exist in the genome and could reflect a difference in the number and locations of exons. This concept is supported by the recent report of Jones et al (13) detailing the structure and possible evolution of a rat casein gene.

All three sequenced β-caseins (human, bovine, ovine), characteristic of caseins in general contain large amounts of proline (ca 40 residues per mole). Over 60% of these prolyl residues are identically situated, showing conservation of the teleological requirement for openness and therefore, maximum digestibility. If the human and bovine β-caseins are aligned as described earlier and their secondary structures compared, the human homologue exhibits even more aperiodicity than the bovine protein (14), previously reported to contain a low proportion of its residues in periodic conformation. Comparison of the hydrophobicity and charged residues profiles reveals no striking differences. This is to be expected since each of these proteins is packaged presumably by protein interaction with κ-casein (4,15) for delivery via the casein micelle described above.

ENDOGENOUS PROTEASES

The presence of endogenous protease activity in human milk has been reported (16,17). Specific plasmin cleaved portions of β-casein, identified in human milk and whey, indicate that the proteolytic activity responsible for the generation of the γ-casein family in the bovine system (18,19) also exists in human milk. In both systems the γ-casein components represent successively smaller carboxyl terminal fragments of β-casein. One group has suggested a method for the quantitation of H-β-Cn using proteolysis by plasmin followed by immunoelectrophoresis (20). Various other enzymes including one with chymotryptic activity have also been reported (17). In fact a whole melange of zymogens, proteases, activators, inhibitors have been observed by many groups (21,22,23). The number of characterized β-casein degradation products continues to increase. In addition to galactothermin (24), the γ-casein system, and temperature sensitive fragments, a 20,000 dalton segment lacking the carboxyl terminal portion has been isolated (5). None of these large pieces has been assigned a functional role as of yet but I would not rule out that possibility. Perhaps the 12,500 dalton protein isolated from human milk by Eckhert (26) that enhances zinc absorption is another fragment of β-casein.

PHYSIOLOGICALLY ACTIVE PEPTIDES

In contrast to the large H-β-Cn proteolytic fragments mentioned above many smaller peptides with their origin in the β-casein molecule have defined physiological activity. The most studied class are the opioid peptides, beta-casomorphins, described first in the bovine system (27,28) and subsequently in relationship to H-β-Cn (29,30). Also in this family are morphiceptin (31), valmuceptin (30), and other derivatives (32), all potent and specific agonists for μ-opiate receptors. These peptides vary from 3 to 8 residues in length and are located in the human protein sequence in the area from positions 50 to 59. An interesting report by Lindstrom et al (33) suggests that certain cases of postpartum psychosis are associated with the occurrence in plasma and CSF of unique opioid peptides probably related to the β-casomorphins. From the same region of H-β-Cn, residues 54-59, Parker et al (34) have identified a hexapeptide which stimulates the phagocytosis of opsonized red blood cells by macrophages. Maruyama et al (35) report the finding of potent inhibitors of angiotensin I-converting enzyme and potentiators of bradykinin activity at still another location in β-casein (residues 177-183 of the bovine protein). This listing is far from complete but illustrates the variety of physiologically active peptides found within the sequence of β-casein.

INFLUENCE OF MATERNAL FACTORS

Once having described the available information on the composition and structure of these human milk proteins it is perhaps worthwhile to look to the well characterized bovine system for additional insight. The finding of polymorphism in the human β-casein molecule brings the genetic factor into consideration. In bovine milk where genetic variants of the caseins and whey proteins and their patterns of inheritance have been carefully examined, relationships have been reported among individual casein or whey protein genotypes and the content of total milk protein, milk yield, or increased or decreased values for individual protein components (37-41). Although protein and casein contents of human milk are much lower, there could still be a relationship between these values and the genetic variants of the individual protein components. We now know there are H-β-Cn polymorphs, there may well be variants of κ-casein, α-lactalbumin, or other whey proteins. In contrast to bovine there is no β-lactoglobulin in human milk (42), one less polymorphic protein to consider.

To carry the analogy one step further, differing genetic variants have been found to affect the coagulation and processing behavior of bovine milk (43,44). Although product development is certainly not a consideration, human milk is processed for preservation and storage in milk banks. Does protein polymorphism affect the heating or freeze/thaw responses of individual human milks? As discussed earlier screening for "silent" genetic variants is quite difficult but as our knowledge of each component grows and analytical techniques continue to advance it will and actually may already be possible. The newest HPLC peptide or protein columns do have the power to resolve molecules differing by one or two residues, charged or uncharged, and to separate components with the same composition but slightly different order of amino acids.

The H-β-Cn multiphosphorylation pattern, whether under genetic control, modulated by stage of lactation, or other maternal factors, is another area worthy of investigation. The micelle is a protein complex held together in part by calcium and phosphate. The varying amounts of the individual phosphate forms and probable associated variation in micellar calcium may play a role in calcium and phosphate availability, in the effective Ca/P ratio, and calcium distribution within the milk system (micellar vs. serum phases). Calcium binds to α-lactalbumin (25), binds and has an effect on the association/dissociation of lactoferrin, and may be involved with other immune and membrane bound components.

Let us assume that the O-P form of H-β-Cn varies under genetic or other control. It is likely that a great deal of this material is non-micellar in nature and found in the milk serum. (This has probably contributed to an underestimation of the β-casein or total casein content of human milk). The amounts of proenzymes, activators, inhibitors at least in the bovine system are known to vary with stage of lactation (45) and may also be genetically regulated. If we put these two factors together we can ask the following questions: Do plasmin and/or other proteolytic enzymes act on non-micellar casein preferentially? Do these enzymes specifically pre digest this β-casein to produce molecules which have a function other than nutritive? Can or do these fragments serve as substrates for further cleavage during the infant digestive process to produce opioid peptides and other bio-active small peptides? Finally, what if anything acts as the regulatory control mechanism governing these events?

Perhaps in the larger view, this can be referred to as "multifunctionality" of human casein. Beta-casein is present as a nutritional protein; it is the major component of micelles, carries and helps modulate phosphate and calcium; it provides an open structure, easily available to proteolysis which supplies physiologically active molecules for the infant. Kappa-casein is present in smaller amounts - necessary and sufficient to permit micelle formation and stability, but here again the carbohydrate moiety and a portion of the protein also serve as the bifidus factor (46).

The foregoing is indeed a speculative, perhaps too simplistic picture of part of the complex system represented by human milk. However, it is a starting point for areas of research which need to be studied further.

Acknowledgement - I wish to thank Alison Pease and Dona Kahn whose continued support made this contribution possible.

REFERENCES

1. R.J. Carroll, J.J. Basch, J.G. Phillips, and H.M. Farrell Jr. Ultrastructural and Biochemical Investigations of Mature Human Milk, Food Microstructure 4:323 (1985)
2. M. Ruegg and B. Blanc. Structure and Properties of the Particulate Constituents of Human Milk. A Review. Food Microstructure 1:25 (1982)
3. R. Greenberg, M.L. Groves, and H.J. Dower. Human β-Casein - Amino Acid Sequence and Identification of Phosphorylation Sites. J. Biol. Chem. 259:5132 (1984)
4. G. Brignon. A. Chtourou, B. Ribadeau-Dumas. Preparation and Amino Acid Sequence of Human κ-Casein. FEBS Lett. 188:48 (1985)
5. N. Azuma, H. Kadoya, and K. Yamauchi. A 20,000 Dalton Casein Fragment in Human Milk. J. Dairy Sci. 68:2176 (1985)
6. N. Azuma, S. Kaminogawa, and K. Yamauichi. Molecular Weight and Conformation of Human κ-Casein and Its Interaction with Other Milk Proteins. Agric. Biol. Chem. 48:771 (1984)
7. M.L. Groves and W.G. Gordon. The Major Component of Human Casein: A Protein Phosphorylated at Different Levels. Arch. Biochem. Biophys. 140:47 (1970)
8. W.N. Eigel, J.E. Butler, C.A. Ernstrom, H.M. Farrell Jr., V.R. Harwalkar, R. Jenness, and R. McL. Whitney. Nomenclature of Proteins of Cow's Milk: Fifth Revision J. Dairy Sci. 67:1599 (1984)
9. R. Greenberg and M.L. Groves. Human β-Casein. J. Dairy Research. 46:235 (1979)

10. J.-C. Mercier. Phosphorylation of Caseins, Present Evidence for Amino Acid Triplet Code Postranslationally Recognized by Specific Kinases. Biochimie 63:1 (1981)
11. B. Ribadeau-Dumas, G. Brignon, F. Grosclaude, and J.-C. Mercier. Structure Primaire de la Caseine β-Bovine- Sequence Complete. Eur. J. Biochem. 25:505 (1972)
12. B.C. Richardson and J.-C. Mercier. The Primary Structure of the Ovine β-Casein. Eur. J. Biochem. 99:285 (1979)
13. W.K. Jones, L. Yu-Lee, S.M. Clift, T.L. Brown, and J.M. Rosen. The Rat Casein Multigene Family- Fine Structure and Evolution of the β-Casein Gene. J. Biol. Chem. 260:7042 (1985)
14. L.K. Creamer, T. Richardson, and D.A.D. Parry. Secondary Structure of Bovine α_{s1}- and β- Casein in Solution. Arch. Biochem. Biophys. 211:689 (1981)
15. J.C. Irlam, C. Holt, S.S. Hasnain, and D.W.L. Hukins. Comparison of the Structure of Micellar Calcium Phosphate in Milk from Six Species by Extended X-ray Absorption Fine Structure Spectroscopy. J. Dairy Research 52:267 (1985)
16. R. Greenberg and M.L. Groves. Plasmin Cleaves Human β-Casein. Biochem. Biophys. Res. Commun. 125:463 (1984)
17. H. Miyashiro. Nippon Shonika Gakkai Zasshi. 82:427 (1978)
18. W.N. Eigel. Formation of γ_1-A^2, γ_2-A^2 and γ_3-A Caseins by in vitro Proteolysis of β-Casein A^2 with Bovine Plasminogen. Int. J. Biochem. 8:187 (1977)
19. W.N. Eigel, C.J. Hofmann, B.A.K. Chibber, J.M. Tomich, T.W. Keenan, and E.T. Mertz. Plasmin Mediated Proteolysis of Casein in Bovine Milk. Biochemistry 76:2244 (1979)
20. M. Korycka-Dahl, B. Ribadeau-Dumas, N. Chene, and J. Martal. Plasmin Activity in Milk. J. Dairy Sci. 66:704 (1983)
21. T. Lindberg. Protease Inhibitors in Human Milk. Pediat. Res. 13:969 (1979)
22. U. Okamoto, N. Horie, Y. Nagamatsu, and J-I. Yamamoto. Plasminogen Activator in Human Early Milk: Its Partial Purification and Characterization. Thrombos. Haemostas. 45:122 (1981)
23. S. Kaminogawa, H. Mizobuchi, and K. Yamauchi. Agric. Biol. Chem. 36:2163 (1972)
24. A.L. Schade and R.W. Reinhart. Galactothermin, A Reversibly Heat-Precipitable Protein of Human Milk at Neutral pH. Biochem. J. 118:181 (1970)
25. B. Lonnerdal and C. Glazier. Calcium Binding by α-Lactalbumin in Human Milk and Bovine Milk. J. Nutr. 115:1209 (1985)
26. C.D. Eckhert. Isolation of a Protein from Human Milk That Enhances Zinc Absorption in Humans. Biochem. Biophys. Res. Commun. 130:264 (1985)
27. V. Brantl, H. Teschemacher, A. Henschen, and F. Lottspeich. Novel Opioid Peptides Derived from Casein (β-Casomorphins) I- Isolation. Hoppe-Seyler's Z. Physiol. Chem. 360:1121 (1979)
28. A. Henschen, F. Lottspeich, V. Brantl, and H. Teschemacher. Novel Opioid Peptides Derived from Casein (β-Casomorphins) II- Structure Hoppe-Seyler's Z. Physiol. Chem. 360:1217 (1979)
29. V. Brantl. Novel Opioid Peptides Derived from Human β-Casein: Human β-Casomorphins. Eur. J. Pharmacology. 106:213 (1984)
30. M. Yoshikawa, T. Yoshimura, and H. Chiba. Opioid Peptides from Human β-Casein. Agric. Biol. Chem. 48:3185 (1984)
31. K-J. Chang, Y.F. Su, D.A. Brent, and J-K. Chang. Isolation of Specific μ-Opiate Receptor Peptide, Morphiceptin from an Enzymatic Digest of Milk Proteins. J. Biol. Chem. 260:9706 (1985)

32. H. Matthies, H. Stark, B. Hartrodt, H-L. Reuthrich, H-T. Spieler, A. Barth, and K. Neubert. Derivatives of β-Casomorphins with High Analgesic Potency. Peptides. 5:463 (1984)
33. L.H. Lindstrom, F. Nyberg, L. Terenius, K. Bauer, G. Besen, L.M. Gunne, S. Lyrenas, G. Willdeck-Lund, and B. Lindberg. CSF and Plasma β-Casomorphin Like Opioid Peptides in Postpartum Psychosis. Am. J. Psychiatry. 141:1059 (1984)
34. F. Parker, D. Migliore-Samour, F. Floch, A. Zerial, G.H. Werner, J. Jolles. M. Casaretto, H. Zahn, and P. Jolles. Immunostimulating Hexapeptide from Human Casein: Amino Acid Sequence, Synthesis and Biological Properties. Eur. J. Biochem. 145:677 (1984)
35. S. Maruyama, K. Nakagomi, N. Tomizuka, and H. Suzuki. Angiotensin I-Converting Enzyme Inhibitor Derived from an Enzymatic Hydrolysate of Casein. II. Isolation and Bradykinin-Potentiating Activity on the Uterus and the Ileum of Rats. Agric. Biol. Chem. 49:1405 (1985)
36. J.C. Monti and P. Jolles. Characterization of a Thermosensitive Protein from Human Milk Whey. Experentia 38:1211 (1982)
37. A. Felenczak, M. Ormian, J. Szarek. Interralationships Between Milk Protein Content and Occurrence of Genetically Determined Protein Fractions. Genetica Polonica 24:355 (1983)
38. E.M. Kroeker, K.F. Ng-Kwai-Hang, J.F. Hayes, and J.E. Moxley. Effects of β-Lactoglobulin Variant and Environmental Factors on Variation in the Detailed Composition of Bovine Milk Serum Proteins. J. Dairy Sci. 68:1637 (1985)
39. E.M. Kroeker, K.F. Ng-Kwai-Hang, J.F. Hayes, and J.E. Moxley. Effects of Environmental Factors with Milk Protein Polymorphism on Composition of Casein Fractions in Bovine Milk. J. Dairy Sci. 68:1752 (1985)
40. K.F. Ng-Kwai-Hang, J.F. Hayes J.E. Moxley, and H.G. Monardes. Association of Genetic Variants of Casein and Milk Serum Proteins with Milk, Fat, and Protein Production by Dairy Cattle. J. Dairy Sci. 67:835 (1984)
41. D.M. McLean, E.R.B. Grahman, R.W. Ponzoni. Effects of Milk Protein Genetic Variants on Milk Yield and Composition. J. Dairy Research. 51:531 (1984)
42. G. Brignon, A. Chtourou, and B. Ribadeau-Dumas. Does β-Lactoglobulin Occur in Human Milk? J. Dairy Research. 52:249 (1985)
43. J. Schaar. Effects of κ-Casein Genetic Variants and Lactation Number on the Renneting Properties of Individual Milks. J. Dairy Research. 51:397 (1984)
44. J. Schaar. Effects of Genetic Variants of κ-Casein and β-Lactoglobulin on Cheesemaking. J. Dairy Research. 52:429 (1985)
45. J. Schaar. Plasmin Activity and Proteose-Peptone Content of Individual Milks. J. Dairy Research. 52:369 (1985)
46. N. Azuma, K. Yamauchi, and T. Mitsuoka. Bifidus Growth-Promoting Activity of a Glycomacropeptide Derived from Human κ-Casein. Agric. Biol. Chem. 48:2159 (1984)

THYROID HORMONES IN MILK

Linda V. Oberkotter

Associate Research Professor of Biological Sciences

Florida Institute of Technology

Investigations related to the thyroid hormone content of milk and its effect upon the suckling neonate have spanned nearly thirty years, and over that time, many conflicting reports have arisen. Rigorous clinical data are sparse, and from all the biochemical analyses to date, no widely-adopted methodology has evolved. As a result, significant issues such as cross-cultural differences in milk hormone content, the influence of maternal diet upon milk hormone concentrations, and even longitudinal changes in the thyroid hormone content of both full- and pre-term milk have been addressed in only a fragmentary manner, if at all. The purpose of this presentation is to document the progress made in defining the thyroidal content of non-human and human breast milk.

ANIMAL STUDIES

Quantitation of Thyroid Hormones in Non-Human Milks

Early studies of thyroid hormones in milk focused by methodologic necessity upon gross distribution of protein-bound iodide, and found little evidence for the transfer of thyroxine (T_4) or its major metabolite, triiodothyronine (T_3), from maternal circulation to the suckling neonate. Brown-Grant & Galton (1) and Potter et al. (2) identified monoiodotyrosine (MIT) as the major form of organified iodine in milk from ^{131}I-injected lactating rats; neither group reported the presence of ^{131}I-iodothyronines in radioiodide-injected animals. Potter's group found small amounts of ^{131}I-T_4 in the milk of dams injected with the labelled hormone however, and Brown-Grant & Galton observed two thyronine-like metabolites of altered mobility which they were unable to identify. Vigouroux et al. (3) substantially confirmed the conclusions of those previous studies: that the bulk of milk-born radiolabel was found as MIT, diiodotyrosine (DIT), and iodide, but no ^{125}I-iodothyronines were detected by them.

Subsequently, improved methods of analysis permitted identification of hormonal iodide in rat and human milks; in rat milk radiolabelled _in vivo_, hormonal iodide represented approximately 2% of total ^{125}I recovered (4). However, because of its high sensitivity, radioimmunoassay quickly became the method of choice for quantitation of T_4 in milk.

Karimova et al. (5) using RIA found 2 - 3 μg T_4/dl in rat and rabbit milks (approximately 50% of serum levels), but low to undetectable concentrations in cow milk. Akasha & Anderson (6) reported the presence of both T_3 and T_4 in cow, goat, sheep, and guinea pig milks, but in contrast found total hormone levels in all cases to be less than 1.0 μg/dl. This lack of agreement in the literature (which is particularly acute in human milk studies, below) emphasizes the need for appropriate preparative procedures to insure the absence of interfering or crossreacting substances in the samples analyzed while effecting a reasonable recovery of the hormones, as discussed by Strbak (7).

Thyroid Hormone in Breast Milk: Effects Upon the Suckling Neonate

The mammary gland is second only to the thyroid in the avidity with which it sequesters iodine (8). While thyronine-bound iodine uptake is certainly retarded relative to the inorganic ion (if only due to its higher molecular weight), the presence of even relatively small quantities of exogenous, chronically-administered T_3 or T_4 (e.g. the 2% of total iodine uptake which we estimate to be hormonal) can effect a wide range of physiological responses in the neonate. Hence, a significant body of research has addressed itself to the suckling animal's response to breast milk thyroid hormone.

Fukuda et al. (9) observed depressed maternal thyroid hormone levels in the lactating rat, accompanied by elevated serum TSH, leading them to hypothesize that lactation induces a state of relative hypothyroidism in the dam. The condition is reversed at weaning, and if the pups are removed prematurely, maternal hormone levels return to normal within a few days. These observations suggested, albeit indirectly, that there is a net loss of maternal thyroid hormone through the milk. Macho et al. (10) reported that premature weaning of rat pups results in a decrease in the sucklings' plasma T_4 levels, followed by an increase of radioiodine uptake and finally an increase in plasma T_4, indicative of a progressive activation of the neonatal thyroid under conditions of early weaning. They further found that thyroid activation was preventable by low doses (1 μg/100 g body weight) of T_4, but not by weaning under a high iodine diet. These data support a role for breast milk in neonatal thyroid regulation, and further clarify the function of organified (and possibly hormonal) iodine in this control. The efficacy of a weaning diet rich in iodotyrosines such as MIT and DIT in preventing neonatal thyroid activation was not tested, however.

Slebodzinski & Cogiel (11) examined serum hormone levels in colostrum-deprived calves, and found significantly-depressed T_4 levels at 3-14 days of life in animals fed a supplemented mature cow's milk vs the colostrum-fed controls; no weight gain data for these experiments were given, however, nor is there evidence that any attempt was made to provide the animals with diets equivalent in iodine content. Neonatal piglets were also studied, but the resultant data were not meaningful because the colostrum-deprived animals developed severe diarrhea and, consistent with caloric deprivation, elevated reverse-T_3 levels.

Another approach to defining the maternal contribution to neonatal thyroid function has been to alter thyroid function in the lactating animal. Thyroidectomy or induction of chemical hypothyroidism is frequently associated with poor lactational performance (12); this then becomes a confounding variable which can interfere with data interpretation in such studies (13). Furthermore, no published data are available regarding how the absence of maternal thyroid hormones might adversely affect the nutrient composition of breast milk. Hence, the method of choice for such investigations has been chemical induction of hyperthyroidism. All of these studies have been performed in rats.

Vigouroux et al. (3) found that when lactating dams received 50 μg LT_4 for 4 days, 6-10 days post-partum (resulting in a tripling of maternal serum T_4 levels) mean T_4 levels in 10 day-old pups of the experimental animals were not significantly different from those of the control pups. We repeated these experiments, examining by paired data analysis both serum T_4 and T_3 levels achieved in 10-day old sucklings with pretreatment values on day 6 for the respective groups. We found that T_3 (but not T_4) concentrations in the pups of T_4-treated dams increased significantly over this period, as seen in Table I, whereas the thyroxinemia of the offspring of control (vehicle-injected) dams displayed no such increase (14). Koldovsky et al. (15) injected massive pharmacological doses (1.25 mg/100g body wt) of T_3 into lactating dams on days 11-15, effecting a 500-fold increase in circulating T_3. This resulted in a 14-fold increase in circulating T_3 of the suckling rats; it also induced a precocious increase in jejunal sucrase and liver acid ß- glucosidases. The latter two experiments clearly indicate that both physiologic and pharmacologic alterations in maternal thyroid status can affect the thyroid economy of the suckling neonate.

While interspecies studies can provide significant insights into the metabolism of radioactive precursors of thyroid hormones in the mammary gland, interpretation of effects upon the suckling's thyroid economy such as those described above must take into consideration both the maturity of the neonate relative to the human infant and specifically, the degree of autonomy achieved by the thyroid axis within that period. Hence, the remainder of this section focuses upon studies in the human.

TABLE I. THYROID HORMONE CONCENTRATIONS IN CONTROL- AND T_4 - TREATED DAMS AND THEIR LITTERS

	Serum T_4, μg/dl		Serum T_3, ng/dl	
	Dams	Pups	Dams	Pups
CONTROLS	2.9*	2.3	41.9	10.7
	±0.2	±0.5	±14.1	±7.8
T_4-INJECTED	7.8	2.7	79.2	44.8
	±2.3	±0.5	±9.5	±9.9
p	<0.0025	NS	<0.0025	<0.0025

*Mean ± SD, n=6 in all cases.

HUMAN STUDIES

Quantitation of Thyroid Hormones in Human Milk

Table II summarizes the major reports of T_4 in human milk; Table III summarizes the same for T_3. The few longitudinal studies (5, 16, 17) performed suggest that both T_3 and T_4 increase over time post-partum up to 4-6 weeks, and then decline. Changes in the physicochemical composition of breast milk over this period could influence the extractability of the hormone, however, and it does not appear that this issue has been addressed.

The most striking aspect of the T_4 data is the lack of agreement found. Scandinavian (21, 22) and Japanese (19) estimates of milk thyroid hormone content are uniformly low, the American (4, 18) and Israeli (17) intermediate, and Eastern European reports (5, 16) highest, but there is little doubt that this discordance reflects foremost the absence of a uniform method of analysis rather than genuine cross-cultural differences. Iodine intake (e.g. via diets derived largely from marine environments could certainly account for differences in milk iodothyronines, but no such comparative studies have thus far been undertaken.

Most investigations have been performed using mature milk samples, for which highest estimates of T_4 content (16) are 60-fold greater than the lowest (detectable) estimate (20). In an attempt to develop an accurate and reproducible procedure for measuring milk T_4 and T_3, we have found proteolysis followed by extraction to be an appropriate preparative procedure (4). Injection of the extract onto a reverse-phase HPLC column followed by RIA of the evaporated fractions co-eluting with internal radiolabelled standards then permits a highly selective quantitation of milk thyroid hormones. We continue to investigate the efficacy of various digestive enzymes in liberating free thyroid hormones from the insoluble fractions at various times post-partum.

Proteolysis appears to liberate measurable concentrations of T_3 from binding proteins in milk (4). Most investigators who have attempted to quantify T_3 in human milk (regardless of method), however, have found at least physiologic concentrations of this hormone (Table III) vis à vis the largely sub-physiologic levels of T_4 recently reported. This likely reflects in part the ten-fold lower affinity of T_3 for serum binding proteins, as this reduced affinity facilitates penetration of the capillary barriers by T_3 as free hormone into the interstitial fluid within breast tissue. Protein-bound T_4, in contrast, requires three times longer (72 hrs) to cross this barrier (23).

Preliminary studies from our laboratory suggest that pre-term milk specimens contain elevated thyroid hormone levels relative to full-term samples at comparable times post-partum, but a sufficient patient population has not yet been amassed for a critical evaluation of these results. Our HPLC data further indicate the presence of a variety of related metabolites in both full- and pre-term milks: thyromimetic substances other than the native hormones themselves, capable of evoking metabolic responses. A qualitative and quantitative study of these components in pre- and full-term colostrum and milk in various clinical populations should help to resolve some of the apparent discrepancies between the reported hormonal

TABLE II. DETERMINATIONS OF T_4 CONTENT IN FULL-TERM MILK: SUMMARY OF MAJOR STUDIES

STUDY	METHODS USED	T_4 ug/dl ± SD						
		DAY 1	3-5	6-8	14-21	22-30	31-60	>60
Strbak et al. (1976) (Czechoslovakia)	Competitive Protein Binding Assay	-	1.3 ±1.3	4.0 -	7.6 ±3.8	7.8 -	12.8 ±3.3	9.5 ±1.8
Sack et al. (1977) (Israel)	Whey Isolate; Radioimmunoassay	-	0.4 ±0.2			4.27 ±1.90		1.11 ±0.8
Varma et al. (1978)	Ethanol extraction; Radioimmunoassay	← 0.8 - 1.3 (4/88 samples) →						
Sato & Suzuki (1979) (Japan)	Radioimmunoassay of Ethanolic Samples	-	-	-	N.D.	-	-	-
Mallol et al. (1982) (Spain)	Ethanol extraction; Exchange Resin; Radioimmunoassay	-	-	-	-	-	-	<0.2
Oberkotter & Tenore (1983) (U.S.A.)	Proteolysis; Ethanol extract; LH-20 Chromatography; RIA	-	-	-	-	-	-	1.21 ±0.48
Karimova et al. (1983) (U.S.S.R.)	"Modified" Radioimmunoassay	3.9 ±0.3	5.1 ±0.5	10.6 ±1.2	-	-	-	-
Jansson et al. (1983) (Sweden)	Diethylether extract; Radioimmunoassay	-	-	-	-	-	-	N.D.
Moller et al. (1983)	Gas Chromatography; Mass Spectroscopy	-	-	-	-	≤0.4	-	-

TABLE III. DETERMINATIONS OF T_3 CONTENT IN FULL-TERM MILK: SUMMARY OF MAJOR STUDIES

STUDY	T_3 ng/dl ± SD						
	DAY 1	2	3	4	5	6	Mature
Varma et al. (1978)	85 ±118 (10-320)*	40 ±59 (10-247)	-	133 ±150 (10-375)	-	-	238 ±146 (10-500)
Sato & Suzuki (1979)	←			10 ±9 (0-40)			→
Oberkotter & Tenore (1983)	-	-	-	-	-	-	275 ±132 (80-560)
Karimova et al. (1983)	33 ±5 §	-	61 ±11	-	-	199 ±15	-
Jansson et al. (1983)	-	-	-	52 ±34 (13-104)	-	-	78 ±27 (39-140)

*Range is given in parentheses where noted by the author.

§SD or SEM not specified in text.

OTHER SUBSTANCES RELATED TO THYROID HORMONE REGULATION FOUND IN BREAST MILK

In addition to T_4 and T_3, rat and human breast milk contain thyroid-stimulating hormone (TSH, thyrotropin) and human milk contains reverse-T_3 (rT_3) and a protein analogous to serum thyroxine-binding globulin (TBG).

Thyrotropin (TSH)

Krulich et al. (24) first observed the presence of TSH in rat milk. They found comparable serum and milk TSH levels in euthyroid (200 ng/ml) and hyperthyroid (70 ng/ml) animals. The intact absorption of biologically-active (bovine) TSH by the suckling, but not weaned, rat gut (25) demonstrates maturative differences in gastrointestinal uptake of milk-borne polypeptide hormones. The data further suggest differences in the manner by which the pre- and full-term human gut may absorb this hormone via its mother's milk, since TSH is also present in mature human milk (26). As in the rat, TSH concentrations in term milk from euthyroid mothers are comparable to those found in serum, i.e. 1.5 - 5 μU/ml. Assuming a TSH secretion rate of approximately 50 mU/day and milk consumption of 1,000 ml/day, it is unlikely that maternal TSH is likely to play a dominant role in thyroid regulation of the full-term euthyroid neonate. No data are presently available regarding the thyrotropin content of premature milk however, and thus the potential hormonal and metabolic impact of exogenous (maternal) TSH upon these infants awaits further investigation.

Reverse-T_3 (rT_3)

This metabolite of thyroxine results from alpha- (inner ring) as opposed to beta- (outer ring) monodeiodination of T_4, and is considered to be physiologically inactive. Varma et al. (18) reported levels of <40 ng/dl in both colostrum and mature milk, while Sata & Suzuki (19) were unable to detect rT_3 in any of their samples.

Thyroxine-Binding Globulin (TBG)

In normal human serum, >99.95% of total T_4 is protein-bound form. Three proteins (in order of decreasing affinities) function to bind T_4: thyroxine-binding globulin (TBG), thyroxine-binding prealbumin (TBPA), and albumin (27). Human milk contains in its soluble fraction a T_4-binding protein ("TBG ") similar to serum TBG. In mature milk specimens, mean TBG levels of 29.0 ± 8.0 μg/dl, or approximately 1% of serum TBG levels are found in normal, puerperally lactating women*. In addition, albumin functions as a low-affinity carrier of thyroxine in human milk (28). Significantly higher levels of TBG (both in absolute terms and as a percentage of serum TBG) are found early in lactation. A strong correlation between serum and milk T_4-binding protein levels exists (29), suggesting that the maternal circulation is likely the source of TBG concentrations. We have further found TBG concentrations in the milk of mothers delivering prematurely to be significantly higher than those of full-term mothers within the first month post-partum (Table IV).

* Karimova et al. (5) also reported the presence of TBG in human milk, but in much higher concentrations. No details regarding the method of preparation nor assay employed were given in their publication.

TABLE IV. TBG_w CONCENTRATIONS IN FULL- AND PRE- TERM MILK

	< 2 WKS	< 5 WKS	≤ 8 WKS
FULL-TERM*			
x	79.3**	53.1	35.5
± SD	13.4	6.0	6.7
(n)	(7)	(5)	(13)
PRE-TERM+			
x	104.2	68.6	
± SD	13.7	10.7	
(n)	(7)	(6)	
p	< 0.01	< 0.02	

*Data from Oberkotter & Farber (1984)

**All values expressed as μg TBG/dl

+Mean gestational age: 32.4 ± 1.2 wks

CONCLUDING REMARKS

Thyroid hormones and their metabolites are present in human milk. There is wide disparity with regard to reported levels of T_4: this is likely due in part to a high affinity for its binding proteins, and to the varied success of investigators in preparing suitable samples for analysis. There is considerable evidence that mature milk contains ≤2 ug T_4/dl, but presently insufficient data to indicate whether thyroxine concentrations in colostrum have been appropriately quantified. T_3, on the other hand, is transferred to breast milk in levels which approach or exceed those found in the maternal circulation. Preliminary data suggest hormone levels in preterm breast milk to be elevated within the first month post-partum. Full- and pre-term human milk also contains thyroxine-binding globulins in concentrations which decrease with time post-partum.

A broad spectrum of maturative processes are either controlled directly or influenced by thyroid hormones. Additional laboratory studies aimed at defining the full complement of thyromimetic and thyrostimulatory substances contained in human milk at its various stages, coupled with appropriately-controlled clinical studies should elucidate the contributory role of these breast milk components in optimizing neonatal development.

ACKNOWLEDGEMENT

These studies were supported in part by grants (HD-12531, HD-21227) from the National Institute of Child Health and Human Development, National Institutes of Health.

REFERENCES

1. K. Brown-Grant, V. A. Galton, 1958, Iodinated compound in milk after radioiodide administration, Biochim Biophys Acta, 27:422-423.
2. G. D. Potter, W. A. Tong, I. L. Chaikoff, 1959, The metabolism of I^{131}-labelled iodine, thyroxine, and triiodothyronine in the mammary gland of the lactating rat, J Biol Chem, 234:350-354.
3. E. Vigouroux, N. Rostaqui, J. M. Fenerole, 1980, Estimation of hormonal and non-hormonal iodine uptake from maternal milk in suckling rats, Acta Endocrinol (Kbh), 93:332-338.
4. L. V. Oberkotter, A. Tenore, 1983, Separation and radioimmunoassay of T_3 and T_4 in human breast milk, Hormone Res, 17:11-18.
5. S. F. Karimova, Y. K. Turakulov, N. S. Salakhova, F. Y. Gulamova, 1983, Content of thyroid hormones in human and animal milk and in cow milk based infant formulas, Endocr Exper, 17:237-242.
6. M. Akasha, R. R. Anderson, 1984, Thyroxine and triiodothyronine in milk of cows, goats, sheep, and guinea pigs, Proc Soc Exp Biol Med 177:360-371.
7. V. Strbak, 1985, The role of maternal milk in endocrine regulation of sucklings, Medical Treatises xxll/2, Bratislava, Veda Publishing House of the Slovak Academy of Sciences, 9-10.
8. K. Brown-Grant, 1961, Extrathyroidal iodide concentrating mechanisms, Physiol Rev, 41:189-213.
9. H. Fukuda, K. Ohsima, M. Mori, I. Kobayashi, M. A. Greer, 1980, Sequential changes in the pituitary thyroid axis during pregnancy and lactation in the rat, Endocrinology, 107:1711-1716.
10. L. Macho, V. Strbak, A. Strazovcova, 1970, Thyroid and adrenal function in prematurely weaned rats, Physiol Bohemoslov, 19:77-82.
11. A. B. Slebodzinski, F. Cogiel, 1983, Serum thyroid hormone levels in colostrum deprived piglets and calves, Endocr Exper, 17:263-270.
12. B. K. Vonderhaar, A. E. Greco, 1979, Lobulo-alveolar development of mouse mammary glands is regulated by thyroid hormones, Endocrinology, 104:409-418.
13. G. F. Glasscock, C. S. Nicoll, 1983, Hormonal control of growth in the infant rat: further evidence that neither thyrotropin nor thyroid hormones are transferred via milk to suckling pups, Endocrinology, 112:800-805.
14. L. V. Oberkotter, 1986, Maternal hyperthyroidism during lactation influences thyroid function in suckling rat pups, Manuscript in preparation.

15. O. Koldovsky, L. Krulich, A. Tenore, J. Jumawan, C. Horowitz, H. Lau, 1980, Effect of triiodothyronine injection on levels of triiodothyronine and and thyroid-stimulating hormone in sera and milk of lactating rats and in sera of their sucklings; precious development of jejunal -disaccharidases in the sucklings, Biol Neonate, 37:103-108.
16. V. Strbak, L. Macho, P. Kovak, M. Skultetyova, J. Michalickova, 1976, 1976, Thyroxine (by competitive protein binding analysis) in human and cow milk and in infant formulas, Endocr Exp, 10:167-174.
17. J. Sack, O. Amado, B. Lunenfeld, 1977, Thyroxine concentration in human milk, J Clin Endocrinol Metab, 45:171-173.
18. S. K. Varma, M. Collins, A. Row, W. S. Haller, K. Varma, 1978, Thyroxine, tri-iodothyronine, and reverse tri-iodothyronine concentrations in human milk, J Pediatr, 93:803-806.
19. T. Sato, Y. Suzuki, 1979, Presence of triiodothyronine, no detectable thyroxine and reverse triiodothyronine in human milk, Endocrinol Jpn, 26:507-514.
20. J. Mallol, J. Obregon, G. Morreale de Escobar, 1982, Analytical artifacts in radioimmunoassay of L-thyroxin in human milk, Clin Chem, 28:1277-1282.
21. L. Jansson, S. Ivarsson, I. Larsson, R. Ekman, 1983, Tri-iodothyronine and thyroxine in human milk, Acta Paediatr Scand, 72:703-705.
22. B. Moller, I. Bjorkhem, O. Falk, O. Lantto, A. Larsson, 1983, Identification of thyroxine in human breast milk by gas chromatography-mass spectrometry, J Clin Endocrinol Metab, 56:30-34.
23. J. T. Nicoloff, 1978, Thyroid hormone transport and metabolism: pathophysiologic implications. In: Werner, SC, Ingbar, SH, eds., The Thyroid, 4th ed., Hagerstown, MD, Harper & Row, 93.
24. L. Krulich, O. Koldovsky, J. Jumawan, H. Lau, C. Horowitz, 1977, TSH in serum and milk of normal, thyroidectomized and hyperthyroid lactating rats, Proc Soc Exp Biol Med, 155:599-601.
25. A. Tenore, J. S. Parks, M. Gasparo, O. Koldovsky, 1980, Thyroidal response to pre-oral TSH in suckling and weaned rats, Am J Physiol, E238:428-430.
26. A. Tenore, L. V. Oberkotter, O. Koldovsky, J. S. Parks, C. M. Vandenberg, 1981, Thyrotropin in human breast milk, Hormone Res, 193-200.
27. K. Woeber, S. H. Ingbar, 1974, Interactions of thyroid hormones with binding proteins, In: Greer, M. A., Solomon, D. H., eds., Handbook of Physiology, Vol. III, The Thyroid, Baltimore: Williams & Wilkins, 187-196.
28. L. V. Oberkotter, A. Tenore, P. S. Pasquariello, W. Zavod, 1983, Thyroxine-binding protein in human breast milk similar to serum thyroxine-binding globulin, J Clin Endocrinol Metab, 57:1133-1139.
29. L. V. Oberkotter, M. Farber, 1984, Thyroxine-binding globulin in serum and milk specimens from puerperal lactating women, Obstet Gynecol, 64:244-247.

EFFECTS OF LOW MATERNAL DIETARY INTAKE OF CALCIUM, SELENIUM AND VITAMIN B-6 UPON BREAST MILK COMPOSITION IN NEPAL

Robert D. Reynolds, Suniti Acharya, James E. Leklem and Phylis B. Moser

U.S. Department of Agriculture, Beltsville, Maryland 20705; Ministry of Health, Kathmandu, Nepal; Oregon State University, Corvallis, Oregon 97331; University of Maryland, College Park, Maryland 20742

ABSTRACT

During October and November 1983, an intensive health and nutrition study was conducted on 26 lactating women and their infants in six villages in the Kathmandu valley of Nepal. During the study period, a 24-hour duplicate food composite was collected and subsequently analyzed for various nutrients. Fasting blood, urine and breast milk samples were obtained from the mothers as well as a blood sample from the infants. Analyses of these dietary composites indicated that the mothers consumed very low amounts of calcium and selenium and an amount of vitamin B-6 comparable to that consumed by lactating women in the U.S. Whereas the maternal plasma and breast milk calcium concentration was comparable to those of American lactating women, the Nepalese mothers excreted in their urine more than twice as high a hydroxyproline/creatinine concentration, suggesting that the Nepalese women were undergoing substantially greater bone demineralization during lactation. The selenium intake is the second lowest reported anywhere in the world. However, their low intake of selenium resulted in only a low-normal concentration of maternal plasma and breast milk selenium and an infant plasma selenium concentration higher than levels reported in healthy infants from Finland, another country with a low dietary selenium intake. Maternal plasma pyridoxal 5'-phosphate (PLP), an indicator of vitamin B-6 status, remained low throughout lactation whereas the concentration of breast milk total vitamin B-6 was equivalent to that in American women. The Nepalese infants had a lower plasma PLP compared to American infants. The presence of a poorly utilizable glucoside derivative of vitamin B-6 in the diets and in the breast milk of the mothers would partially account for the apparent discrepancy in vitamin B-6 intake and status of the infants.

INTRODUCTION

Due to cultural, economic or climatological influences, study of the dietary intake and status of various cultures in the developing countries can teach us much about the effects of specific nutrient imbalances upon the health of the individuals involved. Although several specific nutrient imbalances may be common in the particular culture being studied, it may be difficult to experimentally induce equivalent imbalances in various at-risk populations in Western cultures. For this reason as well as being able to develop nutrition guidelines for the specific cultures involved, it is desirable to study these cultures before their way of life changes. Nepal was chosen for the current study due to their practice of prolonged lactation and their reliance on dietary choices which have been relatively unaffected by Western influences.

METHODS AND MATERIALS

During October and November, 1983, 26 lactating women and their infants in six villages in the Kathmandu valley of Nepal were recruited as subjects by Nepalese Public Health Workers from the Department of Family Planning, Ministry of Health. All women were two to six months postpartum and had given birth to a single child. In-depth details of the subjects are described elsewhere (1). Informed verbal consent was obtained from all women prior to their acceptance into the study.

With the assistance of the Nepalese Public Health Workers, each subject collected a duplicate composite of all foods consumed in a 24-hour period. The following morning, a fasting urine, blood and breast milk sample was obtained from the mothers and a blood sample was obtained from the infants. Due to the practice of breast feeding upon demand, the infant blood samples were not necessarily collected after an overnight fast.

All samples were collected in trace mineral-free containers and processed under conditions designed to reduce contamination to a level equivalent to that which occurs during similar experiments in the Beltsville area. Aliquots of the food composites were frozen at -20° and blood, milk and urine samples were frozen in liquid nitrogen and shipped to the U.S. for analysis. Details of analytical procedures are presented elsewhere (1-4).

RESULTS AND DISCUSSION

Direct analysis of nutrients in the duplicate food composites revealed an extremely low dietary intake of calcium and selenium compared to that consumed by lactating women in the Annapolis, Maryland area (5), and a nearly equivalent intake of vitamin B-6 (6) (Table 1). Intakes of other nutrients are reported elsewhere (1-4).

<u>Calcium</u>. The very low dietary calcium intake of the Nepalese is approximately 40% the RDA of 1200 mg for lactating women in the U.S. (7). Furthermore, 40% of the Nepalese subjects consumed less than 300 mg per day. This raises the question of what detrimental effects, if any, this low calcium intake would have on the health of both the lactating mother and her breast-fed infant. Although the Nepalese women we studied were considerably smaller in stature than the average American women (1,7), the Nepalese were consuming less calcium per body weight or per meter height than were their American counterparts (unpublished observations).

Although the Nepalese lactating women consumed low amounts of dietary calcium, their plasma calcium concentrations were maintained at levels slightly above that observed in American lactating women (Table 2). This maintenance of plasma calcium by the Nepalese women was somewhat unusual when the vitamin D status of the women is considered, as shown by the low concentration of plasma 25-OH vitamin D_3 (Table 2). Even with the low calcium intake and low vitamin D status, the breast milk calcium concentration was maintained at levels comparable to that in the Annapolis lactating women (Table 3). Although the volume of breast milk consumed by the Nepalese infants was not determined, the adequate growth of the infants, as reported by Moser et al. elsewhere in the Proceedings, implied that the infants were receiving adequate milk volume and this milk contained adequate calcium to support their growth.

Table 1. Daily Dietary Intakes of Selected Nutrients by American and Nepalese Lactating Women

	Annapolis, MD	Nepal
Calcium (mg)	1,110[a]	482 ± 249[d]
Selenium (ug)	80[b]	23 ± 16
Vitamin B-6 (mg)	1.5[c]	1.7 ± 0.6

[a]Unpublished observations.
[b]Data from Reference 5.
[c]Data from Reference 6.
[d]Mean ± SD.

Table 2. Maternal Plasma Calcium Status Indicators

Months Postpartum	Calcium US[a]	Calcium Nepal	25-OH Vitamin D_3 US[a]	25-OH Vitamin D_3 Nepal
	(mg/100 ml)		(ng/ml)	
2	8.6 ± 0.2[b]	11.0 ± 0.8	33	15 ± 6
3	9.2 ± 0.2	10.5 ± 0.2	32	11 ± 3
4	--	11.0 ± 0.7	--	14 ± 5
5	--	10.5 ± 0.5	--	17 ± 6
6	9.6 ± 0.3	10.1 ± 0.3	28	18 ± 6

[a]Data from Reference 8, serum values instead of plasma.
[b]Mean ± SD.

Table 3. Maternal Calcium Status Indicators

	Breast Milk Calcium		Urinary Hydroxyproline/creatinine	
	Annapolis, MD[a]	Nepal	Annapolis, MD[a]	Nepal
	(mg/100 ml)		(molar ratio*1,000)	
Mean	24.3	26.4	36	74
Range	19.1-36.3	21.0-33.0	5-131	17-208

[a]Unpublished observations.

Assuming a maximum milk volume of 900 ml per day (9), the amount of calcium secreted in the milk would be approximately 240 mg per day, or approximately 50% of that contained in the diet. Estimated urinary losses of calcium in the Nepalese mothers are 55 mg/day, based on a mean analyzed urinary calcium concentration of 55 ug/ml and an estimated urinary volume of 1 liter per day (data not shown). Due to circadian and daily variations in urinary calcium and uncertainty of daily urine volume output, this value of 55 mg/day must be viewed with caution, but it is useful in providing an approximate estimate of urinary calcium losses. Thus, the total breast milk and urinary losses of calcium would be approximately 295 mg, or 61% of the dietary intake. It is not known whether adults with a low vitamin D status are capable of intestinal calcium absorption rates as high as 60%.

If the Nepalese women were maintaining normal concentrations of both plasma and breast milk calcium during a very low dietary calcium intake and a low vitamin D status, the question arises as to whether there were any parameters which might indicate that this low dietary intake was, in fact, detrimental to either the mother or the infant. Since calcium is so critical to bone formation and remodeling, an index of bone mineral status would be useful in answering this question. When bone is undergoing demineralization, hydroxyproline, one of the constituents of the collagen matrix, is excreted in the urine (10). Thus, the concentration of hydroxyproline, expressed as a function of the urinary creatinine concentration, is a measure of the extent of bone demineralization taking place (11). As shown in Table 3, the Nepalese women excreted over twice as much hydroxyproline as did the Annapolis lactating women. When one considers that urinary hydroxyproline can be derived from either bone demineralization or from the dietary consumption of collagen-containing foods (meat, gelatins, etc.), this difference in hydroxyproline excretion from bone demineralization would be in excess of twice as great for the Nepalese women because their diets did not contain any meat or meat-derived foods whereas the diets of the Annapolis women did. A better estimate of the relative bone structures and strengths of these two populations would be to perform a bone density scan.

Selenium Compared to the diets consumed by lactating women in the Annapolis area, the Nepalese women consumed about 1/4 the amount of dietary selenium (Table 1). This mean dietary intake is less than half the lowest level in the RDA safe and adequate range of 50-200 ug/day (7). The data in Table 4 show that this is the second lowest reported dietary intake of selenium in the world. The only location which has reported a lower daily intake is the Keshan disease area of China (12). The intake in these areas is so low as to precipitate a characteristic cardiomyopathy, especially in young women and children, referred to as Keshan Disease. From extensive studies of such populations, it is estimated that an average selenium intake of 14 ug/day for adult women is required to prevent onset of the disease. Approximately 40% of the Nepalese daily diets contained less than 14 ug selenium, ranging as low as 7.4 ug (data not shown). Nepal has been reported to have the highest frequency of cardio-pulmonary insufficiency in the world (13), a symptom which is consistent with the occurrence of Keshan Disease.

The effects of this very low selenium intake on maternal plasma and breast milk selenium concentrations are shown in Table 5. The maternal plasma selenium is slightly higher than that reported in Finland, even though the dietary intake for the Nepalese was somewhat less than that of the Finns (Table 4). American lactating women who consume nearly four times as much selenium as do the Nepalese have approximately a two-fold greater concentration of plasma selenium. The concentration of selenium in the breast milk of Nepalese mothers is comparable to that of the Finnish women (14) and at the lower end of the range observed for American women (5). We did not observe a decrease in milk selenium concentrations with increasing duration of lactation, as was reported for the Finnish women (14). Surprisingly, the concentration of selenium in the plasma of the Nepalese infants is nearly twice that observed in Finnish infants, even though the concentration in the breast milk of the mothers was comparable. When compared to the plasma concentrations of their mothers, the Nepalese infants had plasma selenium concentrations of 72% compared to only 46% for the Finnish mother-infant pairs. This lower concentration of selenium in the serum of infants compared to adults has been observed previously (15).

Table 4. Worldwide Dietary Selenium Intakes[a]

Country	Dietary Se Intake (ug/day)
China (Keshan Disease Area)	11
Nepal (Kathmandu)	23
New Zealand	28
Finland	30
USA	62-216
Venezuela	218
China (Endemic Selenosis Area)	4,900

[a]Adapted from Reference 12.

The reason for the large discrepancy between the selenium intake and the resulting plasma and breast milk concentrations of the Nepalese and the Finns is not immediately apparent. One possible explanation would be that the Nepalese mothers and infants were exposed to substantial amounts of toxic heavy metals (16). It has been shown (17) that simultaneous administration of selenium and mercury results in an elevated plasma selenium. To resolve this discrepancy between low intake and adequate plasma and milk concentrations, further investigation will be required.

Table 5. Selenium Status Indicators of Lactating Women and Their Breast Fed Infants

	Maternal Plasma Se	Breast Milk Se	Infant Plasma Se
	(ng/ml)	(ng/ml)	(ng/ml)
Nepal	65 ± 26[c]	9.7 ± 3.8	46.5 ± 23.1
Finland[a]	54 ± 1	10.7 (1st Month) 5.8 (3rd Month)	25
USA[b]	110 ± 2	7-33	

[a]Data from Reference 14.
[b]Data from Reference 12.
[c]Mean ± SD.

Table 6. Maternal and Infant Vitamin B-6 Status Indicators

Months Post-Partum	Maternal Plasma Pyridoxal 5'-Phosphate		Breast Milk Total Vitamin B-6		Infant Plasma Pyridoxal 5'-Phosphate	
	US[a]	Nepal	US[a]	Nepal	US[b]	Nepal
	(nM)					
1	16	--	630	--	90	-
2	--	14 ± 5[c]	--	915 ± 227	-	17 ± 7
3	29	19 ± 22	839	859 ± 645	-	22 ± 14
4	--	14 ± 4	--	951 ± 428	110	19 ± 8
5	--	14 ± 8	--	856 ± 265	-	37 ± 23
6	40	9 ± 3	1,008	864 ± 120	125	16 ± 8

[a]Unpublished observations.
[b]Data from Reference 20.
[c]Mean ± SD.

Vitamin B-6 The daily dietary intake of vitamin B-6 of the Nepalese women, as measured by a standard microbiological assay (18), was similar to that of the Annapolis lactating women (Table 1). However, the concentration of maternal plasma pyridoxal 5'-phosphate (PLP), currently accepted as the best indicator of vitamin B-6 status (19), failed to increase in the Nepalese women as lactation proceeded (Table 6). By six months postpartum, the concentration of plasma PLP in the Nepalese women was approximately 1/4 that in their American counterparts. Although the Nepalese women had a lower plasma PLP concentration, indicative of a lower vitamin B-6 status, the concentration of total vitamin B-6 in the breast milk of the two populations was similar (Table 6). Although we did not measure milk volume in either population, the adequate growth of the

Nepalese infants implies that sufficient milk was produced to support growth. However, when the plasma PLP of the Nepalese infants was compared to the concentration in a group of American breast-fed infants (20), the Nepalese infants had a considerably lower vitamin B-6 status (Table 6). It is important to note that the American infants were breast feeding from mothers who were supplemented with 2.5 mg vitamin B-6 above their normal dietary intakes (20). This would result in a total vitamin B-6 intake 2.4-fold greater in the American women as compared to the Nepalese women. However, this increased dietary intake of the American women would not account for the entire difference observed in the vitamin B-6 status of the infants (unpublished observation).

Recently, several papers have described the presence of a glycosylated form of vitamin B-6 in a variety of plant products, including rice and legumes (21, 22). The glycosylated form of the vitamin appears to be absorbed intact in rats (23) and humans (22) and then excreted in the urine without undergoing further metabolism (22). Gregory and coworkers have stated that they believe the presence of the glycosylated vitamin B-6 is the major contributing factor to low bioavailability of vitamin B-6 in many foods (23). Since rice and legumes constitute the vast majority of the diet of the Nepalese (estimated at 80-85% of the calories), one explanation for the relatively low vitamin B-6 status of both the Nepalese mothers and infants would be due to a moderately high dietary intake of the glycosylated form by the mothers and then a subsequent secretion of the poorly utilizable form into the breast milk. The Nepalese diet composites have been analyzed for the amount of glycosylated vitamin B-6 and were found to contain an average of 15% of the total vitamin B-6 in the form of the glycoside (21). The breast milk samples were also analyzed for content of the glycosylated vitamin B-6 (21) and were also found to contain an average of 15% of the total vitamin B-6 in the form of the poorly utilizable glycoside. These data could account for an additional portion of the difference in the vitamin B-6 status of Nepalese and American infants. Presumably, the American lactating women would be consuming foods which contained a lower amount of the glycosylated form of the vitamin. At this time, the influence of a vegetarian diet, as consumed in the US, upon the maternal and infant vitamin B-6 status is unknown, but will be investigated in the future.

SUMMARY

Investigations on the dietary intake of Nepalese lactating women and the resulting biochemical parameters in both mothers and infants suggested that low maternal dietary calcium intakes and low vitamin D status resulted in significant maternal bone demineralization during lactation without affecting the calcium intake of the infant from breast milk. The low dietary consumption of selenium by the Nepalese mothers is not reflected in the plasma selenium concentrations of the mothers or the infants, prompting speculation on possible exposure of the Nepalese mothers and infants to toxic heavy metals. The presence of the biologically poorly utilizable glycoside form of vitamin B-6 in the diets of the Nepalese mothers is reflected in its presence in the breast milk and in the resulting low vitamin B-6 status of the mothers and their infants. This observation raises the question of the adequacy of vitamin B-6 in vegetarian diets consumed in all countries of the world. Thus, more research on appropriate populations are required in order to resolve the questions and discrepancies raised by the present data.

REFERENCES

1. R.D. Reynolds, S. Acharya, W. McConnell, M.B. Andon, M.P. Howard, and P.B. Moser, Nutritional and medical status of lactating women and their infants in the Kathmandu valley of Nepal, (submitted).
2. P.B. Moser, S. Acharya, M.B. Andon, M.P. Howard, and R.D. Reynolds, Nutritional intakes and status of calcium and magnesium in Nepalese lactating women and their breast-fed infants, (submitted).
3. P.B. Moser, S. Acharya, M.B. Howard, M.B. Andon, S. Lewis, and R.D. Reynolds, Nutritional intake and status of selected trace elements in Nepalese lactating women and their breast-fed infants, (submitted).
4. R.D. Reynolds, S. Acharya, M.B. Andon, M.P. Howard, J.E. Leklem, and P.B. Moser, Nutritional intake and status of vitamin B-6 in Nepalese lactating women and their breast-fed infants, (submitted).
5. O.A. Levander, V.C. Morris, and P.B. Moser, Dietary selenium (Se) intake and Se content of breast milk and plasma of lactating and nonlactating women, Fed. Proc. 40:890 (1981) (abstract).
6. R.D. Reynolds, M. Polansky, and P.B. Moser, Analyzed vitamin B-6 intakes of pregnant and postpartum lactating and nonlactating women, J. Am. Dietet. Assoc. 84:1339-1344 (1984) .
7. National Research Council. Recommended Dietary Allowances, 9th ed., Washington, DC, Natl Acad Sci, (1980).
8. F.R. Greer, R.C. Tsang, J.E. Searcy, R.S. Levin, and J.J. Steichen, Mineral homeostasis during lactation-relationship to serum 1,25-dihydroxy vitamin D, 25-hydroxyvitamin D, parathyroid hormone, and calcitonin, Am. J. Clin. Nutr. 38:431-437 (1982).
9. R.G. Whitehead and A.A. Paul, Infant growth and human milk requirements, Lancet ii:161-163 (1981).
10. J.D. Smiley and M. Ziff, Urinary hydroxyproline excretion and growth, Physiol. Rev. 44:30-44 (1964).
11. D.S. Allison, A. Walker, and Q.T. Smith, Urinary hydroxyproline: creatinine ratio of normal humans at various ages, Clin. Chim. Acta 14:729-734 (1966).
12. O.A. Levander, Clinical consequences of low selenium intake and its relationship to vitamin E, NY Acad. Sci. 393:70-82 (1982).
13. I.M. Kozlof, Public Health in Nepal. Leningrad, USSR, Meditsina, (1976).
14. J. Kumpulainen, L. Salmenpera, M.A. Siimes, P. Koivistoinen and J. Perheentupa. Selenium status of exclusively breast-fed infants as influenced by maternal organic or inorganic selenium supplementation, Am. J. Clin. Nutr. 42:829-835 (1985).
15. I. Lombeck, K. Kasperek, L.E. Feinendegen, and H.J. Bremer, Low selenium state in children, in: "Selenium in Biology and Medicine", J.E. Spallholz, J.L. Martin, and H.E. Ganther, ed, AVI Publishing Co, Westport, CT, pp 269-282 (1981).
16. C.I. Davidson, T.C. Grimm, and M.A. Nasta, Airborne lead and other elements derived from local fires in the Himalayas, Science 214:1344-1346 (1981).
17. R.F. Burk, K.A. Foster, P.M. Greenfield, and K.W. Kiker, Binding of simultaneously administered inorganic selenium and mercury to a rat plasma protein, Proc. Soc. Exptl. Biol. Med. 145:782-785 (1974).
18. M. Polansky, Microbiological assay of vitamin B-6 in foods, in: "Methods in Vitamin B-6 Nutrition", J.E. Leklem and R.D. Reynolds, eds., Plenum Press, New York, NY, pp 21-44 (1981).

19. T.-K. Li and L. Lumeng, Plasma PLP as an indicator of nutritional status: Relationship to tissue vitamin B-6 content and hepatic metabolism, *in*: "Methods in Vitamin B-6 Nutrition", J.E. Leklem and R.D. Reynolds, eds., Plenum Press, New York, NY, pp 289-296 (1981).
20. M.W. Borschel, A. Kirksey, and R.E. Hannemann, Effects of vitamin B-6 intake on nutriture and growth of young infants, *Am. J. Clin. Nutr.* 43:7-15 (1986).
21. H. Kabir, J. Leklem, and L.T. Miller, Measurement of glycosylated vitamin B-6 in foods, *J. Food Sci.* 48:1422-1425 (1983).
22. H. Kabir, J.E. Leklem, and L.T. Miller, Relationship of the glycosylated vitamin B-6 content of foods to vitamin B-6 bioavailability in humans, *Nutr. Rep. Internat.* 28:709-716 (1983).
23. S.L. Ink, J.F. Gregory and D.F Sartain, Bioavailability of pyridoxine-beta-glucoside in the rat, *Fed. Proc.* 44:776 (1985) (abstract).

ASSESSMENT OF LACTATION PERFORMANCE IN WOMEN

P.E. Hartmann and P.G. Arthur

Department of Biochemistry
University of Western Australia
Perth WA 6009
Australia

INTRODUCTION

Successful reproduction in animals requires an adequate supply of food for the young to grow and develop into an adult. In many species of birds and reptiles, the adults can thrive in environments which lack suitable foods for their young. Thus vertebrates which bring food to the nest can only breed successfully if they can find sufficient quantities of food suitable for the growth and development of their young. In contrast, mammals nourish their young with milk which is synthesized from the products of digestion. Therefore, mammals can reproduce successfully without a requirement for access to an environment which has special kinds of food for their young. Furthermore, because mammals have the ability to deplete their body reserves of fat, protein and minerals to supply the precursors for milk synthesis, temporary fluctuations in food gathering by the mother do not interrupt the food supply of the neonate.

The two main features of mammalian reproduction are viviparity and lactation, however, only lactation is both unique to mammals and occurs in all living species of mammal. It has been argued[1] that one of the main advantages which the evolution of lactation conferred on early mammals was the ability to successfully reproduce whereever the adults could thrive. In man, as with other mammals, lactation is imperative to ensure the survival of the neonate. Although during the last 100 years, animal milks have been "humanized" to facilitate the hand feeding of human infants, these products only can be used in communities where a high level of sterility can be maintained and the risk of infection is low [2].

Breast feeding not only provides a source of nourishment uniquely adapted to the digestive and metabolic requirements of the human infant, but also provides the infant with protection against pathogenic micro-organisms, facilitates the establishment of a strong relationship between mother and infant, suppresses maternal fertility, reduces the likehood of the infant developing allergies to foreign antigens and may exercise a degree of control over the infant's metabolism[3]. This complex multi-faceted role of lactation has been ignored in the consideration of lactation performance in women. Nevertheless, the most important function of human milk is the provision of nutrients for the growing infant and it is claimed that the ultimate test of the adequacy of lactation in any mother is the growth and health of her infant[4]. Therefore qualitative and semi-quantitative measures of lactation performance include the duration of lactation, sucking frequency, the length of time breast milk is retained as the sole nutrient source for the infant, the time of introduction of supplementary foods to the infant, the rate of growth of the infant and the health status of the infant. On the other hand, the yield and composition of breast milk are considered to be quantitative measures of lactation performance.

Duration of Lactation and Sucking Frequency

The duration of lactation and the frequency of sucking varies considerably even amongst relatively closely related mammals. For example, the harp seal has a lactation period of about nine days, but during this short period of lactation the harp seal pup increases in weight from about 10 to 34 kg. In contrast, the Antarctic fur seal suckles her pup every 6 h for the first 7-8 days of lactation and then makes on average 17 trips to sea to feed (average duration 4.3 days) which are interspersed with visits to shore (average duration 2.1 days) to suckle her pup[5]. The weight of the fur seal pup increases from 6 to 17 kg during the 117 days of lactation[6]. At the other extreme the young of the kangaroo remain firmly attached to the teat for at least the first month of lactation, then release the teat and re-attach at will until they are weaned at about 12 months of lactation[7]. These observations together with those in other mammals such as pigs[8], suggest that, as with all other phases of the reproductive cycle in mammals, consistent and defined patterns of behaviour exist during lactation for both the mother and the young. However, the behaviour patterns observed for lactation in different human societies exhibit extreme variation and it is impossible to establish a consistent cross cultural pattern for either the duration of lactation or the sucking frequency.

Developing Countries. In developing countries the average length of lactation ranges from over 30 months in Bangladesh to under 6 months in Costa Rica[9]. In a critical review of the literature on trends in infant feeding in developing countries Notzon[10] concluded that the existing information on the duration of breast feeding was inadequate and that the overall trends in infant feeding practices in the developing world could not be established. Only seven countries had reliable data on the trends in breast feeding for all major population subgroups and these countries could not be considered to be representative because the majority (Taiwan, Malaysia, Thailand, Korea and Singapore) were in a single region and amongst the most modern of the developing countries. However, Notzon[10] was able to identify certain common elements. Sharp to moderate declines in breast feeding were evident in six of the seven countries (Singapore was the exception), however the pattern of decline varied markedly from country to country. In Taiwan and Malaysia, both the proportion of mothers commencing to breast feed their babies and the duration of lactation in those mothers who commenced breast feeding declined. In Thailand, Korea and Panama most of the decline was due to a reduction in the duration of lactation. Whereas in Mexico contradictory patterns were found with a small decline in the proportion of women commencing to breast feed being offset by inconsistent changes in the proportion of infants breast fed at different ages.

Within each of these countries the relative rate of decline in breast feeding appeared to be greatest in the social groups which had the greatest exposure to modern influences, that is, among the wealthy and the educated in urban areas. Despite the common belief that most of the change in the pattern of breast feeding has occurred in urban populations, declines in breast feeding also were observed in rural areas. In Panama nearly all the recent decline has resulted from changes in breast feeding patterns in the rural population. Studies on the prevalence of breast feeding in Indonesia have revealed that the proportion of women breast feeding in rural areas was much higher than in urban areas. Djumadias and Enoch[11] reported that in Jakarta 21% of 595 mothers investigated did not breast feed their babies whereas in a peri-urban area only 6% of 250 mothers did not breast feed. Furthermore studies conducted at the Child Health Consultation Bureau, Gajah Mada University in Yogyakarta revealed that only 50% of mothers breast fed for one year or more, whereas 93% of mothers breast feed for one year or more in Ngaglik, a rural area[12].

Developed Countries. Major changes in the duration of lactation also have occurred in developed countries. Crawford[13] has reviewed adult attitudes to child care in the first year of life in the seventeenth century in England and concluded that there was no clearly agreed age for weaning a child, but the consensus of advice at that time favoured weaning nearer to twelve rather than eighteen months. Most physicians considered that breast milk was the only food which would keep a child alive and that infants weaned too early had less chance of survival.

Medical advisors during the seventeenth century considered that the baby should not be breast fed at all for the first day of life and they prescribed treacle, sugar, and honey and fresh oil of almonds as the first nutrient for a new born infant. They advised that ideally a baby should be put to the breast of another mother from the second to the eighth day or so (Moses and Hippocrates recommended the forty-second day). Colostrum was observed to be wheyish, foul, turbid and curdy and therefore considered to be very inferior. If the mother insisted in breast feeding her own baby or if poor mothers had no alternative they were advised to have their breasts sucked and emptied of colostrum by either another person or an older child. Preachers and physicians campaigned strenuously against wet nursing and arguments against breast feeding, such as that it either ruined the breasts, was ageing, or noisome to the clothes were discounted. Nevertheless many wealthy women employed wet nurses to breast feed their babies. This practice may have been related more to necessity than desire as it must have been extremely difficult for mothers to discard their colostrum and re-establish lactation eight days or more after delivery.

Furthermore Crawford[13] noted that during the seventeenth century it was assumed that mothers knew how to breast feed their babies, therefore medical advisers did not provide detailed instruction to women about techniques of breast feeding. Most advisors showed a compassionate attitude to the baby, urged adults to heed the baby's cry and advised mothers to satisfy their babies. At first this conclusion seems at odds with other historians[14,15] who have deduced from the harshness and cruelty of infant care practices that mothers did not form strong emotional ties with their babies at this time. However, Crawford (1987) disputes this conclusion as she has found many expressions of mothers' affection for their babies from the limited writings of women in the seventeenth century. Furthermore, this latter conclusion is consistent with the strong bonding which occurs between the mother and newborn of all other species of mammal[16].

Few of the early British women chosen to settle in Australia were literate, therefore there are no accounts of how they fed and weaned their babies in a hot and unfamiliar climate, with limited dietary resources, inadequate fresh water and poor housing[17]. However, it seems that throughout the nineteenth century women in Australia expected to breast feed their infants. Indeed infants and children appeared to occupy a more prominent position in families in Australia than in Britain, presumably because of the lack of suitable women to employ as either wet nurses or nurse maids [18]. The diaries and letters of women living in Western Australia during the mid-nineteenth century suggest that it was usual for women to breast feed for from nine to eighteen months[19]. However, despite the dependence on maternal breast feeding, poor weaning foods, and the general harshness of the environment, infant survival was higher in all the early Australian settlements than in contemporary London[18].

By the beginning of the twentieth century pediatricians agreed that maternal breast feeding was the best way to nourish a baby, but they attempted to regulate natural lactation in ways which impeded successful breast feeding[20,21]. The advice to the mother was harsh; after birth the infant was separated from the mother for a minimum of 12 hours as it was considered that both required rest. Thereafter, under the pretext of improving hygiene, the infant remained separated from the mother between breast feeds. Both the intervals between breast feeds and the duration of sucking at each breast was regimented[21]. Muskett[22] advised Australian mothers to induce regular habits in their babies by, if possible at the very beginning, breaking their babies into a plan of not being breast fed from 11.00 pm until 6.00 am, limiting each breast feed to a maximum of twenty minutes, and breast feeding every two hours during the day for the first 8 weeks after birth and extending this interval to every three hours thereafter. Aided by the support of influential people such as the New Zealander Sir Fredrick Truby King[23], breast feeding at four hourly intervals became entrenched during the early and mid-twentieth century. For

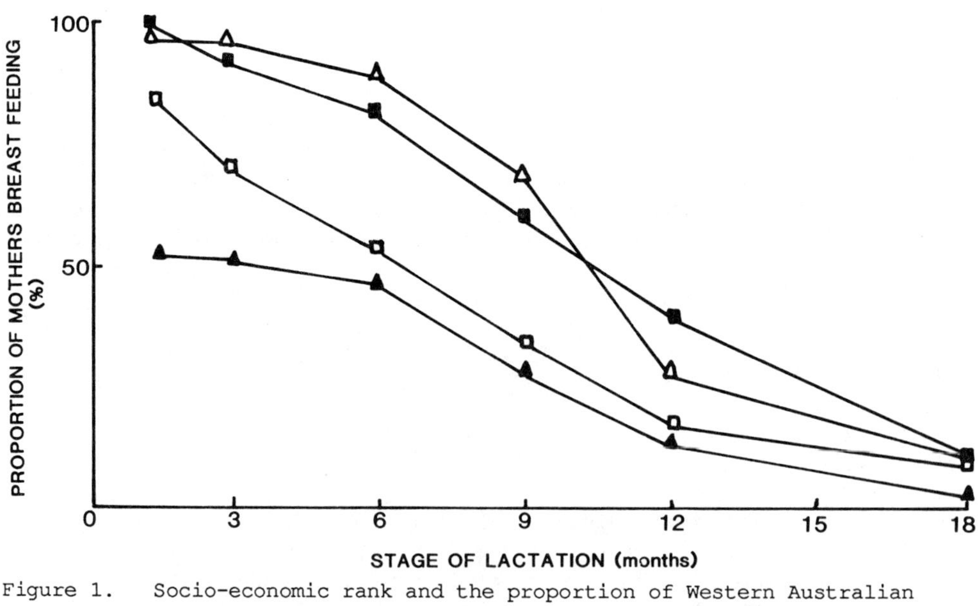

Figure 1. Socio-economic rank and the proportion of Western Australian mothers breast feeding their infants from birth to 18 months post partum. The population was divided into 4 socio-economic groups in decreasing rank (Δ), (˙), (˙) and (Δ), respectively. Data from Hitchcock et al.[26].

example, Harper[24] advised mothers that babies must be fed regularly (preferably four hourly at 6 am, 10 am, 2 pm, 6 pm, and 10 pm) rather than simply because they cry, and once a time-table had been arranged the baby should be kept to it absolutely. Despite the unphysiological nature of this advice, scheduled breast feeding is still practiced in developed countries. For example Aono et al.[25] state in their study of the relationship between prolactin secretion and milk yield in Japanese women that "Mothers started to nurse their babies from the first postpartum day (the day after delivery) and breast-fed babies for approximately 20 min on a 24-h schedule from 0800 h (4 times a day)".

The first national survey of infant feeding in Britain was made in 1946[27,28]. The average duration of lactation was 4.2 months and 53%, 36%, 28%, 6%, and 0.3% of infants were breast fed at 2, 5, 7, 10, and 48 months of age, respectively. By 1960 Newson and Newson[29] found that the proportion of infants who were breast fed had declined to 54%, and 13% at 1 and 6 months of age, respectively. In Australia the proportion of infants breast fed at 3 months of age was 55%, 33%, and 26% in 1943, 1963 and 1964, respectively[30]. Indeed, a similar decline in breast feeding has been reported for most other western countries[3] including the USA where Hendershot[31] concluded from a comprehensive review of the trends in infant feeding that before World War 2 about 75% of women commenced breast feeding, whereas by 1971 this figure had decreased to 25%. There was also a concomitant decline in the duration of lactation during this period. Thus it can be argued that at this time in the USA it was "abnormal" for women to breast feed their babies.

The decline in breast feeding in developed countries reached a nadir by 1972 and over the last 14 years there has been a resurgence of interest in breast feeding[31]. Currently, Australia has the highest incidence of breast feeding of any western country[3,26,32]. This high incidence of breast feeding is most evident in Perth, Western Australia where Hitchcock et al.[26], observed that in 1979, 88% of infants of mothers from the highest of the four socio-economic groups[33] were breast fed at 6 months of age and 25% of all normal infants were breast fed at 12 months of age (Figure 1). This revival of breast feeding has been characterised by mothers feeding their babies on demand and the duration of breast feeding in some of these mothers has approached that reported for primitive societies.

Hunter Gatherers

Although few detailed behavioural studies have been carried out on the few remaining hunter gatherer societies, the essential features of breast feeding among the !Kung hunter gatherers in Botswana and Namibia have been described by Konner and Worthman[34]. Observations from dawn to dusk revealed that breast feeding occurred for a few minutes at a time several times each hour. The infants were always in close physical proximity to their mothers and separations were brief until the age of 3.5 years, when they were weaned.

This pattern of breast feeding results in a long period of lactational amenorrhea and an average birth interval of approximately 4.1 years with an average of 4.7 children during the reproductive life of these women. Since a similar pattern of frequency and duration of lactation has been found among the hunter gatherers in Papua New Guinea, Short[9] suggested that this represented the "normal" pattern of behaviour for human lactation. This pattern of breast feeding is in keeping with the biochemical composition of human milk which is low in fat, protein and dry matter[35]. Furthermore, the casein in human milk, unlike that in cow's milk, forms a soft curd which readily breaks down in the infant's stomach and passes into the small intestine. Moreover it is now generally agreed that the minimum safe birth interval for women is two years[36]. In this connection it is of interest that man's closest living relatives, the chimpanzee and the gorilla, also suckle their young several times each hour in the wild, secrete milk quite similar in composition to human milk, sleep with the infant at the breast at night and have a birth interval of four to five years[9]. Perhaps normal lactation in women should extend for 3 to 4 years and infants should be permitted to breast feed according to need (breast feed on demand). However, it would be incorrect to assume that the hunter gatherers have perfected the art of breast feeding their babies as these societies would be just as vulnerable to illogical taboos and ill informed advice as were seventeenth-century English women[13] and even current western societies[37].

The average duration of lactation in women from either different social groups or at different stages in history span the entire range for the duration of lactation which has been observed in all other mammals [38]. Furthermore, the "normal" sucking frequency of infants ranged from several times each hour to several times each day. Thus the only positive conclusion which can be made about lactation performance from a consideration of the duration of lactation and sucking frequency, is that human lactation exhibits extraordinary flexibility and resilience.

SUPPLEMENTATION

The introduction of supplementary foods (ie the beginning of weaning) to breast fed infants has occurred at a wide range of ages during the past 300 years. Although in the seventeenth century in England infants were given some supplementary foods for the first day or so after birth, most writers suggested that infants should be gradually introduced to other foods at around two to three months of age[13]. These foods were called pap and consisted of either wheat flour, breadcrumbs or barley bread with or without eggs and sugar and mixed with either cow's milk, water or clear ale.

The advice given to Australian and New Zealand mothers on weaning during the early twentieth century is of particular interest. Muskett[22] and James[39] considered that, normally, nothing but breast milk was required until the baby was 6 to 8 months old and stressed that if it could be avoided no baby should be weaned during the hot weather. Truby King[23] also strongly advocated complete breast feeding until the babies' 9th month unless this time fell in the hot summer months in which case he advised that gradual weaning should be delayed for 1 to 2 months. However, by 1929 health authorities recommended that weaning should begin at 5 to 6 months of age[40]. As the proportion of women choosing to breast feed declined during the mid twentieth century women introduced supplementary foods at an earlier and earlier age[41]. Although many infants were fed solid foods within the 1st month after birth[42,43], others were not given solids until they were almost 6 months old[42]. Similar trends for the introduction of solid foods into the infant's diet were observed in other developed countries and, as with the revival of breast feeding over the past decade in these countries, the change in medical advice followed rather than directed these changes in infant feeding practices[44].

Supplementary foods may be introduced as early as two to three months to in excess of six months after birth in developing countries[45]. However, whereas in some communities the most common reason given for the introduction of supplementary foods was the inadequacy of the mother's supply of breast milk[46], in other communities insufficient breast milk was only of minor importance[47].

There is considerable variation in the time after birth at which supplementary foods have been introduced into the infant's diet in both developing and developed societies and, in general, the timing of the introduction of these foods has depended more on cultural beliefs than upon nutritional need. Therefore the time of the introduction and the quantity of supplementary foods given to breast fed infants in both developing and developed countries are not particularly sensitive indicators of maternal lactation performance.

INFANT GROWTH

Before discussing the relationship between infant feeding and infant growth it is necessary to consider some of the obvious but rarely stated difficulties in the study of human nutrition in general, and infant nutrition in particular[48]. The nutrition of domestic animals has been defined as the transformation of food elements into body elements[49] and can be quantitated by the measurement of the formation of economically valuable products (meat, milk, wool etc.). Thus the efficiency of conversion of particular food elements into a livestock product provides a sensitive measure for the determination of optimal nutrition for a domestic animal.

In contrast, human "produce" is not as easily quantitated. The optimal diet for man has been defined as a diet consistent with the attainment of freedom from disease, a desirable life span, an optimal rate of physical development and an optimal rate of intellectual development[50]. Since these criteria are either almost impossible to quantitate, have a widely accepted normal range or are influenced greatly by non-nutritional factors which cannot be definitively separated from nutritional effects, it is impossible to apply most of the definitive experimental techniques used for domestic animals to studies of human nutrition. These difficulties are clearly illustrated in studies of the relationship between infant feeding and infant growth.

Recently, Seward and Serdula[45] in an extensive and critical review of the relationship between infant feeding and infant growth pointed out that all available growth references are based on infants who were predominantly artificially fed, were given early introduction to solid foods and grew faster than breast fed infants in the first 6 months of life. Therefore they questioned the use of these references for exclusively breast fed infants, infants who were small for gestational age and for infants in developing countries. In addition changes in the rate of linear growth frequently occur during infancy as birth length correlates poorly with eventual height at 2 years of age. Thus a healthy baby whose birth length is near the 50th percentile and decreases to the 3rd percentile during infancy may be adjusting to his or her genetic potential for growth in stature and expressing normal growth[51]. Obviously accepted normal ranges of this magnitude limit the sensitivity of any comparison of infant growth to lactation performance. The complex interactions between both dietary and non dietary factors with growth further complicate the interpretation of infant growth studies[45].

Nevertheless, Seward and Serdula[45] were able to conclude from careful analysis of studies on the growth of either exclusively or predominantly breast fed infants in developed countries that "in an ideal situation, where both the mother and infant are well nourished and healthy, breast milk alone will usually enable growth parallel to all established references (for artificially fed babies) from 0 to 3 months and growth with small deviation from some established references between 3 and 6 months". In contrast in developing countries either exclusively or predominantly breast fed infants have incremental weight gains which are slightly greater during the first 3 months and slightly less in the second 3 months of life than those of breast fed babies in developed countries. In developing countries with one exception all studies reviewed showed a clear benefit for breast feeding over artificial feeding during the first 6 months.

These conclusions are indeed remarkable as they show that it is only under an "ideal situation" that the lactation performance of women in developed countries can match that of poorly nourished women in developing countries. That is, the stresses experienced by most women in developed countries must cause a greater inhibition of lactation performance than the sum of nutritional and other stresses experienced by women in developing countries.

Normal growth up to 12 months of age has been reported for some exclusively breast fed infants[52,53]. However, from 6 to 12 months of age supplementary foods normally provide an increasing proportion of the infant's diet in both developed and developing countries and in latter countries this transitional period is often characterised by an increased number of infections. Thus growth in the second half of infancy is a very poor indicator of lactation performance.

INFANT HEALTH AND DEVELOPMENT

There is mounting evidence that breast milk not only contains components which have a major role in protecting the infant against pathogenic micro-organisms but also contains growth factors and hormones which may beneficially influence the physiological development of the infant[3,54,55]. Protection against pathogenic micro-organisms is clearly an important component of lactation performance in developing countries[45], and it may be shown to be of similar importance in developed countries when more precise methods for the assessment of lactation performance are developed.

Attempts to define adequate lactation performance usually have been restricted to a consideration of breast milk as a source of macro and micro nutrients for infant growth [56]. However, optimal nutrition includes not only an optimal rate of physical development (growth) but also freedom from disease, a desirable life span, and an optimal rate of intellectual development[50]. Indeed, in the future the assessment of lactation performance in terms of health and intellectual development of the infant rather than by the infant's rate of growth alone, may prove to be a far more effective semi-quantitative measure of lactation performance in both developing and developed countries.

MILK YIELD

The yield of breast milk has been measured in an attempt to obtain quantitative information on lactation performance in women. However, the measurement of milk yield in any sucking mammal is difficult, and studies in women pose additional restrictions because of the limitations on the nature of the techniques which can be used. Although methods as divergent as calculations based on infant growth rate to isotopic tracer techniques have been used, the most common method used for the determination of milk yield in women is test weighing[57]. The limitations of these techniques have been reviewed recently by Hartmann and Saint[57] and Seward and Serdula[45].

The test weighing method involves weighing either the infant or the mother before and after a breast feed, and taking the difference between the two weights to be the yield of breast milk. The development of electronic balances has greatly increased the accuracy of weighing and now the weight change in either the infant or the mother can be measured with the same high degree of precision. Since maternal test weighing and infant test weighing are two independent methods for measuring milk yield, we have compared the values obtained by each of these methods to validate the test weighing procedure. However, there was relatively poor agreement between these two methods unless the weight losses were corrected for the evaporative weight losses of the mother and infant, respectively. These studies demonstrated that in ambient temperature of 15° to 25°C failure to correct for evaporative weight losses resulted in the over estimation of milk yield by about 15% when the mother was test weighed (Figure 2) and an underestimation of milk yield by about 10% when the infant was test weighed.

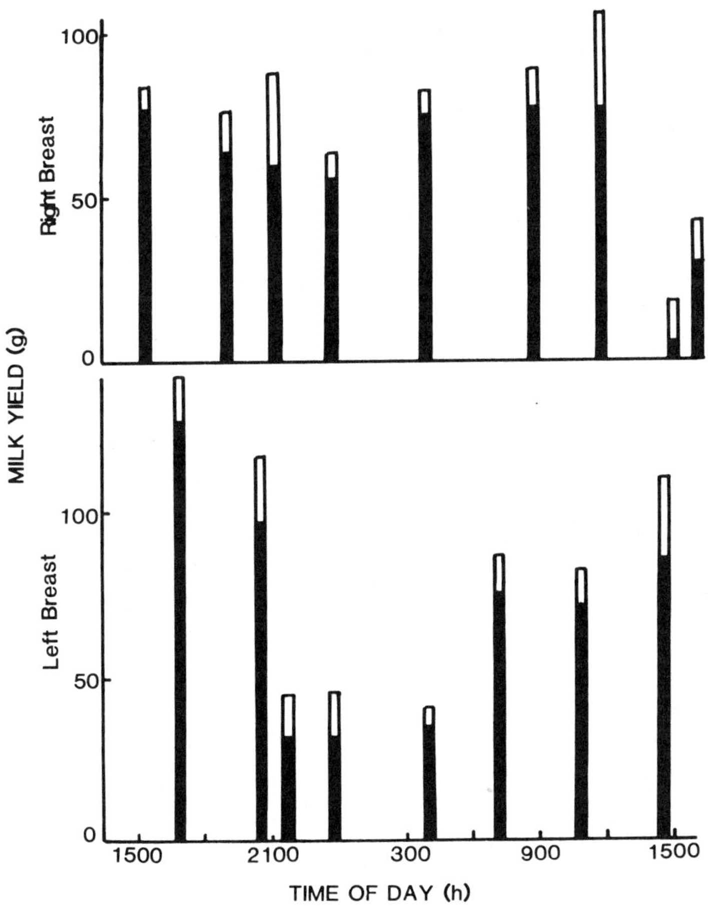

Figure 2. Milk yield over a period of 24h for the right (444 g/24h) and left (543 g/24h) breast of a woman breast feeding a 7 month old infant. The solid section of the histograms represents the corrected milk yield and the open section of the histograms represents the mother's evaporative weight loss during each breast feed.

It is possible that the poor accuracy of mechanical balances, variations in the interval between weighings, variations in the environmental temperature and physiological factors controlling evaporative weight loss could have masked many real effects of various treatments on milk yield in the past. However, it must be stressed that even the accurate measurement of milk yield in mothers still only provides a measure of the amount of milk consumed by the infant and that milk yield may provide a measure of the infant's appetite rather than the mother's potential to synthesize breast milk. Indeed, in Western Australia about 30% of mothers complain of problems of over production during their lactations.

We have reviewed the yield of breast milk from women of different socio-economic backgrounds[58,59]. It is of interest that most contemporary studies using the method of test weighing the infant show that women in developing countries can produce almost as much breast milk as women in developed countries. Since most of the studies in developing countries were carried out in hot environments the evaporative weight loss may have been greater in these infants and the true milk yield may be relatively higher for these women. Indeed, Rowland[60] using the deuterium oxide-to-mother method reported an average milk yield of about 900 ml/24h (range 600 to 1250 ml/24h) of mothers exclusively breast feeding their infants in Bakau, a relatively well off urban area in The Gambia. It is taken for granted that the lactation performance of mothers in developing countries is under considerable stress but, as with infant growth, studies on milk yield suggest that the lactation performance of most women in developed countries must be subjected to just as many stresses. In this connection, Whitehead[56] in a refreshing reappraisal of the lactation performance required to meet the infant's developmental demands for nutrients, presented data which clearly showed that for Cambridge mothers the problem is not their capacity to synthesize milk but rather their ability to maintain production beyond 3 months post partum.

MILK COMPOSITION

Nutritional Components

Any generalisations on the composition of breast milk of a particular species of mammal in relation to the nutritional needs of their young must be made with some reservation because of the 4027 species of mammal, milk analysis has only been carried out on 194 species and of these only 55 species have had 10 or more samples analysed[35]. However it is now accepted that the milk of each species is a complex secretion[61] tailored to the physiological requirements for the optimal development of its young.

The composition of breast milk has long been of interest to man and one of the oldest methods used to determine the quality of breast milk was termed the "nail test"[62]. This test involved placing a drop of breast milk onto a finger nail and observing the colour and viscosity of the milk. Currently knowledge of the complex composition of breast milk is expanding rapidly and has been reviewed in detail by Casey and Hambridge[4], Hartmann and Prosser[58] and Hartmann et al.[59].

The assessment of lactation performance by measuring composition of breast milk is difficult[45,56] because relatively large normal ranges are accepted for most components and few studies have attempted to collect milk samples in a way which can be directly related to the infant breast fed on demand. For example, the concentration of fat in breast milk varies greatly during a breast feed and the milk fat concentrations obtained by the current recommended collection procedures for lipid analysis[63] cannot be extrapolated to the demand fed infant. It is particularly difficult to obtain a composite sample of milk from women who are breast feeding their infants. This in turn means that lactation performance as judged by the energy intake of the breast fed infant may be in considerable error depending on the value taken to be the average concentration of fat in the milk consumed by the infant. Now that it is possible to measure milk yield accurately in mothers breast feeding their infants on demand, further studies are required to develop sampling protocols which permit the accurate quantitation of the nutrient intake of the breast fed infant.

Metabolic Components

The lactating breast is metabolically the most active organ in the body capable of producing in excess of 700 kcal/24h in mothers breast feeding single infants[53] and double this output in mothers breast feeding twins[64]. Despite this, the normal function of the breast has been almost totally ignored by medical science[65]. Indeed the breast must be the only major organ in the human body devoid of routine clinical biochemical tests for the assessment of its normal function. Other organs are usually assessed by the detection of marker biochemicals in either blood or urine. However breast milk bears a more direct association with the breast than either blood or urine and it would seem logical to attempt to develop clinical tests for the assessment of breast function (ie lactation performance) by detailed analysis of breast milk for both the end products of metabolic pathways and the metabolites, coenzymes and enzymes involved in their synthesis. In this connection Faulkner[66] has demonstrated that it is possible to carry out enzyme kinetic analysis of lactose synthesis from the measurement of milk yield and milk composition.

FUTURE CONSIDERATIONS

Previous studies comparing breast feeding to artificial methods of infant feeding must be critically reassessed giving due consideration to the limitations of the methods used to measure lactation performance. It is amazing that authoritative bodies are prepared to proclaim that there is little to choose between breast feeding and artifical feeding in developed countries without heeding the accuracy and precision of the techniques used to provide the data on which they base their proclamations.

Now that accurate methods are available for the measurement of milk yield, future developments should concentrate on differentiating between the potential of the mother to produce milk (ie the synthetic capacity of the breast) and the ability of the infant to consume the milk produced by the mother (ie the infant's appetite). This goal may be achieved by detailed metabolic investigations of the function of the mammary epithelial cells. The urgency of such studies cannot be underestimated. Indeed the fact that there are no routine clinical biochemical tests available to assess normal breast function demonstrates the dimension of medical science's neglect of the importance of human lactation.

Scant progress has been made in defining what constitutes optimum lactation performance and only either crude or unreliable analytical techniques have been available for the assessment of the lactation performance in women. This conclusion is supported, somewhat despairingly, by Whitehead's[67] suggestion that the mother was probably the best judge of what her baby needed and his advice that mothers should follow their instincts rather than be unnecessarily influenced by the opinions of experts. Similarly, over thirty years ago Wickes[20] concluded that the history of infant feeding could be regarded as a chronicle of man-made errors and that when mothers followed their natural instincts successful lactation would ensue. We doubt that much new knowledge will be gained about the biology of human lactation from further studies using semi-quantitative methods for the assessment of lactation performance. Nevertheless, we look to the future with optimism. The normal function of the human breast is at the beginning of a new and exciting era of fundamental research and this research must ultimately lead to the development of accurate methods for the assessment of lactation performance. This in turn will provide a basis for the proper medical care of lactating women in both developed and developing countries.

SUMMARY

Breast milk provides a source of nourishment uniquely adapted to the digestive and metabolic requirements of the human infant, protects the infant against pathogenic micro-organisms, facilitates the establishment of a strong relationship between mother and child, suppresses maternal fertility, reduces the likelihood of the infant developing allergies to foreign antigens and may exercise a degree of control over the infant's metabolism. Therefore, lactation performance should be considered in terms of this complex multi-faceted function of breast feeding.

The simplest qualitative measures of lactation performance are the duration of lactation and sucking frequency. In contrast to other mammals which exhibit defined and consistent behavioural patterns for lactation, the sucking frequency of infants in different social groups varies from 3 to 4 times an hour to only 4 times a day. Furthermore, the variation in the duration of lactation in different social groups of women spans the entire range observed for all other species of mammals.

Other measures of lactation performance have included simple observations such as the length of time that breast milk was the sole source of nutrients for the infant, the amount, timing and nature of supplementary foods consumed by the breast fed infant, and indices of the health and well being of the infant. In addition, the rate of growth of the infant often has been used to assess lactation performance of women. However, all of these measures of lactation performance can be greatly influenced by factors other than the quantity and quality of mother's milk. Therefore, these methods can be considered to provide only a semi-quantitative evaluation of lactation performance. The yield and composition of breast milk has been measured in an attempt to obtain quantitative information on lactation performance in women. However, most of the methods used to measure milk yield have not been rigorously validated and are so inaccurate that they are unlikely to provide a significant improvement over semi-quantitative methods.

The fact that there are no clinical biochemical tests available to assess breast function demonstrates the dimension of medical science's neglect of the importance of human lactation. Methods must be developed to differentiate between the potential of the mother to produce milk (rate of milk synthesis) and the ability of the baby to consume the milk produced by the mother (baby's appetite). Furthermore studies comparing breast feeding to artificial methods of infant feeding must be critically reassessed giving due consideration to the limitations of current methods of measuring lactation performance.

ACKNOWLEDGEMENTS

We wish to thank the National Health and Medical Research Council, the King Edward Memorial Hospital for Women Research Foundation and the Nursing Mothers Association of Australia for their support.

REFERENCES

1. Pond, C. M., 1984, Pysiological and Ecological Importance of Energy Storage in the Evolution of Lactation, in: "Physiological Strategies in Lactation," M. Peaker, R. G. Vernon, C. H. Knight, ed., Academic Press, London.
2. Jelliffe, D. B., and Jelliffe, E. F., 1978, The Weanling's Dilemma, Lancet, i:611.
3. Hartmann, P. E., Rattigan, S., Prosser, C. G., Saint, L., and Arthur, P. G., 1984, Human Lactation: Back to Nature, in: "Physiological Strategies in Lactation," M. Peaker, R. G. Vernon, C. H. Knight, ed., Academic Press, London.
4. Casey, C. E., and Hambridge, K. M., 1983, Nutritional Aspects of Human Lactation, in: "Lactation," M. C. Neville and M. R. Neifert, ed., Plenum Press, New York and London.
5. Bonner, W.N., 1984, Lactation Strategies in Pinnipeds: Problems for a Marine Mammalian Group, in: "Physiological Strategies in Lactation," M. Peaker, R. G. Vernon, C. H. Knight, ed., Academic Press, London.
6. Payne, M. R.,1979, Growth in the Antartic fur seal Arctocephalus gazella, J. Zool., Lond. , 187:1-20.
7. Findlay, L., and Renfree, M., 1984, Growth, Development and Secretion of the Mammary Gland of Macropodid Marsupials, in: "Physiological Strategies in Lactation," M. Peaker, R. G. Vernon, C. H. Knight, ed., Academic Press, London.
8. Hartmann, P. E., McCauley, I., Gooneratne, A. D., and Whitely, J. L., 1984, Inadequacies of Sow lactation: Survival of the Fittest, in: "Physiological Strategies in Lactation," M. Peaker, R. G. Vernon, C. H. Knight, ed., Academic Press, London.
9. Short, R. V., 1984, Breast Feeding, Sci. Am. , 250:35.
10. Notzon, F., 1984, Trends in Infant Feeding in Developing Countries, Pediatrics , 74:648.
11. Djumadias, A., and Enoch, M., 1978, Comparison of breast feeding, weaning and nutritional status of infants in urban and peri-urban Jakarta, Proceeding of National Pediatrics Congress , KONIKA, IV:55-57.
12. Inam, S., Soehadi, Sadjimin, T., Boediman, D., and Ismangun, 1979, Breast milk, weaning and child growth, in "Breastfeeding the biological option," Suharyono and G. J. Ebrahim, Yayasan Essentia Media, Yogyakarta.
13. Crawford, P., 1987, The Suckling Child, Continuity and Change, forthcoming.
14. Wickes, I. G., 1953b, A history of infant feeding: II. Seventeenth and eighteenth centuries, Arch. Dis. Child. , 28:232-240.
15. DeMause, L., 1974, "The History of Childhood," The Psychohistory Press, New York.

16. Walser, E. S., 1976, Maternal Behaviour in Mammals, in: "Comparative Aspects of Lactation," M. Peaker, ed., Academic Press, London.
17. Hitchcock, N., 1983, "Feeding Practises and Growth of Australian Infants," MSc Thesis, University of Western Australia.
18. Gandevia, B., 1978, "Tears often shed. Child health and welfare in Australia from 1788," Pergamon Press, Australia.
19. Grelier, M., 1981, in: "A new history of Western Australia," C. T. Stannage, ed., University of Western Australia Press, Perth.
20. Wickes, I.G., 1953, A history of infant feeding: V. Nineteenth Century concluded and twentieth century, Arch.Dis.Child., 28: 495-502
21. Vis, H. L., and Hennart, P., 1978, Decline in breast feeding: About some of its causes, Acta Paediat. Belgm., 31:195-206.
22. Muskett, P. E., 1903, "Australian Medical Guide," William Brooks & Co., Sydney.
23. Truby King, M., 1941, "Mothercraft," 9th ed., Whitcombe and Tombs Ltd., Sydney.
24. Harper, M. H., 1927, "The Parent's Book," 4th ed., Angus and Robertson, Sydney.
25. Aono, T., Shiozi, T., Shoda, T., and Kurachi, K., 1977, The initiaion of human lactation and prolactin response to suckling, J. Clin. Endocrin. Metab., 44:1101-1106.
26. Hitchcock, N., Gracey, M., Gilmour, A. I., and Owles, E. N., 1986, "Nutrition and growth in infancy and early childhood," Karger, Basel.
27. Douglas, J. W. B., 1950a, The extent of breast feeding in Great Britain in 1946, with special reference to the health and survival of children: II. Infant feeding in relation to survival, health and development, J. Obstet. Gynaecol., 57:349-361.
28. Douglas, J. W. B., 1950b, The extent of breast feeding in Great Britain in 1946, with special reference to the health and survival of children: II. Infant feeding in relation to survival, health and development. J. Obstet. Gynaecol., 57:349-361.
29. Newson, L. J., and Newson, E., 1962, Breast feeding in decline, Br. Med. J., 2:1744-1745.
30. Newton, D. B., 1966, The future of breast feeding, Med. J. Aust., 2:842-844.
31. Hendershot, G. E., 1984, Trends in Breast-Feeding, Pediatrics, 74:591.
32. Coy, J. F., Longmore, E. A., Mair, C. H., and Ratkowsky, D. A., 1976, Tasmanian infant feeding survey, Aust. Paediat. J., 12:171-175.
33. Congalton, A. A., 1969, "Status and Prestige in Australia," Cheshire, Melbourne.
34. Konner, M., and Worthman, C., 1980, Nursing frequency, gonadal function, and birth spacing among !Kung hunter-gatherers, Science, 207:788-791.
35. Oftedal, O. T., 1984,Milk Composition Milk Yield and energy Output at Peak Lactation: A Comparative Review, in: "Physiological Strategies in Lactation," M. Peaker, R. G. Vernon, C. H. Knight, ed., Academic Press, London.
36. Sai, F. T., 1983, Family planning and its relation to nutritional well-being and to maternal and child health, in: "Maternal Diet, Breast-feeding Capacity, and Lactational Infertility," R. G., Whitehead, ed., The United Nations University, Tokyo.
37. Segal, W., 1978, "Food and nutrition - facts and fallacies," Segal, Perth.
38. Peaker, M., Vernon, R. G., and Knight, C. H., ed., 1984,"Physiological Strategies in lactation," Academic Press, 1984.

39. James, H. W., 1912, "Home Nursing and ailments of children: A hand book for mothers," Signs Publishing Co., Warburton.
40. Scantlebury Brown, V., and Campbell, K., 1950, "A Guide to the Care of the Young Child," Government Printer, Melbourne.
41. McMahon, R. A., and Woodhill, J. M., 1959, Evaluation of the health of infants fed full strength cow's milk, Med. J. Aust. , 11:519-520.
42. Hankin, M. E., 1965, Infant feeding, Food and Nutr. Notes and Rev. , 22:47-55.
42. Wickes, I. G., 1953c, A history of infant feeding: V. Nineteenth century concluded and twentieth century, Arch. Dis. Child. , 28:495-502.
43. Allen, J., and Heywood, P., 1979, Infant feeding practices in Sydney, 1976-77, Aust. Paediatr. J. , 15:113-117.
44. Fomon, S. J., 1974, "Infant Nutrition," W.B. Saunders Co., London.
45. Seward, J.F., Serdula, M. K., Infant feeding and infant growth, Pediatrics , 74:728.
46. Kanaaneh H., 1972, The relationship of bottle feeeding to malnutrition and gastroenteritis in a pre-industrial setting, J Trop. Pediatr. and Environ. Child Health , 18:302-306.
47. Lambert, J., and Basford, J., 1977, Port Moresby infant feeding survey, Papua new Guinea Med. J. , 20:175-179.
48. Hartmann, P. E., 1977, "Feed'em, weigh'em" - An unsubstantiated basis for infant nutrition, Proc. Nutr. Soc. Aust. , 2:61.
49. Maynard, L. A., ad Loosli, J. K., 1956, "Animal Nutrition," 4th ed., McGraw-Hill Book Co., London.
50. Davidson, S., Passmore, R., and Brock, J. F., 1972, "Human Nutrition and Dietetics," 5th ed., Churchill Livingstone, London.
51. Smith, D. W., Truog, W., and Rogers, J. E., 1976, Shifting linear growth during infancy: Illustration of genetic factors in growth from fetal life through infancy, J. Pediatr. , 89:225-230.
52. Ahn, C. H., and Maclean, W. C., 1980, Growth of the exclusively breast fed infant, Am. J. Clin. Nutr. , 33:183-192.
53. Rattigan, S., Ghisalberti, A.V., and Hartmann, P.E., 1981, The yield and nutrient content of colostrum and milk of women from giving birth to 1 month post-partum, Br. J. Nutr. , 45:243-249.
54. Hayward, A. R., 1983, The Immunology of Breast MIlk, in: "Lactation," M. C. Neville, and M. R. Neifert, ed., Plenum Press, New York and London.
55. Strbak, V., 1985, "The role of maternal milk in endocrine regulation of sucklings," Veda, Bratislava.
56. Whitehead, R. G., 1985, Infant physiology, nutritional requirements, and lactational adequacy, The Am. J. Clin. Nutr. , 41:447-458.
57. Hartmann, P. E., and Saint, L., 1984, Measurement of Milk Yield in Women, J.Pediatric Gastroenterology and Nutrition , 3:270-274.
58. Hartmann, P. E., and Prosser, C. G., 1984, Physiological basis of longitudinal changes in human milk yield and composition, Federation Proc. , 43:2448-2453.
59. Hartmann, P. E., Rattigan, S., Saint, L., and Supriyana, O., 1985, Variation in the yield and composition of human milk, Oxford Rev. Reprod. Biology , 7:118.
60. Rowland, M. G. M., 1985, The "why" and "when" of introducing food to infants: growth in young breast-fed infants and some nutritional implications, Am. J. Clin. Nutr. , 41:459-463.
61. Davies, D. T., Holt, C., and Christie, W. W., 1983, The composition of milk, in: "Biochemistry of Lactation," T. B. Mepham, ed., Elsevier, Amsterdam.

62. Wickes, I. G., 1953a, A history of infant feeding: I. Primitive peoples, ancient works, renaissance writers, Arch. Dis. Child. 28:151-158.

63. Ferris, M., and Jensen, R. G., 1984, Lipids in Human Milk: A Review. 1: Sampling, Determination, and Content, J. of Pediatric Gastroenterology and Nutrition, 3:108-122.

64. Saint, L., Maggiore, P., and Hartmann, P.E., 1985, Yield and nutrient content of milk in eight women breast feeding twins and one woman breast feeding triplets, Br. J. Nutr. , in press.

65. Minchin, M.K., 1985, "Breastfeeding Matters" Alma Publications, Melbourne.

66. Faulkner, A., 1985, Glucose availability and lactose synthesis in the goat, Biochemical Society Transactions , 13:1985.

67. Whitehead, R. G., 1983, "Maternal Diet, Breast-feeding Capacity, and Lactational Infertility," The United Nations University, Tokyo.

APPROACHES TO THE STUDY OF COLOSTRUM-THE ONSET OF LACTATION

Stuart Patton, Gail E. Huston, *Pamela A. Montgomery and *Ronald V. Josephson

School of Medicine
University of California, San Diego
La Jolla, California 92093
*School of Family Studies and Consumer Sciences
San Diego State University
San Diego, California 92182

INTRODUCTION

As an aspect of lactation, the colostrum period, or so-called onset, presents a challenge to the new mother, her pediatrician and the lactation researcher. It is a time of profound change. The mammary epithelium is fully differentiated; the breasts progress quickly from a state of little or no secretion to production of a unique and transitory substance (colostrum), and then to voluminous mature milk of quite stable composition and properties. We have just completed a study of daily breast secretions from 5 donors starting with the first day that any material could be expressed from their glands following delivery to 5 days postpartum. The study, details of which are being published (1), raised fundamental questions such as: Precisely when is colstrum? How does one sample it? What are colostral lipids a sample of and are they an absolute good for the neonate? We attempt to analyze some of these issues here. Observations on the ultrastructure of colostrum are included.

METHODS

The following summarizes procedures used in our study of colostrum:

Sampling. Efforts to obtain samples from the 5 donors commenced on their days of delivery. Only one was able to express secretion on that day, two others could pump a sample on the next day and the other two on the second day following parturition. Samples, all obtained during mornings by pump, averaged 13.3 ml and ranged from 5 to 31 ml. In addition to those supplied by the 5 donors, we have obtained other colostrum samples for fractionation studies, pigment analyses and ultrastructural investigations.

Fractionation. Fat globules were isolated from colostrum by centrifuging them out of the colostrum through an overlayer of buffer (2). Skim milk phase of colostrum was prepared by centrifuging the sample at 2000 x g for 15 min after removing the cells. Skim milk was withdrawn by suction from under the resulting cream layer.

Analysis. Total protein was analyzed by modifications of the Lowry procedure (3). Total cholesterol was assayed as by Bachman et al. (4). Total lipids were obtained by Roese-Gottleib solvent extraction (5) and quantified by solvent evaporation and gravimetry. Total phospholipids were determined using the procedure of Rouser et al. (6) after their isolation from neutral lipids on thin layer chromatography plates. Carotenoids in total lipids were measured spectrophotometrically in 19:1 chloroform/methanol at a wavelength of 460 nm using β-carotene (Sigma) as a standard (7). Sodium dodecylsulfate-polyacrylamide gel electrophoresis (SDS-PAGE) of colostrum samples and fractions was carried out by established procedures (8-10) using authentic human milk proteins (Sigma) as references. For details on application of these methods, see our earlier reports (1-3,11,12).

Ultrastructure. The first colostral sample from each donor was prepared for electron microscopy by fixation with 3% glutaraldehyde in 0.15 M sodium cacodylate (pH 7.1). The three earlier (days 0 and 1) samples solidified) upon addition of glutaraldehyde. One drop of warm (50°) agarose was added to the two remaining samples (day 2) to provide structure. The solidified samples were cut into 1 mm^2 pieces, post-fixed in 1% osmium tetroxide for 2 hr, post-stained in 2% uranyl acetate overnight, dehydrated in ethanol/acetone and embedded in epon-araldite. Thin sections were stained conventually with uranyl acetate and lead citrate after which they were viewed on a JOEL 100B electron microscope.

Additional colostrum samples were processed for electron microscopy by the same protocol discussed above. Agar was added to provide structure when needed.

RESULTS AND DISCUSSION

Table 1 summarizes data on phospholipid and cholesterol content of first-day colostrum from 5 donors of our study in comparison with such data for mature milks from an earlier study (12). Using the two lipids as criteria of membrane material, it can be seen that colostrum and its fractions contain substantially more membrane than does mature milk and its corresponding parts. This is true even though the colostrum samples averaged considerably less in total lipid, 14.4 mg/ml as compared to 25.4 mg/ml for the mature milk. A major difference lies in the fact that approximately 70% of the phospholipid and 50% of the cholesterol in colostrum are contained in the skim milk. Mature human milk has only about 20% of its phospholipid and cholesterol in the skim milk (Table 1). We are investigating the identity of this increased quantity of membrane material in colostral skim milk. Using cholesterol and phospholipid contents as criteria, Bitman et al. (13) also detected higher levels of membrane material in human colostrum as compared to milk.

The membrane material in milk, around fat globules and in the form of vesicles and cell fragments in the skim milk phase, represents a complex mixture of biologically important molecules (enzymes, cell surface receptors, glycoproteins, glycolipids, phospholipids, etc.). To our knowledge there have been no studies evaluating the contribution of membrane material to nutrition of the newborn. The assumption seems to be that this material is digested and utilized nutritionally according to the conventional understanding even though it is well established that the neonatal gut at birth is in a partially developed state and does not function as it will in the more mature animal (14).

The data for colostrum in Table 1 are derived from samples taken on the first day secretion could be pumped from donor's breasts following delivery

Table 1. A Comparison of Lipid, Protein, Phospholipid and Total Cholesterol Contents of Human Colostrums and Its Fractions with Those Components of Mature Human Milk and Fractions Thereof.[a]

	Lipid	Protein	Phospholipid	Cholesterol
	mg/ml		g/ml	
Whole Sample				
Colostrum	14.4±11.3	73.0±44.0	298±158	228±120
Mature Milk	25.4± 5.4	9.8± 0.8	176±158	107± 21
Skim Milk				
Colostrum	-------	67.0±42.0	205± 93	111± 74
Mature Milk	-------	9.1± 0.7	37±9.5	19±4.7
Fat Globules[b]				
Colostrum	-------	33.0±11.0	13.2±8.6	8.0±2.8
Mature Milk	-------	13.2± 3.8	5.8±0.6	3.6±0.3

[a]Data are from recent studies (1,12). Five colostrum samples were taken from each of 5 donors on their first postpartal days that breast secretion became available. Mature milks were approximately monthly samples from 2 (other) donors during their second through ninth month of lactation.
[b]All data for fat globules are mg/g of globules.

of their babies. This is, in our opinion, most typically colostrum because even a matter of hours, composition and volume of the secretion will change. There seems to be considerable variability between individuals as to when colostrum will become available, how much of it there will be and how long it will persist. Figure 1 reproduces an SDS-gel of proteins (skim milk) in breast secretions of one donor sampled on her day of delivery and on each of the next 4 days. The pattern of samples for the first two days are virtually identical but the third day reveals a transition and the forth- and fifth- day samples have a pattern resembling mature milk. The characteristic band of α-lactalbumin (E) has become a major component and the cluster of bands (C) due to casein micelles has emerged. At the same time the broad bands due to heavy (HC) and light chains (LC) of sIgA have faded. This latter change accounts for the decided drop in protein content of breast secretion as colostrum wanes and milk increases. Some of our donors exhibited the typical SDS-gel pattern of colostrum on only the first day that secretion was available. By the next day their patterns resembled those of mature milk.

SDS-PAGE data for fat globule proteins during the colostral period are shown in Figure 2. These were obtained from the corresponding samples of Figure 1. It is evident that globule proteins on the first and second day of sampling are quite different from those on the third, fourth and fifth days. It appears that fat globules on the first two days were heavily decorated with sIgA, whereas the later samples have taken on the characteristic protein pattern of mature milk fat globules. The progressive appearance of 2 of the major bands, corresponding to xanthine oxidase and butyrophilin, can be seen opposite the arrowheads (upper right).

The relatively large standard deviations for all of our colostrum data categories in Table 1 attest to variations we encountered in the first and

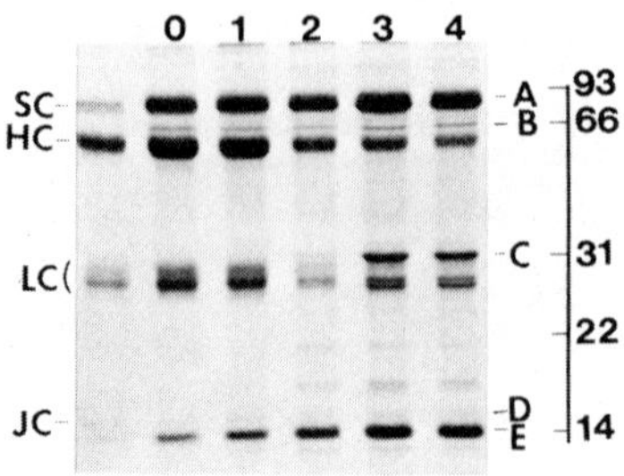

Figure 1. SDS-polyacrylamide gel electrophoresis patterns of skim milk phases from daily samples of a donor's colostrum on her day of delivery (lane 0) and the next 4 days (lanes 1-4). Each sample contained 30 μg of protein. Undesignated lane (left) shows separation of authentic sIgA (5 μg) from human milk into secretory chain (SC), heavy chain (HC), light chain (LC) and J chain (JC). Reference Mr's x 10^{-3} are at right and adjoining it are positions of the major human milk proteins: A- lactoferrin, B- serum albumin, C- β-casein, D- lysozyme, E- α-lactalbumin. The gel was 12.5% acrylamide, 1.5 mm thick and stained with Coomassie blue. Data from ref. 15.

second day samples. After that much greater uniformity in values was obtained. According to Neville et al. (16), the term colostrum is commonly used to describe the breast secretion during the first 4 or 5 days postpartum. That of the next 5 days is called transitional milk. They state further that the composition of colostrum can not be defined because it is rapidly changing. While not disputing that statement, we feel that a concerted effort is needed to specify sampling conditions for colostrum so that data for different donors and between laboratories can be compared and the product better understood. It is evident from our observations and those of others (17), that the product from most donors by the third day breast secretion has been available, assuming that the baby has been nursing, will be largely milk and not colostrum. Perhaps cutoff criteria in the form of certain markers for milk, such as casein or lactose, might be useful.

Another distinctive characteristic of human colostrum in comparison to mature milk is its relatively intense yellow color which is attributed to β-carotene (provitamin A) (18). We have confirmed that the absorption spectrum of the pigment resembles that of β-carotene, although some oxygenated derivatives appear to be present as well (1). Like some other colostral

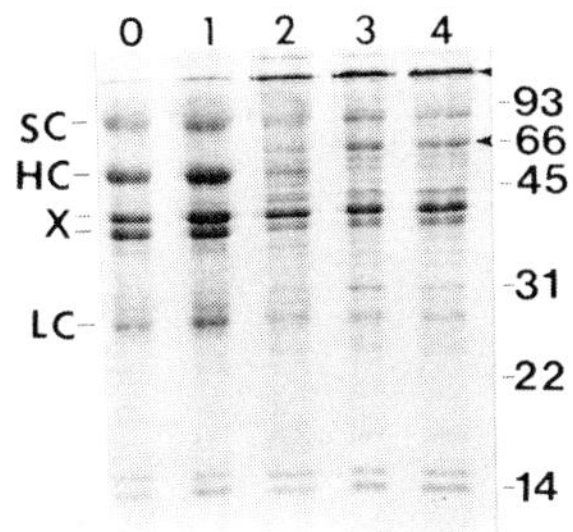

Figure 2. SDS-polyacrylamide gel electrophoresis patterns of fat globules isolated from daily samples of a donor's colostrum (see also the corrosponding skim milks, Figure 1). For designations right, left and top of gel plates, see Figure 1. X denotes two unknown bands of colostrum which are less intense or absent from fat globules of mature milk. Samples contained 50 μg of protein. Gel conditions were as in Figure 1. Data from ref. 1.

components the yellow pigment dissipates rather rapidly during early lactation. Data on carotenoid content of breast secretion samples from our 5 donors during their first five days of lactation are shown in Figure 3. From analyses of mature milks we found a mean carotene value of 4 μg/g of lipid which is shown for purposes of comparison at $>$30 days in the figure. The data of Figure 3 agree well with those of Chapell et al. (19) for carotene in human colostrum and milk.

The yellow color of colostrum appears to be associated exclusively with the fat globules. Diet must be an important factor in determining its intensity since carotenoids are of plant origin. The high concentration of carotenoids in globules of colostrum as compared to that in milk fat globules indicates prepartum accumulation and storage of the pigment in breast tissue. Indeed, tissue (adipose) removed from the breast by surgery is yellow. These observations suggest the idea of colostrum as a means of sampling breast lipid material that has been stored there for weeks and possibly much longer. This concept leads to a number of considerations. One concerns emptying of accumulated undesirable molecules such as environmental contaiminants and lipid oxidation products in colostrum, and whether ingestion of such material by an infant is without risk. For example, see Figure 1, reference 20 (herein). The presence of carotenoids in breast tissue, colostrum and milk also may be of significance in light of indications that the carotenes are cancer antagonists (21-23). Moreover, they have a capacity

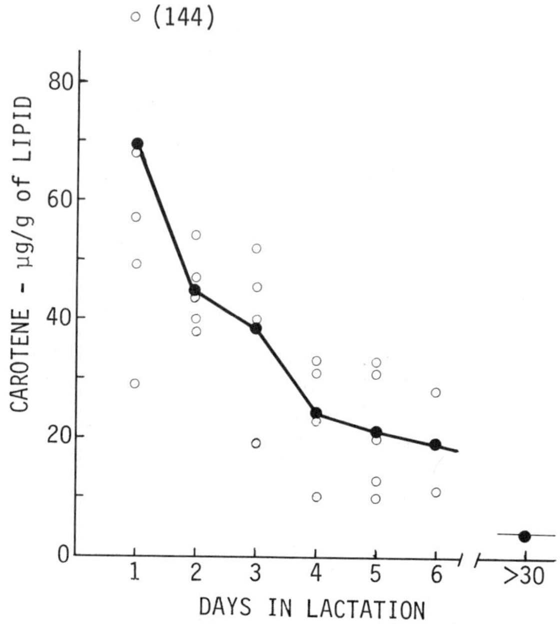

Figure 3. Carotenoid content of daily colostrum samples from 5 donors starting with the first day that breast seretion was available. Values for individuals (O) and means (●) are shown, as well as the mean for 4 mature milks (> 30 days of lactation). Carotenoids were measured at a wavelength of 460 nm in 19:1 chloroform/methanol using β-carotene as a standard.

to inhibit transformation of mouse mammary cells by carcinogens (24,25). While many factors are involved in breast cancer, it is interesting that both gestation (26) and lactation (27) reduce the risk of breast cancer, and both processes entrain carotenoids into mammary epithelial cells, the site of malignant transformation. Of course this relationship may be purely coincidental. Gestation and lactation may also induce turnover of faulty genetic material as well as of carcinogens which have found their way to or developed in the gland. On the otherhand, it appears that colostrum does offer a unique opportunity to gain further insight on carotenoid storage, transport and metabolism in the breast.

The ultrastructural composition of a colostrum sample collected on the same day as delivery is shown in Figure 4. Most notable is the osmiophilic background and the patches of highly stained, densely packed material (arrows). Closer inspection of these areas revealed them to be of the same composition as the background material simply tighter packed. While this phenomena was most striking in the three colostrum samples that solidified upon fixation, it was present but to a much less degree in the two later (day 2) samples. We believe this material to be immunoglobulins which have cross-linked in the presence of glutaraldehyde, the fixative. The substantially higher protein content of the three colostrum samples further substantiates this belief. The other components of colostrum are as expected: fat globules of varying sizes (FG), membrane bound vesicles (V) and whole, seemingly viable (with a nucleus) cells (upper right).

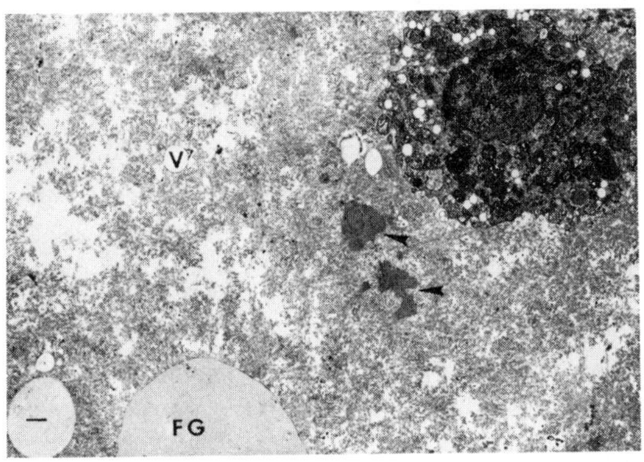

Figure 4. Electron micrograph of human colostrum collected on the day of parturition. Note the presence of fat globules (FG), membrane-bound vesicles (V), whole cells (upper right) and the osmiophilic background material which aggregates into dense patches (arrows). Bar in lower left denotes 1 μm

Two interesting questions have arisen with respect to the ultrastructure of colostrum: one concerns the nature of membrane material in colostral skim milk, and the other involves differences between fat globules in colostrum as compared to those in mature milk. As pointed out in our study (1), there is a time, usually about the third day of lactation, when the colostrum-milk contain two kinds of fat globules: more intensely yellow ones and relatively white ones. These can be differentiated by centrifuging the sample, the yellow globules compacting above the white ones in the cream layer. Earlier samples show only yellow globules, later samples progressively more white globules. We are attempting to resolve these questions with observations on additional samples of colostrum.

SUMMARY

Colostrum is a unique, transitory, imprecisely defined secretion of the breast that becomes available to the neonate at or shortly after parturition. Our recent study (1) confirms that colostrum contains greater amounts of membrane material, especially in the skim milk phase, and much higher concentrations of carotenoids than mature milk. It is not known whether membranes have any special dietary significance to the newborn. Colostrum represents a means of sampling lipids that have been stored in the breast. It also affords an opportunity to evaluate carotenoid storage, transport and metabolism and the possible role of carotene as a breast cancer antagonist. Colostrum in relatively pure form is secreted for at most a day or two after-which it is progressively diluted by increasing milk production. Development of an acceptable sampling protocol for colostrum would facilitate research on this important secretion of the human breast. Initial ultrastructural evaluation of colostrum has not immediately revealed the source of increased membrane. It has, however, shown a cross-linking of globulins with fixation to the point of solidification in the earliest samples. Additonal ultra-structural evaluation of colostrum and fractions thereof at different stages should bring further insight into the question of membrane identity.

ACKNOWLEDGEMENTS

We thank Suzanne D. Dixon and Patricia F. Mooney of the UCSD Medical Center and area mothers for assistance in obtaining colostrum samples. Support for the preparation of this paper and for our research on colostrum is from Contract N01-HD-2-2819 with the National Institute of Child Health and Human Development.

REFERENCES

1. S. Patton and G. E. Huston, Trends in fat, protein, phospholipid, cholesterol and carotenoids of human milk (colostrum) at onset of lactation, Gastroenterol Nutr (1986) (in press).
2. S. Patton and G. E. Huston, A method for isolation of milk fat globules, Lipids 21:170 (1986).
3. S. Patton and G. E. Huston, A procedure for the determination of total protein in human milk, Nutr Rep Int 30:1401 (1984).
4. K. C. Bachman, J-H. Lin and C. J. Wilcox, Sensitive colorimetric determination of cholesterol in dairy products, JAOAC 59:1146 (1976).
5. W. Horowitz, ed., "Official Methods of Analysis; Association of Official Analytical Chemists," Association of Official Analytical Chemists, Washington D.C. (1975).
6. G. Rouser, A. N. Siakatos and S. Fleischer, Quantitative analysis of phospholipids by thin-layer chromatography and phosphorus analysis of spots, Lipids 1:85 (1966).
7. S. Patton, J. J. Kelly and T. W. Keenan, Carotene in bovine milk fat globules: Observations on origin and high content in tissue mito-chondria, Lipids 15:33 (1980).
8. K. Weber and M. Osborn, The reliability of molecular weight determi-nations by dodecylsulfate-polyacrylamide gel electrophoresis, J Biol Chem 255:4406 (1969).
9. U. K. Laemmli, Cleavage of structural proteins during the assembly of the head of bacteriophage T4, Nature 227:680 (1970).
10. G. Fairbanks, T. L. Steck and D. F. H. Wallach, Electrophoretic analysis of the major polypeptides of the human erythrocyte membrane, Biochemistry 10:2606 (1971).
11. G. E. Huston and S. Patton, Membrane distribution in human milks as revealed by phospholipid and cholesterol analysis, in: "Human Lac-tation: Milk Components and Methodologies," R. G. Jensen and M. Neville, ed., Plenum Press, New York (1985).
12. G. E. Huston and S. Patton, Membrane distribution in human milks throughout lactation as revealed by phopholipid and cholesterol analyses, Gastroenterol Nutr (1986) (in press).

13. J. Bitman, L. Wood, M. Hamosh, P. Hamosh and N. R. Mehta, Comparison of term and preterm infants, Am J Clin Nutr 38:300 (1983).
14. W. A. Walker, Antigen handling by the gut, Arch Dis Child 53:527 (1978).
15. P. A. Montgomery, S. Patton, G. E. Huston and D. V. Josephson, Gel electrophoretic analysis of proteins in human milk and colostrum, Comp Biochem Physiol (1986) (submitted).
16. M. C. Neville, J. C. Allen and C. Watters, The mechanisms of milk secretion, in: "Lactation: Physiology, Nutrition and Breastfeeding," M. C. Neville and M. R. Neifert, ed., Academic Press, New York (1983).
17. J. K. Kulski and P. E. Harmann, Changes in human milk composition during initiation of lactation, Aust J Exp Biol Med Sci 59:101 (1981).
18. H. Vorherr, "The Breast: Morphology, Physiology and Lactation," Academic Press, New York (1984).
19. J. E. Chapell, T. Francis and M. T. Clandinin, Vitamin A and E content of human milk at early stages of lactation, Early Hum Dev 11:157 (1985).
20. J. S. Patton, Cellular pathways in the movement of lipophilic xenobiotics from GI tract to breast milk, in: "Human Lactation - Effect of Maternal Environmental Factors," M. Hamosh and P. Hamosh, ed., Plenum Press, New York (1986).
21. R. Peto, R. Doll, J. D. Buckley and M. B. Sporn, Can dietary beta carotene materially reduce human cancer rates?, Nature 290:201 (1981).
22. R. B. Skekelle, S. Liu, W. J. Raymor, M. Lepper, C. Maliza and A. H. Rosoff, Dietary vitamin A and risk of cancer in the Western Electric Study, Lancet II:1185 (1981).
23. National Research Council Committee, "Diet, Nutrition and Cancer," National Academy Press, Washington D.C. (1982).
24. S. Som, M. Chaterjee and M. R. Banerjee, β-carotene inhibition of 7'12-dimethylbenxanthracene-induced transformation of murine mammary cells in vitro, Carcinogenesis 5:937 (1984).
25. K. Manoharan and M. R. Banerjee, β-carotene reduces sister chromatid exchanges induced by chemical carcinogens in mouse mammary cells in organ culture, Cell Biol Int Rep 9:783 (1985).
26. M. Brennan, Lactation and the breast cancer process, in: "Lactation: A Comprehensive Treatise," Vol IV, B. L. Larson, ed., Academic Press, New York (1978).
27. T. Byers, S. Graham, T. Rzeptka and J. Marshall, Lactation and breast cancer: Evidence for a negative association in premenopausal women, Am J Epidemiol 121:664 (1985).

REGULATION OF THE RATE OF LACTOSE PRODUCTION

Margaret C. Neville, Jonathan C. Allen and Clare E. Casey

Departments of Physiology and Pediatrics
University of Colorado School of Medicine
Denver, Colorado 80262

SUMMARY

The rate of lactose synthesis during the declining phase of lactation was examined relative to the concentrations of ionized calcium, glucose and alpha-lactalbumin in human milk. Ionized calcium was found to remain constant at about 2.5 mM or to increase slightly during the declining phase of milk production in 5 subjects. Alpha-lactalbumin concentrations in milk increased or remained constant during the declining phase of lactation in four women. If the concentrations of ionized calcium and alpha-lactalbumin in milk are representative of their concentrations in the Golgi system, the site of lactose synthesis, it is unlikely that either plays a regulatory role in lactose synthesis during the declining phase of lactation. Glucose concentration decreased when the milk yield fell below about 300 g/day and was linearly related to the lactose secretion rate under this condition. A possible relation between milk glucose and the lactose synthesis rate is discussed.

INTRODUCTION

Lactose is synthesized in the Golgi vesicles of the mammary alveolar cell (1,2) and transferred to the lumen of the mammary gland along with a number of other milk components by the process of exocytosis (Fig. 1). Because lactose, at a concentration around 200 mM, makes up two-thirds of the osmotic activity of human milk, the rate of milk secretion is largely determined by the rate of lactose synthesis and secretion. While both the reactions by which lactose synthesis takes place (Fig. 2) and their ultrastructural localization are well-understood, the regulation of these reactions under physiological circumstances is not.

Among the several factors that have been suggested to play a role in the regulation of lactose synthesis (3), three will be assessed in this paper:

1. In goats the concentration of glucose in milk has been observed to increase as the rate of milk secretion increases (4,5). Since glucose is the precursor for lactose, it has been suggested (3,5-8) that the supply of glucose to the mammary alveolar cell is limiting for lactose synthesis. If this is the case regulation of glucose entry into the alveolar cell could regulate the rate of milk secretion.

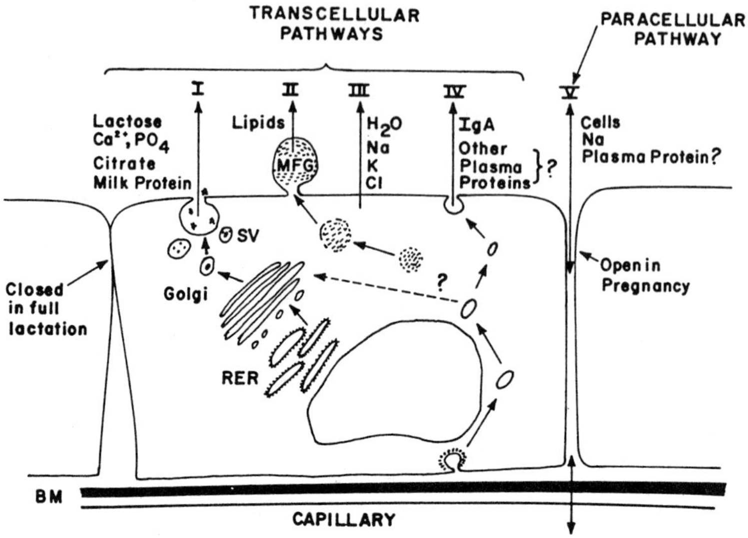

Fig. 1. **The mechanisms of milk secretion.** The upper surface represent the alveolar lumen. (I) Exocytosis of milk proteins, lactose, citrate, calcium and phosphate. (II) Milk fat secretion via the membrane-bound particle, the milk fat globule. (III) The equilibration of water, and monovalent ions across the apical membrane. Glucose likely also equilibrates across this membrane (4,5). (IV) Vesicular transport of IgA. (V) The paracellular pathway which is open in pregnancy and allows components of the extracellular space to enter the milk space. SV, secretory vesicle; RER, rough endoplasmic reticulum; BM, basement membrane; MFG, milk fat globule. From ref. 7; used by permission.

2. Powell and Brew (9), in a study of the ionic dependence of lactose synthetase, found that micromolar concentrations of manganese activated the enzyme system in the presence of millimolar concentrations of calcium, leading them to suggest that *the availability of calcium in the Golgi compartment* regulated the rate of lactose synthesis.

3. Palmiter (10) observed a correlation between the alpha-lactalbumin concentration and the lactose content of the milk of various species leading him to propose that *the availability of the coenzyme, alpha-lactalbumin,* might regulate lactose secretion. The observation of Nicholas *et al.* (11) that the lactose and alpha-lactalbumin concentrations of rat milk are correlated throughout the first 20 days of lactation in the rat was taken as support for this conclusion. A sharp increase in the alpha-lactalbumin concentration in mouse mammary gland coinciding with lactogenesis provides further support for some such mechanism (12). Against this hypothesis is the finding of Lönnerdal et al (13) that the alpha-lactalbumin concentration in human milk decreases during lactogenesis.

In order to investigate these hypotheses we have examined the concentration of glucose, ionized calcium, and alpha-lactalbumin in the milk of 5 lactating women during gradual weaning, when the rate of milk secretion

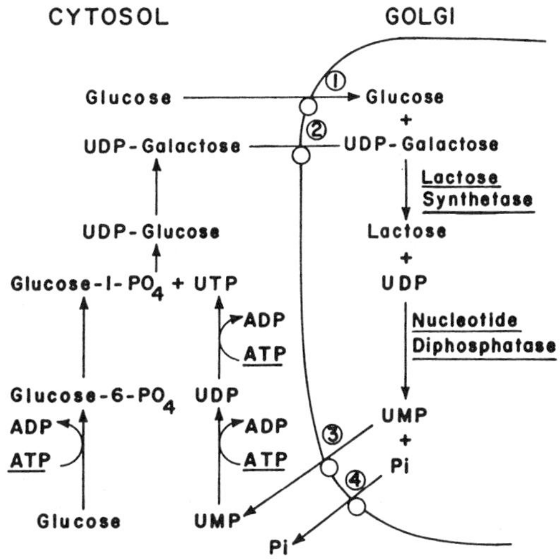

Fig. 2. **The pathways for lactose synthesis.** Note that UDP-galactose is synthesized from glucose and UTP in the cytoplasm while the final synthesis of lactose from UDP-galactose and glucose takes place within the lumen of the Golgi system. The Golgi membrane is not permeable to lactose, so the disaccharide is trapped within the membrane system. The lactose synthetase complex is composed of the membrane-bound enzyme, galactosyl transferase, and the soluble protein, alpha-lactalbumin. From ref. 7; used by permission.

declined from more than 600 g/day to less than 100 g/day over a period of 5 to 10 months. Assuming that the concentration of these substances in the milk reflects their concentration in the Golgi system, our results lead to the conclusion that none of these factors is the primary regulator of lactose synthesis during the declining phase of lactation.

METHODS

Subjects

The subject pool for this study has been described (14). The five subjects described during the declining phase of lactation in this paper decided to wean during the course of a longer study and gradually began substituting beikost for breast feeds at some point after six months of lactation. Data from five subjects during the rising phase of lactation are also given. Data from these subjects were chosen for presentation because of the completeness of the data sets during these periods.

Analytical methods

The measurement of milk yield, collection and storage of milk samples and analysis of milk glucose and lactose have been described previously (14). The ionized calcium content of milk was measured on samples which were taken directly from the breast into a capillary tube which was then sealed to prevent loss of carbon dioxide. The measurement of ionized calcium was carried out with a Radiometer ICA1 calcium electrode as described previously (15). Alpha-lactalbumin was analyzed by radioimmunoassay using rabbit antiserum raised against purified human alpha-lactalbumin (Sigma) at a dilution of 1:300. The antiserum showed no cross reactivity with human IgA, lactoferrin, human serum albumin or lysozyme. The assay buffer was 100 mM sodium phosphate, pH 7.1, with 0.1% bovine serum albumin and 1 mM EGTA. Varying amounts of buffer and test sample were added to 50 ul I^{125}-alpha-lactalbumin (iodinated by the Iodobead^{R} method) containing 5000-10000 counts/minute and 100 ul diluted antiserum. After overnight incubation at $0^{o}C$ 100 ul of goat antirabbit

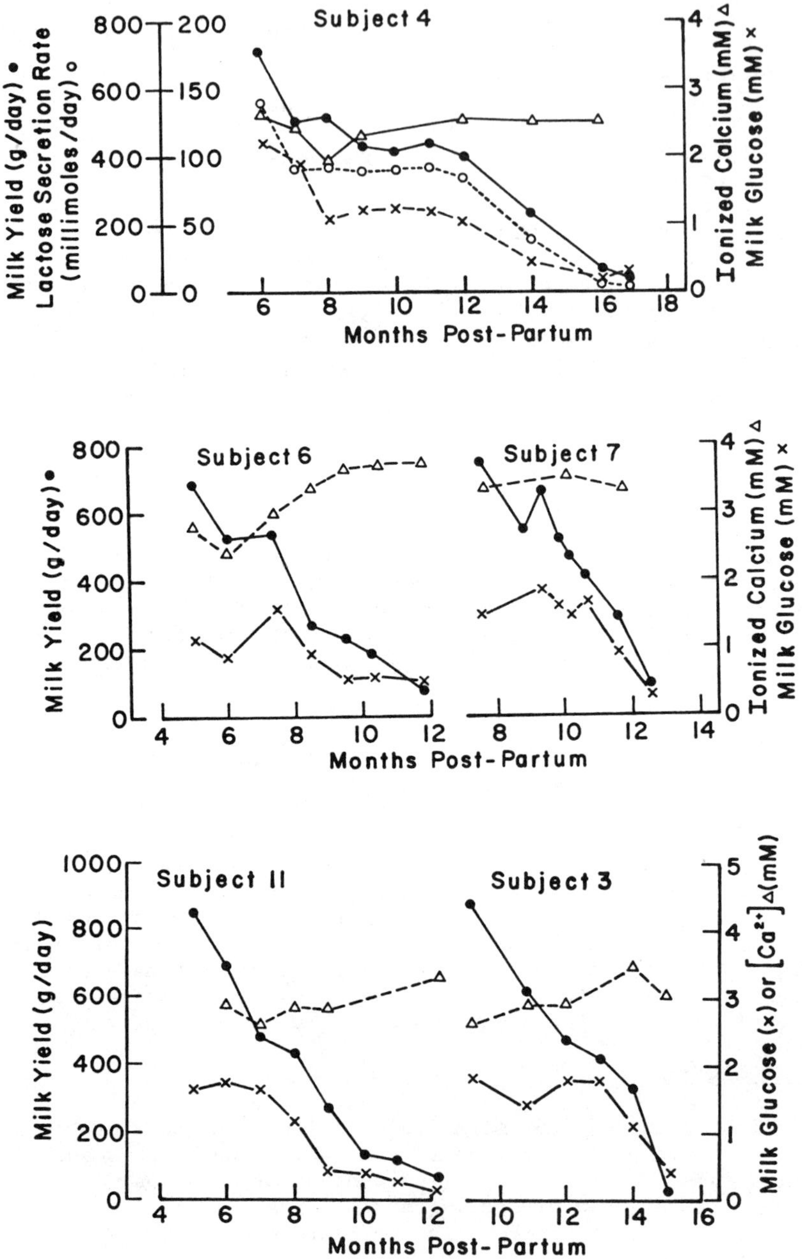

Fig. 3. **Milk yield, ionized calcium and glucose in 5 subjects undergoing gradual weaning.** The lactose secretion rate, calculated as the product of the milk yield and the lactose content of the milk on the corresponding day, are shown for subject 4. Each graph represents data from a single subject.

antiserum was added to the reaction tube and the mixture incubated an additional 2 hours at 37°C. The immune complex was separated by centrifugation and counted in a Beckman gamma counter. A standard curve was run with every assay and used to calculate the concentration of alpha-lactalbumin. Three dilutions of each sample were assayed.

RESULTS

The graphs in Fig. 3 show the milk yield, glucose concentration and ionized calcium in the milk for 5 women studied during the declining phase of lactation. The data for subject 4 are shown in greatest detail: At six months with the addition of some solid food the milk yield declined from about 700 g/day to about 500 g/day and remained near this level until 12 months when the mother made a concerted effort to wean the child, gradually decreasing the number of feeds per day until the yield declined below 100 ml at 16 months. This graph demonstrates the parallel decline in milk yield and lactose secretion rate. This was true in all four subjects since the lactose concentration remained quite constant until the yield fell below 100 g/day (14). During this entire interval the ionized calcium remained approximately constant at 2.5 mM. The glucose concentration fell approximately in parallel with the lactose secretion rate. Similar results were seen in four other subjects (Fig. 3, subjects 6,7,11 and 3) except that the glucose concentration remained approximately constant until the milk yield dropped below 300 g/day.

The lactose secretion rate is shown as a function of the ionized calcium in the milk in Fig. 4. There is no apparent relationship between the two parameters (slope:$P > 0.2$), suggesting that, if the calcium concentration in milk reflects that in the Golgi system, ionized calcium does not play a role in the regulation of lactose synthesis during the declining phase of lactation.

Fig. 5 shows the relation between milk glucose and the lactose secretion rate during the declining phase of lactation. The relation appears to be linear with a slope of 71 millimoles of lactose per day per mM

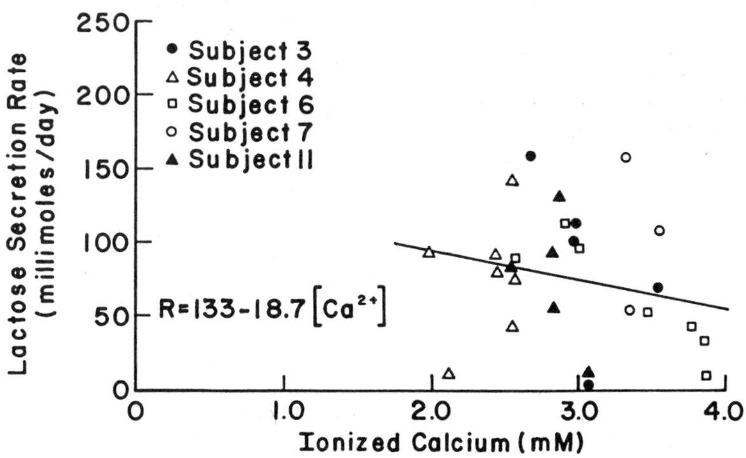

Fig. 4. The relation between ionized calcium and lactose secretion rate during the declining phase of lactation.

glucose. Fig. 6 shows similar data obtained during the rising phase of milk secretion days 1 to 7 postpartum. Again there appears to be a linear relation between the rate of lactose secretion and the glucose concentration. In fact the slopes in Figs 5 and 6 are equal. At first sight this finding would appear to support the hypothesis that the glucose

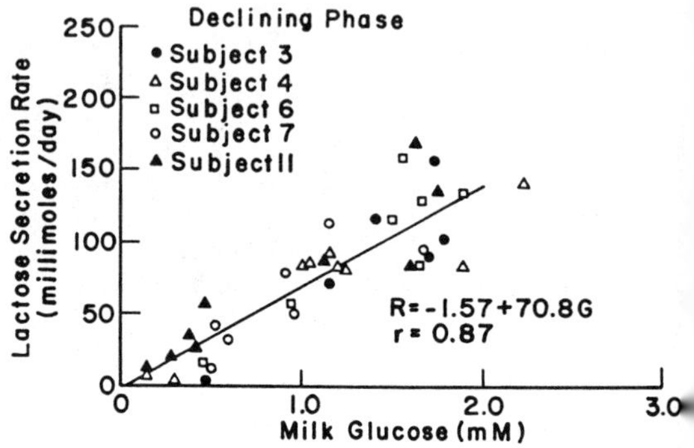

Fig. 5. **The relation between the lactose secretion rate and the milk glucose concentration during the declining phase of lactation.** The best linear fit is given by the equation on the graph where R is the lactose secretion rate and G the glucose concentration. r is the correlation coefficient.

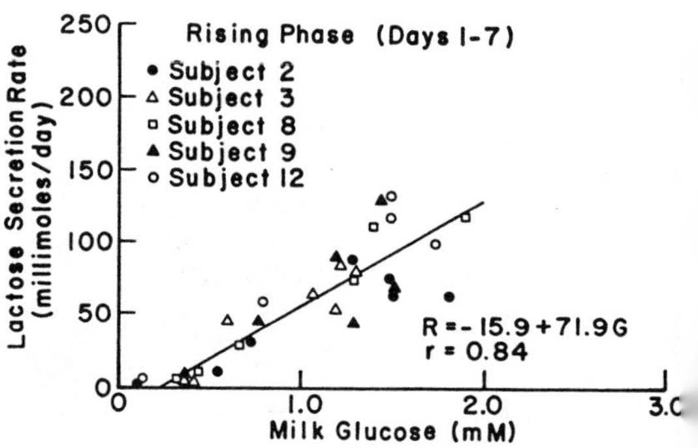

Fig. 6. **The relation between the lactose secretion rate and the milk glucose concentration during the rising phase of lactation (days 1-7 postpartum).** The meaning of the coefficients is given in the legend to Fig. 5.

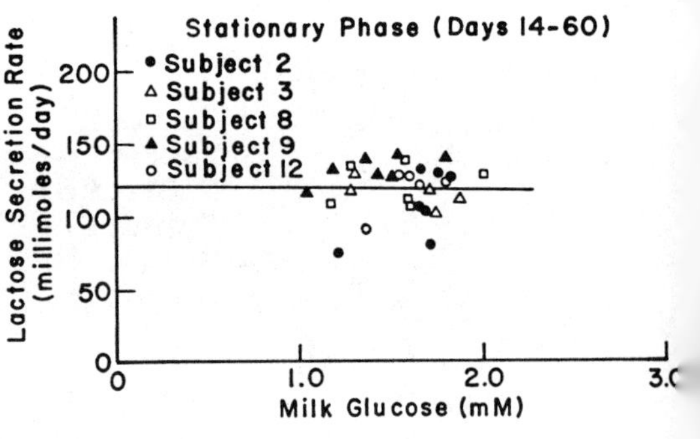

Fig. 7. **The relation between the lactose secretion rate and the milk glucose during the stationary phase of lactation** (Days 14-60 post partum).

supply regulates the lactose synthesis rate. However, attempts to fit the curve of Fig. 5 with Michaelis Menton kinetics failed. Further, during the stationary phase of lactation from days 14 to 60, the lactose secretion rate appeared to be unaffected by the concentration of milk glucose (Fig. 7). This problem is discussed further below.

Fig. 8 shows alpha-lactalbumin concentrations in the milks of four weaning subjects. The amount of milk sample remaining for the fifth subject was insufficient for the assay. In these subjects alpha-lactalbumin appears to be highly variable at about 2 mg/ml around the time of parturition declining to an average value of about 1.5 mg/ml at 6 months and then rising again during the declining phase of lactation in three (subjects 4,6, and 11) of the four subjects. In the fourth subject (subject 7) the alpha lactalbumin appeared to remain constant during the declining phase. These data suggest that a decrease in alpha-lactalbumin is not associated with a decrease in the lactose secretion rate.

DISCUSSION

Milk composition and lactose synthesis

In assessing the significance of the results presented in this report it is important to answer the question "To what extent does the composition of milk provide a window on the function of the mammary alveolar cell?" More specifically we need to know whether the concentrations of glucose, ionized calcium and alpha-lactalbumin are representative of their concentrations at the site of lactose synthesis, thought to be the terminal cisternae of the Golgi apparatus (2,16). Experimental evidence on this point has been obtained by infusing solutions into the udders of goats and examining changes in composition over time. Except for monovalent ions (17), glucose, and galactose (18), it appears that the rate of secretion of most milk components including lactose, sucrose, calcium, phosphate, protein and citrate (17,19-20, Neville and Peaker, unpublished) is unchanged once they are secreted into the the milk space. For this reason the composition of milk is likely to be similar to the composition of the solution within the secretory vesicles responsible for secretion of the aqueous phase of milk.

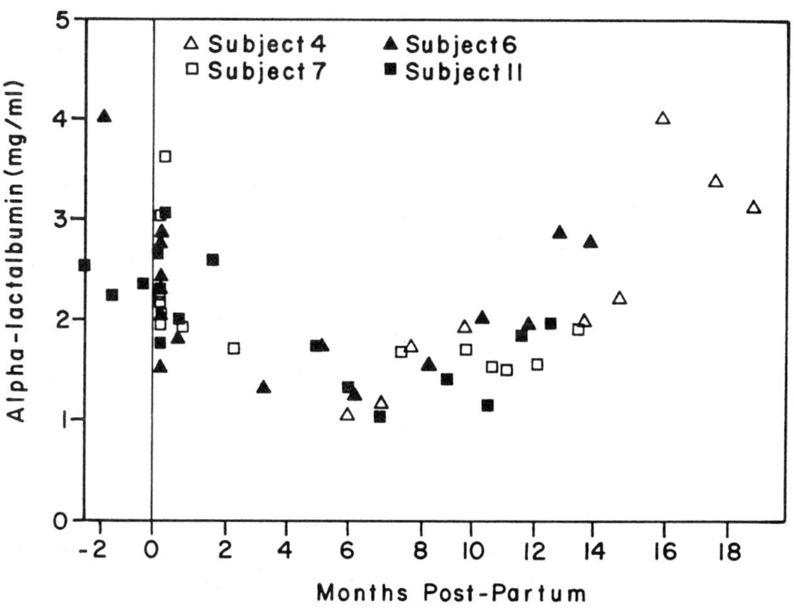

Fig. 8. Milk alpha lactalbumin concentration as a function of duration of lactation in four subjects who practiced gradual weaning after six months lactation. The points at negative times represent prepartum samples.

The question of whether the concentration of milk components within the secretory vesicles is similar to their concentrations within the terminal cisternae of the Golgi is more difficult to resolve. The assembly of the casein micelle, which requires millimolar activities of calcium, has been observed with the electron microscope to take place in the terminal cisternae of the Golgi apparatus and the secretory vesicles (21-22). This suggests that the calcium activity within these compartments may be similar to that in the milk (however, see footnote 1). Glucose has recently been shown to permeate the apical membrane rather freely (18). Further, there is considerable evidence suggesting that its concentration within the milk is similar to its concentration within the cytoplasm (4,23). Since glucose is thought to permeate the Golgi membrane easily (24) its concentration in milk may be representative of its concentration at the site of lactose synthesis. It is more difficult to make inferences about alpha-lactalbumin because of the possibility that some sort of retention takes place within the Golgi compartment. Because it is a soluble protein it seems less likely to be sorted or retained within the Golgi than would be membrane proteins, for example, galactosyl transferase. Further the concentration of alpha-lactalbumin within milk, ~1 mg/ml is sufficient to produce maximal activation of lactose synthesis (3) suggesting that the cofactor may not be conserved within the Golgi. We conclude that the concentrations of ionized calcium, glucose and alpha-lactalbumin within the milk may be at least be proportional to, if not representative of, their concentrations at the site of lactose synthesis.

The role of ionized calcium in the control of lactose synthesis

Powell and Brew (9) found that millimolar concentrations of calcium stimulated lactose synthesis by galactosyl transferase and alpha-lactalbumin derived from cow's milk in the presence of micromolar concentrations of Mn^{++}. On the basis of this finding they suggested that the calcium concentration within the Golgi regulated lactose synthesis. The finding that the ionized calcium concentration in milk, presumably reflecting the ionized calcium concentration within the Golgi, is unchanged during the declining phase of lactation suggests that calcium is not a regulatory agent during gradual weaning. Consistent with this conclusion we observed little change in the ionized calcium during the rising phase of lactation immediately post-partum (Allen and Neville, unpublished). Further, significant stimulation of galactosyl transferase by calcium is not observed in all species. We have recently observed in a vesicular preparation derived from mouse mammary gland that 5-10 mM calcium actually inhibits lactose synthesis at micromolar manganese concentrations (25, Neville and Witsel, unpublished). These data suggest that ionized calcium does not play a physiological role in the regulation of lactose synthesis.[1]

Alpha-lactalbumin and the control of lactose synthesis

In previous studies the concentration of alpha-lactalbumin was found to be related to the concentration of lactose both across species (10)

[1] Kuhn (personal communication) has recently suggested that lactose synthesis may be complete prior to the entry of calcium into the Golgi compartment. If this is the case, its concentration in milk could not be representative of its concentration at the site of lactose synthesis. On the other hand the question of calcium activation of galactosyl transferase is moot.

and over the course of lactation within one species (11) The lactose concentration in milk is a function, not only of the lactose secretion rate, but also of the rate of entry of other substances into the milk. In humans, for example, the lactose concentration does not change with decreases in milk volume until volumes have fallen below 100 g/day (14), that is, until the tight junctions between the alveolar cells have opened admitting much larger quantities of sodium and chloride into the milk. For this reason it is not clear what the significance of a relation between alpha-lactalbumin concentration and lactose concentration as opposed to lactose synthesis rate might be. In the present study the concentration of alpha-lactalbumin actually increased with decreasing lactose synthesis, strongly suggesting that the concentration of this co-factor within the Golgi is not a mechanism for regulation of lactose synthesis. Lönnerdal et al (13) reached a similar conclusion from studies of alpha-lactalbumin and lactose concentrations during lactogenesis in women. Although there is a general proportionality between the rate of alpha-lactalbumin secretion and the rate of lactose secretion, the present evidence indicates that this is not mediated by changes in alpha-lactalbumin concentration.

The role of glucose in lactose synthesis

The linear relation between milk glucose concentration and the lactose synthesis rate during the rising phase of lactation might suggest that glucose supply does play a regulatory role in lactose synthesis. A similar suggestion has been made for the goat by Faulkner and her colleagues (4) on the basis that the relation between lactose synthesis rate and milk glucose was a rectangular hyperbola as expected if Michealis-Menten kinetics are obeyed. This relationship does not fit our data in the human. Further there appears to be no consistent relation between the level of milk glucose and the lactose synthesis rate during the constant phase of lactation (Figs 3 and 7). Finally in the course of glucose clamp experiments on lactating women (26) we were able to increase the milk glucose from about 1.3 mM to 4.0 mM by doubling the plasma glucose. This increase had a minimal on the lactose synthesis rate. All these data suggest that glucose supply is not limiting for lactose synthesis in full lactation. It is not clear that the same is true in the face of low milk yields, but it does indicate that glucose access to the Golgi may not be a major regulator of lactose synthesis at least in humans.

One other point should be made here. The linear relation between the lactose synthesis rate and the milk glucose concentration suggests that the latter can be used as a rough index of the rate of milk secretion during the rising and declining phase of lactation. This could be a useful index of the adequacy of milk secretion under conditions where it is not possible to measure milk volume production in women.

What regulates lactose secretion?

The bottom line is that we do not know what regulates lactose secretion. There is indirect evidence from studies with rats in Kuhn's laboratory (personal communication) and from studies with mice in our own laboratory (Witsell and Neville, unpublished) that there is an unknown factor within the Golgi which stimulates lactose synthesis. Although Kuhn's data suggests an organic cation to be this unknown factor, its role in the regulation of lactose synthesis is unknown.

ACKNOWLEDGEMENT

The research reported here was supported by NIH contract HD 2-2801 and NIH grant HD 19547. We give our most sincere thanks to our subjects who gave unstintingly of their time and energy over the course of more than a year. Without their devotion to increasing our knowledge of human lactation this study would not have been possible.

REFERENCES

1. K. Brew and R.L. Hill, Lactose Biosynthesis. Rev. Physiol. Biochem. Pharmacol. 72:103-158 (1975).
2. N.J. Kuhn and A. White, The topography of lactose synthesis. Biochem. J. 148:77-84 (1975).
3. N.J. Kuhn, Lactose Synthesis: The Possibilities of Regulation, J. Dairy Sci. 63:328-336 (1980).
4. A. Faulkner, N. Chaiyabutr, M. Peaker, D.T. Carrick, and N.J.Kuhn, Metabolic significance of milk glucose. J. Dairy Res. 48: 51-56 (1981).
5. A. Faulkner, Glucose availability and lactose synthesis in the goat. Biochim. Soc. Trtans. 13: 496-497 (1985).
6. L.C. Threadgold, H.G. Coore, and N.J. Kuhn, Monosaccharide transport into lactating-rat mammary acini. Biochem.J. 204:493-501 (1982).
7. M.C. Neville, J.C. Allen, and C. Watters, C. The Mechanisms of Milk Secretion, in Lactation: Physiology, Nutrition and Breast-feeding. M.C. Neville and M.R. Neifert, Eds. Plenum, N.Y. pp. 49-102 (1983).
8. C.G. Prosser, L. Saint, and P.E. Hartmann, Mammary gland function during gradual weaning and early gestation in women. Aust.J. Exp. Biol. Med. Sci. 62:215-228 (1984).
9. J.T. Powell and K. Brew, Metal ion activation of galctosyltransferase. J. Biol. Chem. 251:3645-3652 (1976).
10. R.D. Palmiter, What regulates lactose content in milk? Nature 221:912-917 (1969).
11. K.R. Nicholas, P.E. Hartmann and B.L. McDonald, 1981, Alpha-lactalbumin and lactose concentrations in rat milk during lactation. Biochem. J. 194:149-154 (1981).
12. R.W. Turkington, K. Brew, T.C. Vanaman and R.L. Hill. The hormonal control of lactose synthetase in the developing mouse mammary gland. J. Biol. Chem. 243:3382-3386 (1968).
13. B. Lönnerdal, E. Forsum, and L. Hambraeus. A longitudinal study of the protein nitrogen and lactose contentsd of human milk from Swedish well-nourished mothers. Am.J.Clin.Nutr. 929:1127-1134 (1976).
14. M.C. Neville, C.E. Casey, R.P. Keller, and P. Archer, Changes in milk composition after six months of lactation: the effects of duration of lactation and gradual weaning. in Human Lactation: Effects of Maternal Factors on Milk Composition and Volume. M. Hamosh and A. Goldman, Eds. Plenum, N.Y. pp (1986).
15. J.C. Allen, and M.C. Neville, Ionized calcium in human milk determined with a calcium-selective electrode. Clin. Chem. 29:858-861 (1983).
16. J. Roth and E.G. Berger, Immunocytochemical localization of gtalactosyltransferase in HeLa cells: Codistribution with thiamine pyrophosphatase in trans-Golgi cisternae. J.Cell Biol. 93: 223-229 (1982).
17. J.L. Linzell and M. Peaker, Changes in colostrum composition and in the permeability of the mammary epithelium at about the time of parturition in the goat. J. Physiol. 243:129-151 (1974).

18. A. Faulkner, D.R. Blatchford and H.T. Pollock, The transport of hexoses across the apical membrane of the mammary gland of the goat. Biochem.Soc.Trans. 13: 69=89-690 (1985.)

19. M.C. Neville and M. Peaker, The secretion of calcium and phosphorus into milk, J. Physiol. 290:59-67 (1979).

20. A. Faulkner and M. Peaker, Reviews of the progress of dairy science: secretion of citrate into milk. J. Dairy Res. 49: 159-69 (1982).

21. R.J.Carroll, M.P. Thompson, and H.M. Farrell, Jr., Formation and structure of casein micelles in lactating mammary tissue, 28th Annual Proceedings Electron Microscopy Society of America, p 150. (1970).

22. C.W. Heald, and R.G. Sacke, Cytological comparison of milk protein synthesis of rat mammary tissue in vivo and in vitro. J. Dairy Science. 55:612-625 (1972).

23. L.C. Threadgold, and N.J. Kuhn, Monosaccharide transport in the mammary gland of the intact lactating rat. Biochem. J. 218:213-219 (1984).

24. M.D. White, W. Ward, and N.J. Kuhn, Pore properties of the Golgi membrane from lactating-rat mammary gland. Effects of pH and temperature and reconstitution into phospholipid vesicles. Biochem. J. 218: 213-219 (1984).

25. D. Witsel, P. Staiert, M.C. Neville. Metal ion activation of solubilized and vesicular galactosyl transferase from mouse mammary gland. Fed. Proc. 44:1516 (1985).

26. M.C. Neville, W.W. Hay, V. Lutes and L. Coughlin, Glucose clamp studies in lactating women: effects of glucose and insulin on milk glucose and lactose secretion. Fed. Proc. 45:901 (1986).

FEEDING THE PREMATURE INFANT: METHODS TO ASSESS LACTATION PERFORMANCE

Cutberto Garza, Richard Schanler, Judy Hopkinson, Gary Silber, Kathleen Motil, David Hachey, Nancy Butte, and Edward Emken

USDA/ARS Children's Nutrition Research Center
Department of Pediatrics, Baylor College of
Medicine and Texas Children's Hospital, Houston, TX

INTRODUCTION

The potential nutritional and immunologic benefits of human milk comprise the basis for its use in the feeding of premature infants. The prevailing consensus is that premature infants should be provided milk from their mothers. Early milk produced by women who deliver prematurely is likely to be more appropriate nutritionally, and perhaps immunologically, than is milk from later stages of lactation or milk produced by women who deliver at term. The implementation of this recommendation is complicated, however, by limits in the understanding of basic lactation physiology.

Nutrient Composition of Milk

Numerous studies have investigated the composition of milks produced by women who deliver at term or prematurely (1-6). Differences in the concentrations of protein, fat, Na, Mg, Ca, P, and Fe have been reported between preterm and term milks. Although most investigators agree that the concentrations of protein and Na are higher in the milks of women who deliver prematurely, there is less accord regarding relative and absolute differences in the concentrations of the other nutrients. The lack of agreement may result, in part, from the decreases in the concentrations of many nutrients as lactation progresses. Published data on this topic are difficult to interpret because of complicated perceptions of the manner in which nutrient concentrations are regulated. For example, stimulation to the mammary gland and maternal endocrine changes in the early postpartum period are anticipated to have interactive effects on the secretions of the mammary gland, yet specific interactions remain obscure. In addition, there are at least four sources of variability in nutrient concentrations which are of concern: within day, between day, interindividual, and experimental. Although exceptions exist, most published estimates of the variability of nutrient concentrations do not partition observed variabilities (7,8). There are few insights regarding the basis of this variability other than experimental error.

Immunologic Composition of Milk

The immunologic composition of milk produced by women who deliver prematurely also is distinct from that of women who deliver at term (9).

In a longitudinal study (10) of the effect of prematurity on selected immune components in human milk, we found that the mean concentrations of lactoferrin, lysozyme, and SIgA were higher in preterm milk. The patterns of change as lactation progressed were similar to those observed in term milk for lactoferrin and lysozyme concentrations. The concentration of total and secretory IgA, however, rose linearly during the sixth through the twelfth week in preterm milk, but did not change in term milk during the same period. The significance of these differences is unknown. The duration of pregnancy and lactation appears to be important in the regulation of the immunologic system of human milk. Conditions which initiate premature delivery, the incomplete maturation of the biochemical and endocrine changes associated with term pregnancy, or differences in the management of lactation (e.g., absence of a suckling infant and duration and frequency of milk expression) may each be important in the regulation of immune components in preterm milk.

Practical Concerns

Feeding maternal milk as opposed to donor milk to the premature infant requires that sufficient milk of an appropriate composition be produced to meet the infant's nutritional needs. Few data are available, however, that evaluate lactation performance in women who deliver prematurely. The remainder of this discussion will identify measures of lactation performance and describe techniques used in our laboratories to 1) aid in the quantitation of relationships between lactation performance and specific strategies to initiate and maintain lactation, 2) provide an improved understanding of the factors that regulate milk composition, and 3) evaluate the effects of lactation on maternal well-being.

MEASURES OF LACTATION PERFORMANCE

Milk Volume and Composition

Lactation performance may be evaluated from the quantity and quality of milk that is produced, the infant's growth or the duration that an exclusively breast-fed infant maintains a normal growth pattern, and the effects of lactation on maternal well-being. Of these parameters, daily milk volume may be the most sensitive indicator of lactation performance (11). This judgment is based on the apparent stability of the gross composition of milk from women with widely differing diets and energy stores. In contrast, a falling or inadequate milk volume more commonly is recognized as an early indicator of suboptimal lactation performance in women with a marginal or inadequate nutritional status. Although detailed studies may identify subtle changes in milk composition when milk volumes appear inadequate, available data suggest that after the third or fourth month of lactation, gross changes in human milk composition normally occur only after the initiation of glandular involution. An improved understanding of the regulation of milk composition will help assess the validity of this hypothesis.

Infant Growth

Measures of lactation performance that rely on infant growth are difficult to use because of unresolved questions about the adequacy of available growth standards, characteristics of "normal" growth patterns in human milk-fed infants, inferences which may be drawn from cross-sectional vs longitudinal approaches to the analysis of growth data, and influences other than diet on growth (12). These issues will not be discussed further.

Maternal Well-being

There is very little information available about the effects of lactation on maternal well-being. Most reported studies have dealt with issues of either maternal fertility or body composition. A few studies have addressed the effects of lactation on maternal bone mineral status (13,14). The need for more functional assessments is clear.

PRELIMINARY FINDINGS OF RECENT STUDIES ASSESSING LACTATION PERFORMANCE

Milk Volume and Lactation Management

Factors expected to influence lactation performance include reproductive history, diet and nutrient stores, length of pregnancy, physiologic maturation of the mammary gland during pregnancy and after delivery, feeding behaviors of the infant, general maternal physiologic status (e.g., maternal age, psychological stress, illness, and living conditions), individual characteristics (e.g., genetic make-up and endocrine-diet responses), and lactation management. In the absence of the stimulation provided normally by a suckling infant, lactation management takes on added importance because the frequency and duration of milk expression are determined solely by the mother.

We have estimated the effects of frequency and duration of milk expression on lactation performance in women who deliver prematurely. Thirty-five women who delivered healthy, appropriate for gestational age, VLBW infants between 28 and 30 weeks gestation were enrolled (15). The clinical course of these infants has been reported (16). Two of the 35 women were excluded from these preliminary analyses because of failure to comply with protocol requirements. Subjects were enrolled within 1 week of delivery, provided with an Egnell breast pump (Egnell, Inc., Cary IL), and aided in lactation management by a support team based in the hospital caring for their infants.

Generally, subjects were asked to empty both breasts 6 to 8 times per day. The subjects recorded the time and duration of milk expression and the volume of milk expressed for up to 60 days after delivery. Twenty-two women also provided 24-hr pools of milk. An aliquot of the 24-hr pool was reserved weekly for nutrient and immunologic analyses. Twenty-four-hour volumes of milk collected at 15 and 30 days have been regressed against the interval between delivery and the initiation of milk expression and the daily frequency and duration of milk expression. Parity, gravidity, prior nursing experience, and maternal age also have been examined for their associations with milk volume.

Milk volume on day 15 ($r = -0.44$, $p < 0.02$), but not day 30, was correlated negatively with the interval between delivery and initiation of milk expression. The change in milk volume between days 15 and 30 was related significantly to the average frequency of milk expression between day 15 and 30 (ΔVol = -344 + 68.5 [frequency/day]) and the daily average duration of pump use during the same interval (ΔVol = -76.8 + 1.24 [# min/24 hours]). The change in daily frequency of milk expression between days 15 and 30 was related positively to the net change in milk volume during this interval (ΔVol = 35.1 + 76.7 [frequency/day]). Maternal age also correlated positively with the change in milk volume during the indicated interval. Whether maternal age is a significant variable that is independent of parity, gravidity, and previous breastfeeding experience remains to be determined.

The relative efficacy of altering milk volume by changing either the frequency or duration of milk expression can be approximated cautiously from these relationships if one accounts for the mean duration of a single milk expression, approximately 20 minutes. The regression coefficients relating these management variables to the change in milk volume suggest that a change in the frequency of milk expression is approximately two to three times more effective in altering milk volume than is a change in the duration of milk expression. Importantly, adverse effects on milk volume due to delays in initiating milk expression can be overcome more easily by increasing the frequency of milk expression than by increasing the duration of milk expression. Additional studies are needed to determine whether changes in milk volume can be achieved by increases in the frequency of milk expression even if the breast is not emptied each time milk is expressed. Although changes in milk volume were related to these management variables, significant relationships seldom were observed between the variables and the absolute volume of milk produced.

Although multiple endocrine factors are likely contributors to the regulation of milk production, prolactin is believed to be the principal mediator of the positive association between milk volume and the frequency of milk expression. Most available data have been obtained in subjects who delivered term infants; however, similar responses are likely in women who deliver prematurely. Postpartum prolactin levels fall rapidly in women who feed their infants less than four to six times per day (17). The fall in prolactin levels appears most exaggerated in women who adopt this infrequent pattern of feeding during the first three months of lactation.

Regulation of Milk Composition

Milk volume can be altered substantially by changes in lactation management; milk composition, however, appears more stable. The effects of diet, for example, on milk composition can be summarized briefly (18). The consequences of dietary vitamin intakes are variable; the concentrations of water soluble vitamins appear to be influenced by recent dietary intake more easily than those of minerals and fat-soluble vitamins. The concentrations of protein nitrogen, lactose, and fat generally are less responsive to broad differences in diet, although the levels of specific milk proteins may be influenced by the amount of dietary protein (19). In contrast, alterations in the dietary pattern or content of fatty acids and carbohydrates will influence markedly the fatty acid composition of human milk (20). The picture of general stability in human milk composition is bolstered by observations of significant "tracking" of nutrient concentrations in milks of individual women. The concentrations of total N, protein N, lactose, fat, and calories were observed to correlate significantly (r ranged from 0.42 to 0.74, $p < 0.01$) with their subsequent monthly values (21). When mineral concentrations were evaluated, analogous r values ranged from 0.33 to 0.90 for Na, K, Mg, Ca, P, and Zn (22). Correlation coefficients above 0.7 were observed for Ca and Zn.

We have tested two approaches to identify factors which account for this relative stability. The first was used to evaluate the influence of feeding patterns on the energy concentration of milk (unpublished observations).

Milk samples were collected throughout the day from women exclusively breastfeeding their infants on demand. Subjects gave birth to term, healthy infants; the characteristics of these subjects have been reported (23). Subjects were followed monthly for the first four months of lactation. At each nursing over a 24-hr period, infants were offered one breast and milk was expressed from the other using an Egnell electrical breast pump. Subjects were asked not to exceed 15 minutes of pumping and to stop sooner if milk flow were reduced markedly. Feeding and pumping were done at alternate breasts at successive nursings. The gross energy content of milk was determined in an adiabatic bomb calorimeter (Parr Instruments, Moline, IL). As has been reported by others (24, 25) we found linear ($p < 0.01$) and quadratic ($p < 0.07$) trends when the energy content of milk was regressed against the time of day at which the milk was collected. In our study population, the mean energy content (kcal/L) of milk tended to increase throughout the day with the lowest values observed in the early morning. The energy content of milk, however, was related negatively to the volume of milk that was expressed and to the time interval preceding each milk expression. Furthermore, the time interval preceding each milk expression was correlated positively with the volume of milk expressed. The opposite effects of time lapse on the volume and energy content of milk probably result from the synthesis and/or secretion of fat. Lactose, the other major caloric constituent in human milk, is unlikely to be responsible because its osmotic role requires that its production and secretion be related closely to volume (26).

Further exploration of the dietary and mammary physiologic factors that regulate milk volume and fat content are required before these relationships may be understood adequately. In collaboration with Dr. M.R. Thomas, we have addressed this problem by assessing fat transport to the mammary gland and synthesis and transport of fat by the mammary gland. Two preliminary experiments have been conducted (27-29). The first involved the oral administration of three deuterium-labeled triglycerides, tripalmitin-9-10-$^2H_2$, triolein-14, 14, 15, 15, 17, 18-$^2H_6$, and trilinolein-15, 15, 16, 16, -$^2H_4$ (26). Milk and blood samples were collected from 3 women for 72 hours at specified intervals after the ingestion of the labeled triglycerides. Samples were analyzed by gas chromatography and gas chromatography-mass spectrometry. A 10-hour delay was observed between the test meal and the peak occurrence of the deuterated fatty acids in milk triglycerides (Fig. 1). This delay is unlikely to be accounted for by delayed gastrointestinal absorption since peak triglyceride enrichments in chylomicrons, very low density lipoproteins, and low density lipoproteins were observed before four hours, the earliest lipoprotein sampling point. Preliminary results obtained in this experiment suggest that the chylomicron is quantitatively the most important immediate source of dietary lipids in the mammary gland. These results also support the selective conservation of palmitate 2-monoglycerides across the blood into the alveolar lumen. Integration of results obtained over the 72-hr period suggests that approximately 8 to 16% of the administered label was secreted milk.

The synthesis of fatty acids by the mammary gland has been explored in preliminary experiments utilizing dietary manipulations (28) and ^2H_2O administration (29). Fatty acid synthesis by the mammary gland is accomplished by the usual mechanisms observed in other tissues with one important exception. In most tissues, thioesterase I terminates the growth of acyl chains on fatty acid synthase at fats of 16 carbon length. In the mammary gland, thioesterase II modifies the usual product specificity by interacting with the fatty acid synthase complex. Thioesterase II catalyzes the hydrolysis of the thioester linkages of medium chain acyl moieties to the multienzyme complex (30). The outcome of this modification is evident from the work of Insull et al. (20) on a single lactating subject. When the subject consumed a fat-free diet at an energy level approximately 1/3 above her estimated requirement, lauric and myristic acids made up 39% of the fat on a molar basis compared with 20% when the subject was on a conventional diet. We have recently assessed the effects of 5% fat, 15% protein, and 80% carbohydrate diets on the fat composition of milk produced by women who delivered premature infants. Subjects were placed on the diet 9 to 12 days following delivery. Energy levels were set at each subject's usual intake unless levels were below 2300 kcal/day, the minimum intake the protocol allowed. During the dietary period, lauric and myristic acid concentrations rose compared with prediet values (Table 1).

Based on observations reported by Rittenberg and Schoenheimer (31), we have conducted studies to demonstrate that middle chain-length fatty acids secreted in milk can be labeled successfully following the oral administration of ^2H_2O. Fat synthesis may be evaluated by this technique because the majority of hydrogens on newly synthesized saturated fats appear to be derived from body H_2O. We anticipate that these techniques will allow us to explore the influence of maternal-diet-endocrine-lactation management relationships on the fat content of human milk.

Maternal Well-being

Most measures of lactation performance focus on either the infant or the milk that is produced. Few studies have been directed at the effect of lactation on maternal health. We have begun such studies by obtaining baseline data on protein kinetics in women who are not at any apparent nutritional risk. Accordingly, 12 healthy women (32) have been studied at 1, 5, and 12 months postpartum. Dietary protein was set at 1.0 g/kg/day and dietary energy intakes were set at maintenance levels as determined by 3-day diet records. This constant diet was consumed for 7 days. Maternal milk production was estimated by test-weighing the infant for a minimum of 72 consecutive hours. At the end of the dietary interval, a 96-hour nitrogen balance was conducted and a primed, constant, intravenous infusion of 1-^{13}C leucine was performed in the fasted state. The enrichment of ^{13}C in plasma leucine and expired CO_2 was determined by gas chromatography-mass spectrometry and isotope-ratio mass spectrometry, respectively. When adjusted for the stage of lactation, significant associations were observed between the rate of leucine incorporation into proteins synthesized by the mother and the volume of milk consumed by the infant. Energy and nitrogen outputs in milk also were related positively to the rate of leucine incorporation into total body protein synthesized by the mother (Table 2). These initial results relating maternal protein metabolism to conventional indices of lactation performance have identified avenues for future work. These techniques can be used to explore adaptations of protein metabolism during lactation in women in distinct nutritional states.

SUMMARY

The current preference to feed human milk to premature infants is impeded by our inadequate understanding of basic lactation physiology. Although some of the problems stem from a lack of knowledge of the premature infant's nutrient needs, the incomplete understanding of maternal factors that govern milk composition and volume is also a significant shortcoming. We have conducted studies to quantitate the relationships between milk production and specific management variables. We also have explored tracer methodologies to study the regulation of milk composition and the effects of lactation on maternal metabolism in women who deliver at term and prematurely.

Incorporation of Oleic Acid-d6 into selected plasma and milk triglycerides

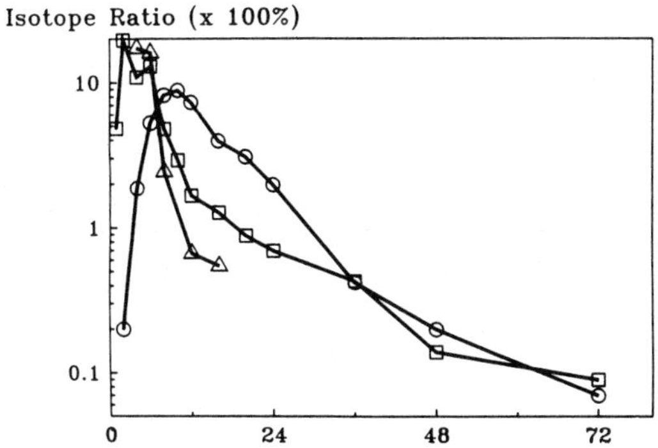

Fig. 1. Mean deuterium enrichment in milk triglycerides (-o-), total plasma triglycerides (-□-), and chylomicrons (-△-). Representative data obtained in one of the three lactating women are presented.

TABLE 1. Lauric and Myristic Acid Content of Human Milk Before and During Controlled Dietary Period[a]

Subject	Prediet (%)	Day 4 (%)
1	13	24
2	10	14
3	7	15
4	11	14
5	12	17

[a] Expressed as % total fat. Changes between prediet and controlled period, significant at $p < 0.05$.

Table 2 Relationship Between Maternal Leucine Metabolism and Milk Production

$$VOL = 0.51 + 0.18\ LI - 0.44\ PPA^{a}$$
$$N = 4.18 + 0.30\ LI - 1.12\ PPA^{a}$$
$$E = 1.41 + 0.15\ LI - 0.32\ PPA^{b}$$
$$N = -8.44 + 0.37\ LQ - 0.79\ PPA^{c}$$

Where: Vol = Milk volume (g/kg maternal body wt/day)
N = Milk nitrogen (mg/kg maternal body wt/day)
E = Milk energy (kcal/kg maternal body wt/day)
LI = Leucine incorporation (mol/kg/hr)
LQ = leucine flux (mol/kg/hr)
PPA = time since delivery (months)

$^{a}p < 0.01$, $^{b}\ p < 0.01$, $^{c}\ p < 0.02$

ACKNOWLEDGMENTS

This research is supported by a contract (NO1-HD-2-2814) from the National Institutes of Health and by the USDA/ARS Children's Nutrition Research Center, Department of Pediatrics, Baylor College of Medicine and Texas Children's Hospital, Houston, TX. This project has been funded in part with Federal funds from the U.S. Department of Agriculture, Agriculture Research Service under Cooperative Agreement number 58-7MNI-6-100. The contents of this publication do not necessarily reflect the views or policies of the U.S. Department of Agriculture, nor does mention of trade names, commercial products, or organizations imply endorsement by the U.S. Government.

REFERENCES

1. S.A. Atkinson, M.H. Bryan, and G.H. Anderson, Difference in nitrogen concentration in milk from mothers of term and premature infants, J. Pediatr. 93:67 (1978).
2. J.A. Lemons, L. Moye, D. Hall, and M. Simmons, Differences in the composition of preterm and term human milk during early lactation, Pediatr. Res. 16:113 (1982).
3. S.A. Atkinson, I.C. Radde, G.W. Chance, M.H. Bryan, and G.H. Anderson, Macromineral content of milk obtained during early lactation from mothers of premature infants, Early Hum. Dev. 4:5 (1980).
4. R.J. Schanler and W. Oh, Composition of breast milk obtained from mothers of premature infants as compared to breast milk obtained from donors, J. Pediatr. 96:679 (1980).
5. S.J. Gross, R.J. David, L. Bauman, and R.M. Tomarelli, Nutritional composition of milk produced by mothers delivering preterm, J. Pediatr. 96:641 (1980).
6. N.F. Butte, C. Garza, C.A. Johnson, E.O. Smith, and B.L. Nichols, Longitudinal changes in milk composition of mothers delivering preterm and term infants, Early Hum. Dev. 9:153 (1984).
7. M.F. Picciano and H.A. Guthrie, Copper, iron, and zinc contents of mature human milk, Am. J. Clin. Nutr. 29:242-254, 1976.

8. M.C. Neville, R.P. Keller, J. Seacat, C.E. Casey, J.C. Allen, and P. Archer, Studies on human lactation. I. Within-feed and between-breast variation in selected components of human milk, Am. J. Clin. Nutr. 40:635 (1984).
9. S.J. Gross, R.H. Buckley, S.S. Wakii, D.C. McAllister, R.J. David, and R.G. Faix, Elevated IgA concentration in milk produced by mothers delivered of preterm infants, J. Pediatr. 99:389 (1981).
10. A.S. Goldman, C. Garza, B.L. Nichols, C.A. Johnson, E.O. Smith, and R.M. Goldblum, Effects of prematurity on the immunologic system in human milk, J. Pediatr. 101:901 (1982).
11. C. Garza and N.F. Butte, The effect of maternal nutrition on lactational performance, in: "Proceedings on the Symposium on Frontiers in Clinical Nutrition," N. Kretchmer, ed., Aspen Press, Rockville, Maryland (1985).
12. R.G. Whitehead and A.A. Paul, Growth charts and the assessment of infant feeding practices in the western world and in developing countries, Early Hum. Dev. 9:187 (1984).
13. G.M Chan, N. Ronald, P. Slater, J. Hollis, and M.R. Thomas, Decreased bone mineral status in lactating adolescent mothers, J. Pediatr. 101:767 (1982).
14. P.J. Atkinson and R.R. West, Loss of skeletal calcium in lactating women, J. Obstet. Gynecol. 77:555 (1970).
15. J. Hopkinson, R.J. Schanler, and C. Garza, Milk production in mothers of preterm infants, (abstr) Am. J. Clin. Nutr. 41:852(1985).
16. R.J. Schanler, C. Garza, and B.L. Nichols, Fortified mothers' milk for very low birthweight infants: results of growth and nutrient balance studies, J. Pediatr. 107:437 (1985).
17. P. Delovoye, M. Demaegd, J. Delogne-Desnoeck, and C. Robyn, The influence of the frequency of nursing and of previous lactation experience on serum prolactin in lactating mothers, J. Biosoc. Sci. 9:447 (1977).
18. B.L. Nichols, and V. Nichols, Nutrition in pregnancy and lactation, Nutr. Abstr. Rev. 53:259 (1983).
19. A.K. Deb and H.R. Cama, Studies on human lactation. Dietary nitrogen utilization during lactation, and distribution of nitrogen in mother's milk, Br. J. Nutr. 16:65 (1962).
20. W. Insull, J. Hirsch, T. James, and E.H. Ahrens, Jr., The fatty acids of human milk II: Alterations produced by manipulation of caloric balance and exchange of dietary fats, J. Clin. Invest. 38:443 (1959).
21. N.F. Butte, C. Garza, E.O. Smith, and B.L. Nichols, Human milk intake and growth performance of exclusively breast-fed infants, J. Pediatr. 104:187 (1984).
22. N.F. Butte, C. Garza, E.O. Smith, and B.L. Nichols, Milk and mineral intakes of 45 exclusively breast-fed infants, (abstr) Fed. Proc. 43:667 (1984).
23. N.F. Butte, C. Garza, J.E. Stuff, E.O. Smith, and B.L. Nichols, Effect of maternal diet and body composition on lactational performance, Am. J. Clin. Nutr. 39:296 (1984).
24. F.E. Hytten, Clinical and chemical studies in human lactation II: Diurnal variations in major constituents of milk, Br. J. Med. 1:179 (1954).
25. A. Prentice, A.M. Prentice, and R.G. Whitehead, Breast-milk fat concentrations of rural African women I: Short-term variations within individuals, Br. J. Nutr. 45:483 (1981).
26. N.J. Kuhn, D.T. Carrick, and C.J. Wilde, Lactose synthesis: the possibilities of regulation, J. Dairy Sci. 63:328 (1980).
27. D.L. Hachey, E.A. Emken, M.R. Thomas, L. Brown, R.O. Adloff, C. Garza, B.L. Nichols, and P.D. Klein, Incorporation of deuterium-labeled dietary lipids into specific milk lipid fractions of human milk, in: "Abstracts of 2nd Int. Cong: Essential Fatty Acids," (1983).

28. G. Silber, J. Hopkinson, D. Hachey, and C. Garza, Modification of fatty acid composition in human milk, (abstr) Am. J. Clin. Nutr. 43:688 (1986).

29. D.L. Hachey, G. Silber, L. Brown-Booth, W. Wong, L. Lee, C. Garza, and P.D. Klein, Endogenous fatty acid synthesis by the mammary gland, (abstr) Am. J. Clin. Nutr. 43:687 (1986).

30. C. Garza and J. Hopkinson, Human milk synthesis and secretion, in: "The Theory and Practice of Nutrition in Pediatrics," R. Grand and J.L. Sutphen, eds, Butterworth, (In press 1985).

31. D. Rittenberg and R. Schoenheimer, Deuterium as an indicator in the study of intermediary metabolism XI: Further studies in the biological uptake of deuterium into organic substrates, with special reference to fat and cholesterol formation, J. Biol. Chem. 121:235 (1937).

32. K.J. Motil, C.M. Montandon, D. Hachey, T. Boutton, P.D. Klein, and C. Garza, The relationship between whole body leucine metabolism and milk production in lactating women (abstr), Am. J. Clin. Nutr. 43:678 (1986).

RELATIONSHIP OF MATERNAL AGE TO BREAST MILK VOLUME AND COMPOSITION

K. G. Dewey, D. A. Finley, M. A. Strode and B. Lönnerdal

Department of Nutrition
University of California
Davis, CA 95616

INTRODUCTION

There is at present little information regarding the relationship of maternal age to breast milk volume and composition. In the 1950's, Hytten reported that "the clinical impression is certainly widespread that the elderly primipara is particularly liable to experience difficulty in establishing and maintaining lactation" (1, p. 844). He noted that few reports had distinguished between the effect of age and that of parity, but cited several studies of milk output during the first 7 to 10 days postpartum that controlled for parity. Those data and his own showed that "older" primiparae (24 yrs or older) produced less milk in the first week postpartum than younger primiparae (16-23 yrs). He speculated that milk yield is "dependent on the amount of functional tissue in the breasts," which may decrease with age due to "disuse atrophy." He suggested that lactational capacity is greatest before age 20, and declines thereafter. However, the data presented were limited to milk production during the first week or two of lactation. In Wallgren's pioneering study in Sweden (2) in which breast milk intake during the first six months was measured, no relationship was found between maternal age and milk intake. Unfortunately, the data to support this finding were not shown, nor was the age range of the mothers indicated. More recently, Butte et al. (3) reported no significant association between maternal age and milk volume during the first four months. However, there was not a wide range in maternal age (28.0 ± 3.1 yr) in the study population.

Even fewer data are available with regard to the effect of maternal age on milk composition. Hytten (1) found no association between maternal age and milk fat content on day 7 post-partum. In a review of studies prior to 1952, Morrison (4) reported a tendency for total nitrogen content to decrease and for fat content to increase with maternal age. However, it is difficult to separate the effect of parity from that of age, given the data presented.

Our interest in the relationship of maternal age and lactational performance originally stemmed from concern about the ability of teenaged mothers to successfully breast-feed their infants. Because of the lack of information on this subject, we initiated a study of 25 lactating mothers, 14-20 years of age, from four Sacramento, California, area school programs for pregnant teens and teen parents. Since the diets of teenage girls may be nutritionally inadequate in several respects (5) and a variety of physiological and psychological factors may compete with the demands of lactation at this age (6-7), our objectives were to examine dietary intake, infant feeding patterns, breast milk composition, and infant growth (as an indicator of the adequacy of milk production).

In order to examine the influence of maternal age over a wider range of age, data from the teen study (8) were subsequently pooled with data from four other lactation studies among adult mothers (9-12). The information presented below is derived from the teen study and the composite data analysis.

METHODS

Detailed methodology for the teen study is described elsewhere (8). Subjects were visited 1-9 times (mean 3.7 visits) during months 1-10 of lactation. At each monthly visit, the infant's weight and length were recorded, a 24-hr dietary recall of foods eaten by the mother was completed, and a milk sample was collected.

For the composite analysis, information on milk composition was included for infants 6-26 wks of age and for milk volume (measured by test-weighing) only for those 6-18 wks of age. (Milk volume is generally unchanged between one and four months [9]). Milk volume data were included only if at least 2 complete days of test-weighing had been completed. Infants consuming more than approximately 80 Kcal/day from sources other than breast milk were excluded. In cases where the subject was a participant in an experimental study (10,12) only data from the "baseline" period were utilized.

Milk composition data were based on milk samples collected between 6 a.m. and 1 p.m. by complete expression of one breast. In most cases, more than one milk sample per mother was collected and fit our selection criteria. Analysis of milk for protein, fat, lactose, and fatty acid composition is described elsewhere (9,11). Except for fatty acid data, composition data were averaged for each mother for statistical comparisons relating to maternal age and other variables. Because our longitudinal study (9) had shown little change in protein, fat, or lactose concentrations between 6 and 26 wks, we did not adjust for month of lactation in calculating these means.

Data analysis was performed using SPSSX subprograms for Pearson correlation, partial correlation, and Student t test.

RESULTS AND DISCUSSION

For the composite analysis, suitable data were available from 102 mothers for milk composition and from 53 mothers for milk volume. Characteristics of all 102 subjects are listed in Table 1. Maternal age ranged from 15 to 37 yrs, with a mean of 27.5 yrs. Mothers were generally well-nourished, as reflected by an average percent of ideal weight of 110 and a pregnancy weight gain of 36.7 lb. Number of feedings per day averaged 7, ranging from 4 to 11.

Table 1. Characteristics of subjects

	Mean	SD	Range
Maternal age (yr)	27.5	5.4	15-37
Pregravid weight-for-height (% of ideal)	103	14	76-153
Pregnancy weight gain (lb)	36.7	9.7	4-68
Current weight-for-height (% of ideal)	110	17	85-177
Nursing frequency	7.0	1.6	4-11

Figure 1 illustrates the association between maternal age and milk volume, measured among women 21-37 yrs of age. The relationship is not statistically significant ($r = 0.16$, $p > 0.10$). These results are consistent with those of Wallgren (2) and Butte et al. (3), and refute the idea that older mothers produce less milk than younger mothers. However, it is possible that maximum potential milk output could vary with age; Hytten and other early investigators measured milk output by extraction rather than by test-weighing. Our data cannot be used to determine maximum milk output. Furthermore, it should be noted that our subjects were those who were still successfully breast-feeding at 6-18 wks post-partum. Those with lower milk volumes would not have been eligible for our study if their infants were supplemented. The percentage of mothers who initiate breast-feeding and subsequently experience true inadequacy of milk production, and the proportion of those mothers who are "older," is unknown.

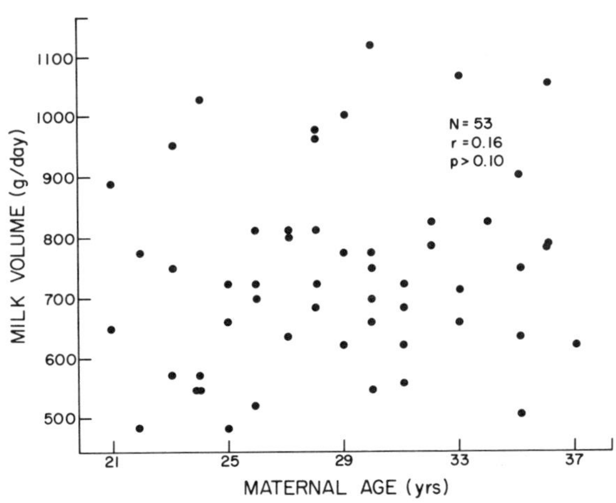

Fig. 1. Relationship between breast milk volume and maternal age.

Growth patterns of infants of teenaged mothers are shown in Fig 2. Fourteen infants were exclusively breast-fed for 3 or more months; none of these were below the 25th percentile of weight-for-age at 3-6 months. Of 11 infants supplemented with formula before 3 months, poor growth was cited as a reason for supplementation in three cases. Milk volume thus appeared adequate for 88% of the teenaged mothers.

It should be noted that the teenagers in our study were probably unusual in several respects, due to the influence of the teen parent programs in which they were enrolled. Two of the programs placed a strong emphasis on nutrition, and students were encouraged to gain a large amount of weight (about 35 lb) during pregnancy. The other two programs also

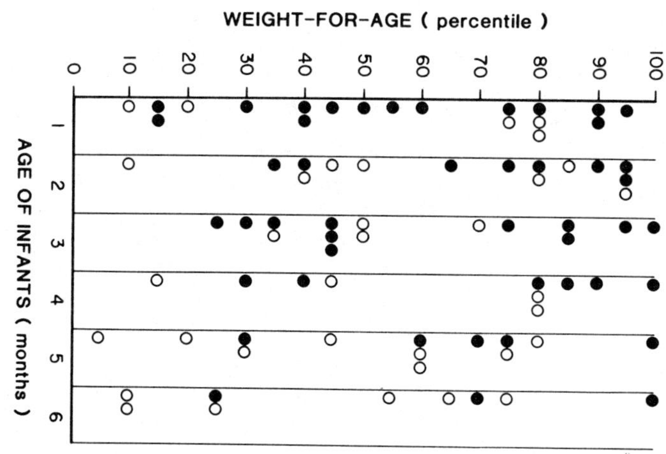

Fig. 2. Weight-for-age of infants of teenaged mothers.

offered nutrition education as part of their prenatal classes. Table 2 lists the average dietary intake of these subjects. Mean energy intake was quite high: 2,897 Kcal/day. In addition, social support for breast-feeding was strong among both teachers and peers. Nonetheless, the data indicate that teenaged mothers are generally capable of providing sufficient breast milk for their infants.

The relationship of maternal age to the lactose, protein, and fat content of breast milk is shown in Figures 3-5. Lactose concentration was positively correlated with maternal age, even when controlling for parity ($r = 0.55$, $p = 0.00001$). The lower values (6.4-7.2 g/100 ml) were found primarily in milk of teenaged mothers. (A subset of their milk samples was reanalyzed to ensure that the observed difference was not a "batch" effect reflecting laboratory variation in the assay). One possible explanation for these low values is that mammary gland development of

Table 2. Dietary intake of lactating teenagers (N=25)

	Mean	SD	Mean % RDA
Energy (kcal)[a]	2,897	699	112
Protein (g)	115	27	176
Fat (g)	144	40	---
Carbohydrate (g)	290	87	---
Fiber (g)	3.18	1.74	---
Calcium (mg)	1,640	601	110
Phosphorus (mg)	2,005	588	134
Iron (mg)	15.0	3.8	84
Potassium (mg)	3,594	1,128	---
Vitamin A (IU)	5,995	2,839	101
Thiamine (mg)	1.49	0.44	94
Riboflavin (mg)	2.88	0.91	161
Niacin (mg)	20.0	5.0	106
Vitamin C (mg)	155.9	136	157

[a] Energy breakdown: 16% of kcal from protein; 40% of kcal from carbohydrate; 44% of kcal from fat.

younger mothers might be less mature, with greater transfer through "leaky" junctions and a consequently lower lactose concentration in the milk (13). However, we also observed somewhat lower concentrations of sodium and potassium in milk from teenagers, which would not be consistent with this explanation. Another possibility is that some glucose is being diverted to other tissues to be used as energy for growth, as a low glucose concentration is one factor that may limit lactose production (14). The significance of the lower lactose concentration among teens is unclear, but it is unlikely to adversely affect infant health to any great extent.

Protein concentration was unrelated to maternal age (Fig 4). Fat concentration was negatively correlated with maternal age, even when controlling for parity ($r = -0.25$, $p < 0.05$). However, since milk samples were collected at only one feeding during the day and diurnal patterns of fat concentration may vary among mothers, the significance of this association is unclear.

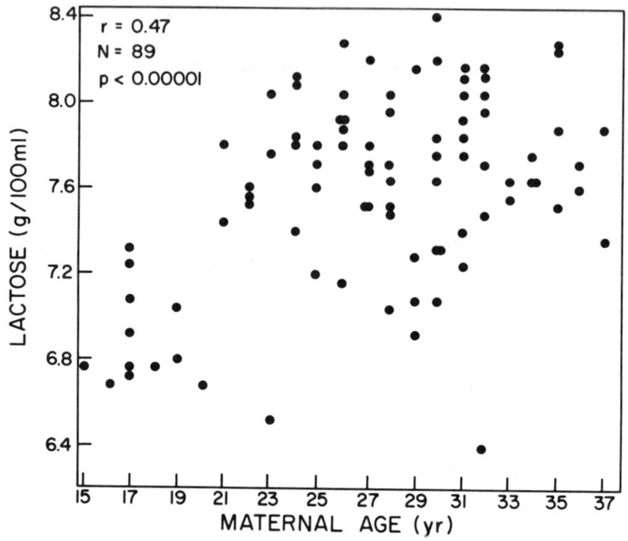

Fig. 3. Relationship between milk lactose concentration and maternal age.

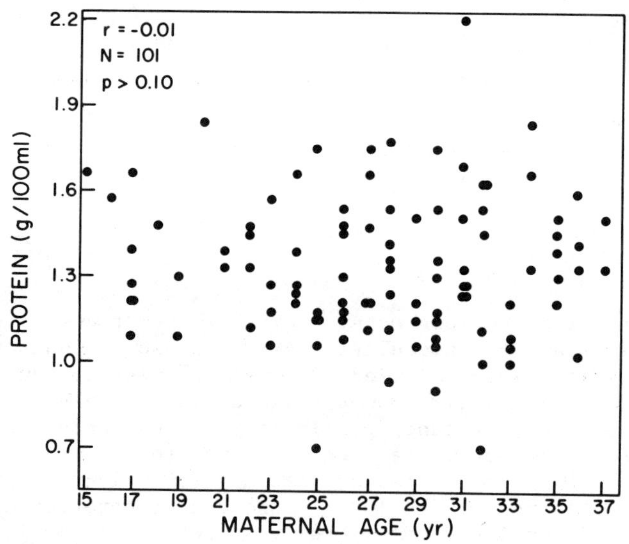

Fig. 4. Relationship between milk protein concentration and maternal age.

In a subsample of women 22-37 yrs of age, fatty acid composition of samples was determined. Table 3 shows the partial correlations of these constituents with maternal age, controlling for month of lactation. Fatty acids C16:1 and C18:1, expressed as percent of total fat, decreased with age, while fatty acids C8:0 and C20:3 increased with age. The latter two fatty acids must be synthesized in the mammary gland, whereas the former

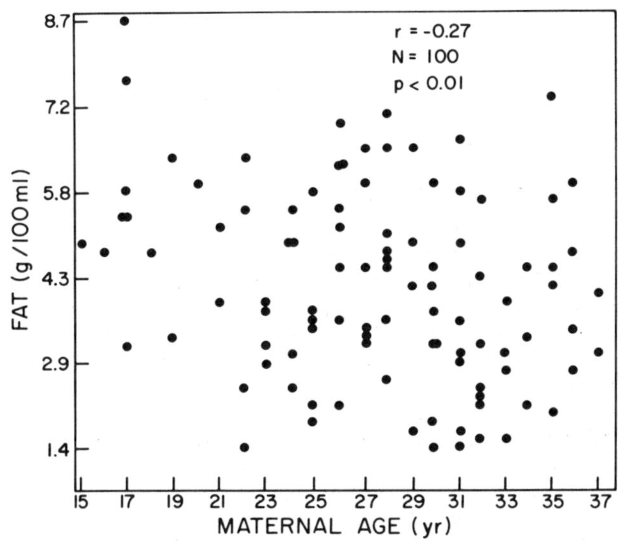

Fig. 5. Relationship between milk fat concentration and maternal age.

two are derived from fat stores or diet. However, when examining the influence of parity, it was found that the level of C18:1 was significantly lower in multiparous women (32.6 vs. 30.9% of fat, $p < 0.01$). The only other fatty acid that was related to parity was C10:0, which was higher in multiparous women (1.0 vs. 1.2% of fat, $p < 0.05$). When controlling for parity, the correlations of C8:0, C16:1, and C20:3 with maternal age were still significant, but that of C18:1 with age was no longer significant. The correlation of C8:0 with maternal age is somewhat artificial, however, because three of the older mothers had unusually high levels of C8:0; when those values are deleted, the correlation is not significant.

Table 3. Partial correlation of maternal age with milk fatty acid composition (as percent of total fat), controlling for month of lactation (1-6 mo.)

	R	N (samples)	P
C8:0	0.24	64	0.03
C10:0	0.00	74	NS
C12:0	-0.05	74	NS
C14:0	0.11	89	NS
C16:0	0.10	89	NS
C16:1	-0.19	89	0.03
C18:0	0.09	89	NS
C18:1	-0.20	89	0.03
C18:2	0.03	89	NS
C18:3	0.07	89	NS
C20:2	0.03	87	NS
C20:3	0.20	87	0.03
C20:4	0.06	87	NS
C22:6	-0.06	80	NS

Several other maternal factors were examined in relation to milk volume and composition, including parity, pregravid percent of ideal weight, pregnancy weight gain, current percent of ideal weight, and nursing frequency. A comparison of primiparous and multiparous mothers 20 yrs of age or older is shown in Table 4. No significant differences were found in milk volume or composition. Rattigan et al. (15) and Butte et al. (3) also reported no effect of parity on milk volume among Australian and American women, respectively. However, Prentice (16) recently reported a marked decrease in milk volume in Gambian mothers with ten or more children. Milk fat concentrations were also significantly lower among multiparous women, in agreement with reports of earlier investigators (17). This effect was apparently independent of maternal fat stores. It is likely that the range in parity among mothers in our studies is too small to detect a parity effect, as most of our multiparous mothers had only two or three children.

Table 4. Relationship of parity with milk volume and composition among women 20 yrs (Mean ± SD)

	Primiparous	Multiparous
Milk volume (g/day)	729 ± 140 (N=30)	755 ± 177 (N=23)
Protein (g/100 ml)	1.37 ± 0.24 (N=52)	1.38 ± 0.28 (N=38)
Fat (g/100 ml)	4.21 ± 1.61 (N=51)	3.75 ± 1.44 (N=38)
Lactose (g/100 ml)	7.62 ± 0.40 (N=46)	7.74 ± 0.39 (N=32)

The other maternal factors examined are shown in Table 5. None of these was significantly associated with milk volume or macronutrient composition, except for a positive correlation between protein concentration and pregnancy weight gain. Similarly, Butte et al. (3) found no association between several maternal anthropometric indices and milk quantity or quality. Among Gambian women, Prentice et al. observed no relationship between maternal subcutaneous fat deposits, as measured by triceps skinfold thickness, and milk volume (16), but they did report a positive correlation with milk fat concentration. In a subsequent supplementation study of Gambian mothers (18), milk protein and fat concentrations increased slightly in supplemented mothers. The range of maternal nutritional status in our studies and in the study of Butte et al. is undoubtedly much narrower than would be encountered in a less privileged population, making it unlikely to observe any effect of maternal malnutrition on lactational performance.

Table 5. Correlations between maternal factors and milk volume and composition

	Milk Volume	Protein	Fat	Lactose
Pregravid weight-for-height	0.16	0.03	-0.01	0.13
Pregnancy weight gain	-0.08	0.25*	0.09	-0.16
Current weight-for-height	-0.07	0.06	-0.01	0.08
Nursing frequency	-0.02	-0.07	-0.06	-0.01
Protein	-0.34**	---	---	---
Fat	-0.10	0.33***	---	---
Lactose	-0.13	0.06	-0.16	---

* $p < 0.05$
** $p < 0.01$
*** $p < 0.001$

Among mothers in our studies, there was no association between nursing frequency and milk volume or composition. In contrast, Rattigan et al. (15) found a positive correlation between feeding frequency and milk production, but their study included both exclusively and partially breast-fed infants 1 to 15 months of age. Within exclusively breast-feeding mothers, nursing frequency does not appear to be related to milk volume, once milk production has been established (in the first few weeks). This is not to imply that milk volume could not be altered by changing nursing frequency by individual mothers.

Table 5 also shows the relationships we found between milk volume and macronutrient composition. It should be kept in mind that milk samples were taken on days other than the test-weighing days, and that both milk volume and composition data are average values for each mother.

Nonetheless, we observed a negative correlation between protein concentration and milk volume, which is in agreement with the findings of Saint et al. (19). Those authors also reported a positive association between lactose concentration and milk volume for the first five days post-partum. We did not find such a relationship, but our samples were mature milk, in which lactose concentrations show much less change. Fat concentration was unrelated to milk volume, which is consistent with the reports of Saint et al. (19) and Prentice et al. (16).

Protein and fat concentrations were positively associated, while lactose showed an inverse trend with fat concentration ($r = 0.16$, $p = 0.066$). The relationships among milk constituents remain unclear, but it is interesting that these associations are consistent with the increase in protein and fat, but decrease in lactose concentrations following supplementation of Gambian women (18). Because the influence of maternal diet on lactational performance will be covered in other reports, it will not be discussed herein.

SUMMARY

To summarize, we found no evidence that maternal age or parity have any effect on breast milk volume in our study population. Teenaged mothers are capable of successful lactation, though milk lactose concentrations are lower. Most of the variation in milk volume and macronutrient composition in relatively well-nourished populations is unrelated to maternal age or anthropometric indicators.

REFERENCES

1. F. E. Hytten, Clinical and chemical studies in human lactation. VIII. Relationship of the age, physique, and nutritional status of the mother to the yield and composition of her milk, Brit. Med. J. 2:844 (1954).
2. A. Wallgren, Breast milk consumption of healthy full term infants, Acta. Paediet. 32:778 (1944).
3. N. F. Butte, C. Garza, J. Stuff, E. O. Smith and B. L. Nichols, Effect of maternal diet and body composition on lactational performance, Am. J. Clin. Nutr. 39(2):296 (1984).
4. S. D. Morrison, Human milk: Yield, proximate principles and inorganic constituents, Technical Communication No. 18, Commonwealth Bureau of Animal Nutrition, Rowett Research Institute, Bucksburn, Aberdeenshire, Scotland (1952).
5. D. D. Marino and J. C. King, Nutritional concerns during adolescence, Pediatr. Clin. North Am. 27(1):125 (1980).
6. L. E. Feinfeld and M. L. Speller, Children bearing children: adolescent pregnancy, Pa. Med. 83:16 (1980).
7. E. R. McAnarney, Adolescent pregnancy--a national priority, Am. J. Dis. Child. 132:125 (1978).
8. S. Lipsman, K. G. Dewey and B. Lonnerdal, Breast-feeding among teenage mothers: milk composition, infant growth and maternal dietary intake, J. Pediatr. Gastroent. Nutr. 4:426 (1985).
9. K. G. Dewey and B. Lonnerdal, Milk and nutrient intake of breast-fed infants from one to six months: relation to growth and fatness, J. Pediatr. Gastroent. Nutr. 2:497 (1983).
10. M. A. Strode, K. G. Dewey and B. Lonnerdal, Effects of short-term caloric restriction on lactational performance of well-nourished women, Acta. Paediat. Scand., in press.
11. D. A. Finley, B. Lonnerdal, K. G. Dewey and L. E. Grivetti, Breast milk composition: fat content and fatty acid composition in vegetarians and non-vegetarians, Am. J. Clin. Nutr. 41:787 (1985).

12. K. G. Dewey and B. Lonnerdal. Infant self-regulation of breast milk intake, in submission.
13. M. C. Neville and M. R. Neifert, eds., "Lactation: physiology, nutrition and breast-feeding," Plenum Press, New York (1983).
14. E. A. Jones, Lactose biosynthesis, in: "Lactation: a comprehensive treatise," B. L. Larson, ed., Academic Press, New York (1978).
15. S. Rattigan, A. V. Ghisalberti and P. E. Hartmann, Breast-milk production in Australian women, *Br. J. Nutr.* 45:243 (1981).
16. A. Prentice, The effect of maternal parity on lactational performance in a rural African community, in: "Human Lactation - Effect of Maternal Environmental Factors," M. Hamosh and A. Goldman, eds., Plenum Publishing Corp., New York (1986).
17. B. Belavady and C. Gopalan, Chemical composition of human milk in poor Indian women, *Ind. J. Med. Res.* 47:234 (1959).
18. A. M. Prentice et al., Dietary supplementation of lactating Gambian women. I. Effect on breast milk volume and quality, *Hum. Nutr.:Clin. Nutr.* 37C:53 (1983).
19. L. Saint, M. Smith and P. E. Hartmann, The yield and nutrient content of colostrum and milk of women from giving birth to 1 month post-partum, *Brit. J. Nutr.* 52:87 (1984).

MILK LETDOWN AND THE CONCENTRATION OF FAT IN BREAST MILK

P.E. Hartmann, S.E.G. Morgan and P.G. Arthur

Department of Biochemistry
University of Western Australia
Perth WA 6009
Australia

INTRODUCTION

Fat contributes 54% of the gross energy content of human milk[1] but is by far the most variable component of breast milk. Although the concentration of milk fat has been reported to vary over the course of 24 h [2,3,4,5] by far the largest changes in the concentration of fat in milk occur between the beginning and the end of a single breast feed[3]. Indeed, visible compositional changes occur, with fore milk at the beginning of a breast feed usually appearing a watery bluish-white and hind milk at the end of a breast feed usually appearing white and creamy.

The change in milk fat during milk withdrawal poses no difficulties in investigation of mammary function in dairy species where it is possible to obtain a mixed sample of milk during the milking process. In women it is extremely difficult to obtain a representative sample of mixed milk during normal suckings. Consequently, the concentration of fat quoted for human milk may be subject to considerable error depending upon which values are taken to be representative of the average concentration of fat in the milk consumed by the infant during a breast feed.

Although a number of theories have been advanced to explain the change in the concentration of fat in milk during milk withdrawal[3,6,7,8,9,10,11] no one theory has been universally accepted. However, the modified filtration theory of Whittlestone[7] has the most general acceptance. Irrespective of the explanations which have been advanced, it is clear that the changes which are observed in the concentration of fat during milk withdrawal eventuate from a complex interaction between the physiology of the milk ejection reflex, the physical nature of the milk fat globules and the mechanics of milk withdrawal.

The present study was undertaken to determine the relationship between the change in the concentration of fat during a breast feed with the volume of milk taken during a feed and the time interval between breast feeds. To ensure that physiologically meaningful results were obtained, the mothers were studied in their homes and milk yield was determined independently for each breast over a period of 26 h.

METHODS

Subjects

The five lactating women who participated in this study were demand feeding their infants. The women were at the 4,5,7,11 and 12 months of lactation and breast feeding their 4th, 1st, 2nd, 1st and 2nd child, respectively.

Analytical Methods

Milk yield was determined independently for each breast over a period of about 26h. The method involved test weighing the mother on an accurate electronic balance (Sauter Model EC 240, ED 3300, FSE Scientific, Perth) and correcting the mother's loss in weight during each breast feed for the evaporative weight losses of the mother over the period of the breast feed. The women collected small samples (<2.0 ml) of breast milk before and after each breast feed during the period that the milk yield was measured. Milk fat was measured by a modification of the method of Martin[12]. Milk was diluted (1:20 v/v in isopropanol) and the milk triacylglycerols extracted and hydrolyzed. The glycerol moiety was then quantitated colourmetrically against a trioleate standard.

RESULTS

Milk Yield

The milk yield for both breasts for the women at 4,5,7,11 and 12 months of lactation was 816, 907, 374, 987, 466, 793 g/24h, respectively. The milk yield at each feed for each breast over the 24 h period for the mother at 4 months of lactation and the mother at 11 months of lactation are shown in Figure 1 and 2, respectively. The milk yield from the right breast was from 45-59% of the total yield of both breasts for the five mothers.

Milk Fat

The average concentration of fat in the fore and hind milk samples for each of the five mothers is presented in Table 1. The average concentration of fat in the fore milk ranged from 29% to 83% of the concentration of fat in the hind milk for each of the mothers with an overall mean of 56%. The mean (± SD) for the concentration of fat in the fore and hind milk samples was 22.4, 19.6, 24.3, 25.6 and 26.7 g/l for the mothers at 4,5,7,11, and 12 months of lactation respectively, and the overall average concentration of fat in the milk from the five mothers was 23.6 g/l.

The changes in the concentration of fat between fore and hind milk at each feed for right and left breasts for the mothers at 4 and 11 months of lactation are presented in Figures 1 and 2, respectively. Whereas 14 of 16 and 12 of 14 of the fore and hind samples showed a distinct increase in the concentration of fat for the mothers at 4 and 11 months of lactation respectively, the other samples either showed no change or a decrease in fat concentration. A similar trend was observed in the other mothers and in total, 66 breast feeds showed an increase, 3 showed no change and 5 showed a decrease in the concentration of milk fat between fore and hind milk samples.

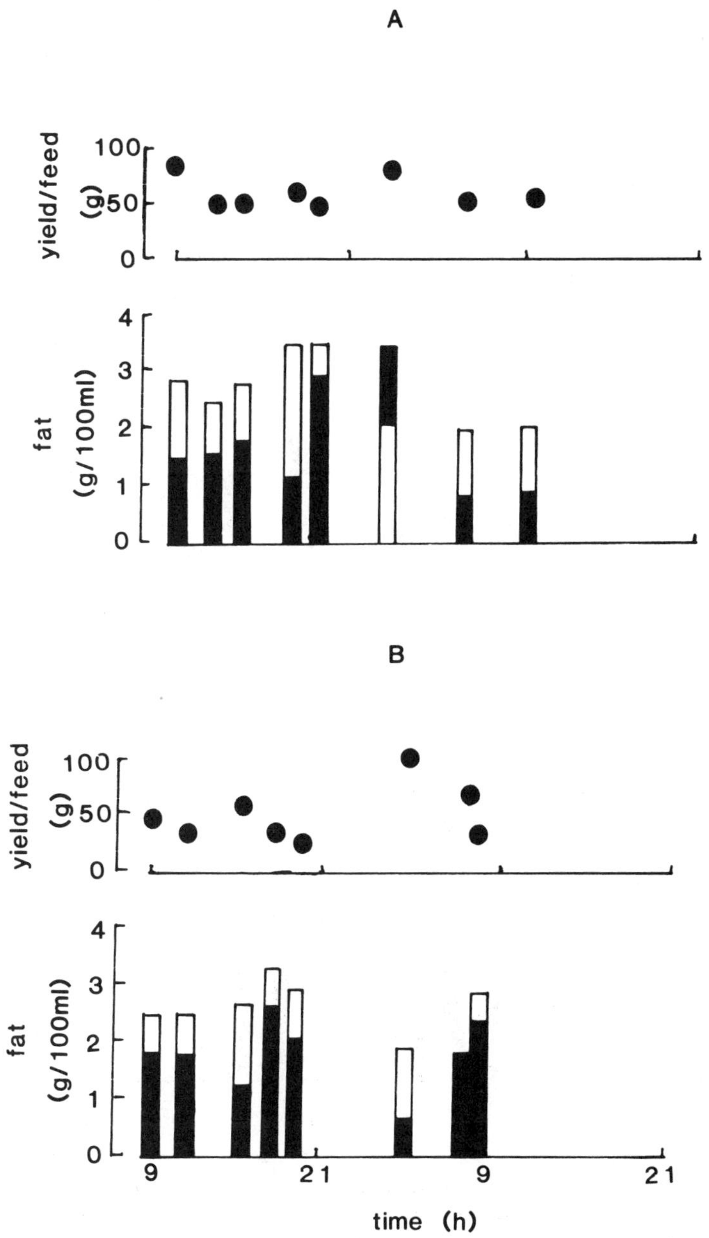

Figure 1. The yield of milk (o) from the right (A, 445 g/24h) and left (B, 371 g/24h) breasts at each breast feed over a period of 24h for the mother at 4 months of lactation together with the concentration of fat in fore milk (solid section of histogram) and hind milk (open section of histogram).

There were significant positive correlations between milk yield and the increase in the concentration of fat at each breast feed for the left breast of the mother at 4 months of lactation (r = 0.93) and right breast of the mother at 11 months of lactation (r = 0.81). In total of the 10 breasts studied only

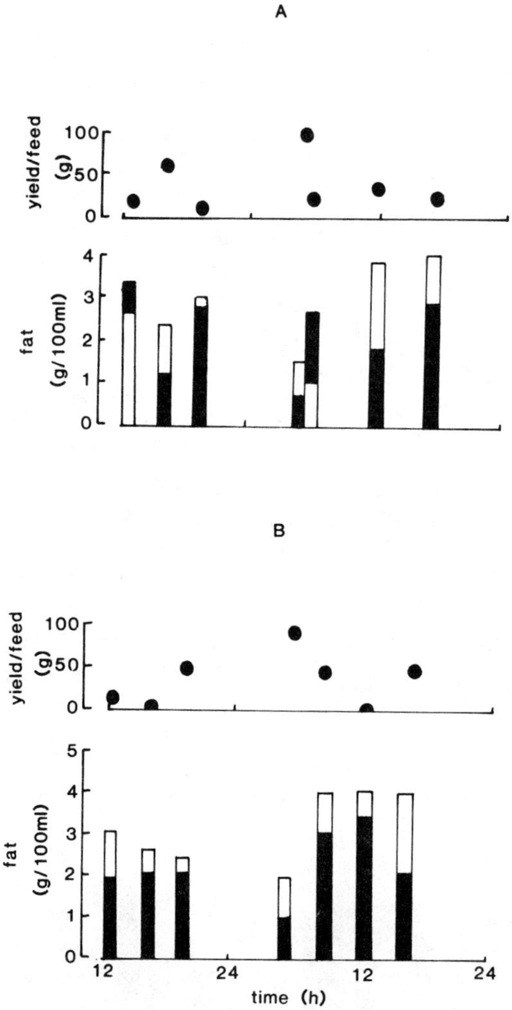

Figure 2. The yield of milk (o) from the right (A, 264 g/24h) and left (B, 182 g/24h) breasts at each breast feed over a period of 24h for the mother at 11 months of lactation together with the concentration of fat in fore milk (solid section of histogram) and hind milk (open section of histogram).

3 showed a significant correlation between milk yield and the increase in the concentration of fat during a breast feed. However, none of the women showed any relationship between the interval between breast feeds and change in the concentration of fat in the hind milk of one breast feed and the fore milk of the next breast feed.

DISCUSSION

Milk yield for each breast at each breast feed was determined by weighing the mother before and after breast feeding and again 20 min after the breast feed using an accurate electronic balance. The weight change during the 20 min period after the breast feed was used to calculate the rate of evaporative weight loss of the mother. The evaporative weight loss of the mother during breast feeding was then estimated and the change in weight of the mother during the breast feed was corrected for evaporative weight loss. We found that failure to correct for evaporative weight loss resulted in an over estimation of milk yield by about 15% if the mother was test weighed and an under estimation of milk yield by about 10% if the infant was test weighed.

Table 1. The concentration of fat (g/l) in fore and hind milk samples for each breast for each of the five mothers. The values presented are the means (± SD) for the milk samples collected at each breast feed during a 24h period.

Mother	Right Breast		Left Breast	
	Fore	Hind	Fore	Hind
4 mth	17 ±9	27 ±6	17 ±6	26 ±4
5 mth	12 ±9	24 ±10	12 ±6	27 ±5
7 mth	17 ±6	29 ±8	20 ±12	32 ±11
11 mth	22 ±10	27 ±8	22 ±8	32 ±9
12 mth	12 ±7	42 ±15	14 ±12	38 ±12

The concentration of fat in fore milk was considerably less than that in hind milk (Table 1) and this finding is in agreement with those of a number of other workers[3,4,13,14,15,16]. However, as with the observations of Dorea et al.[14], during some breast feeds there was a decrease in the concentration of fat between fore and hind milk.

We have calculated the average concentration of fat in the milk taken in by the infant by taking the mean of the concentration of fat in the fore and hind milk. However, Watson et al.[17], have demonstrated that the sequential changes in the concentration of fat during milk withdrawal in women is not linear, with the concentration of fat in milk increasing more rapidly as increasing volumes of milk were withdrawn from the breast. Thus it is likely that the true average concentration of fat in the milk taken in by the infant in the present study was closer to the concentration in hind milk rather than that in fore milk. Human milk is usually considered to contain from about 40 g/l fat[1] based on analysis of milk samples collected by evacuation of the breast either manually or by breast pump. It is apparent that the average concentration of fat in the milk taken in by the demand fed infants in the current study (Table 1) was considerably less than 40 g/l. Part of this difference may have been due to the underestimation of the concentration of fat in milk by the use of the triolean standard in the current study[18].

Prentice et al.[4] suggested that the concentration of fat in breast milk collected by either breast pump or manual expression from both breasts may bear little relationship to the concentration of fat in milk ingested by a breast fed infant during normal lactation especially in communities where demand feeding is practiced. However, to assess the effects of milk yield and interval between breast feeds on the change in the concentration of fat in fore and hind milk in demand fed infants it is not only necessary to collect fore and hind milk samples from each breast at each breast feed over a period of 24h, but it is also essential to measure milk yield from individual breasts as the concentration of fat can differ between breasts of an individual at any one breast feed [3,10]. Whereas Prentice et al.[4] reported that the within feed and between feed changes in the concentration of fat in breast milk were largely explained by differences in the volume of milk ingested by the infant at each feed and the time interval between feeds, no strong relationship was found between these factors in the present study. It is of interest that Prentice et al.[4] observed that the highest circadian concentrations of fat in milk occurred during the early morning at a time when the milk yield was lowest. Such a change would be expected from the observations of Watson et al.[17] if proportionally more milk was withdrawn from the breast of the women at this time. In contrast, in Western Australian women a circadian pattern in the concentration of fat in breast milk is not apparent (Figures 1 and 2) and milk intake may be related to the infant's appetite more than to the mother's ability to synthesize milk[19]. These factors may explain the difference between the present study and that of Prentice et al.[4].

SUMMARY

The yield and concentration of fat in breast milk in milk collected at the beginning (fore) and end (hind) of each breast feed from each breast were determined over a period of 24h for 5 mothers. The mothers were feeding their infants on demand and were at 4,5,7,11 and 12 months of lactation and milk yield was measured by test weighing the mothers before and after each breast feed and correcting the mother's weight change for evaporative weight loss during the duration of each breast feed.

The milk yield for both breasts for the women at 4,5,7,11 and 12 months of lactation was 816, 907, 374, 987, 466, 793 g/24h, respectively, and the yield of milk from the right breast was 45-59% of the total yield. The mean (±SD) concentration of fat in fore milk for each breast of each of the mothers ranged from 12 ±7 to 22 ±10 g/l and that in hind milk from 26 ±4 to 42 ±15 g/l. However, the change in the concentration of fat between fore and hind milk was not closely related to either milk yield or the interval between breast feeds. These findings are compared to previous observations on women in developing countries breast feeding on demand and to those on women who have fully expressed their breast milk.

ACKNOWLEDGEMENTS

We wish to thank the members of the Nursing Mothers' Association of Australia for participating in the study and the National Health and Medical Research Council for financial support.

REFERENCES

1. Oftedal, O. T., 1984, Milk composition, milk yield and energy output at peak lactation: A Comparative Review, in: "Physiological Strategies in Lactation," M. Peaker, R. G. Vernon, C. H. Knight, ed., Academic Press, London.
2. Gunther, M. and Stanier, J. E., 1949, Diurnal variation in the fat content of milk, Lancet, 2:235-237.
3. Hytten, F. E., 1954, Clinical and chemical studies in human lactation, Brit. Med. J. , 1:175-182.
4. Prentice, A., Prentice, A. M., and Whitehead, R. G., 1981, Breast-milk fat concentrations of rural African women. 1. Short-term variation within individuals, Br. J. Nutr. , 45:483-494.
5. Harzer, G., Haug, M., Dieterich, I., and Gentner, P. R., 1983, Changing patterns of human milk lipids in the course of lactation and during the day, Am. J. Clin. Nutr. , 37:612-621.
6. Hammond, J., 1936, The physiology of milk and butterfat secretion, Vet. Rec. , 16:519-535.
7. Whittlestone, W. G., 1953, Variations in the fat content of milk throughout the milking process, J. Dairy Res. , 20:146-153.
8. Zaks, M. G., 1962, The relationships between milk removal and synthesis, in: "Motor apparatus of the mammary gland," A. T. Cowie,ed., Oliver and Boyd, Edinburgh.
9. Hall, B., 1975, Changing composition of human milk and early development of appetite control, Lancet , 1:779-781.
10. Hall, B., 1979, Uniformity of milk, Am. J. Clin. Nutr. , 32:304-312.
11. Woolridge, M. W., Baum, J. D., and Drewett, R. F., 1980, Does a change in the composition of human milk affect sucking patterns and milk intake, Lancet, ii:1292-1293.
12. Martin, P. J., 1975, A quick inexpensive method for serum triglycerides, Clinica Chimica Acta , 62:79-88.
13. Forsum, E., and Lonnerdal, B., 1979, Variation in the contents of nutrients of breast milk during one feeding., Nutr. Rep. Int. , 19:815-820.
14. Dorea, J. G., Horner, M. R., and Lucia, V., 1982, Correlation between changeable human milk constituents and milk intake in breast-fed babies, J. Pediatrics , 101: 80-83.
15. Neville, M. C., Keller, R. P., Seacat, J., Casey, C. E., Allen, J. C., and Archer, P., 1984, Studies on human lactation. I. Within-feed and between -breast variation in selected components of human milk, Am. J. Clin. Nutr. , 40:635-646.
16. Saner, G., and Yuzbasiyan, V., 1984, Diurnal and longitudinal variatons in fat, energy and trace element content of human milk, Nutr. Rep. Int. , 29:1181.
17. Watson, M. A., Alford, E. S., Dill, C. W., Richter, R. L., and Garza, C., 1982, Compositional changes during sequential sampling of human milk, Nutr. Rep. Int. , 26:1105.
18. Anderson, G. H., Atkison, S. A., and Bryan, M. H., 1981, Energy and macronutrient content of human milk during lactation from mothers giving birth prematurely and at term., Am.J.Clin.Nutr., 34:258-265.
19. Saint, L., Maggiore, P., and Hartmann, P.E., 1986, Yield and nutrient content of milk in eight women breast feeding twins and one woman breast feeding triplets, Br. J. Nutr. , in press.

MATERNAL FACTORS IN LACTATION FAILURE

Ruth A. Lawrence

University of Rochester School of Medicine
Division of Neonatology
Rochester, N.Y.

Lactation failure is not clearly defined in the literature and has been given a variety of definitions which can be summarized as: (a) failure of the breasts to produce minimum of milk for example 200 cc per day, (b) failure to thrive in the infant i.e. failure to sustain growth in a normal infant within 2 standard deviations of the norm for that infant, and (c) failure of the mother to achieve her pre-set goal for duration of lactation (1).

For the purpose of this discussion we will use the first definition modified to be failure to produce adequate milk to maintain growth in the infant.

Lactation failure has been attributed in modern literature predominantly to psychosocial interference with the release of milk (2,3). In the human it has been suggested that all post partum women can produce milk. On close inspection, however, it is apparent that this is not true and indeed there are women who can not produce milk. No systematic study of lactation failure has been reported to date, although isolated case reports support the fact that some women can not produce milk.

If the animal model is explored first, there are more data as the production of milk has been the focus of much study especially in the dairy species (4). Lactation failures are rare in most other mammals as the off spring is dependent upon milk for survival and thus the trait is not transmitted because the young are starved to death. The role of infection of the mammary gland and the endometrium in causing agalactia has been demonstrated in sows (5). Although it has been suggested that infection causes low levels of prolactin and oxytocin to be secreted by the pituitary, the association is not well understood. Dairy species are bred for milk production and treated vigorously for infection in order to ensure maximum milk production.

Although the exact hormonal mechanisms are not well described, it is acknowledged in the literature reporting bovine research that the milk yield of a cow is influenced by her individual temperament, by her behavioral response to other members of the herd, and by the interactions with the herdsmen as well (6). Proper attention to these concerns have influenced milk yields and been credited with increased productivity. Much of what has been recommended to enhance human production has simulated this approach of creating a tranquil environment for the mother while nursing her infant.

Primary inhibition of milk secretion is associated with decreased levels of prolactin in non-ruminants. The association of stress to failure to let-down led to the study of adrenaline and its impact on milk production and release. The first observations by Ely and Petersen reported that adrenaline inhibited the contractile responses of the mammary alveoli to oxytocin (7). This was subsequently thought to be mediated by the affect of adrenaline on the mammary blood vessels causing vasoconstriction and restriction of flow of oxytocin to the myo-epitheleal cells (8). Adrenaline was also noted to compete for receptor sites on the myoepithelium. The site of central inhibition of release of oxytocin is still under discussion while the peripheral affects of adrenaline on the myoepithelium are thought to be pharmacological (4).

In addition to stress, ergot derivatives are also known to depress or stop lactation in non-ruminants by inhibiting the release of prolactin from the anterior pituitary (9). Interference with the transport and discharge phases of the secretory process resulting in the retention of milk within the alveolar cells has been attributed to certain plant alkaloids and lethins (10). Colchicine, vincristine, vinblastine, and concanavalin are known examples (11). These plant alkaloids are available to grazing animals.

The mechanisms involved in lactation failure in the human are complex, but can be defined in three main categories:

(a) depression or inhibition of anterior pituitary functions reasonable for the milk synthesis in the alveolar cells;

(b) depression or inhibition of the transport and discharge of the synthesized products from the cells into the alveolar lumen;

(c) depression or inhibition of the milk-ejection reflex which results in back pressure within the alveoli and ultimately cessation of synthesis (12) (see Figure 1).

In human, lactation function is measured indirectly by the growth of the off spring. In dairy animals the product is "milk", but in the human, the product is "the infant." Maternal factors associated with lactation failure can be separated into two major headings: those causes associated with poor production of milk and those associated with poor let-down or release of milk. For generations it has been stated that all women can make milk, but some can not release it - this is not true, indeed, some will fail to produce adequate milk (13). There is no data on the true incidence of production failure, although Raphael claims that only 5 percent of the world's women can not breastfeed for physical reasons. It is probably in the range of one percent of women from our own estimates. Our experience in Rochester is unique because we see only the severe cases that have resulted in failure to thrive in the infant. Usually when feeding does not go well, the infant is switched to formula and no analysis is made regarding lactation failure. It is only when the mother perseveres, that the true problem is exposed as the infant fails to grow in spite of all efforts.

"Insufficient milk" is given by mothers as well as by professionals, as the number one reason for cessation of breastfeeding in most studies on length of breastfeeding (14). In a study of the "Insufficient Milk Syndrome," Gussler and Briesemeister provide a biocultural explanation demonstrating complex transcultural etiology for the inability of some women to produce sufficient milk. They suggest that the syndrome stems from the spread of non-biological breastfeeding patterns in industrialized and urbanized societies (15) (see Figure 2).

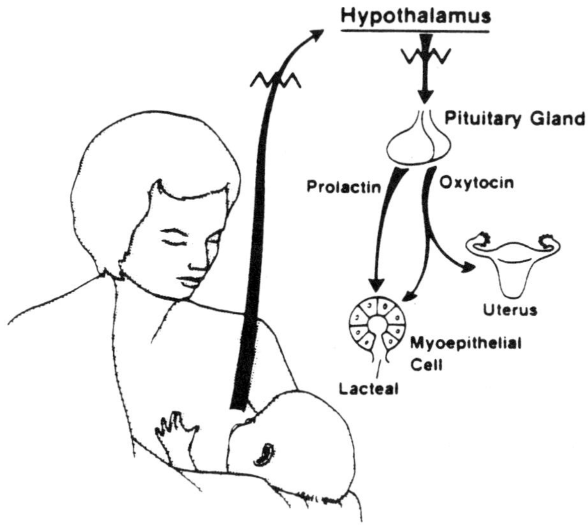

Figure 1. Diagrammatic outline of ejection reflex arc. When infant suckles breast, he stimulates mechanoreceptors in nipple and areola that send stimulus along nerve pathways to hypothalamus, which stimulates the posterior pituitary to release oxytocin. It is carried via bloodstream to breast and uterus. Oxytocin stimulates myoepithelial cell in breast to contract and eject milk from alveolus. Prolactin is responsible for milk production in alveolus. It is secreted by anterior pituitary gland in response to suckling. Stress such as pain and anxiety can inhibit letdown reflex. The sight or cry of infant can stimulate it.
R.A. Lawrence, "Breastfeeding: A Guide for the Medical Profession," 2nd edition, The C.V. Mosby Company, St. Louis, Toronto, Princeton (1985).

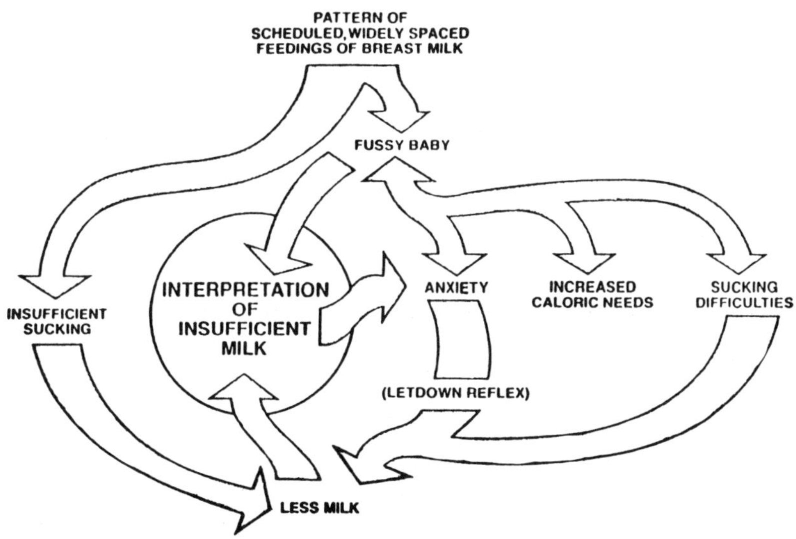

Figure 2. Implications of Non-Biologic Breast Feeding.
J.D. Gussler, and L.H. Briesemeister, The Insufficient milk syndrome: A biocultural explanation, Medic. Anthrop. 4:1-24 (1980).

The amount of sucking directly affects the quantity of milk produced. When the number of feedings are increased, the amount of milk produced is increased according to studies by Egli and Newton in 1961 (16) and by multiple investigators since that time (17, 18). Gussler and Briesemeister propose that (see Figure 2) the modern pattern of infrequent feeds may, therefore, provide a direct pathway to reduced milk production, perceived and reported by mothers as insufficient milk because of the behavior of the crying, fussy, hungry infant, who is fed arbitrarily by the clock (15). The anxious mother correctly interprets the cries as hunger but then assumes it is her milk that is inadequate. Instead of increasing feedings, a bottle is interjected. The bottle may produce quiet and satiation only confirming the mother's suspicions, i.e. her milk is at fault. The further reduction in sucking results in lower milk production and an increase in maternal anxiety which in turn inhibits let down. "Nonbiological breastfeeding results in real or perceived milk insufficiency and often early termination of breastfeeding." (15)

If one examines the lactation process as the interaction of mother and infant then the problem of lactation failure will have infant causes and maternal causes. The clinician is usually confronted with the question of "failure-to-thrive" in the infant instead of "failure to produce by the mother" or lactation failure. The diagramatic outline of such a diagnostic dilemma entails looking to the infant and to the mother (see Figure 3). We can quickly see that some of the infant causes pertain solely to the infant who received adequate milk and nutrients but has decreased absorption, decreased utilization or increased needs. A small number of infants have inadequate sucking mechanism and thus inadequately stimulate the breast to produce and release milk. This is a secondary cause of lactation failure that can be investigated by examining the infant for neurological, structural, or scheduling abnormalities (see Table 1). It should be pointed out that infants who are depressed at birth due to maternal anesthesia or analgesia may well suck poorly for several days and then will be underfed because of diminished stimulation to the breast. This inadequate intake weakens the infant by starvation to further perpetuate the problem unless appropriate management intervenes (19). Similarly the infant with hypoxia, low apgars, or hypoglycemia is unable to adequately stimulate milk production at first and then is slowly starved as milk supply dwindles and the infant is too weak to complain.

Infants with structural problems such as cleft lip or cleft palate may also have difficulty adequately stimulating the breast, either because of inability to create a seal and negative pressure, or inability to control tongue motions (2).

When we direct our attention to solely maternal causes, the etiologies of poor production may be hormonal, nutritional, pharmacological, and psychological, in addition to anatomical. Both production and release of milk can be affected (20). Production can be limited by inadequate glandular tissue as are described by Niefert in this volume (18). Gross deficiencies of precursor substances under relative starvation can influence productivity, but as described earlier by Hartmann and Lonnerdal, actually diminished production in less well fed women is actually uncommon and does not occur until an absolute lack of nutrients has been reached (21).

Poor production can be caused by illness in the mother (22). Chronic illness, such as diabetes, need not be a cause since the diabetic usually does very well, given the increased calories and insulin. The diabetic is capable of producing sufficient milk. Other chronic disease in the mother need not be a problem in milk production. The illness that does interfer with lactation may be the vague nondescript state of "unwellness" that goes undiagnosed and untreated. Illness represents an added stress or drain on productivity. The most widely recognized deterent to ·ood milk production

TABLE 1

Conditions Associated with or Causing Disorders Of Sucking and Swallowing

Absent or diminished suck	Mechanical factors interfering with sucking	Disorders of the swallowing mechanism (not including esophageal abnormalities)
Maternal anesthesia or analgesia	Macroglossia	Choanal atresia
Anoxia or hypoxia	Cleft lip	Cleft palate
Prematurity	Fusion of gums	Micrognathia
Trisomy 21	Tumors of mouth or gums	Postintubation dysphagia
Trisomy 13-15	Temporomandibular ankylosis or hypoplasia	Palatal paralysis
Hypothyroidism		Pharyngeal tumors
Neuromuscular abnormalities		Pharyngeal diverticula
Kernicterus		Familial dysautonomia
Werdnig-Hoffmann disease		
Neonatal myasthenia gravis		
Congenital muscular dystrophy		
Infections of the CNS		
Toxoplasmosis		
Cytomegalovirus infection		
Bacterial meningitis		

Modified From:

J. Gryboski, Philadelphia, 1975 W. B. Saunders Co. from R. E. Behrman, J. M. Driscoll, Jr., and A. E. Seeds eds., Neonatal-perinatal medicine: diseases of the fetus and infant, ed. 2, St. Louis, 1977, the C. V. Mosby Co.

is failure to let down milk due to stress especially fatigue or more appropriately exhausion. Release of prolactin has been found to be influenced by stress (23). Newton and Newton demonstrated the relationship of stress to the amount of milk a women produced at a given feeding. They also demonstrated the therapeutic effect of giving the woman oxytocin following the stress with an associated return to normal of the milk ejected (14).

In industrial societies, motherhood receives no special privileges, and a women is expected to resume all other responsibilities promptly which may interfere with establishment of lactation due to stress. It must be acknowledged, however, that this desire to escape the influence and assistance of parents and relatives, has led nuclear families to isolate themselves from help and support by their own choice. Some women, in their quest for natural and home-like birth, have fled the supportive hospital within hours to assume total responsibility for the new baby before lactation becomes established. In most tradiational cultures, however, there is a mechanism for supporting the new mother, leaving her only to nourish the infant and recover her strength (15). In modern society, however, there are women who are unable to continue the excessive pace and care for a new baby 24 hours a day. They have not learned to pace themselves and carefully monitor their own rest and recuperation. The result is lactation failure.

In 1840, Sir Astley P. Cooper noted that "the secretion of milk proceeds best in a tranquil state of mind and with a cheerful temper," in his volume on the anatomy of the breast (24). Cooper had recognized the destructive influence of stress and fatigue on lactation.

With increased information available about the hormonal control of milk production, it has been suggested that hormone deficiency can lead to lactation failure (25). Clinically, the best example is Sheehan's Syndrome, a well described entity known to obstetricians to be associated with obstetrical catastrophe and shock. It is considered that the pituitary is selectively compromised by the shock and rendered inactive or unresponsive to stimuli. The condition may lead to total pituitary atrophy or in some cases only long term hypopituitarism. Clinically, first signs of the syndrome are a failure of the breasts to fill or become engorged with or without the infant suckling. This is the cardinal sign looked for by the obstetrician.

A study of cases which represent a clinical situation of endocrine failure may assist the understanding of lactation failure due to hormonal cause. A case of Sheehan's Syndrome at the University of Rochester was treated with replacement oxytocin by nasal Syntocin at each pumping or feeding for 3 weeks post partum. Milk production gradually began and increased until the mother was totally sustaining the infant on breastmilk and the Syntocin could be withdrawn. The infant was successfully breastfed following this hormone replacement therapy for over six months. A second case involved a mother's chronic collagen disease which was treated with plasmaphoresis just prior to delivery. She showed no signs of engorgement or milk production after delivery. She too was started on oxytocin replacement therapy by nasal Syntocin. She was able to develop and increase her supply of milk over the next two weeks. She ultimately discontinued the Syntocin and lactated successfully for six months, sustaining her infant solely on breastfeeding. It was speculated that her own prolactin levels had returned to normal in two weeks.

Summary

Maternal causes of lactation failure are not well studied. The animal model has served to explore the hormonal control of lactation and influences

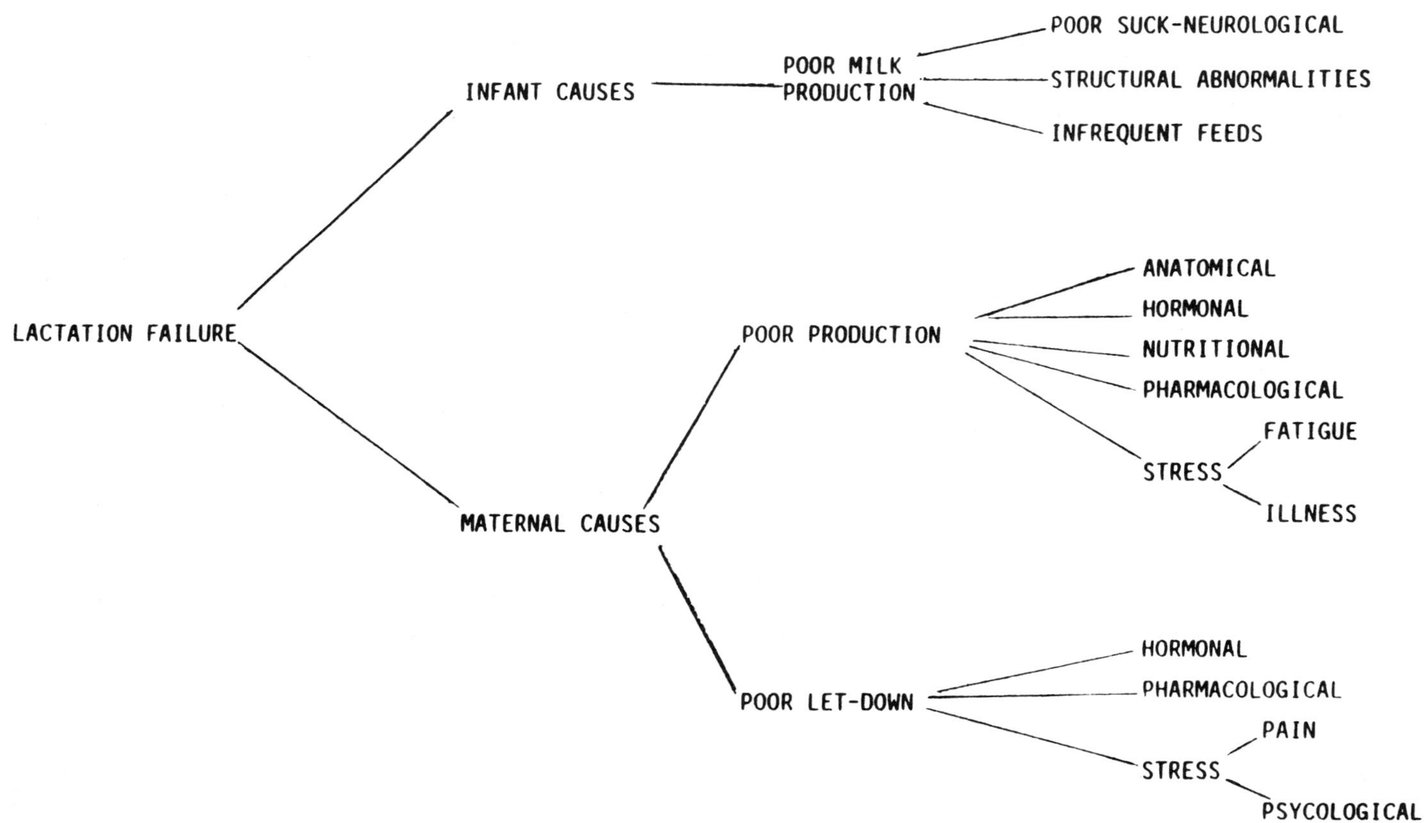

Figure 3. Infant and Maternal Causes of Lactation Failure

Modified From: R.A. Lawrence, "Breastfeeding: A guide for the Medical Profession," 2nd edition, the C.V. Mosby Company, St. Louis, Toronto, Princeton (1985).

of the absence of natural hormonal stimulus. The human model has not been systematically studied and present knowledge stems from observations in disease states. In order to develop a systematic data base, the definition of lactation failure should be agreed upon. Clinical cases of lactation failure should be studied in an organized manner, perhaps in a multicentered study using the same protocol which could lead to some valuable observations and interpretable data. Some women do fail to lactate adequately for various anatomical, physiological and psychological reasons that require further critical study.

REFERENCES

1. D. Rassin, Personnel communication (1986).
2. R. A. Lawrence, "Breastfeeding: A Guide for the Medical Profession," 2nd edition, The C. V. Mosby Company, St. Louis, Toronto, Princeton (1985).
3. H. Vorherr, Human lactation and breast feeding, in: "Lactation," B. L. Larson, ed., Academic Press, New York, London (1978).
4. J. S. Tindal, Neuroendocrine control of lactation, in: "Lactation," B. L. Larson, ed., Academic Press, New York, London (1978).
5. W. R. Threlfall, H. E. Dale, and C. E. Martin, Serum and adenohyophyseal concentrations of prolactin in sows affected with agalactia, Am. J. Vet. Res. 35:313-315 (1974).
6. I. A. Baryshnikov, and E. P. Kokorina, Higher nervous activity of cattle, Dairy Sci. Abst. 26:97-115 (1964).
7. F. Ely, and W. E. Petersen, Factors involved in the ejection of milk, J. Dairy Sci. 24:211-223 (1941).
8. B. A. Cross, Neural control of lactation, in: "Milk: The Mammary Gland and its Secretion," S. K. Kon, A. T. Cowie, eds., Academic Press, New York, London (1961).
9. A. W. Nordskog, and R. T. Clark, Ergotism in pregnant sows, female rats and guinea pigs, Am. J. Vet. Res. 6:107-116 (1945).
10. S. Patton, Milk secretion at the cellular level: a unique approach to mechanism of exocytosis, J. Dairy Sci. 61:643-650 (1978).
11. E. Flückiger, M. Marko, W. Doepfner, W. Niederer, Effects of ergot alkaloids on the hypothalmicpituitary axis, Med. J., 52:(Suppl. 1), 57-61 (1976b).
12. A. T. Cowie, I. A. Forsyth, and I. C. Hart, "Hormonal Control of Lactation," Springer-Verlag, Berlin, Heidelberg, New York (1980).
13. M. Newton, Human lactation, in: "The Mammary Gland and Its Secretion," S. K. Kon, A. T. Cowie, eds., Academic Press, New York (1961).
14. M. Newton, and N. R. Newton, The let-down reflex in human lactation, J. Pediatr. 33:698-704 (1948).
15. J. D. Gussler, and L. H. Briesemeister, The insufficient milk syndrome: A biocultural explanation, Medic. Anthrop. 4:1-24 (1980).
16. G. E. Egli, and M. Newton, The influence of the number of breastfeedings on milk production, Pediatr. 27:314 (1961).
17. A. S. McNeilly, and J. McNeilly, Spontaneous milk ejection during lactation and its possible relevance to success of breastfeeding, Br. Med. J. 2:466-468 (1978).
18. M. C. Neville, and M. R. Neifert, "Lactation Physiology, Nutrition, and Breast-feeding," Plenum Press, New York (1983).
19. C. E. Weichert, Lactational reflex recovery in breastfeeding failure, Pediatr. 63:799 (1979).
20. R. A. Lawrence, Successful breastfeeding, Am. J. Dis. Child. 135:595 (1981).
21. F. E. Hytten, and A. M. Thomson, Nutrition of the lactating women, in: "Milk: The Mammary Gland and its Secretion," S. K. Kon, A. T. Cowie, eds., Vol. 2, Academic Press, New York, London (1961).
22. R. A. Lawrence, Infant nutrition, Ped. Review 5:133 (1983).

23. G. L. Noel, H. K. Suh, J. G. Stone, and A. G. Frantz, Human prolactin and growth hormone release during surgery and other conditions of stress, J. Clin. Endocrinol. Metab. 35:840-851 (1972).
24. Sir A. P. Cooper, "On the Anatomy of the Breast," London: Longman, Orme, Green, Brow and Longman (1840).
25. G. Clarke, D. W. Lincoln, and P. V. D. Schoot, Neuropharmacological studies on the central inhibition of oxytocin release, Br. J. Pharmacol. 62:424P (1978).

MAMMARY GLAND ANOMALIES AND LACTATION FAILURE

Marianne R. Neifert and Joy M. Seacat

Lactation Program, Women's Hospital at AMI Saint Luke's and
University of Colorado School of Medicine
Denver, Colorado

INTRODUCTION

Human milk is universally recognized as optimal infant nutrition, and international attention is being focused on strategies to increase the present incidence and duration of lactation. Despite both professional and lay enthusiasm for breast-feeding, many women experience lactation difficulties, most often attributable to breast-feeding mismanagement. However, primary and secondary breast anatomical problems remain infrequently acknowledged causes of lactation insufficiency. Unfortunately, such causes often go unrecognized since a thorough examination of the breast, with emphasis on its functional potential, is frequently overlooked in routine prenatal care.

INVERTED NIPPLES

Although the normal nipple may be somewhat flat at first inspection, it is composed of erectile fibromuscular tissue and becomes erect with manipulation. In the normal course of breast-feeding, the infant's exploratory mouthing and licking of the nipple help make it more projectile and easier to grasp.

Inverted nipples are among the most common breast anomalies. They can be secondary to trauma or inflammation, but usually are congenital in origin, occuring either unilaterally or bilaterally. An inverted nipple may appear grossly normal or be obviously everted at the tip. Instead of protruding outward upon manipulation, however, the inverted nipple retracts into a sulcus beneath the areola when pinched between the thumb and forefinger. Microscopically the inverted nipple has less dense fibrous tissue than the normal nipple.[1]

This anomaly presents a two-fold problem. First, inverted nipples are difficult for the infant to grasp correctly, particularly when the child has experienced repeated exposure to the long, relatively stiff rubber nipple on a bottle. Without bedside guidance by an experienced nurse or midwife, the initiation of breast-feeding is often undermined by inverted nipples.

A second problem which can be associated with marked nipple inversion is mechanical obstruction to milk flow during infant suckling. Thus the nursing infant may be unable to effectively extract milk. Abnormal ducts, documented by microscopic pathology in severely inverted nipples, may contribute to difficulties in milk flow.[2] A breast pump which successfully everts the nipple during each suction phase of the pump action may allow milk to be mechanically expressed.

If inverted nipples are detected early in pregnancy, it is usually possible to prepare them for nursing by regularly performing prenatal exercises designed to enhance nipple protractility. Hoffman's exercises originated with an obstetrician who found them efficacious in clinical practice.[3] The maneuver is performed by placing the forefingers at opposite locations on the areolar margins and then pulling away from the nipple. The procedure should be repeated dozens of times daily and at various points around the areola.

Breast shields or milk cups, and newer devices known as breast shells, are also helpful adjuvants to the therapy of inverted nipples.[4] These dome shaped devices with a central opening are worn over the inverted nipple inside the nursing bra. They provide even pressure on the areola, eventually causing the nipple to evert through the opening and gradually stretching its attachment to the deep structures of the breast. Breast shells are preferable to the other devices fully enclosing the nipple, as the former have multiple openings to permit circulation of air. Breast shells should be worn for the greater part of the day throughout the last trimester. The pressure should be firm but not uncomfortable. These measures can also prove helpful in making a normal, but very flat, nipple more suitable for nursing.

Often, inverted nipples are overlooked during pregnancy and not discovered until the infant is born. Or, despite prenatal preparation, the nipples remain inverted at the time of delivery. In such cases, Hoffman's exercises should be performed regularly post partum and breast shells worn between feedings as long as necessary.

A method of surgically correcting inverted nipples without disrupting the integrity of the lactiferous ducts has recently been described.[1] The procedure involves raising the inverted nipple by freeing it from the surrounding areolar tissue by vertical and horizontal undermining. The nipple is elevated by applying traction on holding sutures and then stabilized in the new position by a purse-string suture at the base. Although ability to nurse is alleged to be preserved by this technique, successful breast-feeding post-operatively was not documented in the original report of the procedure. The authors are aware of a gravida 5 woman with severe congenital inverted nipples who elected to undergo the described method of surgical correction at approximately 32 weeks gestation. The immediate result appeared much improved, but the woman experienced severe nipple tenderness when initiating breast-feeding and was unable to continue nursing beyond the first week. A year later, the post-operative appearance of the nipples was more inverted than before surgery.

In summary, inverted nipples should be diagnosed early by prenatal manipulation of the nipple. Anecdotally, Hoffman's exercises and breast shells are useful in preparing inverted nipples for nursing. It remains unclear whether surgical correction of severe nipple inversion is a practical therapeutic modality for facilitating breast-feeding.

BREAST REDUCTION

Mammary hypertrophy can cause a woman to be embarrassed about her appearance, to suffer from chronic backaches, or to have difficulty obtaining properly fitting clothing. Reduction mammoplasty may be elected by a self-conscious, nulliparous young woman who has not yet contemplated infant feeding. Radical reduction techniques involving autotransplantation of the nipple preclude normal lactation.[5] Disrupted innervation of the nipple-areola complex interferes with the neuro-humeral pathways involved in breast-feeding, and severing the lactiferous ducts as they enter the nipple prevents normal milk drainage. Tyson obtained baseline and post-nursing prolactin levels on the seventh and fourteenth post partum days in a woman who had previously undergone reduction mammoplasty with nipple autotransplantation. Repeated suckling by the child for fifteen minutes at each breast failed to raise the woman's serum prolactin levels.[6] Two women who previously underwent reduction mammoplasty and nipple autotransplantation experienced subsequent lactation insufficiency and were evaluated by the authors, one at two weeks and one at six weeks post partum. Baseline serum prolactin levels were 28 ng/ml and 5 ng/ml respectively, with no rise in serum prolactin after 20 minutes of infant suckling.

Reduction mammoplasty can also be accomplished by techniques that leave the nipple and areola attached to the underlying parenchyma, moving it to its new location on superior or inferior breast tissue. By leaving the nipple ducts and innervation intact, the potential for lactation may be preserved.[5]

It is important for plastic surgeons performing reduction procedures involving nipple autotransplantation to emphasize to women that full lactation will not be possible post-operatively. Also, obstetricians need to carefully examine the breasts prenatally and recognize the surgical incisions from reduction procedures in order to appropriately counsel pregnant women about their lactation potential.

It should be emphasized that while full lactation may not be possible, breast-feeding can still be achieved by using the Supplemental Nutrition System*. This device allows the infant to obtain formula supplement simultaneously while breast-feeding by means of a thin tubing laid next to the maternal nipple. The tubing is attached to a plastic bottle of formula which is suspended around the mother's neck. This mechanism has allowed breast-feeding to continue uninterrupted in numerous cases of insufficient milk supply secondary to a variety of causes.

BREAST AUGMENTATION

Thousands of women each year elect to have their breasts enlarged to enhance their self-image. Unlike reduction mammoplasty, augmentation procedures do not result in the destruction of breast tissue, the disruption of ducts, or the interruption of the blood supply to the nipple.

It is generally accepted that successful breast-feeding is possible following augmentation. In fact, most patient education materials on augmentation make no reference to organ function following the procedure. Among the more than 250 papers on the use of breast implants for augmentation mammoplasty published in the last 20 years, only 2 have addressed lactation.[7] While it is true that many women have breast-fed successfully following breast augmentation, data is lacking to support the generalization that every woman can. The nerve supply to the nipple-areola complex, provided by the third, fourth, and fifth lateral intercostal nerves, is not routinely identified during surgery.[8] Inadvertant operative nerve damage, suggested by altered nipple sensation post-operatively, is not uncommon.

*Medela, Inc., P.O. Box 386, Crystal Lake, IL 60014 (800-435-8316)

The authors recently evaluated a woman who experienced bilateral breast anesthesia immediately following breast augmentation, performed during an early, unrecognized pregnancy. Over the ensueing months, the woman noted gradual return of sensation to parts of each breast and to one nipple. She had successfully breast-fed three previous children and was extremely anxious about her lactation potential. She was advised to begin feedings after delivery on the breast with intact nipple sensation to help stimulate the let-down reflex in both breasts and effect prolactin rise. In addition, the use of synthetic oxytocin (Syntocinon Nasal Spray) prior to feedings was recommended to augment the let-down response. Following delivery, the woman initiated breast-feeding, but daily formula supplement was required for many months to maintain satisfactory infant weight gain.

In assessing breast function following augmentation mammoplasty, initial breast appearance and lactation potential should be considered. For example, augmentation performed in a nulliparous woman with bilateral primary breast hypoplasia should not be blamed for her subsequent lactation failure. On the other hand, a woman who previously breast-fed successfully, then experienced insufficient lactation after undergoing breast augmentation, should raise questions about the impact of the procedure on her lactation performance. In evaluating women with lactation insufficiency who have previously undergone augmentation mammoplasty, the original appearance of the breasts should be considered, previous breast-feeding history should be explored, post-operative alterations in nipple sensation should be elicited, and prolactin response to suckling should be determined whenever nerve damage is suspected. Oxytocin nasal spray can be prescribed to facilitate the let-down response if necessary. Prospective studies are warranted to examine lactation performance among women with previous breast-feeding success who have undergone augmentation mammoplasty. Isolated anecdotal accounts of successful breast-feeding following the procedure should not be used to argue that breast-feeding is never impaired by such breast surgery.

SYNDROME OF INSUFFICIENT MAMMARY GLANDULAR DEVELOPMENT

Increasing evidence exists that primary lactation failure can occur despite adequate maternal knowledge, motivation, and breast-feeding technique. Yet, such causes of insufficient lactation have received little attention. While it would never be assumed that every woman can conceive, carry an infant to term, or deliver vaginally, it is still supposed that "every woman can breast-feed" and that every breast can potentially produce adequate milk. For virtually every other organ, an obvious association has been made between external appearance and function. Yet, prenatal assurance by well-meaning obstetricians that every woman's breasts, without regard to appearance, are "absolutely perfect" for breast-feeding is still advocated to enhance maternal confidence.[9] The authors recently reported three cases in which lactation insufficiency was associated with abnormal external appearance of the breasts (marked asymmetry). In addition, light scanning of the breasts provided suggestive evidence of diminished glandular tissue presence.[10] It is possible that abnormal external appearance of the breasts is associated with internal breast anomalies affecting function.

Following the initial three case reports, 14 women subsequently have been identified who appear to have a syndrome of insufficient mammary glandular tissue. In each of the seventeen women now recognized, lactation insufficiency occurred despite nursing a term, healthy infant and adhering to optimal breast-feeding routines. Maternal serum prolactin levels were obtained and ruled out prolactin deficiency states in the women. Women ranged in age from 23 to 39 years (mean 31.5 years).

Infant age at the time of evaluation ranged from 5 days to 111 days.

None of the infants established adequate weight gain with exclusive breast-feeding. Fourteen babies were either continuing to lose weight by 10 days or were still below birth weight by 16 days of age. Maximum percent weight loss from birth was 22% (in one infant) and maximum duration of failure to thrive prior to intervention was 6 weeks (in two infants still under birth weight). All infants gained weight satisfactorily once formula supplementation was instituted, thus ruling out infant pathology causing failure to thrive.

Lactation consultations included a detailed lactation history using a standard questionnaire, a complete physical examination of each infant, an examination of the maternal breasts and the observation of a breast-feeding. Maternal milk yields were determined by test-weighing the infant before and after nursing, using the Sartorius integrating balance (accurate to 0.1 gram) and adding post-nursing milk volumes obtained by the Medela electric breast pump. Milk yields were calculated in milliliters/hour since the last feeding and compared with published normal values for the specific post partum interval. A baseline maternal serum prolactin level was drawn at least three hours after last breast-feeding. A post-nursing level was also obtained, and a third level drawn after pumping the breasts for ten minutes with the Medela electric breast pump.

Breast diaphanography, or light scanning, was performed in twelve cases in an attempt to objectively assess the presence of breast glandular tissue. Diaphanography uses visible and infrared light to non-invasively examine the breasts.[11] Scans of non-pregnant, non-lactating breasts transmit light readily, permitting the nipple and superficial and deep venous structures to be visualized. During early lactation, the breast is so dense that no light transmission is evident on the scan, resulting in a totally dark absorptive pattern.

Contrary to typical responses among successfully lactating women, fourteen of sixteen women reported little or no prenatal breast enlargement and fifteen recalled minimal post partum breast engorgement. Several women offered that they had been able to wear their prepregnant bra size throughout pregnancy and commented that "their milk had never come in." One woman was not asked about breast changes.

Milk yields among study women ranged from 3% to 43% (mean 24%) of published normal values for the specific post partum interval. Mean baseline maternal serum prolactin level was 84 ng/ml; after nursing and after pumping values were 164 and 168 ng/ml respectively.

Ten of sixteen women in whom the breasts were examined had marked asymmetry in breast size. Seven had patchy areas of breast fullness prior to feeding. Four had disproportionately large nipples, and one had tubular shaped breasts.

Among the twelve light scans performed, ten were interpreted by the consulting radiologist as abnormal, demonstrating increased transmission of light and overall diminished density of the breasts, often with patchy areas of light absorption corresponding to clinically palpable glandular tissue.

Although it was interpreted to these women that full lactation would not be possible, 15/17 elected to continue breast-feeding while supplementing the infant with formula, either by bottle or with the Lact-Aid or Supplemental Nutrition System. Each woman expressed relief after being told that her insufficient lactation was primary in nature and did not stem from inadequate technique or lack of effort on her part.

A syndrome of inadequate mammary glandular tissue is proposed, with suggestive evidence provided by: failure of the infant ever to establish weight gain with exclusive breast-feeding; lack of prenatal breast changes; minimal or no post partum breast engorgement; minimal or patchy breast fullness prior to feedings; and unusual appearance of the breasts. Although primary lactation failure due to inadequate glandular structures has not been previously reported, Waller described insufficient glandular tissue in postmortem examinations of the breasts of some post partum women dying of unrelated causes.[12]

A classification system for breast asymmetries was recently proposed in a report of 150 cases.[13] Precocious primary asymmetry of the breast, presenting at puberty, accounted for 65 of the cases. Although operative approaches were addressed, lactation ability among women with primary breast asymmetry unfortunately was not mentioned.

A large prospective study is warranted to determine the incidence of this entity and the predictive value of the clinical features described.

SUMMARY

Much emphasis has been placed on the prevention and alleviation of common breast-feeding difficulties by appropriate education and optimal clinical management of lactation. However, primary and secondary anatomical breast problems have received little attention, and the importance of routine prenatal examination of the breast to assess its lactation potential, has been underemphasized. The recognition and investigation of anatomical breast abnormalities should help broaden the present understanding of maternal factors influencing lactation performance. In addition, some cases of failure to thrive among breast-fed infants may be averted by acknowledging that every every breast may NOT be the perfect breast for breast-feeding.

REFERENCES

1. Hauben, D. and Mahler, D., 1982, A simple method for the correction of the inverted nipple. _Plast. Reconst. Surg_. 71:556.
2. Rayner, C., 1980, The correction of permanently inverted nipples. _Br. J. Plast. Surg._ 33:413.
3. Hoffman, J., 1953, A suggested treatment for inverted nipples. _Am. J. Obstet. Gynecol_. 66:346.
4. Waller, H., 1946, The early failure of breast feeding. _Arch. Dis. Child_. 21:1.
5. Bostwick, J., 1983, Breast reduction, _in_ "Aesthetic and Reconstructive Breast Surgery," C.V. Mosby Co., St. Louis.
6. Tyson, J.E., 1977, Nursing and prolactin secretion: Principal determinants in the mediation of puerperal infertility, _in_ "Prolactin and Human Response," P.G. Crosignani & C. Robyn, eds, Academic Press, New York.
7. McGrath, M. and Burkhardt, B., 1984, The safety and efficacy of breast implants for augmentation mammaplasty. _Plast. Reconst. Surg_.74:550.
8. Bostwick, J., 1983, Breast augmentation, _in_ "Aesthetic and Reconstructive Breast Surgery," C.V. Mosby Co., St. Louis.
9. Rawlins, C., 1980, Antenatal preparation for breast-feeding, _in_ "Counseling the Mother on Breast-Feeding." Report of the Eleventh Ross Roundtable, Ross Laboratories.
10. Neifert, M., Seacat, J., Jobe, W., 1985, Lactation failure due to insufficient glandular development of the breast. _Pediatr_. 76:823.

11. Ohlsson, B., 1980, Diaphanography--A new method for investigation of the breast. World J. Surg. 4:701.
12. Waller, H., 1957, "The Breasts and Breast Feeding," William Heinemann Medical Books, Ltd., London, pg. 28.
13. Vandenbussche, F., 1984, Asymmetries of the breast: A classification system, Aesth. Plast. Surg. 8:27.

EFFECTS OF MATERNAL NUTRITION ON HUMAN LACTATION

Bo Lönnerdal

Department of Nutrition
University of California
Davis, CA 95616

INTRODUCTION

Although a decline in breast-feeding has been evident in many industrialized countries during the last decades, human milk is a major source of nutrition for the infant in most parts of the world. The many benefits provided by human milk, beyond being a source of nutrients, are now well-recognized. Components with physiological activity include immunoglobulins (especially secretory IgA), enzymes (such as lipases and lysozyme), growth factors and oligosaccharides with anti-adhesive function (inhibiting attachment of bacteria). Having recognized the significance of human milk in providing nutrition and functional components to the growing and vulnerable infant, it is logical to be concerned about the possibility that poor maternal nutrition may compromise the quantity and quality of human milk. Furthermore, if milk yield and composition can be affected by maternal nutrition, will dietary supplementation of the mother overcome any shortcomings? Such information will aid in designing effective relief programs in areas of poor nutrition and in nutrition counseling to less educated and poor mothers in areas of otherwise adequate food supply.

Information on effects of maternal diet on levels of nutrients in milk is also important in order to establish normative data on nutrient intakes of breast-fed infants. Such data are the foundation for recommendations of nutrient intakes of non-breast-fed infants, i.e., when designing infant formulas. Finally, the plasticity of the mammary gland to respond to low or high intakes of specific nutrients will provide insights into regulation of nutrient transport through the cells of the mammary gland.

The term "plane of maternal nutrition" has gained increasing acceptance to describe the complexity as well as the history of maternal dietary intake. In an ideal situation, the researcher prefers a situation in which the intake of an individual is more or less constant ("steady state") and nutrient levels in milk can be studied at low, "normal" and high maternal intakes. In developing countries, such a situation is exceedingly rare. The supply of various food items and overall dietary intake vary significantly with the seasons. Droughts, flooding, regional conflicts, etc. can have sudden effects on food supply. Diseases affect food intake and metabolism in the mothers and affect nursing capacity of the infant thereby affecting milk output by the mother. Relief programs may bring in specific supplements with some nutrients such as proteins and vitamins, while other nutrients are missing. Overall, the situation facing the researcher working in the field in a developing country is highly complex and far from the ideal one. Studying the effects of high intakes of nutrients by the mother is less complex. Studies can be performed in well-nourished women who receive single or multiple nutrient supplements. It should be emphasized, however, that many interactions among nutrients occur and consequently the whole plane of nutrition needs to be considered. For example, dietary protein deficiency can affect milk niacin levels. If a mother is reducing her energy intake significantly, mobilization of nutrients (and toxicants) from body stores may occur and be reflected in the milk. Therefore, a multifaceted approach needs to be made, focusing in detail on many aspects of maternal intake, weight loss, health etc. in order to enable sensible interpretation of the results obtained.

DAILY MILK VOLUME

Studies on lactation performance of well-nourished as well as malnourished women during the last decades have demonstrated a remarkable consistency in daily milk volumes consumed by the infant (Fig. 1). For example,

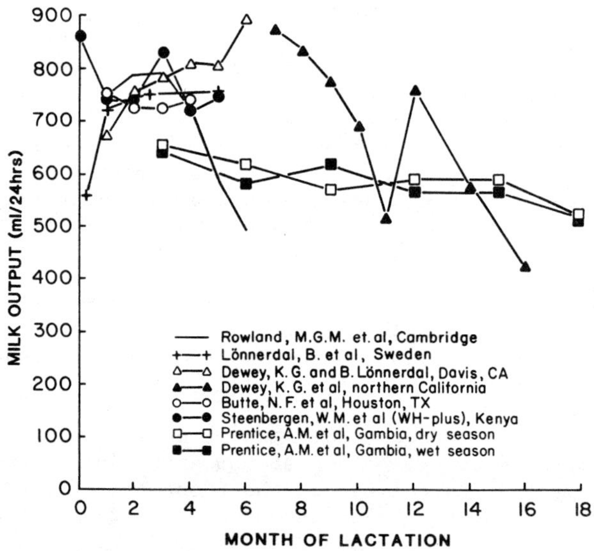

Fig. 1: Daily Milk Volume.

detailed and long-term studies of women with very poor nutritional status in the Gambia have demonstrated that daily milk volumes produced are similar to those of well-nourished women in England, Sweden and the U.S. The question then arises how milk quantity can be maintained in the face of severely compromised maternal nutrition. The research group in Gambia (Prentice et al.) measured serum prolactin levels in the groups of women investigated and found significantly higher prolactin levels in mothers of poorest nutritional status (wet season, Gambia) as compared to the same population of women during the season of higher availability of food (dry season) and, in turn, well nourished women in England. The differences in prolactin levels were evident from early lactation throughout the lactation period. When mothers of poor nutrition received a supplement of calories and micronutrients, prolactin levels became lower and more similar to those of English women. Although the high prolactin levels in Gambian women in part may be due to a higher frequency of nursing than in Cambridge women (Hennart et al., 1985), this would not explain the differences between the Gambian women. Therefore, it is feasible that there is a compensatory mechanism to stimulate milk synthesis via the action of prolactin. A recent study on the effect of maternal caloric restriction ("dieting") in well-nourished women demonstrated that in mothers with a caloric intake less than 1500 kcal/day, serum prolactin levels were increased one week after the introduction of this diet, while in control (non-dieting) women prolactin levels decreased during the same time. Although there appears to be an effect of maternal dietary intake on serum prolactin levels, our knowledge regarding the mechanisms behind this effect is very limited.

If mechanisms exist to compensate for inadequacies in maternal nutrient intake and status, the question arises whether there is a threshold below which the metabolic capacity of the mother is inadequate to provide such a response. There are some reports from developing countries in which low milk volumes have been reported (Hennart & Vis, 1980), although methodological problems in assessing milk volume cannot properly be ruled out. Roberts et al. (1985) have recently addressed this question in a primate animal model. Lactating baboons were allowed to consume an ad libitum diet or 80 or 60% of the same caloric intake. No effect on milk volume was observed in the group ingesting 80% of the control group's caloric intake while a significant decrease in milk volume was observed in the group receiving only 60% of the control group's intake. Thus, there may be a level below which the maternal organism is unable to produce a normal quantity of milk. It is interesting to consider this possibility and to apply the results of Roberts et al. (1985) to the Gambian women in the study by Prentice et al. (1983). The Gambian ad libitum group consumed about 1,700 kcal/day; i.e., 80% of this would be about 1,360 kcal/day which is higher than the 1,200 kcal/day consumed by the Gambian women during the wet season. In this group no effect on milk volume was observed. A caloric intake of 60% of ad libitum intake would correspond to about 1,020 kcal/day or an intake below that of the women during the wet season. Consequently the latter group of women may have been above a threshold level under which an effect on milk volume is observed. There is no evidence that the information gained on the lactating baboon can be applied to the lactating woman, however, the hypothetical reasoning should rather emphasize that the possibility of drastically reduced maternal dietary intake affecting milk yield in the human cannot be ruled out. Belavady and Gopalan (1960) showed a significant increase in daily milk volume in poor Indian women were given a protein supplement, while protein levels were not affected. Similarly, Edozien et al. (1976) demonstrated increased milk volumes in women receiving protein supplements. It is feasible that this supplement provided enough energy to affect an already impaired milk synthesis.

PROTEIN CONCENTRATION AND COMPOSITION

Malnutrition in lactating women does not appear to have a significant effect on the protein concentration of human milk (Table 1). If values obtained by Kjeldahl nitrogen analysis are transformed to "true protein" with a correction for $\sim$25% nitrogen being non-protein nitrogen, it is evident that in most studies the protein concentration of mature human milk is 0.8-1.0%, regardless of maternal nutrition. Some studies, however, show higher concentrations of proteins which is most likely due to problems with protein standards when using colorimetric assays (Lönnerdal et al., 1984). There is no evidence that high protein or energy intake was the cause of these high protein levels. The studies cited in Table 1 were predominately

Table 1. Malnutrition and Protein Concentration.

Country	Concentration(%)	Months	Source
India	0.9±0.1	3-4	Karmarkar & Ramakrishnan, 1960
India	0.8±0.1	2-6	Belavady & Gopalan, 1960
India	0.7±0.1	1-3	Karmarkar et al., 1963
Pakistan	1.1±0.1	1.5	Underwood et al., 1970
Pakistan	0.8±0.1	4-6	Lindblad & Rahimtoola, 1974
New Guinea	0.8-1.0	1-12(?)	Bailey, 1965
New Guinea	0.8-1.0	3-9	Becroft, 1967
Egypt, healthy	0.8±0.1	?	Hanafy et al., 1972
Egypt, malnourished	0.7±0.1	?	Hanafy et al., 1972
Nigeria	0.9-1.2	2-6(?)	Edozien et al., 1976
Ethiopia	0.9±0.1	1.5-4	Lönnerdal et al., 1976b
Gambia	0.7±0.1	4	Prentice, 1979
Ivory Coast	1.0-1.1	2-4	Lauber & Reinhardt, 1979
Brazil	0.8-1.0	1-3	Carneiro & Oliveira, 1973

performed in women which had been malnourished for long periods of time. There appears to be some conditions under which milk protein levels may be affected by maternal diet. Karmarkar et al. (1963) reported that protein supplements given to Indian women with a low protein (21 g/day) and energy (1300 kcal/day) intake, increased milk protein concentration from 0.92% (no supplement) to 1.34% (40 g protein supplement/day). The increases observed were dose-dependent and specific for protein supplementation as no changes in milk protein concentration was observed when fat supplements were given. Hanafy et al. (1972) also reported low protein values in severely malnourished Ethiopian women. It is possible that protein and energy stores of these women were so depleted that a significant effect of protein supplementation was observed although methodological problems cannot be ruled out. In the Gambian study (Prentice et al., 1983) a very modest effect (+7%) throughout lactation on milk protein concentration was observed when the women were supplemented. This difference in the magnitude of response may be due to differences in long-term nutritional status, depletion of stores, etc. We have observed that a re-distribution of calories (at the same energy intake) to high and low protein intakes had a highly significant effect on total and individual proteins in human milk (Forsum & Lönnerdal, 1980). This study was of short-term nature (4 days on each diet; cross-over design for each individual) and it is possible that sudden drastic changes in the diet of the well-nourished woman may affect milk composition, while long-term consumption of diets high or low in nutrient levels may trigger compensatory mechanisms.

The individual proteins of human milk have received some attention lately. In our study in Ethiopia (Lönnerdal et al., 1976) we found high levels of lactoferrin especially in milk from poorly nourished women. Miranda et al. (1983) observed significantly higher levels of lysozyme and serum albumin in milk from malnourished women, while no significant effect was observed on other milk proteins. Prentice et al. (1984) found elevated levels of immunoglobulins and some other bacteriostatic proteins in milk of poorly nourished women. Thus, it is evident that although total protein content may be little affected, some components may be increased and others decreased.

LIPIDS

Dietary fat intake does not appear to affect significantly the total concentration of lipid in human milk (Lammi-Keefe and Jensen, 1984). Regulation of lipid metabolism by mobilization from stress, deposition into adipose tissue etc. may explain this lack of effect. However, similar to the effect of protein supplements on milk composition, under some circumstances, it is possible that if stores are depleted and energy intake is low, supplementation with fat may have an effect on milk synthesis. This was indicated in the study by Karmarkar et al. (1963), in which Indian women with low energy and fat (18 g/day) intake were given supplements. Increasing daily fat intakes stepwise from 0 to 45 g/day, increased milk fat from 3.78% to 4.71%.

Fatty acid composition of human milk fat is responsive to the fatty acid composition of the maternal diet. Important insights into the effects of diet on milk fat were obtained by the studies of Insull et al. (1959). Albeit only one mother was studied, the controlled diet and the drastic changes in fat intake and composition provided useful data for further studies. It was evident that intake of polyunsaturated fatty acids (18:2+3) was reflected in milk concentrations of these fatty acids. When a high calorie, low fat diet was introduced, *de novo* fatty acid synthesis was stimulated and concentrations of medium chain (12:0, 14:0) fatty acids in milk increased. A low caloric intake combined with low fat intake resulted in a fatty acid pattern similar to that of body fat of humans consuming a mixed diet, presumably reflecting mobilization of fatty acids from stores in adipose tissue. Several studies have subsequently shown that maternal fat intake and composition is affecting milk fatty acid composition (Guthrie et al., 1977; Sanders et al., 1978; Mellies et al., 1979; Vuori et al., 1982; Finley et al., 1985a; Kneebone et al., 1985). The high carbohydrate, low calorie diet common in many developing countries is reflected in high levels of C12:0 and C14:0 as compared to milk from women in industrialized countries (Lauber & Reinhardt, 1979). This is further exemplified by the effect of maternal intake of *trans* fatty acids (products of industrial processing) on milk levels of these fatty acids (Aitchison et al., 1977; Finley et al., 1985a; Chapell et al., 1985). The effect of low energy intake (= negative energy balance) was recently demonstrated by the study of Chapell et al. (1985) in which higher levels of *trans* fatty acids were found in mothers rapidly losing weight than in those losing no weight or slowly losing weight.

Concentrations of long-chain polyunsaturated fatty acids, such as docosahexenoic acid (DHA; 22:6w3), with potential physiological significance are also affected by maternal diet. Harris et al. (1985) showed that daily fish oil supplements could increase the concentration of DHA in human milk significantly. Finley et al. (1985a) also demonstrated that fish intake was correlated to milk DHA concentration.

Cholesterol concentration of human milk does not seem to be affected by maternal cholesterol intake. This is not surprising considering our knowledge of the metabolism and transport of cholesterol. Mellies et al. (1978) showed in a cross-over design that milk cholesterol levels were similar, whether high (520 mg/day) or low (190 mg/day) cholesterol diets were fed. In contrast, these investigators found an effect of maternal phytosterol (plant sterols) intake on milk levels of this class of compounds. This finding has been questioned by Jensen (see this volume), who did not detect amounts of phytosterols in human milk.

LACTOSE

It is generally considered that lactose concentration of human milk is resistant to varying maternal nutritional status (Coward et al., 1984).

Lactose concentrations obtained in most studies are remarkably similar. However, there may be conditions under which lactose concentrations can be affected. Prentice (1979) showed that milk lactose levels were higher in milk from Gambian women during the wet season (poorest nutrition) as compared to the dry season. It is possible that maternal mobilization of stores, as evidenced by weight loss, affected milk lactose synthesis. When the poorly nourished Gambian women were given a dietary supplement, lactose concentration decreased (Prentice et al., 1983). A study by Harzer et al. (1984) is difficult to interpret as the values observed are so strikingly different from other studies. When mothers were fed a low fat, high carbohydrate diet, lactose concentration was 4.0-4.5% and when the diet was switched to a high fat, low carbohydrate diet, lactose concentration increased to 6.0-6.5%. A reciprocal change in milk fat was observed. Not only were the initial lactose concentrations unusually low but also the change was of a magnitude hitherto unseen. The number of women studied was very low and methodological problems cannot be excluded.

FAT-SOLUBLE VITAMINS

Our knowledge of the effects of maternal intake of fat-soluble vitamins on their concentrations in milk is limited and detailed information has only recently been published. This is largely due to the fact that methods to analyze various forms and metabolites of these vitamins, which often are present in very low absolute amounts, were not developed until the last few years.

Vitamin A

It was early found that very high doses of vitamin A given during pregnancy (50,000-200,000 IU daily) increased milk vitamin A levels (Hrubetz et al., 1945). These levels, however, are toxic and not generally given to human subjects. It should be recognized that prepartum vitamin A intake is important as this vitamin is stored in the body. Ajans et al. (1965) also found an effect of water dispersable vitamin A (600,000 IU in a single dose), given to mothers shortly before delivery, on milk vitamin A levels. The effect was most pronounced in colostrum and samples from early lactation. No effect was observed when vitamin A was given intramuscularly instead of using oral supplementation. Belavady and Gopalan (1960) did not find any significant difference in milk of Indian women given vitamin A supplements of 2,000-10,000 IU/day as compared to unsupplemented women. However, when 30,000 IU of vitamin A were given daily, colostrum and milk levels of vitamin A were higher than those of unsupplemented women (Venkatachalam et al., 1962). Tarjan et al. (1963) demonstrated that when vitamin A was given to lactating women in the form of liver (55,000-130,000 IU), milk vitamin A levels increased. Maximum milk level was found 14 hours after ingestion of the liver meal. A modest increase in carotenoid levels in milk was found by feeding large amounts of raw carrots (200 g). Gebre-Medhin et al. (1976) showed that vitamin A concentration of milk from poor Ethiopian women was lower than those of well-nourished Ethiopian and Swedish women. Low serum levels of retinol-binding protein (RBP) were also found in the group of poor Ethiopian women. On the other hand, milk β-carotene levels were higher in the Ethiopian women as compared to Swedish women, possibly reflecting a higher intake of carotenoids among Ethiopian women.

Vitamin D

Several factors affect the concentrations of vitamin D and its metabolites in milk (Hollis et al., 1983). Pronounced vitamin D deficiency leads to low levels of vitamin D and 25-hydroxyvitamin D (25-OHD) in milk. Race can affect milk vitamin D levels; blacks were found to have significantly lower levels of vitamin D in milk than whites (Specker et al., 1985). In the same study, total vitamin D in milk, but not 25-OHD, was found to be correlated to maternal diet. The over-riding effect of exposure to sunshine should not be underestimated. Ala-Houhala (1985) and Specker et al. (1985) did not find any correlation of maternal vitamin D status or intake on serum 25-OHD in the nursing infants, most likely because of the effect of the infants' exposure to sunlight. Maternal UV-treatment has been shown to increase serum and milk vitamin D_3 levels with a peak level within 48 hours after exposure (Greer et al., 1984a). Very high levels of vitamin D given to women with hypothyroidism were also found to increase milk vitamin D levels significantly (Greer et al., 1984b).

Vitamin E

Limited information is available on the effects of maternal diet on vitamin E in human milk. In a study by Kramer et al. (1965), mothers were given a vitamin E rich sunflower oil and milk vitamin E (total) level increased from 250 μg/L to 380 μg/L. The maximum level was found six days after introduction of the sunflower oil and baseline levels were achieved about the same time after exclusion of this oil from the diet. Jansson et al. (1981) demonstrated that α-tocopherol is the predominant form of vitamin E in human milk and that total tocopherol concentration in milk is correlated to the linoleic acid concentration. Since an effect of maternal diet on polyunsaturated fatty acids, such as linoleic acid, was documented above, the findings of Jansson et al. implies a dietary effect on milk vitamin E levels.

Vitamin K

A method for analyzing the various forms of vitamin K in human milk was developed only recently (Haroon et al., 1982). In this study, which established a mean value of 2.1 μg/L of phylloquinone in mature human milk, one mother was given a high dose of phylloquinone (20 mg). The level of vitamin K_1 increased to 140 μg/L after 12 hours and was about twice the normal value at 48 hours. This suggests that maternal supplementation with vitamin K may be an indirect route of supplementing the infant. The normal values in this study were obtained by high performance liquid chromatography (HPLC). These values were considerably lower than previously published values which were obtained by chicken bioassay methods. Standards used and lack of sensitivity of the chick assay may explain these discrepancies.

WATER-SOLUBLE VITAMINS

In several early studies, water soluble vitamins were assayed in human milk before and after supplementation. While it is easy to disregard some of these studies because of a general lack of sophisticated laboratory methods for analysis at that time, it should be recognized that many of these vitamins still are assayed with the same or very similar techniques. Therefore it is interesting to compare some of the early studies with information gained in recent studies (Table 2). It can be noted that in many cases, results obtained two decades ago or earlier are similar to those obtained today. New chromatographic techniques based on HPLC are being developed, but it should be recognized that the major advantage of these methods is to separate vitamers, increase speed and sensitivity; the values obtained for total vitamin content may still be similar to values published earlier. Exceptions to this may be folic acid, biotin and vitamin B_{12} since assays may not have analyzed bound forms of these vitamins.

Table 2. Water Soluble Vitamins in Human Milk.

	India[a]		Gambia[b]			Others
	unsuppl.	suppl.	dry	wet	suppl.	
Thiamin (mg/L)	0.11	0.27	0.18	0.16	0.22	0.21±0.03[c]
Riboflavin (mg/L)	0.20	0.74	0.23	0.21	0.28	0.24±0.03[c]
Pantothenic acid (mg/L)	1.0	3.0	2.7	2.0	2.3	1.8–16.7[d] ($\bar{x}$=6.7)
Vitamin B_6 (mg/L)	0.08	0.16	0.09	0.12	0.10	0.09–0.41[e]
Nicotinic acid (mg/L)	0.99	2.75	1.49	1.13	1.62	
Vitamin B_{12} (μg/L)	0.08	0.10	0.29	0.16	0.12	0.33–3.20[f] ($\bar{x}$=0.97)
Folic acid (μg/L)	2.0	5.6	54	38	47	62–280[g] ($\bar{x}$=141)
Biotin (μg/L)	1.6	5.0	10.3	9.0	7.2	
Ascorbic acid (mg/L)	23	61	55–60	20–40	45–50	44–158[h]

a) Deodhar et al., 1964
b) Prentice, 1979; Prentice et al., 1983
c) Thomas et al., 1980a
d) Johnston et al., 1981
e) Styslinger & Kirksey, 1985
f) Sandberg et al., 1981
g) Tamura et al., 1980
h) Byerley & Kirksey, 1985

Thiamin

Poor nutritional status and consequently low intakes of thiamin appears to lead to low milk levels of this vitamin. Deodhar et al. (1964) found that unsupplemented Indian women of poor nutritional status had milk thiamin levels of 0.11 mg/L and that thiamin supplementation could increase the level up to 0.27 mg/L. The dietary thiamin intake of these women at the beginning of the study was 0.25 mg/day and the highest level of supplementation was 20 mg/day. Prentice et al. (1983) did not find any significant difference in milk thiamin levels during periods of food availability (dry season) and shortage (wet season), while dietary supplementation resulted in an increase of milk thiamin from 0.16 to 0.22 mg/L. The dietary supplement provided at least 70% of the RDA for thiamin. In women of adequate nutritional status, thiamin supplementation does not appear to affect milk concentrations significantly (Nail et al., 1980; Thomas et al., 1980a). The thiamin intake of these women was 1.5 mg/day and a supplement of 1.7 mg was given daily for 6 months. Milk levels of non-supplemented and supplemented women were 0.21 and 0.22 mg/L, respectively, which is close to the levels found in supplemented Indian and Gambian women. There may therefore be a threshold for the thiamin level of human milk.

Riboflavin

Similar to thiamin, riboflavin levels in milk of poorly nourished women are low. In Indian women with a daily riboflavin intake of 0.18 mg, milk riboflavin concentration was found to be 0.20 mg/L (Deodhar et al., 1964). Supplementation with increasing amount of riboflavin (up to 10 mg/day) increased milk levels to 0.74 mg/L. Bates et al. (1982a) found in Gambian women having a daily intake of 0.5 mg riboflavin that a supplement of 2 mg riboflavin per day significantly increased milk levels from 0.16 to 0.23 mg/L. Poor riboflavin status among the subjects at the beginning of the study and improvement by treatment was demonstrated by the change in activation coefficient of erythrocyte glutathione reductase (EGR). The magnitude of the increase in milk riboflavin levels was larger in the Indian women at the same level of supplementation (1.5 mg/day; 0.45 mg riboflavin/L in milk) than in Gambian women. It is not known if this difference in response is caused by methodological problems, maternal overall nutritional status or health. Nail et al. (1980) found that riboflavin supplements of 2 mg/day given to well-nourished U.S. women could increase milk riboflavin levels from 0.37 to 0.88 mg/L. The higher levels achieved by supplementation are similar to those found by Deodhar et al., indicating that the level of riboflavin in milk from the supplemented Gambian women may not have reached their potential maximum.

Vitamin B_6

There does not appear to be a threshold level for the concentration of vitamin B_6 in human milk; however, there may be a limit which the supplementation of the mother should not exceed since vitamin B_6 in high dosages has been shown to inhibit lactation (Foukas, 1973; Greentree, 1979). In the previously mentioned study on Indian women, pyridoxine level of milk was 0.08 mg/L initially and was increased to 0.16 mg/L with maternal supplementation. Initial daily intake of pyridoxine was 0.35 mg and the level of supplementation 40 mg/day. In comparison, Gambian women had a level of 0.12 mg/L, which did not increase with a daily supplement of 0.71 mg pyridoxine (Prentice et al., 1983). Thomas et al. (1980b) showed that when well-nourished U.S. women were consuming 5.1 mg vitamin B_6/day, milk pyridoxine levels were 0.24 mg/L as compared to 0.20 mg/L in control women consuming 0.8 mg vitamin B_6/day. When the same investigators examined a group of women of low socioeconomic status, the milk vitamin B_6 level was 0.12 mg/L (Sneed et al., 1981). A high EGPT index in these women indicated low vitamin B_6 status. In a recent study of U.S. women having a daily vitamin B_6 intake of 1.8 mg, the milk vitamin B_6 level was found to be 0.09 mg/L (Styslinger & Kirksey, 1985). Supplementation with 2.5, 10 and 20 mg vitamin B_6 per day increased milk vitamin B_6 levels to 0.19, 0.25 and 0.41 mg/L, respectively. The difference in magnitude of response of the supplementation in Indian and U.S. women may be of methodological origin or that repletion of stores/utilization of vitamin B_6 in energy metabolism in the Indian women limited the availability of the vitamin for transfer into milk. The transfer rate of vitamin B_6 into milk appears to be rapid, peak levels occurred about 4 hours post-supplementation (Styslinger & Kirksey, 1985).

Niacin

Few studies have systematically addressed the question of whether maternal nutrition affects milk levels of this vitamin. Not only nicotinic acid intake, but also tryptophan (= dietary protein) intake need to be taken in consideration. Indian women with a low protein and niacin intake (2.4 mg/day) had milk niacin levels of 0.99 mg/L (Deodhar et al., 1964). Supplementing the mother with niacin up to 60 mg/day increased the milk level of niacin to 2.75 mg/L. Milk from unsupplemented Gambian women had a niacin concentration of 1.13 mg/L (Prentice et al., 1983). Supplementation with protein and niacin (19 mg/day) increased milk niacin levels to 1.62 mg/L.

Pantothenic acid

The concentration of pantothenic acid appears to be strongly affected by maternal diet. Prentice (1979) observed lower pantothenic acid levels (2.0 mg/L) in milk from women during the wet season than during the dry season (2.7 mg/L). This is consistent with results from poorly nourished Indian women that had milk pantothenic acid levels of 1.0 mg/L which would be increased to 3.0 mg/L by dietary supplementation (Deodhar et al., 1964). However, when Gambian women were supplemented, no significant increase in milk pantothenic acid levels were observed (Prentice et al., 1983). This may be explained by the fact that the supplement given was 50 mg/day in the Indian study but only 2.3 mg/day in the Gambian study. It should be noted that a supplement of $\sim$2 mg/day in the Indian study caused an increase in milk pantothenic acid similar to that found in the Gambian study. Johnston et al. (1981) found a milk pantothenic acid level of 6.7 mg/L in U.S. women with a mean dietary pantothenic acid intake of 7.6 mg/day. They also found a positive correlation between maternal intake of pantothenic acid and milk levels of the vitamin. The milk concentrations of pantothenic acid found by Johnston et al. were considerably higher than values obtained in previous studies, which may be explained by inadequate release of the vitamin from bound forms by enzymatic treatment.

Biotin

Limited information is available on biotin levels in human milk and factors affecting it. Prentice et al. (1983) found no effect of biotin supplementation on milk biotin levels. Similarly, season and therefore maternal dietary intake of biotin did not affect the level of biotin in milk which was found to be 9.0-13.0 µg/L (Prentice, 1979). Again, vitamin supplementation was found to be effective in increasing milk biotin levels in Indian women (Deodhar et al., 1964). Initial milk biotin concentration was 1.6 µg/L and supplementation increased the level to 5.0 µg/L. The difference in milk biotin levels between the two studies is likely of methodological nature.

Folate

Poor nutritional status appears to affect milk folate levels. Prentice (1979) found that the folate concentration in milk from Gambian women during the wet season was significantly lower (38 µg/L) than during the dry season (54 µg/L). It should be noted that no significant increase in milk folate concentration was observed when lactating women were given a supplement containing folate. The level of folate (5.7 µg) given per day was relatively modest and it is possible that depleted maternal stores were filled before an effect on milk folate could be observed. Also, the milk folate levels were higher (47 µg/L) in the supplemented group although no statistical difference was established. It is possible that with prolonged supplementation milk folate levels could have increased to a higher level. The "normal" concentration of folate in human milk appears to be around 70-140 µg/L (Tamura et al., 1980; Ek, 1983; Smith et al., 1983). It should be recognized that these values were given for total folate, i.e., the folates had been treated with conjugase to release the monoglutamate which is recognized by the assay microorganism (Smith et al., 1983). About half of the total folate in human milk is present in the polyglutamate form, which is not assayed unless subjected to hydrolysis. Previous studies omitting this necessary precaution have therefore given falsely low values (Deodhar et al., 1964). In the studies mentioned above (Tamura et al., 1980; Ek, 1983; Smith et al., 1983), no effect of maternal folate intake on milk levels could be noted even though maternal serum and RBC folate levels were increased. Cooperman et al. (1982) found lower folate levels in milk than most other investigators and found no correlation between maternal folate status and milk folate levels. Interestingly, these investigators found an exception from this "general" rule; a folate deficient mother was found to have low milk folate levels and these were found to increase when the mother was given folate supplements. Metz et al. (1968) had earlier shown that high levels of folate (100-200 μg daily) given to two lactating women with megaloblastic anemia significantly increased milk folate levels. The low folate levels found in the study by Cooperman et al. are most likely explained by the method used; casein and whey proteins were precipitated by rennin treatment and acid, respectively, prior to conjugase treatment. Thus, folate bound to its binding protein(s) would not be measured. This error is also likely to explain the low levels of milk folate found by Sneed et al. (1981). These investigators found a folate level of 42.8 μg/L in mothers of low socioeconomic status; this level increased to 49.4 μg/L with a folate supplement of 800 μg/day.

While little is known about mechanisms for nutrient transport into milk, Selhub et al (1984) have discussed the various possibilities for folate transport. These investigators found a positive correlation between the level of folate and that of folate-binding protein in human milk. Since a major part of milk folate is comprised of folylpolyglutamate, which does not cross biological membranes, it was hypothesized that folate is secreted as the polyglutamate bound to the folate-binding protein. The complex must be formed just before secretion since plasma folate, mainly 5-methyltetrahydropteroylglutamate, must be modified after entry into the cell and this cannot occur when bound to the folate-binding protein. Complexation after secretion was ruled out as folylpolyglutamates cannot cross the cell membrane. Since Ek (1983) observed that plasma and milk folate levels were maintained in lactating women in negative folate balance at the expense of red cell folate incorporation, this may be a "trapping" mechanism to assure adequate milk folate levels. However, if a sufficiently low folate diet is consumed, plasma folate levels will eventually fall and, as a consequence, so will milk folate levels.

Vitamin B_{12}

Methodological problems in many assays of vitamin B_{12} that earlier have been used makes it difficult to evaluate the effects of maternal vitamin B_{12} status and intake on milk vitamin B_{12} concentration. Sandberg et al. (1981) were able to show that vitamin B_{12} in human milk is virtually exclusively bound to a binding protein. These investigators also showed that this binding protein is identical or similar to the R binder of saliva and gastric juice. Very little, if any, vitamin B_{12} was bound to the small amount of transcobalamin II present in human milk. Since vitamin B_{12} is bound to the R binder and there is a large excess of apo R binder, competitive binding assays will not yield correct results without digestion of the R protein by proteolytic enzymes (such as pepsin). Using a digestion step, Sandberg et al. found the level of vitamin B_{12} in milk from U.S. women to be 0.97 μg/L (range: 0.33-3.20 μg/L). No correlation was found between cobalamin intake by diet or supplements. This is in agreement with a study in India by Jathar et al. (1970). However, in two studies on vitamin B_{12} deficient women, there was a correlation between serum and milk vitamin B_{12} levels (Baker et al., 1962; Srikantia & Reddy, 1967). Therefore, there may be mechanisms controlling transport of vitamin B_{12} from serum to milk that are saturable beyond a certain level.

Deodhar et al. (1964) and Prentice et al. (1983) did not find a significant effect of maternal vitamin B_{12} supplementation on milk vitamin B_{12} levels (Table 2). The reported values were low, though, indicating that possibly only free vitamin B_{12} was assayed. Thomas et al. (1980b) described higher milk vitamin B_{12} levels in milk from supplemented women as compared to non-supplemented women at 1.5 months of lactation although serum vitamin B_{12} levels were similar in the two groups. Milk samples had not been treated enzymatically in this study and the accuracy of the values is uncertain.

Vitamin C

The increasing use of vitamin C supplements at high levels raises the question of whether this would affect milk vitamin C levels. In a recent study, Byerley and Kirksey (1985) did not find any significant effect of supplementation of 250, 500 or 1000 mg ascorbic acid/day on milk ascorbic acid levels, nor was a correlation found between maternal intake of this vitamin and its level in milk. Since urinary levels of vitamin C increased at high intakes of ascorbic acid, these investigators speculated that tissue saturation had been reached and that a regulatory mechanism prevents transfer of ascorbic acid into milk beyond a certain level (100-120 mg/L). In the study by Deodhar et al. (1964), milk vitamin C levels of Indian women were low initially but increased with supplementation. Therefore, if tissue and circulatory levels of vitamin C are depleted, milk levels can be reduced. Bates et al. (1982b) did not find a significant effect of vitamin C supplementation of Gambian women during the period of low vitamin C intake. However, an increasing trend was seen for milk vitamin C levels and it is possible that the level of supplementation was inadequate to fulfill tissue needs of vitamin C.

MINERALS

Calcium

In several studies no correlation has been found between maternal calcium intake and the concentration of calcium in human milk (Vaughan et al., 1979; Feeley et al., 1983a; Finley et al., 1985). This is not surprising since homeostatic mechanisms control serum calcium levels at a constant level. However, in one study, milk calcium levels of lactating teenagers tended to be lower than those of older (control) women (Lipsman et al., 1985). Since these teenagers had not fully completed their growth spurt, it is possible that demands of calcium for other tissues such as bone could compete with mammary transfer of calcium. It has been reported that this group of women is at risk for calcium deficiency since bone demineralization can be found (Chan et al., 1982).

Greer et al. (1982) found a weak correlation between milk calcium level and maternal calcium intake, but not milk maternal serum calcium. Since serum calcium in these women increased with lactation time to reach prepregnancy values, while serum ionized calcium remained unchanged, it was suggested that the increase in calcium was mediated by an increase in serum protein. It is possible that the calcium intake of the women was correlated to protein intake and that the increase in milk calcium was correlated to increased protein-bound calcium in serum. This reasoning is largely conjectural, since the mechanisms of calcium transport into milk and the factors affecting it remain to be studied in detail.

Poor nutritional status in lactating women in developing countries does not appear to affect milk calcium levels, although their calcium intake often also is low (Belavady & Gopalan, 1959; Lindblad & Rahimtoola, 1974). Methodological problems to measure calcium accurately could explain the finding of low (Jansen et al., 1960; Bailey, 1965) and high (Carneiro & de Oliveira, 1973) milk calcium levels. In neither study was it indicated that the methods used compensated for matrix interference.

Magnesium

Dietary intake of magnesium does not appear to affect milk levels of this mineral (Vaughan et al., 1979; Greer et al., 1982; Feeley et al., 1983a; Finley et al., 1985b). Similar to calcium, serum magnesium is normally controlled within a fairly narrow range. However, there can be exceptions when pharmacological doses are given. Cruikshank et al. (1982) studied women that were treated for preeclampsia with magnesium sulfate. Immediately after birth, a bolus dose (4 g) of magnesium sulfate followed by repeated doses of 1 g per hour were given to nursing women. Colostrum levels of magnesium were higher in treated women than in controls although these higher milk magnesium values were still in the normal range. The milk levels were correlated to the increased serum levels of magnesium and once treatment was stopped and serum magnesium returned to normal, milk magnesium rapidly returned to a level similar to control women.

Phosphate

Few studies have attempted to investigate the correlation between dietary phosphate and milk phosphate in detail. In most reports to date, no effects of phosphate intake on phosphate in milk have been observed (Greer et al., 1982; Finley et al., 1985b).

Sodium and potassium

There does not appear to be an effect of maternal sodium intake on milk sodium concentration (De Filippi et al., 1981; Keenan et al., 1982). Giving a low sodium diet to lactating women did not affect milk sodium or potassium levels (Keenan et al., 1982). Similarly, a short-term study using low and high sodium diets failed to show effects on milk sodium or potassium (Dewey et al., 1986). In this latter study, post-prandial effects on milk sodium and potassium were investigated as it was expected that hormonal control of sodium/potassium excretion would regulate serum levels in long-term studies.

Chlorine

The level of chlorine in human milk does not appear to be affected by maternal diet although very few studies have addressed this issue. Chlorine deficiency has been described in a breast-fed infant, but maternal serum and milk chlorine levels were found to be normal (Asnes et al., 1982).

Iodine and fluorine

Studies on the effect of maternal iodine intake on iodine concentration of human milk are conflicting (Bruhn & Franke, 1983; Gushurst et al., 1984). It is possible that this discrepancy may be explained by different effects of various sources of dietary iodine. For example, Gushurst et al. (1984) found an effect of intake of iodized salt on human milk iodine, while iodine provided by cow's milk, bread or seafood (all high in iodine) was not correlated to milk iodine. It has been shown that iodine used in medical preparations can affect milk iodine concentrations (Postellon & Aronow, 1982).

While the benefits of fluorine on development of teeth in the infant and their resistance against caries now are well-recognized, there have been few studies on the effect of maternal fluorine intake and milk fluorine. In Finland, Esala et al. (1982) found that women in areas of high water fluorine levels had higher milk fluorine concentration (11 μg/L) than women in areas of lower water fluorine (7 μg/L). In another study, however, such an effect was not found (Backer-Dirks et al., 1974) possibly because of a smaller difference in fluorine levels between the study groups. Plasma fluorine levels can be reflected in milk when pharmacological levels are used; Ekstrand et al. (1984) found that plasma fluorine had a peak 2 h after intake of a larger dose of fluorine, and milk fluorine also increased but not to the same extent.

TRACE ELEMENTS

There does not appear to be a pronounced effect of maternal trace element status or intake on milk levels of these elements. The only exception is selenium, the metabolism of which is quite different from that of other trace elements and more closely related to protein metabolism. It should be noted, though, that in few studies have situations of deficiency and supplementation been investigated in detail (Lönnerdal et al., 1981). The increasingly popular use of supplements of trace elements that earlier might have been judged pharmacological may widen the range of levels to be studied. Since interactions among trace elements can occur at several levels (e.g., absorptive pathways, liver metabolism), the potential effects of one trace element on others should be considered as well (Lönnerdal & Keen, 1983).

Iron

For this element, the situations of maternal deficiency and excess certainly are common. Iron deficiency anemia is prevalent in many developing countries and supplementation with high levels of iron during pregnancy and lactation is common in many industrialized countries. Consequently, wide differences in circulating levels of iron can be expected to occur.

Several studies have failed to find a correlation between poor maternal iron status and milk iron (Karmarkar & Ramakrishnan, 1960; Murray et al., 1978; Celada et al., 1982). Fransson et al. (1985), however, found higher concentrations of iron in milk from anemic Indian women. These higher milk iron levels were paralleled by higher milk lactoferrin levels, possibly indicating some compensatory mechanisms of iron transfer into milk. Dietary intake of iron seems to have little effect on milk iron (Picciano & Guthrie, 1976; Kirksey et al., 1979; Vaughan et al., 1979; Vuori et al., 1980; Feeley et al., 1983b; Fransson et al., 1984; Finley et al., 1985b). (For further details on iron in milk, see another chapter in this volume.)

Zinc

Maternal dietary zinc intake does not appear to affect milk zinc concentration (Kirksey et al., 1979; Vaughan et al., 1979; Vuori et al., 1980; Feeley et al., 1983b). In a case study by Zimmerman and Hambidge (1980), low zinc levels in milk from women delivering prematurely were not correlated to low maternal serum zinc levels nor did maternal zinc supplementation increase milk zinc concentrations. In a recent study by the same group (Krebs et al., 1985), maternal zinc supplementation (13 mg/day) had a slight effect on milk zinc levels after 6 months of supplementation. However, Moser and Reynolds (1983) did not find an effect of maternal zinc supplementation on milk zinc levels. It is possible that these populations were different with regard to zinc status and that they therefore responded differently to the supplementation. Preferably, a population of women with documented suboptimal zinc status should be investigated. (For further details on zinc in milk, see another chapter in this volume.)

Copper

Dietary intake of copper does not appear to affect milk copper concentration (Kirksey et al., 1979; Vaughan et al., 1979; Vuori et al., 1980; Feeley et al., 1983b). Increased serum copper levels in women using oral contraceptives did not appear to affect milk copper levels (Kirksey et al., 1979). In a study of questionable ethics, intravenous copper injections were found to have no effect on milk copper (Munch-Petersen, 1950). Few studies have investigated low maternal copper status and milk copper.

Manganese

Very few studies have attempted to correlate maternal manganese intake to milk manganese concentration. This is most likely explained by methodological difficulties, since the manganese concentration of human milk is very low (4-8 μg/L). Vuori et al. (1980) found an effect of manganese intake during lactation on milk manganese. The study by Vaughan et al. (1979) also indicated an effect of maternal dietary manganese on the level of manganese in milk. However, our limited knowledge of manganese absorption, status and homeostasis makes it difficult to evaluate or interpret these findings.

Selenium

While our knowledge of selenium metabolism still is limited, it is known that selenium in biological tissues and fluids is primarily bound to proteins as selenocysteine and selenomethionine. Selenium concentration of soil varies significantly in different regions of the world and within countries, and it is known that these differences are reflected in plant foods and meats produced in these different areas. An early study by Shearer and Hadjimarkos (1975) demonstrated that geographic location has a significant effect on levels of selenium in human milk. This effect was most likely due to the consumption of foods with different selenium content. More recently, Kumpulainen et al. (1985) found low selenium levels in milk from women in Finland, an area with low soil and food selenium concentration. Supplementation of the women with selenium (100 μg/d) as selenite or in yeast increased milk selenium concentration from 9-11 μg/L to 13-14 μg/L when yeast was given. The increase in milk selenium was lower when selenite was used. The changes observed in milk were paralleled by similar changes in maternal serum. It is possible that an organic form of selenium (yeast) is better absorbed than an inorganic salt (selenite), or that selenomethionine and selenocysteine from yeast is incorporated into milk proteins to a larger extent than selenite. (For further details on selenium in milk, see another chapter in this volume.)

CONCLUSIONS

There appears to be little effect, if any, of maternal nutrition on milk volume, although there may be a lower limit below which energy will be inadequate for milk production. In general, milk lipids such as fatty acids and phospholipids, but with the exception of cholesterol, are affected by maternal diet. Fat-soluble vitamins are also affected by maternal diet. The situation is more variable for the water-soluble vitamins, most likely due to differences in transport mechanisms into milk. Also there appear to be upper limits with regard to transfer of water-soluble vitamins but not of fat-soluble vitamins. Proteins and non-protein nitrogen compounds may be affected by maternal nutrition under some conditions, although these differences appear to be of small magnitude. Carbohydrates, minerals, trace elements (with the exception of selenium) and electrolytes are not significantly affected by maternal diet, judging from the literature to date. It is hoped that further studies in this area will enhance our knowledge with regard to the quantitative effects of maternal diet on milk composition as well as the mechanisms regulating nutrient transport across the mammary epithelium.

REFERENCES

Aitchison, J. M., Dunkley, W. L., Canolty, N. L. & Smith, L. M. (1977) Influence of diet on trans fatty acids in human milk. Am. J. Clin. Nutr. 30, 2006-2015.

Ajans, Z. A., Sarrif & Husbands, M. (1965) Influence of Vit A on human colostrum and early milk. Am. J. Clin. Nutr. 17, 139-142.

Ala-Houhala, M. (1985) 25-Hydroxyvitamin D levels during breast-feeding with or without maternal or infantile supplementation of vitamin D. J. Pediatr. Gastroenterol. Nutr. 4, 220-226.

Asnes, R. S., Wisotsky, D. H., Migel, P. F., Seigle, R. L. & Levy, J. (1982) The dietary chloride deficiency syndrome occurring in a breast-fed infant. J. Pediatr. 100, 923-924.

Backer-Dirks, O., Jongeling-Eijndhoven, J. M. P. A., Flissebaalje, T. D. & Gedelia, I. (1974) Total and free ionic fluoride in human and cow's milk as determined by gas-liquid chromatography and the fluoride electrode. Caries Res. 8, 181-186.

Bailey, K. V. (1965) Quantity and composition of breastmilk in some New Guinean populations. J. Trop. Pediatr. 11, 35-49.

Baker, S. J., Jacob, E., Rajan, R. T. & Swaminathan, S. P. (1962) Vitamin B_{12} deficiency in pregnancy and the puerperium. Br. Med. J. 1, 1658-1661.

Bates, C. J., Phil, D., Prentice, A. M., Watkinson, M., Morrell, P., Sutcliffe, B. A., Foord, F. A. & Whitehead, R. G. (1982a) Riboflavin requirements of lactating Gambian women: A controlled supplementation trial. Am. J. Clin. Nutr. 135, 701-709.

Bates, C. J., Prentice, A. M., Prentice, A., Paul, A. M. & Whitehead, R. G. (1982b) Seasonal variations in ascorbic acid status and breast milk ascorbic acid levels in rural Gambian women in relation to dietary intake. Trans. Royal Soc. Trop. Med. Hyg. 76, 341-347.

Becroft, T. C. (1967) Child-rearing practices in the highlands of New Guinea: a longitudinal study of breast-feeding. Med. J. Austr. 2, 596-601.

Belavady, B. & Gopalan, C. (1959) Chemical composition of human milk in poor Indian women. Ind. J. Med. Res. 47, 234-235.

Belavady, B. & Gopalan, C. (1960) Effects of dietary supplementation on the composition of breast milk. Ind. J. Med. Res. 48, 518-523.

Bruhn, J. C. & Franke, A. A. (1983) Iodine in human milk. J. Dairy Sci. 66, 1396-1398.

Butte, N. F., Garza, C., Stuff, J. E., O'Brian Smith, E. & Nichols, B. L. (1984) Effect of maternal diet and body composition on lactational performance. Am. J. Clin. Nutr. 39, 296-306.

Byerley, L. O. & Kirksey, A. (1985) Effects of different levels of vitamin C intake on the vitamin C concentration in human milk and the vitamin C intakes of breast-fed infants. Am. J. Clin. Nutr. 41, 665-671.

Carneiro, T. A., & Dutra de Oliveira, J. E. (1973) Nutritional studies in human lactation in Brazil. I. Chemical composition of breast milk. J. Trop. Pediatr. Environ. Child. Health 19, 284-387.

Celada, A., Brusset, R., Gutierrez, J. & Herreros, V. (1982) No correlation between iron concentration in breast milk and maternal iron stores. Helv. Paediatr. Acta 37, 11-16.

Chan, G. M., Ronald, N., Salter, P., Hollis, J. & Thomas, M. R. (1982) Decreased bone mineral status in lactating adolescent mothers. J. Pediatr. 101, 767-770.

Chappell, J. E., Clandinin, M. T. & Kearney-Volpe, C. (1985) Trans fatty acids in human milk lipids: influence of maternal diet and weight loss. Am. J. Clin. Nutr. 42, 49-56.

Cooperman, J. M., Dweck, H. S., Newman, L. J., Garbarino, C. & Lopez, R. (1982) The folate in human milk. Am. J. Clin. Nutr. 36, 576-580.

Coward, W. A., Paul, A. A. & Prentice, A. M. (1984) The impact of malnutrition on human lactation: Observations from community studies. Fed. Proc. 43, 2432-2437.

Cruikshank, D. P., Varner, M. W. & Pitkin, R. M. (1982) Breast milk magnesium and calcium concentrations following magnesium sulfate treatment. Am. J. Obstet. Gynecol. 143, 685-688.

De Filippi, J. P., Kaanders, H. & Hofman, A. (1981) Sodium in the diet and milk of breast feeding women. Acta Paediatr. Scand. 70, 417-418.

Deodhar, A. O., Rajalakshmi, R. & Ramakrishnan, C. V. (1964) Studies on human lactation. Part III. Effect of dietary vitamin contents of breast milk. Acta Pediatr. 53, 42-48.

Dewey, K. G., Ereman, R. R. & Lönnerdal, B. (1986) Does maternal sodium intake affect postprandial sodium concentrations in breast milk? Fed. Proc. 45, in press.

Dewey. K. G., Finley, D. A. & Lönnerdal, B. (1984) Breast milk volume and composition during late lactation (7-10 months). J. Pediatr. Gastroenterol. Nutr. 3, 713-720.

Dewey, K. G. & Lönnerdal, B. (1983) Milk and nutrient intake of breast-fed infants from 1 to 6 months: Relation to growth and fatness. J. Pediatr. Gastroenterol. Nutr. 2, 497-506.

Edozien, J. C., Khan, M. A. R. & Waslien, C. I. (1976) Human protein deficiency: Results of a Nigerian village study. J. Nutr. 106, 312-328.

Ek, J. (1983) Plasma, red cell, and breast milk folacin concentrations in lactating women. Am. J. Clin. Nutr. 38, 929-935.

Ekstrand, J., Spak, C.-J., Falch, J., Afseth, J. & Ulvestad, H. (1984) Distribution of fluoride to human breast milk following intake of high doses of fluoride. Caries Res. 18, 93-95.

Esala, S., Vuori, E. & Helle, A. (1982) Effect of maternal fluorine intake on breast milk fluorine content. Br. J. Nutr. 48, 201-204.

Feeley, R. M., Eitenmiller, R. R., Benton Jones, Jr., J. and Barnhart, H. (1983a) Calcium, phosphorus and magnesium contents of human milk during early lactation. J. Pediatr. Gastroenterol. Nutr. 2, 262-267.

Feeley, R. M., Eitenmiller, R. R., Jones Jr., J. B. & Barnhart, H. (1983b) Copper, iron and zinc contents of human milk and early stages of lactation. Am. J. Clin. Nutr. 37, 443-448.

Finley, D. A., Lönnerdal, B., Dewey, K. G. & Grivetti, L. E. (1985a) Breast milk composition: Fat content and fatty acid composition in vegetarians and non-vegetarians. Am. J. Clin. Nutr. 41, 787-800.

Finley, D. A., Lönnerdal, B., Dewey, K. G. & Grivetti, L. E. (1985b) Inorganic constituents of breast milk from vegetarians and non-vegetarians: Relationships with each other and with organic constituents. J. Nutr. 115, 772-781.

Forsum, E. & Lönnerdal, B. (1980) Effect of protein intake on protein and nitrogen composition of breast milk. Am. J. Clin. Nutr. 33, 1809-1813.

Foukas, M. D. (1973) An antilactogenic effect of pyridoxine. J. Obstet. Gynecol. Br. Commonw. 80, 718-720.

Fransson, G.-B., Agarwal, K. N., Gebre-Medhin, M. & Hambraeus, L. (1985) Increased breast milk iron in severe maternal anemia. Physiological trapping or leakage? Acta Paediatr. Scand. 74, 290-291.

Fransson, G.-B., Gebre-Medhin, M. & Hambraeus, L. (1984) The human milk contents of iron, copper, zinc, calcium and magnesium in a population with a habitually high intake of iron. Acta Paediatr. Scand. 73, 471-476.

Gebre-Medhin, M., Vahlquist, A., Hofvander, Y., Uppsäll, L., Vahlquist, B. (1976) Breast milk composition in Ethiopian and Swedish mothers. I. Vitamin A and β-carotene. Am. J. Clin. Nutr. 29, 441-451.

Greentree, L. B. (1979) Dangers of vitamin B_6 in nursing mothers. N. Engl. J. Med. 300, 141-142.

Greer, F. R., Hollis, B. W., Cripps, D. J. & Tsang, R. C. (1984a) Effects of maternal ultraviolet B irradiation on vitamin D content of human milk. J. Pediatr. 105, 431-433.

Greer, F. R., Hollis, B. W. & Napoli, J. L. (1984b) High concentrations of vitamin D_2 in human milk associated with pharmacologic doses of vitamin D_2. J. Pédiatr. 105, 61-63.

Greer, F. R., Tsang, R. C., Levin, R. S., Searcy, J. E., Wu, R. & Steichen, J. J. (1982) Increasing serum calcium and magnesium concentrations in breast-fed infants: Longitudinal studies of minerals in human milk and in sera of nursing mothers and their infants. J. Pediatr. 100, 59-64.

Gushurst, C. A., Mueller, J. A., Green, J. A. & Sedor, F. (1984) Breast milk iodide: Reassessment in the 1980's. Pediatrics 73, 354-357.

Guthrie, H. A., Picciano, M. F. & Sheehe, D. (1977) Fatty acid patterns of human milk. J. Pediatr. 90, 39-41.

Hanafy, M. M., Morsey, M. R. A., Seddick, Y., Habib, Y. A. & el Lozy, E. (1972) Maternal nutrition and lactation performance. J. Trop. Pediatr. Environ. Child. Health 18, 187-191.

Haroon, Y., Shearer, M. J., Rahim, S., Gunn, W. G., McEnery, G. & Barkham, P. (1982) The content of phylloquinone (vitamin K_1) in human milk, cow's milk and infant formula foods determined by high-performance liquid chromatography. J. Nutr. 112, 1105-1117.

Harris, W. S., Conner, W. E. & Lindsey, S. (1984) Will dietary ω-3 fatty acids change the composition of human milk? Am. J. Clin. Nutr. 40, 780-785.

Harzer, G., Dieterich, I. & Haug, M. (1984) Effects of the diet on the composition of human milk. Ann. Nutr. Metab. 28, 231-239.

Hennart, P., Hofvander, Y., Vis, H. & Robyn, C. (1985) Comparative study of nursing mothers in Africa (Zaire) and in Europe (Sweden): breast-feeding behavior, nutritional status, lactational hyperprolactinaemia and status of the menstrual cycle. Clin. Endocrinol. 22, 179-187.

Hennart, P. & Vis, H. L. (1980) Breast-feeding and post partum amenorrhoea in Central Africa. I. Milk production in rural areas. J. Trop. Ped. 26, 177-183.

Hollis, B. W., Lambert, P. W. & Horst, R. L. (1983) Factors affecting the antirachitic sterol content of native milk. In: Perinatal Calcium and Phosphorus Metabolism (Holick, M. F., Gray, T. K. & Anast, C. S., eds.). pp. 157-182.

Hrubetz, M. C., Devel, Jr., H. J. & Hanley, B. J. (1945) Studies on carotenoid metabolism. V. The effect of a high vitamin A intake on the composition of human milk. J. Nutr. 29, 245-254.

Insull, W., Hersch, J., James, T. & Ahrens, E. H. (1959) The fatty acids of human milk. II. Alterations produced by manipulation of caloric balance and exchange of dietary fats. J. Clin. Invest. 38, 443-450.

Jansen, A. A. J., Luyken, R., Malcolm, S. H. & Willems, J. J. L. (1960) Quantity and composition of breast milk in Biak Island (Neth. New Guinea). Trop. Geog. Med. 2, 138-144.

Jansson, L., Åkesson, B. & Holmberg, L. (1981) Vitamin E and fatty acid composition of human milk. Am. J. Clin. Nutr. 34, 8-13.

Jathar, V. S., Kamath, S. A., Parikh, M. N., Rege, D. V. and Satoskar, R. S. (1970) Maternal milk and serum vitamin B_{12}, folic acid, and protein levels in Indian subjects. Arch. Dis. Child. 45, 236-241.

Johnston, L., Vaughan, L. & Fox, H. M. (1981) Pantothenic acid content of human milk. Am. J. Clin. Nutr. 34, 2205-2209.

Karmarkar, M. G., Rajalakshmi, R. & Ramakrishnan, C. V. (1963) Studies on human lactation. I. Effects of dietary protein and fat supplementation on protein, fat, and essential amino acid contents of breast milk. Acta Paediatr. 52, 473-480.

Karmarkar, M. G. & Ramakrishnan, C. V. (1960) Studies on lactation. Relation between the dietary intake of lactating women and the chemical composition of milk with regard to principle and certain inorganic constituents. Acta Paediatr. 49, 599-604.

Keenan, B. S., Buzek, S. W., Garza, C., Potts, E. & Nichols, B. L. (1982) Diurnal and longitudinal variations in human milk sodium and potassium:

Implications for nutrition and physiology. Am. J. Clin. Nutr. 35, 527-534.

Kirksey, A., Ernst, J. A., Roepke, J. L. & Tsai, T.-L. (1979) Influence of mineral intake and use of oral contraceptives before pregnancy on the mineral content of human colostrum and of more mature milk. Am. J. Clin. Nutr. 32, 30-39.

Kneebone, G. M., Kneebone, R. & Gibson, R. A. (1985) Fatty acid composition of breast milk from three racial groups from Penang, Malaysia. Am. J. Clin. Nutr. 41, 765-769.

Kramer, M., Szöke, K., Lindner, K. & Tarjan, R. (1965) The effect of different factors on the composition of human milk and its variations. III. Effect of dietary fats on the lipid composition of human milk. Nutr. Dieta. 7, 71-79.

Krebs, N. F., Hambidge, K. M., Jacobs, M. A. & Rasbach, J. D. (1985) The effects of a dietary zinc supplement during lactation on longitudinal changes in maternal zinc status and milk zinc concentrations. Am. J. Clin. Nutr. 41, 560-570.

Kumpulainen, J., Salmenperä, L., Siimes, M. A., Koivistoinen, P. & Perheentupa, J. (1985) Selenium supplementation of breast-fed infants via the mother. Am. J. Clin. Nutr. 42, 829-835.

Lammi-Keefe, C. J. & Jensen, R. G. (1984) Lipids in human milk: A Review. 2. Composition and fat soluble vitamins. J. Pediatr. Gastroenterol. Nutr. 3, 172-198.

Lauber, E. & Reinhardt, M. (1979) Studies on the quality of breast milk during 23 months of lactation in a rural community of the Ivory Coast. Am. J. Clin. Nutr. 32, 1159-1173.

Lindblad, B. S. & Rahimtoola, R. J. (1974) A pilot study of the quality of human milk in a lower socioeconomic group in Karachi, Pakistan. Acta Paediat. Scand. 63, 125-128.

Lipsman, S., Dewey, K. G. & Lönnerdal, B. (1985) Breast-feeding among teenage mothers: milk composition, infant growth and maternal dietary intake. J. Pediatr. Gastroenterol. Nutr. 4, 426-434.

Lönnerdal, B., Forsum, E. & Hambraeus, L. (1976a) A longitudinal study of the protein, nitrogen and lactose contents of human milk from Swedish well-nourished mothers. Am. J. Clin. Nutr. 29, 1127-1133.

Lönnerdal, B., Forsum, E., Gebre-Medhin, M. & Hambraeus, L. (1976b) Breast milk composition in Ethiopian and Swedish mothers. II. Lactose, nitrogen, and protein contents. Am. J. Clin. Nutr. 29, 1134-1141.

Lönnerdal, B., Keen, C. L. & Hurley, L. S. (1981) Iron, copper, zinc and manganese in milk. Ann. Rev. Nutr. 1, 149-174.

Lönnerdal, B. & Keen, C. L. (1983) Trace element absorption in infants: Potentials and limitations. In: Reproductive and Developmental Toxicity of Metals (Clarkson, T. W., Nordberg, G. F. & Sager, P. R., eds.), pp. 759-776, Plenum Press, New York.

Lönnerdal, B., Smith, C. & Keen, C. L. (1984) Analysis of breast milk: Current methodologies and future needs. J. Pediatr. Gastroenterol. Nutr. 3, 290-295.

Mellies, M. J., Ishikawa, T. T., Gartside, P., Burton, K., MacGee, J., Allen, K., Steiner, P. M., Brady, D. & Glueck, C. J. (1978) Effects of varying maternal dietary cholesterol and phytosterol in lactating women and their infants. Am. J. Clin. Nutr. 31, 1347-1354.

Mellies, M. J., Ishikawa, T. T., Gartside, P. S., Burton, K., MacGee, J., Allen, K., Steiner, P. M., Brady, D. & Glueck, C. J. (1979) Effects of varying maternal dietary fatty acids in lactating women and their infants. Am. J. Clin. Nutr. 32, 299-303.

Metz, J., Zalusky, R. & Herbert, V. (1968) Folic acid binding by serum and milk. Am. J. Clin. Nutr. 21, 289-294.

Miranda, R., Saravia, N. G., Ackerman, R., Murphy, N., Berman, S. & McMurray, D. N. (1983) Effect of maternal nutritional statuses on immunological substances in human colostrum and milk. Am. J. Clin. Nutr. 37, 632-640.

Moser, P. B. & Reynolds, R. D. (1983) Dietary zinc intake and zinc concentrations of plasma, erythrocytes, and breast milk in antepartum and postpartum lactating and nonlactating women: A longitudinal study. Am. J. Clin. Nutr. 38, 101-108.

Munch-Petersen, S. On the copper content in mother's milk before and after intravenous copper administration. Acta Paediatr. 39, 378-387.

Murray, M. J., Murray, A. B., Murray, N. J. & Murray, M. B. (1978) The effect of iron status of Nigerian mothers on that of their infants at birth and 6 months, and on the concentration of Fe in breast milk. Br. J. Nutr. 39, 627-630.

Nail, P. A., Thomas, M. R. & Eakin, R. (1980) The effect of thiamin and riboflavin supplementation on the level of those vitamins in human breast milk and urine. Am. J. Clin. Nutr. 33, 198-204.

Picciano, M. F. & Guthrie, H. A. (1976) Copper, iron, and zinc contents of mature human milk. Am. J. Clin. Nutr. 29, 242-254.

Postellon, D. C. & Aronow, R. (1982) Iodine in mother's milk. JAMA 247, 463-464.

Prentice, A. M. (1979) Variations in maternal dietary intake, birthweight and breast-milk output in the Gambia. In: Maternal Nutrition During Pregnancy and Lactation (Aebi, H., & Whitehead, R., eds.), pp. 167-182, Hans Huber Publishing.

Prentice, A., Prentice, A. M., Cole, J. J., Paul, A. A. & Whitehead R. G. (1984) Breast-milk antimicrobial factors of rural Gambian mothers. I. Influence of stage of lactation and maternal plane of nutrition. Acta Paediatr. Scand. 73, 796-802.

Prentice, A. M., Roberts, S. B., Prentice, A., Paul, A. A., Watkinson, P. M., Watkinson, A. A. & Whitehead, R. G. (1983) Dietary supplementation of lactating Gambian women. I. Effect on breast-milk volume and quality. Human Nutr.: Clin. Nutr. 37C, 53-64.

Roberts, S. B., Cole, T. J. & Coward W. A. (1985) Lactational performance in relation to energy intake in the baboon. Am. J. Clin. Nutr. 41, 1270-1276.

Rowland, M. G. M., Paul, A. A. & Whitehead, R. G. (1981) Lactation and infant nutrition. Br. Med. Bull. 37, 77-82.

Sandberg, D. P., Begley, J. A. & Hall, C. A. (1981) The content, binding and forms of vitamin B_{12} in milk. Am. J. Clin. Nutr. 34, 1717-1724.

Sanders, T. A. B., Ellis, F. R., Path, F. R. C. & Dickerson, J. W. T. (1978) Studies of vegans: The fatty acid composition of plasma choline phosphoglycerides, erythrocytes, adipose tissue, and breast milk, and some indicators of susceptibility to eschemic heart disease in vegans and omnivore controls. Am. J. Clin. Nutr. 31, 805-813.

Selhub, J., Arnold, R., Smith, A. M. & Picciano, M. F. (1984) Milk folate binding protein (FBP): A secretory protein for folate. Nutr. Res. 4, 181-187.

Shearer, T. R. & Hadjimarkos, D. M. (1975) Geographic distribution of selenium in human milk. Arch. Environ. Health 30, 230-233.

Smith, A. M., Picciano, M. F. & Deering, R. H. (1983) Folate supplementation during lactation: maternal folate status, human milk folate content, and their relationship to infant folate status. J. Pediatr. Gastroenterol. Nutr. 2, 622-628.

Sneed, S. M., Zane, C. & Thomas, M. R. (1981) The effects of ascorbic acid, vitamin B_6, vitamin B_{12} and folic acid supplementation on the breast milk and maternal nutritional status of low socioeconomic lactating women. Am. J. Clin. Nutr. 34, 1338-1346.

Specker, B. L., Tsang, R. C. & Hollis, B. W. (1985) Effect of race and diet on human-milk vitamin D and 25-hydroxyvitamin D. Am. J. Dis. Child 139, 1134-1137.

Srikantia, S. G. & Reddy, V. (1967) Megaloblastic anaemia of infancy and vitamin B_{12}. Br. J. Haemat. 13, 949-953.

Styslinger, L. & Kirksey, A. (1985) Effects of different levels of vitamin B-6 supplementation on vitamin B-6 concentrations in human milk and vitamin B-6 intakes of breastfed infants. Am. J. Clin. Nutr. 41, 21-31.

Tamura, T., Yoshimura, Y. & Arakawa, T. (1980) Human milk folate and folate status in lactating mothers and their infants. Am. J. Clin. Nutr. 33, 193-197.

Tarjan, R., Kramer, M., Szöker, K. & Lindner, K. (1963) The effect of different factors on the composition of human milk and its variations. I. The effect of vitamin-rich foods on the composition of human milk. Nutr. Dieta 5, 12-29.

Thomas, M. R., Sneed, S. M., Wei, C., Nail, P. A., Wilon, M. & Sprinkle III, E. E. (1980a) The effects of vitamin C, vitamin B_6, vitamin B_{12}, folic acid, riboflavin, and thiamin on the breast milk and maternal status of well-nourished women at 6 months postpartum. Am. J. Clin. Nutr. 33, 2151-2156.

Thomas, M. R., Kawamoto, J., Sneed, S. M. & Eakin, R. (1980b) The effects of vitamin C, vitamin B_6 and vitamin B_{12} supplementation on the breast milk and maternal status of well-nourished women. Am. J. Clin. Nutr. 32, 1679-1685.

Underwood, B. A., Hepner, R. & Abdullah, H. (1970) Protein, lipid, and fatty acids of human milk from Pakistani women during prolonged periods of lactation. Am. J. Clin. Nutr. 23, 400-407.

Van Steenbergen, W. M., Kusin, J. A., De With, C., Lacko, E. & Jansen, A. A. J. (1983) Lactation performance of mothers with contrasting nutritional studies in rural Kenya. Acta Paediatr. Scand. 72, 805-810.

Vaughan, L. A., Weber, C. W. & Kemberling, S. R. (1979) Longitudinal changes in the mineral content of human milk. Am. J. Clin. Nutr. 32, 2301-2306.

Venkatachalam, P. S., Belavady, B. & Gopalan, C. (1962) Studies on vitamin A nutritional status of mothers and infants in poor communities of India. Trop. Pediatr. 61, 262-266.

Vuori, E., Mäkinen, S. M., Kara, R. & Kuitunen, P. (1980) The effects of the dietary intakes of copper, iron, manganese and zinc on the trace element content of human milk. Am. J. Clin. Nutr. 33, 227-231.

Vuori, E., Kiuru, K., Mäkinen, S. M., Väyrynen, P., Kara, R. & Kuitunen, P. (1982) Maternal diet and fatty acid pattern of breast milk. Acta Paediatr. Scand. 71, 959-963.

Zimmerman, A. W. & Hambidge, K. M. (1980) Low zinc in mothers' milk and zinc deficiency syndrome in breast-fed premature infants. Am. J. Clin. Nutr. 33, 951 (Abstr.).

EFFECT OF DIET ON THE LIPID

COMPOSITION OF HUMAN MILK

Robert G. Jensen

Nutritional Sciences Department
University of Connecticut
Storrs, CT. 06268

INTRODUCTION

Sosa et al (1) have stated, "Feed the mother: thereby the infant". The quotation embodies the belief, well supported by extensive research with cows (2), that diet affects lactation performance (quantity) and composition (quality) of human milk. The effects could be caused by insufficient levels of dietary nutrients, primarily protein and energy, changes in amounts of dietary nutrients and supplementation. Most of the studies have been done with ad lib diets and were not well controlled, although in the comparisons of regions, diets differed markedly. Further, sampling was often done improperly and volumes of milk and lipid contents were not reported. Finally, the effects of parasitism and mastitis have not been considered.

It is well documented that the lipid content of human milk is the most variable major constituent (3,4). The content varies within a nursing, from breast-to-breast, diurnally, longitudinally and among individuals. Further, the weight loss enjoyed by some nursing women mobilizes fatty acids from adipose tissue and these will appear in milk fat (3). Because of the variability, it is extremely important that a standardized sampling procedure be followed to isolate the influence of diet. A sampling procedure (4) and methods for determination of total lipids have been described (5).

In this review I will present and discuss the information available on alterations in diet and their effects on the contents of total lipids, phospholipids, sterols and fatty acids in human milk.

TOTAL LIPIDS

There are few controlled studies available on alterations in total lipids due to diet, but, in general, the amounts of energy, protein, lactose and fat are little changed by variations, within limits, in the nutritional status or dietary intake of the mother (6). In contrast, Karmarkar et al (7) observed a rise in milk fat contents from 3.78 to 4.71% with dietary supplementation of up to 45g of fat per day. However, control of sampling with inadequate in that foremilk was taken. This alone negates

Scientific Contribution No. , Storrs Agricultural Experiment Station
Storrs, CT 06268

Table 1. Dietary regimens used to induce changes and the changes found in the fatty acid composition of human milk lipids[a]

	Dietary period and days postpartum						
	I 5-11	II 12-18	III 19-26	IV 27-33	V 34-43	VI 44-48	VII 49-52
Caloric intake	ad libitum	2750	3750	1838	3750	2938	2938
Fat calories (% of total)		40	-	-	70	70	40
Fat intake (g/day)		123	3.0	1.4	292	228	131
Type of fat fed		Lard	Cow's milk	Cow's milk	Corn oil	Corn oil	Corn oil
Fatty acids in milk fat wt%							
12:0	6.0	4.6	15.0	7.9	3.0	3.0	4.9
14:0	9.0	9.3	22.0	9.0	2.3	2.0	4.3
16:0	25.0	23.8	25.0	23.5	13.1	14.0	12.7
16:1	2.0	3.1	5.0	6.8	1.4	1.0	1.5
18:0	8.0	7.8	3.0	3.2	3.0	3.0	2.9
18:1	34.0	42.6	24.0	36.9	31.4	31.0	28.7
18:2+3	9.0	10.3	1.0	7.3	43.0	45.0	42.0
Daily milk fat production g/24h	24	25	24.3	23.8	30	23	27

[a]Insull et al (9)

the findings. The subjects' diets before supplementation had 1300 kcal, an amount deficient by Western standards. It is likely that supplementation of malnourished women might increase the fat content, although this was not seen by Prentice et al (8) who were careful about sampling.

In one of the few controlled studies, Insull et al (9) fed the diets in Table 1 to one subject. The amounts of fat produced/24h are also given. The peak of about 30g on day 44 coincides with an increased milk volume at that time. Did the corn oil diet cause either increase or was it a physiological or analytical anomaly? Most likely, the latter. Otherwise the fat contents were stable.

Harzer et al (10) conducted a two-week crossover study with three nursing women (Table 2). During the first week, one mother was on a low fat-high carbohydrate diet (B). The other two subjects were on the reverse regimen. In diet A, about 15% of the calories were from fat, 20% from protein and 65% from carbohydrate. With diet B, the contributions were: fat, 50%; protein, 15% and carbohydrate, 35%. Both contained about 2500 kcal. A drastic reduction in triacylglycerol content, 4.1 to 2.6% and an increase in lactose amounts, 5.2 to 6.4%, occurred with the subjects were switched from diet A to B. These results are extraordinary and inexplicable, since lactose is the most stable component in milk and there is no physiological explanation for the decrease in fat.

Table 2. Influence of dietary changes in selected milk constituents, calculated from the results at day 3 and day 10 of the trial, respectively (n=3)[a]

Constituents	Low fat/high (A) carbohydrate	High fat/low (B) carbohydrate
Milk		
Lactose, g/100 ml	5.2	6.4
Protein, g/100 ml	1.7	1.5
Chol, mg/100 ml	37.5	20.8
PL, mg/100 ml	45.3	26.4
TG, g/100	4.1	2.6
FA, weight %		
12:0	5.01	3.90
14:0	7.61	6.10
18:1n9	36.34	38.32
18:2n6	10.81	15.38
20:4n6	0.26	0.21

[a]Harzer et al (10) Diets were fed to one and two subjects for one week and then switched.

My conclusion is that there are almost no reliable data showing changes in fat content of human milk due to dietary alterations. The studies were not and probably could not be controlled. The evidence suggests that the amounts of fat are maintained at or near normal levels regardless of the nutritional status of the mother.

STEROLS AND PHOSPHOLIPIDS

Most of the data indicate that diet does not affect the cholesterol content of milk. Potter and Nestel (11) found that significant dietary induced changes in plasma cholesterol in lactating women were not correlated with changes in milk cholesterol or lipids. These results were confirmed by Mellies et al (12) when they sequentially fed low and high cholesterol diets. However, they also reported a large increase in phytosterol content. The presence of phytosterols in human milk was not confirmed by us (13) using gas-liquid chromatography and mass-spectrometry nor by Haug and Harzer (14) with high-performance liquid chromatography. In their study on the effects of diet on the composition of milk described above, Harzer et al (10) noted the change in cholesterol and phospholipid contents in Table 2. These changes correlate with the decrease in fat content from 4.1 to 2.6% and these are suspect. Again, cholesterol and phospholipids are not likely to be changed by diet and phytosterols are present only in trace amounts.

FATTY ACIDS

Triacylglycerols account for about 98% of the lipids in human milk and fatty acids 85% of these. The fatty acids are the most responsive of the major components to diet. There are three sources: diet, biosynthesis in the mammary gland and mobilization from other sites, primarily adipose tissue. The fatty acids in adipose tissue in the lactating women will be a mixture from the diet and endogenous synthesis dependent upon the caloric balance and type of diet. The peak secretion of isotopically labelled dietary lipids into human milk is about 10h (15). However, in those women who are losing weight, mobilization from adipose tissue is an important source of fatty acids. With trans fatty acids (mostly 18:1), both immediate and long term dietary effects have been noted (16). The shorter fatty acids, 10:0-14:0, found in human milk are synthesized in the mammary gland. Thompson and Smith (17) found that 85% of the fatty acids with less than 16 carbons are synthesized in the gland and noted that stimulation of this pathway is triggered by a low fat-high carbohydrate diet.

Insull et al (9) were the first not only to analyze human milk fatty acids by gas-liquid chromatography, but also to apply the method to analysis of dietary effects. The dietary regimen used and the results are in Table 1 as are the fatty acid compositions of the milk lipids. The 18:2 + 18:3 content of the milk increased as a result of feeding corn oil while 12:0 responded reciprocally. In dietary period III, when the 12:0 content of milk was highest, the excess dietary calories (3750 kcal) were carbohydrate. These changes were not caused by normalization to percent, since the fat content was 3.5% throughout except for period V. The response to diet and the reciprocal relationship between 12:0 and 18:2 has been confirmed in later investigations. Other than for 18:2, changes were not observed. Read et al (18) investigated the influence of dietary carbohydrates and fat on fatty acids of mature milks in four ethnic groups who consumed widely differing diets. Their results are in Table 3. When most of the calories were derived from carbohydrates, e.g., in the diet of the Tanganyikan mothers, the content of 12:0 was 16.5% and 18:2 only 1.0%. It is likely that if the infants consumed this milk for any length of time, they might show symptoms of essential fatty acid deficiency. Again the reciprocal relationship between 12:0 and 18:2 is evident.

The effect of vegetarian diets on the fatty acid composition of breast milk has been determined. Sanders et al (19) compared the milks of four vegan and four omnivore controls. The major differences (Table 4) were: vegan, lower contents of 16:0, 16:1 and 18:0 than the omnivores. The quantities of 18:2 were almost five times higher (31.7%) in the vegan milks as compared to the omnivore samples (6.9%). Lauric acid (12:0) contents were similar: 3.9 and 3.3%. Finley et al (20) analyzed the milks from 109 vegetarian and 100 nonvegetarian lactating women. They noted that except for more 18:2 (18.38%) in the vegetarian as compared to the non-vegetarian milk (14.65%), the differences were small.

Table 3. The major fatty acid components of human milk in relation to diet from four ethnic groups[a]

	ETHNIC GROUPS			
	Tanganyikan	Jordanian	Bedouin	Lebanese
	No. of Samples			
FATTY ACIDS	17	31	9	19
12:0	16.5±6.0[b]	7.2±4.0	5.0±2.0	5.8±2.1
14:0	12.7±4.1	9.7±5.4	8.5±2.9	7.0±3.2
16:0	17.5±5.5	22.2±4.9	26.7±4.1	24.0±2.8
16:1	1.4±0.8	3.0±1.1	4.5±1.5	2.0±0.5
18:0	6.0±1.2	4.3±2.1	7.9±2.4	7.1±1.9
18:1	39.6±8.6	33.5±9.3	35.4±6.5	39.6±5.5
18:2	1.0±0.5	15.2±7.2	6.3±1.8	11.3±3.4
Total calories	2800	1500-2000	1500-2000	2350
Percent calories as fat	7	30-40	40	51
Remarks	75% of calories derived from carbohydrates, dietary fat mainly vegetable	Fat mainly vegetable, including varying amounts of soya oil	Fat mainly animal in origin	Fat about 70% vegetable, main source olive oil

[a]Read et al (18)

[b]Mean ± SD as wt%

Table 4. Breast milk fatty acids in vegans and omnivore controls[a]

Methyl esters	Vegans Mean	Vegans SE	Controls Mean	Controls SE
12:0	39	12.5	33	7.1
14:0	68	17.0	80	5.3
16:0	166[b]	14.4	276	10.5
18:0	52[b]	5.9	108	8.5
16:1	12[b]	0.9	36	5.3
18:1	313	25.0	353	11.1
18:2n6	317[b]	44.5	69	8.1
18:3n3	15[b]	2.4	8	0.5
20:2n6	5.1[b]	0.7	1.8	0.3
20:3n6	3.1	0.8	2.3	0.2
20:4n6	7.2	2.1	5.4	1.3
22:4n6	1.4	0.5	0.8	0.3
22:5n6	0.9	0.4	1.5	1.2
20:4n3	0.3[b]	0.1	0.9	0.2
20:5n3	0.4	0.1	2.0	0.8
22:5n3	2.7	1.4	5.2	2.7
22:6n3	2.3	1.1	5.9	2.3

[a]Mean values expressed as mg/g total methyl esters for four vegans and four omnivore controls. Vegans do not eat food from animal sources. Adapted from Sanders et al (19).

[b]Statistical significance of difference between means shown at the level of $p<0.05$.

Table 5. Major fatty acids of total acyl lipids in human milk samples obtained during the consumption of partially (H) and nonhvdrogenated fats (NH)[a]

Day	Dietary period	12:0	14:0	16:0	16:1c	18:0	18:1t	18:1c	18:2cc
		Fatty acid							
		% of total fatty acid							
1	H	3.48	5.14	23.61	2.33	8.45	4.23	33.24	13.93
	NH	3.71	6.18	25.50	2.40	8.53	3.93	32.28	12.59
2	H	3.00	5.95	24.05	2.44	7.39	6.09[x]	31.94	13.16
	NH	3.14	7.12	27.56	2.59	7.50	2.32[y]	30.76	15.52
3	H	2.79	4.64[x]	24.99	2.79	7.52	6.70[x]	33.30[a]	11.85
	NH	3.57	6.94[y]	27.96	3.03	6.88	1.78[y]	30.70[b]	14.28
4	H	2.92	5.04	23.66[a]	2.54	7.01	5.49[x]	35.14	12.99
	NH	3.13	5.58	28.55[b]	2.91	7.08	1.71[y]	33.14	15.00
5	H	2.26	4.44[x]	24.15[a]	2.65	7.50	5.63[x]	33.31	12.96
	NH	3.54	6.99[y]	29.23[b]	2.81	7.49	1.64[y]	31.41	13.30
6	H	2.32[a]	4.05[x]	22.63	2.23[x]	7.25	9.04[x]	33.02	13.00
	NH	4.23[b]	6.22[y]	25.66	2.92[y]	6.42	1.69[y]	31.91	15.45
SEM (common)		0.48	0.42	1.34	0.14	0.45	0.40	0.80	0.98
Mean (days 2-6)	H	2.66	4.24[x]	23.93[x]	2.54[a]	7.34	6.53[x]	33.35[a]	12.98
	NH	3.52	6.58[y]	27.85[y]	2.85[b]	7.09	1.84[y]	31.57[b]	14.40
SEM (common)		0.30	0.23	0.87	0.07	0.35	0.33	0.46	0.85

[a]Treatment means with days, within fatty acids with different letters are different (a,b=p<0.05), (x,y=p<0.01); n=8 except for day 6 where n = 7.

[b]Craig-Schmidt et al (22).

The trans isomers of fatty acids in partially hydrogenated food fats and oils consumed by women who nurse appear in their milk (21). The isomers are either derived directly from the diets or indirectly by mobilization from adipose tissue during weight loss. In one of the two controlled studies on the influence of diet on the amounts of trans acids in milk, Craig-Schmidt et al (22) fed diets containing non (NH) and partially hydrogenated (H) fats to nursing mothers. Their data are in Table 5. In the relatively short feeding period, the total 18:1t content rose from 4.23 to 9.04% as a result of the H diet, and dropped from 3.93 to 1.69% on the NH diet. Weight loss of the mothers, if any, was not given. The changes in 18:2cc were small and an average of 0.69%, 18:2tt was found.

Chappell et al (16) studied the effects of lactational stage, gestational age and diet on the trans fatty acid contents of human milk. For the dietary study, they fed 7 term mothers sequentially (2 weeks each), margarines containing low (0%), high (35%) and medium (13%) amounts of trans acids. The 18:2 contents were 58, 6 and 44%. The quantities of both acids in milk from these donors directly reflected the contents in the diet. However, when influences of weight loss and diet on 18:1t contents were combined, the effect of weight loss was independent of maternal diet. Milks from a group of donors who lost 4-7 kg contained about 3.3% 18:1t and the 0-2 kg group, 1.8%. There were no apparent differences in these groups in expressed milk volume, energy intake or food selection. While lactational stage and gestational age affected the patterns of trans fatty acids in milk, rate of maternal weight loss was the most important influence.

I have mentioned several of the investigations in which the 18:2 content of milk has been manipulated by alterations in maternal diet. Note that trials in which there was even reasonable control are few. Linoleic acid (18:2) contents of from 1 to 43% were reported, the latter on a high corn oil diet and the former on a high carbohydrate, low fat diet. A range for Western mothers is 10-14%. An investigation by Mellies et al (23) had a degree of dietary control. Fourteen mothers took an ad lib diet for 30 days after delivery, then were randomly assigned to a polyunsaturate-rich diet (P/S 1.8, 190 mg cholesterol per day). The P rich diet was the then named National Heart, Lung, Blood Institute type II diet. They remained on these regimens for 4 weeks, and crossed over to the other for another 4 weeks. The changes in 18:2 were pronounced: ad lib, 14.5%; P diet, 24.4 and S diet, 10.1. It has been adequately proven that the 18:2 content of human milk is positively responsive to dietary manipulation.

Recently, aware of the role of docosahexanoic acid (DHA, 22:6n-3) in infantile nerve and brain tissue and retinal development, Harris et al (24), evaluated fish oil as a means of increasing DHA in milk. A fish oil concentrate containing 11% W-3 fatty acids was used as the supplement. Six lactating women took 5 g/day for 28 days; five 10 g/day for 14 days and one 47 g/day for 8 days. Each intake level produced dose-dependent responses in the DHA contents of blood and milk. While some of these increases may have been statistically significant, the problem of precisely measuring small amounts of fatty acids is always a problem. Again, sampling was not controlled and amounts of fat and milk were not reported. The amount of fish oil fed in the study provided 0.5 and 1.0g of DHA per day. Harris et al say that these amounts could be obtained by eating 350-700 g of low fat fish or 75-150 g of high fat fish per day. These intakes, they continue, are not unrealistic or unachievable.

SUMMARY

There is no compelling evidence that the total lipid, cholesterol or phospholipid contents can be altered by diet. The contents of the de novo synthesized acids; 8:0, 10:0, 12:0 and 14:0 can be increased by a high carbohydrate diet. Consumption of oils rich in 18:2, 18:1t and long-chain polyunsaturated fatty acids increases the quantities of these acids in milk.

REFERENCES

1. R. Sosa, M.Klaus and J.J. Urrutia, Feed the nursing mother: thereby the infant, J. Pediatr., 88:668 (1976).
2. W.W. Christie, The effects of diet and other factors on the lipid composition of ruminant tissues and milk, Progr. Lipid Res., 17:245 (1979).
3. L. Hambraeus, Maternal diet and human milk composition, in Maternal Nutrition During Pregnancy and Lactation, H. Aebi and R. Whitehead, eds., Hans Huber Publ., Bern (1980).
4. A.M. Ferris, and R.G. Jensen, Lipids in human milk: A review. I: Sampling, determination and content, J. Pediatr. Gastroenterol. Nutr., 3:108 (1984).
5. R.G. Jensen, R.M.Clark, J. Bitman, L. Wood, M. Hamosh, and M.T. Clandinin, Methods for the sampling and analysis of human milk lipids, in: Human Lactation. I. Milk Components and Methodologies, R.G. Jensen and M.C. Neville, eds, Plenum Press, New York, 1985.
6. World Health Organization, The Quantity and Quality of Breast Milk, WHO, (1985).
7. M.G. Karmarkar, R. Rajalakshmi, and C.V. Ramakrishnan, Studies on human lactation. I. Effect of dietary protein and fat supplementation on protein, fat and essential amino acid contents of breast milk, Acta Pediatr. 52:473 (1963).
8. A.M. Prentice, S.B. Roberts, A. Prentice, A.A.Paul, M. Watkinson, A.A. Watkinson, and R.G. Whitehead, Dietary supplementation of lactating Gambian women. I. Effect on breast milk volume and quality, Hum. Nutr. Clin. Nutr., 37C:53 (1983).
9. W. Insull, Jr., J. Hirsch, T. James, E.H. Ahrens, Jr., The fatty acids of human milk. II. Alterations produced by manipulation of caloric balance and exchange of dietary fats, J. Clin. Invest., 38:443 (1959).
10. G. Harzer, I. Dieterich, and M. Haug, Effects of the diet on the composition of human milk, Ann. Nutr. Metab., 28:231 (1984).
11. J.M. Potter, P.J. Nestel, The effects of dietary fatty acids and cholesterol on the milk lipids of lactating women and the plasma cholesterol of breast-fed infants, Am. J. Clin. Nutr., 29:60 (1976).
12. M.J. Mellies, T.T. Ishikawa, P. Gartside, K. Burton, J. Macbee, K. Allen, P.M. Steiner, D. Brady, and C.J. Glueck, Effects of varying maternal dietary cholesterol and phytosterol in lactating women and their infants. Am. J. Clin. Nutr., 31:1347 (1978).
13. R.M. Clark, M.B. Fey, and R.G. Jensen, Desmosterol in human milk, Lipids, 18:264 (1983).
14. M. Haug, and G. Harzer, Cholesterol and other sterols in milk, J. Pediatr. Gastroenterol. Nutr., 3:816 (1984).
15. C. Garza, D.L. Hachey, N.L. Butte, P.D. Klein, and E. Emken, Maternal variables and the secretion of lipids in human milk, J. Am. Oil Chem. Soc., 62:637, Abstr 177 (1985).
16. J.E. Chappell, M.T. Clandinin, and C. Kearney-Volpe, Trans fatty acids in human milk lipids: Influence of maternal diet and weight loss, Am. J. Clin. Nutr., 42:49 (1985).
17. B.J. Thompson, and S. Smith, Biosynthesis of fatty acids by lactating human breast epithelial cells: An evaluation of the contribution to the overall composition of human milk fat, Pediatr. Res., 19:139 (1985).

18. W.W.C. Read, P.G. Lutz, and A. Tashjian, Human milk lipids. II. The influence of dietary carbohydrates and fat on the fatty acids of mature milk. A study in four ethnic groups, Am. J. Clin. Nutr., 17:180 (1965).
19. T.A.B. Sanders, F.R. Ellis, and J.W.T. Dickerson, Studies of vegans: The fatty acid compositions of plasma choline phosphoglycerides, erythrocytes, adipose tissue, and breast milk and some indicators of susceptibility to ischemic heart disease in vegans and omnivore controls, Am. J. Clin. Nutr., 31:805 (1978).
20. D.A. Finley, B. Lonnerdal, K.G. Dewey, and L.E. Grivetti, Breast milk composition:fat content and fatty acid composition in vegetarians and non-vegetarians, Am. J. Clin. Nutr., 41:587 (1985).
21. C.J. Lammi-Keefe, and R.G. Jensen, Lipids in human milk. 2: Composition and fat-soluble vitamins, J. Pediatr. Gastroenterol. Nutr., 3:172 (1984).
22. M.C. Craig-Schmidt, J.D. Weete, S.A. Faircloth, M.A. Wickwire and E.J. Livant, The effect of hydrogenated fat in the diet of nursing mothers on lipid composition and prostaglandin content of human milk, Am. J. Clin. Nutr., 39:778 (1984).
23. M.J. Mellies, T.T. Ishikawa, P.S. Gartside, K. Burton, J. MacGee, K. Allen, P.M. Steiner, D. Brady and C.J. Glueck, Effects of varying maternal dietary fatty acids in lactating women and their infants, Am. J. Clin. Nutr., 32:299 (1979).
24. W.S. Harris, W.E. Connor and S. Lindsay, Will dietary n-3 fatty acids change the composition of human milk? Am. J. Clin. Nutr., 40:780 (1984).

HUMAN MILK CARNITINE

P. R. Borum*, J. J. Chapman**, M. J. Macey**
and M. Keegan**

*Food Science & Human Nutrition Department
University of Florida
Gainesville, FL

**School of Nursing
Vanderbilt University
Nashville, TN

INTRODUCTION

Carnitine is critically important in the energy metabolism of the neonate. It is well established that carnitine is required for the transport of long chain fatty acids into the matrix of the mitochondron which is the site for β-oxidation[1]. Since the newborn experiences a metabolic shift from carbohydrate to lipid as the major fuel source, an adequate concentration of tissue carnitine is needed during the newborn period. The tissue stores of carnitine in the newborn are limited[2]. Milk appears to be the major source of carnitine for the newborn[3]. The total carnitine concentrations of milk are reported for samples taken from a group of healthy women at different stages of lactation.

MATERIALS AND METHODS

Healthy women with no chronic diseases who were planning to breast feed for a least four months and were between the ages of 18 and 35 years were entered into the study. The protocol was approved by the Institutional Review Board and participants signed an informed consent form. The study participants collected the complete expression of one breast at the first feeding time of the day and fed the infant from the other breast. Milk samples were obtained at the following days of lactation: birth to 3 days, 7 to 13 days, 14 to 20 days, 28 to 34 days, 56 to 62 days, and 112 to 118 days. Milk samples were placed on ice after collection, transported to the laboratory, and frozen at -70 degrees centigrade until assayed for carnitine. Milk samples were assayed for carnitine using a modification[4] of the radioisotopic method developed by Cederblad and Lindstedt[5] which is termed Method 1, and by a modification of the radioisotopic assay developed for milk samples[6] which is termed Method 2. The major difference between the two methods is that Method 2 has a filtration step added as part of the protein removal process in sample preparation. The filtration step removes particulate material.

RESULTS

Table 1 lists the milk carnitine concentrations of samples obtained at different stages of lactation. The samples were assayed by Method 1 and again by Method 2 when the sample volume permitted. The mean milk carnitine concentrations were higher at each stage of lactation when Method 2 was used. The milk carnitine concentration increased during the first two weeks of lactation and then decreased to values similar to that of colostrum.

Table 1. Milk Total Carnitine Concentrations

Days of Lactation	Assay Methodology	No. of Mothers	Mean $\pm$ Std.Dev. (nmol/ml)
Birth-3 days	Method 1	56	60.4 $\pm$ 29.5
	Method 2	44	66.9 $\pm$ 29.2
7-13 days	Method 1	55	84.5 $\pm$ 26.0
	Method 2	55	98.2 $\pm$ 26.0
14-20 days	Method 1	54	69.4 $\pm$ 17.7
	Method 2	53	80.9 $\pm$ 19.1
28-34 days	Method 1	51	68.6 $\pm$ 18.8
	Method 2	51	75.4 $\pm$ 23.9
56-62 days	Method 1	49	57.7 $\pm$ 16.4
	Method 2	48	66.1 $\pm$ 18.7
112-118 days	Method 1	39	57.5 $\pm$ 33.0
	Method 2	37	62.3 $\pm$ 21.2

DISCUSSION

Milk samples from all species investigated to date contain significant quantities of carnitine. The carnitine assay methodology used for blood appears to underestimate the concentration in milk. It has been reported[7] that the spectrophotometric assay[8] underestimates the milk carnitine concentration when compared to the radioisotopic assay methodology. The present study indicates that the radioisotopic assay methodology will also underestimate the milk carnitine concentration unless a filtration step is included to remove particulate material.

The decrease in milk carnitine concentrations during the second month of lactation has been observed by other investigators[7]. However the same investigators have not observed the increase in milk carnitine concentration during the first two weeks of lactation[7]. One possible explanation is that only fore milk was collected in the previous report[7] and our sampling technique obtained the complete expression of milk from one breast.

SUMMARY

Milk carnitine concentrations increase and then decrease with a peak carnitine concentration at approximately two weeks of lactation. Carnitine must be carefully assayed using methodology developed for the complex matrix of milk in order to avoid underestimation of the milk carnitine concentration.

ACKNOWLEDGEMENT

This work was supported in part by NIH Contract HD-2-2818. The authors thank Mrs. Robin Adkins for assistance in data analyses and manuscript preparation.

REFERENCES

1. P. R. Borum, Carnitine, Ann. Rev. Nutr. 3:233-259, (1983).
2. J. P. Shenai and P. R. Borum, Tissue Carnitine Reserves of Newborn Infants, Pediatr. Res. 18:679-681, (1984).
3. C. Robles-Valdes, J. D. McGarry and D. W. Foster, Maternal-fetal Carnitine Relationships and Neonatal Ketosis in the Rat, J. Biol. Chem. 251:6007-6012, (1976).
4. P. R. Borum, C. M. York and S. G. Bennett, Carnitine Concentration of Red Blood Cells, Am. J. Clin. Nutr. 41:653-656, (1985).
5. G. Cederblad and S. Lindstedt, A Method For the Determination of Carnitine in the Picomole Range, Clin. Chim. Acta 37:235-243, (1972).
6. P. R. Borum, S. A. Atkinson, A. M. Ferris, L. Hambraeus, M. C. Neville and T. A. Picone, Carbohydrates, Amino Acids, Metabolic Intermediates, And All Other Nutrients, in: "Human Lactation, Milk Components and Methodologies" R. G. Jensen and M. C. Neville, ed., Plenum Press, New York and London, (1985).
7. A. Sandor, K. Pecsuvac, J. Kerner and I. Alkonyi, On Carnitine Content of the Human Breast Milk, Pediatr. Res. 16:89-91, (1982).
8. D. J. Pearson, P. K. Tubbs and J. F. A. Chase, Carnitine and Acylcarnitines, in: "Methods of Enzymatic Analysis", H. V. Bergmeyer, ed., Vehag Chemie Weinheim, (1974).

EFFECTS OF VITAMIN SUPPLEMENTATION ON VITAMIN LEVELS IN HUMAN MILK: VITAMIN B-6, VITAMIN C AND FOLACIN

Avanelle Kirksey

Department Foods and Nutrition
Purdue University
West Lafayette, IN 47907

INTRODUCTION

The nutritional needs of lactating women for several of the water-soluble vitamins have been established provisionally by national and international groups[1-5]. Increases of one-fourth to two-thirds the vitamin levels recommended for non-lactating women have been proposed to meet the needs of milk production for the infant as well as to protect against maternal deficiencies. These recommendations represent scientific judgements based on attaining what is presumed to be adequate levels of nutrients in milk for breastfeeding, and on meeting the metabolic needs associated with additional nutrient intakes and/or nutrient conversions during lactation[5].

Unfortunately, simple relationships between nutrient intake and lactational performance can be confounded by a multiplicity of variables. If lactation studies are to provide useful and comparable data for examination of these relationships, many factors in the investigation should be carefully controlled and described. These include nutritional state of mother; dietary intake; time, amount/type and frequency of supplementation; use of drugs; stage of lactation; time of milk sampling; collection from right and/or left breast; completeness of sample collection; sampling variation within/between feeds; handling and storage of samples; and analytical procedures. Some supplementation studies have employed a few massive doses; others have used small doses approximating the recommended allowances for extended periods of time. Data from supplementation studies are most reliable when subjects take supplements in the presence of the experimenter.

Levels of several water soluble vitamins in breast milk can be raised or lowered in apparently well-nourished women by a change in intake. Whether maintenance of high levels of these vitamins in breast milk through the use of supplementation is beneficial or protective to the infant remains speculative. Obviously vitamin requirements for lactation should be related both to the health of the mother and to the level of vitamin in milk that meets the nutritional needs of the infant.

VITAMIN B-6

Effect of Level of Supplementation

Early observations of Karlin[6] showed that following oral administration of a single large dose of pyridoxine (500 or 1000 mg) to lactating women, the vitamin passed rapidly into milk and in approximately 3h peaked at about 100 times the initial level. The vitamin level decreased rapidly in the next 9h. These findings were supported by later work in this laboratory[7-9] in which small doses of PN·HCl ranging from 2.5 to 20 mg/day showed peak concentrations in milk at 3 to 5h post-ingestion of the supplement.

Several studies from this laboratory[7-12] have demonstrated clearly that levels of vitamin B-6 in milk of lactating women parallel their intake of the vitamin. In two of these studies[9,10], samples of fore milk were obtained at each feeding during a 24h period either monthly or bimonthly for 6 months of lactation. Mothers were supplemented daily from delivery with different levels of PN·HCl ranging from 0 to 15 mg/day. Levels of vitamin B-6 in milk and in maternal plasma, vitamin B-6 intakes and plasma PLP levels of breastfed infants were found to parallel maternal intakes of vitamin B-6. Each of these parameters was significantly influenced by the highest levels of PN·HCl supplementation, 10 or 15 mg/day.

Marked diurnal variation in B-6 concentrations was observed in milk, especially following supplementation[7,8]. Variability in the concentration of vitamin B-6 in breast milk whether related to the level of intake of the vitamin, stage of lactation, length of gestation, use of drugs or other factors, contraindicates the use of a random sample of milk as a basis for evaluating the adequacy of the level of vitamin B-6 in breast milk for the infant. Presently, the use of vitamin B-6 supplementation during human lactation is controversial with regards to special benefits to healthy mothers and breastfed infants.

Forms and Distribution of B-6 Vitamers Following Supplementation

The major forms and distribution of the B-6 vitamers, PL, PLP, PM, PN and PMP, in human milk have been investigated by reverse-phase HPLC prior to and following PN·HCl supplementation when the concentration of total vitamin B-6 in milk showed marked changes. Total vitamin B-6 levels in milk from women supplemented with 15 mg PN·HCl/day were significantly higher at each of the four time periods studied compared to values for women supplemented with 2.5 mg. The peak concentration was observed at approximately 3 to 8h post-supplementation (Figure 1).

Mean distribution of the B-6 vitamers in milk, determined by reverse-phase HPLC and expressed as percent of total vitamin B-6 concentration, was 81%, PL; 7%, PLP; 5%, PM; 5%, PN and 2% PMP[13]. Distribution of the B-6 vitamers in milk of women supplemented with 2.5 or 15 mg PN HCl daily were similar at each time period studied for PMP, PM, PLP and PN). However the percentage of PL was significantly higher at two time periods in milk of women supplemented with 15 mg PN·HCl/day compared to values for the 2.5 mg group.

Effect of Time of Supplementation

The time of supplementation influences diurnal variations observed in vitamin B-6 levels in breast milk as well as the intake of the vitamin by the infant. Possible beneficial effects of supplementation for the breastfed infant were most obvious when the supplement was taken in the morning[10]. This was related to the finding that most infants consumed their largest volume of milk during daytime and early evening hours. Infants were generally fed only a few times during the night and this increased the chances of missing the elevation of vitamin B-6 in milk due to the supplement.

Effects of Megadoses of Vitamin B-6

The influence of pharmacologic doses of vitamin B-6 ($\geq$600 mg/day) on lactation has been a source of controversy for the last 10 years. The controversy about megadoses concerns quantitative (milk volume) rather than qualitative influences of the vitamin on milk. Foukas[14] first proposed that PN was an effective lactation inhibitor. Studies by Marcus[15] and McIntosh[16] confirmed that 600 mg vitamin B-6/day suppressed lactation and lowered prolactin levels. Most recent human studies[17,18] have failed to confirm the findings of earlier investigators and suggest that megadoses of vitamin B-6 have no effect either on lactation or on levels of prolactin. The decarboxylase which converts dopa to dopamine also converts 5-hydroxytryptophan to serotonin; therefore, the lack of effect of PN on prolactin levels may be due to the simultaneous stimulation of both dopaminergic and serotonergic activities. Also, the quantity of PN in supplements (1-20 mg) is 30 times less than the levels used in studies of lactation inhibition. Findings from our laboratory[8] show that 4-20 mg PN·HCl/day did not significantly affect the milk volume of nursing mothers. Also, Andon et al.[19] found that prolactin levels in lactating women were not affected by supplementation of 4 mg PN·HCl/day.

Mechanism of B-6 Vitamer Transport Into Mammary Cells

The mechanism of B-6 vitamer transport from the circulatory system

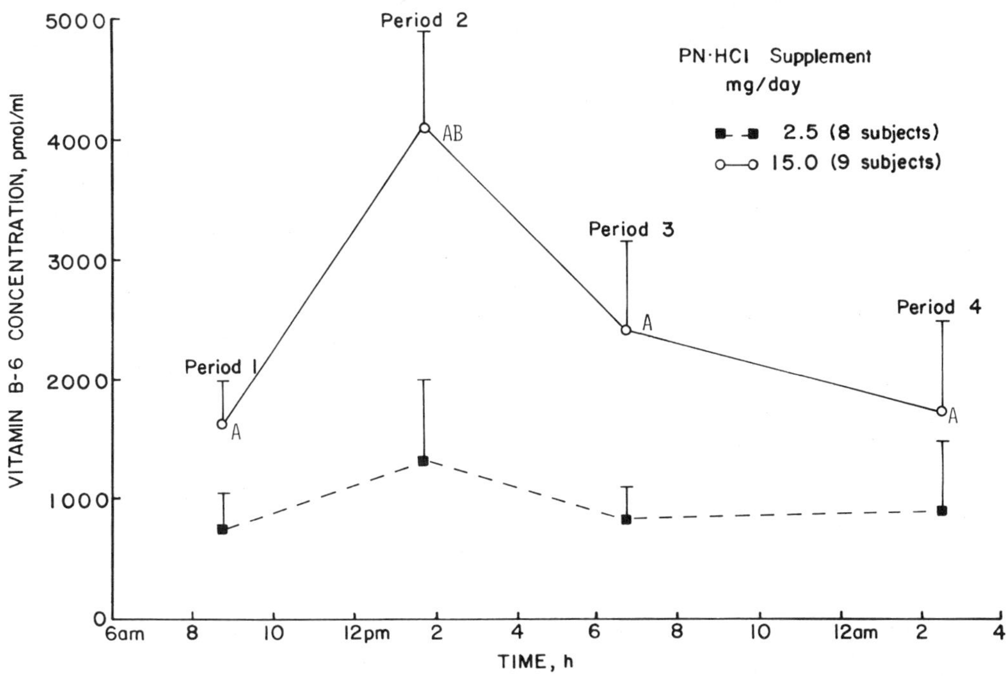

Fig. 1. Vitamin B-6 concentrations in milk at four time periods before and following PN·HCl supplementation. Period 1 is before supplementation; period 2 is highest observed concentration, 3 to 8h post-supplementation; periods 3 and 4 are lowest observed concentrations 2 to 5h and 5 to 15h, respectively following the peak observed at period 2.

into the mammary gland is not well established. However, the vitamin has been observed to pass freely from plasma to milk. Following vitamin B-6 supplementation concentrations of all B-6 vitamers in human milk, except PMP, paralleled total vitamin B-6 concentration and vitamin B-6 intake. Contrary to these findings in human milk, Lumeng et al.[20] found that only PL and PLP levels increased in plasma following an oral dose of PN·HCl. These investigators reported that vitamin B-6 in plasma is comprised of 62% PLP and 14% PL. Our findings show a predominance of PL (75-85%) in human milk suggesting that a dephosphorylating mechanism is present at the blood:mammary gland barrier[13]. This observation is consistent with other reports that the dephosphorylated forms of the vitamin are those that most readily cross physiological barriers and/or cell membranes[20,21].

VITAMIN C

Effect of Level of Supplement

In recent years, ascorbic acid supplements have been used extensively, but their effects on the vitamin C levels of human milk and intakes of infants have not been demonstrated conclusively. Studies[22-24] conducted during the 1930's indicated that vitamin C content in milk paralleled vitamin C intake and possibly reached a maximum concentration at around 80 mg/l milk[22-24]. The level of dietary vitamin C intake of the women who participated in those studies was reported to be not more than 20 mg/d prior to the studies. Also Deodhar et al.[25] found that ascorbic acid supplementation increased the level of vitamin C in the milk from 25 to 61 mg/l in lactating Indian women who consumed approximately 23 mg vitamin C daily. Recently Bates et al.[26] reported that increased intakes of vitamin C from 34 to 103 mg/d by undernourished lactating women in a West African rural community were paralleled by increased levels of vitamin C in their milk from 34 to 55 mg/l. At the higher levels of vitamin C intake, the concentration of this vitamin in milk appeared to plateau.

The parallel between vitamin C intake and levels of the vitamin in breast milk observed in undernourished lactating women has not been observed in adequately nourished women. Observations from our laboratory indicated that vitamin C intakes as high as 1200 mg/d did not significantly effect the levels of vitamin C in milk of well-nourished mothers (Figure 2). Also, Thomas et al.[27] reported no significant changes in the vitamin C content in milk of well-nourished lactating women who were given daily supplements of 90 mg ascorbic acid; however, total intake of vitamin C from diet plus supplements did not differ significantly between the non-supplemented and supplemented group. Sneed et al.[28] found that concentrations of vitamin C in milk did not change significantly when a supplement of 90 mg ascorbic acid/day was given to lactating women from a low socioeconomic group who had habitually consumed approximately 100 mg of vitamin C daily. In agreement with findings from these studies, data from our laboratory[29] showed that short-term supplementation with ascorbic acid levels of 250, 500 or 1000 mg/day did not significantly affect the concentration of vitamin C in milk of well-nourished lactating women.

Differences in individual responses to vitamin C supplementation during lactation appeared to reflect differences in vitamin C nutritional status. Vitamin C concentration in milk and urinary excretion of the vitamin were extremely low for an individual who consumed only 9 mg vitamin C/day (Figure 3). The level of vitamin C in her milk increased each day a 1000 mg supplement of ascorbic acid was taken and urinary excretion of the vitamin was minimal. In contrast, the same levels of ascorbic acid supplementation did not significantly affect the vitamin C concentration in milk of an individual who consumed >100 mg vitamin C daily but urinary excretion

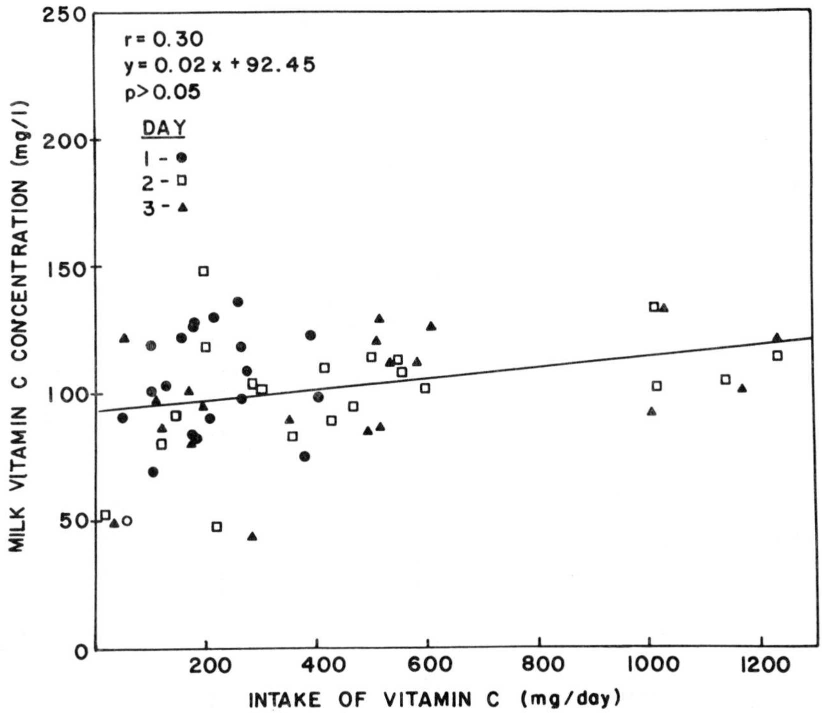

Fig. 2. Relationship between vitamin C intake from diet and supplements on the vitamin C level in milk from 24 women on 3 consecutive days at 3 months of lactation.

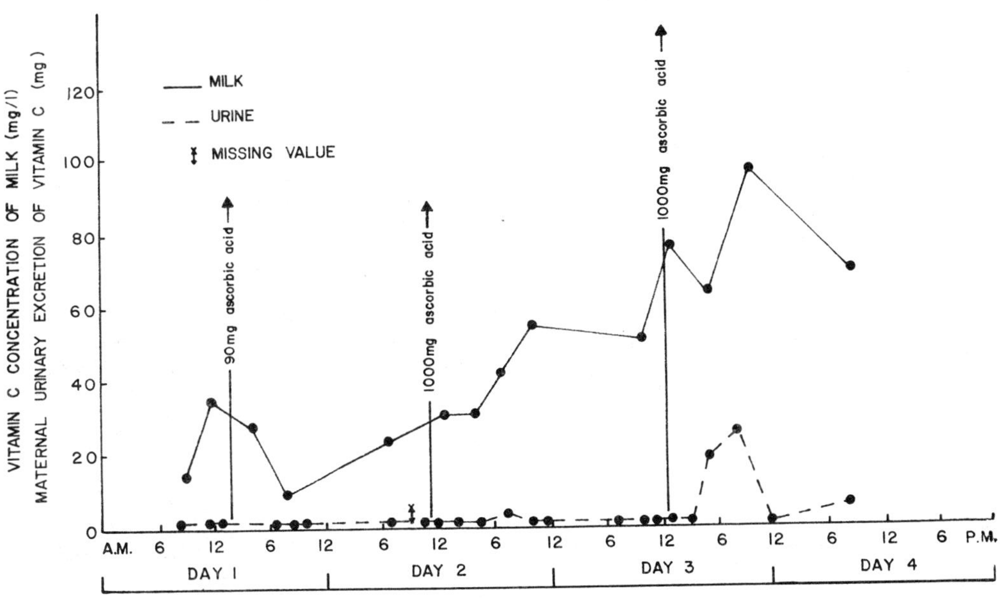

Fig. 3. Effects of vitamin C supplementation on the vitamin C levels in milk and urinary excretion of the vitamin by a subject who routinely consumed <10 mg vitamin C/day.

increased markedly in response to the supplement. These individual cases support the hypothesis that ascorbic acid supplementation increases the vitamin C levels in milk of women who habitually consume inadequate amounts of the vitamin but does not appreciably effect the vitamin C levels in milk from women who are adequately nourished.

Mechanism of Vitamin C Transport Into Mammary Cells

A regulatory mechanism in mammary cells appears to control the concentration of vitamin C in human milk. In support of this postulation levels of vitamin C in milk of well-nourished lactating women did not respond to an increased intake of the vitamin ranging from 100 to >1200 mg/day whereas urinary excretion of the vitamin increased significantly[29]. Thus in healthy lactating women, vitamin C content in milk failed to respond significantly to more than ten-fold increases in vitamin C intake. These observations suggested that mammary tissue was saturated with the vitamin and that excess vitamin was excreted.

Adequacy of Vitamin C Levels in Human Milk

In recent years, greater awareness of vitamin C, the widespread availability of citrus fruits, and increased use of prenatal supplements has undoubtedly led to improved ascorbic acid nutriture among many lactating women. This in turn appears to be reflected in the higher levels of vitamin C which are currently observed in human milk. Data from this laboratory[29] indicated that women who routinely consumed levels of vitamin C $\geq$100 mg/day had significantly higher concentrations of vitamin C in their milk and higher excretion of the vitamin in urine than women who habitually consumed <100 mg vitamin C daily. Regardless of the level of maternal intake of vitamin C ranging from 100 to >1200 mg/day, data from this laboratory indicated that the mean vitamin C concentration in milk of well-nourished lactating women was approximately 100 mg/l (Figure 2). This level is about twice the minimum level recommended for infant formulas and also, is approximately twice the vitamin C concentration in certain infant formulas.

FOLACIN

A variety of factors influences the folacin status of lactating mothers and consequently the folacin levels in breast milk. Evaluation of the nutritional status of mother-infant pairs is a necessary first step in order to establish folacin requirements and develop recommended allowances.

Effect of Folic Acid Supplementation in Well-Nourished Lactating Women

A recent report by Ek[30] indicated that dietary folacin intakes of 91 Norwegian women were adequate to meet the requirements of lactation and that routine folic acid supplementation was unnecessary. The criteria used were maternal plasma and red cell folacin concentrations and the peripheral blood picture. Tamura et al.[31] observed no significant increase in folacin levels in milk of well-nourished lactating women after 4 weeks of supplementation with 1 mg of folic acid daily. Also Thomas et al.[27] reported that supplementation with 0.8 mg/day of folacin at 6 months postpartum did not affect folacin concentration in milk or the nutritional status of well-nourished mothers. Findings from our laboratory (Figure 4) indicated that folacin concentrations in milk of well-nourished women were not significantly changed by short term folic acid supplementation of 100 to 800 µg/day, levels which are used frequently in vitamin-mineral supplements. Furthermore, a 30-day period with no folic acid supplementation did not affect the level of folacin in milk of these women.

Recent observations of Smith et al. indicated that[32] folic acid supplementation was unnecessary to maintain folacin levels in milk, but could be essential for maintenance of normal levels of folacin in plasma and erythrocytes especially during prolonged lactation. Findings from this laboratory[33] indicated that folacin levels in milk of well-nourished lactating women were maintained even after 12 months of no supplementation and that both plasma and RBC folacin were well above the lower limit of the normal range. However data for one mother who had breastfed for 15 months suggested that folacin levels in her milk responded to folate supplementation. The practice of routine supplementation with folic acid during pregnancy, often with an amount in excess of maternal needs, may provide the nursing mother with adequate folate for even prolonged lactation. However, studies of lactating women following extended lactation appear warranted to examine whether folacin levels in their milk will respond to folic acid supplementation.

Effect of Folic Acid Supplementation in Malnourished Lactating Women

A number of investigators[34-36] have reported that folacin is preferentially supplied to milk at the expense of the undernourished mother and that lactation is, therefore, a conditioning factor for folacin deficiency. In non-lactating patients with megaloblastic anemia, daily supplements of 100 μg of folic acid induced a hematologic response whereas in lactating women, 400 μg folic acid daily were needed to produce significant reticulocytosis[37]. In lactating women suffering from megaloblastic anemia, Metz[34] observed that folic acid supplementation increased the levels of folacin in their milk prior to a hematological response. Subsequently Metz[35] observed that in lactating women fed diets low in folate, levels of folacin in their milk did not change whereas concentrations of folacin in their serum fell rapidly suggesting that levels in milk were maintained at the expense of maternal stores.

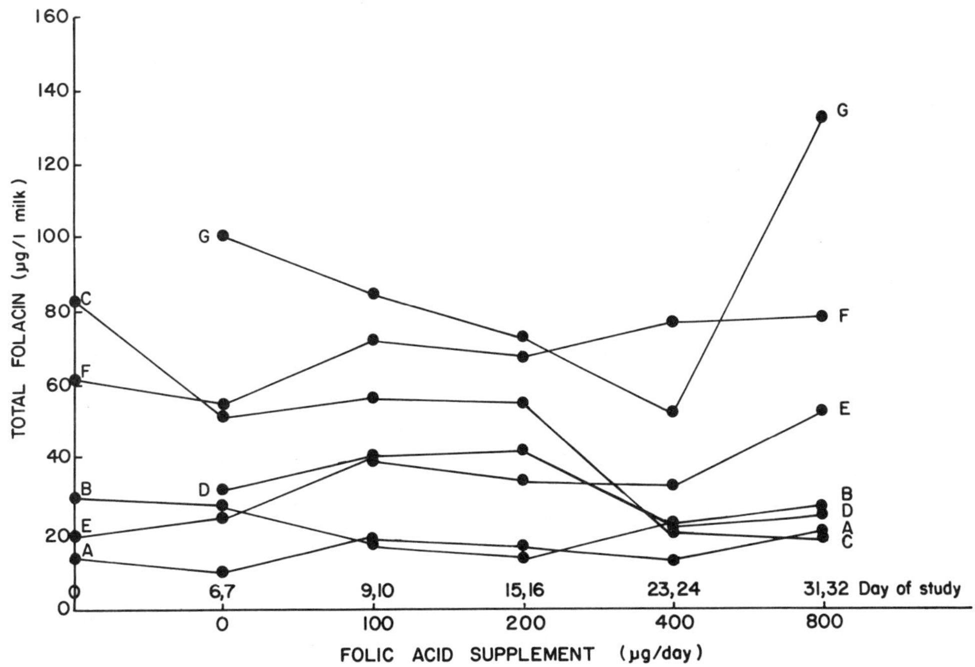

Fig. 4. Effects of different amounts of folic acid supplementation on the levels of folacin in milk collected from 6 women at the beginning of each feeding during two consecutive 24h periods at 6 intervals during a 32 day study.

Deodhar et al.[25] observed in lactating women of low nutritional status that folacin levels in their milk were not appreciably changed by folic acid supplements of up to 1.0 mg/day but were increased when supplements between 1.5 and 10 mg/day were given. Each level of supplement was given for a month before the next increment was given. Sneed and co-workers[28] observed significant increases in folacin levels from 41 to 49 μg/l in breast milk from women of low socioeconomic status following folic acid supplementation with 0.8 mg/day for about 6 weeks. Prentice et al.[38] reported increases in mean folacin concentration from 38 μg to 47 μg/l milk after supplementation of diets of lactating Gambian women who were of low nutritional status.

Regulatory Mechanism for Folacin Levels in Milk

Several observations have led researchers[30,31,34] to suggest the presence of a regulatory mechanism in mammary cells which controls the level of folacin in human milk. Most studies of the effects of supplementation on folacin levels in breast milk are based on long-term supplementation with levels of folic acid as high as 10 mg/day; only recently have lower levels of folic acid and shorter periods of supplementation been examined.

Investigations of proteins in human milk[39-41] indicate the presence of a folate binding protein (FBP) which accumulates folacin from the blood. Antony et al.[42] have recently reported that human milk contains a particulate and a soluble FBP which binds one mole of folate per mole of protein. Also Selhub et al.[43] reported that the concentration of FBP paralleled folacin concentrations in milk. Both of these reports suggested that secretion of folacin into human milk is coordinated with that of FBP. Furthermore, after the binding protein is saturated with folacin, the level of folacin in human milk appears to resist change.

REFERENCES

1. WHO Report of a Scientific Group, Physiology of lactation, World Health Organization Technical Report Series, No. 305 (1965).
2. American Academy of Pediatrics, Committee on Nutrition, Commentary on breast-feeding and infant formulas, including proposed standards for formulas, Pediatrics 57:278 (1976).
3. WHO/UNICEF, Meeting on infant and young child feeding, Food and Nutrition, 5:36 (1979).
4. American Academy of Pediatrics, Committee on Nutrition, Breast Feeding, Pediatrics 62:591 (1978).
5. Recommended Dietary Allowances (9th ed.), Washington, D.C., Food and Nutrition Board, National Academy of Sciences (1980).
6. M. K. Karlin, Effect d-un enrichissement en pyridoxine sur la teneur en vitamine B-6 du lait de femme, Bull. Soc. Chem. Biol. 41:1085 (1959).
7. A. Kirksey and K. D. West, Relationship between vitamin B-6 intake and the content of the vitamin in human milk, in: "Human Vitamin B-6 Requirements," National Academy of Sciences, Washington (1978).
8. L. Styslinger and A. Kirksey, Effects of different levels of vitamin B-6 supplementation on vitamin B-6 concentrations in human milk and vitamin B-6 intakes of breastfed infants, Am. J. Clin. Nutr. 41:21 (1985).
9. J. L. Steiner, Factors influencing the vitamin B-6 status of mothers and their breastfed infants during the first six months of lactation, Master of Science Thesis, Purdue University, West Lafayette, Indiana (1985).
10. M. W. Borschel, A. Kirksey, and R. E. Hannemann, Effects of vitamin B-6 intake on nutriture and growth of young infants, Am. J. Clin. Nutr. 43:7 (1986).
11. A Kirksey, J. L. B. Roepke, and L. M. Styslinger, The vitamin B-6

content in human milk, in: "Methods in Vitamin B-6 Nutrition," J. E. Leklem and R. E. Reynolds, eds., Plenum Press, New York (1981).

12. J. L. B. Ropeke and A. Kirksey, Vitamin B-6 nutriture during pregnancy and lactation. II. The effect of long term use of oral contraceptives, Am. J. Clin. Nutr. 32:2257 (1979).
13. B. Hamaker, A. Kirksey, A. Ekanayake, and M. Borschel, Analysis of B-6 vitamers in human milk by reverse-phase liquid chromatography, Am. J. Clin. Nutr. 42:650 (1985).
14. M. D. Foukas, An antilactogenic effect of pyridoxine, J. Obstet. Gynecol. 80:718 (1973).
15. R. G. Marcus, Suppression of lactation with high doses of pyridoxine, S. Afr. Med. J. 6:2155 (1975).
16. E. M. McIntosh, Treatment of women with galactorrhea-amenorrhea syndrome with pyridoxine (vit B-6), J. Clin. Endocrin. Metab. 42:1192 (1976).
17. G. Tolis, R. Laliberte, H. Guyda, and F. Naftolin, Ineffectiveness of pyridoxine (B-6) to alter secretion of growth hormone and prolactin and absence of therapeutic effects of galactorrhea-amenorrhea syndrome, J. Clin. Metab. 44:1197 (1977).
18. T. J. Goodenow and W. B. Malarky, Ineffectiveness of pyridoxine in evaluation and treatment of hyperprolactinemic amenorrhea-galactorrhea syndrome, Am. J. Obstet. Gynec. 133:161 (1979).
19. M. B. Andon, M. P. Howard, P. B. Moser, and R. D. Reynolds, Supplementation of lactating women with vitamin B-6 does not suppress plasma prolactin, Pediatrics 76:769 (1985).
20. L. Lumeng, R. E. Brashear, and T. K. Li, Pyridoxal 5'-phosphate in plasma: source, protein-binding, and cellular transport, J. Lab. Clin. Med. 84:334 (1974).
21. R. Spector, Vitamin B-6 transport in the central nervous system: in vivo studies, J. Neurochem. 30:881 (1978).
22. I. Selleg and C. G. King, The vitamin C content of human milk and its variation with diet, J. Nutr. 11:599 (1936).
23. R. H. Ingalls, R. Draper, and H. M. Teel, Vitamin C in human pregnancy and lactation: II. Studies during lactation, Am. J. Dis. Child. 56:1011 (1938).
24. F. T. Chu and C. Sung, Effect of vitamin C administration on vitamin C of milk and urine of lactating mothers, Proc. Soc. Exp. Biol. Med. 35:171 (1936).
25. A. D. Deodhar, R. Rajalakshmi, and C. Ramakrishman, Effect of dietary vitamin supplementation on vitamin contents of breast milk, Acta. Paediatr. 53:42 (1964).
26. C. J. Bates, A. M. Prentice, A. Prentice, W. H. Lamb, and R. G. Whitehead, The effect of vitamin C supplementation on lactating women in Keneba, a West African rural community, Internat. J. Vit. Res. 53:68 (1983).
27. W. R. Thomas, J. Kawamoto, S. M. Sneed, and R. Eakin, The effects of vitamin C, vitamin B-6, and vitamin B-12 supplementation on the breast milk and maternal status of well-nourished women, Am. J. Clin. Nutr. 32:1679 (1979).
28. S. M. Sneed, C. Zane, and M.R. Thomas, The effects of ascorbic acid, vitamin B-6, vitamin B-12, and folic acid supplementation on the breast milk and maternal nutritional status of low socioeconomic lactating women, Am. J. Clin. Nutr. 34:1338 (1981).
29. L. O. Byerley and A. Kirksey, Effects of different levels of vitamin C intake on the vitamin C concentration in human milk and the vitamin C intakes of breastfed infants, Am. J. Clin. Nutr. 41:665 (1985).
30. J. Ek, Plasma, red cell and breast milk folacin concentrations in lactating women, Am. J. Clin. Nutr. 38:929 (1983).
31. T. Tamura, Y. Yoshimura, and T. Arakawa, Human milk folate and folate status in lactating mothers and their infants, Am. J. Clin. Nutr. 33:193 (1980).

32. A. M. Smith, M. F. Picciano, and R. H. Deering, Folate supplementation during lactation: Maternal folate status, human milk folate content, and their relationsip to infant folate status, J. Pediat. Gastroenterol. Nutr. 2:622 (1983).
33. S. A. Udipi, Factors influencing the folacin nutriture of lactating mothers and their breastfed infants, Ph.D. Thesis, Purdue University, West Lafayette, Indiana (1984).
34. J. Metz, R. Zalusky, and V. Herbert, Folic acid binding by serum and milk, Am. J. Clin. Nutr. 21:289 (1968).
35. J. Metz, Folate deficiency conditioned by lactation, Am. J. Clin. Nutr. 23:843 (1970).
36. J. Shapiro, H. W. Alberts, P. Welch, and J. Metz, Folate and vitamin B-12 deficiency associated with lactation, Br. J. Haematol. 11:498 (1965).
37. V. Herbert, Current concepts in therapy: megaloblastic anemia, N. Engl. J. Med. 268:201,268,368 (1963).
38. A. M. Prentice, S. B. Roberts, A. Prentice, A. H. Paul, M. Watkinson, A. A. Watkinson, and R. G. Whitehead, Dietary supplementation of lactating Gambian women. I. Effect of breast-milk volume and quality, Hum. Nutr. Clin. Nutr. 37C:53 (1983).
39. Folic Acid:Proceedings of a Workshop on Human Folate Requirement, Washington (1977).
40. J. E. Ford, Some observations on the possible nutritional significance of vitamin B-12 and folate-binding proteins in milk, Br. J. Nutr. 31:243 (1974).
41. J. Ghitis, The folate binding in milk, Am. J. Clin. Nutr. 20:1 (1967).
42. A. C. Antony, C. S. Utley, P. D. Marcel, J. F. Kolhouse, Isolation, characterization, and comparison of the solubilized particulate and soluble folate binding proteins from human milk, J. Biol. Chem. 257: 10081 (1982).
43. J. Selhub, R. Arnold, A. M. Smith, and M. F. Picciano, Milk folate binding protein (FBP): A secretory protein for folate?, Nutr. Res. 4:181 (1984).

MATERNAL FACTORS AFFECTING THE VITAMIN D CONTENT OF HUMAN MILK

Bruce W. Hollis

Department of Pediatrics
Medical University of South Carolina
171 Ashley Avenue
Charleston, South Carolina 29425

INTRODUCTION

The antirachitic activity of human milk has been estimated using a variety of techniques during the past several years (1-9). The earlier studies were dependent upon the rat line biological assay to provide crude estimates of total antirachitic activity (1-3). Later studies utilized chemical methods that proved to be totally unreliable in estimating the vitamin D content of human milk (4-6). Only recently has the actual vitamin D content of human milk been determined using procedures based on high-performance liquid chromatography (HPLC) and/or competitive protein binding assay (CPBA) (7-13). These techniques have demonstrated: 1) that vitamin D sulfate does not contribute to the antirachitic activity of human milk; 2) that many vitamin D compounds exist in human milk; 3) of the vitamin D compounds in human milk 25-hydroxyvitamin D (25-OH-D) contributes the vast majority of antirachitic activity; 4) that maternal factors such as diet, ultraviolet light exposure and race greatly affect the vitamin D content of human milk. This last aspect, the effect of maternal vitamin D status on the vitamin D content of her milk, is relatively new and has not been reported in great detail. Thus, it is the purpose of this report to provide a detailed and comprehensive review of this area of nutritional investigation.

MATERNAL DIETARY INFLUENCE

For many years, the possibility of improving the vitamin D content of human milk by direct vitamin supplementation of the mother has been a source of controversy (1-3). A significant amount of the controversy could be attributed to the bioassay methodology utilized, since bioassays tend to be more qualitative than quantitative. Polskin et al (2) reported that the antirachitic quality of human milk could be improved if the mother ingested large amounts of fish liver oil.

From the standpoint of infant nutrition, it is important to know how the supplementation of the mother with vitamin D effects the antirachitic properties of her milk in a quantitative manner. Hollis et al (7) furnished the first direct assessment of vitamin D and its metabolites in human milk. This investigation revealed that although a variety of vitamin D compounds were present in human milk, 25-OH-D accounted for the majority of the antirachitic activity in this fluid. This study was later confirmed by Reeve et al (10). Both studies revealed that human milk normally contains 20-60 IU/L of vitamin D activity. Later studies involving larger numbers of lactating mothers (14) supported the results of these two earlier studies. Table 1 lists the amount of antirachitic activity in human milk accounted for by vitamin D_2, vitamin D_3, 25-OH-D_2 and 25-OH-D_3. As can be seen from this data, 25-OH-D is the major contributer to human milk vitamin D content.

Specker et al (13) have recently demonstrated that breast milk vitamin D is correlated to maternal vitamin D intake. This data is presented in Figure 1. Other studies have provided evidence that milk vitamin D content is responsive to dietary supplementation. Hollis (8) demonstrated that the vitamin D content of human milk increased following maternal supplementation with various amounts of vitamin D. In a recent case study Greer et al (12) reported that potentially toxic amounts of vitamin D could occur in human milk following administration of pharmacological doses of vitamin D_2. These investigators demonstrated that a subject ingesting 100,000 IU vitamin D_2/day for the maintenance of plasma calcium provided milk which contained in excess of 7,000 IU/L of antirachitic activity. Thus it appears quite clear from the data presented that the maternal dietary intake of vitamin D directly affects the antirachitic properties of native milk.

INFLUENCE OF MATERNAL ULTRAVIOLET EXPOSURE

Prior to the discovery of vitamin D, Park (15) stated that rickets was due to either a lack of sunlight or the lack of an unknown dietary factor. Until recently, little work had been performed with respect to the effect of ultraviolet exposure on the plasma levels of vitamin D. Adams et al (16) first demonstrated that direct ultraviolet exposure greatly increased the plasma level of vitamin D_3. This increase of vitamin D_3 was maximal at 24-48 hrs post-exposure and then rapidly declined to near baseline levels at 7 days. On the other hand, plasma 25-OH-D_3, levels in these patients didn't start to increase until 3 days post-exposure and remained elevated several weeks following treatment. Based on the above observations, Hollis et al (17) investigated the effect of maternal ultraviolet exposure on the vitamin D content of maternal plasma and milk. These preliminary studies confirmed the findings of Adams et al (16) and for the first time, provided direct evidence that maternal ultraviolet exposure increased the vitamin D_3 content of her milk. These preliminary studies were followed by a more detailed study (11) which substantiated the preliminary results (17). Figure 2 depicts the results obtained from Greer et al (11) which clearly demonstrate the effect of maternal ultraviolet exposure on maternal plasma and milk vitamin D_3 levels. It is important to note here that the major increase in milk vitamin D activity under these conditions is due to the parent compound, vitamin D_3, and not to its hepatic product, 25-OH-D_3.

Clemons et al (18) made an important observation with relation to epidermal vitamin D_3 synthesis, that being the role of skin pigment as a regulating factor in vitamin D activation. These investigators demonstrated that, compared to white subjects, black individuals required substantially greater exposure to ultraviolet irradiation in order to achieve equivalent plasma vitamin D_3 levels. This observation, coupled with a recent report by Hollis and Pittard (19), which demonstrated that black mothers have significantly lower plasma levels of both vitamin D_3 and 25-OH-D_3 than white mothers, presented an important question. Does milk from black mothers contain less vitamin D activity than milk from white mothers? This important question was addressed by Specker et al (13), These investigators determined that milk from black mothers contained significantly less vitamin D activity (36 IU/L) as compared to white subjects (69 IU/L). This racial difference in the milk content of vitamin D may in part explain why rickets in the U.S. is most often observed in the black breast-fed infant.

Table 1. Summary of vitamins D_2, D_3, 25-OH-D_2, 25-OH-D_3 and vitamin D-binding protein in plasma and milk from lactating mothers.

Compound	Plasma Concentration (x ± S.E., n=51)	Milk Concentration (x ± S.E., n=51)	Contribution to Milk Vitamin D Activity (IU/liter)		
			A*	B**	C***
Vitamin D_2, ng/ml	0.65 ± 0.10	0.20 ± 0.03	8.0	8.0	8.0
Vitamin D_3, ng/ml	1.93 ± 0.22	0.26 ± 0.04	10.4	10.4	10.4
25-OH-D_2, ng/ml	6.3 ± 0.5	0.09 ± 0.01	5.4	18.0	24.0
25-OH-D_3, ng/ml	20.4 ± 1.4	0.16 ± 0.01	9.6	32.0	42.7
DBP, ug/ml	346 ± 12	11.4 ± 0.6	-	-	-

* Based on the relative abilities of vitamin D and 25-OH-D_3 to heal rickets as judged by the rat line-test (25).

** Based on the relative abilities of vitamin D and 25-OH-D_3 to maintain serum calcium and stimulate growth in rats on low calcium diet (25) or based on the ability of 25-OH-D_3 to stimulate intestinal calcium transport (10).

*** Based on the relative abilities of vitamin D and 25-OH-D_3 to increase plasma 25-OH-D levels in term infants (26).

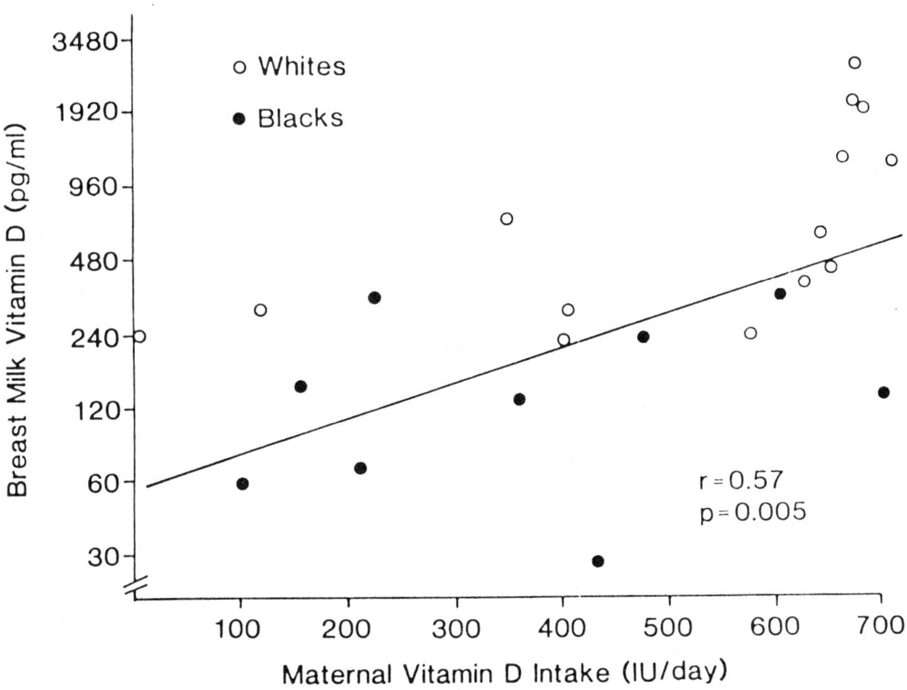

Figure 1. Relationship between milk vitamin D intake (IU/day). From Specker et al (13).

INFLUENCE OF MATERNAL CIRCULATING CONCENTRATION OF VITAMIN D AND 25-OH-D ON THEIR MILK CONCENTRATION

From the previous sections, it is quite clear that circulating maternal vitamin D levels must directly influence the vitamin D content of milk. A recent study by Hollis et al (14) has addressed this relationship. In this study, the concentrations of vitamin D_2, vitamin D_3, 25-OH-D_3 and vitamin D-binding protein were determined in serum and corresponding

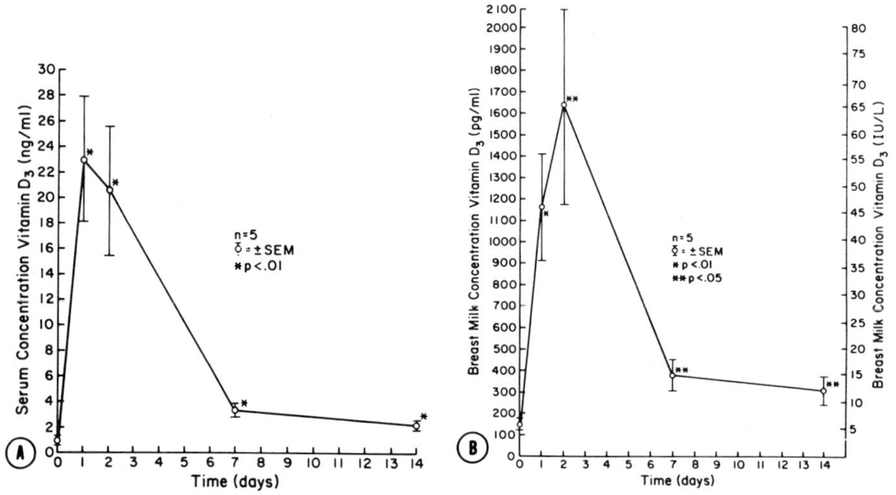

Figure 2. Serum (A) and milk (B) concentrations of vitamin D_3 in five white lactating women before and after 1.5 minimal erythemic dose of total body ultraviolet B irradiation. From Greer et al. (11).

milk samples from 51 women. Figure 3A and 3B depict the relationship observed between plasma and milk levels of vitamin D_2 and D_3, respectively. It is clear from these figures that circulating vitamin D to a large degree controls the amount of vitamin D entering the milk. A similar type of relationship was also observed for 25-OH-D_2 and 25-OH-D_3 (Figure 4). However, a close inspection of Figures 3 and 4 reveal that vitamin D and 25-OH-D cannot enter the milk from the circulation in an equivalent manner.

Vitamin D_2 and D_3 were much more effective in gaining access into the milk as compared to their 25-hydroxylated metabolites (Table 1, Figures 3 and 4). For instance, vitamin D_2 in milk was 30% of that observed in plasma while 25-OH-D_2 in milk was approximately 1% of that observed in the circulation. A similar trend was observed between vitamin D_3 and 25-OH-D_3. In contrast, the vitamin D binding protein levels in plasma and milk were not significantly related (Figure 5). Thus, differential transport of vitamin D and 25-OH-D exists from blood into milk and this process may well be controlled by the vitamin D-binding protein in circulation. The mechanism by which the vitamin D-binding protein controls the translocation of these compounds from blood to milk likely involves the affinity with which these compounds bind to the vitamin D-binding protein. The vitamin D-binding protein is known to have a greater affinity towards 25-OH-D than it does toward the parent compound (20,21). This differential affinity has also been observed between 25-OH-D_2, 25-OH-D_3 and vitamin D_2, D_3 (21-23). In these cases, the vitamin D-binding protein always exhibits a greater affinity toward the vitamin D_3 compound (21-23). As a

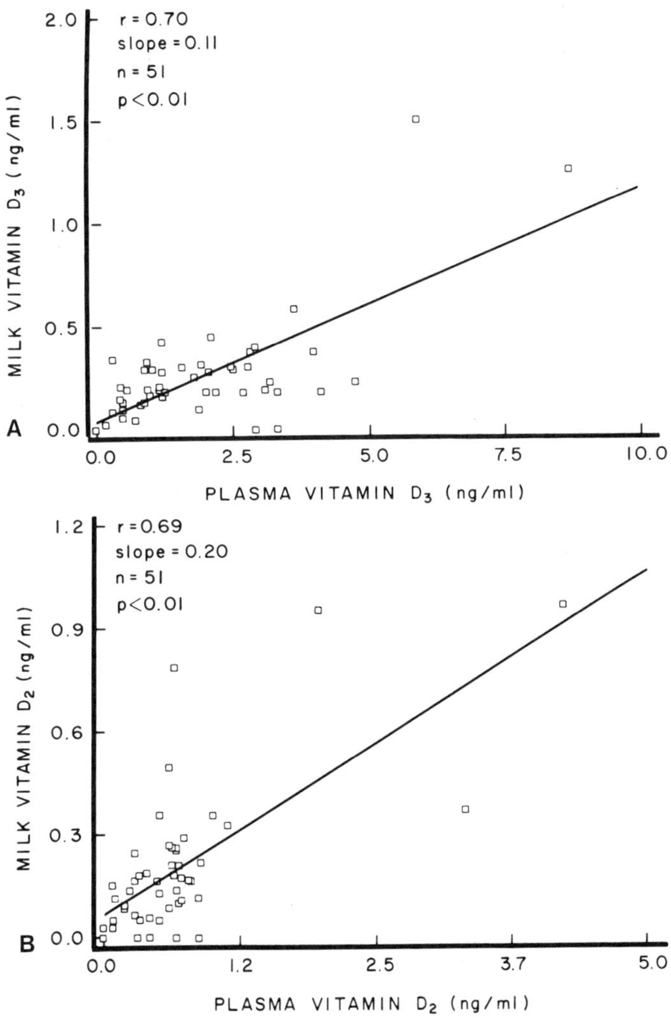

Figure 3. Regression of milk vitamin D concentration on plasma vitamin D concentrations from 51 lactating women. (A) vitamin D_2, (B) vitamin D_3. From Hollis et al. (14).

result, the compounds exhibiting the lowest affinity toward the vitamin D-binding protein would achieve the greatest relative free concentration in the circulation (24), and thus, would occur at the highest relative concentration in the milk. As a result, vitamin D_2 and its metabolites will more readily gain access into milk as compared to vitamin D_3 compounds.

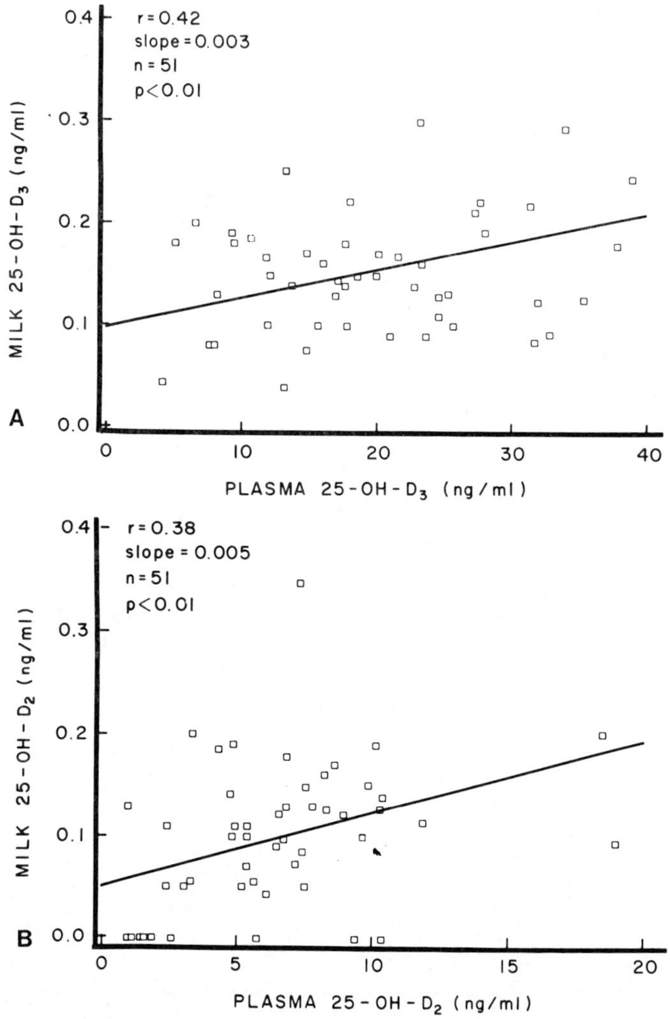

Figure 4. Regression of milk 25-OH-D concentration on plasma 25-OH-D concentration from 51 lactating women. (A) 25-OH-D_2, (B) 25-OH-D_3. From Hollis et al. (14).

PRACTICAL CONSIDERATIONS

From a practical standpoint, the studies presented have a clear implication. The vitamin D content of human milk is directly related to the lactating mothers' vitamin D status. In a normal population we found human milk to contain 33-85 IU/liter of vitamin D activity (Table 1). These calculations are based on various conversion factors for the biologic activity of 25-OH-D. All biological assays are based on the parent vitamins containing 1 IU of activity per 25 ng (25). However, the agreement ends here. For instance, the biological potential of 25-OH-

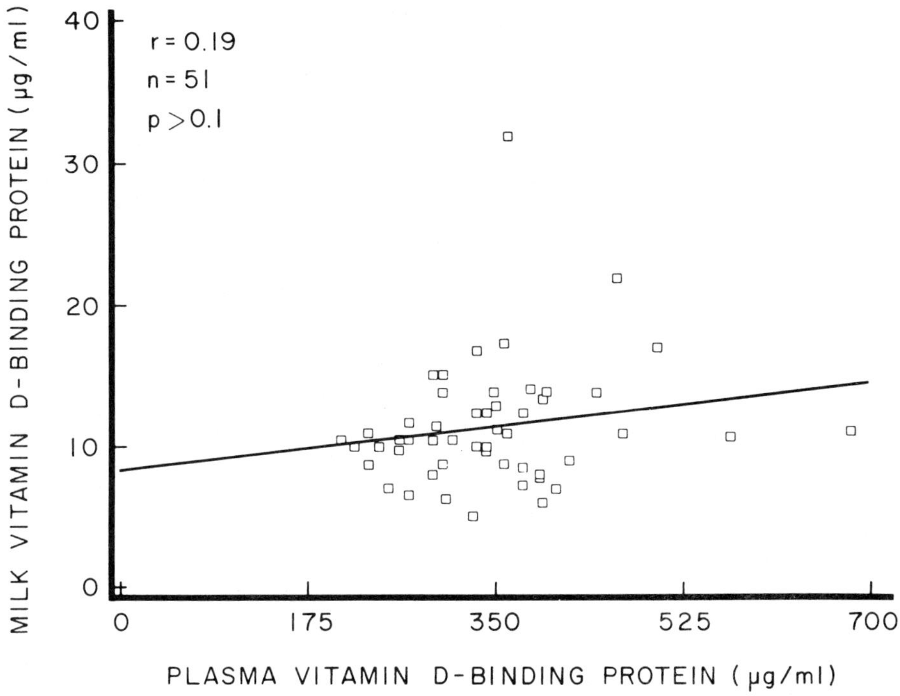

Figure 5. Regression of milk vitamin D-binding protein concentration on plasma vitamin D-binding protein concentration from 51 lactating women.

D is 1 IU/18 ng based on the rat-line test (25), but changes of 1 IU/5 ng if maintenance of plasma calcium and growth are assessed in rats on a low calcium diet (25). Moreover, by still another criteria, 25-OH-D_3 has been shown to be 5-10 times more active than the parent compound in elevating plasma levels of 25-OH-D in term infants (26). This last observation could be very important in neonates, especially preterm newborns, who appear to have difficulty in maintaining plasma levels of 25-OH-D (27). Whether this amount of vitamin D and 25-OH-D in human milk is sufficient to satisfy the growing infants' requirement is unknown at this time, however, studies to resolve this question are underway.

ACKNOWLEDGEMENT

This work was supported in part by grant HD-16510 and Research Career Development Award HD-000479 from the NIH. I gratefully acknowledge Pamela Woodruff for the typing of this manuscript.

REFERENCES

1. Adams, J.S., Clemens, T.L., Parrish, J.A., Holick, M.F., 1982, Vitamin D synthesis and metabolism after ultraviolet irradiation of normal and vitamin D-deficient subjects, N. Engl. J. Med., 306:722-25.
2. Belsey, R., Clark, M.B., Dernat, M., Glowacki, J., Holick, M.F., DeLuca, H.F., Potts, J.T., 1974, The physiologic significance of plasma transport of vitamin D and metabolites, Amer. J. Med., 57:50-6.
3. Bouillon, R., VanBaelen, H., 1981, Transport of vitamin D: significance of free and total concentrations of the vitamin D metabolites, Calcif. Tiss. Internatl., 33:451-33.
4. Clemens, T.L., Henderson, S.L., Adams, J.S., Holick, M.F., 1982, Increased skin pigment reduces the capacity of skin to synthesize vitamin D_3, Lancet 8263:74-6.
5. Drummond, J.C., Gray, C.H., Richardson, N.E.G., 1939, The antirachitic value of human milk, Br. Med. J., 2:757-60.
6. Greer, F.R., Hollis, B.W., Cripps, D.J., Tsang, R.C., 1984, Effects of maternal ultraviolet irradiation on vitamin D content of human milk, J. Pediat., 105:431-33.
7. Greer, F.R., Hollis, B.W., Napoli, J.L., 1984, High concentrations of vitamin D_2 in human milk associated with pharmacologic doses of vitamin D_2, J. Pediat., 105:61-4.
8. Haddad, J.G., Walgate, J., 1976, 25-Hydroxyvitamin D transport in human plasma: isolation and partial characterization of calcifidiol-binding protein, J. Biol. Chem., 251:4803-809.
9. Harris, R.S., Bunker, J.W., 1939, Vitamin D potency of human breast milk, J. Publ. Health, 29:744-7.
10. Hoff, N., Haddad, J., Teitelbaum, S., McAlister, W., Hillman, L., 1979, Serum concentrations of 25-hydroxyvitamin D in rickets of extremely premature infants, J. Pediat, 94:460-66.
11. Hollis, B.W., 1984, Comparison of equilibrium and disequilibrium assay conditions for ergocalciferol, cholecalciferol and their major metabolites, J. Steroid Biochem, 21:81-6.
12. Hollis, B.W., 1983, Individual quantitation of vitamin D_2, vitamin D_3, 25-hydroxyvitamin D_2 and 25-hydroxyvitamin D_3 in human milk. Anal. Biochem., 131:311-19.
13. Hollis, B.W., Greer, F.R., Tsang, R.C., 1982, The effects of oral vitamin D supplementation and ultraviolet phototherapy on the antirachitic sterol content of human milk, Calci. Tiss. Internatl., 34-552 (abst).
14. Hollis, B.W., Pittard, W.B., 1984, Evaluation of the total fetomaternal vitamin D relationships at term: evidence for racial differences, J. Clin. Endocrinol. Metab., 59:652-57.
15. Hollis, B.W., Pittard, W.B., 1985, Mineral metabolic parameters in the serum of term infants following their supplementation with vitamin D_2, D_3 or 25-hydroxyvitamin D_3, Pediat. Res, 19:312A (abst).
16. Hollis, B.W., Pittard, W.B., Reinhardt, T.A., 1986, Relationships between vitamin D, 25-hydroxyvitamin D and vitamin D-binding protein concentrations in the plasma and milk of human subjects, J. Clin. Endocrinol. Metab., 62:41-44.
17. Hollis, B.W., Roos, B.A., Draper, H.H., Lambert, P.W., 1981, Occurence of vitamin D sulfate in human milk whey, J. Nutr., 111:384-90.
18. Hollis, B.W., Roos, B.A., Draper, H.H., Lambert, P.W., 1981, Vitamin D and its metabolites in human and bovine milk, J. Nutr.,

19. Horst, R.L., Reinhardt, T.A., Beitz, D.C., Littledike, E.T., 1981, A sensitive competitive protein binding assay for vitamin D in plasma, Steroids, 37:581-91.

20. Lakdawala, D.R., Widdowson, E.M., 1977, Vitamin D in human milk, Lancet, i:167-8.

21. LeBoulch, N., Gulat-Marnay, C., Raoul, Y., 1974, Derives de la vitamin D_3 des laits de femme et de vache: ester sulfate de cholecalciferol et hydroxy-25-cholecalciferol, Int. J. Nutr. Res., 44:167-79.

22. Park, E., 1923, The etiology of rickets, 3:106-19.

23. Polskin, L.J., Kramer, B., Sobel, H.E., 1945, Secretion of vitamin D in milks of women fed fish liver oil, J. Nutr., 30:451-66.

24. Reeve, L.E., Chesney, R.W., DeLuca, H.F., 1982, Vitamin D of human milk: identification of biologically active forms, Am. J. Clin. Nutr., 36:122-26.

25. Sashi, Y., Suzuki, T., Higaki, M., Ansano, T., 1967, Metabolism of vitamin D in animals. V. Isolation of vitamin D sulfate from mammalian milk, J. Nutr. Sci., Vitaminol., 13:33-6.

26. Specker, B.L., Tsang, R.C., Hollis, B.W., 1985, Effect of race and maternal diet on breast milk vitamin D and 25-hydroxyvitamin D concentrations, Am. J. Dis. Child., 139:1134-1137.

27. Tanaka, Y., Frank, H., DeLuca, H.F., 1973, Biological activity of 1,25-hydroxy-vitamin D_3 in the rat, Endocrinol., 92:417-22.

CHANGES IN MILK CONCENTRATIONS WITH DURATION OF LACTATION IN RELATION TO ZINC REQUIREMENTS OF BREAST FED INFANTS

Nancy F. Krebs and K. Michael Hambidge

Department of Pediatrics School of Medicine, University of Colorado Health Sciences Center
4200 East Ninth Avenue, Box C233, Denver, Colorado 80262

INTRODUCTION

The rate of decline in the zinc concentration of human milk associated with the duration of lactation is notably rapid compared with the longitudinal changes in the concentrations of other nutrients (1). The relatively low zinc concentrations in mature human milk have led to concern that the zinc intake of the fully breast fed infant may be suboptimal with prolonged lactation (2). Intakes are indisputably low in relation to the estimated requirements established by a World Health Organization Expert Committee (3). However, recent re-evaluation of zinc requirements during the first year of life (4) suggests that these earlier estimates were unduly high and that the infant's needs for zinc actually may follow a declining pattern similar to that observed for milk zinc concentrations.

The objectives of this paper are to examine the progressive decline in milk zinc concentrations with duration of lactation in relation to changes in the estimated zinc requirements of infants, and to consider how differences in maternal zinc intake may affect the adequacy of infant zinc intakes.

SOURCES OF DATA

Zinc intakes of fully breast fed infants have been calculated using a standard milk volume of 750 ml/day (5) and milk zinc concentrations have been taken from a recently completed longitudinal study in this laboratory (1). The subjects in that study included one group of women who received no zinc supplements (NZS) and whose mean dietary zinc intake was 11 mg/day, and a second group who received a daily zinc supplement (ZS) and whose total mean zinc intake was 25 mg/day. Milk zinc concentrations at mid monthly intervals (to correspond with requirement data) have been calculated by taking the mean of the concentration for the two adjacent months at each interval from our study (1). These values are similar to other recent data in the literature. The basis for the estimates of zinc requirements has been described elsewhere (4). Briefly, figures for increases in lean body mass have been derived form data compiled by Fomon et al (6); a concentration of 30 ug zinc/g lean body mass has been assumed (3,7); and a figure of 10 ug zinc/kg body weight/day has been used for both urinary and sweat zinc losses (4). The estimate for urine zinc excretion is lower than some literature values, but has received support from the results of recent measurements in this center of 24 hour urine zinc excretion rates for three breast-fed infants aged 4,7, and 9 months (7.5,9.9, and 5.6 ug/kg/day, respectively).

RESULTS AND DISCUSSION

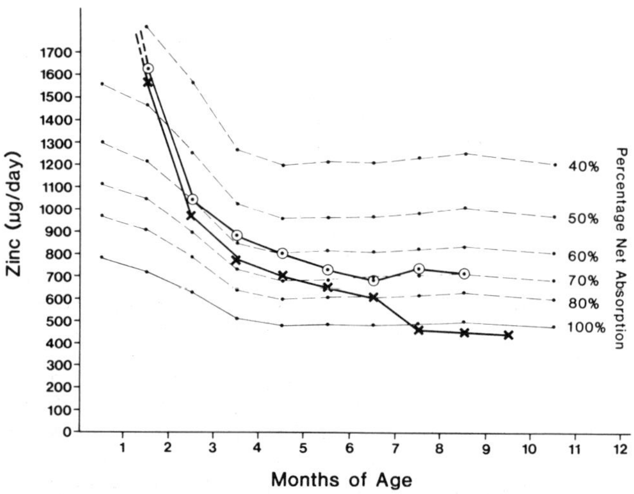

FIGURE 1: Calculated zinc intakes of fully breast fed infants compared with estimated dietary zinc requirements of male infants. X-----X based on milk zinc concentration data from mothers who did not receive a zinc supplement. O-----O based on milk zinc concentration data from mothers who received a zinc supplement (reference 1). 100% percentage net absorption line indicates estimate of zinc required for growth and to replace losses in urine and sweat.

Results of the various calculations are summarized in Figure 1. The rapid decline in calculated zinc intake by the fully breast fed infant is illustrated. From other observations in this center (8) it is known that this decline begins as early as 8 days of lactation, though it is quite gradual during the first month; calculated zinc intakes at one month (not shown) were approximately 2 mg/day. The calculated intakes for the infants of the ZS mothers are higher (than those of infants of NZS mothers) at every month of lactation. During the first 6 months this difference averages about 100 ug day, but during the seventh month there is a rapid decline in calculated zinc intake of infants of NZS mothers which is not paralleled by infants of the ZS mothers. Hence, the difference in mean calculated intake between infants of NZS and ZS mothers increases to approximately 250 ug/day after 7 months. During the 8th and 9th months mean calculated intakes of fully breast fed infants of

ZS mothers are more than 50% higher than those of NZS mothers.

Estimated requirements for growth and to replace urine and sweat losses in the male infant from the first to the 12th month are depicted by the solid "100% net absorption line in the figure. The percentage absorption of breast milk zinc necessary to meet those estimated requirements during months 1 and 2 is less than 50% for infants of both groups of women. For infants of NZS mothers this increases to 65 - 75% between months 2 and 6, rising to over 80% in the 7th month, and then to over 100% in the 8th, 9th and 10th month. Hence, these calculations indicate that fully breast fed male infants of mothers whose dietary zinc intake averaged about 11 mg/day would not meet estimated requirements after the 7th month even if they achieved 100% net absorption. On the other hand, infants of ZS mothers would not have needed more than 60% absorption until the 6th month, and an average of 69% for the next 4 months would have been sufficient. These differences could be of practical significance for infants whose major source of nutrients continues to be breast milk after the first 6 months, as is typical in many developing countries (9).

Because of slower growth rates, estimated requirements for female infants are less than for males. Hence, assuming a similar volume of milk intake (which is not necessarily true (10)), the percentage net absorption of dietary zinc necessary to meet requirements will be correspondingly less. The overall difference has been calculated to average 13%. These differences could conceivably explain the sex related differences in infant growth response to zinc supplements that have been observed in two studies in this center (11,12).

CONCLUDING REMARKS

Definitive interpretation of the absorption data discussed here must await the results of zinc absorption studies on normal term breast fed infants. Such studies are now feasible with stable isotope methodology. Meanwhile, the calculated percentage absorption values necessary to meet requirements are clearly attainable in early lactation and are maintained within what is probably a realistic range with prolonged lactation, provided maternal zinc intake is adequate. Thus, it is concluded that this decline in milk zinc content could provide a physiological mechanism for conserving maternal zinc while continuing to meet the needs of the fully breast fed infant.

ACKNOWLEDGEMENTS: Supported be grant 5 RR2 AM12432 from NIAMKDD and by grant #RR-69 from NIH, General Clinical Research Centers.

REFERENCES

1. Krebs NF, Hambidge KM, Jacobs MA, Rasbach JO. The effects of a dietary zinc supplement during lactation on lonogitudinal changes in maternal zinc status and milk zinc concentrations. Am J Clin Nutr 41:560-71 (1985).
2. Dewey KG, Finley DA, Lonnerdal B. Breast milk volume and composition during late lactation (7-20 months). J Ped Gastr Nutr 3:713-20 (1984).
3. World Health Organization, Report of a WHO Expert Committee, Technical Report Series No. 532, Trace Elements in Human Nutrition, Geneva, (1973).
4. Krebs NF, Hambidge KM. Zinc requirements and zinc intakes of breast fed infants. Am J Clin Nutr 43:288-292 (1986).

5. Casey CE, Hambidge KM. Nutritional aspects of human lactation. In: Lactation: Physiology, Nutrition and Breast Feeding, Neville MC, Neifert MA, eds., Plenum Publishing Corporation, 1983.
6. Fomon SJ, Haschke F, Ziegler EE, Nelson SE. Body composition of reference children from birth to age 10 years. Am J Clin Nutr 1169-75 (1982).
7. Hambidge KM, Krebs NF, Casey CE. Zinc. In: Underwood's Trace Elements in Human and Animal Nutrition, W Mertz ed., 5th Edition, Academic Press, Florida, 2:1-137 (1986).
8. Casey CE, Hambidge KM, Neville MC. Studies in human lactation: Zinc, copper, manganese and chromium in human milk in the first month of lactation. Am J Clin Nutr 41:1193-1200 (1985).
9. World Health Organization, Contemporary Patterns of Breast Feeding, Report on the WHO Collaborative Study on Breast-feeding, Geneva, (1981).
10. Dewey KG, Strode MA, Lonnerdal B. Maternal vs infant factors related to breast milk volume. Fed Proc 44:1675A (1985).
11. Walravens PA, Hambidge KM. Growth of infants fed a zinc supplemented formula. Am J Clin Nutr 29:1114-21 (1976)
12. Walravens PA, Koepfer DM, Hambidge KM, Casey CE. Zinc supplementation in infants with failure to thrive: Effects on weight gain. Clin Res 33:134A. (1985).

EFFECT OF MATERNAL IRON STATUS ON IRON IN HUMAN MILK

Bo Lönnerdal

Department of Nutrition
University of California
Davis, CA

INTRODUCTION

Iron deficiency anemia is common during infancy and childhood. In some developing countries, the incidence has been reported to be as high as 60-80%[1]. The effects of this iron deficiency are several; immune function is impaired and recent reports suggest many non-hematological manifestations including changes in level of catecholamines and impairment of carbohydrate and energy metabolism. Prolonged deficiency may affect brain function and learning ability[2,3]. Breast-feeding has traditionally been thought to protect against iron deficiency anemia. The occurrence of iron deficiency in breast-fed infants in Finland was nil at 4 months of age, while that of infants fed an unsupplemented formula was 4%[4]. However, the iron provided by breast milk is not sufficient indefinitely. At 9 months of age a similar incidence of anemia, 4%, was observed in breast-fed while at 12 months of age 7% of the breast-fed and 4% of the formula-fed infants were iron deficient. In addition, Siimes et al.[5] have shown that although anemia was not found in breast-fed infants at 9 months of age, they had a higher incidence of iron deficiency than iron-supplemented infants. In the U.S. anemia in infancy is uncommon, possibly due to the frequency of breast-feeding and/or the feeding of iron-supplemented formula. Duncan et al.[6] have shown adequate iron status of exclusively breast-fed U.S. infants at 6 months of age. Recently, infants, after exhibiting frequent low-grade infections (colds, diarrhea, otitis media, etc.), were studied and found to have a higher incidence of anemia than healthy infants regardless of their diet[7]. Therefore, it seems that not much of an insult is needed to precipitate an anemia in this age group. In conclusion, the quantity of iron provided by breast milk may not be much above the minimum amount required for appropriate hematopoiesis.

Assuming that there is a strong need for iron during rapid growth, an increased supply beyond that provided by breast milk could be beneficial and aid in the build-up of iron stores. There are two avenues that could be taken to meet this need: 1) to supply extra iron by oral supplementation of the breast-fed infant and 2) to attempt to increase the amount of iron in breast milk by maternal supplementation. The first approach has met with resistance because of the potential negative effects iron supplements may have on the anti-infective mechanisms of breast milk[8]. Lactoferrin, a protein present in high concentration in breast milk but low in cow's milk or formula, is a major iron-binding compartment. *In vitro*, most of the bacteriostatic activity of breast milk, specifically lactoferrin, against several pathogens such as *Vibrio cholerae*, *Pseudomonas aeroginosa* and *P. pyocyaneus*, *Candida albicans* and *Streptococcus mutans* is inhibited by the addition of iron[9,10]. These bacteria require iron for growth; however, the binding affinity of lactoferrin for iron is much higher than most bacterial siderophores, and consequently lactoferrin, which is present in breast milk in an unsaturated form, can successfully compete with bacteria and inhibit their growth. Therefore, when iron is abundant, lactoferrin becomes saturated with iron and its bacteriostatic properties are inhibited. Analogous to this phenomenon in milk, it has been demonstrated that iron supplements given to iron deficient subjects can trigger several diseases, possibly by inhibiting similar anti-infective properties of transferrin[3]. It should be recognized that there is little direct *in vivo* data supporting a bacteriostatic role for lactoferrin in the infant; field studies on iron and infection have been ambiguous. Nevertheless, such circumstantial evidence has been used to dissuade routine iron-supplementation of breast-fed infants. Recently it has also been suggested that supplemental iron may have a negative effect on zinc absorption[11]. However, when oral iron supplements were given to infants during the first year of life there were no negative effects on zinc status as assessed by plasma zinc[12].

The alternative pathway, supplementing the mother with iron to increase milk iron concentration, remains to be proven. It has been assumed that the iron content of breast milk is comparatively resistant to differences in iron supply. This has been based on a limited number of reports of more circumstantial nature rather than directly designed studies to investigate the hypothesis that iron concentration of breast milk is not changed by maternal iron status.

Effect of Iron Intake on Milk Iron

Several studies have attempted to correlate dietary iron intake of lactating women to the iron concentration in their milk. No such correlation has been found, although in most studies the women were taking oral iron supplements at comparatively high dosages[13,14]. However, Karmarkar and Ramakrishnan[15] studied Indian women who had been lactating for 3-4 months and analyzed their dietary intake of iron. Women were classified into four groups (each containing eight women) dependent on iron intakes (8-14, 14-21, 21-28 and 28-40 mg/ day). Iron concentration of milk samples varied between 0.17 and 0.21 mg/ 100 ml and no significant difference was found between groups. It should be noted, however, that unless the concentration measure was given erroneously (mg/100 ml instead of mg/L), the analyzed values appear to be about ten times higher than most other data for this stage of lactation (Table 1). Therefore, firm conclusions from this study are impossible to make.

No effect of iron intake on milk iron concentration was found in the study by Picciano and Guthrie[18]. These women were receiving at least 30 mg of iron per day and 74% of them were taking iron supplements. Iron levels in the milk samples analyzed were generally low (Table 1), which the authors

Table 1. Iron concentration of human milk (mg/L)

0-0.5	0.5-3	3-6	> 6 months of lactation	References
		1.7-2.1		Karmarkar & Ramakrishnan, 1960[15]
0.59				Cavell & Widdowson, 1964[16]
0.36-0.41				Nassi et al., 1974[17]
	0.20-0.23			Picciano & Guthrie, 1976[18]
	0.86			Anonymous, 1977[19]
1.15-1.23				Murray et al., 1977[20]
0.56	0.37-0.51		0.28-0.36	Siimes et al., 1979[21]
	0.49	0.43	0.38-0.42	Vaughan et al., 1979[22]
0.33-0.46				Kirksey et al., 1979[23]
		0.41		Fransson & Lönnerdal, 1980[24]
0.40				Celada et al., 1982[25]
	0.22-0.31	0.20-0.22		Dewey & Lönnerdal, 1983[26]
0.85-0.96	0.76			Feeley et al., 1983[27]
0.43-0.72	0.30-0.50	0.22-0.40	0.24-0.26	Palma et al., 1983[28]
0.46-0.50				Fransson et al., 1984[29]
	0.19-0.34	0.16-0.22	0.22	Finley et al., 1985[30]

explain by the use of collected fore-milk samples. Iron concentration of human milk samples has been shown to vary significantly within a feed, with lower values in the beginning and high levels of iron at the end[24]. Vaughan et al.[22] investigated iron concentration of milk samples from women who had nursed for 1-31 months post partum. Iron intake was high (39-65 mg/day) and no correlation between diet and milk iron was found. Similarly, Vuori et al.[31] did not find a correlation between iron intake of lactating women and the iron concentration of their milk. In their study, 60% of the women were taking oral iron supplements. In a recent study by Finley et al.[30], mean iron intake of the women participating in the study was more than 200% of the RDA; no correlation between iron intake and milk iron was found.

While all the above studies investigated women that mostly were taking oral iron supplements during lactation, another factor needs to be taken into account. Even if the women were not taking iron supplements while lactating, it is very likely that they were taking iron supplements during pregnancy and consequently their iron stores would have been adequate for an extended time post partum. Kirksey et al.[23] and Feeley et al.[27] analyzed milk iron during early lactation and did not attempt to correlate iron intake to milk iron since > 96% of the women had been taking prenatal iron supplements of 50-175 mg/day. This consideration is important to keep in mind when examining data from human milk samples obtained in early lactation (see below).

The effect of very high levels of dietary iron intake was investigated by Fransson et al.[29]. In this study, Ethiopian women, who commonly had daily iron intakes of more than 200 mg, provided milk samples from 4-5 days of lactation. Milk iron concentrations were similar to those of milk samples from Swedish women; however, iron status was not assessed. It should also be noted that even if dietary iron intake was high, the major source of this iron was a contamination of a major cereal, teff, with iron-rich soil. It has been shown that iron provided in this form may have a very low bioavailability[32]; consequently, only a small proportion of this iron may be absorbed. However, it is known that unprivileged Ethiopian women with poor nutritional status have an excellent iron status, indicating an adequate iron utilization from this diet. In conclusion, it is difficult to evaluate the effect of excess iron intake on iron stores, hematology and circulating iron in this population and the consequences on milk iron concentration.

Effect of Maternal Iron Deficiency on Milk Iron

Few studies have investigated the effects of poor maternal iron status on the iron concentration of human milk. Murray et al.[20] analyzed milk iron in samples collected from lactating Nigerian women that neither received iron supplements nor consumed meat. Meat consumption is important to consider since iron bound to heme is absorbed to a much higher extent than from most other iron sources[33] and consequently even if iron intake is low, the amount absorbed can be comparatively high if it is provided in meat. The women were separated into three groups: a deficient group with Hb $\leq$ 10 g/dl; an "overloaded" group with Hb > 12 g/dl; and an intermediate ("normal") group. Transferrin saturation was widely different among the groups; 6, 27 and 64%, respectively. At 2 weeks and 6 months post partum, no significant differences in milk iron concentrations were found among the groups. However, the concentrations given for milk iron at 2 weeks of lactation were very high (1.2 mg/L) compared to most other investigations (Table 1), possibly because of analytical problems. Even if absolute values were over-estimated, it appears that very low levels of circulating iron do not have an adverse effect on milk iron concentration.

Celada et al.[25] investigated hemoglobin levels, serum ferritin and transferrin in Swiss women and found no correlation between these parameters and milk iron concentration. Transferrin saturation in these women was 11.9% and mean hemoglobin concentration was 13.1 g/dl with a range of 11-15 g/dl; therefore, this group of women is comparatively homogenous and iron status was much better than the deficient group in the study by Murray et al.[20]. It should also be recognized that these women had been taking 100 mg of supplemental iron during pregnancy and the milk samples were collected 10 days post partum. Therefore, the data provided may be of limited value when assessing effects of iron status on milk iron.

A recent study in India by Fransson et al.[34] implies a positive effect of iron deficiency on milk iron concentration. Anemic women with Hb < 8.0 g/dl had a milk iron concentration of 1.4 mg/L which was significantly higher than that of milk from women with Hb > 11.0 g/dl. In addition, the concentration of lactoferrin, the major iron-binding protein of human milk[24], was significantly higher in milk of anemic women than from non-anemic women. However, the hematological parameters were assessed at delivery and milk samples were taken at $\leq$ 2 weeks post partum. It was not stated in the paper, but it is very likely from an ethical point of view that women found severely anemic at delivery were immediately given iron supplements. While hemoglobin levels would not be affected at the time of milk sampling, circulatory levels and therefore transferrin saturation would be. The mechanisms of iron transport from serum to milk are largely unknown, but Moutafchiev et al.[35] have described receptors for transferrin on the plasma membrane of cells from lactating rabbit mammary glands. Therefore, a sudden increase in transferrin receptor saturation may have led to a significantly higher transfer of iron into the milk.

Effect of iron status on milk iron concentration in experimental animals

There are limits to the degrees of deficiency and excess of iron that can be investigated in humans. In addition, use of various modes of iron supplementation is restricted because of the uncertainty of safety during long-term use. Therefore, some of the fundamental questions concerning regulation of milk iron must be addressed in experimental animals.

Dietary iron deficiency in rats was shown by Sherman et al.[36] to significantly decrease milk iron concentration at day 18 of lactation. The dams were fed 5 μg of iron/g diet from conception and iron concentration was 3.1 mg/L in milk from deficient dams and 9.4 mg/L in control dams that received 300 μg of iron/g diet. Anaokar and Garry[37] also showed that milk iron concentration is decreased in iron-deficient rats as compared to control dams. The iron content of the deficient diet was not given but the level of the control diet was 250 μg iron/g diet. Diets were introduced at day 3 of lactation and at days 11-12 and 19-20, milk, blood and liver samples were collected from dams and pups. Liver and plasma ferritin, TIBC and hemoglobin levels were lower in iron deficient dams than in control dams at both time points. Iron concentration was ∿ 3.5 mg/L in milk from iron-deficient dams and ∿ 8.0 mg/L in control dams at 19 days of lactation. In conclusion, in both these studies iron concentration of milk from iron-deficient rats could be reduced to less than 50% of control values, even if the iron-deficient diet was not introduced until lactation. Ezekiel and Morgan[38] have shown that iron deficiency caused by repeated bleeding can also lead to decreased milk iron concentration. By day 16 of lactation, bled rats with a hemoglobin level of 11 g/dl had a milk iron concentration of ∿ 3 mg/L while milk from control rats had an iron concentration of ∿ 4.5 mg/L (Hb = 13 g/dl). It should be noted, however, that independent of the manner in which circulating iron levels were reduced, the large number of mammary glands and the high rate of milk production makes milk iron assimilation a much more demanding process in the rat as compared to the human.

Iron supplementation of the diet can increase the concentration of iron in rat milk. In the study of Ezekiel and Morgan[38], a group of rats received iron in the form of ferrous ammonium sulfate in the drinking water. The lactating rats, being overloaded by the high intake of iron (0.3 g/L) produced a milk with an iron concentration of ∿ 8 mg/L as compared to ∿ 4.5 mg/L in milk from control rats. However, tissue iron concentrations were not were not higher in pups of overloaded dams as compared to control pups. Keen et al.[39] added iron (0.9 g/L) chelated to nitrilotriacetic acid (NTA) to the drinking water of lactating rats. Liver iron concentration of lactating dams and suckling pups were significantly higher than those of control rats. Iron concentration was ∿ 7 mg/L at 19 days of lactation in milk from supplemented dams as compared to ∿ 4 mg/L in milk from control dams. Although transferrin saturation was not determined in this study, NTA is known to be an excellent donor of iron to transferrin and it can be assumed that circulating iron levels and transferrin saturation were high. The study by Anaokar and Garry[37] also included a group of rats fed a high level of dietary iron 2500 μg of iron/g diet. Liver and plasma ferritin were higher and TIBC lower in iron supplemented dams and pups at day 19 of lactation as compared to control rats. Iron concentration was ∿ 12 mg/L in milk from supplemented dams and ∿ 8 mg/L in milk from control dams. In conclusion, iron concentration of rat milk can be increased by both a high level of iron in the solid diet and a high concentration of chelated iron (in soluble form) introduced by drinking water.

Concluding remarks

Iron concentration of milk from lactating experimental animals can be affected by iron status of the mother. Such effects have not yet been conclusively shown in humans; existing studies are not adequate to rule out that similar mechanisms could exist. It is possible that the extent of iron deficiency and excess needed to affect milk iron in humans is quite pronounced as compared to other species such as the rat and that such conditions are unlikely to occur in humans. Further studies on mechanisms of iron transfer into milk and how they are affected by iron status are clearly needed to resolve some of these questions.

REFERENCES

1. R. F. Florentino and R. M. Guirriec, Prevalence of nutritional anemia in infancy and childhood with emphasis on developing countries, _in_: "Iron Nutrition in Infancy and Childhood," A. Stekel, ed., Nestle, Vevey/Raven Press, New York, pp. 61-72 (1984).
2. B. Lozoff, G. M. Brittenham, F. E. Viteri, A. W. Wolf, and J. J. Urrutia, The effects of short-term oral iron therapy on developmental deficit in iron-deficient anemic infants, _J. Pediatr._ 100:351 (1982).
3. D. Vyas and R. K. Chandra, Functional implications of iron deficiency, _in_: "Iron Nutrition in Infancy and Childhood," A. Stekel, ed., Nestle, Vevey/Raven Press, New York, pp. 45-59 (1984).
4. U. M. Saarinen, Need for iron supplementation in infants on prolonged breast feeding, _J. Pediatr._ 93:177 (1978).

5. M. A. Siimes, L. Salmenperä, and J. Perheentupa, Exclusive breast-feeding for 9 months: risk of iron deficiency, J. Pediatr. 104:196 (1984).
6. B. Duncan, R. B. Schifman, J. J. Corrigan, and C. Schaefer, Iron and the exclusively breast-fed infant from birth to six months, J. Pediatr. Gastroenterol. Nutr. 4:421 (1985).
7. J. D. Reeves, R. Yip, V. A. Kyley, and P. R. Dallman, Iron deficiency in infants: the influence of mild anticedent infection, J. Pediatr. 105:874 (1985).
8. J. J. Bullen, H. J. Rogers, and L. Leigh, Iron-binding proteins in milk and resistance to Escherichia coli infection in infants, Br. Med. J. 1:69 (1972).
9. R. R. Arnold, M. F. Cole, and J. R. McGhee, A bactericidal effect for human milk lactoferrin, Science 197:263 (1977).
10. G. Spik, A. Cheron, J. Montreuil, and J. M. Dolby, Bacteriostasis of a milk-sensitive strain of Escherichia coli by immunoglobulins and iron-binding proteins in association, Immunology 35:663 (1978).
11. N. W. Solomons and R. A. Jacobs, Studies of the bioavailability of zinc in man. IV. Effects of heme and non-heme iron on the absorption of zinc, Am. J. Clin. Nutr. 34:475 (1981).
12. R. Yip, J. D. Reeves, B. Lönnerdal, C. L. Keen, and P. R. Dallman, Does iron supplementation compromise zinc nutrition in healthy infants? Am. J. Clin. Nutr. 42:683 (1985).
13. B. Lönnerdal, C. L. Keen, and L. S. Hurley, Iron, copper, zinc and manganese in milk, Ann. Rev. Nutr. 1:149 (1981).
14. B. Lönnerdal, Iron in breast milk, in: "Iron Nutrition in Infancy and Childhood," A. Stekel, ed., Nestle, Vevey/Raven Press, New York, pp. 95-118 (1984).
15. M. G. Karmarkar and C. V. Ramakrishnan, Studies on lactation. Relation between the dietary intake of lactating women and the chemical composition of milk with regard to principle and certain inorganic constituents, Acta Paediatr. 49:599 (1960).
16. P. A. Cavell and E. M. Widdowson, Intakes and excretions of iron, copper and zinc in the neonatal period, Arch. Dis. Child. 39:496 (1964).
17. L. Nassi, G. Poggini, C. Vecchi, and P. Galvan, Considerazioni sul contenuto di zinco, di rame e di ferro nel colostro e nel latte umano, Minerva Pediatr. 26:832 (1974).
18. M. F. Picciano and H. A. Guthrie, Copper, iron, and zinc contents of mature human milk, Am. J. Clin. Nutr. 29:242 (1976).
19. Anonymous, The composition of mature human milk. Report on Health and Social Subjects, No. 12, Her Majesty's Stationery Office, London, (1977).
20. M. J. Murray, A. B. Murray, N. J. Murray, and M. B. Murray, The effect of iron status of Nigerien mothers on that of their infants at birth and 6 months, and on the concentration of Fe in breast milk, Br. J. Nutr. 39:627 (1978).
21. M. A. Siimes, E. Vuori, and P. Kuitunen, Breast milk iron -- a declining concentration during the course of lactation, Acta Paediatr. Scand. 68:29 (1979).
22. L. A. Vaughan, C. W. Weber, and S. R. Kemberling, Longitudinal changes in the mineral content of human milk, Am. J. Clin. Nutr. 32:2301 (1979).
23. A. Kirksey, J. A. Ernst, J. L. Roepke, and T.-L. Tsai, Influence of mineral intake and use of oral contraceptives before pregnancy on the mineral content of human colostrum and of more mature milk, Am. J. Clin. Nutr. 32:30 (1979).
24. G.-B. Fransson, K. N. Agarwal, M. Gebre-Medhin, and L. Hambraeus, Increased breast milk iron in severe maternal anemia: Physiological "trapping" or leakage?, Acta Paediatr. Scand. 74:290 (1985).

25. A. Celada, R. Brusset, J. Gutierrez, and V. Herreros, No correlation between iron concentration in breast milk and maternal iron stores, Helv. Paediatr. Acta 37:11 (1982).
26. K. G. Dewey and B. Lönnerdal, Milk and nutrient intake of breast-fed infants from one to six months: relation to growth and fatness, J. Pediatr. Gastroenterol. Nutr. 2:497 (1983).
27. R. M. Feeley, R. R. Eitenmiller, J. B. Jones, Jr., and H. Barnhart, Copper, iron and zinc contents of human milk and early stages of lactation, Am. J. Clin. Nutr. 37:443 (1983).
28. P. A. Palma, W. E. Seifert, R. M. Caprioli, and R. R. Howell, X-ray fluorescence spectrometry in the analysis of trace elements in human milk, J. Lab. Clin. Med. 102:88 (1983).
29. G.-B. Fransson, M. Gebre-Medhin, and L. Hambraeus, The human milk contents of iron, copper, zinc, calcium and magnesium in a population with a habitually high intake of iron, Acta Paediatr. Scand. 73:471 (1984).
30. D. A. Finley, B. Lönnerdal, K. G. Dewey, and L. E. Grivetti, Inorganic constituents of breast milk from vegetarians and non-vegetarians: Relationships with each other and with organic constituents, J. Nutr. 115:772 (1985).
31. E. Vuori, S. M. Makinen, R. Kara, and P. Kuitunen, The effects of the dietary intakes of copper, iron, manganese and zinc on the trace element content of human milk, Am. J. Clin. Nutr. 33:227 (1980).
32. L. Hallberg, E. Björn-Rasmussen, L. Rossander, R. Suwanik, R. Pleehachinda, and M. Tuntawiroon, Iron absorption from some Asian meals containing contamination iron, Am. J. Clin. Nutr. 37:272 (1983).
33. L. Hallberg, Bioavailability of dietary iron in man, Ann. Rev. Nutr. 1:123 (1981).
34. G.-B. Fransson and B. Lönnerdal, Iron in human milk, J. Pediatr. 96:380 (1980).
35. D. A. Moutafchiev, A. C. Shishera, and L. M. Sirakov, Binding of transferrin-iron to the plasma membrane of a lactating rabbit mammary gland cell, Int. J. Biochem. 15:755 (1983).
36. A. R. Sherman, H. A. Guthrie, I. Wolinsky, and I. M. Zulak, Iron deficiency hyperlipidemia in 18-day-old rat pups: effects on milk lipids, lipoprotein lipase, and triglyceride synthesis, J. Nutr. 108:152 (1978).
37. S. G. Anaokar and P. J. Garry, Effects of maternal iron nutrition during lactation on milk iron and rat neonatal iron status, Am. J. Clin. Nutr. 34:1505 (1981).
38. E. Ezekiel and E. H. Morgan, Milk iron and its metabolism in the lactating rat, J. Physiol. 165:336 (1963).
39. C. L. Keen, B. Lönnerdal, M. V. Sloan, and L. S. Hurley, Effect of dietary iron, copper, and zinc chelates of nitrilotriacetic acid (NTA) on trace metal concentrations in rat milk and maternal and pup tissues, J. Nutr. 110:897 (1980).

EFFECT OF MATERNAL SELENIUM NUTRITION ON HUMAN MILK CONTENT AND FORM

Mary Frances Picciano and Sayeeda Mannan

University of Illinois at Urbana-Champaign
College of Agriculture
Division of Nutritional Sciences
Department of Foods and Nutrition
Urbana, Illinois 61801

INTRODUCTION

Selenium (Se) was recognized as an essential trace element in animal nutrition in 1957 by Schwarz and Foltz.[1] The discovery of the seleno-enzyme, glutathione peroxidase (GSH-Px), in human blood[2] and in placenta[3] has served to focus attention on the role of Se in human nutrition. Glutathione peroxidase protects the cell from oxidative damage by hydrogen peroxides or lipid peroxides.[4] In recent years, a large body of evidence has accumulated which links Se nutrition to a number of diseases and pathological conditions in infants and children as well as in adults.[5-8]

During infancy, milk is the principal source of energy and nutrients and the milk of all species is low in Se.[9,10] There is evidence that human milk Se concentration displays a geographical pattern of variation. Women living in countries where Se content of soil and crops are low, such as in Finland[11] and in New Zealand,[12] have lower milk Se concentrations than women living in high Se areas in the United States,[9] Germany,[10] and Japan.[13] These observations suggest that human milk Se content is dependent on maternal Se nutrition. Animal studies from our laboratory show a direct effect of maternal selenium intake on milk content.[14] However, human data are conflicting. A very strong positive relationship ($r = 0.81$, $p < 0.001$) was observed between Se concentration of human milk and whole blood Se concentration of New Zealand women.[12] Yet no such relationship was evident between Se concentration of milk and plasma for women living in Maryland[15] or between milk and serum for women in Japan.[13]

The purpose of this study was to determine whether there are any relationships among maternal indices of Se status and concentration of Se and activity of GSH-Px in human milk. Specific indices of maternal Se nutrition evaluated were plasma and erythrocyte Se concentrations and plasma activity of GSH-Px. Whether milk sampling procedure and/or stage of lactation influenced Se concentration and activity of GSH-Px in human milk samples were also assessed.

Materials and Methods

Subjects. Ten lactating women living in the Champaign-Urbana, Illinois area provided milk and blood samples for analysis. Mean age of lactating women was 30 ± 5.6 yr. From occupation and years of formal education, socioeconomic status (SES) was determined using the method of Green.[16] The range of possible SES scores was 30 to 85. The mean SES score was 70.0 ± 3.2 indicating that subjects were at or near the top of the scale. Two subjects were primiparae and eight were multiparae. All subjects were apparently healthy and had uncomplicated pregnancies. Infants born to subjects were full-term and had 5 min Apgar score ≥ 8. All mothers reported taking vitamin and mineral supplements, EN-CEBRIN F (Eli-Lilly and Company, Indianapolis, IN), once a day during the last two trimesters of pregnancy and during the study. None received supplemental Se either during pregnancy or lactation. Two subjects discontinued lactation after 8 wk; one for employment reasons and the other because of recurrent mastitis. The use of human subjects in this study was reviewed and approved by the Institutional Review Boards of the University of Illinois and Carle Foundation Hospital and Clinic. Blood samples were also collected from eight nonpregnant, nonlactating women to provide control values for this population. Mean age of the control group was 29.1 ± 6.2 yr and mean SES score was 71.5 ± 0.1.

Milk and Blood Sample Collection

All samples were collected between June, 1984 and February, 1985. At 4 and 8 wk postpartum (± 3 days), 10 ml of heparinized fasting blood were drawn from subjects and immediately transported on ice to the laboratory. Plasma and erythrocytes were separated and a portion of plasma was used immediately for measurement of GSH-Px activity. The remaining plasma and erythrocytes were stored at -70°C for subsequent Se and protein analyses. Milk samples were obtained at 4, 8, 12, and 16 wk (± 3 days) postpartum. A total of 72 milk samples was collected, 2 at each time frame from each participant. Milk samples were collected via mechanical pump between the hours of 7 a.m. and 11 a.m., one of foremilk and the other of hindmilk at a single nursing period. All sample collection equipment was acid washed to prevent Se contamination. Aliquots of fresh milk were transported to the laboratory on ice and analyzed immediately for GSH-Px activity. Remaining milk was dispensed into plastic vials, frozen immediately in liquid nitrogen and transported to the laboratory in the frozen state. Frozen milk samples were stored at -70°C for subsequent analyses.

Analytical Procedures

Activity of GSH-Px in human milk and plasma was measured by modifications of the coupled assay of Paglia and Valentine using t-butylhydroperoxide.[12,17] Milk samples were defatted by centrifugation prior to assay and defatted and heat treated milk samples were used as blanks.[12] One mUnit of GSH-Px activity is defined as one nanomole of NADPH oxidized/min. The effect of storage on GSH-Px activity in human milk was evaluated by comparing values obtained on fresh samples with frozen samples stored at -70°C for 4 months. Mean GSH-Px activity of the frozen samples (65.23 ± 24.05) did not differ significantly from fresh samples (77.10 ± 27.09). In this study, values obtained from fresh samples are reported. Selenium concentration of milk, plasma and erythrocytes was measured by the method of McCarthy et al.[18] using a gas chromatograph (Hewlett-Packard model 5710A, Avondale, PA) equipped with an electron capture detector (model 5709A) and an automatic sample injector (model 7671A). The accuracy of the Se method was tested using Bovine Non-Fat Milk Powder (National Bureau of Standards reference material #1549, Gaithersburg, MD). The mean Se concentration obtained for the reference standard was 0.12 ± 0.015 ug/g compared to the certified value of 0.11 ± 0.01 ug/g. Protein concentration in plasma was measured by the method of Lowry et al.[19] using lysozyme (Sigma Chemical Co., St. Louis, MO) as the reference standard.

Statistical Analyses

Repeated measure analysis of variance, paired "t" test, and correlational statistics were used in data evaluation. Repeated measure analysis of variance was applied to data on Se concentration and GSH-Px activity of milk samples collected at 4, 8, 12, and 16 wk postpartum. Paired "t" tests were applied to data on fore- and hindmilk samples and to blood values of control and lactating women. Correlational statistics were used to assess possible relationships between Se concentration and GSH-Px activity in blood and milk samples. A value of $p < 0.05$ was considered statistically significant.

RESULTS

Mean plasma and erythrocyte Se concentrations and plasma GSH-Px activity of control and lactating subjects are presented in Table 1. Since blood values did not differ from wk 4 to 8 of lactation, data were pooled for presentation. Mean concentration of plasma Se of the lactating women, 97 (range 63-132) ng/ml, was significantly lower ($p < 0.05$) than mean concentration of control women, 122 (range 87-172) ng/ml. Mean plasma GSH-Px activity of lactating subjects, 2.29 (range 1.5-3.0) mUnit/mg protein, was approximately 22% lower ($p < 0.05$) than plasma GSH-Px activity, 2.93 (range 2.5-3.4) mUnit/mg protein, of control subjects. The difference between lactating and control women was most evident for erythrocyte Se content. Mean erythrocyte Se concentration was approximately 40% lower ($p < 0.005$) for lactating (173 ng/ml) than for control (305 ng/ml) women. Plasma Se concentration of lactating women was linearly correlated with plasma GSH-Px activity ($r = 0.53$, $p < 0.01$) but not for control women.

Table 1. Blood Indices of Selenium Status of Lactating and Control Women[1]

Parameter	Control Women	Lactating Women
Selenium (ng/ml)		
Plasma	122 ± 9.2	97 ± 6.0*
Erythrocytes	305 ± 21.9	173 ± 6.4†
GSH-Px activity (mUnit/mg protein)		
Plasma	2.93 ± 0.1	2.29 ± 0.1*

[1]Values are expressed as mean ± S.E., n=8 for control women and n=10 for lactating women.
*Significantly lower than control values at $p < 0.05$.
†Significantly lower than control values at $p < 0.005$.

Data on milk selenium concentration and GSH-Px activity are summarized in Table 2. Mean concentration of milk Se was 16.75 while values ranged from 11.50 to 27.25 ng/ml. The samples of hindmilk analyzed contained significantly higher ($p < 0.05$) amounts of Se (18.10 ng/ml) than samples of foremilk (15.56 ng/ml) collected at the same nursing. Glutathione peroxidase activity of milk samples followed the same pattern as milk Se concentration. Mean GSH-Px activity of all milk samples was 77.10 and values ranged from 32.92 to 185.00 mUnit/ml. Mean activity of GSH-Px of hindmilk samples, 90.44 mUnit/ml, was significantly higher ($p < 0.05$) than of foremilk samples, 68.10 mUnit/ml. A highly significant positive correlation ($r = 0.81$, $p < 0.001$) between human milk Se concentration and milk GSH-Px activity was observed (Fig. 1).

Correlational analyses were also performed between maternal indices of Se status and milk parameters. Results of these analyses are tabulated in Table 3. Positive relationships were observed between plasma concentration of Se with both milk Se concentration and GSH-Px activity ($p < 0.01$). Plasma activity of GSH-Px was also positively correlated with both milk Se concentration and activity of GSH-Px ($p < 0.05$). However, erythrocyte Se concentration neither correlated with milk Se concentration nor with GSH-Px activity.

DISCUSSION

The results of this study clearly indicate a direct effect of maternal Se status on quantity of this trace element and GSH-Px activity in human milk. Plasma Se concentration was positively correlated with milk Se concentration (Table 3). Similarly, Williams[12] noted a strong relationship ($r = 0.81$, $p < 0.001$) between Se in human milk and whole blood samples of New Zealand women. This investigator also reported that Se concentration in whole blood of lactating subjects was lower than values typical for this population. We observed significantly lower values for concentrations of Se in plasma and erythrocytes and for activity of GSH-Px in plasma of lactating subjects compared to controls. Differences in blood indices of Se status between our lactating and

Table 2. Selenium Concentration and GSH-Px Activity in Fore- and Hindmilk Samples Collected at 4, 8, 12 and 16 Weeks of Lactation[1]

Stage of Lactation (weeks)	Se Concentration (ng/ml)		GSH-Px Activity (mUnit/ml)	
	Foremilk	Hindmilk	Foremilk	Hindmilk
4	15.6 ± 1.5	18.6 ± 1.5*	77.4 ± 9.2	103.4 ± 11.4*
8	15.2 ± 1.4	17.9 ± 1.1*	64.9 ± 5.7	87.1 ± 6.4*
12	15.1 ± 0.5	17.5 ± 0.6*	60.6 ± 7.4	82.3 ± 5.4*
16	15.3 ± 0.5	17.6 ± 0.7*	63.5 ± 4.2	82.6 ± 4.6*

[1]Values are expressed as mean ± S.E. Ten subjects (at 4 and 8 weeks) and 8 subjects (at 12 and 16 weeks) provided samples for analysis.
*Significantly higher than foremilk ($p < 0.05$).

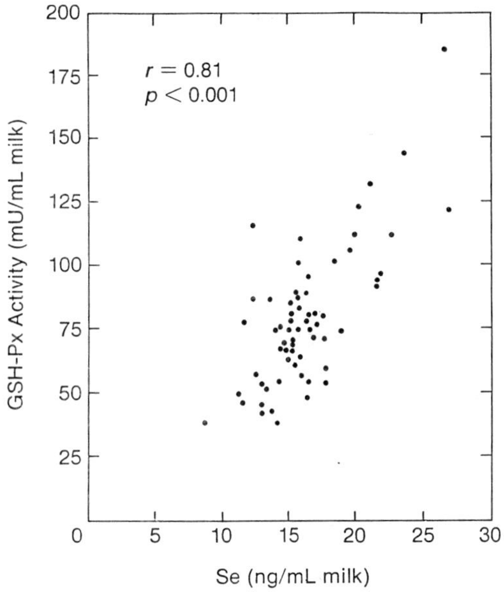

Fig. 1. Correlation between Se concentration and GSH-Px activity in human milk samples (n=72) collected at 4, 8, 12 and 16 weeks postpartum.

Table 3. Relationships of Maternal Blood Indices of Se Status and Milk Se Concentration and Activity of GSH-Px[1]

	Correlation Coefficient (r)	p-value
Plasma Se concentration with		
Milk Se	0.61	0.01
Milk GSH-Px	0.51	0.01
Plasma GSH-Px activity with		
Milk Se	0.40	0.05
Milk GSH-Px	0.39	0.05
Erythrocyte Se concentration with		
Milk Se	0.23	NS
Milk GSH-Px	0.25	NS

[1]Correlational statistics are each based on 20 observations.

control subjects suggest that maximal plasma activity of the Se-dependent enzyme was not achieved by lactating women and the increased quantity of Se needed for milk production was not provided by the diet. This possibility is supported by our findings of significant relationship between plasma Se concentration and GSH-Px activity ($p < 0.01$) for lactating but not for control subjects. Levander et al.[15] observed a 10% lower plasma Se concentration for lactating than for control subjects in their study of Maryland women in spite of an increased intake of dietary Se by the lactating subjects. However, these investigators did not find any relationship between Se in milk and plasma. Higashi et al.[13] reported that serum Se concentration of lactating Japanese women was similar to that of controls and not related to milk content of this element. Differences in maternal Se status among population studied may account for apparently contradictory findings for lactating women. Mean serum Se concentration of Japanese subjects, 148 ng/ml, is about 50% higher than plasma values we observed for mothers living in Central Illinois. Unfortunately, actual plasma Se values were not reported for Maryland women. The difference in plasma Se concentration between Japanese and Illinois lactating women does indicate that depressed values are not characteristic of lactation and that compromised Se nutrition is responsible. Animal data from our laboratory[14] support this conclusion since maternal Se intake is directly related to milk Se concentration of rats. Increased dietary demand for Se during lactation was also evident from these animal studies since Se concentration and GSH-Px activity in blood and tissues of lactating dams were consistently lower than age and sex-matched control animals. Depressed plasma GSH-Px activity of rats during lactation was also reported by Behne et al.[20]

The mean Se concentration in milk found in this study, 16.8 ng/ml, is strikingly similar to the mean value obtained in a previous study from our laboratory, 16.3 ng/ml.[9] It is interesting to note that the concentration of Se in milk is approximately 7 times lower than in plasma. For other trace elements, i.e., copper and zinc, concentrations are higher in milk than in serum.[21] The mechanism of transfer of Se from blood to mammary gland and to milk has not yet been studied. Milk activity of

GSH-Px activity was also assayed in this study and the same pattern of variation as milk Se concentration was noted, i.e., consistently higher in hindmilk than in foremilk. Mean GSH-Px activity of milk samples, 77.0 mUnit/ml, was more than twice that of milk from New Zealand women, 31 mUnit/ml.[12] This is not surprising considering that the mean Se concentration of milk samples from New Zealand was 7.6 ng/ml, less than one-half of the mean value we observed. The strong positive correlation ($r = 0.81$, $p < 0.001$) between milk Se concentration and milk GSH-Px activity that we observed suggests that a large portion of the Se in human milk is present as part of this enzyme. That this is indeed the case was verified by subsequent chromatographic analyses of human milk samples.[22,23] Further study is needed to determine to what extent Se, as part of the enzyme GSH-Px, is available to the nursing infant and whether or not bioavailability is influenced by processing procedures. Hojo[24] reported that bovine milk exhibits GSH-Px activity. It follows that bovine milk-based formulas would furnish some Se as part of the enzyme but possibly in a denatured form. However, the form of Se in other infant formula is unknown.

Animal data[14] clearly indicate a higher dietary Se requirement during lactation. However, comparable work has not been performed with human beings. Based on our milk values for Se and an average daily yield of 600-700 ml,[25] Illinois lactating women excrete an additional 10-12 ug of Se per day. Kumpulainen et al.[26] reported that 50 ug Se/day was sufficient to prevent a decline in milk Se concentration of Finnish women. In the present study, we did not observe a decline in milk Se concentration but maternal Se status was compromised as indicated by measured blood indices. Mean dietary Se intake reported for Maryland women, 80 ± 37 ug/day (14), is higher than the estimated intake of Finnish women[26] yet plasma Se values were lower in lactating than in nonlactating controls. Assuming a 70% absorption rate for Se,[27] an additional dietary intake of 14-17 ug Se/day is needed to merely replace that used for milk production. There are indications that urinary excretion of Se decreases with low Se intake in both rats and human beings;[28] however, it is not known whether such adaptive mechanisms can totally compensate for the extra demand for Se during lactation.

SUMMARY

Although the essentiality of selenium in animals has been documented for several decades, the importance of selenium in human nutrition has been indicated only recently. Results from both animal and human studies support an increased selenium requirement during reproduction. The quantity of selenium in human milk displays a geographical pattern of variation and is directly related to indices of maternal selenium status. Since the nursing neonate is totally dependent on human milk for nourishment, the need to define maternal dietary factors exerting an influence cannot be overstressed. A portion of human milk selenium is present as part of the enzyme glutathione peroxidase. Bioavailability of selenium from human milk and other milks used in infant feeding is unknown.

ACKNOWLEDGMENT

The participation of subjects and Carle Clinic Hospital and Clinic, Urbana, Illinois are acknowledged. This research was supported in part by the National Institute of Child Health and Human Development (#HD 18689) and by the Illinois Agricultural Experiment Station (#60-334).

REFERENCES

1. K. Schwarz and C. M. Foltz, Selenium as an integral part of factor 3 against dietary necrotic liver degeneration, J. Amer. Chem. Soc. 79:3292-93 (1957).
2. G. C. Mills, The purification and properties of glutathione peroxidase of erythrocytes, J. Biol. Chem. 234:502-6 (1959).
3. Y. C. Awasthi and D. D. Dao, Purification and properties of glutathione peroxidase from human placenta, Fed. Proc. 37:1340 (1978).
4. A. M. Michelson, O. Dangeon, K. Puget, P. Durosay, B. Perdereau, and C. Barbaroux, Comparative studies of glutathione peroxidase as free enzyme or liposome encapsulated in rats and rabbits, Mol. Phys. 3:27-34 (1983).
5. Keshan Disease Research Group of the Chinese Academy of Medical Sciences. Observations on effect of sodium selenite in prevention of Keshan disease, Chin. Med. J. 92:471-6 (1979).
6. A. M. Van Rij, C. D. Thomson, J. M. McKenzie, and M. F. Robinson, Selenium deficiency in total parenteral nutrition, Am. J. Clin. Nutr. 32:2076-85 (1979).
7. J. T. Salonen, G. Atfathan, J. K. Hutlunen, B. Pikkarainen, and C. Barbaroux, Comparative studies of glutathione peroxidase as free enzyme or liposome encapsulated in rats and rabbits, Mol. Phys. 3:27-34 (1983).
8. A. S. Majaj and L. L. Hopkins, Selenium and Kwashiorkor, Lancet 2:592-97 (1966).
9. A. M. Smith, M. F. Picciano, and J. A. Milner, Selenium intakes and status of human milk and formula fed infants, Am. J. Clin. Nutr. 35:521-26 (1981).
10. I. Lombeck, K. Kasperek, B. Bonnermann, L. E. Fienendegen, and H. J. Bremer, Selenium content of human milk, cow's milk and cow's milk infant formulas, Eur. J. Pead. 129:139-49 (1978).
11. J. Kumpulainen, E. Vuori, P. Kuitunen, S. Makinen, and R. Kara, Longitudinal study on the dietary selenium intake of exclusively breast-fed infants and their mothers in Finland, Internat. J. Vit. Nutr. 53:420-26 (1983).
12. M.M.F. Williams, Selenium and glutathione peroxidase in mature human milk, Proc. Univ. Otago. Med. Sch. Dunedin 61:20-21 (1983).
13. T. H. Higashi, Y. Kuroki, and I. Matsuda, Longitudinal changes in selenium content of breast milk, Acta Paediatr. Scand. 72:433-36 (1983).
14. A. M. Smith and M. F. Picciano, Dietary selenium requirement during reproduction: evidence for an increase during lactation, Fed. Proc. 44:1504 (Abstr) (1985).
15. O. A. Levander, V. C. Morris, and P. B. Moster, Dietary selenium (Se) intake and Se content of breast milk and plasma of lactating and non-lactating women, Fed. Proc. 40:890 (Abstr) (1981).
16. L. W. Green, Manual for scoring socioeconomic status for research on health behavior, Public Health Rep. 85:815-27 (1970).
17. D. E. Paglia and W. N. Valentine, Studies on the quantitative and qualitative characterization of the erythrocyte glutathione peroxidase, J. Lab. Clin. Med. 70:158-69 (1967).
18. T. P. McCarthy, B. Brodie, J. A. Milner, and R. F. Bevill, Improved method for selenium determination in biological samples by gas chromatography, J. Chromatography 225:9-16 (1981).
19. O. H. Lowry, N. J. Roberrough, A. L. Farr, and R. J. Randall, Protein measurement with the folin phenol reagent, J. Biol. Chem. 193:265-67 (1951).
20. D. Behne, R. V. Berswordt-Wallrabe, W. Elger, and W. Wolters, Glutathione peroxidase in erythrocytes and plasma of rats during pregnancy and lactation, Experentia 34:986-87 (1978).

21. S. Hatano, K. Aihara, Y. Nishi, and T. Usui, Trace elements (copper, zinc, manganese, and selenium) in plasma and erythrocytes in relation to dietary intake during infancy, J. Pedeatr. Gastroenterology Nutr. 4:87-92 (1985).
22. J. A. Milner, L. Sherman, A. M. Smith, and M. F. Picciano, Characterization of forms of selenium in human milk, presented at the XIII International Congress of Nutrition, Brighton, United Kingdom, August (1985)
23. M. F. Picciano and J. A. Milner, Selenium in human milk: Factors exerting an influence, form and distribution, in: "Composition and Physiological Properties of Human Milk," J. Schaub, ed., Elsevier Science Publishers, Amsterdam (1985).
24. Y. Hojo, Selenium concentration and glutathione peroxidase activity in cow's milk, Biol. Trace Elem. Res. 4:233-39 (1982).
25. R. Matheny and M. F. Picciano, Feeding and growth characteristics of human milk-fed infants, J. Am. Diet. Assoc. 86:327-31 (1986).
26. J. Kumpulainen, E. Vouri, and M. A. Simes, Effect of maternal dietary selenium intake on selenium levels in breast milk, Internat. J. Vit. Nutr. Res 54:251-55 (1984).
27. C. D. Thomson and R.D.H. Stewart, Measurement of intestinal absorption of selenium, Proc. Univ. Otago. Med. Sch. 50:63-64 (1972).
28. R. F. Burk, Selenium in man, in: "Trace Elements in Human Health and Disease," A. S. Prasad, ed., Academic Press, New York (1976).

DISTRIBUTION OF SELENIUM IN HUMAN MILK

J.A. Milner, L. Sherman-Martin and M.F. Picciano

University of Illinois at Urbana-Champaign
College of Agriculture
Department of Food Science and Division of Nutritional Sciences
University of Illinois, Urbana, IL 61801

INTRODUCTION

Selenium is a trace element which possesses a strong metabolic similarity to sulfur. Early investigators suggested this element was highly toxic and possibly carcinogenic (1,2). However, during the early 1960's increasing evidence indicated that selenium was an essential nutrient, especially in production animals where supplementation prevented a wide array of disorders (3). More recent support for the essentiality of selenium comes from its ability to maximize growth of mammalian cells in culture, including the clonal growth of normal human fibroblasts (4). Generally, the concentration of selenium needed to stimulate cellular growth is about 50 nM.

In 1973, Rotruck et al. (5) reported the only known metabolic role of this trace element, which is as an active component of the enzyme, glutathione peroxidase. This enzyme is involved in the destruction of hydroperoxides (6). While other seleno-proteins have been isolated in mammalian cells their metabolic function remains unknown (7).

The importance of selenium in human nutrition is becoming increasingly apparent. The association of low intakes of selenium with increased susceptibility to cardiac myopathy (8) and various types of cancer (9) serve to emphasize the need for understanding the dietary requirements and physiological action of selenium. Unfortunately, the human requirement for selenium, especially in the growing years, has not been defined. For adults, a range of safe and adequate dietary intakes of selenium has been estimated primarily from extrapolations of requirements of animals. These extrapolations are based on the assumption that dietary concentrations adequate for animals will also meet human requirements. Results from controlled feeding studies by Levander (10) support such approximations for adults. For infants and children, similar studies are not available and dietary recommendations do not reflect the measured intakes of infants in the United States. Our recent data (11) show that approximately 60% of human milk fed and 95% of formula fed infants had selenium intakes below the 10 to 40 ug/day proposed by the National Research Council for infants 0-6 months of age.

The content of selenium in food is known to increase with increasing soil content. Blood concentrations of selenium likewise increase with increasing dietary intakes. Milk from women living in countries where the soil content of selenium is low, such as Finland and New Zealand, have lower selenium concentrations than milk obtained from women residing in the United States, Germany or Japan, where the soil content of selenium is higher (11-15). Thus, geographic variations in the selenium content of human milk suggest that dietary selenium can influence milk concentrations of this element in humans, as observed in other mammals (16).

Selenium intakes and the associated selenium status of totally breast-fed infants should serve as the basis for recommendations for this trace element in infant feeding. Human milk is known to contain about twice as much selenium as normal cow's milk. Millar and Sheppard (17) reported human milk samples from five areas in New Zealand had selenium concentrations ranging from 11.5 to 14.5 ng/ml, compared to 5 ng/ml for cow's milk. These values compare well to the 13-53 ng/ml range reported by Shearer and Hadjimarkos (18) and 8-34 ng/ml range reported in our laboratory for mature human milk (11).

While the quantity of a nutrient in milk can determine the infants' status, other factors may likewise modify a nutrient's overall utilization or bioavailability. Therefore, molecular form and location of an element in a food source can be a major determinant of its bioavailability. To date, little information is available on the distribution of selenium in human milk. Therefore, there is a need to identify the nature of compounds binding selenium in human milk. The present studies were designed to characterize the chemical forms and distribution of selenium in human milk.

MATERIALS AND METHODS

Subjects

Milk specimens from healthy lactating mothers were collected for the present studies. All subjects lived in or near Champaign-Urbana, Illinois. The mothers ranged in age from 20 to 35 years. Of the 19 mothers the average number of children was 2.1. The use of human subjects in this investigation was annually reviewed and approved by the Institutional Review Board of the University of Illinois. Eighteen mothers reported taking a daily multivitamin and mineral supplement during pregnancy, and they continued taking the supplement for the duration of the study. No subject reported taking supplements containing selenium during pregnancy or during lactation.

Milk was collected by the subjects by hand expression into acid-washed containers and either immediately frozen in liquid nitrogen or kept on ice until placed in a -70°C freezer. All samples were stored at -70°C. Milk samples were thawed in an ice water bath and used immediately for all procedures. Whole milk or defatted milk, produced by centrifugation at 10,000 x g for 90 min. were used in the various methods described below.

Selenium and Glutathione Peroxidase Analysis

A gas chromatograph equipped with an electron capture detector was used for all selenium analyses (19). This method of analysis has been shown to yield values that are comparable to those obtained fluorometrically, yet utilizes considerably less sample; 0.2 ml of whole milk or dialyzed milk was analyzed for selenium. Three ml of each fraction from the Sephadex columns was analyzed for selenium. For all types of samples the reproducibility of the selenium analysis was within 5% and recovery of added selenium was always in the range of 95 to 110%.

The activity of glutathione peroxidase (GPx) in human whole or skim milk was measured by modifications of the coupled assay of Paglia and Valentine using t-butylhydroperoxide (14,20). Heat treated milk samples were used as blanks. One mUnit of GPx activity is defined as one nanomole of NADPH oxidized/min.

Dialysis and Precipitation

Whole milk was dialyzed to determine the amount of selenium which was associated with low molecular weight components. Milk was placed in membrane tubing (Spectrum Labware, New York) with a molecular weight cut-off of 6-8 KDal. The milk was dialyzed at 4°C against deionized water (Nanopure) for seven days. The water was replaced once daily. In a separate experiment, milk was dialyzed against mercaptoethanol (0.5 M) for 24 h.

Total breast milk macromolecules were precipitated with 55% ice cold acetone. Twenty ml of milk were slowly added to 1.1 volumes of acetone, kept on ice for 1 h, and centrifuged at 10,000 x g for 30 min. at 4°C. The resultant pellet was resuspended in 20 ml of 10 mM tris buffer (pH 7.6) containing 1mM GSH. Analysis of the dialysis buffer indicated minimal selenium contamination. Breast milk macromolecules were also selectively precipitated using ammonium sulfate. In this method, one volume of saturated ammonium sulfate was slowly added to skim milk while maintained on ice. After twenty four hours, the mixture was centrifuged at 10,000 x g for 30 min. at 4°C. The supernate solution was decanted and saturated ammonium sulfate was added to obtain a 65% salt solution which was treated as described for the 50% solution. The resultant pellets were resuspended in deionized water and dialyzed for 7 days against 10 mM tris buffer (pH 7.6) containing 1 mM glutathione. An aliquot of each dialyzed sample was assayed for selenium.

Method of Specimen Handling

In a separate study, milk from 5 women was collected to evaluate the impact of collection procedures on selenium content and distribution. For each subject two milk specimens were collected and kept on ice while a third sample was placed immediately in liquid nitrogen until returned to the laboratory. One sample which had been kept on ice was analyzed immediately (fresh) for selenium, glutathione peroxidase activity and the percent dialyzable selenium. The second sample which had been maintained on ice was placed in a -70°C freezer for one month (slow frozen) before analysis. The liquid nitrogen frozen sample (fast frozen) was also placed in the -70°C freezer for one month before being analyzed.

Column Chromatography

Dialyzed and nondialyzed milk was centrifuged at 10,000 x g for 90 min. at 4°C to separate the lipids. The fat was removed by aspiration and any partial casein pellet was resuspended in the supernate solution. Fifteen ml of the resultant milk was applied to a Sephadex G-100 (Pharmacia, Piscataway NJ) (2.5 cm x 50 cm) column maintained at room temperature. The milk macromolecules were eluted by gravity with 10 mM tris buffer containing 1 mM glutathione, pH 7.6. The column was calibrated using blue dextran and molecular weight standards (Sigma, St. Louis, MO). Five ml fractions were collected and each fraction was monitored for relative absorbance at 280 nm, selenium content, and when applicable, glutathione peroxidase activity.

Samples assayed for glutathione peroxidase were separated on a Sephadex G-150 column at 4°C. The elution buffer was as described above. In the GPx assays, whole milk was diluted 10 fold with reaction buffer, and a 10 fold dilution of boiled milk was used as a blank. Column fractions were assayed undiluted using the elution buffer as a blank.

RESULTS

Approximately 5% of the total selenium in human milk was associated with the lipid fraction separated by centrifugation (Table 1). Acetone (55 %) treatment of whole milk was found to precipitate all of the selenium. The proportion of selenium in whole milk that was precipitated increased with the addition of increasing quantities of ammonium sulfate (Table 1). Subsequent studies revealed that in most milk specimens some

TABLE 1

Influence of Various Procedures on Milk Selenium[1]

Treatment	Whole Milk Se (%)
None	100
Centrifugation Supernatant (10,000 xg)	95
Acetone (55%) Precipitate	100
$(NH_4)_2SO_4$ (50%) Precipitate	47
(65%) Precipitate	54
Dialysis - H_2O	66
" " - Mercaptoethanol	67

[1]Percentages were determined from a minimum of triplicate analysis.

of the selenium could be removed by dialysis (Table 1). Dialysis against water or mercaptoethanol (0.5 M) resulted in comparable quantities of selenium associated with the low molecular weight fraction. In the first set of milk samples analyzed, an average of 34%, with a range of 0 to 40%, of the selenium was removed by dialysis.

Results of a study designed to determine if method of collection modified the percentage dialyzable selenium are presented in Table 2. No significant differences in the percentage of dialyzable selenium were observed among fresh, fast frozen and slow frozen specimens. Freezing likewise did not significantly modify the glutathione peroxidase activity of these specimens. Dialysis decreased glutathione peroxidase activity by approximately 60% in both fresh and frozen milk samples (Table 2).

Table 2

Influence of Dialysis and Freezing on Selenium and Glutathione Peroxidase Activities[1]

	Undialyzed	Dialyzed
Selenium (ng/ml)		
Fresh	14.4 ± 1.53	11.2 ± 0.9
Fast Frozen		12.2 ± 1.5
Slow Frozen		11.5 ± 1.5
Glutathione Peroxidase (mU/ml)		
Fresh	136.3 + 9.2	48.4 + 21.0
Fast Frozen	147.3 + 15.7	62.6 + 28.9
Slow Frozen	122.2 + 23.9	57.8 + 25.0

[1]Milk samples were analyzed immediately (fresh), after storage on ice and freezing for one month (slow freezing) or after immediate freezing in liquid nitrogen and storage for one month (fast frozen). Values are means ± SEM for five samples per collection method.

Figure 1 depicts the quantity of nondialyzable selenium in 34 milk specimens evaluated as a function of time of lactation. Mean percent dialyzable selenium at 1, 2, 3 and 4 months of lactation were: 18.3, 7.9, 19.4, and 23.1, respectively, with a pooled standard error of 8.9%. In cross-sectional samples no significant effect of stage of lactation on the percentage dialyzable selenium was observed. Likewise, in longitudinal samples no significant effect of stage of lactation on the percentage dialyzable selenium was detected.

A scatter plot of nondialyzable selenium as a function of total milk selenium is given in Figure 2. This figure illustrates that the percentage of nondialyzable selenium in human milk increases proportionally (r = 0.71) to the total milk selenium content. These data reveal that the amount of dialyzable selenium increases as the total quantity of selenium in the milk increases.

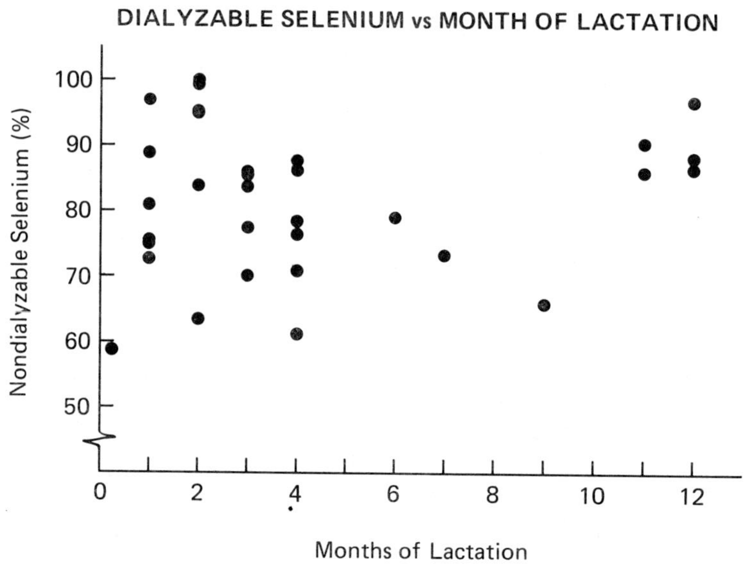

Figure 1. Influence of stage of lactation on the quantity of nondialyzable selenium in human milk. Five ml of milk from fourteen subjects was dialyzed to determine the quantity of nondialyzable selenium in milk after 1-12 months of lactation. Each point is a mean of at least three determinations.

Elution profiles of nondialyzed and dialyzed skim milk applied to a Sephadex G-100 column is presented in Figures 3 and 4. The chromatograms of both the dialyzed and nondialyzed milk were similar. Absorption at 280 nm revealed three major protein fractions in both dialyzed and nondialyzed samples.

The nondialyzed milk sample shown in Figure 3 contained 16.15 ng Se/ml. The recovery of selenium from the column was 97%. Only three predominate selenium fractions could be identified when nondialyzed milk was applied to the Sephadex column (Figure 3). These three peaks corresponded to molecular weights of approximately 150 KDal, 30 KDal and 10 KDal, respectively. The largest fraction was associated with proteins in 150 KDal range.

SELENIUM IN DIALYZED AND NONDIALYZED HUMAN MILK

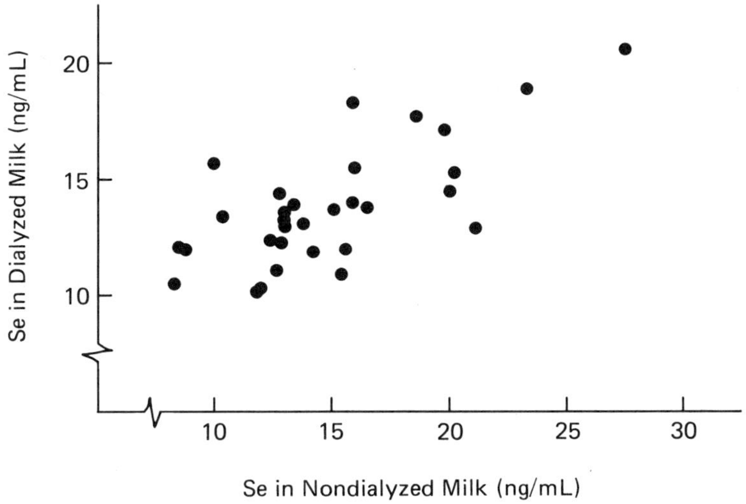

Figure 2. Influence of total milk selenium on the proportion of nondialyzable selenium. Each point represent the mean of duplicate analysis of 5 ml milk samples.

NONDIALYZED MILK PROTEINS

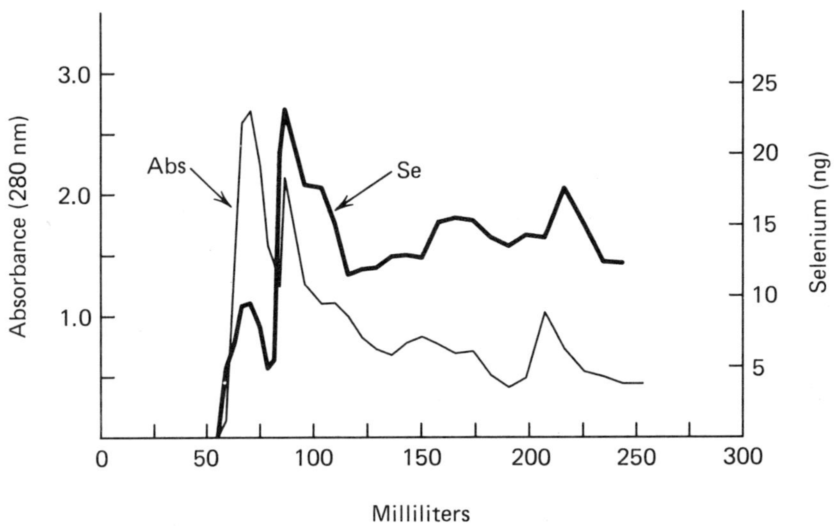

Figure 3. Selenoproteins in 10 ml of pooled defatted milk separated on a Sephadex G-100 column and eluted with 10 mM tris buffer containing 0.02% sodium azide and 1 mM glutathione. Milliliters refers to elution volumes.

An elution profile of the selenoproteins in the milk sample shown in Figure 3 following dialysis is presented in Figure 4. Preliminary studies indicated that dialysis of milk against tris or phosphate buffer resulted in identical chromatographic profiles. Again the quantity of selenium recovered from the column was 97%. In this dialyzed milk sample at least nine selenium containing proteins were identified. These proteins ranged in molecular weight from approximately 150 KDal to approximately 6 KDal (Fig. 4).

The separation of glutathione peroxidase on a Sephadex G-150 column was also undertaken. Preliminary studies revealed a loss of enzymatic activity in separation occurred at room temperature. Therefore, separations of glutathione peroxidase were conducted at 4°C. Using tert-butyl hydroperoxide three peaks of activity were detected (Figure 5). The minor peak occurring early in the separation probably represents

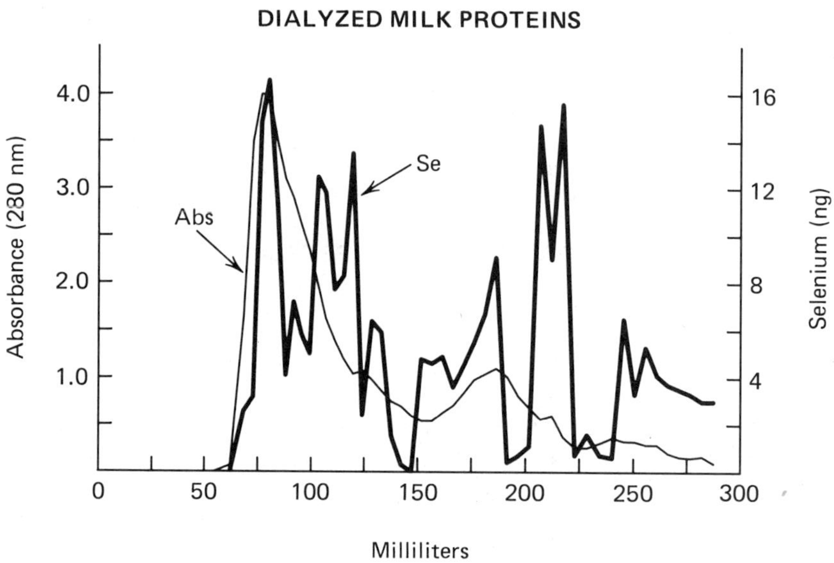

Figure 4. Selenoproteins in 10 ml of pooled defatted and dialyzed milk separated on a Sephadex G-100 column and eluted with 10 mM tris buffer containing 0.02% sodium azide and 1 mM glutathione. Milliliters refers to elution volumes.

a polymer of glutathione peroxidase. The first major peak occurs at a position of the molecular weight of glutathione peroxidase. The second major peak possibly represents glutathione S-transferase activity since this enzyme is also known to utilize the substrate used for these analyses. The last peak of enzymatic activity may also represent a subunit of glutathione peroxidase that has activity against the substrate used.

DISCUSSION

Human milk is the natural source of nutrients for the infant. However, cow's milk and infant formulas have been used successfully for infant feeding for several decades. Young mammals are born at widely different stages of physiological maturity. Since the milk of mammals also varies greatly in its composition, it is easy to teleologically reason the milk of a given species is best adapted to the nutritional

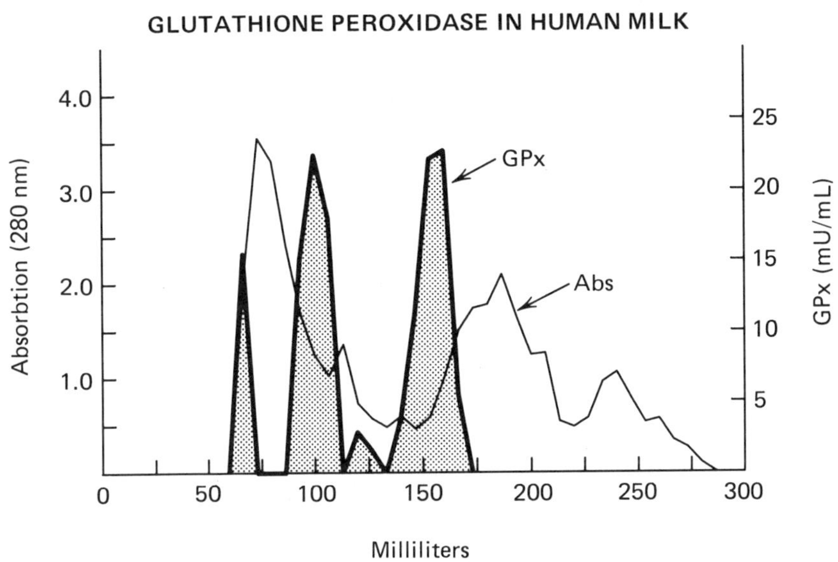

Figure 5. Total peroxidase activity in human milk. Enzymatic activity was determined as described in the materials and methods section after separation on a Sephadex G-150 column. Milliliters refers to elution volumes.

needs of the young of that species. However, it is difficult to prove that this is the case and that the nutritive requirements of the young have exerted a selective force in the evolution of milk composition. Nevertheless, considerable evidence has demonstrated that the bioavailability of some nutrients is not identical between human and cow milk (21,22).

The present studies have shown that most of the selenium in human milk is bound to macromolecules. Most of the selenium separated with these macromolecules was associated with proteins. Both the dialyzable and nondialyzable selenium content increase with increasing selenium content of the whole milk. The quantity of dialyzable selenium was variable and ranged from 0 to 40 %. The reason for this variation is unknown but possibly related to the dietary habits of each subject.

Only a small fraction (5%) of the selenium was associated with the lipid component of human milk. Selenium was present at a lower percentage than has been found with some other trace elements such as manganese, iron, zinc and copper which are found at approximately 20, 30, 44 and 37 % in the lipid fraction of human milk (23-26). The selenium in the lipid fraction is likely associated with outer membrane proteins surrounding the fat globule as observed with iron.

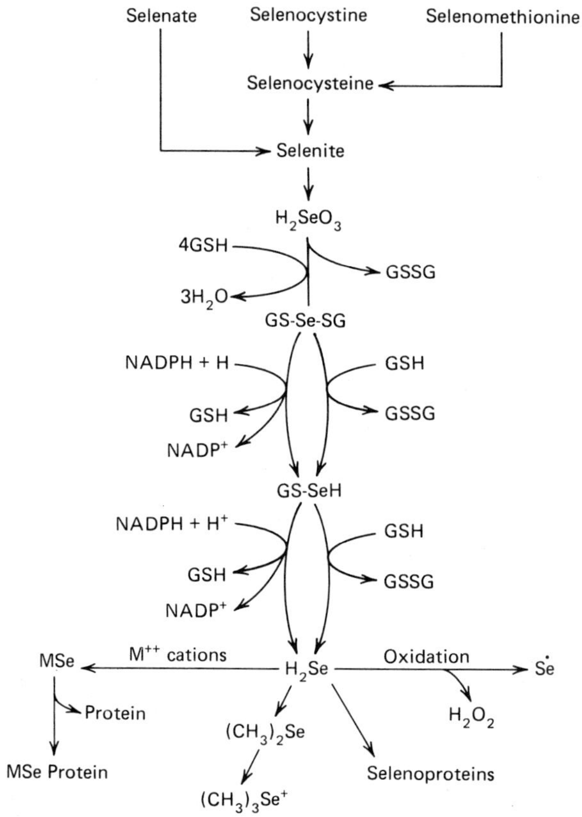

Figure 6. Proposed pathway for selenium metabolism and detoxification in mammalian cells.

These studies show that dialysis removes low molecular weight seleno-compounds that are not separated by gel chromatography. After dialysis, at least nine selenoproteins could be identified in human milk. One of the peaks in the chromatogram of dialyzed milk corresponded to the molecular weight of glutathione peroxidase, which has a molecular weight of about 95 KDal in human erythrocytes (27). However, major selenium peaks also occurred at molecular weights greater than 150 KDal and 8-10 KDal. A small (about 10 KDal) selenoprotein has also been shown to be present in muscle tissue of lambs fed a selenium adequate diet but absent in lambs fed limiting quantities of selenium (28).

The ratio of Se to GPx activity in a solution of crystalline GPx is 0.131 (29). Although variability in individual samples was evident, using this value the selenium associated with glutathione peroxidase only accounted for about 15 to 30 percent of the total selenium in milk. This percentage is consistent with the quantity of selenium found in the fraction corresponding to the molecular weight of glutathione peroxidase and is consistent with estimations of Hojo (30). Thus of the selenium associated with proteins only a small percentage could be accounted for by its association with this only known biologically active form of selenium. The presence of two major peroxidase activity peaks following gel chromatography of human milk may indicate the presence of glutathione peroxidase and glutathione S-transferase. Additional studies are needed to determine if this represents the activity of a second enzyme or a subunit of glutathione peroxidase.

The GSH/glutathione reductase/NADPH pathway involved in the reduction of selenite to selenide has been well characterized, as has the excretory methylation of selenide (Figure 6) (31).

Hydrogen selenide appears to be a central compound in selenium metabolism and detoxification. Selenide is methylated to form $(CH_3)Se^+$ (trimethyl selenonium ion) and excreted in the urine or dimethylselenide and eliminated in the breath. Selenide may be the form that binds to a number of proteins. Hydrogen selenide or a close metabolite has been suggested to be the form inserted post-translationally into a pre-glutathione peroxidase polypeptide to form the active glutathione peroxidase subunits (32). Such incorporation may explain the number of selenoproteins isolated in human milk. However, these selenoproteins may also arise from the direct incorporations of seleno-amino acids into cellular proteins. Selenomethionine or selenocysteine can be incorporated into general body proteins in place of methionine or cysteine directly or via degradation through the transsulfuration pathway forming selenocysteine. Alternatively, selenomethionine may be transaminated and decarboxylated, with final release of methane selenol in a manner similar to the methionine transamination pathway. Methane selenol catabolism would yield methane and selenide. Selenocysteine may also be degraded to release selenite in a manner similar to the degradation of cysteine. However the high reduction potential of selenocysteine should favor the direct release of selenide. Whether some of the selenoproteins present in milk represent the utilization of selenomethionine or selenocysteine in place of methionine or cysteine remains to be determined. Studies are needed to determine the impact of form of supplemental selenium on the distribution of selenium in human milk.

Milk facilitates the bioavailability of several essential nutrients by providing them in an appropriate molecular form (21,24,33,34). A number of studies have shown that the quality or chemical state and not necessarily the quantity is the major factor affecting the function or availability of a molecule in living organisms. Whether this is the case for selenium is unknown, but clearly deserves investigation. Investigation of the characteristics of the different compounds binding selenium in human milk may aid in the understanding of this trace element's absorption and utilization. Such knowledge is essential for the design of formulas in order to optimize the availability of trace elements.

SUMMARY

The present studies were designed to characterize the distribution of selenium in human milk. These studies reveal that the majority of the selenium in human milk is protein bound. The quantity of dialyzable selenium increased proportionally with increasing total selenium content of the milk but did not correlate with the stage of lactation. Neither rate of freezing nor frozen storage of samples for one month influenced the selenium distribution profiles. At least nine selenoproteins were detected in dialyzed milk samples following molecular sieve (Sephadex) chromatography. Glutathione peroxidase in these molecular profiles accounted for approximately 15 to 30% of the selenium found in milk. Approximately half of the peroxidase activity of human milk was associated with selenium dependent glutathione peroxidase activity. Additional studies are presently underway to determine the influence of dietary supplementation of selenium on the distribution and form of this trace element in human milk.

REFERENCES

1. A. T. Diplock, Metabolic aspects of selenium action and toxicity, CRC Crit Rev Toxicol, 4:271 (1976).
2. A. A. Nelson, O. G. Fitzburgh and H.O. Calvery, Liver tumors following cirrhosis caused by selenium in rats, Cancer Res, 3:230 (1943).
3. R. J. Shamberger, Selenium Deficiency Diseases in Animals, in: "Biochemistry of Selenium" pp 31-58. Plenum Press, New York (1983).
4. W. L. McKeehan, W. G. Hamilton, and R. G. Ham, Selenium is an essential trace nutrient for growth of WI-38 diploid human fibroblasts, Proc. Natl. Acad. Sci. USA, 73:2023 (1976).
5. J. T. Rotruck, A. L. Pope, H. E. Ganther, A. B. Swanson, D. G. Hafeman, and W. G. Hoekstra, Selenium: Biochemical role as a component of glutathione peroxidase, Science, 179:588 (1973).
6. C. Little, R. Olinescu, K. G. Reid, and P. J. O'Brien, Properties and regulation of glutathione peroxidase, J Biol Chem, 245:3632 (1970).
7. R. F. Burk, and P. E. Gregory, Some characteristics of 75-Se-P, A selenoprotein found in rat liver and plasma, and comparison of it with selenoglutathione peroxidase, Arch Biochem Biophys, 213:73 (1982).
8. Keshan Disease Research Group of the Chinese Academy of Medical Sciences. Observations on effect of sodium selenite in prevention of Keshan disease, Chin Med J, 92:471 (1979).
9. J. A. Milner, Selenium and Carcinogenesis, in: "Xenobiotic Metabolism: Nutritional Effects," J. W. Finley and D. E. Schwass, ed., American Chemical Society, Washington, D.C. (1985).
10. O. Levander, and V. C. Morris, Dietary selenium levels needed to maintain balance in North American adults consuming self-selected diets, Am J Clin Nutr, 39:809 (1984).
11. A. M. Smith, M. F. Picciano, and J.A. Milner, Selenium intakes and status of human milk and formula fed infants, Am J Clin Nutr, 35:521 (1981).
12. J. Kumpulainen, E. Vuori, P. Kuitunen, S. Makinen, and R. Kara, Longitudinal study on the dietary selenium intake of exclusively breast-fed infants and their mothers in Finland, Internat J Vit Nutr, 53:420 (1983).
13. I. Lombeck, K. Kasperek, B. Bonnermann, L. E. Fienendegen, and H. J. Bremer, Selenium content of human milk, cow's milk and cow's milk infant formulas, Eur J Pead, 129:139 (1978).

14. M. M. F. Williams, Selenium and glutathione peroxidase in mature human milk, Proc Univ Otago Med Sch Dunedin, 61:20 (1983).
15. T. H. Higashi, Y. Kuroki, and I. Matsuda, Longitudinal changes in selenium content of breast milk, Acta Paediatr Scand, 72:433 (1983).
16. H. R. Conrad, and A. L. Moxon, Transfer of dietary selenium to milk, J Dairy Sci, 62:404 (1979).
17. K. R. Millar, and A. D. Sheppard, Alpha-tocopherol and selenium levels in human and cow's milk, N Z J Sci, 15:3 (1972).
18. T. R. Shearer, and D. M. Hadjimarkos, Geographic Distribution of Selenium in Human Milk, Arch Environ Health, 30:230 (1973).
19. T. P. McCarthy, B. Brodie, J. A. Milner, and R. F. Bevill, Improved method for selenium determination in biological samples by gas chromatography, J. Chromatography, 225:9 (1981).
20. D. E. Paglia, and W. N. Valentine, Studies on the quantitative and qualitative characterization of the erythrocyte glutathione peroxidase, J Lab Clin Med, 70:158 (1967).
21. P. E. Johnson, and G. Evans, Relative zinc bioavailability in human breast milk, infant formulas, and cow's milk, Amer J Clin Nutr, 31:416 (1978).
22. B. Lonnerdal, C. L. Keen, and L. S. Hurley, Iron, copper, zinc and manganese in milk, Ann Rev Nutr, 1:149 (1978).
23. B. Lonnerdal, C. L. Keen, and L. S. Hurley, Manganese binding proteins in human and cow's milk, Amer J Clin Nutr, 41:550 (1985).
24. U. M. Saarinen, M. A. Siimes and P. R. Dallman, Iron absorption in infants: high bioavailability of breast milk iron as indicated by the extrinsic tag method of iron absorption and by the concentration of serum ferritin, J Pediatr, 91:36 (1977).
25. B. Lonnerdal, B. Hoffman, and L.S. Hurley, Zinc and copper binding proteins in human milk, Amer J Clin Nutr, 36:1170 (1982).
26. G. B. Fransson, and B. Lonnerdal, Iron in human milk, J Pediatr, 96:380 (1982).
27. Y. C. Awasthi, E. Beutler, and S. K. Srivastava, Purification and properties of human erythrocyte glutathione peroxidase, J Biol Chem, 250:5144 (1975).
28. N. D. Pedersen, P. D. Whanger, P. H. Weswig, and O. H. Muth, Selenium binding proteins in tissues of normal and selenium-responsive myopathic lambs, Bioinorg Chem, 2:33 (1972).
29. L. Flohe, and W. A. Gunzler, Glutathione peroxidase. in: "Glutathione," L. Flohe, H. C. Benohr, H. Sies, H. D. Waller, and A. Wendei, ed. pp 133, Academic Press, New York (1974).
30. Y. Hojo, Selenium concentration and glutathione peroxidase activity in cow's milk, Biol Trace Elem Res, 4:233 (1982).
31. H. E. Ganther, Enzymatic synthesis of dimethyl selenide from sodium selenite in mouse liver extracts, Biochemistry, 5:1089 (1966).
32. R.A. Sunde, The biochemistry of selenoproteins, JAOCS, 61:1891 (1984).
33. J. A. McMillan, S. A. Landaw, and F. A. Oski, Iron sufficiency in breast fed infants and the availability of iron from human milk, Pediatrics, 58:686 (1976).
34. G. B. Fransson, and B. Lonnerdal, Distribution of trace elements and minerals in human and cow's milk, Pediat Res, 17:912 (1983).

A COMPREHENSIVE ASSESSMENT OF DRUGS AND CHEMICAL TOXINS EXCRETED IN BREAST MILK

John T. Wilson, James L. Hinson, R. Don Brown and Iain J. Smith

Section on Clinical Pharmacology
Departments of Pharmacology and Therapeutics and Pediatrics
Louisiana State University Medical Center
1501 Kings Highway
Shreveport, Louisiana 71130

INTRODUCTION

Inherent difficulties of opportunistic approaches have contributed to the existing paucity of information about drug excretion in human breast milk. This situation prevails for new drugs and also for post marketing surveillance of drugs. Most anecdotal or purely descriptive studies have offered too little understanding about fundamental mechanisms which in turn allow accurate quantitative estimations of the milk/plasma (M/P) drug concentration ratio after single and/or repeated doses or even during a dosing interval. Few studies have sufficient numbers of women to address this M/P ratio, or even amount of drug in milk, with regard to interindividual variation. The practical importance of an accurate, widely applicable but drug specific M/P ratio is recognized because it captures the net effect of maternal dose, dose interval, and drug disposition to give a ratio for calculation of dose delivered to the infant via breast milk.

Extrapolation of existing data on drugs in breast milk for use by the general population is difficult if not impossible. To further confound the situation, we have little reported data to propose or confirm a pharmacokinetic model for certain drugs. No animal has received the rigorous comparative pharmacologic evaluations necessary to deem it suitable for assessment of the amount of drug excreted in milk.

Let us highlight our current dilemma by developing a perspective of a cogent but elementary nature - one which will form the basis for a detailed and comprehensive approach to understanding drug excretion in human milk. We recognize that the excretion of drugs into breast milk is important only if:

1. Women breast feed: They do and their numbers are increasing with encouragement by public health officials, physicians and lay organizations.

2. Breast feeding women ingest drugs: They do, both on a need and incidental or preference basis.

3. Drugs are excreted in breast milk: They are and it is just a matter of how much and for how long.

4. Nursing infants are affected by drugs in breast milk: They are and it is a matter of risk and extent for each chemical.

Incidence of breast feeding

In an earlier review it was observed that the incidence of breast feeding differed from country to country (1). In the western developed world 53% of U.S. women in 1976, 35% of Canadian women in 1978 and 70% of Swedish women in 1975 were breast feeding at the time of discharge from hospital.

A more recent global report published by the World Health Organization (2) cites the incidence of breast feeding in 6 countries. These countries represent the developed, developing and semi-developed nations. In Hungary and Sweden, between 93 and 97% of all women attempted to breast feed one child. In India 96-100% of all women attempted breast feeding as did 91-100% of Ethiopian women. However, in Guatemala and the Phillipines, the incidence fell in economically advantaged women to 77 and 68%, respectively, but rose to 98 and 94% in rural communities. At the time of hospital discharge in Norway and Northern Ireland, a respective 97.5% and 33% women were breast feeding (2a). The duration of breast feeding was also reported (2). In Sweden and Hungary, 30 and 32% respectively were still breast feeding at 6 months. Ninety per cent of India and all the Ethiopian women were still feeding at 6 months; in fact, 65% were still feeding at 18 months. Of the women of the Phillipines and Guatemala, 66% of infants were fully weaned by 6 months.

National and international policy statements highlight the unique usefulness of human breast milk for infant nutrition (3-10). In accordance with these emerging statements, it is both necessary and prudent to provide information about the risk of drug excretion in breast milk. Without this information, it is unlikely that we will meet the Surgeon General's goal of 75% incidence for breast feeding. It is also unlikely that mothers who require medicines for their health care needs will continue to breast feed when the consequences to the nursing infant remain unknown.

Prevalence of drugs in women breast feeding (or those of child bearing age)

There are very little data on the drug ingestion rates for lactating women. Lack of information makes it difficult to estimate the potential magnitude of the problem. However, it is possible to give some approximate figures for drug usage in this group of women.

In the U.S. in 1983, there were approximately 3.614 million births (11). It can be assumed, therefore, that 3.5 million women were available to breast feed. However, this is a minimum estimate of breast feeding women since it does not include those continuing from the previous year. It is a maximum in that the number actually beginning or continuing is not known. From the WHO data now available (2) and from previously cited reports (1), it can be estimated that 70% of these women would breast feed, i.e., 2.5 million.

It has been reported that between 71-98.6% of pregnant women will consume between 2.3 and 11 drugs per pregnancy (12-16). If we extrapolate this drug consumption into the lactation period (2a), then one can estimate that approximately 2.3 million U.S. women in 1983 consumed two or more drugs during lactation. Numerically, therefore, for each country the potential problem is large, and with increasing pressure to increase the numbers breast feeding, the size of this problem will undoubtedly be magnified in the future.

The presence of environmental toxins e.g., hexachlorobenzene, aldrin and dieldrin is largely determined by geographical considerations (17). Only if the lactating women moves from one area to another may the exposure risk change and even then only slightly, because these compounds tend to accumulate in biological systems over a prolonged period. The difficulty in assessing the problem for toxins is that both dose and duration of dosing are often unknown. The "at risk" population is not well defined and, in many cases, little can be done about a prior, or even a current, exposure. It appears prudent to focus attention on exposure of lactating women to drugs so that the extent of this problem can be estimated.

Drugs excreted in breast milk

A recent clinical summary regarding guidelines for drug use during lactation (18) as well as reviews of work in man (1) have clearly shown that a large number of drugs are excreted in breast milk. Little is known, however, about the amount of drug in milk or the fundamental processes underlying the time-course aspects of its appearance in milk.

Effects on nursing infants

Drug effects on the infant can be overt or covert, immediate or delayed, transient or permanent, minor or major. The etiologic basis for these effects includes:

1. Pharmacology inherent to the drug (i.e., specific effect of the chemical on biologic systems).

2. Amount (i.e., dose) of drug in milk.

3. Immaturity of infant systems which predispose to vulnerability (i.e., drug toxicity) and to decreased drug elimination.

The recent review (18) by the American Academy of Pediatrics highlights this etiologic basis for the practical decision to use, or not, a drug in the breast feeding woman. Item 1 (Pharmacology) is often known and of predictive value. We now respect item 3 (immaturity) even though it is seldom studied as a logical endpoint of investigations on dosing of drug in milk. How then, are we to address item 2 (dose in milk) so that the dose of a drug in milk can be estimated with regard to fundamental processes responsible for its excretion.

A comprehensive approach is needed. The question asked must be broad in scope. It is not just:

How much drug is in the mother, i.e., maternal drug disposition?

How much drug is in the milk, i.e., mammary drug disposition?

How much drug is in the infant, i.e., infant drug disposition?

But rather, we must ask how much drug is in each of the above as a succeeding function of the other, and also over what period of time? The comprehensive approach includes investigation of the maternal-mammary-infant unit of drug disposition (Figure 1).

This maternal-mammary-infant unit is linked pharmacokinetically such that a study of one demands a study of the other two when the question addresses drug excretion in breast milk. How can this seemingly complex

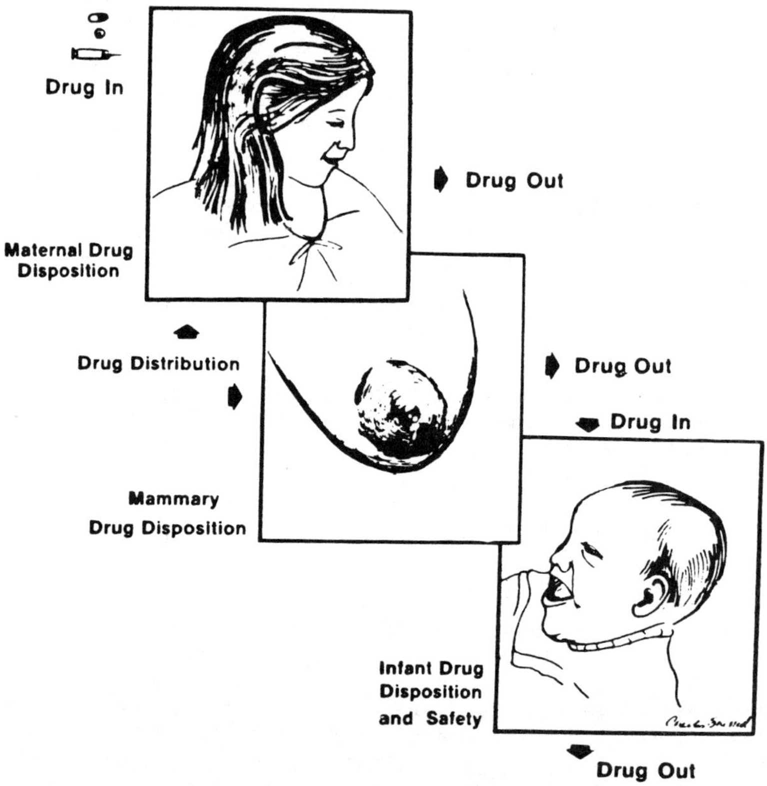

Figure 1. The maternal-mammary-infant unit of drug disposition. This chain which starts with maternal drug administration and ends with infant drug elimination must be understood in order to accurately make predictions about infant safety.

issue be conceptualized to give a framework for approaches which yield both fundamental understanding of mechanisms as well as clinically usable information? The following discussion addresses a critical appraisal of one approach.

MATERNAL DRUG DISPOSITION

Concept

The human female shows a sequence of well defined biologic events, each with likely impact on drug disposition. These events are called states and each is accompanied by unique physiologic changes. In women of child bearing age they are maternal sequential states (Figure 2). With regard to their influence on drug disposition, they include state specific and co-existing variables. State specific variables are those parameters altered by the state and which, in turn, alter drug disposition. Examples include hormonal changes in liver drug metabolism or protein binding. Co-existing variables include those of a genetic, age or disease nature. Associated with a state are integral components of drug disposition. Examples are drug disposition in the utero-fetal or mammary components. Component specific variables may change (vary) while the state itself remains relatively stable. For lactation these variables include milk volume, composition, suckling pattern, etc.

Drug disposition in the female must be described with reference to a particular state so that the global influence of the state is known. The disposition of a drug in the non pregnant woman may be quite different than that in the lactating woman. This is important because it is this drug disposition that determines the proportion of a dose which is actually presented to the breast for transfer into milk. Conclusions developed for one state may lead to erroneous assumptions when applied to

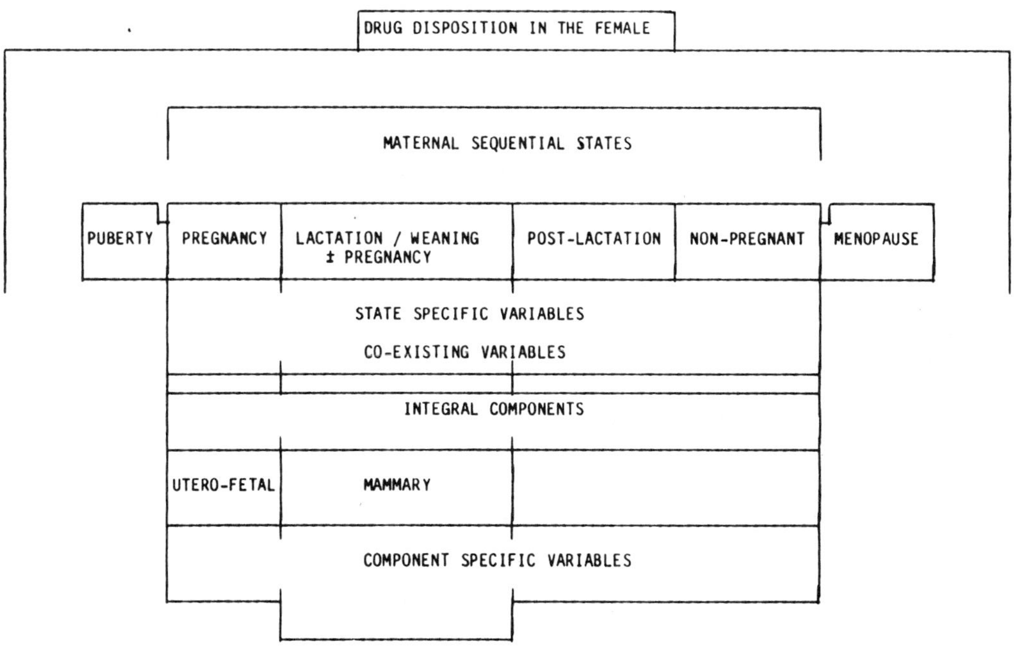

Figure 2. Maternal sequential states. Every female cycles through several maternal specific states which possess variables specific for that state. Drug disposition during a maternal state is governed by the variables of that state.

another. Lactation is of particular note as a maternal sequential state with obvious impact on drug disposition and hence amount of drug available to the breast for excretion in breast milk. Maternal drug disposition is discussed in the context of the state of lactation. Mammary drug disposition is discussed later as an integral component of that state.

State of Lactation

The state of lactation presents several unique features for drug disposition. Milk excretion provides an additional route for drug elimination. By means of breast enlargement and milk production, a dormant "collapsed" compartment is opened for drug distribution. Breast tissue per se may metabolize certain drugs. Hormonal and other events associated with the state of lactation may influence the normal distribution or elimination of drugs. The meager amount of information on these aspects of lactation has been reviewed (19) and is briefly summarized. This summary emphasizes the need for a systematic pharmacokinetic approach which regards lactation as a state requiring full characterization if we are to understand the mechanism of drug excretion in breast milk.

Some overlap is expected for the states of pregnancy and lactation such that drug disposition during the latter part of pregnancy may be similar to that of early lactation. These two states which are discussed together as one (late pregnancy) may influence findings in the other (lactation). More is known about drug disposition during pregnancy or at the time of delivery than during lactation. Extrapolations from data in pregnant women may give some estimate of drug disposition changes which impact on the amount of drug in milk. They are only useful, however, until investigations provide validating (or not) data in the state of lactation. The following state specific variables are pertinent to maternal drug disposition during lactation.

Protein binding

At term, salicylic acid is bound less extensively to plasma protein as compared with nonpregnant women (20, 21). This may be a consequence of higher fatty acid or lipoprotein concentration in maternal blood (and other endogenous substances) and resultant displacement of protein binding for some drugs (22, 23). Free drug diffuses into a body water space which is an average of 3.2 liters larger in the pregnant woman (not including conceptus) (24, 25). Mammary gland water increases from 135 gm at 20 weeks to 304 gm at 40 weeks of pregnancy (24, 26). The total amount of drug in the plasma space may be higher in pregnancy because of the 50% expansion of plasma volume.

Serum drug protein binding has recently been studied in pregnant, postpartum and nonpregnant women by using a non-longitudinal, cross section design (27). In general, the serum free fraction of three weakly acidic drugs (salicylic acid, sulfisoxazole and phenytoin), a base (diazepam) and one steroid (dexamethasone) rose during pregnancy and for 1-5 days postpartum. The acidic drugs showed the greatest change in binding. The most quantitative effect was found for sulfisoxazole, diazepam and salicylic acid. [Similar changes have been shown for the rat during late pregnancy and early postpartum (28)]. Plasma protein binding of these drugs returned to normal about 5-7 weeks after parturition. Except for dexamethasone, the free fraction of these drugs showed a negative correlation with serum albumin concentration during pregnancy. Recent studies confirm the decreased serum protein binding of phenytoin (29), diazepam (30, 31) and salicylate (31), while that of warfarin and propranolol (31) did not change during pregnancy. An increase in the unbound fraction of valproic acid, phenobarbital, pethedine, and lignocaine has been summarized (32). Some of these changes are a result of decreased serum albumin and/or a change in drug site specific capacity and affinity (31). Pregnancy associated endogenous competitors may also be responsible for decreased binding of some drugs. The clinical impact of an increase in the unbound fraction of drug is that of increased distribution to breast (and milk) and an observed lower total concentration in serum (32, 33). Both conceivably influence the milk/plasma (M/P) drug concentration ratio (34).

Non-pregnant women taking oral contraceptives showed a decreased plasma protein binding (for salicylic acid) or no change in drug binding (phenytoin, sulfonamide) (27, 20, and 33). The combined effects on plasma drug protein binding of oral contraceptives, lactation and the observed postpartum changes in binding are not known.

Blood flow

An organ specific increase in blood flow occurs during the state of pregnancy with regard to renal, pulmonary, and uterine but not hepatic flow (35). The increased cardiac output of pregnancy increases further during delivery. These hemodynamic changes would be expected to deliver more drug to the breast during the puerperium.

Routes/rates of elimination

Creatinine clearance is increased about 50% during the state of pregnancy and this may apply to drugs dependent on renal elimination such that their clearance would be increased (35). For example the important role of pregnancy associated changes in renal plasma flow and glomerular filtration rate is illustrated by finding a rapid clearance of sotolol in this state as compared with drug clearance in non-lactating women six months post-partum (36). Progesterone and estrogen levels of pregnancy may either stimulate or inhibit hepatic drug metabolism (37). Estrogen related cholestasis could impair hepatic excretion of drugs and their metabolites (38). A review of pregnancy effects on disposition of specific drugs has appeared recently (39). The extent and duration of physiologic alterations associated with pregnancy in regard to their post-partum influence on drug disposition during early lactation are not known.

Recent reviews highlight changes in antibiotic disposition during pregnancy (40, 41). In general, antibiotic serum levels decreased and t 1/2 changes were variable. Volume of distribution and clearance of oxacillin and ampicillin were increased. Maternal changes in antibiotic disposition must be considered when milk and plasma concentrations are evaluated during early and later periods of lactation (42).

Hepatic mixed function oxidase and glucuronide conjugating activity are apparently increased for several drugs during the state of pregnancy. Indirect evidence for this comes from the decreased plasma steady state levels of phenytoin (as much as two fold), phenobarbital (43-46) and carbamazepine (43, 44). (Changes in protein binding may explain some of this decrease.) An increase in anticonvulsant drug dose was needed to control seizures during pregnancy. Plasma levels of these drugs rose during the puerperium over several weeks to months. Other metabolized drugs showed an increased t 1/2 (noramidopyrine methane sulfonate sodium, methaqualone, aminophenazone) in women intrapartum as compared with controls (41). The oral dose clearance of metoprolol was increased in pregnancy, apparently as a result of enhanced hepatic metabolism of the drug (47). Glucaric acid excretion in urine increased during pregnancy and returned to normal by the sixth postpartum week (37). Without reference to concomitant controls, studies of milk and plasma elimination rates in lactating women reveal similarities to population averages for acetaminophen (48, 49) and theophylline (28, 50).

A change in plasma drug concentration per dosage ratio indicates a difference in rate of drug elimination. This is one disposition factor altered by lactation (or pregnancy) as compared with the non-lactating state. Phenytoin dose requirements increase during pregnancy, and phenytoin clearance was found to be about double that of non-pregnant women (51). The metabolism of propranolol to naphthoxylacetic acid appears to be decreased in the third trimester of pregnancy as compared to the third month post partum (52). The pharmacokinetic profile of other major metabolites of propranolol was similar for these two periods. Antipyrine clearance in epileptic women was lower during late pregnancy (at term) as compared with that at 3 months post partum (53). Phenobarbital clearance, while variable, was similar in pregnant and non-pregnant women (54).

Metoprolol clearance during the third trimester of pregnancy was increased as compared to that in the same women studied 3-6 months after delivery (55). Increased hepatic metabolism of the drug apparently occured during pregnancy. Other drugs showing increased clearance during pregnancy include phenytoin (56) and ampicillin (57).

It is probable that maternal disposition of drugs would show the greatest changes in the immediate postpartum period due to the stress of labor and delivery and the lingering effects of pregnancy (39, 53). More intensive drug monitoring during this period would be worthwhile. Values for milk and plasma drug levels obtained several weeks after birth may not be applicable for a maternal drug dose given soon after birth with regard to estimated amount appearing in milk especially if maternal drug disposition undergoes changes during this time. (This compounds any effects of immature milk on drug excretion. Maturity of milk is a component specific variable of mammary drug disposition).

Drug metabolites

The excretion of drug metabolites in breast milk should be examined with an approach not unlike that used for the parent drug. Metabolites in breast milk have been shown for the following drugs: disopyramide (58), procainamide (59), salicylazosulfapyridine (60, 61), isoniazid (62), and prazepam (63). Metabolites of antipyrine (64) and acetaminophen (65) were not found in breast milk. An extensive analysis (66) revealed multiple drug metabolites in breast milk after administration of a combination drug product containing aspirin, caffeine, phenacetin and codeine. The M/P ratio of these drugs and their respective metabolites did not necessarily correspond with regard to value or time dependent profile. [We have recently found the glucuronide metabolite of acetaminophen in milk of the Rhesus monkey (unpublished)]. The dose of drug metabolites in breast milk is important if such metabolites are pharmacologically active and/or require excretion by immature systems in the nursing infant.

States co-existing with lactation

The influence of parity or age on drug disposition during lactation has not been assessed. These are of conceivable importance from the standpoint of maternal and mammary pharmacokinetics. Disease effects co-existing with lactation are also important, especially with regard to those affecting the liver or kidney. The drug disposition profile - in plasma or milk - has not been systematically studied during weaning even though breast tissue and hormonal changes during this time suggest marked effects (19). The state of pregnancy may co-exist with lactation thereby allowing two states to influence drug disposition.

The genetic variable always co-exists with lactation and contributes to the observed differences in drug disposition. These differences are often expressed as variation in the M/P ratio as well as in the elimination rate constant. That interindividual variation in the M/P ratio likely exists is shown by the wide range of percent of maternal dose in milk values for antipyrine (0.56-2.38%) (64). Other drugs show interindividual variation in either breast milk drug concentrations or the M/P ratio when it is assumed that data were collected under similar conditions for each subject. Such drugs include atenolol and propranolol (67), methyldopa (68), lormetazepam (69), phenytoin, (70), valproic acid (71, 72), dyphylline (73), metoclopramide (both early and late puerperium) (74) butorphanol (by either the oral or intramuscular route) (75), suprofen (for 8 hours after a single oral dose) (76) and for both flufenamic acid and mefenamic acid (early and near steady state conditions) (77, 78). These few existing population studies highlight the weakness of a M/P ratio derived from a single case report. The studies also emphasize the importance of interindividual variation as a variable co-existing with the state of lactation. Biologic aspects of lactation must be standardized in any investigation designed to assess the co-existing but distinct role of genetic and lactation states.

Other states

The state of pregnancy was discussed above. The role of pregnancy as it influences drug transfer to the fetus is clearly recognized (79, 80). Residual effects of pregnancy extending through to early lactation are of equal importance for drug transfer into milk. Drug disposition in each of these states (pregnancy and lactation) is essential to the understanding of drug excretion in milk. To confound the issue further, pregnancy can occur with lactation.

The state of post-lactation addresses a data base which presupposes estrous cycle influences as well as interindividual differences. Interindividual (genetically determined) differences in drug disposition have been shown for many drugs studied in adult males. That these differences exist also in females is apparent, but the extent has not been defined. It is important, however, to examine interindividual differences in pharmacokinetic profiles (and models) from a sufficient number of lactating and non-lactating subjects so that the influence of this state dependent variable (i.e., post or non-lactation) on drug excretion in breast milk can be ascertained. Extrapolations made from a larger existing data base in non-lactating women to lactating women also requires this type of information.

MAMMARY DRUG DISPOSITION

Concept

The breast (and milk) is an integral component of the state of lactation. Mammary drug disposition includes both drug distribution (to and from other maternal components) and elimination (both by in situ metabolism and excretion in milk). From the standpoint of overall drug transfer and excretion in milk, it is appropriate to emphasize the mammary component specific variables. Some of these variables are

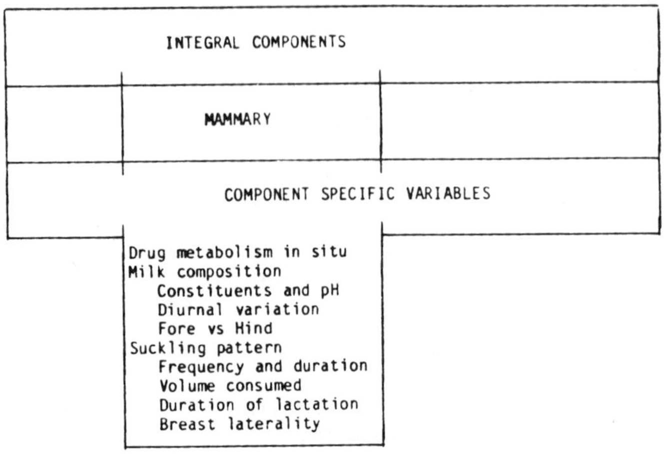

Figure 3. Integral components of lactation and their component specific variables. Mammary component specific variables such as breast and milk impact upon drug disposition directly (i.e., metabolism) and indirectly (i.e., diurnal variation).

summarized (Figure 3). Their influence must be evaluated to appropriately qualify any proposed pharmacokinetic model.

Component specific variables

Drug metabolism in situ

While drug metabolism by the breast may also be an important determinant of dose delivered to the infant, such metabolism has only been shown for N-acetylation of sulfanilamide (81). Xenobiotic metabolism by breast tissue has been demonstrated for several carcinogens both in vivo and in vitro. For example, quantitative differences were noted for metabolites of 7,12-dimethylbenzanthracene formed by breast tissue and both organ and chemical induced selectivity was shown for induction of metabolite formation in animals (82). Both 7,12-dimethylbenzanthracene and benzo (a) pyrene are metabolized by monolayer cultures of epithelial cell aggregates derived from human mammary tissue (83). It is thus probable that breast tissue has the capability for biotransformation of some drugs. The extent of this metabolism, selective production of metabolites at risk for the suckling infant, and the effect of lactation on biotransformation rates or routes remain unknown.

Milk composition

Variation in the daily yield of breast milk and changes in its composition and pH are likely determinants of the amount of drug which is excreted in breast milk. They are major specific variables of mammary drug disposition. The daily yield of human milk is estimated at 600-840 ml (84) such that a 4 kg infant ingests about 150 ml/kg/d. A direct linear relationship exists for blood flow to the breast and milk yield (85). Excretion of a high clearance and/or highly lipid soluble drug in breast milk probably shows a similar relationship to blood flow. A marked interindividual difference in milk yield, fat and protein content has been shown for term and preterm infants (86). A decrease in average milk volume occurs for about the first 7-14 days postpartum regardless of the gestational age. Fat content is low in preterm milk but then increases and remains at about the same average concentration for 28 days postpartum. Protein is high in colostrum for about the first week and the average protein concentration remains higher for preterm infants. Individual values for these parameters, however, may vary on each postpartum day. Furthermore, other studies have shown that the coefficient of variation is large for diurnal changes in breast milk components for each individual woman (86). Fat content and milk yield show the most pronounced diurnal changes. Fat content is highest for the morning feeds (87) as is the yield; these then reach a nadir about 6 to 10 p.m. Simulations of drug excretion in breast milk indicate an effect of both lipid (1) and pKa (34).

Variations in yield and composition also occur during a feeding (88). Most of the milk volume is consumed in the first 10-15 minutes of a feeding. Hindmilk contains more fat than foremilk. Notable are the changes in milk pH with foremilk being more acidic. Some have found a milk pH of 6.35-7.65 (50). The pH of milk varies within a narrow range (6.6-6.95) as a function of months post partum (1-16 months) (Neville; Personal Communication). Little variation in pH was found among values from 10 women. In general, milk is acidic to plasma when an anaerobic collection technique is used (Matheson; Personal Communication).

The impact of a pH difference between milk and plasma on the ultrafiltrate M/P ratio for drugs with various pKa's is shown (Figure 4).

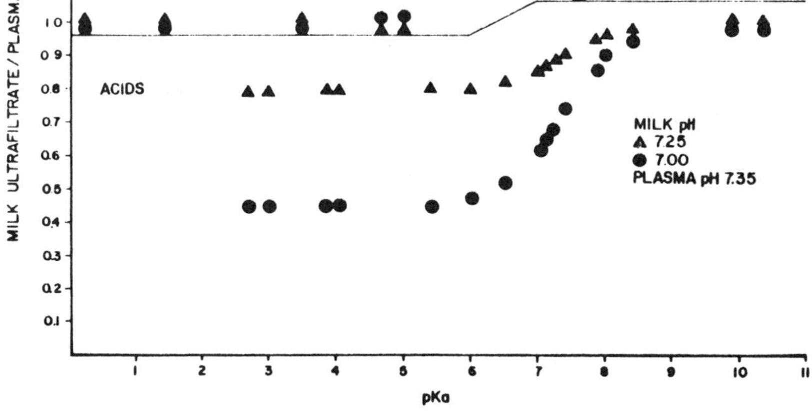

Figure 4. Estimated M/P ratio for a drug in human milk and plasma based upon the pK_a of the drug. See Figure 9 of reference 34 for details about calculation of the M/P ratio.

Suckling pattern:

The frequency and duration of suckling have not been systematically studied for their effects on drug excretion in breast milk. Volume of a milk sample (taken or consumed) may influence either the amount of drug in milk or kinetics of its transfer, if this volume is large relative to the volume of milk residing in the breast or produced per unit time. Data are not available on this variable. Personal communications of unpublished data reveal differences in drug excretion when amounts are compared in milk from right and left breasts. Others, however, have not observed this "breast laterality" for drug excretion (89). Milk composition also apparently varies in some women with regard to the breast sampled. This "breast laterality" for drug excretion needs to be substantiated and explained to assess its role as a component specific variable. The duration of lactation may influence drug excretion in milk but too few longitudinal studies are available to establish a pattern for this variable. Other variables, as they may affect milk composition and flow, include seasonal variations, minor fluctations in diet and psychological or drug mediated influences on milk let-down.

MILK/PLASMA (M/P) RATIO: INTEGRATION OF MATERNAL AND MAMMARY DRUG DISPOSITION

Concept:

The milk to plasma (M/P) ratio captures the net effect of drug disposition differences with regard to both maternal and mammary drug

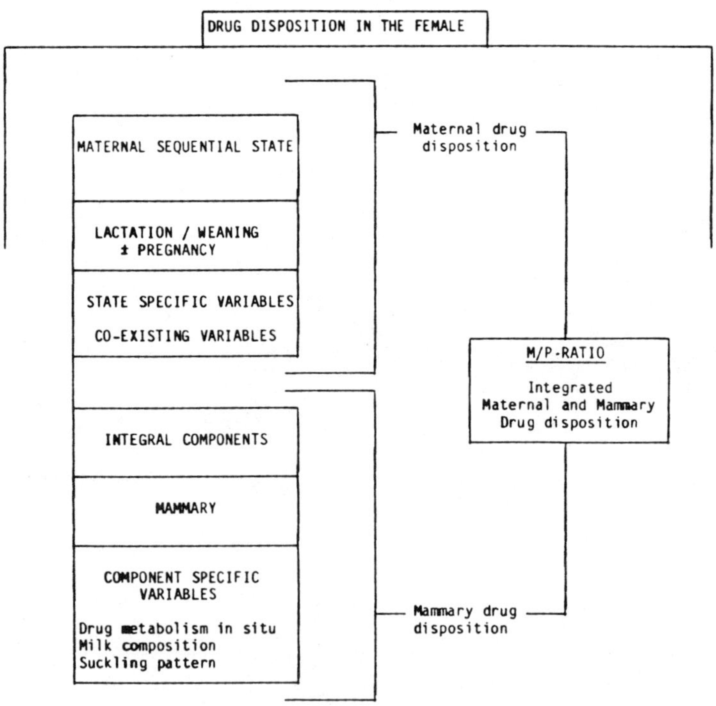

Figure 5. Drug disposition in the female. The M/P ratio integrates the maternal and mammary drug disposition into one concise measure of drug effects.

disposition (Figure 5). This assumption is only valid, however, if the M/P ratio is invariant for a particular drug. If not, then it must be appropriately qualified under conditions of its application. Qualifications are both biologic (state and component specific variables) and pharmacologic (dosing,etc.) in nature. This is appreciated by considering use of the M/P ratio to estimate the dose of maternal drug delivered via breast milk to the infant. An accurate ratio applicable to different dose strengths and to chronicity of dosing is very useful when the concentration of drug in mother's plasma, but not in milk, is known. This ratio can be used to estimate amount of drug excreted in breast milk at the time of nursing. An inaccurate ratio, or one which cannot be used under the intended or desired clinical circumstances, produces erroneous estimates of the amount of drug in milk.

The M/P ratio is a derived parameter dependent on two kinetically distinct profiles. Accordingly, pitfalls exist in estimation of the M/P ratio. The most common pitfall is an implicit assumption that milk and plasma drug concentrations parallel each other throughout dosing, i.e., that a concurrence exists for the milk and plasma concentration profiles. Another error arises when either lactation or component specific variables are unassessed for their effect on a M/P ratio described for a given set of circumstances. Maternal plasma drug concentrations extrapolated from one state to another can also cause errors. Importance of these M/P ratio pitfalls is shown by describing pharmacokinetic models, simulating illustrations, and citing human studies reported for a few drugs. It will be shown that the M/P ratio captures the net effect of differences in maternal and mammary drug disposition. This ratio is thus dependent on the pharmacokinetic model and inherent transfer mechanisms operative for each drug. Knowledge of the model enables accurate prediction of the M/P ratio and also the amount of drug in breast milk.

Use of the M/P ratio

The M/P ratio is essentially used to estimate the dose of drug in milk as a function of maternal plasma drug concentration. The M/P ratio adjusts for those factors which can change this concentration in either fluid. For example, an increase in maternal dose or use of multiple doses is expected to produce a higher concentration of drug in plasma, and hence in milk, than a lower or single dose. The ratio between milk and plasma concentrations expresses these changes without need for a nomogram of maternal drug dose versus concentration of drug in milk. Usefulness of a nomogram would be limited by the multiple influences on maternal drug disposition. The M/P ratio captures the net result of maternal drug dosing and disposition, i.e., the resultant plasma concentration, and the transfer of drug into milk. The M/P ratio, however, is not necessarily invariant under all conditions and at all times after dosing of a particular drug. The ratio may be affected by factors which are biologic (state and component sepcific variables) or pharmacologic [e.g., dosing, deep compartment distribution behavior or physicochemical properties of drug (pKa)]. These may perturb the expected concurrence of the milk and plasma drug concentration profiles and hence destabilize a M/P ratio determined under conditions dissimilar to those used originally for estimation of that ratio.

The practical consequence of an inaccurate M/P ratio is apparent. Consider a M/P ratio that varies with time during a dosing interval (Figure 6). For an acidic drug, early or late assessment may produce a M/P of 0.1 or 1.0 respectively. For a basic drug, the same assessment may yield a ratio of 1 or 10. Table 1 shows that these different M/P ratios could influence the estimate of drug excreted in breast milk.

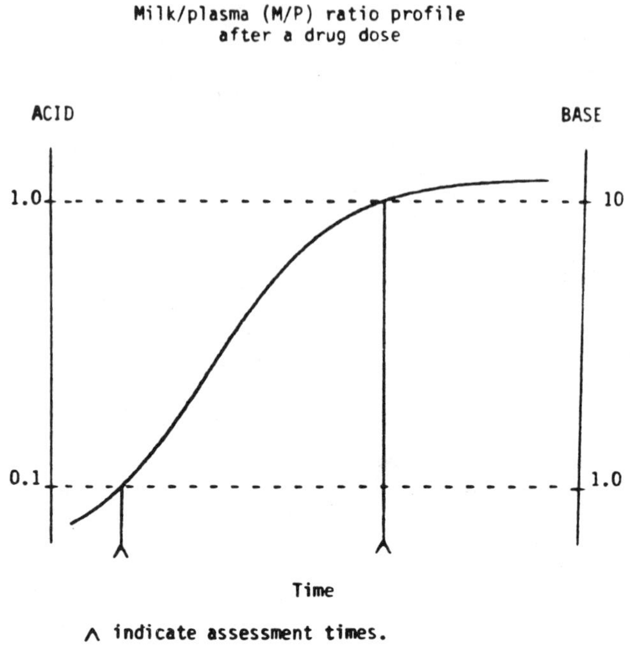

Figure 6. Milk plasma ratio versus time. Because the M/P ratio after a drug dose varies with time, the assessment time is crucial and has profound effects on the obtained value of the M/P ratio.

The role of the M/P ratio is magnified by its placement high in a cascade of events starting with the excretion of a drug in breast milk and ending with assessment of safety for the nursing infant (34). Milk is seldom analyzed for drug concentration in the individual case, so estimates are usually derived from maternal plasma levels and a reported value for the M/P ratio. It is apparent that an error in the estimation of drug concentration in milk confounds an evaluation of safety, unless plasma drug concentrations are analyzed in the infant. Such analyses should be done at the time of predicted steady state conditions in the infant or else drug concentrations will be underestimated. When only the

Table 1. M/P Ratio based estimates of drug in breast milk.

General equation:			
M/P X	Maternal plasma concentration X	milk volume/day	
M/P X	20 ug/ml	X 600 ml	
Acidic drug:			
M/P	Amount calculated (mg/d)		
0.1	1.2		
1.0	12.0		
Basic Drug:			
1.0	12		
10	120		

calculated dose in milk is used as a guide, then an accurate M/P ratio is crucial.

Use of a single point in time M/P ratio or an average ratio calculated with single dose area under the curve (AUC) data is not sufficient for all drugs. Neither ratio attests to the importance of the time dependent variation of drug concentration in milk. This time dependency presents pitfalls in determination of an accurate M/P ratio as well as estimates of drug dose in milk at the time of infant suckling.

Illustrated pitfalls of the M/P ratio

Applicable models and simulated profiles of the M/P ratio

The M/P ratio is a function of the model which best describes maternal drug distribution and elimination. Drug profiles were simulated for several pharmacokinetic models including the one, two, three (mamillary or sequential) and four compartment (mixed) open models. See details in our previous work (34). These showed model dependent effects on the M/P ratio and illustrated the pharmacokinetic nature of pitfalls in estimation of the ratio. From these models we choose to illustrate the resulting M/P ratio by the sequential three compartment in Figure 7. Statements about this model are generally applicable to the other models referenced.

For these models oral dosing is used and the absorption rate constant is k_a. The overall elimination rate constant is k_{10}. Simulations of each model utilized equations which were solved for **amount** of drug in a compartment. Conversion to drug concentration units requires information about the apparent drug distribution volume of each compartment and is not necessary for the simulations. The M/P ratios reported for the simulations illustrate effects of particular combinations of pharmacokinetic rate constants on amounts of drug. The resultant **trend** of M/P ratios for drug amounts should correspond closely to the trend of M/P ratios for drug concentrations in these models. However, the value of the M/P ratio for drug concentrations may not be the same as that for the M/P ratio for drug amount (unless the apparent volumes of distribution for the two compartments were the same). We haveassumed that infant suckling (k_{30}) does not occur or has no effect on the simulated profile.

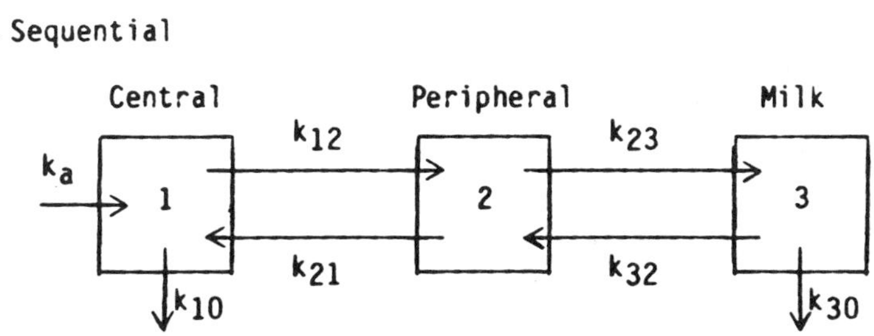

Figure 7. Sequential three compartment model. In this pharmacokinetic model, elimination may occur from the milk compartment (k_{30}) as well as the central compartment (k_{10}).

The M/P ratio for this and the referenced simulations is determined solely by the pharmacokinetic parameters without regard to drug partitioning characteristics between fluids of different pH. It is quite likely that the distribution rate constants incorporate (or are largely a function of) the ion partitioning characteristics of a drug. Observation of a similarity between the predicted and observed ultrafiltrate M/P ratio may require determination of the M/P ratio under post distribution conditions. This is apparent from review of the following simulations which emphasizes the relative time dependency rather than absolute M/P ratio.

In this model, the milk compartment #3 has a drug amount which is limited by that of compartment #2. This model was suggested previously as was the mamillary model (1). This model allows the depth (and capacity) of the milk compartment to be estimated in a manner which distinguishes it from other compartments. This is advantageous since breast blood flow and milk production may alter characteristics of the milk compartment irrespective of other compartments during various periods of lactation. Analysis of drug concentration in both plasma and milk at various post dose intervals may allow each compartment to be distinguished so that a model which best fits the data can be selected. Simulations of profiles for the sequential three compartment open model are shown in Figure 8. In panel A of the figure the amount of drug in milk exhibits deep compartment behavior. This exaggerates the dose interval variation in the M/P ratio.

The M/P ratio is a function of transfer kinetics operative for all three compartments and this produces a time dependency of the M/P ratio after a single dose. A dose number dependency can also occur for this model (Figure 9). In each compartment model that we have simulated, we have noted a variable M/P ratio. The M/P ratio varies primarily with time, dose number and interval between doses.

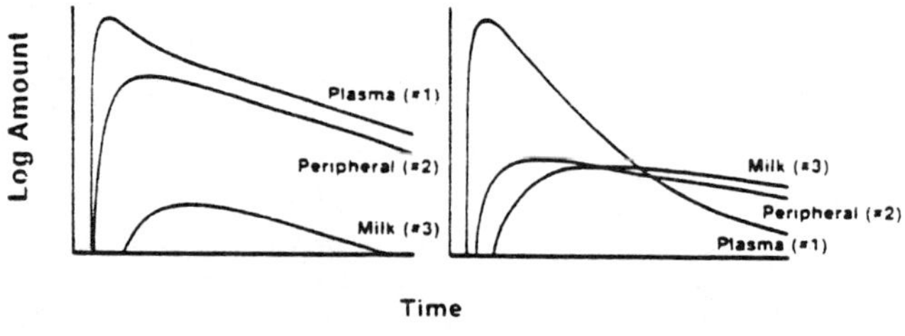

Figure 8. Simulated profiles of milk and plasma drug amounts and the derived M/P ratios. These profiles are based upon a sequential three compartment open model after a single oral dose.

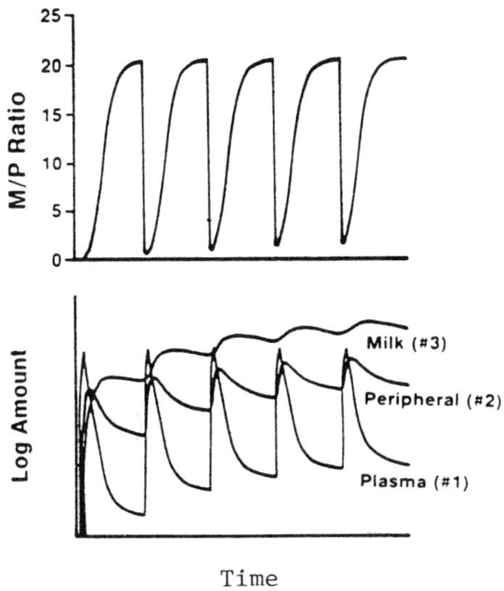

Figure 9. Simulated multiple dose profiles of milk and plasma drug amounts for a sequential three compartment open model. Dose number and interval dependency of the M/P ratio are illustrated.

Reported profiles of milk and plasma drug concentration

A perturbed concurrence between milk and plasma drug concentrations has been reported for several drugs. This illustrates variance of the M/P ratio with regard to time after drug administration (34). The concentration of drug in milk and the timing of breast feeding to deliver the lowest amount of drug are affected accordingly. A notable example of pitfalls in the M/P ratio caused by a lack of concurrent drug concentration profiles is that of hydrochlorothiazide concentration in milk and plasma after a single dose (90). Nadolol milk and plasma concentrations showed a marked difference with multiple dosing and after the drug was discontinued (91). A similar single vs chronic dose discrepancy was found for cimetidine such that the drug appeared to accumulate in milk more than in plasma after multiple doses (92).

The milk/plasma ratios derived from reported milk and plasma drug concentration profiles are summarized in a previous report (34). The data were arbitrarily grouped for M/P ratios <0.2, 0.2 - 1 and >1.Several observations of practical importance emerged from analysis of M/P ratios for a wide variety of drugs. First, most drugs showed a variable M/P ratio during the early periods following a dose. The variability appeared to be less for those drugs with a M/P ratio <1. Second, a discrepancy in the single vs multiple dose M/P ratio was found for nadolol, propranolol, and cimetidine (74). This discrepancy was apparent with pharmacokinetic parameters used in our multiple dose simulations wherein a dose number dependency was observed. Some drugs, notably those with a M/P ratio >1, may have milk distribution characteristics which enhance this discrepancy in single versus multiple dose M/P ratios. These are the drugs which may produce the highest concentrations in milk after multiple doses and hence may pose a risk to the infant. Overall, the derived M/P ratios (34) need to be defined according to the post dose interval and, presumably, also in regard to the single or multiple dose conditions. This need also applies to dose interval variance in the M/P ratio reported for cefotaxime (93) and ceftriaxone (94). The third point of emphasis is that only eleven of the studies had data for more than one subject. It is difficult to apply a single subject derived M/P ratio to the general population. Studies of appropriate design and in a sufficient number of lactating subjects are needed so that proposed models can be validated and so that generally applicable drug dose-in-milk calculations can be made.

Effect of other variables on the M/P ratio

We have summarized the evidence for (or against) effects of maternal and mammary variables on the M/P ratio and hence any model derived from data collected under a standard set of biologic conditions. Other factors which potentially confound our proposed temporal variance in the M/P ratio under certain biologic conditions are pharmacologic in nature. Their role is conceptualized as shown in Figure 10. We have recently examined their role in the lactating goat (95), and clinical evidence exists concerning the influence of these pharmacologic factors on the M/P ratio.

A review of reported studies supports the variance of the M/P ratio with time but offers conflicting evidence about dosing factors. When equal doses of aztreonam were administered by two separate routes, intramuscularly and intravenously, to two groups of women the resultant M/P ratios were indistinguishable in time (96). The ratios obtained after oral or intramuscular administration of butorphanol (75) were clearly different; this was confounded by the increase in dose for the oral route.

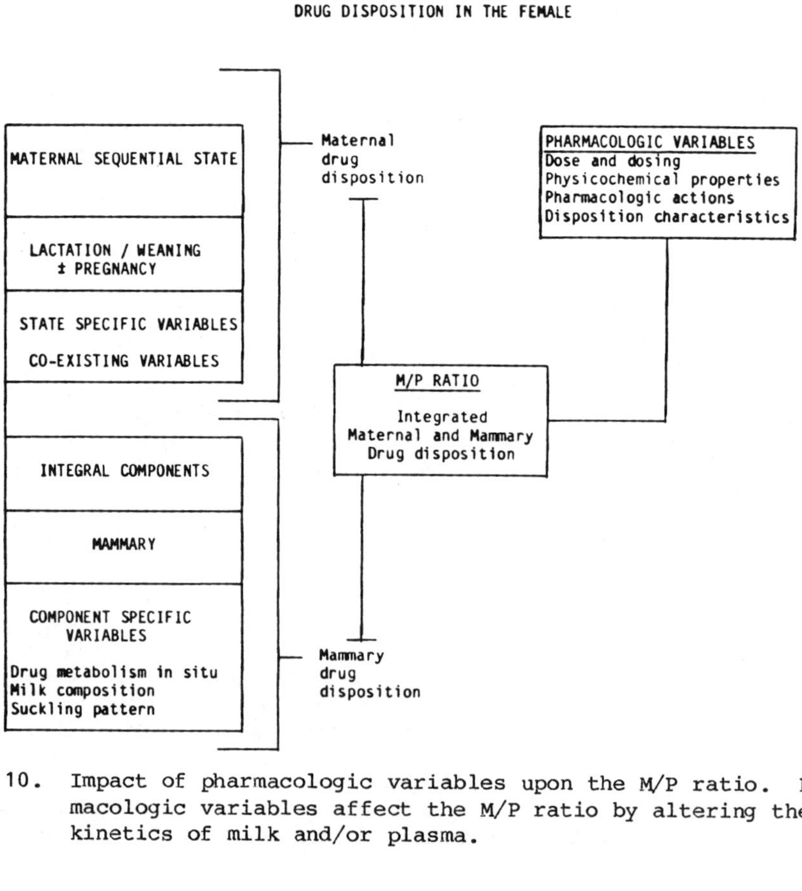

Figure 10. Impact of pharmacologic variables upon the M/P ratio. Pharmacologic variables affect the M/P ratio by altering the drug kinetics of milk and/or plasma.

Increasing the dose and keeping the route of administration constant appeared to increase the M/P ratio for naproxen (97) and perturb that for prednisolone (89). Increasing the dose of phenytoin appears to increase the M/P ratio (70).

Several reports consider the M/P ratio after single dosing only (48, 49, 98, 99, 100). For those reports that measure the ratio after multiple dosing the changes in ratio are unpredictable. The M/P ratio appears to be unchanged after increasing the duration of systemic exposure to piroxicam (101),sudoprofen (76) and flufenamic acid (77). The ratio is apparently increased after chronic dosing with mefenamic acid (78), cimetidine (92) and nadolol (91).

In many of the reports there is a clear change in M/P ratio with time after dosing. The ratio appears to fall after administration of procainamide (59) and to rise after dosing with baclofen (102), cimetidine (92),hydrochlorothiazide (103) or aztreonam (96). The change can also be biphasic, increasing with time then declining after 12-16 hours for captopril (104), digoxin (105) and phenytoin (70).

Interpretations about fundamental mechanisms of drug excretion in breast milk require an assessment of pharmacologic variables as they affect the pharmacokinetic model, one also appropriately qualified by the biologic variables. Although such biologic variables may modulate the model toward enhanced accuracy, we expect that evaluation of physicochemical properties of a drug, its pharmacologic actions, and in particular its disposition characteristics (i.e., hepatic metabolized or renal excreted, protein bound or unbound) will produce a unified theory applicable to more drugs than those tested. Unified theories can be tested through predictions of drug excretion in animals and eventually be used for design of studies to produce validating data in man.

UNIFIED THEORY AND PREDICTION

Information about state and component variables in the biologic (animal) model provides a basis for comprehensive interpretation of drug concentration profiles for milk and plasma. An appropriately qualified biologic model is then used to evaluate the role of pharmacologic variables. These variables are integrated into the pharmacokinetic model in order to explain the mechanism of drug transfer into breast milk.

The development of unified theories to explain drug transfer into breast milk proceeds in two steps: (I) the empiric or biologic approach, which involves selection of a pharmacokinetic model and the evaluation of state and component specific variables, and (II) the molecular approach, which involves evaluation of the effect that pharmacologic variables such as drug pKa, protein binding, lipid solubility, etc., have on the models described by Step 1. By using this systematic stepwise approach, we believe that experimental results will produce a fundamental, mechanistic understanding of drug transfer into breast milk and expedite the design of human studies.

Clinically relevant predictions are obtained from the development of unified theories. The empiric or biologic approach yields pharmacokinetic models obtained from a species of animal close to man (i.e., a subhuman primate). This animal model allows prediction of most appropriate models in man for each drug tested. On the other hand, the molecular approach utilizes information about drug specific (pharmacologic) variables and allows predictions of a more generalized nature based on those variables. (For example it may very well be that all of the drugs that have a pK_a of 8.0 follow similar pharmacokinetic profiles). These

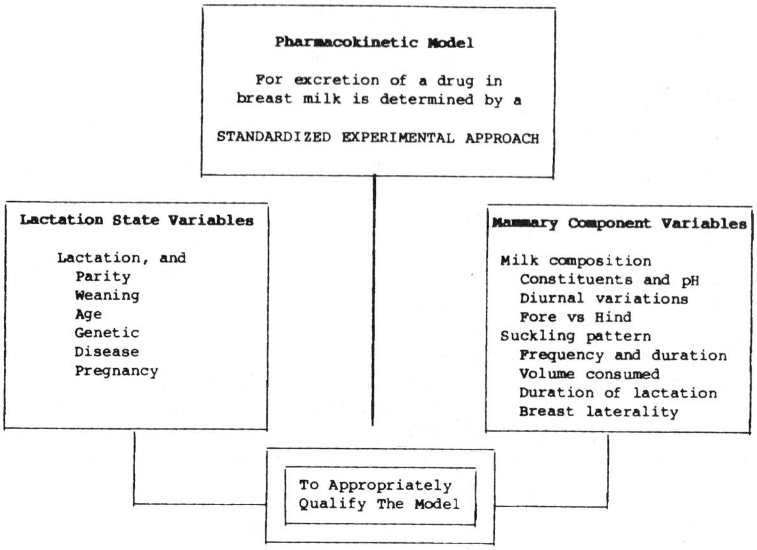

Figure 11. Empiric or biological approach to a unified theory of drug transfer into breast milk. The model developed in this approach is limited to a particular drug and must be appropriately qualified by lactation, state and mammary component variables.

generalized models developed in the primate can be tested in breast feeding women to confirm assumptions about clinical relevance.

The unified theory of drug transfer into breast milk is a collection of statements that can be made in order to relate the various drug specific variables (and combinations of drug specific variables) to the models first described by the biologic approach which used state and component specific variables.

Step 1, empiric or biologic approach is shown in Figure 11. This step is basically a deductive approach to the tabulated biologic data for a certain drug and allows predictions to be made for that drug. However, it is limited in the sense that no generalization can be made to other drugs of the same pharmacologic class or other classes since the physicochemical characteristics of the drug (and other pharmacologic variables) are not involved, per se, in the development of the model up to this point.

The assessment of state and component specific variables allows qualification of a model with two dimensions by which drug transfer into breast milk is evaluated. One may conceive of biologic variables as one-dimensional and spanning through various discrete physiological stages typical of the female. Associated with each state is a particular or "most probable" linear model. Single dose studies furnish the data used to discriminate this model. The impact of mammary component specific variables assessed by single and multiple dose studies add an additional depth, or second dimension, to the model already qualified by lactation state specific variables. The model now becomes a "function"

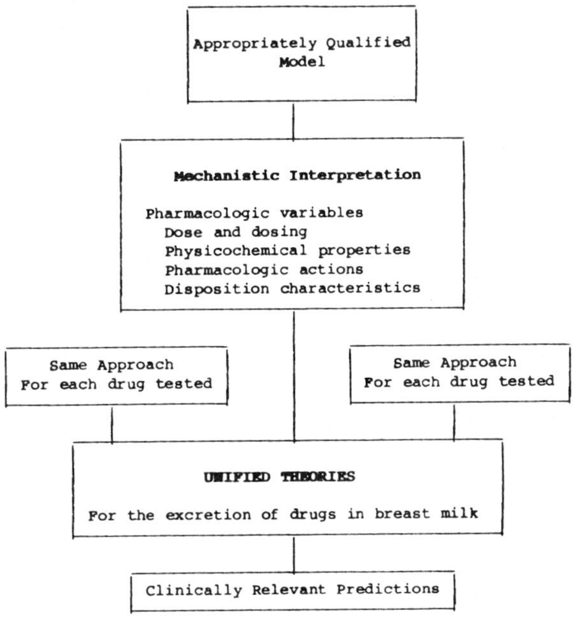

Figure 12. Molecular approach to a unified theory of drug transfer into breast milk. Qualified models from several drugs of different pharmacologic variables are evaluated to establish a unified theory. Such a theory will explain the effects of these variables upon the model.

which can be linked to the mechanisms of drug transfer as determined by the physical or general reality of the pharmacologic variables evaluated in Step II. This Step II, molecular approach, is shown in Figure 12.

Study of two drugs having a common physicochemical characteristic allows inductive reasoning to predict with a reasonable degree of certainty which drugs will fit a similar model or mechanism for their excretion in breast milk. The end result to this approach is to allow predictions about drugs based on their physicochemical characteristics as distinguished from the predictions made after the empiric approach. This empiric approach is restricted to only those drugs studied and therefore suffers the limitations of purely descriptive studies.

We have recently developed mathematical solutions to derive the most appropriate model from empirical data. Computer assisted solutions reveal predicted profiles for drug in milk similar to those actually observed. Animal model validation of our approach (conceptualized by Steps I and II of the unified theory approach) supports our proposed fundamental temporal variance of the M/P ratio. Its temporal dependence has a kinetic basis governed essentially by the pharmacokinetic model. The model, in turn, is modulated by both state and component specific variables. Its general nature is imposed by pharmacologic properties of the drug. The distinct and combined role of these factors for the unified theory is discernable. The means is now clear to investigate the fundamental processes for drug excretion in breast milk.

Table 2. Plasma half-lives of various drugs in neonates and in adults.*

Drug	Plasma half-life (h)	
	Neonates	Adults
Analgesics		
Aminopyrine	30-40	2- 4
Phenylbutazone	21-34	12-30
Indomethacin	14-20	2-11
Pethidine	22	3- 4
Local Anaesthetics		
Bupivacaine	25	1. 3
Mepivacaine	8.7	3. 2
Psycho-active drugs		
Diazepam	25-100	15-25
Nortriptyline	56	18-22
Antiepileptics		
Phenytoin	21	11-29
Carbamazepine	8-28	21-36
Other drugs		
Tolbutamide	10-40	4.4- 9
Amylobarbitone	17-60	12-27
Theophylline	24-36	3- 9

*Adapted from Rane and Thompson, 1980.

DRUG ACCUMULATION IN THE NURSING INFANT

Drug accumulation (and effect) in the infant is the third and final area addressed by a comprehensive approach to drug excretion in breast milk. The drug dose in milk may be a fraction of the maternal dose, or a function of the M/P ratio, but aside from the difference between maternal and infant weight, there may be a marked difference in drug clearance by the infant such that the drug accumulates to higher than expected levels. For example, Table 2 highlights differences in plasma t 1/2 for some commonly used drugs in neonates. These neonate to adult differences in plasma drug t 1/2 are 10-20 fold in some cases. More extensive discussions of these differences (106-112) reveal both metabolic and renal function in immaturity as a cause of decreased drug elimination in young infants.

While some have predicted infant plasma levels based on drug dose in milk and the infant's drug clearance, few studies have undertaken monitoring of breast milk and plasma from infant and mother to confirm predictions. A recent study (70) showed that plasma phenytoin levels of breast fed infants were much below the therapeutic range (Table 3). This was also shown for ethosuximide (79a). The chloramphenicol associated grey baby syndrome, however, reminds us that immature drug clearance can lead to unexpected and toxic drug levels in an infant (113).

Table 3. Phenytoin (DPH) Excretion in Breast Milk.*

Study design:	6 mother-infant pairs at steady state dosing of DPH and sampling for 7-8 hr after a dose; 1-3 months post partum.			
DPH conc:	Plasma		Milk	M/P
(umol/L)	Mother	Infant		
	13-79	0.5, 0.7	0.8-12	0.06-0.18
Estimated dose to infant: 0.03-0.47 mg/kg/d				
Linear relationship existed between milk concentration and either plasma concentration or AUC of DPH.				

* Adapted from data of Steen et al, 1982
DPH pKa 8.3; avg. plasma unbound DPH is 0.15

Pharmacodynamic assessment of drug effects in the infant extends risk evaluation based on infant plasma levels of a drug received via breast milk. For example, warfarin was not detectable in breast milk or in plasma of nursing infants (114). Three of seven infants had prolonged prothrombin time. Recently two nursing infants from mothers treated with warfarin after delivery were studied for 56-130 days (115). Prothrombin time was not abnormal in either infant even though the mothers serum demonstrated an anticoagulant effect. One infant showed no abnormality in factor II and VII/X activities. Longitudinal pharmacodynamic assessments in the nursing infant provide useful data to form guidelines about safety of drugs excreted in breast milk.

CONCLUDING REMARKS

A comprehensive and longitudinal evaluation includes 3 crucial components (maternal, mammary and infant) of drug delivery to infant via breast milk. Simplistic notions about uniformity of a M/P ratio and the role of confounding variables lead to erroneous estimates of drug in milk. Emerging evidence reveals that drug disposition is state dependent. Pharmacokinetics of one state do not necessarily prevail for another. Too little is known about the state of lactation and drug disposition. Future studies must include more women at each defined period of lactation and control for these variables likely to influence the amount of drug found in milk. The effect of dose received by the infant should be confirmed by monitoring infant plasma levels of drug coupled with longitudinal studies to assess immediate and delayed toxicity. Pragmatic approaches to toxicity should be based on pharmacology of the drug and maturational state of the breast feeding infant.

Dose in milk (measured or predicted), infant plasma levels and clinical monitoring are needed to make definitive statements about infant safety in medicated breast feeding women.

ACKNOWLEDGEMENTS

The skillful and dedicated assistance of Mrs. Carole Webb is gratefully acknowledged for preparation of this manuscript. We appreciate the art work prepared by Mr. Charles Fox Sherrod.

REFERENCES

1. J. T. Wilson, R. D. Brown, D. Cherek, J. W. Dailey, B. Hilman, P. C. Jobe, B. R. Manno, J. E. Manno, H. M. Redetzki, and J. J. Stewart. "Drugs in Breast Milk," J. T. Wilson, ed., ADIS Press, Australia (1981).
2. W.H.O. Corraborative Study: Contemporary patterns of breast feeding. World Health Organization (Geneva), 31-46 (1981).
2a. I. Matheson. Drugs taken by mothers in the puerperium. Br. Med. J. 290:1588-1589 (1985).
3. Report of the Surgeon General's Workshop on Breastfeeding and Human Lactation, U.S. Department of Health & Human Services, DHHS Publication No. HRS-D-MC 84-2 (1984).
4. Promoting Breastfeeding: A guide for health professionals working in the WIC and CSF programs, U.S. Department of Agriculture, Food and Nutrition Service, FNS-247.
5. Board of Directors of the Ambulatory Pediatric Association, The World Health Organization code of marketing of breast milk substitutes. Pediatrics 68:432-434 (1981).
6. American Academy of Pediatrics, Policy statement based on task force report: The promotion of breast-feeding. Pediatrics 69: 654-661 (1982).
7. Promotion of breast feeding: Recommendations of the Councils of the Society for Pediatric Research (SPR) and American Pediatric Society (APS), and of the American Academy of Pediatrics (AAP). Pediatr. Res. 16:264-265 (1982).
8. G. A. Martinez, and J. P. Nalezienski. 1980 update: The recent trend in breast-feeding. Pediatrics 67:260-263 (1981).
9. Ameriacan Academy of Pediatrics, Current issues in feeding the normal infant. Pediatrics 75(1 Pt 2):135-215 (1985).
10. Report of the Task Force on the assessment of the scientific evidence relating to infant-feeding practices and infant health. Pediatrics 74(4 pt 2):579-762 (1984).
11. U.S. Bureau of the Census. Statistical Abstract of the U.S. 1985 (105th Edition) Washington, D.C., (1984).
12. J. O. Forfar, and N. M. Nelson. Epidemiology of drugs taken by pregnant women: drugs that may affect the fetus adversely. Clin. Pharmacol. Ther. 14:632-642 (1973).
13. O. P. Heinonen, D. Slone, and S. Shapiro. Birth defects and drugs in pregnancy. Publishing Sciences Group, Inc., Littleton, Mass. Corraborative Perinatal Project of the National Institute of Neurological and Communicative Disorders and Stroke. U.S. Public Health Service.
14. R. M. Hill. Drugs ingested by the pregnant woman. Clin. Pharmacol. Ther. 14:654-659 (1973).
15. W. A. Bleyer, W. Y. Au, W. A. Lange, L. G. Raisz. Studies on the detection of adverse drug reactions in the newborn. I. Fetal exposure to maternal medication. JAMA 213:2046-2048 (1970).
16. T. K. A. B. Eskes, W. S. Nijdam. Epidemiology of drug intake during pregnancy. in: "Drugs and Pregnancy. Maternal Drug Handling - Fetal Drug Exposure". B. Krauer, F. Krauer, F. E. Hytten, E. Pozo, eds., Academic Press, London (1984).
17. W.H.O corraborative study on breast feeding. The quantity and quality of breast milk. World Health Organization (Geneva) 20-21 (1985).
18. A. W. Pruitt, Chairman. Committee on Drugs. The transfer of drugs and other chemicals into human breast milk. Pediatrics 72:375-383 (1983).
19. J. T. Wilson. Determinants and consequences of drug excretion in breast milk. Drug Metab. Rev. 14:619-652 (1983).

20. J. S. Crawford, and H. W. Hooi. Binding of salicylic acid and sulphanilamide in serum from pregnant patients, cord blood and subjects taking oral contraceptives. Br. J. Anasthesiol. 40: 825-833 (1968).
21. G. Levy. Salicylate pharmacokinetics in the human neonate. in: "Basic and Therapeutic Aspects of Perinatal Pharmacology", P. L. Morselli, S. Garattini, F. Sereni, eds., Raven Press, New York.
22. I. Bobok, G. Czako, L. Csernyanszky, and K. Ludmany. Lipoids in maternal cord and newborn blood serum. Acta. Paediatr. Acad Sci. Hungaricae. 15:95-100 (1974).
23. P. Rebond, J. Groulade, P. Groslambert, and M. Colomb. The influence of normal pregnancy and the postpartum state on plasma proteins and lipids. Am. J. Obstet. Gynecol. 86:820-828 (1963).
24. F. E. Hytten, and I. Leitchh. "The Physiology of Human Pregnancy," Blackwell, Oxford (1971).
25. E. G. Robertson. Physiological adjustments in pregnancy: Water metabolism. Clinics Obstet. Gynecol. 2:431-440 (1975).
26. B. Krauer F. Krauer, and F. Hytten. Drug disposition and pharmacokinetics in the maternal-placental-fetal unit. Pharmacol. Ther. 10:301-328 (1980).
27. M. Dean, B. Stock, R. J. Patterson, and G. Levy. Serum protein binding of drugs during and after pregnancy in humans. Clin. Pharmacol. Ther. 28:253-261 (1980).
28. B. Stock, M. Dean, and Levy G. Serum protein binding of drugs during and after pregnancy in rats. J. Pharmacol. Exp. Ther. 212:264-268 (1980).
29. S. S. Chen, E. Perucca, J. N. Lee, A. Richens. Serum protein binding and free concentration of phenytoin and phenobarbitone in pregnancy. Br. J. Clin. Pharmacol. 13:547-552 (1982).
30. J. N. Lee, S. S. Chen, A. Richens, M. Menabawey, and T. Chard. Serum protein binding of diazepam in maternal and foetal serum during pregnancy. Br. J. Clin. Pharmacol. 14:551-554 (1982).
31. T. Yoshikawa, Y. Sugiyama, Y. Sawada, et al. Effect of late pregnancy on salicylate, diazepam, warfarin, and propranolol binding: Use of fluorescent probes. Clin. Pharmacol. Ther. 36:201-208 (1984).
32. E. Perucca, and A. Crema. Plasma protein binding of drugs in pregnancy. Clin. Pharmacokinet. 7:336-352 (1982).
33. W. D. Hooper, F. Bochner, M. J. Eadie,and J. H. Tyrer. Plasma protein binding of diphenylhydantoin: Effects of sex hormones, renal and hepatic disease. Clin. Pharmacol. Ther. 15:276-282 (1974).
34. J. T. Wilson, R. D. Brown, J. L. Hinson, and J. W. Dailey JW. Pharmacokinetic pitfalls in the estimation of the breast milk/plasma ratio for drugs. Ann. Rev. Pharmacol. Toxicol. 25:667-689 (1985).
35. B. Krauer, and F. Krauer. Drug kinetics in pregnancy. Clin. Pharmacokinet. 2:167-181 (1977).
36. M. F. O'Hare, W. Leahey, G. A. Murnaghan, and D. G. McDevitt DG. Pharmacokinetics of sotalol during pregnancy. Eur. J. Clin. Pharmacol. 24:521-524 (1983).
37. M. Davis, C. J. Simmons, B. Dordoni, J. D. Maxwell, and R. Williams. Induction of hepatic enzymes during normal human pregnancy. J. Obstet. Gynaecol. Br. Commonwealth. 80:690-694 (1973).
38. L. I. Harrison, and M. Gibaldi. Influence of cholestasis on drug elimination: Pharmacokinetics. J. Pharm. Sci. 65:1346-1348 (1976).
39. R. L. Nation. Drug kinetics in childbirth. Clin. Pharmacokinet. 5:340-364 (1980).

40. A. Philipson. Pharmacokinetics of antibiotics in pregnancy and labour. Clin. Pharmacokinet. 4:297-309 (1979).

41. H. Noschel, G. Peiker, R. Voigt, et al. Research on pharmacokinetics during pregnancy. Arch. Toxicol. 4:380-384 (1980).

42. R. D. Brown. Antimicrobials. in: "Drugs in Breast Milk," J. T. Wilson, ed., ADIS Press, Australia (1981).

43. M. Dam, J. Christiansen, O. Munck, K. I. Mygind. Antiepileptic drugs: Metabolism in pregnancy. Clin. Pharmacokinet. 4:43-62 (1979).

44. M. J. Eadie, C. M. Lander, and J. H. Tyrer. Plasma drug level monitoring in pregnancy. Clin. Pharmacokinet. 2:427-436 (1977).

45. C. M. Lander, V. E. Edwards, M. J. Eadie, and J. H. Tyrer. Plasma anticonvulsant concentrations during pregnancy. Neurology 77:128-131 (1977)

46. K. I. Mygind, M. Dam, J. Christiansen. Phenytoin and phenobarbitone plasma clearance during pregnancy. Acta Neurol. Scand. 54:160-166 (1976).

47. S. Hogstedt, B. Lindberg, and A. Rane. Increased oral clearance of metoprolol in pregnancy. Eur. J. Clin. Pharmacol. 24:217-220 (1983).

48. C. M. Berlin, S. J. Yaffe, and M. Ragni. Disposition of acetaminophen in milk, saliva, and plasma of lactating women. Pediatr. Pharmacol. 1:135-141(1980).

49. P. O. Bitzen, B. Gustafsson, K. G. Jostell, A. Melander, E. Wahlin-Boll.E. Excretion of paracetamol in human breast milk. Eur. J. Clin. Pharmacol. 20:123-125 (1981).

50. A. M. Yuchak, and W. J. Jusko. Theophylline secretion into breast milk. Pediatrics 57:518-520 (1976).

51. C. M. Lander, M. T. Smith, J. B. Chalk, et al. Bioavailability and pharmacokinetics of phenytoin during pregnancy. Eur. J. Clin. Pharmacol.27:105-110 (1984).

52. M. T. Smith, I. Livingstone, M. J. Eadie, W. D. Hooper, E. J. Triggs. Chronic propranolol administration during pregnancy. Maternal pharmacokinetics. Eur. J. Clin. Pharmacol. 25:481-490 (1983).

53. K. Chiba, T. Ishizaki, T. Tabuchi, T. Wagatsuma, and Y. Nakazawa. Antipyrine disposition in relation to lowered anticonvulsant plasma level during pregnancy. Obstet. Gynecol. 60:620-626 (1982).

54. P. V. Luoma, J. E. Heikkinen, P. R. Ylostalo. Phenobarbital pharmacokinetics and salivary and serum concentrations in pregnancy. Ther. Drug Monit. 4:65-68 (1982).

55. S. Hogstedt. B. Lindberg, D. R. Peng, C. G. Regardh, and A. Rane. Pregnancy-induced increase in metoprolol metabolism. Clin. Pharm. Ther.37:688-692 (1985).

56. M. J. Landon, and M. Kirkley. Metabolism of diphenylhydantoin (phenytoin) during pregnancy. Br. J. Obstet. Gynaecol. 86:125-132 (1979).

57. A. Philipson. Pharmacokinetics of ampicillin during pregnancy. J. Infect. Dis. 136:370-376 (1977).

58. D. B. Barnett, S. A. Hudson, A. McBurney. Disopyramide and its N-monodesalkyl metabolite in breast milk. Br. J. Clin. Pharmacol. 14:310-312 (1982).

59. W. B. Pittard III, and H. Glazier. Procainamide excretion in human milk. J. Pediatr. 102:631-633 (1983).

60. C. M. Berlin, and S. J. Yaffe. Disposition of salicylazosulfapyridine (azulfidine) and metabolites in human breast milk. Dev. Pharmacol. Ther. 1:31-39 (1980).

61. A. K. Azad Khan, and S. C. Truelove. Placental and mammary transfer of sulphasalazine. Br. Med. J. 2:1553 (1979).

62. C. M. Berlin, and C. Lee. Isoniazin and acetylisoniazid disposition in human milk, saliva and plasma. Fed. Proc. 38:426 (1979).

63. R. R. Brodie, L. F. Chasseaud, and T. Taylor. Concentrations of N-descyclopropylmethylprazepam in whole-blood, plasma, and milk after administration of prazepam to humans. Biopharm. Drug Dispos. 2:59-68(1981).
64. Berlin CM. Antipyrine appearance and decay in human breast milk and saliva. Pharmacologist 20:219 (1978).
65. C. M. Berlin, S. J. Yaffe, and M. Ragni. Disposition of acetaminophen in milk, saliva, and plasma of lactating women. Pediatr. Pharmacol. 1:135-141 (1980).
66. J. W. Findlay, R. L. DeAngelis, M. F. Kearney, R. M. Welch, J. M. Findlay. Analgesic drugs in breast milk and plasma. Clin. Pharmacol. Ther. 29:625-633 (1981).
67. K. J. Thorley, and J. McAinsh. Levels of the beta-blockers atenolol and propranolol in the breast milk of women treated for hypertension in pregnancy. Biopharm. Drug Dispos. 4:299-301 (1983).
68. J. C. Allen, M. C. Neville. Ionized calcium in human milk determined with a calcium selective electrode. Clin. Chem. 29:858-861 (1983).
69. M. Humpel, I. Stoppelli, S. Milia, E. Rainer. Pharmacokinetics and biotransformation of the new benzodiazepine, lormetazepam, in man. III. Repeated administration and transfer to neonates via breast milk. Eur. J. Clin. Pharmacol. 21:421-425 (1982).
70. B. Steen, A. Rane, G. Lonnerholm, O. Falk, C. E, Elwin F. Sjoqvist. Phenytoin excretion in human breast milk and plasma levels in nursed infants. Ther. Drug. Monit. 4:331-334 (1982).
71. G. E. von Unruh, W. Froescher, F. Hoffman, and M. Niesen. Valproic acid in breast milk: How much is really there? Ther. Drug. Monit. 6:272-276 (1984).
72. H. Nau, D. Rating, S. Koch, I. Hauser, and H. Helge. Valproic acid and its metabolites: Placental transfer, neonatal pharmacokinetics, transfer via mother's milk and clinical status in neonates of epileptic mothers. J. Pharmacol. Exp. Ther. 219:768-777 (1981).
73. C. H. Jarboe, L. N. Cook, I. Malesic, J. Fleischaker. Dyphylline elimination kinetics in lactating women: Blood to milk transfer. J. Clin. Pharmacol. 21:405-410 (1981).
74. A. Kauppila, P. Arvela, M. Koivisto, S. Kivinen, O. Ylikorkala, and O. Pelkonen. Metoclopramide and breast feeding: Transfer into milk and the newborn. Eur. J. Clin. Pharmacol. 25:819-823 (1983).
75. K. A. Pittman, R. D. Smyth, M. Losada, I. Zighelboim, A. L. Maduska, and A. Sunshine. Human perinatal distribution of butorphanol. Am. J. Obstet. Gynecol. 138:797-800 (1980).
76. P. Chaikin, M. Chasin, B. Kennedy, B. K. Silverman. Suprofen concentrations in human breast milk. J. Clin. Pharmacol. 23: 385-390 (1983).
77. R. A. Buchanan, C. J. Eaton, S. T. Koeff, and A. W. Kinkel. The breast milk excretion of flufenamic acid. Curr. Ther. Res. 11: 533-538 (1969).
78. R. A. Buchanan, C. J. Eaton, S. T. Koeff, and A. W. Kinkel AW. The breast milk excretion of mefenamic acid. Curr. Ther. Res. 10: 592-597 (1968).
79. H. Nau, W. Kuhnz, H. J. Egger, D. Rating, and H. Helge. Anticonvulsants during pregnancy and lactation: Transplacental, maternal and neonatal pharmacokinetics. Clin. Pharmacokinet. 7: 508-543 (1982).
80. H. Nau. Clinical pharmacokinetics in pregnancy and perinatology. I. Placental transfer and fetal side effects of local anaesthetic agents. Dev. Pharmacol. Ther. 8:149-181 (1985).
81. F. Rasmussen, and J. L. Linzell. The acetylation of sulphanilamide by mammary tissue of lactating goats. Biochem. Pharmacol. 16: 16:918-919 (1967).

82. J. Digiovanni, and M. R. Juchau. Biotransformation and bioactivation of 7,12-dimethylbenz(a)anthracene (7,12-DMBA). Drug.Metab. Rev. 11:61-101 (1980).
83. A. D. MacNicoll, G. C. Easty, A. M. Neville, P. L. Grover, and P. Sims. Metabolism and activation of carcinogenic polycyclic hydrocarbons by human mammary cells. Biochem. Biophys. Res. Commun. 95:1599-16-6 (1980).
84. D. B. Jelliffe, and E. F. Jelliffe. The volume and composition of human milk in poorly nourished communities - A review. Am. J. Clin. Nutr. 31:492-515 (1978).
85. J. L. Linzell. Mammary blood flow and methods of identifying and measuring precursors of milk. in: "Lactation," B. L. Larson, and V. R. Smith, eds., Academic Press, New York (1974).
86. S. J. Gross, M. S. Geller, and R. M. Tomarelli. Composition of breast milk from mothers of preterm infants. Pediatrics 68:490-493 (1981).
87. F. E. Hytten. Clinical and chemical studies in human lactation. Br. Med. J. 1:175-182 (1954).
88. B. Hall. Changing composition of human milk and early development of appetite control. Lancet 1:779-781 (1975).
89. L. Ost, G. Wettrell, I. Bjorkhem, and A Rane. Prednisolone excretion in human milk. J. Pediatr. 106:1008-1011 (1985).
90. M. E. Miller, R. D. Cohn, and P. H. Burghart. Hydrochlorothiazide disposition in a mother and her breast fed infant. J. Pediatr. 101:789-791 (1982).
91. R. G. Devlin, K. L. Duchin, P. M. Fleiss. Nadolol in human serum and breast milk. Br. J. Clin. Pharmacol. 12:393-396 (1981).
92. A. Somogyi, and R. Gugler. Cimetidine excretion into breast milk. Br. J. Clin. Pharmacol. 7:627-629 (1979).
93. D. A. Kafetzis, C. V. Lazarides, C. A. Siafas, P. A. Georgakopoulos, C. J. Papadatos. Transfer of cefotaxime in human milk and from mother to foetus. J. Antimicrob. Chemother. (6 suppl A):135-141 (1980).
94. D. A. Kafetzis, D. C. Brater, J. E. Fanourgakis, P. Georgakopoulos. Ceftriaxone distribution between maternal blood and fetal blood and tissues at parturition and between blood and milk postpartum. Antimicrob. Agents Chemother. 23:870-873 (1983).
95. J. T. Wilson, I. J. Smith, J. L. Hinson, T. W. Woods, V. A. Johnson, and R. D. Brown. Fundamental kinetics of drug excretion in breast milk. In press, (1985).
96. P. M. Fleiss, G. A. Richwald, J. Gordon, M. Stern, M. Frantz, and R. G. Devlin. Aztreonam in human serum and breast milk. Br. J. Clin. Pharmacol. 19:509-511 (1985).
97. F. Jamali, and D. R. S. Stevens. Naproxen excretion in milk and its uptake by the infant. Drug Intell. Clin. Pharm. 17:910-911 (1983).
98. D. A. Kafetzis, C. A. Siafas, P. A. Georgakopoulos, and C. J. Papadatos. Passage of cephalosporins and amoxicillin into the breast milk. Acta. Paediatr. Scand. 70:285-288 (1981).
99. J. P. Kampmann, K. Johansen, J. M. Hansen, and J. Helweg. Propylthiouracil in human milk. Lancet 1:736-737 (1980).
100. J. Putter, and F. Held. Quantitative studies on the occurrence of praziquantel in milk and plasma of lactating women. Eur. J. Drug. Metab. Pharmacokinet. 4:193-198 (1979).
101. M. Ostensen. Piroxicam in human breast milk. Eur. J. Clin. Pharmacol. 25:829-830 (1983).
102. G. Eriksson, C. G. Swahn. Concentrations of baclofen in serum and breast milk from a lactating woman. Scand. J. Clin. Lab. Invest. 41:185-187 (1981).
103. M. E. Miller, R. D. Cohn, and P. H. Burghart. Hydrochlorothiazide disposition in a mother and her breast fed infant. J. Pediatr. 101:789-791 (1982).

104. R. G. Devlin, P. M. Fleiss. Captopril in human blood and breast milk. J. Clin. Pharmacol. 21:110-113 (1981).
105. D. Reinhardt, O. Richter, T. Genz, and S. Potthoff. Kinetics of the translactal passage of digoxin from breast feeding mothers to their infants. Eur. J. Pediatr. 138:49-52 (1982).
106. J. T. Wilson. Pediatric pharmacology. in: "Pharmacology in Medicine: Principles and Practice." Pradhan and Maickel, eds., SP Press International, in press.
107. C. M. Berlin. Advances in pediatric pharmacology and toxicology. Adv. Pediatr. 30:221-248 (1983).
108. M. L. Mirkin, ed. "Perinatal pharmacology and therapeutics." Academic Press, New York (1976).
109. S. M. MacLeod, A. B. Okey, and S. P. Speilberg, eds. "Developmental pharmacology", A.R. Liss, Inc., New York (1983).
110. S. J. Yaffe, ed. "Pediatric pharmacology: Therapeutic principles in practice." Grune & Stratton, New York (1980).
111. P. L. Morselli. Clinical pharmacokinetics in neonates, in: "Handbook of Clinical Pharmacokinetics." Adis Health Science Press, New York (1983).
112. H. Braunlich. Excretion of drugs during postnatal development. Pharmacol. Ther. 12:299-320 (1981).
113. A. Mulhall, J. de Louvois, and R. Hurley. Chloramphenicol toxicity in neonates: Its incidence and prevention. Br. Med. J. 287: 1424-1427 (1983).
114. R. McKenna, E. R. Cole, and U. Vasan. Is warfarin sodium contraindicated in the lactating mother? J. Pediatr. 103:325-327 (1983).
115. M. L. Orme, P. J. Lewis, M. deSwiet, et al. May mothers given warfarin breast-feed their infants. Br. Med. J. 1:1564-1565 (1977).

FUNDAMENTAL KINETICS OF DRUG EXCRETION IN BREAST MILK

John T. Wilson, Iain J. Smith, James L. Hinson, Thomas W. Woods, Virginia A. Johnson and R. Don Brown

Section on Clinical Pharmacology
Departments of Pharmacology and Therapeutics and Pediatrics
Louisiana State University Medical Center
1501 Kings Highway
Shreveport, Louisiana 71130

INTRODUCTION

We have emphasized the variance of the M/P ratio with time after dosing (1). This variance is kinetically determined. Accordingly, variance in the M/P ratio may be confounded by factors altering the kinetic profile of drug concentration in the fluid of reference i.e., blood or milk. These factors include dose, route and duration of administration. We have evaluated each of these for their contribution to the temporal variance of the M/P ratio (2). These pharmacological manipulations were performed by using the goat as an animal model and with acetaminophen (APAP) as the test drug. Acetaminophen was chosen because it has a short elimination half-life and can be administered by either the oral or intravenous route in the goat.

MATERIALS AND METHODS

Three 45 kilogram goats were dosed on 7 temporally separate occasions with APAP as detailed below. After dosing, serial blood and milk samples were taken at known time intervals. The blood was taken either from direct puncture of an external jugular vein or from a temporary indwelling jugular venous catheter. The milk samples were stored at 4°C prior to analysis (within 1-2 days). The APAP assay was performed by High Performance Liquid Chromatography. The assay procedure and additional details of animal dosing have been described previously (2) or are shown in the legend of each figure. (It must be appreciated that oral dosing of a drug in the goat may not yield absorption kinetics closely relevant to such dosing in lactating women. Goat forestomach anatomy and rumination may alter the drug absorption profile. For this reason the i.v. route was used in most studies.)

RESULTS

The data from the 7 experiments are summarized in Table 1. For each experiment there is a clear time-lag for the milk peak APAP concentration

Table 1. Acetaminophen excretion into milk after a single dose in the goat.

	Plasma		Milk		Plasma-Milk	M/P Ratio	
	C_{max}	t 1/2	C_{max}	t 1/2	t_{max} Offset	Max	Range
GOAT 1-A	1.05 ug/ml	131 min	1.05 ug/ml	134 min	100.00 min	2.12	0.65 - 2.12
GOAT 1-B	13.05 ug/ml	22.9 min	7.00 ug/ml	31.9 min	40.00 min	6.33	1.01 - 6.33
GOAT 1-C	35.03 ug/ml	19.4 min	11.06 ug/ml	25.7 min	53.00 min	26.05	0.24 - 26.05
GOAT 2-A	28.01 ug/ml	26.6 min	17.09 ug/ml	51.0 min	19.33 min	16.57	0.18 - 16.57
GOAT 2-B†	47.01 ug/ml	18.0 min	50.05 ug/ml	20.4 min	30.05 min	5.92	0.25 - 5.92
GOAT 2-C	3.09 ug/ml	40.3 min	4.06 ug/ml	50.8 min	31.03 min	1.69	0.22 - 1.69
GOAT 3-A	12.99 ug/ml	21.3 min	28.35 ug/ml	39.6 min	0.05 min	8.56	0.12 - 8.56

Each goat is shown by #1, 2 or 3.
A, B, and C refer to different treatment conditions as described in legend of the figures.
† Milked to dryness at each sampling time (others - pooled 2 ml aliquots from each teat).
t 1/2 is for the apparent beta phase of elimination.
Duration of post dose sampling was for 8 hours except for goat 1-A and 1-B (4 hour).

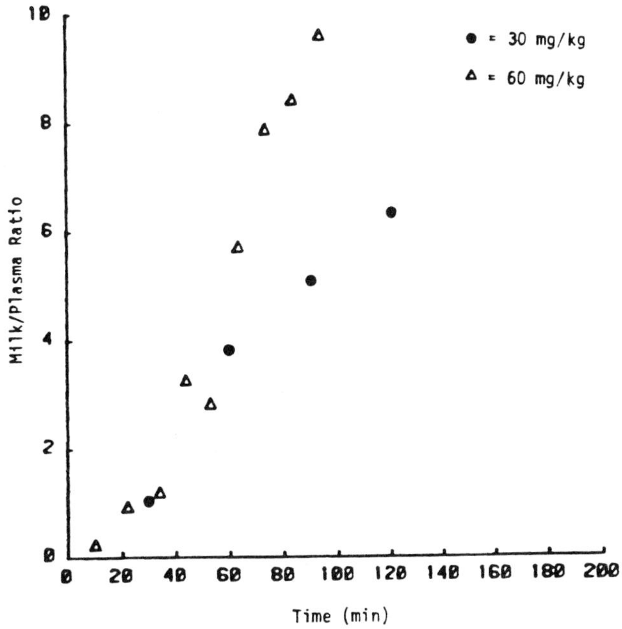

Figure 1. Ratio of acetaminophen (APAP) concentrations in milk and plasma (M/P) of a lactating goat after administration of 2 different doses of APAP by the same route (intravenous) versus time after sampling (Goats 1B and 1C). APAP powder was dissolved in propylene glycol: ethanol: dextrose 5% in a v/v ratio of 45 : 5: 55 (5) and filtered through a 0.2 micron filter. The solution was injected directly into an external jugular vein. The doses given were 30 mg/kg (●) (total dose = 1.3 grams) and 60 mg/kg (△) (total dose = 2.7 grams).

(C_{max}) relative to that of plasma, and this is described by the plasma-milk offset. In general the terminal half-life of plasma APAP showed a trend to be less than that for milk in all cases. Variance in the M/P ratio is shown by the maximum as well as the range of observed ratios. Pharmacological reasons for variance in the ratio were discernable as described below.

M/P ratio as a function of dose (Figure 1)

When 2 different doses (30 mg/kg and 60 mg/kg) were administered by the same route (intravenous), the pattern of the derived M/P ratios was similar. Dose of APAP does not appear to be a confounding factor.

M/P ratio as a function of duration of dosing (Figure 2)

The duration of APAP infusion was associated with a post-dose variance of the M/P ratio after cessation of dosing. The trend of this variance was similar for each infusion. The M/P ratio for the 'bolus' infusion of 2 minutes starts at zero while the 1 hour and the 4 hour infusions start at 1.8 and 2.2 respectively. This difference is expected as a result of accumulation of drug to steady state conditions during the course of a more prolonged infusion.

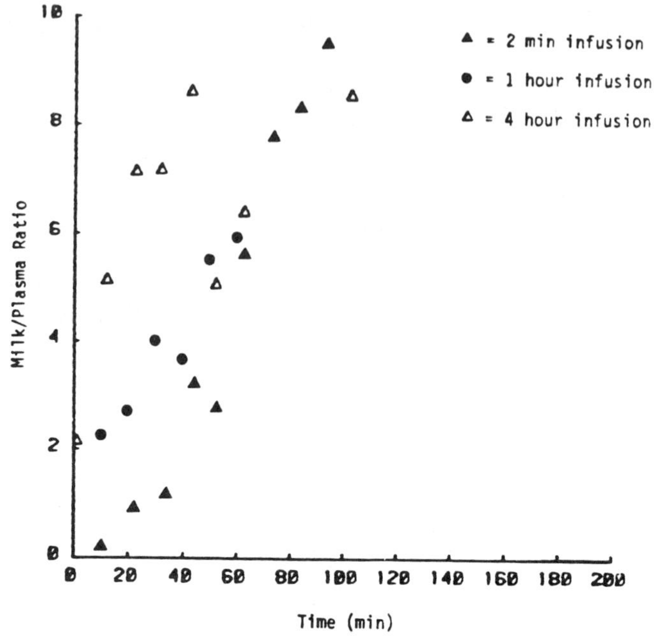

Figure 2. Ratio of acetaminophen (APAP) concentrations in milk and plasma (M/P) in a lactating goat after the administration of APAP by intravenous infusion of 3 different durations vs time after dosing was complete. The APAP solution was prepared as above and was infused for 2 minutes (▲) to a dose of 30 mg/kg/min (Goat 1C), 1 hour (●) to a dose of 1.3 mg/kg/min (Goat 2B) and for 4 hours (△) to a dose of 1.0 mg/kg/min (Goat 3A). The total doses administered were 2.7, 3.6 and 10.8 grams respectively.

M/P ratio as a function of route of administration (Figure 3)

The route of administration was examined for its effect on the temporal variance of the M/P ratio. A marked difference in the pattern of the post-dose ratio was found for oral vs intravenous dosing.

Different patterns of post-dose M/P ratios as a function of various pharmacologic factors is highlighted by the summary (Figure 4). This "shotgun pattern" readily shows the chance for error when using the M/P ratio for a specific drug if both the post-dose time and experimental conditions are not similar to those used for its derivation.

The kinetic basis for temporal variance of the M/P ratio under various pharmacological conditions is illustrated by the parameters derived for a 3-compartment open model (Table 2). The M/P ratio varied with regard to distribution as well as elimination phases of the plasma profile of APAP. This is apparent from the small contribution of the alpha-phase at about 30 minutes after the dose. This and the apparent trend toward a higher elimination rate constant for plasma vs milk (Table 1) illustrates the importance of mammary and maternal drug disposition as individual determinants of variance in the M/P ratio.

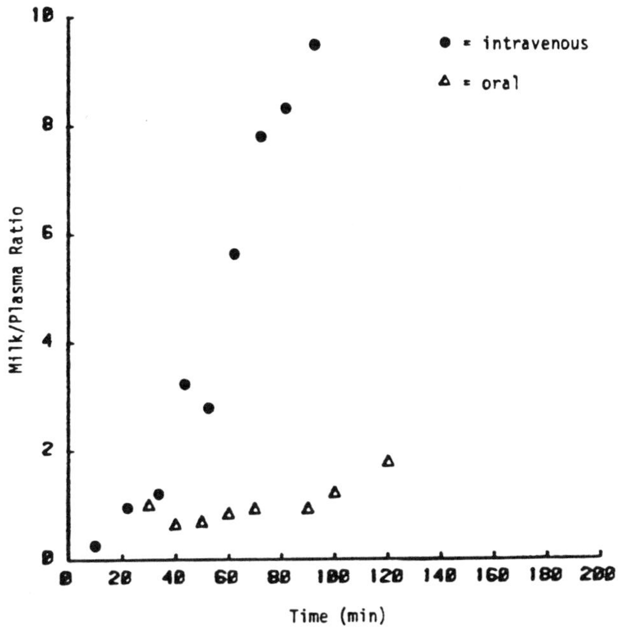

Figure 3. Ratio of acetaminophen concentrations (APAP) in the milk and plasma of a lactating goat after the administration of the same dose of APAP (60 mg/kg) via 2 differing routes (oral Δ and intravenous ●) vs time after dosing. The APAP solution was prepared as above and infused into an external jugular vein over 2 minutes (Goat 1C). APAP elixir (Tylenol®) was instilled directly into the stomach via an oro-ruminal tube (Goat 1A). The total dose given was 2.7 grams.

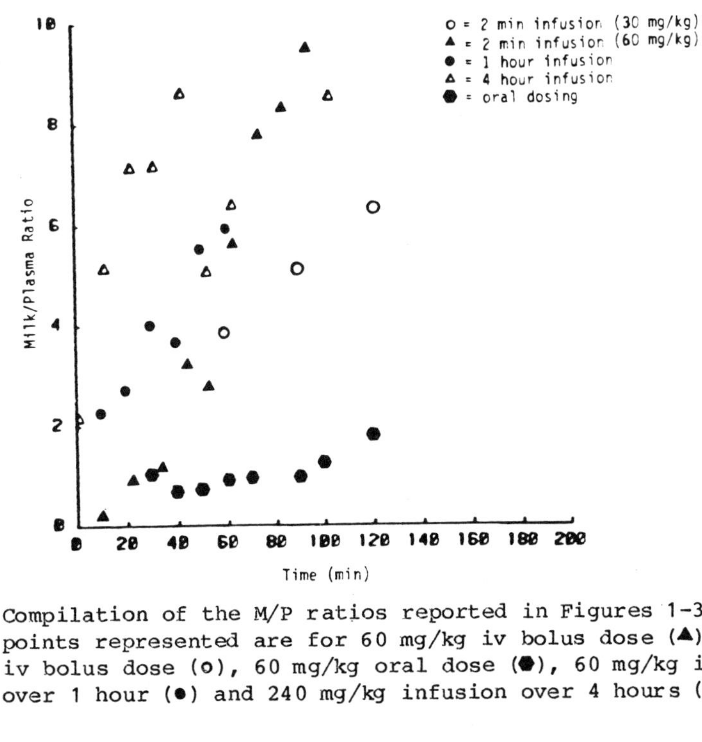

Figure 4. Compilation of the M/P ratios reported in Figures 1-3. The points represented are for 60 mg/kg iv bolus dose (▲), 30 mg/kg iv bolus dose (o), 60 mg/kg oral dose (⬢), 60 mg/kg iv infusion over 1 hour (●) and 240 mg/kg infusion over 4 hours (Δ).

Table 2. **Pharmacokinetic parameters for acetaminophen in the lactating goat.**

Model	Mean Parameter Value (± S.E.)		
	(min^{-1})		
	alpha	beta	gamma
Three compartment			
plasma	0.1222 (0.0224)	0.0516 (0.0061)	0.0255 (0.0030)
milk	0.0835 (0.0231)	0.0415 (0.0069)	0.0202 (0.0025)

DISCUSSION

The amount of drug in breast-milk is essentially time and maternal dose dependent. If the dose is known then the time dependency is a function of maternal drug distribution and elimination i.e., maternal drug disposition, as well as mammary drug disposition. These kinetic parameters are captured by the M/P ratio which is derived from the concentrations of the drug in simultaneously obtained milk and plasma samples. The ratio can also be an average term when the numerical average of several temporally distinct ratios is used. The usefulness of this ratio lies in its calculation of the dose of drug delivered to the nursing infant in the milk (Table 3). It is clear, therefore, that the estimated dose is dependent upon an accurately defined M/P ratio. Variation in the ratio will cause variation in the dose of drug delivered in the milk. A ratio derived immediately before maternal dosing may not give an accurate estimate of the dose delivered to the infant nursing several hours later. Table 4 shows two examples of calculation of dose to the infant based upon the general calculation in Table 3. It is important to examine carefully the means by which a M/P ratio is derived.

The time dependency of the M/P ratio is a function of drug distribution and elimination. These pharmacokinetic terms utilize the concepts of volume and rate. Thus, a drug distributes into a volume yielding a concentration, and the derivation assumes that the drug exists in the same concentration in this apparent volume as it does in plasma. A rate constant (k) helps define the speed with which a drug moves in and out of a compartment. Both volume and rate are conceptualized by pharmacokinetic models. These models utilize the concept of volume compartments which may <u>not</u> correspond to a discrete physiological or anatomical compartment. Compartments are distinguished by pharmacokinetic analysis of drug concentration profiles in a given body fluid, usually blood. This fluid is then used as a reference fluid for all pharmacokinetic calculations, and volume parameters are apparent rather than actual. The concept of a pharmacokinetic model for the breast feeding women is illustrated by Figure 5.

The "kinetic" nature of the model is emphasized by the realization that these compartments are not static in size. This concept is illustrated by consideration of the maternal sequential states of pregnancy and lactation (3). An additional compartment in both anatomical and pharmacokinetic terms opens up in these states, i.e., utero-fetal compartment and the breast-milk compartment. These can be considered as distinct integral pharmacokinetic components of each state with regard to drug disposition. The rate of transfer into and out of these additional compartments is determined both by the condition of physiological membranes, drug transfer processes, and the physicochemical nature of each compartmental fluid as well as pharmacologic characteristics of each drug. Either maternal state exerts potential perturbations in the distribution and elimination of drugs as a consequence of the altered physiological state of the female. A perturbation drug handling capacity impacts on the amount of drug that will be presented to the fetus or breast.

Table 3. Drug dose given to infant via breast milk.

General calculation

C_{avg} x M/P x milk volume (ml/kg/d) = dose (mg/kg/d)

Worse case analysis

C_{max} x M/P x milk volume (ml/kg/d) = dose (mg/kg/d)

C_{avg} and C_{max} are respective averages and maximum drug concentrations in plasma at time of feeding. M/P is the milk to plasma ratio of drug concentration and is assumed to be invariate with regard to time after dosing.

Milk volume average is 150 ml/kg/d.

It is clear that pharmacokinetic changes within the individual female and her breast "compartment" will affect the M/P ratio. It is also clear that these changes need to be accurately defined before any meaningful calculation of the M/P ratio can be used to estimate the dose of a drug that is presented to the nursing infant. To assess the changes we must know the extent of their effect on drug disposition. This requires detailed measurements of drug concentrations in the plasma and milk of appropriate subjects. To validate the changes due to the altered physiological states, longitudinal studies are required to describe these changes in a small but representative group. The states of lactation must be studied with regard to the mammary component specific variables, e.g., milk composition, suckling pattern, etc. We propose that the biological variables associated with maternal and mammary drug disposition can be controlled by using animal models. The appropriate pharmacokinetic model for a certain drug can then be developed with greater precision.

In addition to biological variables of a maternal and mammary nature, those of a pharmacological nature must be described with regard to their effect on the M/P ratio. Categorical pharmacological variables include physicochemical aspects of the drug and dosing characteristics. The latter was studied in the lactating goat under standardized biological conditions. We found that the post dose M/P ratio for APAP was essentially variant with time. Pharmacological influences on this variance were duration of dosing and the route of administration. From these data it is clear that a M/P ratio must be defined in relation to both the biological and pharmacological conditions under which it was determined. Elucidation in animals of the most likely model determining the M/P ratio, as well as its observed variance, will allow restricted or widespread application of the ratio to breast-feeding women consuming a particular drug.

Table 4. Use of the M/P ratio to calculate drug dose in milk.

Drug	Maternal C_{avg} ug/ml	M/P	Milk Volume ml/kg/day	Dose in Milk mg/kg/day	Therapeutic Dose mg/kg/day	RDF*
Phenytoin (7)	16.29	0.14	150	0.342	5-10	14.6
Procainamide (8)	1.10	4.3	150	0.709	28.8	40.6

$$*RDF = \text{relative dose factor} = \frac{\text{Therapeutic dose for child}}{\text{Dose in milk}}$$

Clinical relevance of these findings for APAP in the goat is illustrated by reported human studies. A mixed pattern of temporal variance of the M/P ratio is apparent for various pharmacological factors (Table 5). Work with aztreonam in lactating women emphasizes the

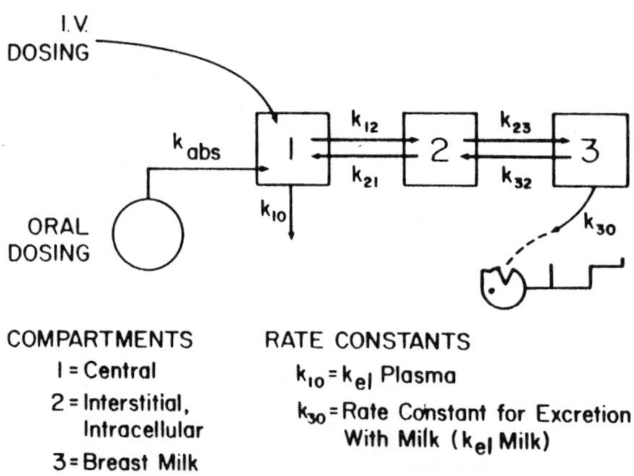

Figure 5. An infant modulated 3-compartment open model for drug excretion into breast milk (6).

temporal variance of the M/P ratio by two parenteral routes (4) (Figure 6). These findings are consistent with our data in the goat in that an upward trend of the ratio is found after an intravenous dose. That these perturbed M/P ratios may be a function of the stage of lactation is being studied.

Table 5. **Reported M/P Ratios in Lactating Women Under Different Pharmacologic Conditions.**

DRUG	DESCRIPTION	DOSE (D) + TIME	M/P RATIO	REFERENCE
Dose				
Prednisolone	10 mg/day x 1	D1 + 1 hr	0.12	(9)
(Steady state)	15 mg/day x 1	D1 + 1 hr	0.10	
(oral)	10 mg/day x 2	D1 + 1 hr	0.11	
	15 mg/day x 2	D1 + 1 hr	0.21	
	45 mg/day x 1	D1 + 1 hr	0.19	
	80 mg/day x 1	D1 + 1 hr	0.25	
Duration of Dosing				
Praziquantel (oral)	50 mg x 1 dose	D1 + 1-24 hr	0.43 - 0.66	(10)
	20 mg x 3 doses in 24 hours	D1 + 2-32 hr	0.138 - 0.12	
Indoprofen (oral)	200 mg x 1 dose 2 patients	D1 + 2 hr	0.013 & 0.018	(11)
	200 mg x 4 doses 4 patients	D4 + 2 hr	0.014, 0.025 0.033, 0.075	
Mefenamic acid	500 mg x 1	D1 + 2 hr	0.178 (mean)	(12)
(oral)	500 mg x 4	D4 + 2 hr	0.134 (mean)	
	500 mg x 7	D7 + 2 hr	0.23 (mean)	
Flufenamic acid	200 mg x 1	D1 + 2 hr	0.016 (mean)	(13)
(oral)	200 mg x 3	D4 + 2 hr	0.18 (mean)	
		D7 + 2 hr	0.007 (mean)	
Captopril	100 mg x 3	D4 + 1 hr	0.38	(14)
(oral)		D9 + 1 hr	0.08	
Propanolol (oral)	40 mg x 1	D1 + 4 hr	0.38 & 0.25*	(15)
	40 mg x 8	D8 + 4 hr	1.97	
Route of Administration + Dose				
Butorphanol	2 mg x 1 I.M.	D1 + 1 hr	000	(16)
		D1 + 6 hr	0.7	
	8 mg x 1 oral	D1 + 1 hr	0.7	
		D1 + 6 hr	1.7	
			2.2	
Aztreonam	1 g x 1 I.M.	D1 + 1.5 hr	0.0005	(4)
		D1 + 8 hr	0.05	
	1 g x 1 I.V.	D1 + 1.5 hr	0.001	
		D1 + 8 hr	0.048	

* 1 Patient dosed on 2 separate occasions.

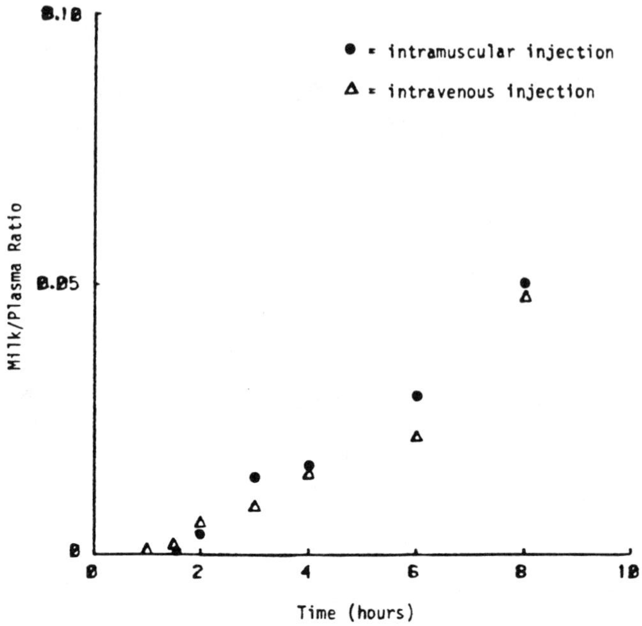

Figure 6. Mean M/P ratios versus time for aztreonam excretion after intramuscular and intravenous injection of the same single dose. This profile is constructed from data of reference (4).

CONCLUDING REMARKS

Investigation of the biological and pharmacological factors modulating the M/P ratio and the underlying pharmacokinetic model is a necessary step in our understanding of the fundamental processes that govern drug excretion in breast milk.

STATEMENT ADDED IN PROOF

A fourth lactating goat was administered a 1 hour infusion of 80 mg/kg APAP on two separate occasions, once with APAP prepared in the alcoholic solution (See Figure 1) and once in water only. The plasma drug levels on both occasions were similar while the milk drug levels of the alcoholic preparation were slightly higher. Half-lives in both plasma and milk on the two occasions were comparable to those reported. Also, the M/P ratios showed the same trends for a one hour infusion as we have discussed indicating that the alcoholic content of our preparations has no impact on our results. The excursion of post infusion M/P ratios was, however, less in this goat. The possible influence of duration of lactation on the extent of change in the M/P ratio is being studied in goats at various lactation periods following parturition.

Acknowledgement

The diligent typing assistance of Mrs. Carole Webb is gratefully acknowledged.

REFERENCES

1. J. T. Wilson, R. D. Brown, J. L. Hinson, and J. W. Dailey. Pharmacokinetic pitfalls in the estimation of the breast milk/plasma ratio for drugs. Ann. Rev. Pharmacol. Toxicol. 25:667-689 (1985).
2. J. T. Wilson, J. L. Hinson, V. A. Johnson, T. W. Woods, I. J. Smith,and R. D. Brown. Pharmacologic factors contributing to variance in the milk to plasma (M/P) ratio for acetaminophen in the goat, (Submitted).
3. J. T. Wilson, J. L. Hinson, R. D. Brown, and I. J. Smith. A comprehensive assessment of drugs and chemical toxins excreted in breast milk. (In press).
4. P. M. Fleiss, G. A. Richwald, J. Gordon, M. Stern, M. Frantz and R. G. Devlin. Aztreonam in human serum and breast milk. Br. J. Clin. Pharmac. 19:509-511 (1985).
5. B. Ameer, M. Divoll, D. R. Abernethy, D. J. Greenblatt, and L. Shargel L. Absolute and relative bioavailability of oral acetaminophen preparations. J. Pharm. Sci. 72:955-958 (1983).
6. J. T. Wilson. Pharmacokinetics of drug excretion, in: "Drugs in Breast Milk," J. T. Wilson, ed., ADIS Press, Australia (1981).
7. B. Steen, A. Rane, G. Lonnerholm, O. Falk, C. E. Elwin and F. Sjoqvist. Phenytoin excretion in human breast milk and plasma levels in nursed infants. Ther. Drug. Monit. 4:331-334 (1982).
8. W. B. Pittard III, and H. Glazier. Procainamide excretion in human milk. J. Pediatr. 102:631-633 (1983).
9. L. Ost, G. Wettrell, I. Bjorkhem, and A. Rane. Prednisolone excretion into human milk. J. Pediatr. 106:1008-1011 (1985).
10. J. Putter, and F. Held. Quantitative studies on the occurrence of praziquantel in milk and plasma of lactating women. Eur. J. Drug Metab. Pharmacokinet. 4:193-198 (1979).
11. D. B. Lakings, C. Lizarraga, W. J. Haggerty, and M. J. Williamson. High performance liquid chromatographic microdetermination of indoprofen in human milk. J. Pharm. Sci. 68:1113-1116 (1979).
12. R. A. Buchanan, C. J. Eaton, S. T. Koeff, and A. W. Kinkel. The breast milk excretion of mefenamic acid. Curr. Ther. Res. 10: 592-597 (1968).
13. R. A. Buchanan, C. J. Eaton, S. T. Koeff, and A. W. Kinkel. Breast milk excretion of flufenamic acid. Curr. Ther. Res. 11:533-538 (1969).
14. R. G. Devlin, and P. M. Fleiss. Captopril in human blood and breast milk. J. Clin. Pharmacol. 21:110-113 (1981).
15. J. H. Bauer, B. Pape, J. Zajicek, and T. Groshong. Propranolol in human plasma and breast milk. Am. J. Cardiol. 43:860-862 (1979).
16. K. A. Pittman, R. D. Smyth, M. Losada, I. Zighelboim, A. L. Maduska and A. Sunshine. Human perinatal distribution of butorphanol. Am. J. Obstet. Gynecol. 138:797-800 (1980).

EPIDEMIOLOGY OF ENVIRONMENTAL CHEMICAL CONTAMINANTS IN BREAST MILK

Walter J. Rogan

Epidemiology Branch
National Institute of Environmental Health Sciences
Research Triangle Park, North Carolina 27709

Human beings are exposed to a wide variety of synthetic and natural chemicals, but acute illnesses due to exposures to most environmental pollutants are unusual. Most of the environmental chemicals to which human beings are exposed are metabolized or excreted, but some are persistent. They are stored in depot tissues such as bone or fat, depending on solubility and other factors. In terms of breast milk contamination, the best studied chemicals are those that are persistent and fat soluble, and thus appear in breast milk at a higher concentration than in serum--milk has about 8 times the fat of serum. The most familiar of these chemicals are the insecticide DDT and the family of the industrial chemicals, the polychlorinated biphenyls, or PCBs. Both of these chemicals are extremely widespread in the environment, exposure to them is essentially universal, and they have been detected repeatedly in the fat of adipose or breast milk samples throughout the world. There is little evidence that these agents cause disease at the levels they have been found in the general population; in fact, few surveys have even attempted to measure morbidity. Besides PCBs and DDT, there are several other fat soluble, persistent chemicals that are close to endemic in their degree of exposure prevalence--they are pesticides, such as dieldrin, chlordane, heptachlor, and benzene hexachloride (BHC).

Besides the very widespread exposures, there have also been epidemics of poisonings in which breast milk contamination has played a part. The largest and best documented of these have been two outbreaks of PCB poisoning in Asia and an outbreak of BHC poisoning in Turkey. In these outbreaks it appears that illness was produced in the children through breast milk exposure. There have also been incidents in which breast milk contamination was documented, but no illness appears to have resulted, such as the polybrominated biphenyl exposure in Michigan in the mid-70's and the heptachlor contamination of dairy herds in Hawaii. Finally, there is the largely theoretical concern that women working around lipophilic substances who are also lactating will absorb and excrete such substances in their milk. Evidence that this actually takes place is scanty, but the concern is real.

The discussion here will be divided into endemic and epidemic exposures. It will be limited for the most part to persistent fat soluble compounds, mostly because there are more data available for them. The volatiles are now beginning to get some attention[1], but the analytic difficulties inherent in quantitative recovery are formidable. There are some data available on metals, such as lead, in human milk, but breast milk does not appear to concentrate metals and so the problems are more those related to the actual intoxication of the mother. Drugs are dealt with elsewhere in this volume. Beverage alcohol and some components of cigarette smoke can contaminate milk, but that is outside the scope here.

ENDEMIC CONTAMINANTS

DDT was first reported in human milk in 1951 by Laug.[2] Since then, a large and fairly coherent body of literature has developed (reviewed in Jensen).[3] The predominant form in which DDT occurs in areas that have ceased spraying is dichlorodiphenyl dichloroethene (DDE), the "environmental" metabolite that is most persistent. Humans metabolize some DDT, but a residue remains. In the US, the ratio of DDE to DDT is about 10 to 1, with some other metabolites, such as dichlorodiphenyl acetic acid (DDA), also present. The source is probably very low level contamination of foods. At this point, almost 15 years after its ban in the US, there is virtually no DDT in air. DDT's role as a water pollutant is complex. It is quite insoluble in water, and is thus not a water pollutant in the classic sense that, say, nitrates and phosphates are. However, bottom sediments and small organisms come into steady state with the very low levels of these kinds of environmental contaminants. From this low level there is bioconcentration at each trophic level, as successive organisms absorb the small amounts in their diets but then do not excrete them. Typically, there is about a 10 fold increase at each trophic level. Thus, large predator fish, such as salmon, and fish eating birds, such as herons, can have tissue levels that are hundreds of times higher than the waters in which they prey (reviewed in Bevenue).[4] Sediments and trash fish are still used as fertilizers, and occasionally as part of protein supplements for meat producing animals. The exposures for human beings produced by such activities is probably in the low micrograms per day range, but since the chemicals cannot be excreted nor metabolized, a body burden eventually builds up. In steady state, these lipophilic chemicals are stored in fat, and appear in the fat of breast milk on simple solubility grounds.

In areas where DDT is still used, there is a higher ratio of DDT to DDE, and levels are in general higher. In some recent WHO data, countries like Mexico and the PRC had DDE levels about 4 fold and DDT levels about 10 fold higher than the US.[5]

In most studies, older women have higher levels than younger, and primiparous women are higher than multiparous. This is consistent with accumulation as the means of achieving a given body burden, and with lactation as a means of excreting the chemicals. In our study of PCBs and DDE in milk in NC, levels decline about 20% with six months of breast feeding.[6]

We find that blacks have higher levels than whites. This has been seen in other studies using adipose tissue as a matrix,[7] and is unexplained. There are no occupational groups thus far reported who have exceptionally high levels, and in our data no occupational grouping stands out as particularly high.

Urban rural gradients depend more on food handling practices than on "urbanity" per se. Rural women who eat food locally grown without the pesticide have lower levels.[8] In general, women from areas that eat about the same foods will have about the same levels. In the US, women in the Southeast have somewhat higher levels than elsewhere, for unknown reasons.[9]

There are no data showing direct absorption of DDT by the child, although there is no reason to believe that orally administered DDT is not absorbed. In passing, it should be noted that cows are lower on the food chain than human beings, and that a dairy cow will secrete literally tons of milk in her career. Thus, cows' milk is essentially free of DDT. The fat in commercial formula is typically coconut oil, which is again pesticide free. Thus, there is substantial contrast between the perinatal exposure of infants fed breast milk or formula.

PCBs

PCBs were first reported in human milk by Jensen in 1966,[10] but they had probably been appearing as interference peaks in the chromatograms of those seeking DDT residues for several years before that. The conceptual difference that is the likely cause for the delay is that PCBs are not pesticides, and they had not been widely applied. Their main use was as the insulating fluid in large electrical transformers, but because they were cheap to manufacture and had excellent electrical insulating, optical, and fire retardant properties, they had achieved a wide array of uses. Small electrical parts, fluorescent ballasts and the like were insulated with PCBs. They were the oily fluid that suspended the pigment in carbonless copy paper, and were the major part of microscope immersion oil. These were all items that were not thought to require any particular care in use or disposal, and PCB containing products were widely dispersed in the environment from the inception of their manufacture in the 1930's to the passage of the Toxic Substances Control Act in the late 70's. Like DDT, PCBs are fat soluble and persistent in the environment. They are not a single chemical, but rather a family that shares the two linked phenyl rings and variable degrees of chlorination. Although some of the less chlorinated congeners can be broken down, most are quite resistant to breakdown, either in the environment or in organisms, and are thus subject to the same bioconcentration as is DDT. Quantitatively, PCBs are the second of the major environmental contaminants of human milk, and in industrialized countries that have not used much DDT, they can be present at higher concentrations than the insecticide.[8]

PCBs can be detected if not well quantified in more than 90% of unselected samples of breast milk worldwide.[3] Detailed comparisons are not justified, since the complex nature of the mixture leads to different estimates of concentrations, depending on the method used. In general, though, the highest levels have been found in Japan, Sweden, the FRG, and the US. Eating fish from contaminated waters is thought to produce higher levels, but this factor does not appear to be a large one.[11,12] Older women and primiparous women have higher levels, as for DDT, and levels decline with time spent breastfeeding at about the same rate. There does not appear to be a relationship with cigarette smoking, but women who drink alcohol regularly have slightly higher levels.[6,13]

There are Japanese data that indirectly imply that women who work around PCBs have relatively higher levels--children of women occupationally exposed were shown to have higher blood PCB levels at ages up to 14 years, with the blood levels related to the duration of breast feeding.[14] There have been few other occupational studies of breast milk directly, but those who work around PCBs are known to have higher blood levels and so would presumably have higher breast milk levels.

Other Chemicals

Dieldrin, chlordane as its oxy metabolite, heptachlor in its epoxide form,[15] and hexachlorobenzene[16] all appear with relatively high frequency in breast milk, although except in special circumstances they are both less prevalent and at lower concentrations than PCBs and DDT. These chemicals are persistent, fat soluble pesticides, some of which are still used. The routes of exposure are probably similar to those for PCBs and DDT, in addition to direct exposure. The general characteristics of distribution in terms of age, parity, etc. are likely similar for these chemicals, but there are fewer data available to document this. These three chemicals have also been involved in specific outbreaks of exposure. These will be discussed below.

EPIDEMIC EXPOSURES

Hexachlorobenzene

The first epidemic exposure in which breast milk contamination was important began in Turkey in 1957. A dermatologist noted an outbreak of porphyria cutanea tarda among patients who had been consuming seed wheat, which had been treated with hexachlorobenzene as a fungicide. About 3000 cases were reported, and the government eventually banned treated seed in 1959.[17] Although there were many childhood cases of porphyria, nurslings did not develop it. Rather, they got pembe yara (pink sore), an annular papular rash, along with weakness and convulsions. Hexachlorobenzene was found to be present in milk, and although a good animal model has not been found, suspicion is high that pembe yara is produced by some combination of breast milk and transplacental exposure. Children were literally wiped out in some villages--the illness carried about a 95% case fatality rate.[18]

The major use of hexachlorobenzene is as a seed treatment. It has been reported as a residue contaminant of fat or breast milk samples in Europe, Japan, and Canada, but not regularly from the US.[16] This incident is known to public health authorities, and treated seed is now dyed striking colors. However, the potential for recurrence is real.

PCBs

There have been two outbreaks of illness due to PCB exposure, one in Japan in 1968[19] and one in Taiwan in 1979.[20] In both instances, the vector was cooking oil that had been heat treated. The heat transfer agents were commercial PCBs, which were run through pipes in the vats of oil. The pipes developed leaks allowing the PCBs to contaminate the product. Since PCBs are clear, oily, and tasteless, the contamination was not detected until people had become ill. This particular use of PCBs leads to a degree of thermal degradation, and over time they became contaminated with terphenyls, quatraphenyls, and furans.[21] These contaminants can be much more toxic than the parent compound; the polychlorinated dibenzofurans include some extremely toxic congeners.

About 1100 cases of Yusho (in Japan) and over 2000 cases of Yucheng (in Taiwan)--both words mean oil disease--are being followed by health authorities. The most prominent symptom is chloracne, a cystic, non-inflammatory acne that lasts for years and is not responsive to usual treatment. Patients also have pigmentation, neuralgia, and abdominal pain. Children born to affected mothers tend to have low birthweight, pigmentation, natal teeth, scalp calcification, and dysmorphic nails.[22] Few samples of breast milk have been analyzed, and of those, levels of PCBs are not much higher than those in the general population of Japan.[23] However, the chromatographic pattern differs,[24] and presumably the more toxic contaminants are present and account for some of the toxicity. Harada[25] reported several cases of Yusho in children that he thought were produced by breast milk exposure alone. We are following the children in the Taiwan outbreak to see if clinical manifestations are more severe among children who had been breast fed.

The Japanese outlawed the use of PCB containing machinery for food processing after the 1968 outbreak. The machine responsible for the Taiwan epidemic was never found, and it is not known how many of these machines are still in Asia. The potential for yet another cooking oil related outbreak is directly proportional to the number of them still in use.

Polybrominated biphenyls

In 1973, Firemaster, a flame retardant, was inadvertently substituted for Nutrimaster, a MgO2 food supplement, in dairy cattle feed in Michigan.[26] PBB is another two ring, halogen substituted compound that differs from PCBs by bromine rather than chlorine substitution. Before the contamination was discovered, cows, chickens and swine that had eaten the food were sold locally and consumed. The contamination was quite widespread in Michigan, and investigators used the fact that the compound would appear in the fat of breast milk to estimate the degree of contamination. Using a random sample of hospitals and volunteer donors, Brilliant[27] found that over 90% of samples of breast milk from the lower peninsula had detectable PBB.

Despite the obvious toxicity in the livestock and many claims of illness, several surveys of Michigan residents were unable to find any specific illness or syndrome that occurred regularly in those with the highest exposures. Two surveys were done of the children.[28,29] Neither showed obvious dose related illness, but one showed a shorter length of breast feeding among the exposed women.[29] This could not be interpreted, however, since the state had offered breast milk analysis to lactating women and advised them not to breast feed if their concentration exceeded a certain level. Another study showed a tendency for children with higher PBB levels in fat to score lower on the McCarthy scales of children's abilities,[30] but breast feeding was not investigated directly.

It is too soon to conclude that the contamination in Michigan resulted in no chemical induced toxicity. There certainly was substantial social and economic disruption that follow on any disaster, natural or man-made. There is no potential for recurrence of this particular contamination, since PBB is no longer made. The circumstances that lead to the contamination are not unique, however.

Heptachlor

Pineapples are a major cash crop in Hawaii, and growers were accustomed to using heptachlor to help control mealybug damage. They had even gotten an exemption to continue using it after other uses had been curtailed by the Environmental Protection Agency. After the pineapples were harvested, the leafy plant parts, called "green chop", were fed to dairy cows. No material that had been sprayed within a year was supposed to be included. Because of this activity, the state health department routinely monitored cow's milk for heptachlor, and in January, 1982, an unexpected amount of heptachlor was found, subsequently to be confirmed by other labs. Retrospective testing of green chop samples showed that contamination had been present back to the previous summer.[31]

Analysis of breast milk samples showed, as expected, the presence of heptachlor epoxide, the stable metabolite of heptachlor. Chemists in Hawaii had been interested in heptachlor, and previous data had shown that levels in Hawaii were quite a bit lower than the mainland.[32,33] The new data showed Hawaii to be at about the levels found in the rest of the US.[15,34]

This posed a problem for those responsible for investigating the possibility of illness in breast fed children. A "heptachlor study" might best be done in the southeastern US, where levels were highest. Even at the levels found there, heptachlor still represented a relatively minor part of the organohalide contaminants in breast milk. However, there was considerable local interest in a Hawaiian study of the children, and several projects were proposed; no results are yet available.

SUMMARY

Fat soluble, persistent chemicals are valuable economically as a class. In fact, their persistence was a desirable characteristic, leading to less frequent applications and longer duration of action. The consequences of their use can be undesirable, however, since very minor but sustained exposure can lead to an appreciable body burden. For the very widespread agents, the circumstances of exposure can be unknown or unknowable, and thus the individual can take no specific action to avoid it.

Thus far, most countries have been spared episodes of illness attributable to breast milk contamination, although outbreaks that were not widespread and severe may well have gone undetected. It is also true that to date, levels high enough to produce illness in the child are accompanied by illness in the mother. Thus, the situation in which a healthy mother has inadvertently poisoned her child has not occurred with these chemicals. This may not be true for the volatiles-there is one case report of a woman whose child developed cholestatic jaundice during breast feeding. The mother lunched daily with her dry cleaner husband, and the solvent, perchlorethylene, was found in her milk. She was not ill.[35]

Analysis of breast milk samples from women without special exposures has thus far not proved useful. Besides the difficulty in deciding on a level at which the supposed hazard might outweigh the benefit, there are analytic difficulties. There are no quality control programs for different laboratories, and thus no assurance that a given lab will come up with the right number, or even the same number on a series of identical samples. In addition, the tests are expensive, and can take up to six weeks to complete. There is some reassurance available from the fact that breast fed children have been studied in many cultures, and they in general do better than their bottle fed counterparts. Several groups are now looking at the question of morbidity from these kinds of chemicals in milk, but there are no reports of major morbidity thus far.

For some chemicals, infants live at the very top of the food chain, and because of their limited diets and developmental state, they may be the group most likely to suffer damage. Continued vigilance is warranted, since the relative absence of major problems in the past is no guarantee for the future.

REFERENCES

1. E. D. Pellizzari, T. D. Hartwell, B. S. H. Harris III, R. D. Waddell, D. A. Whitaker, and M. D. Erickson, Purgeable organic compounds in mother's milk, Bull Environ Contam Toxicol, 28:322-8 (1982).
2. E. P. Laug, F. M. Kunze, and C. S. Prickett, Occurrence of DDT in human fat and milk, Arch Ind Hyg Occup Med, 3:245-6 (1951).
3. A. Jensen, Chemical contaminants in human milk, Residue Rev, 89:1-128 (1983).
4. A. Bevenue, The "bioconcentration" aspects of DDT in the environment, Residue Rev, 61:37-112 (1976).

5. S. A. Slorach and R. Vaz, eds., "Assessment of human exposure to selected organochlorine compounds through biological monitoring," Swedish National Food Administration for the United Nations Environment Program and WHO, Uppsala (1983).
6. W. J. Rogan, B. C. Gladen, J. D. McKinney, N. Carreras, P. Hardy, J. Thullen, J. Tingelstad, and M. Tully, Polychlorinated Biphenyls (PCBs) and Dichlorodiphenyl Dichloroethene (DDE) in Human Milk: Effects of Maternal Factors and Previous Lactation, Am J Public Health, 76:172-177 (1986).
7. J. E. Davies, W. F. Edmundson, A. Raffonelli, J. C. Cassaday, and C. Morgade, The role of social class in human pesticide pollution, Amer J Epidemiol, 96:334-41 (1972).
8. WHO, "Contemporary patterns of breast feeding," WHO, Geneva (1981).
9. E. P. Savage, "National study to determine levels of chlorinated hydrocarbon insecticides in human milk: 1975-1976 and supplementary report to the national human milk study 1975-1976," National Technical Information Services, Accession No, PB-284 393, Springfield (1977)
10. Report of a new chemical hazard, New Scientist, 32:612 (1966).
11. P. M. Schwartz, S. W. Jacobson, G. Fein, J. L. Jacobson, and H. A. Price, Lake Michigan fish consumption as a source of polychlorinated biphenyls in human cord serum, maternal serum, and milk, Am J Public Health, 73:293-6 (1983).
12. H. E. B. Humphrey, Population studies of PCBs in Michigan residents, in: "PCBs: Human and environmental hazards," F. M. D'Itri and M. A. Kamrin, eds., Butterworth Publishers, Boston, 299-310 (1983).
13. G. G. Fein, J. L. Jacobson, S. W. Jacobson, P. M. Schwartz, and J. K. Dowler, Prenatal exposure to polychlorinated biphenyls: effects on birth size and gestational age, J Peds, 105:315-20 (1984).
14. K. Kuwabara, T. Yakushiji, I. Watanabe, S. Yoshida, K. Koyama, N. Kunita, and I. Hara, Relationship between breast feeding and PCB residues in blood of the children whose mothers were occupationally exposed to PCBs, Int Arch Occup Environ Health, 41:189-97 (1978).
15. E. P. Savage, T. J. Keefe, J. D. Tessari, H. W. Wheeler, F. M. Applehans, E. A. Goes, and S. A. Ford, National study of chlorinated hydrocarbon insecticide residues in human milk, USA, Am J Epidemiol, 113:413-22 (1981).
16. K. D. Courtney, Hexachlorobenzene: A review, Environ Res, 20:225-66 (1979).
17. H. A. Peters, S.A.M. Johnson, S. Cam, S. Oral, Y. Muftu, and T. Ergene, Hexachlorobenzene induced porphyria: effects of chelation on the disease, porphyrin and metal metabolism, Am J Public Health, 76:172-177 (1966).
18. D. J. Cripps, A. Gocmen, and H. A. Peters, Porphyria Turcica, Arch Dermatol, 116:46-50 (1980).
19. M. Kuratsune, Yusho, in: "Halogenated biphenyls, terphenyls, napthalenes, dibenzodioxins, and related products," R. D. Kimbrough, ed., Elsevier/North Holland, Amsterdam, 287-302 (1980).
20. S. Hsu, C. Ma, S. K. Hsu, S. Wu, N. H. Hsu, and C. Yeh, Discovery and epidemiology of PCB poisoning in Taiwan, Amer J Ind Med, 5:71-9 (1984).
21. L. R. Kamps, W. J. Trotter, S. J. Young, L. J. Carson, J. A. Roach, J. A. Sphon, J. T. Tanner, and B. McMahon, Polychlorinated quatraphenyls identified in rice oil associated with Japanese Yusho poisoning, Bull Environ Cont Toxicol, 20:589-91 (1978).
22. W. J. Rogan, PCBs and cola colored babies, Teratology, 26:259-62 (1982).
23. Y. Masuda, R. Kagawa, M. Kuratsune, T. Yoshimura, I. Taki, M. Kusuda, F. Yamashita, and M. Hayashi, Transfer of polychlorinated biphenyls from mothers to foetuses and infants, Fd Cosmet Toxicol, 16:543-6 (1978).
24. Y. Masuda, R. Kagawa, and M. Kuratsune, Comparison of polychlorinated biphenyls in Yusho patients and ordinary persons, Bull Environ Contam Toxicol, 11:213-6 (1974).
25. M. Harada, Intrauterine poisoning: clinical and epidemiological studies of the problem, Bull Inst Constitutional Med, (Kumamoto Univ) 25 Sup:1-60 (1976).

26. K. Kay, Polybrominated biphenyls (PBB) environmental contamination in Michigan, 1973-1976, Environ Res, 13:74-93 (1977).
27. L. B. Brilliant, K. Wilcox, G. VanAmburg, J. Eyster, J. Isbister, A. W. Bloomer, H. Humphrey, and H. Price, Breast milk monitoring to measure Michigan's contamination with polybrominated biphenyls, Lancet, 2:8091-5 (1978).
28. M. Barr, Pediatric aspects of the Michigan polybrominated biphenyl contamination, Environ Res, 21:255-274 (1980).
29. W. B. Weil, M. Spencer, and D. Benjamin, The effect of polybrominated biphenyl on infants and young children, J Ped, 98:47-51 (1981).
30. E. W. Seagull, Developmental abilities of children exposed to polybrominated biphenyls (PBB), Am J Public Health, 73:281-5 (1983).
31. R. J. Smith, Hawaiian milk contamination creates alarm, Science, 217:137-140 (1982).
32. L. J. Casarett, G. C. Fryer, W. L. Yanger, and H. W. Klemmer, Organochlorine pesticide residue in human tissue--Hawaii, Arch Environ Health, 17:306-11 (1968).
33. W. Takahashi, D. Saidin, G. Takei, and L. Wong, Organochlorine pesticide residues in human milk in Hawaii, 1979-1980, Bull Environ Toxicol, 27:506-11 (1981).
34. Pesticide Hazard Assessment Project, "Heptachlor epoxide in mother's milk, Oahu, August 1981 - November 1982," University of Hawaii at Manoa, Manoa (1983).
35. P. C. Bagnell and H. A. Ellenberger, Obstructive jaundice due to a chlorinated hydrocarbon in breast milk, Can Med Assoc J, 117:1047-8 (1977).

THE INFLUENCE OF MATERNAL FACTORS ON DRUG LEVELS IN HUMAN MILK

Richard A. Ehrenkranz

Department of Pediatrics and
Obstetrics and Gynecology
Yale University School of Medicine
New Haven, Connecticut 06510

Transfer of drugs into human milk has been shown to be dependent upon the physiochemical properties of the drug and several maternal factors.[1-3] The physiochemical properties include the molecular weight of the drug, its degree of ionization, its solubility in water and lipids, its binding to plasma and milk proteins, and the relative difference between the pH of maternal plasma and milk.[1-5] The plasma drug concentration and mammary gland blood flow are the main maternal factors.[1,2] Of the two, the maternal plasma drug concentration is the most important since it determines the amount of drug that is potentially available for transfer into milk.[2-6]

The maternal plasma drug concentration is a function of the pharmacokinetics of the drug in the mother.[2,5,7] This paper will review the maternal factors that may influence drug pharmacokinetics during the perinatal period and during lactation, and thus may affect drug levels in milk (Figure). The pharmacokinetic process involves drug absorption, distribution, metabolism, and excretion.[7] Since a number of physiological adjustments occur during the perinatal period and during lactation, each of these aspects may be affected.[8,9]

Influence of Perinatal Factors on Maternal Drug Absorption

Although the rate of absorption of oral medications may be decreased by the delay in gastric emptying and by the decreased intestinal motility common in pregnancy, drug absorption might be more complete.[8] However, with the return of normal gastrointestinal function after delivery, drug absorption will return to normal. Drug absorption can also be affected by factors such as concurrent drug use or food intake, and the pharmaceutical preparation used.[7]

Influence of Perinatal Factors on Maternal Drug Distribution

Pregnancy is associated with an increase in the volume of distribution for many drugs because of an increase in maternal plasma volume, body water, and fat. Plasma volume begins to increase in the first trimester and is about 50% higher than non-pregnant levels at term.[8,9] Plasma volume is also related to fetal size, being greater in multiple gestation and less with intrauterine growth retardation. Thus, in most pregnancies, the plasma concentrations of drugs with a normally small apparent volume of distribution will tend to be lower with standard drug dosages.[8,10] Similarly, extravascular water is increased at term, with edematous women accumulating on average an additional 5 liters of extracellular fluid.[8] Since unbound water-soluble drugs can distribute into this extracellular water, their volume of distribution may be even greater. Finally, the volume of distribution for fat-soluble drugs also increases during pregnancy since body fat increases.[1,8] Thus, excessive weight gain augments this potential fat-soluble drug reservoir.

In addition to these influences, drug distribution may also be affected by alterations in plasma protein drug binding that may occur during pregnancy.[8,10] Most drugs are partly bound to circulating proteins, usually albumin, but also to globulins, lipoproteins, and acid glyco-proteins, and an equilibrium is established between the bound and free fractions of the drug in the plasma. Only the free drug fraction is able to bind with active receptor sites, to be metabolized, and to be excreted.[7] Since serum albumin concentration is reduced in normal pregnancy due to an increased plasma volume and an increased rate of catabolism, the fraction of unbound drug may be larger and its volume of distribution increased.[8-10] However, elevated circulatory estrogen levels during pregnancy stimulate the synthesis of some proteins, including alpha and beta globulins, ceruloplasmin, and corticosteroid-binding and thyroid-binding proteins, which may increase potential plasma protein binding sites for certain drugs.[9] With pre-eclampsia, proteinuria may further reduce serum albumin levels and affect protein drug binding.[8]

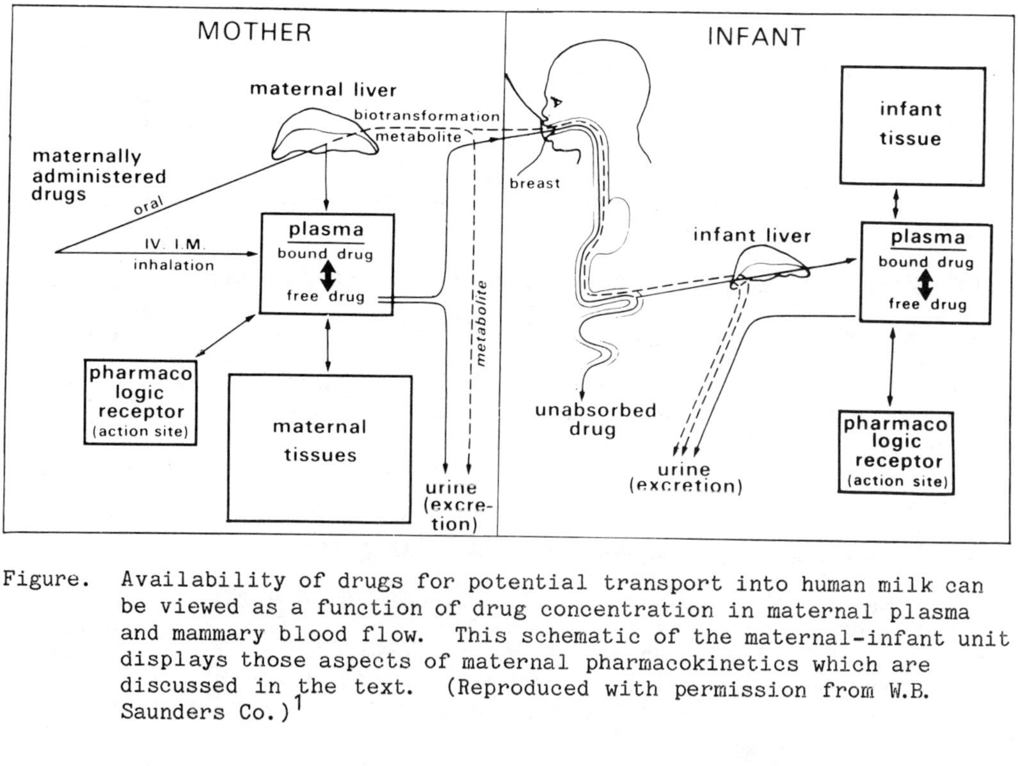

Figure. Availability of drugs for potential transport into human milk can be viewed as a function of drug concentration in maternal plasma and mammary blood flow. This schematic of the maternal-infant unit displays those aspects of maternal pharmacokinetics which are discussed in the text. (Reproduced with permission from W.B. Saunders Co.)[1]

The changes in blood volume, plasma protein levels, and the cardiovascular system that occur during pregnancy return to basal, non-pregnant levels within 6 weeks after delivery, with most of the readjustment completed during the first 2 postpartum weeks.[9] Thus, the effect of an increased plasma volume, an increased total body water and a decreased serum albumin concentration on drug distribution are rapidly dissipated. However, while the majority of women will lose most of their pregnancy-acquired fat quickly, the distribution of lipid-soluble drugs during early lactation may be affected by the extra fat.[1,8]

Influence of Perinatal Factors on Maternal Drug Metabolism

Most drug metabolism occurs in the liver via microsomal oxidation, reduction, hydrolysis, and conjugation reactions.[7] The results of many animal studies demonstrate a marked inhibition of these drug-metabolizing enzyme activities during pregnancy, presumably due to high levels of estrogens and progestagens.[8,11] Although the limited data concerning the effects of human pregnancy on such drug biotransformation reactions do not support such an alteration during normal human pregnancy,[8,10,11] several reports[12-15] have inferred that pregnancy increases hepatic mixed-function oxidase and glucuromide-conjugating activity, since the plasma steady-state levels of several anticonvulsants were decreased beyond that explanable by changes in plasma-binding proteins. Nonetheless, since delivery is followed by a rapid fall in estrogen and progesterone in humans, their influence on drug metabolism during lactation would be quickly dissipated, unless severe liver disease had developed.

In addition to hepatic drug metabolism, drug metabolism by breast tissue during lactation must also be considered. Although such metabolism has only been shown for N-acetylation of sulfanilamide,[16] it is likely that breast tissue has the capability for biotransformation of some drugs.[17]

Influence of Perinatal Factors on Maternal Drug Excretion

The main route of drug excretion is via the kidneys, being a function of glomerular filtration, passive tubular reabsorption, and active tubular secretion.[7] If the total renal clearance of a drug approximates the glomerular filtration rate times the fraction of unbound drug in the plasma, then glomerular filtration is the principal excretion mechanism. However, if the degree of renal clearance of the drug is lower, passive tubular reabsorption is occurring in the proximal and/or distal tubule, while if the degree of renal clearance is greater, then active secretion of the drug is occurring in the proximal tubule. Since renal plasma flow and glomerular filtration rate increase by 60 to 100% during pregnancy, the total renal clearance of a drug would be expected to be increased.[8-10] In addition, this effect may be enhanced by the presence of a larger fraction of unbound drug due to the normally lower serum albumin concentration. However, renal function only influences the rate of drug elimination when the drug or an active metabolite is excreted unchanged in the urine.[7] A substantial loss of protein bound drug may occur with proteinuria from pre-eclampsia.[8,9]

As part of the postpartum physiological readjustment, renal blood flow and glomerular filtration rate promptly return to basal, non-pregnant values.[9] Thus, renal excretion of drugs during lactation should also revert to normal, unless abnormal renal function is present.

Biliary excretion of drugs would also be expected to be normal unless cholestasis was present.[8] However, a recent study in rats demonstrated an increased rate of bile acid secretion during lactation.[18] If such an alteration existed during human lactation, biliary excretion of drugs would be expected to be increased.

Mammary Blood Flow

The volume of mammary blood flow is the other important maternal factor that affects the transfer of drugs into human milk.[1,2] Since mammary blood flow is increased during lactation,[1,19] drug formulations and dosage schedules which maintain elevated plasma concentrations would tend to predispose toward more drug passage or clearance into milk than regimens that would minimize plasma drug concentration.[1,3,5]

Conclusion

In summary, although maternal pharmacokinetics may be altered during pregnancy, physiological readjustments which occur rapidly in the first several weeks postpartum should cause maternal pharmacokinetics during established lactation to be similar to those in non-pregnant women. However, only limited pharmacokinetic data supporting this speculation exist. Nonetheless, availability of drugs for potential transport into human milk can be viewed as a function of drug concentration in maternal plasma and mammary blood flow. The influence of maternal factors on drug transfer may be minimized by selection of drug preparations, dosage regimens, and feeding times which are associated with the lowest plasma drug concentrations.

REFERENCES

1. G. P. Giacoia and C. S. Catz, Drugs and pollutants in breast milk, _Clin Perinatol_ 6:181-196 (1979).
2. L. Beeley, Drugs and breast feeding, _Clin Obstet Gynecol_ 8:291-295 (1981).
3. D. Reinhardt and O. Richter, Pharmacokinetics of translactal passage, _in_: "Clinical Pharmacology in Pregnancy: Fundamentals and Rational Pharmacotherapy," H. P. Kuemmerle and K. Brendel, eds., Thieme-Stratton, Inc., New York (1984). 1984:260-268.
4. D. Pecorari, Translactal passage and pharmacotherapy of lactation, _in_: "Clinical Pharmacology in Pregnancy: Fundamentals and Rational Pharmacotherapy," H. P. Kuemmerle and K. Brendel, eds., Thieme-Stratton, Inc., New York (1984).
5. P. J. Lewis and E. L. Hurden, Drugs and breast feeding, _in_: "Drugs and Pregnancy: Human Teratogenesis and Related Problems," D. F. Hawkins, ed., Churchill Livingstone, Inc., New York (1983).
6. J. T. Wilson, R. D. Brown, J. L. Hinson, and J. W. Dailey, Pharmacokinetic pitfalls in the estimation of the breast milk/plasma ratio for drugs, _Ann Rev Pharmacol Toxicol_ 25:667-689 (1985).
7. E. Fingl and D. M. Woodbury, General Principles, _in_: "The Pharmacological Basis of Therapeutics, Fifth Edition," L.S. Goodman and A. Gilman, eds., MacMillan Publishing Co., Inc., New York (1975).
8. S. M. Wood and F. E. Hytten, The fate of drugs in pregnancy, _Clin Obstet Gynecol_ 8:255-259 (1981).
9. R. Resnik, Gestational changes of the reproductive tract and breasts: The puerperim, _in_: " Maternal-Fetal Medicine: Principles and Practice," R. K. Creasy and R. Resnik, eds., W.B. Saunders Company, Philadelphia (1984).
10. D. G. Grahame-Smith and J. K. Aronson, Drug therapy in the young, in the elderly, and in pregnancy, _in_: "The Oxford Textbook of Clinical Pharmacology and Drug Therapy," Oxford University Press, New York (1984).
11. I. Amon and H. Huller, Drug metabolism in the pregnant woman, _in_: "Clinical Pharmacology in Pregnancy: Fundamentals and Rational Pharmacotherapy," H. P. Kuemmerle and K. Brendel, eds., Thieme-Stratton, Inc., New York (1984).

12. M. Dam, J. Christiansen, O. Munck, and K. I. Bygind, Antiepiletic drugs: Metabolism in pregnancy, Clin Pharmacokinet 4:43-62 (1979).
13. M. J. Eadie, C. M. Lander, and J. H. Tyrer, Plasma drug level monitoring in pregnancy, Clin Pharmacokinet 2:427-436 (1977).
14. C. M. Lander, V. E. Edwards, M. J. Eadie, and J. H. Tyrer, Plasma anticonvulsant concentrations during pregnancy, Neurology 27:128-131 (1977).
15. K. I. Mygind, M. Dam, and J. Christiansen, Phenytoin and phenobarbitone plasma clearance during pregnancy, Acta Neurol Scand 54:160-166 (1976).
16. F. Rasmussen and J. T. Linzell, The acetylation of sulphanilamide by mammary tissue of lactating goats, Biochem Pharmacol 16:918-919 (1967).
17. J. T. Wilson, Determinants and consequences of drug excretion in breast milk, Drug Metab Rev 14:619-652 (1983).
18. M. J. G. Bolt, T. M. Lee, and H. Moltz, Altered bile acid physiology during lactation in the rat, Proc Soc Exp Biol Med 176:164-167 (1984).
19. M. Katz and R. K. Creasy, Mammary blood flow regulation in the nursing rabbit, Am J Obstet Gynecol 150:497-500 (1984).

EFFECT OF ORAL CONTRACEPTIVES ON LACTATION

Bo Lönnerdal

Department of Nutrition
University of California
Davis, CA 95616

INTRODUCTION

The use of oral contraceptive agents (OCAs) has been steadily increasing since their introduction in the 1960's. For women in industrialized countries this has been considered a generally safe method to avoid unplanned pregnancies. It should be recognized, however, that during these years the hormone levels used in OCAs have been decreasing. This has partially been due to some alarming reports of side-effects from the hormonal treatment and partially due to further research showing a high degree of contraceptive effect at levels lower than those originally used. Therefore, studies on the long-term effects of OCAs, besides the intended contraceptive effect, have been limited; the dosages and combinations of hormones have frequently changed[1].

The potential use of OCAs for population control in developing countries was recognized quite early. However, these were introduced later in the developing countries because of the high cost of the hormonal components and an estimation of poor compliance in less educated populations. The tendency to use OCAs has been increasing as the hormone levels have been decreasing (and subsequently, the cost decreasing). These advantages have combined with the initiation of local or international educational-health programs. Although depot injections of contraceptives also are used to avoid the compliance problem, OCAs are increasingly used in developing countries. Consequently, there are an increased number of women using OCAs in all parts of the world.

One of the most desired uses of any contraceptive method is to prevent the birth of the next child from being too close to that of the previous child. In developing countries, the consequences of short child-spacing are well known: a dramatic drain of natural resources in a situation of short nutritional supply and early weaning of breast-fed infants who face inadequate alternatives of feeding[2,3]. While the latter effect would be of less consequence in developed countries, it is still avoided by both gynecologists and women to ensure a "reasonable" space between child births. With the increasing popularity of OCAs, one can predict that lactating women will re-introduce their OCAs soon after birth. While this can easily be done without consulting gynecologists/pediatricians, the advise given when sought can be highly variable. This merely reflects the lack of scientific studies documenting the effects of OCAs on the lactating woman and her infant. This paper will review the literature with regard to the effects of OCAs on lactation performance, milk hormone levels and milk nutrient composition.

CHEMICAL COMPOSITION OF OCAs

A wide variety of hormones and hormone combinations as well as dosages have been used[1,4]. Although progestins have been used alone, a combination of a progestin and the estrogen ethinyl estradiol is most commonly used.

Table 1. Daily Dosages of Progestin-only OCAs

Hydroxyprogesterone acetate	30 mg	Toaff et al., 1969[5]
Chlormadinone diacetate	0.6 mg	Zanartu et al., 1976[6]
Chlormadinone acetate	0.5 mg	Hefnawi et al., 1976[6]
Lynestrenol	0.5 mg	Kamal et al., 1969[7]
Norethisterone	0.35 mg	Toddywalla et al., 1977[9]
Quingestanol acetate	0.3 mg	Guiloff et al., 1974[10]; Hefnawi et al., 1976[7]
Norgestrel	0.075 mg	Task Force, WHO, 1984[11]
Norgestrel	0.05 mg	Gupta et al., 1974[12]
Norgestrel	0.03 mg	Nilsson et al., 1977[13]

For the combination-type OCAs, the trend to decrease both the progestin and the estrogen component has been evident in recent years (Table 2).

The reason for this hormone combination is that the progestin-only OCAs are slightly less effective contraceptives than the combined types and are also more frequently associated with irregular uterine bleeding[1]. The dosages of the progestin-only OCAs vary widely because of differences in their potency (Table 1).

Table 2. Daily Dosages of Combination-type OCAs

Norethindione	10 mg	Mestranol	0.06 mg	Rice-Wray et al., 1963[14]
Quingestanol acetate	5 mg	Quinestrol	2 mg	Guiloff et al., 1970[15]
Norethisterone	5 mg	Mestranol	0.15 mg	Chinnatamby, 1973[16]
Megestrol acetate	4 mg	Ethinyl estradiol	0.05 mg	Nilsson et al., 1977[17]
Norethisterone acetate	4 mg	Ethinyl estradiol	0.05 mg	Chinnatamby, 1973;[16] Koetsawang et al., 1972[18]
Norethynodrel	2.5 mg	Mestranol	0.1 mg	Chinnatamby, 1973[16]
Norethisterone	2.5 mg	Mestranol	0.1 mg	Koetsawang et al., 1972[18]
Norethisterone	2.5 mg	Mestranol	0.075 mg	Chinnatamby, 1973[16]; Kamal et al., 1969[8]
Norethisterone	2 mg	Mestranol	0.1 mg	Koetsawang et al., 1972[18]
Norethisterone	1 mg	Mestranol	0.1 mg	Kamal et al., 1969[8]
Ethynodiol diacetate	1 mg	Mestranol	0.1 mg	Chinnatamby, 1973[16]; Koetsawang et al., 1972[18]
Norethindione	1 mg	Mestranol	0.08 mg	Miller and Hughes, 1970[19]
Norethindione	1 mg	Mestranol	0.05 mg	Kaern, 1967[20]
Norgestrel	0.5 mg	Ethinyl estradiol	0.05 mg	Gupta et al., 1974[12]; Ibrahim and El-Tawil, 1968[21]
Norgestrel	0.25 mg	Ethinyl estradiol	0.05 mg	Nilsson et al., 1977[13]
Norgestrel	0.15 mg	Ethinyl estradiol	0.05 mg	Nilsson et al., 1977[13]

METABOLIC CHANGES INDUCED BY OCAs

Besides their contraceptive effect, several metabolic changes are known to occur with the use of OCAs. Estrogens and progestins yield different responses in the body, therefore progestin-only and combination type OCAs result in different metabolic changes. Because of an implicated correlation between use of OCAs and risk of myocardial infarction, Bradley et al.[22] studied serum levels of high-density-lipoprotein (HDL) cholesterol in a large population of women. Women using progestin-only pills had significantly lower HDL cholesterol levels in serum than control women, while estrogen users had significantly higher levels. Women using combination-type OCAs had serum levels of HDL cholesterol that varied with the relative proportion of progestin to estrogen. It is therefore evident that HDL cholesterol levels can be affected by OCAs; the type of OCA used may be a contributory factor to vascular disorders in women[23].

Protein synthesis and consequently plasma protein levels are increased by OCAs[24]. This is probably the reason for the increased level of plasma vitamin A in OCA users; the concentration of retinol-binding protein (RBP) was also significantly higher in this group of women[25]. The effects were observed in the group of women taking estrogens (norethisterone acetate + ethinyl estradiol) but not in the progestin-only OCA group. This is in agreement with the results of Vahlquist et al.[26] who found an estrogen-stimulated increase in both plasma retinol-binding protein (RBP) and pre-albumin, the plasma protein to which RBP is normally bound.

Trace element metabolism is also affected by the use of OCAs[27-29]. A significant increase in serum copper levels occur in women that have taken OCAs for three months[30]. While some previous studies have found decreased serum zinc levels in women using OCAs as compared to non-users, neither this study nor that of Hinks et al.[31] found any effect of OCAs on plasma or serum zinc. However, other studies have shown an effect on serum zinc levels[28,32-34]. The increase in serum copper appears to be closely correlated to an increase in ceruloplasmin, the major copper binding protein in human serum[24]. Ceruloplasmin synthesis is stimulated by the estrogen component of OCAs[27], while progestins do not seem to affect serum copper or ceruloplasmin[34]. When OCAs were found to effect serum zinc, the decrease was primarily in the albumin-bound zinc pool; both the estrogen and the progestin appeared to cause such an effect[34]. Leukocyte, erythrocyte and hair trace element concentrations have been suggested as representative of long-term status; in the previously mentioned studies by Vir and Love[30] and Hinks et al.[31], no effects of OCAs were found on these parameters although the validity of using these parameters for assessment of trace element status is questionable. It is possible that only the circulating level of copper is affected without much consequence on status. A study by King et al.[35] indicates that absorption of trace elements is not significantly altered by the use of OCAs. If significant changes in trace element status were induced by OCAs, homeostatic regulation of trace element metabolism would have been expected to affect absorptive mechanisms.

EFFECTS OF OCAs ON BREAST MILK VOLUME AND DURATION OF LACTATION

Initially it was feared that OCAs would have negative consequences on lactation such as a decreased output of milk. Milk production and the consumption of milk by the breast-fed infant appears to be under the control of several complex psychological factors[36]. Therefore, the mothers' attitude to the OCAs and their potential effects on lactation may very well affect the results of studies intended to investigate the effects of OCAs on milk volume and composition. For obvious reasons, double-blind studies are ethically impossible to perform and bias of the subjects participating in the studies published to date has to be taken into consideration. One parameter that may be of value and which has been used in some studies, is to compare duration of lactation when using OCAs to previous lactation when not using OCAs. In general, mothers experience less problems with lactation and nurse for longer periods in subsequent lactation periods than in the first one[36].

The time interval postpartum prior to the introduction of OCAs is likely to effect whether or not a reduction in milk volume and lactation performance will occur. In a study by Kaern[20], a combination OCA was given immediately postpartum which led to significantly higher number of women giving complementary feeds to their infants, indicating inadequate milk yield. However, no significant change in infant weight gain was observed. Several studies, in which the postpartum interval prior to introduction of OCAs was not specified, have found negative effects of combination-type OCAs on milk volume and/or duration of lactation. Most of these studies were performed with doses of hormones considerably higher than those used presently[8,12,14-16,18,19,21,37,38]. Decreased milk volume was determined in some of these studies by pumping[8,38] or by test-weighing[12,37]. Contrary to these results, some studies have found no effect of combination-type OCAs on milk volume[5,39,40].

A recent series of studies in Chile using placebo groups[41-43] has focussed on the short- and long-term effects on a low dose combination-type OCA (0.030 mg ethinyl estradiol and 0.15 mg norgestrel). When the OCA was introduced 30 days postpartum, a lower percentage of women were exclusively breast-feeding at 3 months postpartum in the OCA group than in the control group. In addition, infants of OCA treated women had significantly lower weight gain than those of control groups (the control women received either an oral placebo or an injectable placebo). Later in lactation, a lower percentage of OCA treated women were exclusively lactating their infants at 4-10 months than control women. Infant weight data were less conclusive when comparing groups at this time period. When OCAs were introduced at 90 days of lactation, these authors state that a "moderate inhibitory influence" on lactation was noted; fewer OCA-treated women were exclusively breast-feeding and a lower infant weight gain was noted in this group as compared to controls. The overall effects appeared to be of similar magnitude as compared to the earlier introduction of OCAs. It should be noted that in the latter study, only mothers exclusively breast-feeding infants and having infants showing adequate weight gain were included.

Progestin-only OCAs have also been reported to have a negative effect on milk volume[7,9] and duration of lactation[10]. It should be cautioned though that in one study the number of women was low (n=7)[9] and in another the difference in milk yield not statistically significant[10]. Unchanged[5,12] or increased milk yield[7] and increased duration of lactation[44] have also been reported for this type of OCA.

A recent collaborative study by WHO in Thailand and Hungary has addressed several of the questions raised above[11]. In a double-blind design, women were given either a combination-type OCA (0.03 mg ethinyl estradiol + norgestrel) or a progestin-only OCA (0.075 mg d-norgestrel). Women using no contraception or non-hormonal contraception methods served as controls. The combination-type OCA led to a decrease in milk volume within 6 weeks of starting treatment (6 weeks postpartum), while no such decrease was observed in the other groups. Later in lactation (18 weeks of treatment), 42% of the women taking the combination-type OCA experienced a decline in milk volume, as compared to 12% of the progestin-only group and 6% of the control women. No differences were found among the groups for infant weight gain. The investigators concluded that in this population of selected healthy women, combined OCAs can impair milk production although no adverse effect was observed on their infants. It should be cautioned, however, that the composition of the milk produced by these women was not assessed and the mere criterion of infant growth may not reflect changes induced by potential changes in milk composition and/or composition of weight gain of the infants.

TRANSFER OF HORMONES INTO BREAST MILK

The relative proportion of contraceptive steroids that are transferred from maternal plasma into milk and its subsequent absorption and metabolism in the breast-fed infant has received little attention. In early studies[45-47], radiolabelled steroids were used to quantify transfer from the maternal circulation into the milk. A low proportion (highly variable), 0.02-1.52%, of the oral dose was found in the milk samples collected. It should be noted, however, that the milk was collected in very early lactation from mothers that for various reasons had chosen not to nurse their infants. Consequently, milk volumes collected were very low and not truly reflecting normal, fully established lactation. Van der Molen et al.[47] found that 0.02-0.09% of the administered radioactivity in the form of lynestrenol was transferred into milk and calculated that the amount of lynestrenol and its metabolites transfered into the infant with 600 ml per day would be about 0.1% of the dose given to the mother each day. A drawback with all these radiolabel studies is that both the active (intact) steroid as well as its metabolites are being measured together.

More recent studies have determined precise amounts of intact steroids in milk by the use of radioimmunoassays. Nilsson et al.[13] found that in women given OCAs containing 250 or 150 µg d-norgestrel, an average plasma to milk ratio of 100:15 was obtained. Foremilk contained about half the concentration of steroid found in hindmilk, which was suggested by the authors to reflect the lipophilic nature of this steroid as milk lipid concentration is considerably higher in hindmilk than in foremilk. Milk samples from mothers given an OCA containing only 30 µg of d-norgestrel did not contain measurable amounts of this steroid. The proportion of maternal steroid ingested by the mother which was found in the milk was estimated to about 0.1%, which is similar to the study by van der Molen et al.[47]. Plasma levels of d-norgestrel in the nursing infants were found to be similar to those found in plasma of women given this steroid, but it appeared that it was metabolized by the infants.

The same investigators[17] also studied the transfer of megestrol acetate into milk. A significantly higher proportion of this drug was transferred into the milk; the plasma to milk ratio was 100:80. Similar to what was found for d-norgestrel, hindmilk had a significantly higher concentration of megestrol acetate than foremilk. That the steroid is readily transferred into milk was illustrated by following the plasma and milk concentrations after giving the dose. The higher degree of transfer of megestrol acetate into milk as compared to d-norgestrel was explained by a different binding strength to a drug-binding protein in plasma, the so-called sex hormone binding globulin[48]. This protein has a much higher affinity to d-norgestrel than to megestrol acetate; 1.5 g of d-norgestrel will displace testosterone from the binding protein in vitro, while 740 g of megestrol acetate is required. Therefore, a low binding of megestrol acetate to the binding protein may explain why this steroid is more readily transferred into the milk.

The gestagens discussed above have very different biological potency and the dosages used for contraceptive effectiveness are therefore quite different. However, although 4 mg of megestrol acetate and 0.15 or 0.25 mg d-norgestrel was used daily, the absolute concentrations of these steroids in plasma were similar. This may reflect the high affinity of d-norgestrel for the binding protein. For the infant, though, the consequence will be a higher concentration of the less potent megestrol acetate ingested via the milk or a lower concentration of the more potent d-norgestrel. Further studies are clearly needed to determine the fractional absorption of steroids and their potential physiological effects in the infants. Although some studies have implicated OCAs as responsible for breast milk jaundice[49-51] or for infant gynecomastia (breast enlargement)[52-53], these findings are rare and cannot be considered as consistent side effects.

During the menstrual cycle, progesterone levels in milk follow those in plasma and about 12 mg/day of progesterone can be taken in by the infant at peak progesterone concentrations[54]. Estrogens are also transferred into milk of non-OCA users in a regular pattern during the menstruation cycle[55,56]. The quantity of estradiol in 600 ml of milk from mothers not using OCAs is about 3 to 6 ng during anovulatory cycles and 6-12 ng during ovulatory cycles. The amount transferred from mothers taking 50 μg of ethinyl estradiol has been estimated to be around 10 ng; i.e., in a range that can be considered physiological.

EFFECTS OF OCAs ON HUMAN MILK COMPOSITION

Besides the previously described methodological problems which are encountered when studying effects of drugs on lactation, there are several factors that need to be considered when collecting human milk samples. Duration of lactation (length of time postpartum), time of the day, time of prior feeding, fore- or hind-milk, amount expressed from the breast and time interval prior to analysis are all factors that need to be controlled to ensure proper comparisons among study groups. In few studies have these matters been taken into account and our knowledge about the effects of OCAs on the composition of human milk is still very limited.

An early study on the effect of various OCAs and an injectable CA was performed by Abdel Kader et al.[57] in Egypt. Mothers were given two types of combination-type OCAs (2.5 mg lynestrenol + 0.075 mg mestranol or 1.0 mg lynestrenol + 0.2 mg mestranol), one progestin-only OCA (0.5 mg lynestrenol) or an injectable CA (150 mg hydroxypregesterone + 10 mg estradiol enanthate). A control group was given a placebo and an intrauterine contraceptive device (IUCD). The study was stated to have been double-blind, but for obvious reasons this design must have been only the three OCA groups. Although introduction of the OCA was not specified, it is apparent from the milk protein concentrations that they represent very early lactation. It can therefore be assumed that the contraceptive methods were started immediately post partum or shortly thereafter. Milk samples were collected by pumping at specified time periods of the day every two weeks. Milk protein concentration decreased with lactation time in all groups but this decrease was only significant in milk of women using CAs. After 12 weeks, protein concentration of milk from the control group had decreased 5%, while that of the other groups had decreased ∿39-43%. There was no significant difference among the different treatments. Similar results were obtained for milk fat; in control women fat concentration changed little, while significant decreases were found for all treatments. Lactose concentration did not appear to be affected by the treatments. The inorganic constituents calcium, magnesium, sodium and potassium decreased in concentration with time in all groups; this decrease was claimed to be significant for the treatment groups. The effects observed were hypothesized to be mediated via an effect of the gestagens on alveolar cells which are involved in biosynthesis of milk constituents such as fat and most milk proteins. The fact that serum protein concentration increases during gestagen use was claimed as support for the hypothesis. In this study an effect on infant growth was observed and the decrease was found to be most pronounced for the high dose combination OCA and the injected groups.

In a study in Israel[5], two different OCAs were used. While the progestin-group (30 mg hydroxy progesterone acetate) had no change in milk nutrient concentrations, the estrogen (0.3 mg ethinyl estradiol daily) treated mothers had a significantly higher protein content in their milk. Total protein as analyzed by the Biuret-method, was found to be 2.20% for the estrogen-treated group and 1.88% and 1.76% for the progestin-treated group and control women, respectively. The high levels of protein observed in all milk samples is explained by the fact that they were collected on the fifth day after delivery. The OCA treatment had started immediately (1-4 h) after delivery, which may explain some of the effects on milk composition. Ramadan et al.[58] also introduced OCAs (3 mg chlormadinone acetate + 0.1 mg mestranol) early in lactation and followed the mothers for four months. Protein concentration decreased in milk from OCA-treated women, and by separating the milk proteins by chromatographic techniques it was observed that all milk proteins estimated (immunoglobulins, α-lactalbumin, serum albumin and casein subunits) were present in lower concentrations than in milk from women not taking OCAs. Fat concentration increased markedly while there was a minor increase in lactose in milk from women not using OCAs.

Introduction of OCAs was not until 1-9 months of lactation in the study by Barsivala and Virkar[59]. Major nutrients (fat, protein, lactose) as well as calcium and phosphorus were analyzed in women using either a combination-type OCA (0.5 mg norgestrel + 0.05 mg ethinyl estradiol), a progestin-only OCA (0.5 mg megestrol acetate) or conventional contraceptive methods. Each woman acted as her own control and was followed for three consecutive menstrual cycles. The decrease in milk protein, fat and calcium concentration was significantly more pronounced in women using combination-type OCA as compared to the other two groups. Although selection criteria for women participating were set and milk sampling appeared to be standardized, it is not known if the groups were matched with regard to lactation time. The decrease in concentrations of several milk nutrients is considerably more rapid in early lactation than later, and an over-representation of women with short lactation would give a larger decrease than in those with longer lactation time. The finding of similar mean protein concentrations at the start of the study speaks against this. The decrease in protein concentration in the combination-type OCA group appeared substantial (38%) as compared to the other groups (8-10%) after 3 menstrual cycles. Fat decreased by 39% in treated women as compared to 12% in control women and the decrease in calcium was 36% and 10%, respectively.

No effect on milk nutrient composition was observed in a study of Indian women[12]. Three types of OCAs were used and these were initiated at 6 weeks of lactation. It is interesting to note that although a marked decrease was noted in milk yield of women using combination-type OCAs, milk quality was not affected. These findings are similar to those of Koetsawang et al.[18].

Significant increases in milk protein concentration were observed in the studies by Abdel Kader et al.[60] and Toddywalla et al.[9]. In the first study, however, there were differences in milk protein concentration among groups already at the first sampling occasion. Time of introduction of OCAs was not specified but the first measurement was at 1-2 months. It is conceivable that medication was started very early post partum, but selection bias cannot be ruled out. Relative decrease in the groups appeared to be similar throughout the year that the women were followed. Fat and lactose were stated to be unaffected. The study by Toddywalla et al.[9] gives more details with regard to design of the study. Besides, a combination-type OCA (0.35 mg norethisterone + 0.01 ethinyl estradiol) and a low-dose progestagen (0.35 mg norethisterone). two types of injected CAs were used; all of these were compared to a control group. OCAs were introduced at 2 months of lactation and each mother served as her own control. Milk protein decreased to a significantly higher degree in the high-dose injected CA group as compared to the control groups. Of all other treatments, the low-dose progestagen group had the lowest milk protein concentration; the combination-type OCA group had protein levels similar to the control group up to 6 months of lactation. The results for milk fat and calcium were similar to those obtained for milk protein, while lactose and phosphorus concentrations were similar to those of the control group. Thus, it appears that the progestagen effect on milk fat and protein is counteracted by the addition of an estrogen.

Kirksey et al.[61] studied the effect of OCAs on minerals in human milk. In spite of effects on maternal serum copper levels, no effects on milk copper concentrations were observed. Calcium, magnesium, iron and zinc levels were also unaffected by prior maternal use of OCAs. Although an effect of OCAs on milk manganese concentration was reported, all values, including thos of control women, were considerably higher than other reports on manganese in human milk and methodological problems cannot be ruled out.

In our study[62], four different types of OCAs were initiated after 2 months of lactation (3 combination OCAs: HP: 4 mg megestrol acetate + 0.05 mg ethinyl estradiol; MP: 0.25 mg norgestrel + 0.05 mg ethinyl estradiol; LP: 0.15 mg norgestrel + 0.03 mg ethinyl estradiol; and one progestin-only OCA: PO: 0.03 mg norgestrel). HP was withdrawn from the market by the manufacturer early in the study, which limited the data from this group. The mothers were followed throughout lactation and milk volume, protein, non-protein nitrogen, lactose and individual milk proteins (lactoferrin, α-lactalbumin and serum albumin) were analyzed. Significant changes were observed between experimental groups and controls for all parameters studied, although the changes observed were within the physiological variation of human milk of control women. Decreased milk protein concentrations were most pronounced in the MP and LP groups; the PO group had values similar to controls. In the HP group, as long as it was followed, protein concentration as well as milk volume decreased to a significantly higher degree than in the control group. It should be noted that although these women were expecting to successfully nurse (and most of them had previously), had established effective lactation and had a positive attitude to OCAs (these well-educated women had, against advice, decided to use OCAs), 12 out of 21 women had the opinion that the treatments had negatively affected lactation. The volume measurements and the milk composition data supported their opinions.

CONCLUDING REMARKS

There appears to be a negative effect of OCAs on milk volume and that this effect is dose-related, although progestin-only OCAs at lower dosages rarely have been reported to adversely affect milk volume. The latter fact has led to a suggestion of estrogens having a suppressive effect on milk production through its action on prolactin secretion. The effects of OCAs on milk composition are very difficult to evaluate. In the few studies performed to date, widely varying dosages and hormone combinations were used, they were introduced at different time points and collection methods used and parameters analyzed varied considerably. Consequently, apparently conflicting results were obtained which may be explained by the above differences. It is very evident that further studies are needed using present dosages and standardized designs.

REFERENCES

1. Committee on Drugs, American Academy of Pediatrics, Breast-feeding and contraception, Pediatrics 68:138 (1981).
2. D. Wolfers and S. Scrimshaw, Child survival and intervals between pregnancies in Guayaquil, Ecuador, Popul. Stud. 29:479 (1985).
3. J. E. Anderson, J. S. Marks, and T.-K. Park, Breast-feeding, birth interval, and infant health, Pediatrics 74:695 (1984).
4. V. J. Hull, Research on the effects of hormonal contraceptives on lactation: current findings, methodological considerations and future priorities, World Health Stat. Q. 36:168 (1983).
5. R. Toaff, H. Ashkenazi, A. Schwartz, and M. Herzberg, Effects of oestrogen and progestagen on the composition of human milk, J. Reprod. Fert. 19:475 (1969).

6. J. Zanartu, E. Aguilera, and G. Munoz-Pinto, Maintenance of lactation by means of continuous low-dose progestogen given post-partum as a contraceptive, Contraception 13:313 (1976).
7. F. Hefnawi, G. Fawzi, and M. H. H. Badraoui, Effect of some progestational steroids on lactation in Egyptian women. I. Milk yield during the first year of lactation, J. Biosoc. Sci. 8:45 (1976).
8. I. Kamal, E. Hefnawi, M. Ghoneim, et al., Clinical, biochemical, and experimental studies on lactation. II. Clinical effects of gestagens on lactation, Am. J. Obstet. Gynecol. 105:324 (1969).
9. V. S. Toddywalla, L. Joshi, and K. Virkar, Effect of contraceptive steroids on human lactation, Am. J. Obstet. Gynecol. 127:245 (1977).
10. E. Guiloff, A. Ibarra-Polo, J. Zanartu, C. Toscannini, T. Mischler, and C. Gomez-Rogers, Effect of contraception on lactation, Am. J. Obstet. Gynecol. 118:42 (1974).
11. Task Force on Oral Contraceptives, WHO Special Programme of Research, Development and Research Training in Human Reproduction, Effects of hormonal contraceptives on milk volume and infant growth, Contraception 30:505 (1984).
12. A. K. Gupta, V. S. Mathur, and S. K. Garg, Effect of oral contraception on quantity and quality of milk secretion in human beings, Indian J. Med. Res. 62:964 (1974).
13. S. Nilsson, K. G. Nygren, and E. D. B. Johansson, d-Norgestrel concentrations in maternal plasma, milk, and child plasma during administration of oral contraceptives to nursing women, Am. J. Obstet. Gynecol. 128:178 (1977).
14. E. Rice-Wray, J. W. Goldzieher, and A. Aranda-Rosell, Oral progestins in fertility control: a comparative study, Fertil. Steril. 14:402 (1963).
15. E. Guiloff, E. Berman, A. Montiglio, R. Osorio, and C. W. Lloyd, Clinical study of a once-a-month oral contraceptive: quinestrol-quingestanol, Fertil. Steril. 21:110 (1970).
16. S. Chinnatamby, Effects of "Nordiol" on fertility and lactation: some preliminary observations, Curr. Med. Res. Op. 1:376 (1973).
17. S. Nilsson, K. G. Nygren, and E. D. B. Johansson, Megestrol acetate concentrations in plasma and milk during administration of an oral contraceptive containing 4 mg megestrol acetate to nursing women, Contraception 16:615 (1977).
18. S. Koetsawang, P. Bhiraleus, and T. Chiemprajert, Effects of oral contraception on lactation, Fertil. Steril. 23:24 (1972).
19. G. H. Miller and L. R. Hughes, Lactation and genital involution effects of a new low-dose oral contraceptive on breast-feeding mothers and their infants, Obstet. Gynecol. 35:44 (1970).
20. T. Kaern, Effect of an oral contraceptive immediately port partum on initiation of lactation, Br. Med. J. 3:644 (1967).
21. A. Ibrahim and N. Z. El-Tarvil, The effect of a new low-dosage oral contraceptive pill on lactation, Int. Surg. 49:561 (1968).
22. D. D. Bradley, J. Wingerd, D. B. Petitti, R. M. Krauss, and S. Ramcharan, Serum high-density-lipoprotein cholesterol in women using oral contraceptives, estrogens and progestins, N. Engl. J. Med. 299:17 (1978).
23. Collaborative Group for the Study of Stroke in Young Women, Oral contraception and increased risk of cerebral ischemia or thrombosis, N. Engl. J. Med. 288:87 (1973).
24. C.-B. Laurell, S. Kullander, and J. Thorell, Rate of plasma protein normalization after parturition and withdrawal of oral contraceptives, Scand. J. Clin. Lab. Invest. 26:345 (1970).
25. F. J. Cumming and M. H. Briggs, Changes in plasma vitamin A in lactating and non-lactating oral contraceptive users, Br. J. Obstet. Gynecol. 90:73 (1983).

26. A. Vahlquist, A. Johnsson, and K. Nygren, Vitamin A transporting plasma proteins and female sex hormones, Am. J. Clin. Nutr. 32:1433 (1979).
27. M. E. Carruthers, C. B. Hobbs, and R. L. Warren, Raised serum copper and ceruloplasmin levels in subjects taking oral contraceptives, J. Clin. Pathol. 19:498 (1966).
28. J. A. Halsted, B. M. Haddey, and J. C. Smith, Plasma zinc and copper in pregnancy and after oral contraceptives, Lancet 2:278 (1968).
29. J. G. Schenker, S. Hellerstein, E. Jungreis, and W. Z. Polishuk, Serum copper and zinc levels in patients taking oral contraceptives, Fertil. Steril. 22:229 (1971).
30. S. C. Vir and A. H. G. Love, Zinc and copper nutriture of women taking oral contraceptive agents, Am. J. Clin. Nutr. 34:1479 (1981).
31. L. J. Hinks, B. E. Clayton, and R. S. Lloyd, Zinc and copper concentrations in leucocytes and erythrocytes in healthy adults and the effect of oral contraceptives, J. Clin. Pathol., 36:1016 (1983).
32. M. H. Briggs, M. Briggs, and J. Austin, Effects of steroid pharmaceuticals on plasma zinc, Nature 232:480 (1971).
33. A. S. Prasad, D. Oberleas, K. Y. Lei, K. S. Moghissi, and J. C. Stryher, Effect of oral contraceptive agents on nutrients. 1. Minerals, Am. J. Clin. Nutr., 28:377 (1975).
34. D. C. Chilvers, A. Hodgkinson, and M. K. Bahreyni-Toosi, Steroid-induced changes in plasma protein-bound copper and zinc in post-menopausal women, in: "Trace Element - Analytical Chemistry in Medicine and Biology," vol. 2, Berlin, Walter de Gruyter (1983).
35. J. C. King, W. L. Raynolds, and S. Margen, Absorption of stable isotopes of iron, copper, and zinc during oral contraceptive use, Am. J. Clin. Nutr. 31:1198 (1978).
36. D. B. Jelliffe and E. F. P. Jelliffe, Human Milk in the Modern World, Oxford, Oxford University Press (1978).
37. S. J. Kora, Effect of oral contraceptives on lactation, Fert. Ster. 20:419 (1969).
38. N. E. Borglin and L. E. Sandholm, Effect of oral contraceptives on lactation, Fertil. Steril. 22:39 (1971).
39. K. Semm and F. W. Dittmar, Post partum ovulation: inhibition and milk yield, Curr. Therap. Res. 8:48 (1966).
40. I. Kamal, F. Hefnawi, M. Ghoneim, M. Abdallah, and S. Abdel Razeh, Clinical, biochemical, and experimental studies on lactation, Am. J. Clin. Nutr. 108:655 (1970).
41. S. Diaz, O. Peralta, G. Juez, C. Herreros, M. E. Casado, A. M. Salvatierra, P. Miranda, E. Duran, and H. B. Croxatto, Fertility regulation in nursing women: III. Short-term influence of a low-dose combined oral contraceptive upon lactation and infant growth, Contraception 27:1 (1983).
42. H. B. Croxatto, S. Diaz, O. Peralta, G. Juez, C. Herreros, M. E. Casado, A. M. Salvatierra, P. Miranda, and E. Duran, Fertility regulation in nursing women: IV. Long-term influence of a low-dose combined oral contraceptive initiated at day 30 postpartum upon lactation and infant growth, Contraception 27:13 (1983).
43. O. Peralta, S. Diaz, G. Juez, C. Herreros, M. E. Casado, A. M. Salvatierra, P. Miranda, E. Duran, and H. B. Croxatto, Fertility regulation in nursing women: V. Long-term influence of a low-dose combined oral contraceptive initiated at day 90 postpartum upon lactation and infant growth, Contraception 27:27 (1983).
44. J. Zanartu, E. Aguilera, and G. Munoz, Effect of a long-acting contraceptive progestogen on lactation, Obstet. Gynecol. 47:174 (1976).
45. G. Pincus, G. Bialy, D. S. Layne, M. Paniagua, and K. I. H. Williams, Radioactivity in the milk of subjects receiving radioactive 19-norsteroids, Nature 212:924 (1966).
46. K. R. Laumas, P. K. Malkani, S. Bhatnagar, and V. Laumas, Radioactivity in the breast milk of lactating women after oral administration of ^{3}H-norethynodrel, Am. J. Obstet. Gynecol. 98:411 (1967).

47. H. J. van der Molen, P. G. Hart, and H. G. Wijinenga, Studies with 4-^{14}C-lynestrenol in normal and lactating women, Acta. Endocrinol. 61:665 (1969).
48. A. Victor, E. Weiner, and E. D. B. Johansson, Sex hormone binding globulin: the carrier protein for d-norgestrel, J. Clin. Endocrinol. Metab. 43:244 (1976).
49. Y. K. Wong and B. S. Wood, Breast-milk jaundice and oral contraceptives, Br. Med. J. 4:403 (1971).
50. D. Barnardo, et al.,Breast-milk jaundice and the pill, Br. Med. J. 2:348 (1972).
51. J. B. McConnell, et al., Effect on neonatal jaundice of estrogens and progestogens taken before and after conception, Br. Med. J. 3:605 (1973).
52. E. M. Curtis, Oral contraceptive feminization of a normal male infant, Obstet. Gynecol. 23:295 (1964).
53. J. J. Gellen, Fertility regulation during human lactation: Side effects of steroid contraception, J. Biosoc. Sci. 4(suppl.):149 (1977).
54. P. Hartmann and C. G. Prosser, Acute changes in the composition of milk during the ovulatory menstrual cycle in lactating women, J. Physiol. Lond. 324:21 (1982).
55. S. Nilsson, K. G. Nygren, and E. D. B. Johansson, Ethinyl estradiol in human milk and plasma after oral administration, Contraception 17:131 (1978).
56. S. Nilsson, K. G. Nygren, and E. D. B. Johansson, Tranfer of estradiol to human milk, Am. J. Obstet. Gyneol. 132:653 (1978).
57. M. M. Abdel Kader, A. Abdel Hay, S. El-Safouri, M. T. Abdel Aziz, J. Saad-El-Din, I. Kamal, F. Hefnawi, M. Ghoneim, M. Talaat, N. Younis, A. Tagui, and M. Abdulla, Clinical, biochemical, and experimental studies on lactation. III. Biochemical changes induced in human milk by gestagens. Am. J. Obstet. Gynecol. 105:324 (1969).
58. M. A. Ramadan, M. M. Salah, S. Z. Eid, and M. B. Sammour, The effect of the oral contraceptive ovosiston on the composition of human milk, J. Reprod. Med. 9:81 (1972).
59. V. M. Barsivala and K. D. Virkar, The effect of oral contraceptives on concentrations of various components of human milk, Contraception 7:307 (1973).
60. M. M. Abdel Kader, M. T. Abdel Aziz, R. Bahgat, F. Hefnawi, G. Fawzi, and M. H. H. Badraoui, Effect of some progestational steroids on lactation in Egyptian women. II. Chemical composition of milk during the first year of lactation, J. Biosoc. Sci. 8:49 (1976).
61 A. Kirksey, J. A. Ernst, J. L. Roepke, and T.-L. Tsai, Influence of mineral intake and use of oral contraceptives on the mineral content of human colostrum and of more mature milk, Am. J. Clin. Nutr. 32:30 (1979).
62. B. Lonnerdal, E. Forsum, and L. Hambraeus, Effect of oral contraceptives on composition and volume of breast milk, Am. J. Clin. Nutr., 33:816 (1980).

DRUG EXCRETION INTO HUMAN MILK:
ANSWERED AND UNANSWERED QUESTIONS

Cheston M. Berlin, Jr.

Department of Pediatrics
The Pennsylvania State University College of Medicine
The Milton S. Hershey Medical Center
P. O. Box 850
Hershey, Pennsylvania 17033

In the United States, interest in and support of breast feeding grew greatly beginning in the early 1970's. Knowledge of drug and chemical excretion at that time was quite limited. Most studies concerned single case reports with analyses of drugs done at random times after maternal administration. Considerable progress has been made since then, both in studies of groups of lactating women with more complete sampling periods and also in the use of more precise qualitative and quantitative instrumentation. This paper will discuss both results as well as unsolved problems of studies in humans.

QUESTIONS ANSWERED

1. What Type of Compounds Are Excreted Into Human Milk?

Nearly all types. The major factors limiting a drug appearing in human milk are:

a. Molecular weight above 200 (or higher for some lipophilic drugs). Sulfasalazine (M.W.=398) does not appear in human milk although its metabolic sulfapyridine does[1].

b. Degree of binding to maternal plasma proteins. Warfarin is over 90% bound to maternal plasma proteins; it has not been found in milk of mothers on chronic dosing[2]. This factor is also influenced by distribution characteristics of a drug.

c. Degree of ionization at plasma pH of 7.40. Unionized compounds appear to traverse cell membranes easier than ionized compounds. This is accentuated by lipid solubility. A marked exception to this is in the case of the lithium ion which crosses well. Its very small molecular weight may allow it to easily diffuse through membrane pores[3] or it may have a specific membrane transport protein.

d. Lipid solubility. A small molecular weight compound with high lipid solubility and unionized at pH 7.40 will cross easily. Ethanol levels in human milk are identical with simultaneous maternal plasma levels[4].

It is clear that for each drug all of the above have to be considered. Although of a high molecular weight, dieldrin (M.W.=380) and DDT (M.W.=354) are very lipid soluble and are found in most samples of human milk in the United States[5], albeit in very small quantities (about 0.1-0.2 parts per million).

2. How Much Drug Crosses Into Milk?

Studies employing a single maternal dose with subsequent miltiple milk samplings have permitted reasonably accurate estimations for a small number of drugs. Two examples will illustrate this. Assuming that the infant will ingest 90 mls. of milk every three hours after maternal dosing, it has been found that for acetaminophen the mean exposure for an infant is 1 mg in the 24 hours after a single 650 mg maternal dose. No acetaminophen or its metabolites (glucuronide, sulfate) were detected in infants' urine[6]. White et al studied α-methyldopa[7]. Three mothers received chronic α-methyldopa therapy: 2 received 500 mg q.d. and the third received 1000 mg per day. In the 12 hours after a 500 mg maternal dose a nursing infant would be exposed to an estimated dose of 188 μg of a α-methyldopa. In one of three infants the drug was detectable in the infant's plasma at very low levels (0.09 μg/ml) 10 hours after maternal ingestion. Such data are becoming increasingly available for a number of compounds. This allows quantitative estimation of risk to the nursing infant. It must be emphasized that calculation of amount offered to infant in milk cannot predict how much will actually reach the infant. Timing of nursing is the most obvious way of minimizing drug exposure. Erickson et al give a good illustration of this with the drug metronidazole[8]. The authors assumed that if the infant would nurse 165 mls. every six hours starting at two hours following a 2 gm oral dose to mother, he would be exposed to 15.5 mg in the first 12 hours, 21.8 mg in the first 24 hours and only 3.5 mg in the second 24 hours. If nursing is delayed 24 hours after the single dose, very little drug would be excreted in the milk and hence exposure of the infant would be negligible.

3. Are Metabolites Secreted Into Milk?

The answer to this is yes based upon a very small number of studies (summarized by Wilson et al[9]). Limitations appear to be both technical (metabolite concentrations at or below the limit of detection by instrumentation) and a consequence of rapid maternal plasma clearance of the metabolite so that very little is available for passage into milk, e.g. 5-aminosalicylic acid (sulfasalazine metabolite)[1] and acetaminophen glucuronide[6].

4. Are Pharmacokinetics of Drugs in Milk Understandable by Standard Techniques?

The answer is yes as illustrated by the extensive work of Wilson et al[9,10]. Much of their work requires knowledge of milk/plasma ratios which is reported at this Symposium. See unanswered question #4, the answer to which may modify current concepts.

5. Is It Safe for Infants to be Exposed to Milk From a Medicated Mother?

The answer appears to be a qualified yes with some exceptions. The qualification is due to a data base consisting mainly of single case reports[11]. The long-term (years and decades) effects on the nursing infant ingesting milk with trace amounts of drugs or chemicals (e.g. insecticides) are, of course, unknown and may remain so. This leads to a consideration of the unanswered questions of drugs in milk.

QUESTIONS UNANSWERED

1. What is the Amount of Drug Transferred to Milk in Lactating Women on Chronic Drug Therapy?

Most reports deal with single dose studies. No doubt the reason such small amounts are transferred to milk is the rapid decline in maternal plasma concentrations for drugs with a short half-life; after six hours, very little of any drug studied so far is available for transfer.

Figure 1 shows data calculated from the report of the excretion of acetaminophen in human milk[6]. The amount available to this nursing infant in the 24 hours after a single maternal dose of 650 mg is 0.8 mg. However, if sufficient repeated doses of the drug are ingested by mother to keep her

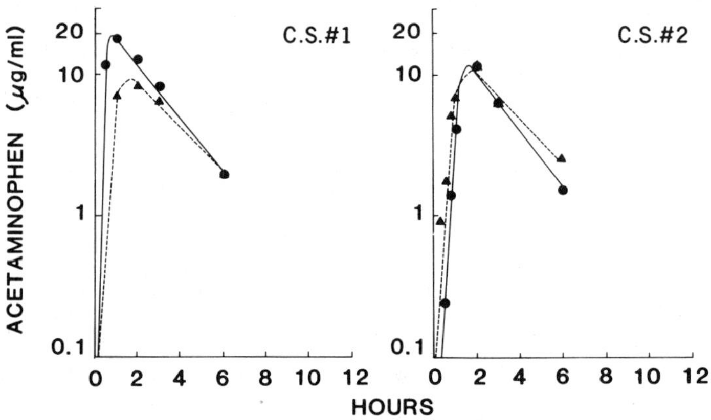

Fig. 1. Time course of the appearance and disappearance of acetaminophen in human milk under two conditions: a single dose of 650 mg of acetaminophen and with multiple dosing such that the plasma (and hence) the milk level is held constant at 15 μg/ml. The mg/24 hr refers to the amount of acetaminophen available to the infant who nurses 90 ml every 3 hr for the 24-hr time period. From: Banbury Report 1982;11:495. Cold Spring Harbor Laboratory. Reproduced by permission.

plasma level at 15 μg/ml, then the amount available for ingestion by the infant is 10.8mg, or a 13.5 fold increase. A case report involving aspirin echoes this increased risk. A 16-day-old infant developed symptomatic salicylism with a serum concentration of 24 mg/dl after nursing from a mother taking 650 mg of aspirin every four hours[12]. Berlin and Yaffe[1] reported an infant with detectable urinary sulfapyridine (3-4 μg/ml urine) nursing from a mother on chronic sulfasalazine therapy (500 mg qid). On the other hand, digoxin was not detected in the plasma of infants whose mothers were on chronic digoxin therapy[13].

Much work needs to be done on sufficient numbers of mother-nursing infant pairs to elucidate with confidence the pattern of drug excretion in mothers on chronic drug therapy.

2. Is There a Difference Between Assaying a Drug in the Relatively Small Samples (About 15-30 ml) Usually Obtained by Expression vs. Completely Emptying the Breast (90-120 ml)?

There are no data on this point in humans. However, Rasmussen, studying the cow, detected no difference[14]. Completely emptying the breast by any means is difficult for some mothers. Possible differences between fore and hind milk need to be clarified.

3. Can Breast Tissue Metabolize Drugs?

Certainly the lactating breast is a very active metabolizing organ synthesizing, for example, in one liter of milk: 10 grams protein, 70 grams lactose and 33 grams of fat. No metabolites have yet been described that could not be explained by prior formation in the liver. Breast tissue may possess the capacity to make unusual, and perhaps, toxic metabolites[15]. New methodology to detect very small quantities of such metabolites may answer this question.

4. Does Back Diffusion Occur Into Maternal Circulation of Drug From Either the Aveolar Lumen or Cell?

This is perhaps the most important unanswered question. It is obviously closely related to question #5 concerning storage of milk in the breast. Decay of drug concentration in parallel with maternal plasma decay (viz. antipyrine, acetaminophen, theophylline) argues for back diffusion (at least relatively rapid back diffusion). But divergent decay curves (e.g. caffeine) may suggest either back diffusion (milk decay more rapid than maternal plasma) or storage (maternal plasma decay more rapid than milk) - perhaps in breast gland fat. Rasmussen has demonstrated back diffusion for a number of compounds in the cow[4]. However, the pharmacokinetic simulations of Wilson et al[9] show different ingress and egress rates for drug transfer in milk.

5. Does Significant Storage of Milk Occur in the Breast Between Feedings?

The above cited studies suggest that when drug concentrations in both milk and maternal plasma decrease in parallel, then there is no storage (accumulation) of the drug in milk, or else the curves should be divergent. Many nursing women report shrinkage of breast size and absence of milk leakage after 4-6 months of nursing. It is intriguing to speculate that for the established lactating woman, milk may be formed (at least the aqueous part) while suckling occurs. Consider an analogy to the kidney; both kidneys filter about 125 ml/min. of fluid with a resultant urine flow of 2-3 ml/min. Thus, during a 20 minute nursing period on each side (40 minutes total) it would be very reasonable for a breast to secrete a total 120 ml or more of milk.

If a mother wishes to minimize drug exposure in her offspring by temporarily stopping nursing until her plasma level has declined to very low or undetectable level, should she pump during this period of time in order to empty the breast of milk and, presumably, stored drug? The only suggestion to an answer to this is seen in Figure 2 (taken from [6]). This

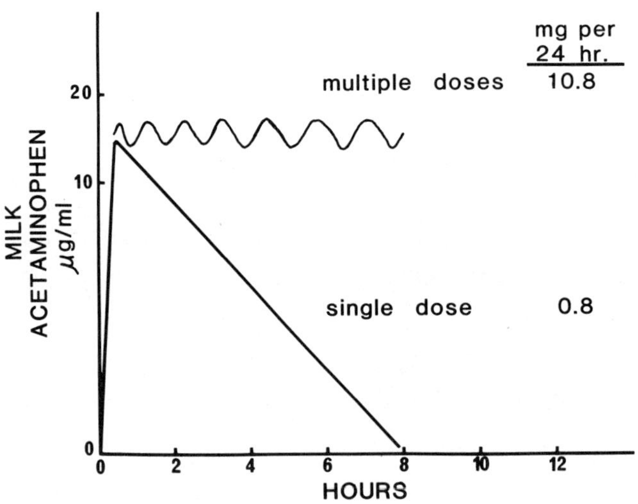

Fig. 2. Appearance and disappearance of acetaminophen in milk following oral dose of 650 mg acetaminophen. CS #1 was actively nursing at the time this study was done. CS #2 was done 2 weeks after weaning. From: Pediatric Pharmacology 1980;1:139. Reproduced by permission.

mother took a single 650 mg dose of acetaminophen on two separate occasions two months apart. The first time she was actively nursing and the second time she had stopped nursing two weeks previously, but was able to express milk samples for analyses. There is little difference in the elimination rate constant. Clearly, the frequency of emptying the breast seemed to have no effect of drug appearance in this subject with this particular drug.

Further studies need to be done to determine the time course changes in the transfer of drugs into human milk. These studies should be done with and without evacuation of milk by the infant.

6. Do Variations in Milk Components Affect Drug Excretion?

There is little variation in protein or lactose concentration, but alterations in fat amount or type may be contributory. Do milk fat globules concentrate lipophilic drugs? (See paper by Patton in this monograph.) Is there preferential binding by milk fat or even milk protein in comparison to plasma free fatty acids or proteins? Perhaps *in vitro* experiments utilizing isotopes could definitively answer this question.

As the above questions point out, answers to questions of pharmacology require answers based in physiology. A clearer understanding of the excretion of drugs in milk will require substantial elucidation of the physiology of lactation, especially the timing of milk formation in relation to drug concentration in plasma. It is most probable that current and future studies will allow careful drug administration to the nursing mother without placing the infant at risk.

REFERENCES

1. C. M. Berlin and S. J. Yaffe, Disposition of salicylazo-sulfapyridine and metabolites in human breast milk, *Develop. Pharmacol. Therap.* 1:31 (1980).
2. M. L. Orne, P. J. Lewis, M. de Swiet, M. J. Serlin, R. Sibeon, J. D. Baty, and A. M. Breckenridge, May mothers given warfarin breast-feed their infants?, *Brit. Med. J.* 1:1564 (1977).
3. M. Schou and A. Amdisen, Lithium and pregnancy-III, Lithium ingestion by children breast-fed by women on lithium treatment, *Brit. Med. J.* 2:138 (1973).

4. Y. A. Kesaniema, Ethanol and acetaldehyde in the milk and peripheral blood of lactating women after ethanol administration, J. Obst. Gynecol. Br. Commonwealth 81:84 (1974).
5. E. P. Savage, T. J. Keefe, J. D. Tessari, H. W. Wheeler, F. M. Applehaus, E. A. Grees, and S. A. Ford, National study of chlorinated hydrocarbon insecticide residues in human milk, USA. I. Geographic distribution of dieldrin, heptachlor, heptachlor epoxide, chlordane, oxychlordane and mirex, Amer. J. Epidem. 113:413, (1981).
6. C. M. Berlin, Jr., S. J. Yaffe, and M. Ragni, Disposition of acetaminophen in milk, saliva, and plasma of lactating women, Pediat. Pharmacol. 1:135 (1980).
7. W. B. White, J. W. Andreoli, and R. D. Cohen, Alpha-methyldopa disposition in mothers with hypertension and in their breast-fed infants, Clin. Pharmacol. Ther. 37:387 (1985).
8. S. H. Erickson, G. L. Oppenheim, and G. H. Smith, Metronidazole in breast milk. Obstet. Gynec. 57:48 (1981).
9. J. T. Wilson, R. D. Brown, J. L. Hinson, and J. W. Dailey, Pharmacokinetic pitfalls in the estimation of the breast milk/plasma ratio for drugs, Ann. Rev. Pharmacol. Toxicol. 25:667 (1985).
10. J. T. Wilson, R. D. Brown, D. R. Cherek, J. W. Dailey, B. Hilman, P. L. Jobe, B. R. Manno, J. E. Manno, H. M. Redetzki, and J. J. Stewart, Drug excretion in human breast milk: Principles, pharmacokinetics and projected consequences, Clin. Pharmacokin. 5:1 (1980).
11. C. M. Berlin, Jr., Pharmacologic considerations of drug use in the lactating mother, Obstet. Gynecol. 58:175 (1981).
12. J. H. Clark and W. G. Wilson, A 16-day-old breast-fed infant with metabolic acidosis caused by salicylate, Clin. Ped. 20:53 (1981).
13. P. M. Loughnan, Digoxin excretion in human breast milk, J. Peds. 92:1019 (1978).
14. F. Rasmussen, Excretion of drugs by milk, in "Concepts in Biochemical Pharmacology Part I. Handbook of Experimental Pharmacology Vol. 28, B. B. Brodie and J. R. Gillette, ed., Springer-Verlag, New York (1971).
15. G. Bruder, A. Fink, and E. D. Jarasch, The B-type cytochrome in endoplasmic reticulum of mammary gland epithelium and milk fat globule membranes consisting of two components, cytochrome b_5 and cytochrome P-420. Exper. Cell Res. 117:207 (1978).

CELLULAR PATHWAYS IN THE MOVEMENT OF LIPOPHILIC XENOBIOTICS FROM GI TRACT TO BREAST MILK

John S. Patton

Department of Pharmacological Sciences
Genentech, Inc., 460 Point San Bruno Boulevard
South San Francisco, CA 94080

INTRODUCTION

Throughout the world human breast milk is contaminated with fat soluble (log octanol/water partition coefficient >5) organic molecules that have originated from industrial synthesis or the pyrolysis of organic matter (lipophilic xenobiotics = LXs). There have been numerous measurements of contaminant levels in human milk (for a review see Jensen 1983) most of which have focused on the lipophilic xenobiotics. On a whole milk basis the concentrations are usually in the parts per billion (ppb) or parts per trillion (ppt) range, which seems miniscule; however, if one adds up the molecules, 100 ml of milk contaminated with 1 ppb DDT contains approximately 17,000,000,000,000 molecules of the pesticide. Although there are many kinds of lipophilic xenobiotics, DDT and PCB contaminants have been the most studied (the use of both is banned in the U.S.A.). PCBs, which have primarily urban and industrial applications, are found in highest levels (ppms) in human milk in urban and industrial areas (Jensen 1983). In contrast, the highest levels of DDT in human milk (ppms) are found in rural agriculture areas where its use as an insecticide is still approved (Campos and Olszyna-Marzys, 1979).

The purpose of this article is to discuss the cellular pathways followed by lipophilic xenobiotics as they move from the diet to breast milk.

MODERN AND ANCIENT XENOBIOTICS

Halogenation of certain organic molecules under extreme conditions (i.e., in some cases, boiling sulfuric acid) has produced a wide variety of modern xenobiotic chemicals that have many unique properties, not the least of which is remarkable stability. Highly fat soluble, these organohalide chemicals have been used as insecticides (i.e., DDT), flame retardants (i.e., polybrominated biphenyls - PBBs), and as electrical insulating material (i.e., polychlorinated biphenyls - PCBs), just to name a very few of their many applications. Worldwide production of them has been enormous. Unfortunately the stability of these new chemicals, coupled with their great affinity for the lipids of organisms has been their "achilles heel". They have permeated the global food chain and some have been shown to be toxic to a variety of organisms, including humans (Rogan et al., 1980). They are aptly classified as xenobiotics, "foreign to biology". Evolution has had very little time to adapt to them; many of them accumulate in organisms because existing enzymes have little, if any, capacity to hydroxylate and conjugate them for excretion.

Another group of fat soluble organic molecules, the polynuclear aromatic hydrocarbons (PAHs) are also called xenobiotics. They too have permeated the global environment but they originate from fossil fuels and are produced when organic material is burned (i.e., in forest fires, or during the high temperature cooking of food). Thus, although organisms do not synthesize PAHs, they have been in the environment for millions of years. Humans have been breathing and ingesting PAHs from their cooking and warming fires for perhaps as long as one million years. Enzymes that rapidly hydroxylate and conjugate PAHs are widespread in animal tissues. PAHs in food and air occur as a complex mixtures of many molecules, all having different numbers of aromatic rings in different isomeric arrangements. Benzo(a)pyrene (BP), a typical PAH, has become the "E. coli" of PAHs and a very large literature is available on its carcinogenicity and metabolism (Jones and Leber, 1979). The PAHs can be thought of as ancient xenobiotics and the organohalides, like the PCBs, as modern xenobiotics. The octanol/water partition coefficients (K_{ow}) of both of these classes of lipophilic xenobiotics are similar (log K_{ow} 4–7).

In addition to the two classes of fat soluble molecules described above there are many others. Nature produces an enormous variety of its own fat soluble organics (Patton, 1981) including long chain fatty acids and alcohols, sterols, long chain hydrocarbons, fat soluble vitamins, wax esters, and countless secondary metabolites, from which numerous drugs have been derived. The octanol/water partition coefficients of many of these molecules are similar to those of the PAHs, DDT and PCBs (Patton et al., 1984).

OVERVIEW

Numerous factors control the transfer of a drug or xenobiotic from the gastrointestinal tract to breast milk (Welsh and Findlay, 1981, Findlay, 1983 and Wilson et al. 1985). The pka of the compound, its protein binding characteristics, lipid/water partition coefficient and rate and degree of metabolism, are some of the most important determinants of its biological fate. In some ways the pharmacokinetics of the lipophilic xenobiotics are easier to predict and study than the pharmacokinetics of more water soluble compounds. Since they are uncharged, pH is not an important factor in their disposition; their high lipophilicity means that their binding to protein and lipid will be maximal, and when their rates of metabolism are slow, as they often are, they persist in organisms for a long time (i.e., days, weeks, months and even years in some cases compared to minutes and hours for most drugs). Because lipophilic xenobiotics equilibrate with body lipid in chronically exposed individuals, their concentration in any tissue parallels the concentration of lipid in that tissue. Thus although whole milk levels of lipophilic xenobiotics are generally ten times that of blood levels (Yakushiji et al., 1978, 1979), on a lipid basis both fluids contain similar concentrations of the xenobiotic. In the absence of metabolism (which usually makes rapid excretion possible) some highly lipophilic xenobiotics that were acquired at one time may theoretically persist in a person in gradually declining concentrations throughout their lifetime (DeWolfe Miller et al., 1984). This is not to say that persistence is a static phenomenon; on the contrary, lipophilic xenobiotics are continually partitioning from tissue lipid into blood lipid and then back to tissue lipid again in a continuous dynamic cycle. One way for an organism to efficiently excrete these persistent lipophilic xenobiotics is to secrete fat. For mothers, lactation represents a rapid excretion pathway for some compounds that would otherwise remain in the body (Yakushiji et al., 1978). Figure 1 shows the decline in total PCBs in mother's blood following delivery and subsequent nursing of a child. Note that before delivery PCB blood levels were relatively constant.

The pharmacokinetics of lipophilic xenobiotics is complicated by the fact that they usually occur in the environment and in food as complex mixtures of many different isomers and homologs, each of which has its own unique pharmacokinetics and partition coefficient (see for example Rapaport and Eisenrich, 1984): some are rapidly metabolized and others are not. Figure 2 shows two typical PCB chromatograms, one from a standard PCB mixture (Figure 2A) and one from the fat of a PCB-exposed worker (Figure 2B) (Wolff et al., 1982). The missing peaks in the workers fat presumably were conjeners that were rapidly metabolized while those present represented conjeners that were slowly metabolized. Figure 3 shows PCB chromatograms of milk and blood from a housewife occupationally exposed to PCBs, and a chromatogram of a commercial PCB mixture that most closely resembled the mothers profile (Yakushijii et al., 1979). Although the composition of PCBs in the milk and blood are similar, many PCB conjeners from the original commercial mixtures, particularly the lower molecular weight compounds, do not persist in human tissues. Numerous factors may affect PCB persistence and disposition including solubility (Wolff et al., 1982) and the induction of mixed function oxidases (MFOs). In general, those PCBs that persist in human fat have relatively low toxicity compared to their rapidly metabolized isomers and conjeners which do not accumulate in fat (J.D. McKinney personal communication, McKinney and Singh, 1981).

The excellent correlations between the toxicity of chlorinated lipophilic xenobiotics and their potencies as MFO inducers (Safe, 1985) raises several questions. Is it the parent compound or its metabolite that is most toxic? Is the greater toxicity of the readily metabolized PCBs

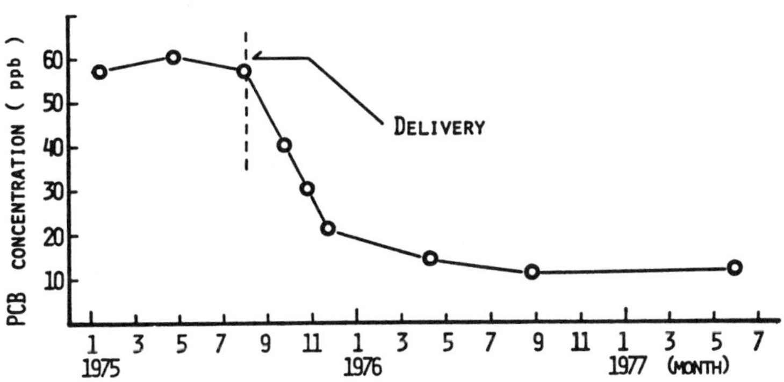

Fig. 1. Decline in concentrations of PCB's in the blood of an occupationally exposed women who worked with PCB's in a capacitor factory. The women delivered her first child nearly 10 years after she ceased working in the factory in 1966. An approximate 76% decrease in PCB levels in the milk were noted 16 months after delivery; 200 mg of PCB's were excreted in about 818 liters of milk for this 16-month period. (From Yakushiji et al., 1978, with permission from the authors and Springer Verlag).

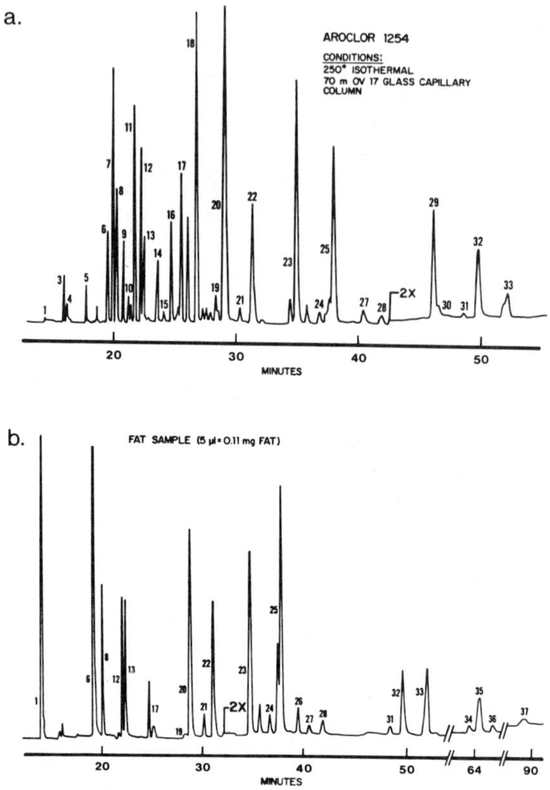

Fig. 2a Typical chromatogram from high resolution gas chromatography analysis of a standard PCB solution (Aroclar 1254). Peak numbers refer to structures designated in Wolff et al. 1982.

Fig. 2b Figure 2b shows a typical chromatogram from an analysis of adipose tissue from a PCB-exposed worker. The peak immediately preceding peak 17 is p.p'.-DDE. (From Wolfe et al., 1982, with permission from the authors and Academic Press).

(relative to their slowly metabolized conjeners) a simple dose effect of the metabolites? Although induction of MFOs by a specific compound usually implies that that compound is then metabolized, this may not always be the case. For example, Dioxin (2,3,7,8, tetrachlorodibenzo-p-dioxin TCDD) is one of the most potent MFO inducers known, yet it is relatively slowly metabolized (J.D. McKinney, personal communication). Because species vary widely in their ability to metabolize xenobiotics, extrapolation of animal studies to humans must be done with caution. Figure 4 shows the concentration of PCB isomers in five species 29 days after a single feeding of an equimolar mixture of five isomers (Sparling and Safe, 1980). Note that in each species, different proportions of the five isomers persist. Although there is little direct information about individual variation in lipophilic xenobiotic metabolism by humans, studies of caffeine metabolism in humans (Grant et al., 1983) have shown that there is, indeed, wide variability in the profile of metabolites among human subjects given the same dose of caffeine.

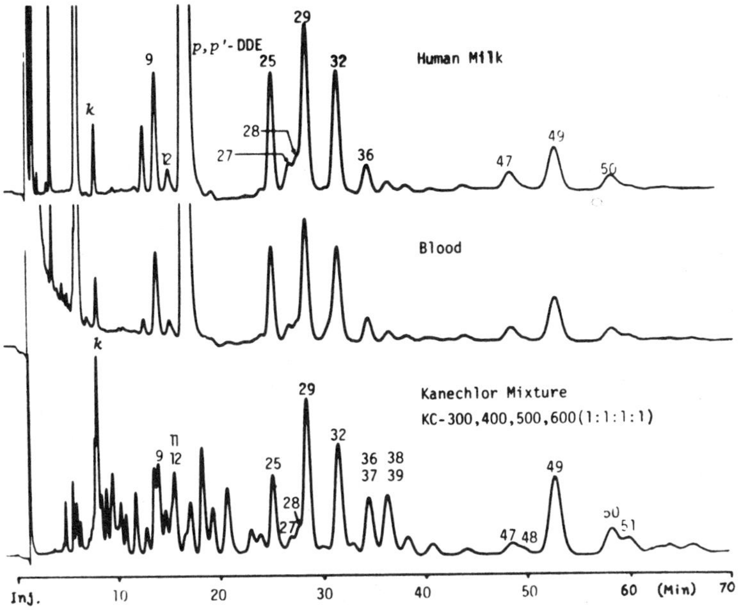

Fig. 3 Typical gas chromatographic separation of PCB residues in the milk and blood from the same mother and a commercial PCB mixture (Kanechlor). This mother was from the general population of an area in Japan where high PCB use occurred (From Yakushiji et al., 1979, with permission from the authors and Springer Verlag).

INTESTINAL EVENTS

Lipophilic xenobiotics (LXs) enter the body primarily by inhalation and by ingestion with food. Much of that which is inhaled is particulate (i.e., diesel particles, indoor air particles) (MacLead, 1981; Schuetzle et al., 1981) and is cleared from the lungs and nose, and deposited in the GI tract by muco-ciliary action (Sun et al., 1984). Lipophilic xenobiotics in food may be dissolved primarily in the fat fraction of the food particularly in animal products, but in plant material they may also occur in the skins and membranes of the fruit or vegetable (Patton, 1981). In general most human foods are contaminated with small amounts of PAHs and

Table 1. Carcinogen Levels in Commercial Margarines and Oils*

Carcinogen	No. Samples	Percent Contaminated	Concentration
Aflatoxin	4	100	98–150 μg/Kg
N-Nitrosodimethylamine	61	30	1– 23 μg/Kg
PAHs	7	100	23–750 μg/Kg
Benzo(a)pyrene	7	100	0.6–105 μg/Kg

*From Fong et al. (1980), Hedler et al. (1978), and Kolarouic and Traitler (1982).

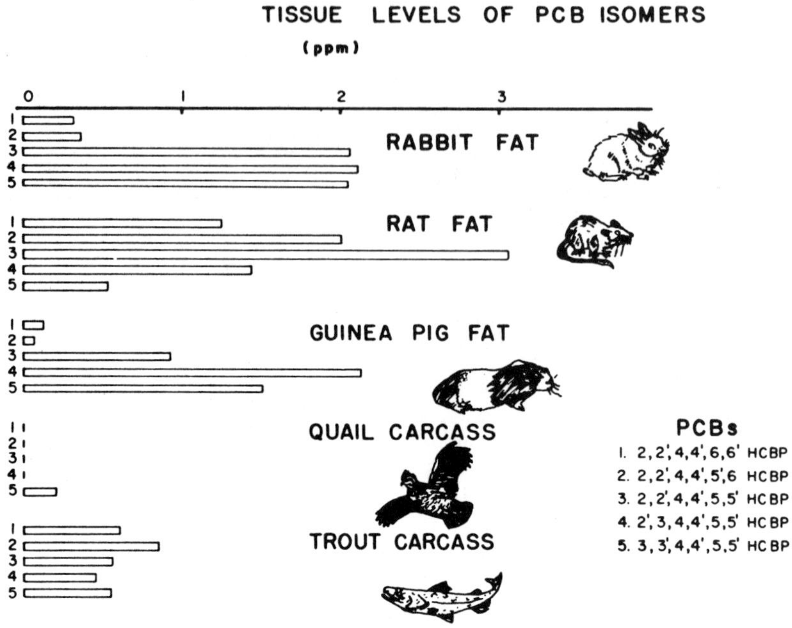

Fig. 4 The concentration of PCB isomers in five animal species 29 days after a single feeding of an equimolar mixture of five isomers (5 mg/kg). Only fatty tissue was examined in rat, guinea pig, and rabbit experiments. Whole carcasses were used in the trout and quail experiments (modified from Sparling and Safe, 1980).

PCBs and some fish may contain "excessive" amounts of PCBs (Dennis et al., 1983; Zabik et al., 1979). Table 1 shows levels of fat soluble carcinogens that have been found in commercial margarines and oils. In the stomach, fat, lipophilic particles from the lungs, plant skins and other food associated lipophilic xenobiotics are mixed together as the macroscopic structure of food is broken down into microscopic particles during the formation of chyme. Although fat digestion begins in the stomach through the action of lingual and gastric lipases (Liao et al., 1984; De Nigris et al., 1985) little fat absorption appears to occur there and virtually nothing is known about lipophilic xenobiotic absorption in the stomach. The main function of gastric fat digestion appears to be to prepare fat for more efficient and complete digestion by pancreatic lipases in the small intestine (Plucinski et al., 1979). Since the concentration of bile salts (detergent) in the stomach is generally very low, fat and its lipolytic products are thought to exist in stomach content primarily as insoluble droplets and particles of lipid. Presumably most LXs are extracted from gastric content by dietary fat and enter the small intestine predissolved in the triglyceride droplets. However, the efficiency of extraction of hydrophobic molecules in gastrointestinal content by dietary fat is poorly understood.

In the small intestine a series of events occur which permit the entry of LXs into the bodies circulatory system. Figure 5 shows a scale model of these events (for a recent review see Kuksis, 1984). In the intestinal lumen the first event (which also occurs in the stomach) is the cosolubilization of LX and dietary fat. The second event 2) is enzymatic hydrolysis of the dietary triglyceride into liquid crystalline and

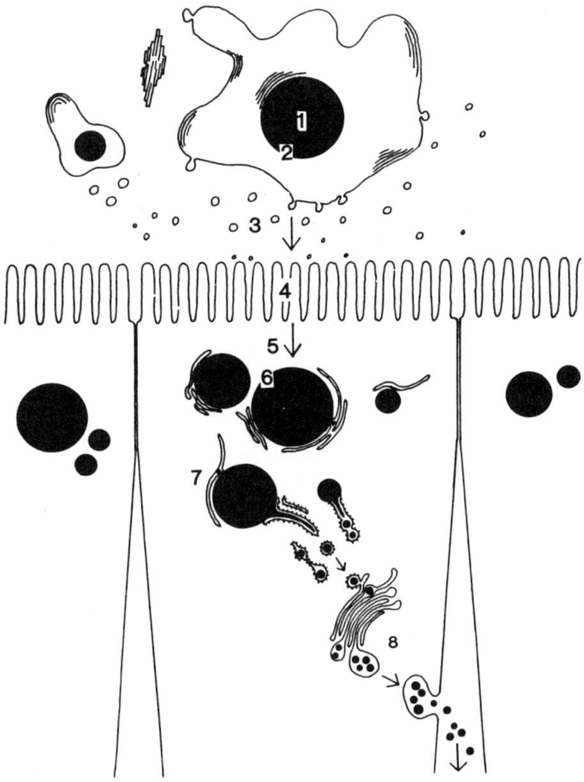

Fig. 5 Steps in the intestinal digestion and absorption of fat 1) Spherical dietary fat droplets act as sinks for lipophilic xenobiotics (LXs) in the intestinal lumen. 2) Lipases act at the oil-water interphase of fat droplets and create amorphous liquid crystalline product phases of fatty acids and monoglycerides. LXs can move quantitatively into the lipase product phases during the digestion of the oil droplets. 3) Lipase product phases are dispersed into vesicles and micelles by bile salts. Micellar dispersion of the products of fat digestion presents a high concentration of digested fat to the absorptive membrane. A portion of the LXs originally dissolved in dietary fat may precipitate during micellar dispersion. 4) Products of fat digestion are transported across the brush border membrane. It is uncertain if specific transport proteins are involved in lipid transport. 5) The transport of LXs and digested fat through the cytosol of the cell may be assisted by intracellular transport proteins. 6) Fat is resynthesized in the apical region of the cell. LXs originally associated with the dietary fat reappear in the newly synthesize fat. 7) Some LXs can be removed from the absorbed fat by MFO enzymes in the endoplasmic reticulum which convert the LX into more water soluble forms. 8) Dietary fat is packaged into lipoprotein particles called chylomicrons which are secreted into the lymph. Unmetabolized LXs remain dissolved in the liquid triglyceride core of these particles.

crystalline phases of fatty acid and monoglyceride (Patton et al., 1985). In the absence of bile salts these product phases can be partially dispersed into vesicles and liposomes. Also in the absence of bile salts LX's originally dissolved in the fat appear to flow quantitatively into the product phases of fat digestion (Patton et al., 1985; Vetter et al., 1985). The third luminal event, 3) is the dispersion of the product phases of fat digestion by bile salts. Figure 6 shows a schematic "zipper" model of these luminal events. On the right of Figure 6 is the oil phase which contains partially digested fat from the stomach and dissolved LXs. The boundary between the triglyceride droplet and the product phases is the site of lipase action in Figure 6 (Step 2, Figure 5). The boundary between the product phases and the bile salt micelles is the site of product phase dispersion. In Figure 6 typical LXs are shown as they move from fat into digested fat into the mixed bile sale micelles along a hydrocarbon continuum (Patton, 1981). The dispersion of product phases by bile salts is a highly dynamic process which produces a solution in which monomers of LX (individual molecules dissolved in water), digested fat (fatty acids and monoglycerides) and bile salts are in rapid equilibrium with micellar aggregates. During this dispersion process some of the LX that was originally dissolved in the dietary fat may not be able to achieve complete solubility in the micellar solution and will precipitate as insoluble crystals or aggregates (Figure 6) and be excreted in the feces.

Once dispersed into mixed lipolytic product-bile salt micelles, relatively high concentrations of LXs can diffuse up to the intestinal brush border membrane where they may be efficiently absorbed. In the absence of dietary fat, LXs will still equilibrate with the micellar phase of intestinal content, however, in the absence of liquid crystalline lipolytic products (i.e., fatty acids and monoglycerides), LXs and other lipophilic molecules such as cholesterol are up to an order of magnitude less soluble in bile salt micelles (Laher and Barrowman, 1983). Thus the products of dietary fat digestion aide dispersion and serve as a delivery vehicle for otherwise poorly soluble LXs and increase their bioavailability at the absorptive surface.

Individual lipid molecules, dissolved in water, yet in rapid equilibrium with the bile salt-lipid micelle, are thought to be the active species that enter the absorptive membrane (Thomson and Dietschy, 1981). The precise manner by which lipophilic molecules cross the brush border membrane (Step 4, Figure 5) of the enterocyte is uncertain (Patton, 1986). Until recently it was generally thought that lipids simply diffused, individually as monomers through the lipid bilayer of the membrane into the cell. Now there is evidence that dietary fatty acids may be transported across the enterocyte plasma membrane by a specific membrane protein (Stremmel et al., 1985a). There is also evidence for such a membrane protein in hepatocyte and adipocyte plasma membranes (Nada et al., 1984; Stremmel et al., 1985b). The fatty acid transporter in the brush border does not bind to cholesterol esters, phospholipids, bile salts or sulfobromophthalein. Whether or not it transports LX's is uncertain at this time.

Once inside the absorptive cell, dietary fatty acids and monoglycerides (and LXs) diffuse to the smooth endoplasmic reticulum (Step 5, Figure 5) where they are resynthesized into triglyceride droplets (Step 6, Figure 5). In the enterocyte the cytosolic transport of absorbed fatty acids and LXs like the PAHs and its metabolites are thought to be assisted by two proteins, fatty acid binding protein (FABP) and ligandin (Ockner and Manning, 1974; Fleischner, 1977) both of which appear to bind one molecule of PAH (or fatty acid) with similar affinities (Tipping et al., 1980).

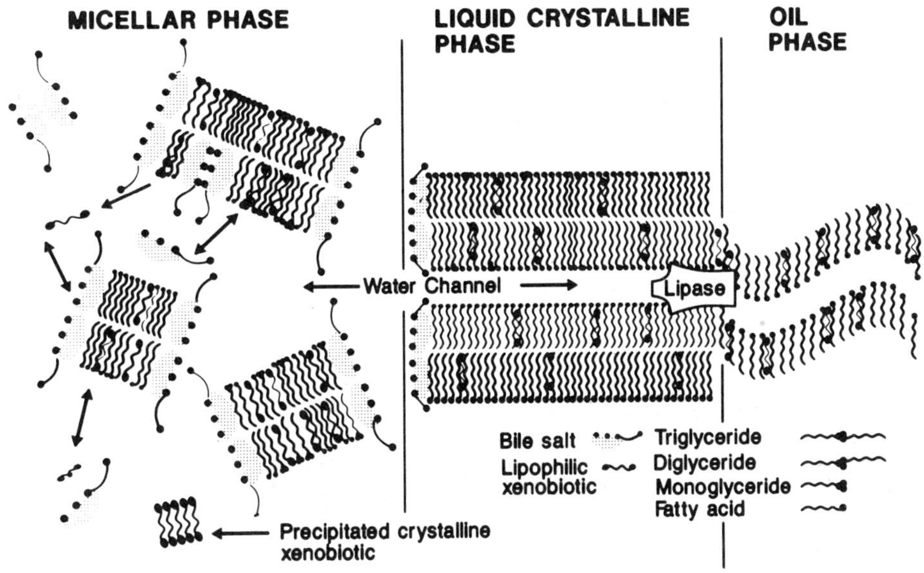

Fig. 6 Schematic zipper model of fat digestion showing a closeup of steps 1-3 from Figure 5. Lipophilic molecules dissolved in the mixture micelle are in rapid equilibrium with monomers dissolved in the water phase (Modified from Patton, 1981).

The cellular concentration of these two proteins have been estimated to be ~10^{-4} M (Ketterer et al., 1978) which is roughly two orders of magnitude lower than the concentration of fatty acid that occurs in intestinal content during digestion of a fatty meal (Hofmann and Borgstrom, 1964). Thus it is unclear whether or not fatty acids are transported through the cytosol as individual monomers or as small aggregates or micelles (with a hydrophobic domain for carrying LX molecules).

The absorption or "downhill" diffusion of digested fat into the enterocyte from the lumen is driven by the continual resynthesis of triglyceride droplets (Step 6, Figure 5) that occurs in the endoplasmic reticulum (Manganaro and Kuksis, 1985). Newly synthesized intracellular oil droplets also serve as a sink for LXs which diffuse "down hill", down a concentration gradient into the enterocyte (Vetter et al., 1985). Up to this point the intestine is rather nonspecific; dietary fat and associated hydrophobic solutes (i.e., LXs) are codigested, codispersed, coabsorbed, and coincorporated into intracellular fat droplets (Vetter et al., 1985). Intestinal absorption of LXs (like cellular uptake in general) appears to be a simple partitioning phenomenon that is controlled by the relative lipid volumes of the donor micelles and acceptor cells (Plant et al., 1985).

Once absorbed and resynthesized, dietary fat is then processed and packaged (Step 7, Figure 5) for secretion (Step 8, Figure 5) as chylomicrons into the lymph. Intestinal fat processing is an important event that determines what percentage of the absorbed LX will enter the general circulation. If the LX is readily metabolizable by the intestinal mixed function oxidase (MFO) system, much of it will be removed from the intracellular fat droplets, hydroxylated, conjugated, secreted from the cell as water soluble metabolites, and transported in the portal blood to the liver. The liver rapidly removes the metabolites from the blood and secretes them into the bile (Vetter et al., 1985). If the LX is poorly metabolized, much of it remains with the dietary fat as it is packaged into chylomicrons. Because of their size (250–500 nm) chylomicrons cannot enter the >10 nm pores (fenestae) of the capillary endothelial cells. Instead of entering the portal blood, chylomicrons are slowly drained from the intestine by the lymphatics and enter the general circulation through the thoracic lymph duct which empties into the left subclavian vein. Thus chylomicron associated LXs escape the first pass metabolism of the intestine and liver and enter the circulation where they interact with blood lipoproteins, albumin and all of the peripheral tissues including the mammary gland. Uptake of chylomicron associated LX by the mammary gland, although the most direct route of LX movement from diet to milk, is only one of several pathways.

The intestine also synthesizes triglyceride rich particles known as very low density lipoproteins (VLDLs). These particles are similar to chylomicrons but can be made in the absence of dietary fat (Havel, 1973). Presumably they can serve as cellular carriers of LXs that are absorbed in the absence of dietary fat (i.e., LXs cleared from the lungs).

Benzo(a)pyrene (BP) is an example of an LX that is readily metabolized by the intestine. Figure 7 shows the fate in the rat of ^{14}C-BP dissolved in dietary fat (Laher et al., 1984). Roughly 80% of the absorbed dose was recovered in the bile (as water soluble metabolites). Only 20% of the dose entered the lymph but in contrast to bile, the BP in lymph was unmetabolized parent compound. The fraction of dietary BP that enters the lymph is controlled by several factors. Evidence suggests that at a

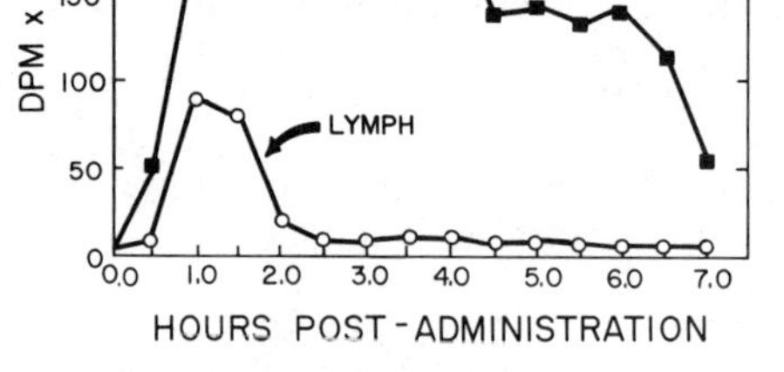

Fig. 7 The recovery of benzo(a)pyrene in the rat following feeding of a single dose (0.4 μmoles) dissolved in 500 μmoles dietary fat. Radioactivity in the bile was BP metabolites while radioactivity in the lymph was primarily unmodified BP. Approximately 17% of the total BP dose was recovered in the total lymph and bile combined. (Modified from Lehar et al., 1984).

constant fat level the percentage of BP entering the lymph increases as the BP concentration decreases (Van Veld et al., 1985). Since MFO activity in the intestine is inducible, the history of exposure of the intestine to LXs may effect their metabolism (Aito et al., 1972; Bock et al., 1979; Van Veld et al., 1985). There are numerous forms of cytochrome P_{450} which serve as the terminal enzymes in the MFOs system and different forms may be selectively induced by different drugs or xenobiotics (Boukousky et al., 1985).

Unfortunately the substrate specificities of the different intestinal cytochrome P_{450}s are poorly understood. Theoretically LXs which are poorly metabolized by the intestinal MFO system should remain preferentially with the chylomicrons (Vost and MacLean, 1984). Unfortunately, with the exception of DDT, there are few studies in this area and the results with DDT are not conclusive. Although it is agreed that 95-99% of lymphatic DDT is parent compound that is dissolved in the chylomicron core (Pocock and Vost, 1984; Sieber et al., 1974) the percentage of total absorbed DDT that was recovered in 24 hr lymph was only as high as 33% in the study of Sieber et al. (1974) and 60% in the 12 hr study by Pocock and Vost (1974). Pocock and Vost suggested that their value of 60% was an underestimate because some of the lymph flowed around the cannula and therefore escaped collection. It is unclear from the study of Sieber et al. where absorbed DDT that was not recovered in lymph resided in the body and how it got there. Both of the studies cited above collected thoracic duct lymph which drains both the liver and intestine, thus it is also uncertain if the DDT in the lymph originated directly from the intestine (Noguchi et al., 1985). Since all LXs partition freely into lipophilic environments, whether they be in fat droplets, membranes or pockets of proteins, partitioning of unmetabolized LXs from the intestine will always occur by both lymphatic and portal blood pathways (intestinal blood flow is roughly 500 x intestinal lymph flow, Sieber et al., 1974). Although chylomicron (or VLDL) transport should be greatly favored by unmetabolized LXs, partitioning of LX into the portal blood will always be a competing pathway that may become significant when lipid secretion by the intestine is low such as with low fat diets or between meals. The quantitative importance of the portal route for unmetabolized LXs remains to be determined.

THE FATE OF CHYLOMICRON ASSOCIATED LXS

After secretion both chylomicrons (and VLDLs) acquire several proteins from high density lipoproteins (HDL) present in lymph and blood (C and E apoproteins) (Havel, 1983). One of the C proteins (Apo C II) permits lipoprotein lipase on the surface of blood capillaries to rapidly hydrolyze chylomicron triglycerides. Figure 8 shows a hypothetical scale model of the interaction of a chylomicron particle with a capillary endothelial cell (Scow et al., 1980). Lipoprotein lipase (LPL) is bound to the endothelial cell by heparin sulfate. Apo C-II, on the chylomicron, binds to LPL, LPL then begins digesting the triglyceride and producing lipolytic products (DG, FA and MG in Figure 8) which, according to Scow's hypothesis, migrate along a membrane continuum into the tissue (Scow et al., 1980, 1983). Figure 9 shows a model of Scow's hypothesis of lipid movement from blood to tissue fat droplet along a membrane continuum. The parenchymal cell is a generalized cell, it could be an adipocyte, muscle cell, mammary cell, etc. (Wetzel and Scow, 1984). An alternative mode of lipid transport from capillary lumen to intracellular fat droplet (or vice versa) may be via a series of membrane and cytosolic transport steps involving membrane transport proteins and cytosolic carriers such as fatty acid binding protein (Scow et al., 1983). Scow's hypothesis is based upon electron microscopic images (which are static) and knowledge of the spreading behavior of fatty acids at interphases. The mechanism of transport within the membrane continuum is not thought to be simple random diffusion but much more rapid and directed mass movement of lipid in "rivers" or channels within the membrane. It is a controversial but elegant hypothesis that has been difficult to prove or disprove. The digestion, absorption, and resynthesis of chylomicron triglyceride by peripheral tissues occurs within minutes, as does fat assimilation in the intestine. Presumably some of the LXs dissolved in chylomicrons, follow the membrane continuum with lipolytic products and are incorporated into tissue lipid stores.

Most of the lipolytic products produced by LPL during chylomicron digestion enter the tissue, however, some fatty acids (~1/3 of the total) bind to albumin in the blood. Other protein and lipid components of the chylomicron are transferred to HDLs, VLDLs, and LDLs in the blood, and some lipid and protein components remain with the remnant chylomicron which is cleared by the liver. It is unclear which of these pathways is favored by a particular LX, however, within minutes most of the LX disappears from the circulation. BP dissolved in chylomicrons and injected into rats exhibited typical biphasic clearance kinetics (Vauhkonen et al., 1980). The initial rapid phase lasted approximately 5 minutes with over 80% of the BP removed from the blood (~70% was removed by 30 seconds). After 5 min. blood cells contained 6% and serum 13% of the total BP. At 30 seconds the serum ^{3}H-BP was found equally distributed between the chylomicron-VLDL remnant fraction and the albumin fraction. During the slow phase, further distribution of BP occurred with most of the label being in low density and very low density lipoproteins. After 60 min. serum contained 5% and blood cells 6% of the total BP (Vauhkonen et al., 1980). Although BP and other hydrocarbons appear to be cleared from the rat circulation simultaneously

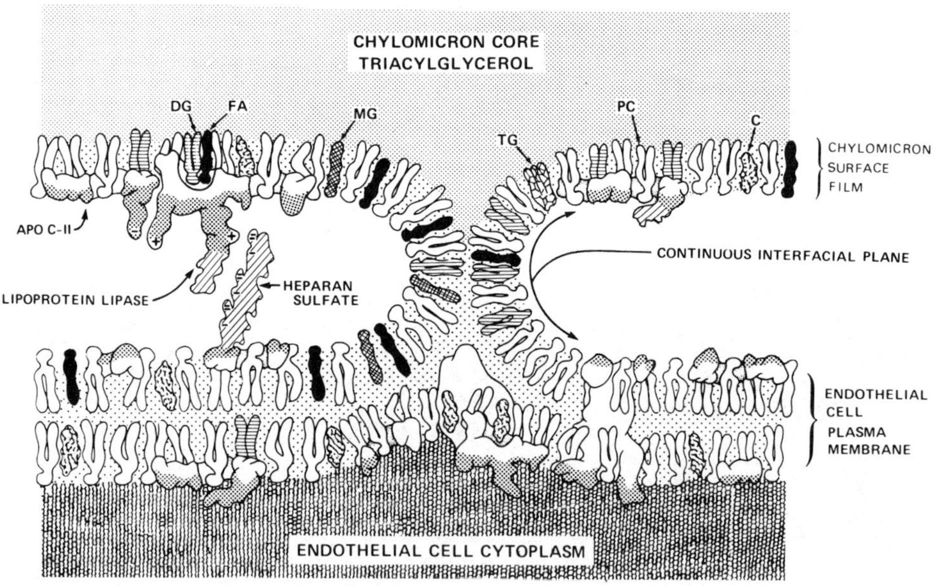

Fig. 8 Schematic diagram showing fusion of chylomicron surface film with the external leaflet of the endothelial cell plasma membrane at the luminal surface of the capillary. C, cholesterol; DG, diglyceride; FA, fatty acid; MG, monoglyceride; PC, phosphatidylcholine; TG, triglyceride (from Smith and Scow, 1979, with permission from the authors and S. Karger AG, Basel).

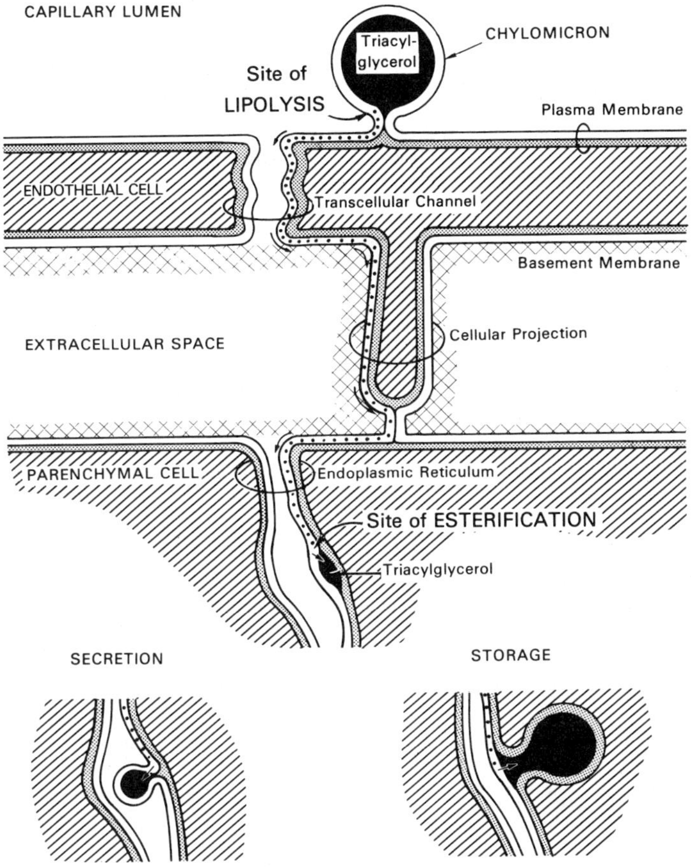

Fig. 9 The model of Scow et al. (1980) for transfer of lipid from a chylomicron to a parenchymal cell in extrahepatic tissue by lateral movement in a continuous water-lipid interfacial plane. The interfacial continuum, represented by the broad white line, consists of the chylomicron surface film, the external leaflets of plasma and vesicle membranes of the endothelial cell, and the external leaflet of the plasma membrane and the luminol (external) leaflet of the endoplasmic reticulum of the parenchymal cell. The cytoplasmic leaflet of membranes is represented by the broad finely stippled line. The dots indicate the route of transit of lipolytic products and LX from the chylomicron to the esterification site in the parenchymal cell. (From Scow et al., 1980 with permission from the authors and the Federation of American Society of Experimental Biologists).

with chylomicrons, DDT appears to be cleared even faster than chylomicrons (Vost and MacLean, 1984; Vauhkonen et al., 1980). Vost and Maclean (1984) suggest that HDLs are major intermediate acceptors of LXs following intravenous injection of LX's in chylomicrons. The important point to be made here, however, is that within seconds most of the LXs associated with chylomicrons disappear from the blood. Following oral administration BP and other PAHs rapidly distribute to all tissues in the body including the mammary gland (Vauhkonen et al., 1980; Gruggs and Moon, 1973; Daniel et al., 1967). Much of the BP that enters the tissues is rapidly metabolized and reappears in the blood bound to albumin. In a detailed pharmacokinetic study of BP clearance in rats, Wiersma and Roth (1983) found that by 20 minutes BP metabolite concentrations in the blood exceeded that of BP itself. The circulating BP metabolites are then cleared by the kidney and liver (Shu and Bymun, 1983). It is uncertain if an albumin receptor on the hepatocyte membrane is required for efficient uptake of BP metabolites by the liver (Ockner et al., 1983; Weisiger 1985). BP metabolites cleared by the kidney are apparently filtered as unbound monomers since albumin cannot pass through the pores in the kidney endothelial cells. Pretreatment of rats with the PAH, 3-methylcholanthrene increased the apparent volume of distribution of BP *in vivo* presumably by increasing the extrahepatic metabolism of BP (i.e., extrahepatic tissues "pulled" more BP out of circulation because the concentration of their BP metabolizing enzymes had been increased by PAH pretreatment) (Wiersma and Roth, 1983). Although the liver hepatocyte is well known for its BP metabolizing ability, most other cell types appear to be capable of metabolizing BP. Human mammary epithelial cells are no exception. Indeed they metabolize BP and form adducts with DNA more readily and at lower concentrations of BP than do fibroblasts from the same breast specimens (Bartley et al., 1982). Compared to BP there has been relatively little work with clearance of the chlorinated hydrocarbons. Like BP, chylomicron associated DDT appears to be initially cleared by the liver (30% of the dose after 14 min) (Vost and Maclean, 1984). The more rapid clearance of chylomicron DDT relative to chylomicron triglyceride (Vost and MacLean, 1984) is an intriguing observation that should be further studied. It is hard to imagine how a lipophilic solute could be cleared faster than the already rapidly cleared triglyceride.

During lactation, through the action of prolactin, uptake of fat by adipose tissue is inhibited and the mammary gland may take up a large percentage of dietary chylomicrons (Hamosh et al., 1970 and Zinder et al., 1974). Scow et al. (1977) found that 60% of the triglyceride fatty acid, 13% of the cholesterol and 6% of the phosphatidylcholine of intravenously injected chylomicrons were taken up within 11 min. by lactating rat mammary gland. Approximately 14% of the triglyceride fatty acid was recovered in the liver, whereas negligible amounts were taken up by adipose tissue. Non-suckling for 44 h decreased markedly uptake of all lipids by mammary gland and retarded clearance of chylomicrons from blood while it increased significantly uptake of triglyceride fatty acids and cholesterol by adipose tissue (Scow et al., 1977). Unfortunately similar experiments as those above with LXs have not been performed.

THE TOTAL BODY LIPID COMPARTMENT

Following a bolus injection of BP-labeled chylomicrons, there is a rapid clearance phase followed by a slow clearance phase (Vauhkonen et al., 1980). Generally, in pharmacokinetics the rapid clearance phase is attributed to the distribution of drug or xenobiotic into the total body volume while the slow clearance rate represents true excretion from the body. Lipophilic xenobiotics, which have lipid/water partition coefficients >100,000/1 distribute overwhelmingly into total body lipid. Simultaneously metabolism of the xenobiotic begins as the dietary fat (in chylomicrons) is hydrolyzed and reassembled or burned for energy. When the lipophilic xenobiotic is diluted into the total body lipid it becomes less accessible to metabolic enzymes. The majority of body lipid consists of triglyceride droplets whose cores do not appear to contain proteins. The remainder of body lipid is comprised of membrane bilayers in which LXs can laterally diffuse and the MFO enzymes reside. Assuming that MFO-xenobiotic reactions follow the law of mass action, then below binding saturation, the lower the concentration of LX the slower will be its rate of metabolism and the longer it will take the body to excrete the compound. Even non-metabolizable LXs are excreted, albeit at very slow rates, in urine, feces and sloughed skin with its associated oils.

Because most humans are constantly ingesting and inhaling a daily dose of LXs, we have achieved a rough steady state concentration in our body's lipid. In the equilibrated human, the concentration of LX in serum lipids is the same as in adipose fat and if total body fat is known, the total body burden of LX can be calculated from serum levels (Brown and Lawton, 1984). The steady state concentration of any LX in our bodies is determined by our daily intake, the metabolizability of the compound, its octanol-water partition coefficient and our total lipid volume (Hutcheon et al., 1983). Human body fat contains about 1 ppb PAH (0.01 ppb BP) and 1000 ppb PCB (Obana et al., 1981). Since both classes of compounds have similar octanol-water partition coefficients (Patton et al., 1984) and PAHs are much more common in the environment than PCBs, the much higher levels of PCBs can be explained by their relative resistance to metabolism compared to PAHs.

REDISTRIBUTION OF LX IN THE BODY TO THE MAMMARY GLAND

Most of this section is speculative. As discussed earlier, through lactation a women can dramatically lower her body burden of LX (Figure 1). Obviously, LX stored in other parts of a womens body redistributes to the mammary gland. The favored transport mechanisms from adipose tissue to mammary gland are not known, however, the extremely rapid partitioning of LX from one lipophilic environment to another (Vomachka et al., 1983, Plant et al., 1985) suggests that LXs partition from the adipose tissue into the blood where lipoproteins carry them to the mammary gland. Most studies suggest that albumin is not as important in this regard as the lipoproteins (Vomachka et al., 1983, Shu and Bymun et al., 1983).

The pathway of lipid movement from adipose tissue to mammary gland is also not well understood. Fatty acid released by hormone sensitive lipase in adipose tissue, binds to albumin in the blood and goes to the liver where it is incorporated into VLDLs, or to other cells to be used for energy or directly to the mammary gland which reesterifies it into triglyceride. VLDL secreted by the liver is then taken up by the mammary epithelium through the LPL pathway. Whether or not adipose LX's accompany adipose fatty acids to the liver and then accompany liver VLDLs or LDLs to the mammary gland is unknown.

EVENTS IN THE MAMMARY GLAND

Milk fat originates from at least three sources, from the diet, from adipose stores and from the mammary gland itself which synthesizes fat from carbohydrate (Prentice et al., 1981; Bussman et al., 1984; and Thompson and Smith, 1985). The relative contribution of each source will depend primarily upon the level of fat in the mother's diet and adipose stores. Figure 10 shows four diagrams of milk producing tissue at progressively larger scale (Patton, 1969). Small fat droplets (less than 1.0 μm) first appear at the base of the lactating cell and grow in size as they move to the secretory (apical) end of the cell where they are eventually enveloped in the apical plasma membrane and released from the cell (Stemberger and

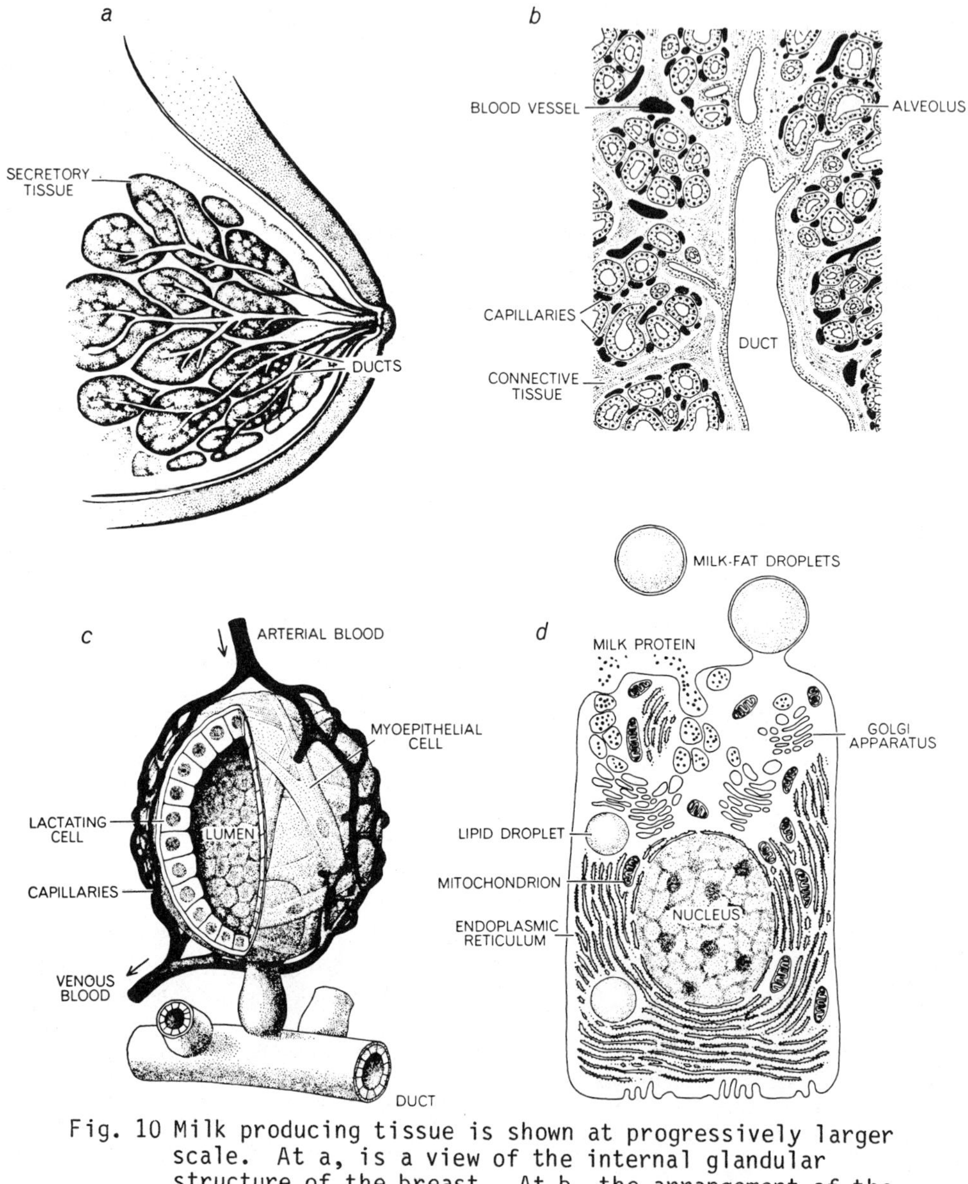

Fig. 10 Milk producing tissue is shown at progressively larger scale. At a, is a view of the internal glandular structure of the breast. At b, the arrangement of the alveoli and duct system that drains them is shown. A single alveolus (c) consists of an elliptical arrangement of lactating cells surrounding the lumen, which is linked to the duct system. A single lactating cell (d) is shown as it discharges a droplet of fat into the lumen. Part of the cell membrane becomes the membranous covering of the fat droplet (Modified from Patton, 1969).

Patton, 1981; Stemberger et al., 1984; and Patton and Keenan, 1975). In the rat, growth and secretion of droplets appears to take up to several hours (Stemberger and Patton, 1981). Milk of most species examined (including humans) contains polydisperse subpopulations of triglyceride droplets with a subpopulation of ~4 μm diameter containing the largest amount of fat (Ruegg and Blanc, 1981).

Total milk fat among Californian vegetarians and non-vegetarians averaged 3.2% in both groups (Finley et al., 1985). Among 120 rural West African women studied over 12 months, milk fat content was a relatively constant value (roughly 10 x that of blood) (Prentice et al., 1981).

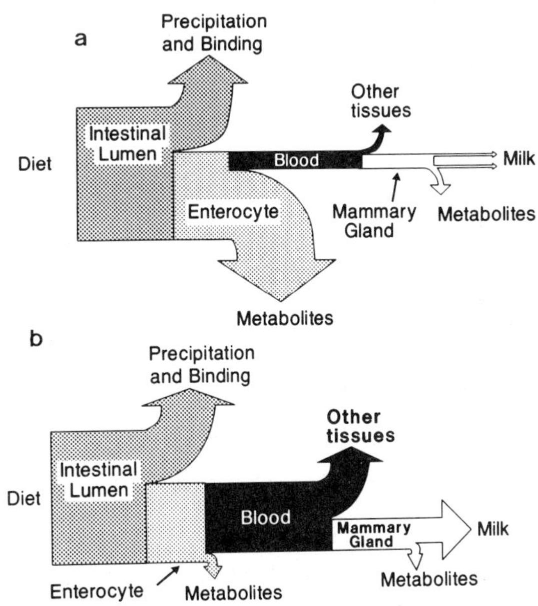

Fig. 11 Semiquantitative schematics of the metabolic fate of a rapidly metabolized dietary lipophilic xenobiotic (a) and a slowly metabolized dietary lipophilic xenobiotic (b).

The movement of lipophilic xenobiotics into the mammary gland may occur as Scow as depicted in Figure 9 or by a series of rapid diffusion steps through membranes and aqueous spaces (mediated by soluble protein carriers). The origin of the milk fat globule is the endoplasmic reticulum which is also rich in xenobiotic metabolizing enzymes (Bruder et al., 1978). As the forming fat droplets move up to the apical region of the cell they probably equilibrate with blood borne LXs. At the same time they maintain contact with the endoplasmic reticulum (Deeny et al., 1985) which may remove LX by metabolism before the droplet is secreted. Albumin in milk arises both from blood and from synthesis in the mammary gland (Phillipy and McCarthy, 1979). Thus, some LXs and their metabolites may be carried into the milk bound to albumin and some may diffuse back into the blood.

SUMMARY

Lipophilic xenobiotics follow dietary fat as it moves from GI tract into the body. In the intestinal lumen fat is digested and some LX is left behind because of binding to nonabsorbed food stuffs and poor solubility. In the intestinal epithelial cell more LX is separated from dietary fat, the amount determined primarily by the metabolizability of the LX. That which is metabolized is excreted by the liver. The twice "cleansed" dietary fat is then passed into the general circulation where it is again digested before it enters the peripheral tissues. Again it is cleansed of LX, as much as possible by the MFO system of the peripheral tissues. The metabolized LXs are excreted by the kidney and liver. Figures 11A and B semiquantitatively summarize the metabolic fate of a rapidly metabolized dietary LX like BP (Figure 11A) and a slowly metabolized dietary LX such as PCB (Figure 11B). Note that Figure 11 does not show the movement of stored LX to the mammary gland.

A steady state level of each LX exists in the body that represents the difference between intake and excretion. The LX in milk fat, blood fat, and adipose fat are all in equilibrium with each other. Lactation is a potent mechanism for LX excretion which allows the body to dramatically lower its steady state level of the most persistent LXs such as the PCBs and DDT.

ACKNOWLEDGEMENTS

This work was supported in part by NIH grants AM27304 and RCDA-AM01076.

REFERENCES

Aito, A., H. Vainio, and O. Hanninea (1972) Enhancement of drug oxidation and conjugation by carcinogens in different rat tissues. FEBS Lett. 24:237-240.

Bartley, J., J.C. Bartholomew, and M.R. Stampfer (1982) Metabolism of bonzo(a)pyrene by human epithelial and fibroblastic cells: Metabolite patterns and DNA adduct formation. J. Cell. Biochem. 18:135-148.

Bock, K.W., U.C.V. Clansbruuch, and D. Winne (1979) Absorption and metabolism of naphthalene and benzo(a)pyrene in the rat jejunum in situ. Med. Biol. 57:262-264.

Boukousky, H.L., H.P. Hauri, U. Marti, R. Gasser, and U.A. Meyer (1985) Cytochrome P_{450} of small intestinal epithelial cells. Gastroenterology 88:458-467.

Brown, J.F. and R.W. Lawton (1984) Polychlorinated biphenyl (PCB) partitioning between adipose tissue and serum. Bull. Environ. Contam. Toxicol. 33:277-280.

Bruder, G., A. Fink, and E.-D. Jarasch (1978) The B-type cytochrome in endoplasmic reticulum of mammary gland epithelium and milk fat globule membranes consist of two components, cytochrome b_5 and cytochrome P-420. Exp. Cell Res. 117:207-217.

Bussman, L.E., S. Ward, and N.J. Kuhn (1984) Lactose and fatty acid synthesis in lactating-rat mammary gland. Biochem. J. 219:173-180.

Daniel, P.M., O.E. Pratt, and M.M.L. Prichard. 1967. Metabolism of labelled carcinogenic hydrocarbons in rats. Nature 215:1142-1146.

DeCampos, M. and A.E. Olszyna-Marzys (1979) Contamination of human milk with chlorinated pesticides in Guatamala and El Salvador. Arch. Environm. Contam. Toxicol. 8:43-58.

Deeny, J.T., Valivullah, H.M., Dapper, C.H., Dylewski, D.P. and Keenan, T.W. (1985) Microlipid droplets in milk secreting mammary epithelial cells: evidence that they originate from endoplasmic reticulum and are precursors of milk lipid globules. Eur. J. Cell. Biol. 38:16-26.

DeNigris, S.J., M. Hamosh, D.K. Kasbekar, C.S. Fink, T.C. Lee and P. Hamosh. 1985. Secretion of human gastric lipase from dispersed gastric glands. Biochim. Biophys. Acta 836:67-72.

DeWolfe Miller, F., L.B. Brilliant, and R. Copeland (1984) Polybrominated biphenyls in lactating Michigan women: Persistence in the population. Bull. Environ. Contam. Toxicol. 32:125-133.

Dennis, M.J., R.C. Massey, D.J. McWeeny, M.E. Knowles and D. Watson. 1983. Analysis of polycyclic aromatic hydrocarbons in UK total diets. Fd. Chem. Toxic. 21:569-574.

Findlay, J.W.A. (1983) The distribution of some commonly used drugs in human breast milk: Drug Metabolism Reviews 14:653-684.

Finley, D.A., B. Lonnerdal, K.G. Dewey, and L.E. Grivetti (1985) Breast milk composition: fat content and fatty acid composition in vegetarians and non-vegetarians. Amer. J. Clin. Nut. 41:787-800.

Fleischner, G.M., J.B. Robbins, and I.M. Arias (1977) Cellular localization of ligandin in rat, hamster and man. Biochem. Biophys. Res. Commun. 74:992-1000.

Fong, L.Y.Y., C.C.T. Ton and P. Koonannwatchaidet (1980) Mutagenicity of peanut oils and effect of repeated cooking. Food. Cosmet. Toxicol. 18:467-470.

Grant, D.M., B.K. Tang, and W. Kalow (1983) Variability in caffeine metabolism. Clin. Pharm. Therap. 33:591-602.

Gruggs, C.J. and R.C. Moon (1973) Transport of orally administered 9,10-dimethyl-1,2-benzanthracene in the Sprague-Dawley rat. Cancer Res. 33:1785-1789.

Havel, R.J. (1983) Dietary regulation of plasma lipoprotein metabolism in humans. Prog. Biochem.-Pharmacol. 19:110-122.

Hamosh, M., T.R. Clary, S.S. Chernick, and R.O. Scow (1970) Lipoprotein lipase activity of adipose and mammary tissue and plasma triglyceride in pregnant and lactating rats. Biochim. Biophys. Acta 210:473-482.

Hedler, L., C. Schurr, and P. Marquardt (1979) Determination of volatile n-nitroso compounds in various samples of edible vegetable oils and margarine. J. Am. Oil Chem. Soc. 56:681-684.

Hofmann, A.F. and B. Borgstrom. 1964. The intraluminal phase of fat digestion in man. The lipid content of the micellar and oil phases of intestinal content obtained during fat digestion and absorption. J. Clin. Invest. 43:247-257.

Hutcheon, D.E., J. Kantrowitz, R.N. Van Gelder, E. Flynn (1983) Factors affecting plasma benzo(a)pyrene levels in environmental studies. Environmental Research 32:104-110.

Jensen, A.A. (1983) Chemical contaminants in human milk. Residue Reviews 89:128.

Jones, P.W. and P. Leber. editors (1979) Polynuclear aromatic hydrocarbons. Third International Symposium on chemistry and biology - Carcinogenesis and mutagenis. Ann Arbor Science Publishers, Inc., Ann Arbor, MI.

Ketterer, B., T.J. Crane, and E. Tipping (1978) Ligandin and protein A: intracellular binding proteins. in: "Transport by Proteins," D.G. Blauer and H. Sund, editors. Walter de Gruyter, Berlin. 78-94.

Kolarouic, L. and H. Traitter (1982) Determination of PAHs in vegetable oils by caffein complexation and glass capillary gas chromatography. J. Chromatog. 237:263-272.

Kuksis, A. (1984) Intestinal digestion and absorption of fat-soluble environmental agents. in: "Intestinal Toxicology," edited by C.M. Schiller, Raven Press, NY. 69-114.

Laher, J.M. and Barrowman, J.A. (1983) Polycyclic hydrocarbon and polychlorinated biphenyl solubilization in aqueous solutions of mixed micelles. Lipids 18:216-222.

Laher, J.M., M.W. Rigler, R.D. Vetter, J.A. Barrowman, and J.S. Patton (1984) Similar bioavailability and lymphatic transport of benzo(a)pyrene when administered to rats in different amounts of dietary fat. J. Lipid Res. 25:1337-1342.

Liao, T.H., P. Hamosh, and M. Hamosh (1984) Fat digestion by lingual lipase: Mechanism of lipolysis in the stomach and upper small intestine. Pediatric Res. 18:402-409.

Macleod, K.E. (1981) Polychlorinated biphenyls in indoor air. Environm. Sci. Technol. 15:926-928.

Manganaro, F. and A. Kuksis (1985) Rapid isolation of a triacylglycerol synthetase complex from rat intestinal mucosa. Can J. Biochem. Cell Biol. 63:107-114.

McKinney, J.D and P. Singh (1981) Structure-activity relationships in halogenated biphenyls: unifying hypothesis for structural specificity. Chem. Biol. Interactions 33:271-283.

Nada, A.A., J.H. Park, C.R. Park (1984) Permeation of long-chain fatty acid into adipocytes. J. Biol. Chem. 259:8945-8953.

Noguchi, T., W.N.A. Charman and V.J. Stella (1985) Lymphatic appearance of DDT in thoracic or mesenteric lymph duct cannulated rats. Internat. J. Pharmaceut. 24:185-192.

Obana, H., S. Hori, T. Kashimoto, and N. Kunita (1981) Polycyclic aromatic hydrocarbons in human fat and liver. Bull. Environm. Contam. Toxicol. 27:23-27.

Ockner, R.K., R.A. Weisiger, J.L. Gollan (1983) Hepatic uptake of albumin-bound substances: albumin receptor concept. Am. J. Physiol. 245: G13-G18.

Ockner, R.K. and J.A. Manning. (1974) Fatty acid-binding protein in small intestine: identification, isolation and evidence for its role in cellular fatty acid transport. J. Clin. Invest. 54:326-338.

Patton, J.S. (1981) Gastrointestinal lipid digestion. In Physiology of the Gastrointestinal Tract. L.R. Johnson, editor, Raven Press, New York 1123-1146.

Patton, J.S., B. Stone, C. Papa, R. Abramowitz and S.H. Yalkowsky. (1984) Solubility of fatty acids and other hydrophobic molecules in liquid triglyceride. J. Lipid Res. 25:189-197.

Patton, J.S. and J.A. Couch (1984) Can tissue anomalies that occur in marine fish implicate specific pollutant chemicals? In Concepts in Marine Pollution Measurements. pp 511-538. Ed. by H.H. White, Maryland Sea Grant Publication, Univ. of Maryland, College Park, MD.

Patton, J.S., Vetter, R.D., Hamosh, M., Borgstrom, B, Lindstrom, M. and Carey, M.C. (1985) The light microscopy of triglyceride digestion. Food Microstructure 4:29-41.

Patton, J.S. (1986) Is the intestinal lipid bilayer freely permeable to lipophilic molecules? In: 25 years of Research on the Brush Border. edited by F. Alvarado and C.H. van Os. Elsevier Press (in press).

Patton, S. (1969) Milk. Sci. American 221:1-11.
Patton, S. and T.W. Keenan (1975) The milk fat globule membrane. Biochim. Biophys. Acta 415:273-309.
Phillippy, B.O. and R.D. McCarthy (1979) Multi-origins of milk serum albumin in the lactating goat. Biochim. Biophys. Acta 584:298-303.
Plant, A.L., D.M. Benson and L.C. Smith. 1985. Cellular uptake and intracellular localization of benzo(a)pyrene by digital fluorescence imaging microscopy. J. Cell. Biol. 100:1295-1308.
Plucinski, T.M., M. Hamosh, and P. Hamosh (1979) Fat digestion in rats: role of lingual lipase. Am. J. Physiol. 237:E541-E547.
Pocock, D.M.E. and A. Vost (1974) DDT absorption and chylomicron transport in rat. Lipids 9:374-381.
Prentice, A., A.M. Prentice and R.G. Whitehead (1981) Breast-milk fat concentrations of rural African women. 2-Long term variations within a community. Br. J. Nutr. 45:495-507.
Rapaport, R.A. and S.J. Eisenrich (1984) Chromatographic determination of octanol-water partition coefficients (Kow's) for 58 polychlorinated biphenyl conjeners. Env. Sci. Technol. 18:163-170.
Rogan, W.J., A. Bagniewska, and T. Damstra (1980) Pollutants in breast milk. New England Journal of Medicine 302:1450-1453.
Ruegg, M. and B. Blanc (1981) The fat globule size distribution in human milk. Biochim. Biophys. Acta. 666: 7-14.
Safe, S. Polychlorinated biphenyls (PCBs) and polybrominated biphenyls (PBBs): Biochemistry, toxicology and mechanism of action. CRC Critical Reviews in Toxicology 13:319-396.
Schuetzle, D. F.S.C. Lee, T.J. Prater, S.B. Tejada (1981) The identification of polynuclear aromatic hydrocarbon (PAH) derivatives fractions of diesel particulate extracts. Intern. J. Environ. Anal. Chem. 9:93-144.
Scow, R.O., E.J. Blanchette-Mackie, and L.C. Smith. (1980) Transport of lipid across capillary endothelium. Fed. Proc. 39:3610-2617.
Scow, R.O., E.J. Blianchette-Mackie, M.G. Wetzel and A. Reinila (1983) Lipid transport in tissue by lateral movement in cell membranes. In: "The Adipocyte and Obesity: Cellular and Molecular Mechanisms," ed. by A. Angel, C.H. Hollenberg and D.A.K. Roncari. Raven Press, N.Y.
Scow, R.O., Chernick, S.S., and Fleck, T.R. (1977) Lipoprotein lipase and uptake of triglyceride cholesterol and phosphatidylcholine from chylomicrons by mammary and adipose tissue of lactating rats in vivo. Biochim. Biophys. Acta 487:297-306.
Shu, H.P. and E.N. Bymun (1983) Systemic excretion of benzo(a)pyrene in the control an microsomally induced rat: The influence of plasma lipoproteins and albumin as carrier molecules. Cancer Res. 43:485-490.
Sieber, S.M., V.H. Cohn, and W.T. Wynn (1974) The entry of foreign compounds into the thoracic duct lymph of the rat. Xenobiotica 4:265-284.
Sparling, J. and S. Safe (1980) The effects of ortho chloro substituents on the retention of PCB isomers in rat, rabbit, Japanese quail, guinea pig and trout. Toxicology Letters 7:23-28.
Stemberger, B.H. and S. Patton (1981) Relationship of size, intracellular location and time required for secretion of milk fat droplets. J. Dairy Sci. 64:422-426.
Stemberger, B.H., R.M. Walsh, and S. Patton. 1984. Morphometric evaluation of lipid droplet associations with secretory vesicles, mitochondria and other components in the lactating cell. Cell Tissue Res. 236:471-475.
Stremmel, W., G. Lotz, G. Strohmeyer and P.D. Berk (1985a) Identification, isolation, and partial characterization of a fatty acid binding protein from rat jejunal microvillus membranes. J. Clin. Invest. 75:1068-1076.

Stremmel, W., G. Strohmeyer, F. Borchard, S. Kochwa, P.D. Berk (1985b) Isolation and partial characterization of a fatty acid binding protein in rat liver plasma membranes. Proc. Natl. Acad. Sci. 82:4-8.
Sun, J.D., R.K. Wolff, G.M. Kanapilly, and R.O. McClellan (1984) Lung retention and metabolic fate of inhaled benzo(a)pyrene associated with diesel exhaust particles. Toxicol. Applied Pharm. 73:48-59.
Thompson, A.B.R. and Dietschy, J.M. (1981) Intestinal lipid absorption: Major extracellular and intracellular events. in: "Physiology of the Gastrointestinal Tract," ed. Johnson, L.R. pp. 1147-1220. Raven Press, NY.
Thompson, B.J. and S. Smith (1985) Biosynthesis of fatty acids by lactating human breast epithelial cells: An evaluation of the contribution to the overall composition of human milk fat. Pediatric Research 19:139-143.
Tipping, E., B.P. Moore, C.A. Jones, G.M. Cohen, B. Ketterer, and J.W. Bridges (1980) Non-covalent binding of benzo(a)pyrene and its hydroxylated metabolites to intracellular proteins and lipid bilayers. Chem. Biol. Interactions 32:291-304.
VanVeld, P.A., R.D. Vetter, R.F. Lee and J.S. Patton (1985) Metabolism of triglyceride-solublized benzo(a)pyrene by the intestine of fish: Influence of triglyceride concentration and cytosolic glutathione transferases. J. Lipid Res. (submitted).
Vauhkonen, M., T. Kuusi and P.K.J. Kinnunen (1980) Serum and tissue distribution of benzo(a)pyrene from intravenously injected chylomicrons in rat in vivo. Cancer Lett. 11:113-119.
Vetter, R.D., M.C. Carey, and J.S. Patton (1985) Coassimilation of dietary fat and benzo(a)pyrene in the small intestine: an absorption model using the killifish. J. Lipid Res. 26:428-434.
Vomachka, M.S., Vodicnik, M.J., and Lech, J.J. (1983) Characteristics of 2,4,5,2',4',5' hexachlorobiphenyl distribution among lipoproteins in vitro. Toxicol and Applied Pharm 70:350-361.
Vost, A. and N. MacLean (1984) Hydrocarbon transport in chylomicrons and high density lipoproteins in rat. Lipids 19:423-435.
Weisiger, R.A. (1985) Dissociation from albumin: a potentially rate-limiting step in the clearance of substances by the liver. Proc. Natl. Acad. Sci. 82:1563-1567.
Welch, R.M. and J.W.A. Findlay (1981) Excretion of drugs in human breast milk. Drug Metabolism Reviews 12:261-277.
Wetzel, M.G. and R.O. Scow (1984) Lipolysis and fatty acid transport in rat heart: electron microscopic study. Am. J. Physiol. 246:C467-C485.
Wiersma, D.A. and R.A. Roth (1983) Total body clearance of circulating benzo(a)pyrene in conscious rats: Effect of pretreatment with 3-methylcholanthrene and the role of liver and lung. J. Pharmacol. Exp. Therap. 226:661-667.
Wilson, J.T., R.D. Brown, J.L. Hinson and J.W. Dailey (1985) Pharmacokinetic pitfalls in the estimation of the breast milk/plasma ratio for drugs. Ann. Rev. Pharmacol. Toxicol. 25:667-689.
Wolff, M.S., J. Thornton, A. Fischbein, R. Lilis and J.J. Selikoff (1982) Disposition of polychlorinated biphenyl conjeners in occupationally exposed persons. Toxicol. Applied Pharm. 62:294-306.
Yakushiji, T., I. Watanabe, K. Kuwabara, S. Yoshida, K. Koyama, I. Hara and N. Kunita (1978) Long term studies of the excretion of polychlorinated biphenyls (PCBs) through the mother's milk of an occupationally exposed worker. Arch. Environm. Contam. Toxicol. 7:493-504.
Yakushiji, T., I. Watanabe, K. Kuwabara, S. Yoshida, K. Koyama and N. Kunita (1979) Levels of polychlorinated biphenyls (PCBs) and organochlorine pesticides in human milk and blood collected in Osaka Prefecture from 1972 to 1977. Int. Arch. Occup. Environ. Health 43:1-15.

Yakushiji, T., I. Watanabe, K. Kuwabara, S. Yoshida, S. Hori, S. Fukushima, T. Kashimoto, K. Koyama, and N. Kunita (1979) Levels organochlorine pesticides and polychlorinated biphenyls (PCBs) in mothers milk collected in Osaka Prefecture from 1969 to 1976. _Arch. Environm. Contam. Toxicol._ 8:59-66.

Zabik, M.E., P. Hoojjat, and C.M. Weaver (1979) Polychlorinated biphenyls, dieldrin, and DDT in lake trout cooked by broiling, roasting, or microwave. _Bull. Environm. Contam. Toxicol._ 21:136-143.

Zinder, O., M. Hamosh, T.R. Fleck and R.O. Scow (1974) Effect of prolactin on lipoprotein lipase in mammary glands and adipose tissue of rats. _Am. J. Physiol._ 226:742-748.

ANTIBODIES IN MILK DIRECTED AGAINST SPECIFIC ENTEROPATHOGENS

Larry K. Pickering and Guillermo Ruiz-Palacios

Program in Infectious Diseases and Clinical Microbiology and Department of Pediatrics, University of Texas Medical School at Houston and Department of Infectious Diseases Institute of Nutrition, Mexico City

INTRODUCTION

Many organisms have been identified as causing diarrhea in infants and children (1). Diarrhea is prevalent when personal hygiene and sanitation are deficient. In addition diarrhea occurs more frequently in infants who are formula fed compared to those who are bottle fed (2-4). Human milk provides a large number of nonspecific and specific

Table 1. Enteropathogens against which antibodies have been reported in human colostrum and milk.

Organisms	Function or antigen against which human milk antibodies reported
Escherichia coli	agglutination (10) somatic (11,15,21) capsular (11) enterotoxin (12,13,17,18) adherence (17)
Vibrio cholerae	enterotoxin (14,19,20) antibacterial (19,20) adherence (16,20)
Clostridium difficile	toxin (30,31)
Salmonella	agglutination (32) somatic (33)
Campylobacter	outer membrane protein (36)
Rotavirus	common antigen (39-41)
Giardia lamblia	capsular antigen (49,51)
Entamoeba histolytica	unknown antigen (53)

protective factors that are present in varying concentrations throughout all stages of lactation (5,6). Total secretory IgA immunoglobulin and specific IgA antibodies to many enteropathogens have been recognized in human milk (table 1) (7,8). Secretory IgA is not absorbed in significant quantity from the human intestine and therefore presumably acts at the mucosal surface of the intestine (8). Secretory IgA is more resistant to acid degradation and to the proteolytic activity of gut enzymes than is serum IgA, and can be found intact in significant quantities in feces (9). It is known that immunoglobulin concentrations and antibody titers are high in colostrum and decrease significantly in mature milk. Little is known about the relation between the presence and concentration of these antibodies and the occurrence of diarrhea due to various enteropathogens.

HUMAN MILK ANTIBODIES TO ENTEROPATHOGENS

Several reports show that human colostrum and milk contain antibodies against specific bacterial enteropathogens or toxins elaborated by them, viruses and parasites (table 1). The concentrations of specific antibodies in milk varies among women in different populations, indicating differences in exposure to various enteropathogens. No changes in the quality and immune capacity of human milk appears to occur in undernourished women, although volume may be decreased.

Escherichia coli and Vibrio cholerae. Antibodies directed against several antigens of *E. coli* and *V. cholerae* have been reported. These antibodies agglutinated common serotypes of *E. coli* (10), were active against both somatic and capsular antigens of *E. coli* (11), and inhibited the induced fluid accumulation in rabbit ileal loops when incubated with *V. cholerae* and *E. coli* enterotoxin (12). Secretory IgA antibody which neutralized *E. coli* toxin was shown to be present in milk from undernourished women from Pakistan, but not from healthy women from Sweden (13). Human milk also has been shown to contain secretory IgA against cholera toxin (14), as well as antibodies to somatic antigens of enteropathogenic *E. coli* (15).

Human milk and colostrum inhibited *E. coli* and *V. cholerae* adhesion to intestinal epithelium and binding of secreted enterotoxins to specific cell membrane receptors (16,17). Part of this inhibitory activity resided in the immunoglobulin fraction; however, the nonimmunoglobulin fraction inhibited both bacterial cell adhesion and enterotoxin binding, usually to a greater extent than did the immunoglobulin fraction. Aust-Kettis, *et al.* (18) showed that antibody titers to *E. coli* LT were present in 33% of milk specimens from Ethiopian women (18). Neutralization tests with cholera enterotoxins were all negative. The inhibitory factor they described may have been something other than antibody to *E. coli* LT. Majumdar *et al.* (19) demonstrated a significant increase in both antibacterial and antitoxin titers in sera and milk of convalescent phase cholera patients. Majumdar and Ghose (20) showed that *V. cholerae* antibacterial and antitoxin titers were significantly higher in colostrum from Indian women than from Swedish women. Colostrum from Indian women inhibited adherence of *V. cholerae* to intestinal slices *in vitro* and induced protection against live vibrio challenge in rabbit ileal loops. Cruz and associates (21) showed that malnourished women were able to produce SIgA in milk against *E. coli* somatic antigens in quantities comparable to those observed in well nourished populations.

Several studies using animal models have shown the protective effect of antibodies in human milk to *E. coli* and *V. cholerae* (12,13,20). The significance of these antibodies in protecting human infants from diarrhea is not known. Epidemiologic studies have shown that human milk protects infants from diarrhea due to specific enteropathogens (2-4). In the majority of these studies it is not known whether such protection is mediated by specific immunologic components, nonspecific defense factors or by decreasing exposure to enteropathogens that may contaminate other food or formula. Nursery outbreaks of diarrhea due to *E. coli* 0111 have been controlled by feeding infants human milk (22). In Guatemala a lower incidence of *E. coli* in breast fed infants than in bottle fed infants was found (23).

In a study by Michael *et al.*, the number of *E. coli* in stools from breast fed infants correlated inversely with the concentration of IgA in the milk being consumed (24), although in studies in which colostrum was successfully used to combat infantile diarrhea caused by *E. coli*, a decrease in the colonization rate by *E. coli* after administration of the colostrum could not be demonstrated (25,26). Rowland, *et al.* (27) evaluated the bacteriostatic properties of milk from Gambian women against *E. coli* and found that the amount of time that infants were ill with diarrhea was inversely related to breast milk activity against *E. coli*.

In a case control study of 61 episodes of diarrhea due to *V. cholerae* in Bahrain, (28) a significantly higher incidence of cholera in nonbreast fed infants was shown, but it could not be determined whether the protection was due to protective factors in milk or lack of exposure to contaminated bottle feedings. In a prospective study of cholera in Bangladesh, breast milk IgA antibodies did not appear to protect children from colonization with *V. cholerae* 01, but did protect the breast fed children against symptomatic cholera illness (29).

Clostridium difficile. Kim and associated (30) showed that milk from 56% of 55 women had neutralizing activity against one or both toxins of *C. difficile*. In suckling mice 65% of milk samples with *in vitro* neutralizing activity against toxin A inhibited fluid accumulation by toxin A and 65% of milk samples with *in vitro* neutralizing activity against toxin A appeared to reside in the secretory IgA fraction. Wade et al (31) showed *in vitro* neutralizing activity of *C. difficile* crude toxin by the aqueous phase of colostral samples. Twenty five percent of colostral samples had neutralizing activity against *C. difficile* crude toxin.

Salmonella. Antibodies which agglutinated *Salmonella typhimurium* have been demonstrated in human milk (32). Antisalmonella O antigen antibodies were reported to be higher in urban rich than in urban poor living in Guatemala (33). France, *et al.* (34) reviewed histories of 253 infants less than 12 months from whom salmonella was identified in stools. Only 5% had ever been breast fed, only one infant had been breast fed near the time of infection and 27% of age matched controls had been breast fed.

Shigella. An investigation of shigellosis in infants under 2 years of age in Bangladesh (35) showed that the need for hospitalization was significantly less in breast fed than in nonbreast fed infants (5% vs 19%), as was the requirement for intravenous fluids (16% vs 38%). These results suggest that diarrhea in breast fed infants may be milder than in nonbreast fed infants. In areas where shigella is endemic, dysentery dramatically increases with weaning (2).

Campylobacter. Antibodies against campylobacter have been

demonstrated in human milk from women in Houston and Mexico City (36). A significant correlation between levels of secretory antibody to *C. jejuni* and prevention of diarreha due to *C. jejuni* was noted.

Rotavirus. It was not until the 1960's that neutralizing activity of human milk against viruses was shown to be mediated by immunoglobulin (37). Since then antibodies to many viral agents have been shown to be present in human colostrum, and in lower dilution in milk (38). Studies involving detection of antibody in human milk to rotavirus, which is the most common viral cause of diarrhea, have shown antibody in colostrum from women from all over the world. Nearly all this activity was in the secretory IgA fraction of colostrum and milk (14,39,40,41). Serum IgG antirotavirus activity is capable of being transferred placentally (41). In a study of 92 women from Australia, the only two milk samples which were negative for IgA to rotavirus were obtained from two IgA deficient women (41). In this series a small amount of antirotavirus activity also was detected in the IgM and IgG fractions of colostrum, and rarely of milk. As with other antiviral antibodies, the concentration of activity decreased with duration of lactation.

The majority of *in vitro* animal work has centered about rotavirus, with multiple groups demonstrating antibody to rotavirus in colostrum and milk from cows, lambs, pigs and mice. In these animals the antibody was present as IgA and also IgG_1 (38). Solid protection against rotavirus diarrhea by breast milk has been shown in infant mice, pigs, cows and lambs.

There are less convincing data regarding the role of human milk antibody in preventing or modifying human rotavirus infection. In newborns breast feeding was associated with a lower rate of neonatal rotavirus infection (22% vs 58%, $p < 0.01$). When infected, breast-fed neonates shed less virus, and it was often clumped (42,43), as shown to occur by antibody *in vitro* (44). In one of the few convincing studies, breast feeding protected neonates against rotavirus infection (45). The protection was correlated both with antirotavirus secretory IgA and anti-trypsin activity of the mother's milk (45). Provision of high titer antirotavirus antisera orally to low-birth-weight infants was shown to delay rotavirus excretion, decrease the amount of excretion and the severity of the diarrhea (46). In a small study in older infants, provision of milk to hospitalized children had no effect on rotavirus excretion but reduced the severity of illness (47). Antirotavirus activity in the milk was not measured. In two immunodeficient children, one with severe combined immunodeficiency and one with agammaglobulinemia, provision of irradiated, lactose-free milk containing antibody to rotavirus seemed to rid the children of their chronic rotavirus excretion and diarrhea (48).

Giardia lamblia. Miotti, *et al*. (49) showed that milk specimens from women from different geographic locations had IgA antibodies to *G. lamblia*. The concentrations of antibody of women living in Mexico were significantly greater than those of women living in the United States. Stevens and Frank (50) showed that infant mice suckling on immune mothers were resistant to infection by orally administered giardia cysts. The resistance was conveyed by suckling immune milk and was independent of the immune status of the infant's natural mother. Andrews and Hewlett (51) extended these data by showing that for infant mice to be protected, they must be suckling immune milk at the time of challenge by *G. muris* and must continue to do so for at least three to five days thereafter. Suckling immune milk did not induce sustained immunity. The immune milk contained specific IgA and IgG antibody to giardia. A study conducted in humans by Islam and associates (52) did not substantiate the protection of milk demonstrated in mice. The human study was unable to establish clear-cut protection related to human milk anti-*G. lamblia* antibodies as measured by immunofluorescence.

Entamoeba histolytica. Using an ELISA procedure, Grundy, *et al*. (53) demonstrated antibodies against *E. histolytica* in 31% of colostral specimens and 14% of sera specimens tested from women living in Kenya. Few women had titers in both milk and serum.

SUMMARY

The control and prevention of diarrhea depends upon improving sanitation in the environment including improvements in water supply, food and personal hygiene, waste disposed and education. Oral rehydration and breast feeding are also critical in the struggle against diarrhea, dehydration and death.

Multiple types of antibodies to bacteria, viruses and parasites have been detected in milk from animals and humans; however, the role of these antibodies is not entirely clear. In animals there is passage of antibody from the intestine to the systemic circulation of the infant. Thus, while protection is afforded by milk, the mechanisms may be either local or systemic. The latter avenue of protection is not available to human infants which absorb little to no antibody though their intestines, due to early "gut closure" to immunoglobulins. Although a significant correlation between levels of secretory antibody to *V. cholerae* and *C. jejuni* and prevention of diarrhea due to these organisms has been reported (29,36), substantiation of protection against other organisms needs to be obtained.

REFERENCES

1. DuPont, H.L., Pickering, L.K. (1980): Infections of the gastrointestinal tract. Plenum Publishing Corp, New York.
2. Kovar, M.G., Serdula, M.K., Marks, J.S., et al. (1984): Review of the epidemiologic evidence for an association between infant feeding and infant health. Pediatric, 74 (suppl.), 615.
3. Jason, J.M., Nieburg, P., Marks, J.S. (1984): Mortality and infectious disease associated with infant-feeding practices in developing countries. Pediatrics, 74 (suppl), 702.
4. Feachem, R.G., Koblinsky, M.A. (1984): Interventions for the control of diarrhoeal diseases among young children: promotion of breast feeding. Bull W H O, 62, 271.
5. Welsh, J.K., May, J.T. (1979): Anti-infective properties of breast milk. J Pediatr, 94, 1.
6. Goldman, A.S., Goldblum, R.M. (1985): Protective properties of human milk in nutrition in pediatrics. In Basic Science and Clinical Application. Ed. W.A. Walker. Little Brown and Co. Boston, MA.
7. Ogra, S.S., Ogra, P.L. (1978): Immunologic aspects of human colostrum and milk. I. Distribution characteristics and concentrations of immunoglobulins at different times after the onset of lactation. J Pediatr, 92, 546.
8. Ammann, A.J., Steihm, E.R. (1966): Immune globulin levels in colostrum and breast milk, and serum from formula- and breast-fed newborns. Proc Soc Exp Biol Med, 122, 1098.
9. Kenny, J.F., Boesman, M.I. Michaels, R.H. (1967): Bacterial and viral coproantibodies in breast-fed infants. Pediatrics, 39, 202.

10. Gindrat, J.J., Gothefors, L., Hanson, L.A., et al. (1972): Antibodies in human milk against E. coli of the serogroups most commonly found in neonatal infections. Acta Paediatr Scand, 61, 587.
11. Hanson, L.A., Carlsson, B., Ahlstedt, S., et al. (1975): Immune defense factors in human milk. Mod Probl Paediatr, 15, 63.
12. Stolier, O.A., Pelley, R.P., Kaniecki-Green, E., et al. (1976): Secretory IgA against enterotoxins in breast milk. Lancet, 1, 1258.
13. Holmgren, J., Hanson, L.A., Carlson, B., et al. (1976): Neutralizing antibody against E. coli and V. cholerae enterotoxins in human milk from a developing country. Scand J Immunol, 5, 867.
14. Simhon, A., Yolken, R.H., Mata, L. (1979): S-IgA cholera toxin and rotavirus antibody in human colostrum. Acta Paediatr Scand, 68, 161.
15. Vardinon, N., Spiner, Z., Goldhar, J., et al. (1979): Human milk anti-E. coli antibodies: relationship to maternal parity. Eur J Pediatr, 130, 173.
16. Holmgren, J., Svennerholm, A-M., Lindblad, M. (1983): Receptor-like glycocompounds in human milk that inhibit classical and El Tor Vibrio cholerae cell adherence (hemagglutination). Infect Immun, 39, 147.
17. Otnaess, A.B., Orstavik, I. (1981): Effect of fractions of Ethiopian and Norwegian colostrum on rotavirus and Escherichia coli heat labile enterotoxin. Infect Immun, 33, 459.
18. Aust-Kettis, A., Gebre-Medhin, M., Habte, D., et al. (1981): Antibiotics to heat-labile Escherichia coli enterotoxins in human milk and sera: a study of Ethiopian and Swedish mothers and their children. Trop Geo Med, 33, 225.
19. Majumdar, A.S., Dutta, P., Dutta, D., et al. (1981): Antibacterial and antitoxins in the serum and milk of cholera patients. Infect Immun, 32, 1.
20. Majumdar, A.S., Ghose, A.C. (1982): Protective properties of anticholera antibodies in human colostrum. Infect Immun, 36, 962.
21. Cruz, J.R., Garcia, C.B., Gebre-Medhin M., et al. (1982): Studies on human milk III. Secretory IgA quantity and antibody levels against Escherichia coli.
22. Svirsky-Gross, S. (1958): Pathogenic strains of E. coli (0111) among prematures and the use of human milk in controlling the outbreak of diarrhea. Ann Paediatr, 190, 109.
23. Mata, L.J., Urrutia, J.J. (1971): Intestinal colonization of breast-fed children in a rural area of low socioeconomical level. Ann NY Acad Sci, 176, 93.
24. Michael, J.C., Ringenback, R., Hottenstein, S. (1971): The antimicrobial activity of human colostral antibody in the newborn. J Infect Dis, 124, 445.
25. Gothefors, L., Carlsson, B., Ahlstedt, S., et al. (1976): Influence of maternal gut flora and colostral and cord serum antibodies on the presence of Escherichia coli in the feces of the newborn infant. Acta Paediatr Scand, 65, 225.
26. Larguia, A.M., Urman, J., Stoliar, O.A., et al. (1977): Fresh human colostrum for the prevention of E. coli diarrhea - a clinical experience. J Trop Pediatr Environ Child Health, 23, 289.
27. Rowland, M.G.M., Cole, T.J., Tully, M. (1980): Bacteriostasis of Escherichia coli by milk. VI The in vitro bacteriostatic property of Gambian mothers' breast milk in relation to the in vivo protection of their infants against diarrheal disease. J Hyg, 85, 403.
28. Gunn, R.A., Kimball, A.M., Pollard, R.A., et al. (1979): Bottle feeding is a risk factor for cholera in infants. Lancet, 2, 730.

29. Glass, R.I., Svennerholm, A., Stoll, B.J., et al. (1983): Milk antibodies protect breast-fed children against cholera. N Engl J Med, 308, 1389.
30. Kim, K., Pickering, L.K., DuPont, H.L., et al. (1984): _In vitro_ and _in vivo_ neutralizing activity of human colostrum and milk against purified toxins A and B of _Clostridium difficile_. J Infect Dis, 150, 57.
31. Wada, N., Nishida, N., Iwaki, S., et al. (1980): Neutralizing activity against _C. difficile_ toxin in the supernatants of cultured colostral cells. Infect Immun, 29, 545.
32. Allardyce, R.A., Shearman, D.J.C., McClelland, D.B.L., et al. (1974): Appearance of specific colostrum antibodies after clinical infection with _Salmonella typhimurium_. Brit Med J, 3, 307.
33. Hanson, L.A., Carlsson, B., Cruz, J.R., et al. (1979): Immune response in the mammary gland: _In_ Immunology of Breast Milk. Ed P.L. Ogra, D Dayton. Raven Press, New York.
34. France, G.L., Marmer, D.J., Steele, R.W. (1980): Breast-feeding and Salmonella infection. Am J Dis Child, 134, 147.
35. Stoll, B.J., Glass, R.I., Hug, M.I. (1982): Epidemiologic and clinical features of patients infected with Shigella who attended a diarrheal disease hospital in Bangladesh. J Infect Dis, 146, 177.
36. Ruiz-Palacios, G.M., Lopez-Vidal, Y., Calva, J., et al. (1986): Impact of breast feeding or diarrhea prevention. Pediatr Res, 20, 320A.
37. Michaels, R.M. (1965): Studies of antiviral factors in human milk and serum. J Immunol, 94, 262.
38. Pickering, L.K., Kohl, S., Cleary, T.G. (1986): Humoral factors in breast milk that protect against diarrhea: _In_ Human Lactation: Milk Components and Methodologies. Ed R.G. Jensen and M.C. Neville. Plenum Publishing Corporation, New York, 63-78.
39. Simhon, A., Mata, L. (1978): Anti-rotavirus antibody in human colostrum. Lancet, 1, 39.
40. Yolken, R.H., Wyatt, R.G., Mata , L., et al. (1978): Secretory antibody directed against rotavirus in human milk - measurement by means of enzyme-linked immunosorbent assay. J Pediatr, 93, 916.
41. McLean, B., Holmes, I.H. (1980): Transfer of anti-rotaviral antibodies from mothers to their infants. J Clin Microbiol, 12, 320.
42. Totterdell, B.M., Chrystie, I.L., Banatvala, J.E. (1976): Rotavirus infections in a maternity unit. Arch Dis Child, 51, 924.
43. Chrystie, I.L., Totterdell, B.M., Banatvala, J.E. (1978): Asymptomatic endemic rotavirus infections in the newborn. Lancet, 1, 1176.
44. Totterdell, B.M., Banatvala, J.E., Chrystie, I.L. (1983): Studies on human lacteal rotavirus antibodies by immuno electron microscope. J Med Virol, 11, 167.
45. McLean, B.S., Holmes, I.H. (1981): Effects of antibodies, trypsin, and trypsin inhibition on susceptibility of neonates to rotavirus infections. J Clin Microbiol, 13, 22.
46. Barnes, G.L., Hewson, P.M., McLellan, J.A., et al. (1983): A randomized trial of oral gammaglobulin in low-birth-weight infants infected with rotavirus. Lancet, 1, 1371.
47. Berger, R., Hadziselimovic, F., Just, M., et al. (1984): Influence of breast milk on nosocomial rotavirus infections in infants. Infection, 12, 171.
48. Saulsbury, F.T., Winkelstein, J.A., Yolken, R.M. (1980): Chronic rotavirus infection in immunodeficiency. J Pediatr, 97, 61.
49. Miotti, P., Gilman, R., Pickering, L.K., et al. (1985): Serum and

milk antibody levels to *Giardia lamblia*. J Infect Dis, 152, 1025.

50. Stevens, D.R., Frand, D.M. (1978): Local immunity in murine giardiasis: is milk protective at the expense of maternal gut? Trans Assoc Am Physicians, 91, 268.
51. Andrews, J.S., Jr., Hewlett, E.L. (1981): Protection against infection with *Giardia muris* by milk containing antibody to *Giardia*. J Infect Dis, 143, 242.
52. Islam, A., Stoll, B.J., Ljungstrom, I., et al. (1983): *Giardia lamblia* infections in a cohort of Bangladeshi mothers and infants followed for one year. J Pediatr, 103, 996.
53. Grundy, M.S., Cartwright-Taylor, L., Lundin, L., et al. (1983): Antibodies against *Entamoeba histolytica* in human milk and serum in Kenya. J Clin Microbiol, 17, 753.

PREGNANCY ASSOCIATED HORMONAL MILLEU AND BRONCHOMAMMARY CELL TRAFFIC

James C. Cumella, and Pearay L. Ogra

Department of Pediatrics and Microbiology, School of Medicine, State University of New York and Division of Infectious Diseases and Microbiology Laboratories Children's Hospital, Buffalo, N.Y. 14222

INTRODUCTION

Previous studies have established that a well defined secretory immune system exists in man and other mammalian species. This system has been analyzed in several recent monographs and reviews (1,2,3,4). Briefly, the secretory immune system refers to immunocompetent lymphoid tissue found in association with many external mucosal surfaces. It includes the gut associated lymphoid tissue (GALT), the bronchus associated lymphoid tisue (BALT), and the lymphoid tissues of male and female external genital tracts, conjunctiva, and mammary glands. Investigations have clearly shown that antigenic exposure in the intestinal and bronchial mucosa results in the appearance of specific secretory IgA locally in the mucosal lumen as well as in more distant secretory sites.

The physiologic, histologic, and functional nature of the mammary glands is quite distinct from that of other external mucosal surfaces such as the respiratory and intestinal tracts. However, sufficient evidence is available to suggest that the mammary glands act as extensions of the gut and bronchus associated immunocompetent lymphoid tissue in man and in other mammalian species (5,6). A number of important immunological events occur during pregnancy, in addition to the functional changes related to the development of lactation, associated with the profound changes that occur in the hormonal milieu. This chapter will review several aspects of bronchus associated lymphoid tissue and its role in the development of immunity in the breast. Information concerning the effects of pregnancy related hormones on immune response during pregnancy and lactation will also be reviewed.

IMMUNOLOGICAL CHANGES ASSOCIATED WITH PREGNANCY

Several distinct immunological changes occur during pregnancy and the immediate post partum period. For example, the concentrations of immunoglobulin A, M and G have been found to be significantly depressed during the second and third trimester (7). Conflicting data exists about the levels of circulating lymphocytes during pregnancy. However, several studies have demonstrated a clear inversion of T/B cell ratio (8,9). Most reports indicate that pregnancy is associated with a reduction in T cell function, as evidenced by decreased lymphoproliferative response to phytohemagglutinin (PHA) (8,10,11) decreased mixed lymphocyte culture (MLC) reactivity and allograph rejection (12,13), decreased response to purified protein derivative (PPD),(14) decreased human T cell colony formation (15) and decreased response to Concanavalin A (Con A)(16). In addition there are reports of polyclonal activation of B cells and increased specific antibody production (17) during pregnancy (18,19,20). Other changes associated with pregnancy include increased phagocytosis (21) and decreased inflammatory response (22). Various serum factors have been implicated in the immunological alteration observed during pregnancy. These include the appearance of alpha-fetoprotein a glycoprotein produced by the yolk sac and fetal liver (23,24,25), human chorionic gonadotropin (HCG) synthesized by the placenta (26,27), human chorionic somatomammotrophins (HCS)(27) and presence of circulating immune complexes (28,29,30). More recent studies have suggested that the immunological alterations associated with pregnancy and the enhanced immunoglobulin activity observed post partum in the products of lactation may also be related to the unique hormonal milieu that occurs during pregnancy. Several studies dealing with the relationship of several specific hormones and immune response are summarized below.

HORMONES AND THE IMMUNE RESPONSE

Sex Hormones. There is evidence to suggest that sex hormones play an important modulating role in isotype specific immunoglobulin responses. The switch of IgM to IgG during the natural course of autoimmune diseases in NZB/NZW F1 mice is strongly influenced by sex hormones (31,32). Animal experimentation has shown that castration of male mice resulted in a significant decline in their serum testosterone levels and an accelerated switch from 19S to 7S autoantibodies to DNA and Poly A. Castration of female mice and treatment with androgens delayed or eliminated such isotype switch (31,32). The levels of IgA and IgG in cervical secretions alter during the menstrual cycle, a period characterized by profound changes in hormonal concentrations (33,34,35,36). A correlation between plasma progesterone and specific isotype response has also been observed (37). Fluctuations in the levels of anti-Candida antibodies correlated with circulating levels of estradiol or progesterone. Studies on antibody formation and antigen induced cell differentiation have demonstrated that IgM production during primary immune response and IgG production during the secondary response is influenced by sex hormones (38). The primary and secondary immune response were evaluated in response to thymus-dependent and independent antigens in normal male and female mice and in castrated male mice. Both IgM antibody production during the primary response and IgG antibody production during the secondary challenge were enhanced in females when compared to males of equivalent age.

Despite numerous observations on induction of immunoregulatory changes induced by sex hormones, the mechanism of their interaction is largely unexplained. To date specific hormone receptors have not been identified in lymphocytes for estrogen and progesterone. It has been reported that the murine as well as bovine thymus glands contain estradiol binding proteins which have the characteristics of steroid receptor proteins. However, it is not clear if the estrogen binding sites exist on lymphoid or epithelial components of the thymus gland (39,40). Recently, a specific enzyme, 20 alpha-hydroxysteroid dehydrogenase (20 SDH) involved in the metabolism of sex hormones has been demonstrated in T lymphocytes and thymocytes. Induction of this enzyme has been shown to be associated with differentiation of T cells

(41,42). These observations raise the possibility of a receptor dependent interaction between sex hormones and immunocompetent cells.

Prolactin. The importance of prolactin in maintaining normal humoral and cellular immunity has been recently explored in rats by Berczi and Nagy. Prolactin has been reported to be important in induction of contact sensitivity (43), in regulating primary and secondary antibody responses, (44) in the development of adjuvant arthritis, (45) and in rejection of allogenic skin grafts (46). The immunospecific functions of prolactin with parasitic infestations has also been explored employing cell transfer procedures (47). The functional activity of mesenteric lymph node cells, as assessed by their capacity to cause parasite rejection, was reduced by the treatment of recipients with prolactin. These results suggest that prolactin may affect a specific component of the immune response. Prolactin receptors have very recently been identified on human T and B lymphocytes (48). These observations raise the possibility that prolactin has an important physiological role in man in the regulation of humoral and cell mediated immune responses.

In preliminary studies carried out in our laboratory, we have observed that the pregnancy related hormones are involved in directing maturation or expansion of IgA-B cells. Several experiments examined the effects of hormones on the lymphocytes of normal adult volunteers employing a modified plaque assay system in agar. We found that *in vitro* stimulation with prolactin resulted in production of IgA and IgM in a dose dependent fashion. Little or no IgG production was observed. Stimulation with estrogen or progesterone on the other hand resulted in enhancement of synthesis of all immunoglobulin isotypes.

To further examine hormone interelationships, a limited number of combination experiments were performed utilizing physiological concentrations of prolactin, estrogen, and progesterone (See Figure 1). For experiments utilizing both steroid hormones in conjunction with prolactin, a selective IgA response was observed for multiple concentrations of prolactin employed. On the other hand, combination of prolactin with either progesterone or estrogen alone, exhibited considerable variability in the nature and the degree of enhancement for specific isotype responses. The lowest concentrations of prolactin with either progesterone or estrogen alone elicited a polyclonal response involving all isotypes while higher doses of prolactin resulted in selective IgA responses with progesterone, and suppression of all isotypes with estrogen. It thus appears that prolactin may selectively enhance IgA production in certain defined concentrations of the hormonal environment.

These preliminary experiments suggest that lactational hormones affect B cell expansion or immunoglobulin release in the absence of other apparent stimuli. Enhancement of IgA and IgM was the predominant effect of all hormones when used alone. Combinations of hormones in certain concentrations enhanced isotype specific plaque formation with a high degree of selectivity and the system could be manipulated to induce a response limited to the IgA isotype.

ORIGIN OF IMMUNOLOGICAL REACTIVITY IN THE BREAST

Human milk contains large amounts of secretory IgA immunoglobulin specific for normally resident organisms or pathogenic microorganisms found either in the gut or the respiratory tract (1-4). The predominance of secretory IgA with defined specificities is consistant with either a process of local synthesis with selective accumulation of IgA producing cells in the mammary gland, or a process of active transport of IgA from GALT and or BALT. There is good evidence to suggest that the immunoglobulin observed in the mammary secretions originates, at least in part, from local synthesis in plasma cells that reside in mammary gland stroma and that these cells are derived from IgA precursors which originate in the lymphoid tissue of GALT or BALT. Consistant with this notion of local production of IgA are the following findings. First, morphological studies in rabbit, mouse, and human mammary glands have demonstrated that the overall number of plasma cells is much higher in the lactating breast than in the resting breast. Weisz-Carrington et. al. 1977, demonstrated that the plasma cell population of the mammary gland increased dramatically during pregnancy and lactation (49). They found that the increase was far in excess of what could be explained solely on the basis of increased size of the mammary gland. The mammary gland had a six fold increase in weight and a 150 fold increase in plasma cells per unit area for a total net increase of about 900 fold. The increase in plasma cells paralled the development of the glandular epithelium. Furthermore, weaning resulted in a sharp decrease in the number of plasma cells and involution of the epithelium. Immunofluorescent staining demonstrated that most of the increase in plasma cells was due to increase in the number of cells staining for IgA. Similar studies were performed by Lee et al in rabbits (50,51). They found few IgA containing cells in virgin animals (20 cells/unit area), but in pregnancy there was a dramatic increase (400-650 cells/unit area). A similar hormonal expansion has been demonstrated in man (52). The greatest increase in plasma cells parallels the fullest extent of glandular development which occurs during lactation. Another line of evidence consistent with the local immunoglobulin production by the IgA plasma cells within the mammary gland is derived from adoptive transfer experiments. Roux et. al. and McDermont et. al. have both demonstrated that mesenteric lymphnode (MLN) lymphoblasts injected intravenously into mice will selectively home to the mammary glands (53,54). The lymphoblasts localize to the mouse mammary glands late in pregnancy and throughout lactation but not in the resting mammary glands. These cells seem to become a rich source of IgA secreting plasma cells that localize in periglandular locations within the breast (52). Experiments that investigate immunoglobulin specificity lend further support for the concept of local synthesis in the breast. Several clinical studies have demonstrated that the secretory IgA antibodies found in human milk and colostrum are directed against intestinal and bronchial microorganisms often in the absence of any specific IgA activity in the circulation. Finally the colonization experiments with *Escherichia coli* 083 in pregnant women carried out by Goldblum and Hanson (1975)(55) have suggested that lymphoid cells in GALT selectively seed the mammary gland where they produce IgA antibodies to the specific microorganisms encountered in the gut. They have shown that oral immunization resulted not only in specific IgA antibody secretion in colostrum but that there were lymphoid cells in these secretions apparently synthesizing specific IgA antibody.

An additional mechanism by which dimeric IgA antibodies specific for enteric or respiratory organisms may enter mammary secretions is via selective transport by the removal of serum IgA that is actually synthesized at distant mucosl sites. Studies in ruminants (Cows and Sheep), in whom serum IgA is predominately derived from plasma cells in the intestinal lamina propria, demonstrate that during several stages of lactation there is a major contribution from serum to the IgA content of milk (56,57). A selective transport mechanism was demonstrated that was probably dependent in the localization of the secretory component.

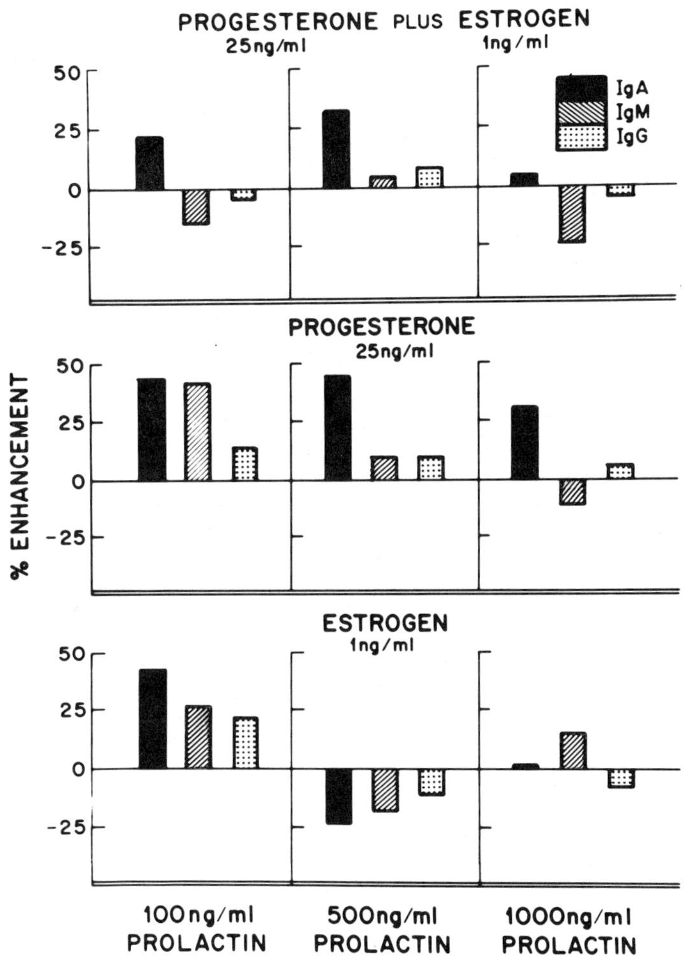

Figure 1. Effect of combinations of lactational hormones (prolactin, estrogen, and progesterone) in different concentrations on the polyclonal IgG, IgM, IgA synthesis. The vertical axis represents enhancement of isotype-specific plaques in presence of the hormones relative to the hormone-free control.

The transfer of IgA from serum into milk has also been demonstrated in the mouse (58,59) and in the sow (60). This route of transport is probably important in animals in whom most of the serum IgA is dimeric such as in ruminants (56) and when the serum IgA is derived from the intestine (61,62). However, studies of Dahlgren et al in rats have demonstrated that there was no transfer of serum IgA into rat milk (63).

On the other hand, the cellular origin of the immunoglobulin in human milk and colostrum has not been clearly defined. It is unlikely that the transfer of serum immunoglobulin into mammary secretions is the predominant source of IgA. There are several findings that make this unlikely. Human blood contains relatively little polymeric IgA. Immunofluorescence studies of the connective tissue stroma of human mammary glands provide little evidence that the glandular stroma acts as a depot for polymeric IgA (52). Furthermore observations previously cited demonstrate that specific IgA antibodies are often found in milk after bronchial or gastrointestinal immunization in the absence of any detectable specific circulating IgA. This strongly favors the transfer of antigen reactive immunoblasts rather than immunoglobulin to mammary glands. A quantitative evaluation of the selective contribution of locally secreted immunoglobulin as opposed to that derived from serum has not been performed in humans.

Since milk may contain as much as 11 gm of IgA per day in 24 hr specimens, it is striking to note a disproportionately sparse number of immunoglobulin producing cells in the lactating breast. The mechanism underlying the disparity between the number of antibody producing cells and the content of immunoglobulin in milk is somewhat puzzling if local synthesis is the sole source for the immunoglobulin. The transfer of some IgA from the serum would help to explain this disparity.

If the transfer of IgA from serum to milk does take place in significant quantities in man, it may also have important implications with respect to exposure of the neonate to antigens since it has been demonstrated that antigen complexed with polymeric IgA may gain entrance into the milk. This may be a mechanism of important immunologic interaction between the neonate and mother.

BRONCHIAL LYMPHOID TISSUE AND MAMMARY GLAND IMMUNOLOGICAL REACTIVITY

Replication of infectious pathogens at exposed mucosal surfaces is an important determinant for the immunological repertoire of the mammary glands. Certain viruses such as rhinovirus, respiratory syncytial virus, myxoviruses and certain types of adenovirus remain localized superfically in the mucosa, where they produce disease, as opposed to other viruses exemplified by poliovirus, echovirus, and measles virus where there is usually viremia and systemic infection. Certain bacteria are also more commonly associated with infections limited to the mucosal surface of the respiratory or intestinal tracts. The restriction of an organism to replication in the respiratory tract make them ideal for examining the role of bronchial mucosal surfaces in relation to the immune responses in the breast. To date specific antibody activity in milk has been demonstrated against a variety of microorganisms (Table 1).

Table 1
Specific Antibody Reactivity in Human Colostrum and Milk

Bacteria	Viruses	Fungi	Others
E. coli (O+K) antigens and enterotoxin)	Rotavirus	Candida albicans	Milk proteins
Salmonella	Poliovirus 1,2,3		Dietary antigens
Shigella	Echovirus 6,9		Other macromolecules
Vibrio cholerae	Coxsackievirus A9,B3		Giardia
Bacteroides fragilis	Respiratory syncytial virus		
Streptococcus pneumoniae	Cytomegalovirus		
Bordetella pertussis	Rubella		
Cornybacterium diphtheriae	Varicella zoster		
Clostridium tetani	Influenza A virus		
Streptococcus mutans	Herpes simlex virus		
	Arboviruses Semlike Forest Ross River Japanese B Dengue		

Earlier studies carried out in rabbits with pneumococcal antigen after bronchial or intestinal immunization have shown the appearance of specific IgA in antibodies in colostrum and milk (64,65). These studies additionally demonstrated that there was no correlation between the high levels of secretory IgA antibodies and serum antibody production. Naturally acquired respiratory viral infections or immunizations via the mucosal route appears to be a very effective means of inducing a secretory IgA antibody response in mammary secretions. Epidemiologic studies carried out by Fishaut et al during a community outbreak of infection with respiratory syncytial virus (RSV) provided a unique opportunity to study the role of bronchial mucosal exposure to a virus on the development of specific immunocompetence in the milk (66). Groups of nursing mothers were sequentially evaluated for the presence or appearance of RSV-specific antibody in the breast milk at different stages of lactation before, during, and towards the end of the RSV epidemic. RSV-specific IgA activity was observed in 75% of the specimens of colostrum and in 40% and 57% of the specimens of milk obtained three months and six months after the onset of lactation (Table 2). The latter increase in frequency of IgA antibody containing milk samples appeared to follow the peak of the RSV infection in the community. Of particular significance was the observation that many subjects documented as having reinfection with RSV during the outbreak manifested an increase in the preexisting IgA antibody titers in milk (66). In view of the fact that the pathogenesis of RSV is characterized by its exquisite restriction of replication to the respiratory tract mucosa, these observations strongly link bronchial immune responsiveness to the mammary gland during conditions of naturally acquired infections.

The characteristics of the class of antibody activity observed in the milk may also be influenced by the dissemination of specific antigens from the mucosal sites to the mammary glands by way of systemic circulation. Unlike RSV, the pathogenesis of rubella virus infection is frequently associated with the development of viremia and involvement of other systemic sites. The mucosal immune response to rubella virus was studied by Losonsky et al in groups of lactating women after immunization with HPV-77 DE5 or RA 27/3 live attenuated rubella virus vaccine administered subcutaneouly or intranasally (68,69). It should be pointed out that HPV-77 vaccine does not replicate in the mucosa when introduced intranasally, while RA 27/3 results in mucosal infection after intranasal as well as parenteral inoculation. Over 69 percent of immunized women shed virus into the milk. A predictable nasopharyngeal IgA and serum IgG response was observed after subcutaneous or intranasal immunization with RA 27/3 vaccine and little or no nasopharyngeal IgA response was detected after subcutaneous immunization with HPV-77 vaccine (Figure 2). HPV-77 vaccine virus was shed only minimally into the respiratory tract after subcutaneous immunization and failed to induce respiratory infection when introducted intranasally. A virus specific IgA response in milk was however seen in all women regardless of the type of immunization. The presence of virus in milk appeared to potentiate the peak IgA antibody activity in the milk. The dichotomy of nasopharyngeal and milk IgA response observed here suggests a potential contribution of local antibody synthesis in the mammary glands secondary to the local availability of the antigen. The appearance of antibody in milk may be partly mediated by the further proliferation of BALT-derived rubella-sensitized IgA cells as a result of local availability of virus in the breast. This possibility is further supported by the observations that IgA rubella activity in the milk was highest in subjects who shed measurable amounts of virus in the nasopharynx as well as milk compared to those who shed the virus only in the nasopharynx or milk (Figure 2). These and other studies have strongly supported the concept of a bronchomammary axis of mucosal immunity.

In order to examine the differential role of bronchial vs gut-associated lymphoreticular tissue, as well as the nature of the antigen (soluble vs particulate, replicating vs non replicating), groups of pregnant rabbits were immunized with RSV or bovine serum albumin (BSA) administered intratracheally, intravenously, or by intragastric intubation (67). The response to RSV was characterized by the regular appearance of IgA anti-RSV in the colostrum, milk, bronchial and intestinal secretions following either oral or intratracheal immunization but not after intravenous immunization. RSV-specific IgG appeared in the colostrum, milk, and serum regardless of the route of immunization. On the other hand, the response to BSA by all three routes of immunization was characterized by the appearance of anti-BSA antibody in serum, colostrum, and milk limited to IgG isotype. No IgA specific anti-BSA response was observed. The anti-BSA antibody response was unaffected during the observed nursing period and did not exhibit any change in response to BSA ingestion before or during pregnancy or

Table 2
Temporal Patterns of Class-Specific Antibody Activity Against RSV in the Colostrum and Milk of Lactating Women

		Subjects with RSV Antibody Response in Colostrum and Milk					
		IgG		IgA		IgM	
Day Postpartum	Number Tested	Number Positive / Percent	RSV Antibody Titer (Mean)	Number Positive / Percent	RSV Antibody Titer (Mean)	Number Positive / Percent	RSV Antibody Titer (Mean)
1-3	24	7 / (29.1)	2.5	18 / (75.0)	6.5	1 / (4.1)	10
8-28	19	0	-	7 / (36.8)	3.1	0	-
85-112	15	0	-	6 / (40.0)	4.3	0	-
>168*	7	0	-	4 / (57.1)	16.8	0	-

*Corresponds to the onset of infection with RSV in the community.

during nursing. These observations suggest that the appearance of IgA antibody response in the mammary gland following mucosal immunization is not uniform for different types of antigen. The presence of mammary IgA antibodies in response to RSV and its absence to BSA following respiratory or intestinal immunization suggests that the physical as well as the chemical nature of the antigens may be important determinants of mammary immune response. Furthermore, the presence of a replicating organisms by influencing the duration of exposure, (prolonging antigenic stimulation) at the mucosal surface and helping to foster the proliferation of antibody producing cell may be important and may influence the nature isotypic specific responses.

Table 3
Distribution of immunohistologic staining for IgG, IgM, and IgA immunoglobulin-containing cells in 9 days post-partum rabbit mammary glands.

Route of immunization	Mean* percentage of immunoglobulin-staining ± SD		
	IgG	IgM	IgA
i.v.	55.4 ± 19.9	5.0 ± 5.7	39.6 ± 16.3
p.o.	31.8 ± 10.8	8.8 ± 5.7	58.4 ± 9.7
i.t.	26.4 ± 10.73	13.2 ± 7.0	60.4 ± 13.8
Post-partum controls	21.3 ± 11.2	12.3 ± 5.3	66.4 ± 15.1

*100 cells counted/specific Ig.

i.v. intravenous
p.o. per oral
i.t. intratracheal

During the course of these investigations, it was also noted that the class of antibody found in milk may also be influenced by the route of antigen exposure. Changes in the proportion of specific IgA isotype bearing cells in the mammary gland were found to occur following intravenous, oral or transtracheal immunization with RSV (67) (see table 3). The mean proportion of IgG staining cells appeared to be higher and IgA staining cells lower in intravenously immunized animals than following oral or transtracheal immunization.

The mechanism underlying the seeding of antigen activated IgA cells from the BALT to the mammary glands is not well understood. Several different mechanisms may interplay to account for the cell traffic patterns that have this far been described. The factors involved in mucosal lymphoblast localization were recently reviewed by Bienstock et al 1983 (70,71).

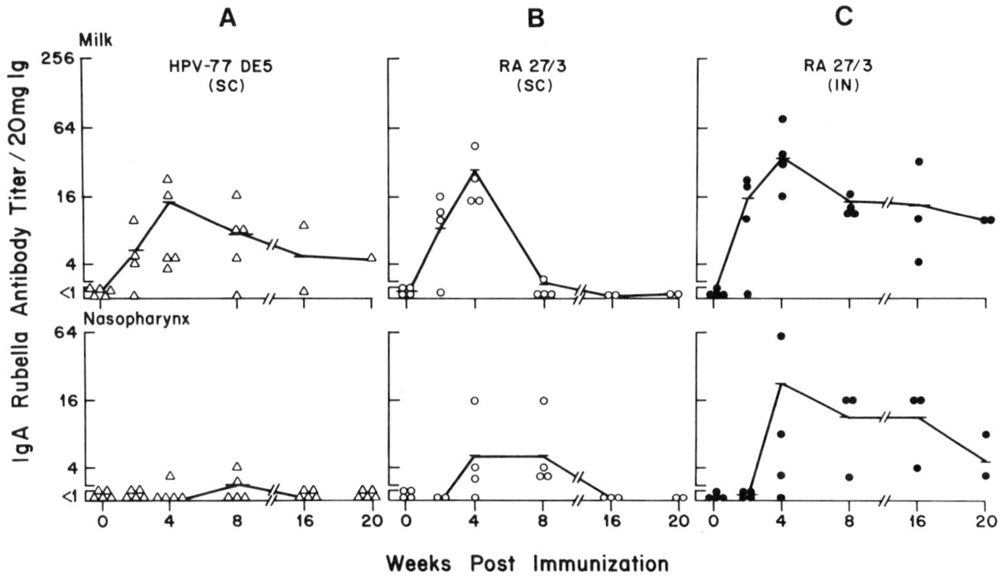

Figure 2. Temporal patterns of IgA-rubella antibody response in the milk and nasopharyngeal secretions after subcutaneous (SC) or intranasal (IN) immunization with HPV-77 DE/5 or RA 27/34 live attenuated rubella virus vaccine.

There is substantial evidence to suggest that in the mammary gland immunoblast traffic appears to be under the control of the endocrine system. Weisz-Carrington et al (49) demonstrated that during pregnancy and early lactation there is an increase in the number of plasma cells in the breast and that by the first week of lactation most are synthesizing IgA. In a study of virgin mice, treatment with gestational hormones resulted in increased content of IgA cells in the mammary glands and the development of the capacity of gut cells to seed mammary tissues (72). They demonstrated that an extended exposure to estrogen, progesterone and prolactin was necessary for maximal increments in IgA-producing plasma cells in the breast. Similarly castrated males exposed to hormones become moderately receptive to mammary gland homing of cells specific for IgA. Testosterone, as would be expected, eliminated female breast reactivity to these cells (72).

In an earlier study on immunoglobulin production in the nonlactating human breast several interesting findings were observed (73). Mononuclear antibody containing cells were present in the nulliporous and parous non lactating breast, with IgA-containing cells predominating. Synthesis of IgA immunoglobulin appeared to be slightly increased in the parous subjects. IgA immunoglobulin was found in the mammary tissues during the proliferative stages of the menstrual cycle for the nulliparous subjects. The number of IgA producing cells in the non-lactating breast was observed to increase with parity. These findings provide further evidence that the immunologic make-up of the nonlactating breast may also be significantly influenced by the hormonal mileu.

The effect of hormones on cell traffic is not limited to the mammary glands. Adoptive transfer experiments in mice with radiolabeled mesenteric lymphoblasts have demonstrated that such antigen sensitized cells also seed the genital tract. The number of cells entering the cervix and the vagina varies with the stage of estrus (proestrus estrus or diestrus)(74). The greatest number of cells were found during proestrus with a marked decline in diestrus phase. These studies are strongly suggestive of the existence of a homing mechanism for the mammary gland and other sex hormone target tissues for class-specific immunoglobulin producing cells, dependent on a specific hormonal milieu. Weisz-Carrington et al have suggested that sex hormones induce a receptor in target tissues that directs B cell localization. Hanson has suggested that lactational hormones may induce Ia antigens coded for by the major histocompatability complex on glandular epithelial cells in the breast and that this may be the signal responsible for the migration of specific IgA committed cells to home to the mammary gland (75). Recently HLA-DR like antigens have been identified in colostral and milk fat globules and in epithelial cells in the products of human lactation (76,77).

Curtis and coworkers have performed a number of experiments that do suggest that histocompatibility antigens may have much to do with lymphocyte adhesion and their eventual localization in the tissues (78,79).

Finally, there is growing evidence on T cells that have specificity for autologous immunoglobulin determinants. Functionally distinct subsets of helper T cells that induce isotype switching from precursor cells and cells that induce terminal differentiation with specificity for isotype determinants have been defined (80,81,82). The detection of IgA class specific T helper cells in Peyers Patches has led to the alternative speculation that the predominance of an IgA response in a given area may depend primarily on its T cell content and that T cells may specificaly home to mucosal tissues where they then determine the B cell traffic and clonal expansion. However, their role in cellular homing mechanisms in the mammary glands remains to be determined.

REFERENCES

1. Bienenstock, J. The lung as an immunological organ. Ann. Rev. Med. 35:49-62,1984.

2. Tomasi, T.B., Jr. Reviews of infectious disease mechanisms of immune regulation at mucosal surfaces. 5:S784,1983.

3. Ogra, P.L., Losonsky, G.A., Fishaut, M. In the secretory immune system. McGhee, J. and Mestecky, J. (eds)., Ann. N.Y. Acad. Sci. 409:81-95,1983.

4. Bienenstock, J., and Befus, A.D. Mucosal immunity. Immunology 41:249,1980.

5. Tomasi, T.B., Jr. The immune system of secretions. Prentice-Hall, Englewood Cliffs, N.J. 1976.

6. Lamm, M.E. Cellular aspects of immunoglobulin A. Adv. Immunol. 22:223,1976.

7. Amino, N., Tanizawa, O., Mizai, K., Tanaka, F. et. al. Changes of serum immunoglobulins IgA, M, G, and E during pregnancy. Obstetrics and Gynecology p.415,1978.

8. Strelkauskas, A.J., Davies, I.J. and Dray, S. Longitudinal studies showing alterations in the levels and functional response of T and B lymphocytes in human pregnancy. Clin. Exp. Immunol. p.531-539,1978.

9. Bulmer, R. and Hancock, K.W. Depletion of circulating T lymphocytes in pregnancy. Clin. Exp. Immunol. 28:302-305,1977.

10. Burrells, C., Wells, P.W. and Sutherland, A.D. Reactivity of ovine lymphocytes to PHA and PWM during pregnancy and the immediate post-partum period. Clin. Exp. Immunol. p.410-415,1978.

11. Ruppert, B. and Richie, E. PHA response of murine spleen cells during pregnancy and inhibition of normal PHA response by pregnancy and post partum serum. Exp. Hemat. p.59-68,1977.

12. Heslap, R.W., Krohn, P.L. and Sparrow, F.M. The effects of pregnancy on the survival of skin homografts in rabbits. J. Endocr. p.332,1954.

13. Anderson, R.H. and Monroe, C.W. Experimental study of the behavior of adult human skin homografts during pregnancy. Am.J. of Gynecol. p.1096,1962.

14. Biakeland, S.A. and Hastleitner, W. Cellular immunity in pregnancy. Clin. Exp. Immunol. 30:408-412,1977.

15. Stahn, R. Fabricius, H. and Jartleitman, W. Suppression of human T cell colony formation during pregnancy. Nature 276:831,1978.

16. Mendelson, J., Multer, M.M. and Bernheim, J.L. Inhibition of human lymphocyte stimulation by steroid hormones. Clin. Exp. Immunol. p.127,1977.

17. Fabris, N. Immunological reactivity during pregnancy in the mouse. Expermentatia 29:610,1973.

18. Fabris, N., Piantanelli, L. anmd Muzziali, M. Differential effect of pregnancy gestagens on humoral and cell mediated immunity. Clin. Exp. Immunol. 28:306,1977.

19. Nossal, J.V., Bussard, A.E., Lewis, H., and Mazie, J.C. Formation of hemolytic plaques by peritoneal cells in vitro. In Developmental Aspects of Antibody Formation and Structure, Czeckoslakia. Acad. Press p.655,1970.

20. Mathur, S., Mathur, R.S., Gourst, J.M., Williamson, H.O., and Fudenberg, H.H. Sex steroid hormones and circulating IgE levels. Clin. Exp. Immunol. 30:403-407,1977.

21. Nicol, T., Bilbery, D.L.J., Cardingley, J.L., and Vernon-Roberts, B. Oestrogen: The natural stimulant of body defense. J. Endocrin. 30:277-291,1964.

22. Carter, J. The effect of progesterone, oestradiol and HCG on cell mediated immunity in pregnant mice. J. Reprod. Fert. 46:2110-216,1976.

23. Murgita, R.A., Goidl, E.A., Konteainea, S., Wizzell, H. Alpha fetoprotein induces suppressor T cells in vitro. Nature p.257,1977.

24. Murzita, R.A. and Tomasi, T.B. Suppressing the immune response by AFP. J. Exp. Med. 141:260-285,1975.

25. Yachinin, S. anmd Lester, E. Inhibition of human lymphocyte transformation by human AFP. Clin. Exp. Immunol. p.484,1976.

26. Adcock, E.W., Teasdale, F. et. al. HCG: Its possible role in maternal lymphocyte suppression. Science p.845,1973.

27. Contractor, S.F., Davies, H. Effect of HCS and HCG on PHA induced lymphocyte transformation. Nature p.284,1973.

28. Buckley, R.H., Schiff, R.I., and Amos, D.B. Blocking of autologous and hemologous leukocyte responses by human alloimmune plasma. J. Immunol. p.34,1972.

29. Rocklin, R.E., Kitzmiller, J.L., Carpenter, C.B., Garavery, M.R., David, J.R. Maternal fetal relation. NEJM p.1209,1976.

30. Kasakura, S. A factor in maternal plasma during pregnancy that suppresses the reactivity of MLC. J. Immunology p.1296,1971.

31. Roubinian, J., Talal, N., Siiteri, P.K., and Sadakian, J.A. Sex hormone modulation of autoimmunity in NZB/NZW mice. Arth and Rheum. 22:1162,1979.

32. Roubinian, J., Papoion, R. and Tabal, N. Androgenic hormones modulate autoantibody responses and improve survival in murine lupus. J. Clin. Invest. 59:1066-1070,1977.

33. Coughlan, B.M., and Shinner, G.R. Concentration of immunoglobulin in cervical mucus in patients with normal and abnormal cervical cytology. Brit. J. Obst. and Gynecol. p129,1977.

34. Schumacher, G.F. Soluble proteins in cervical mucus. Biology of the cervix. Eds. Blandau and Mazhissi. Univ. of Chicago Press p.201,1973.

35. Hulka, J.F., and Omron, W.F. The uterine cervix as a potential local antibody secretor. Am. J. Obst. and Gyn. p.440,1969.

36. Chipperfield, E. and Evans, B. Effect of local infection and oral contraception on immunoglobulin levels in cervical mucus. Infection and Immunity p.215-221,1975.

37. Mathur, S., Mathur, R.S., Gramling, T.S., Landgrebe, S.C., Williamson, H.O., and Fudenberg, H.H. Sex steroid hormones and antibody to Candida albicans. Clin. Exp. Immunol. 33:79-87,1978.

38. Eidinger, D., and Garrett, T. Studies of the regulation effects of the sex hormones on antibody formation and stem cell differentiation. J. Exp. Med. 136:1098,1972.

39. Richmann, M.E. and Villee, C.A. Estradiol binding by rat thymus cytosol. J. Steroid Biochem. p.637,1978.

40. Grossman, C.J., Nathan, P. Specific estrogen receptor in rat and beef thymus (Abstract S119) Fed Proc. p.1236,1977.

41. Weinstein, Y. 20 Alpha-hydroxysteroid dehydrogenase: A T-lymphocyte associated enzyme. J. Immunol. p.1223,1977.

42. Fuks, A.S., and Weinstein, Y. 20 Alpha-hydroxysteroid dehydrogenose activity in New Zealand mice T lymphocytes and bone marrow cells. J. Immunol. 123:1266-1271,1979.

43. Nagy, E., and Berazi, I. Prolactin and contact sensitivity allergy 36:429,1981.

44. Berczi, I., Nagy, E., Keracz, K., Harrath, E. Regulation of humoral immunity in rats by pituitary hormones. Acta Endocrinologica p.506,1981.

45. Berczi, I., and Nagy, E. A possible role of prolactin in adjuvant arthritis. Arth. and Rheum. p.591-4,1982.

46. Berczi, I. and Nagy E. Immunodeficiency in hypophysectomized rats: Restoration by prolactin. Red. Proc. p.1031,1981.

47. Kelly, J.D. amd Dineen, J.K. The suppression of rejection of Nippostronzylus braseliensis in lewis strain rats treated with ovine prolactin. Immunology 24:551,1973.

48. Russell, D.H., Kibler, R., Matrision, L., Larson, D.F., Poulos, B., and Magun, B.E. Prolactin receptors on human T and B lymphocytes. J. Immunol. 134:3027,1985.

49. Weiz-Carrington, P., Roux, M.E., and Lamm, M.E. Plasma cells and epithial immunoglobulins in the mouse mammary gland during pregnancy and lactation. J. Immunology 119:1306,1977.

50. Lee, H., Carey Honly, W., and Knight, K.L. Kinetics of appearance of IgA containing cells in the mammary glands of pregnant rabbits. Fed. Proc. 36:1310.

51. Lee, H., and Carey Honly, W. Relationship of glandular development to development of Ig cell systems in rabbit mammary tissues. Fed. Proc. 37:1744.

52. Brandtzaeg, P. The secretory immune system of lactating human mammary glands compared with other exocrine organs: In: The Secretory Immune System, ed. by J.R. McGhee and J. Mestecky NYAS 409:353-380,1983.

53. Roux, M.E., McWiliams, M., Phillips-Quagliata, J.M., Weisz-Carrington, P., and Lamm, M.E. Origin of IgA-secreting plasma cells in the mammary gland. J. Exp. Med. 146:1311,1977.

54. McDermott, M.R., Bienstock, J. Evidence for a common mucosal immunologic system I. J Immunol. 122:1892,1979.

55. Goldblum, R.M., Ahlstedt, S., Carlsson, B., et. al. Antibody forming cells in human colostrum after oral immunization. Nature 257:787,1975.

56. Sheldrake, R.F., Husband, A.J., Watson, D.L., and Cripps, A.W. Selective transport of serum-derived IgA into mucosal secretions. J. Immunology 132:363,1984.

57. Newly, T.J., and Bourne, J. The nature of the local immune system of the bovine mammary gland. J. Immunology 118:461,1977.

58. Halsey, J.F., Johnson, B.H., and Cebra, J.J. Transport of immunoglobulins from serum into colostrum. J. Exp. Med. p.767-772,1980.

59. Halsey, J.F., Mitchell, C., Meyer, R. and Cebra, J.J. Metabolism of immunoglobulin A in lactating mice: origins of immunoglobulin A in milk. Eur. J. Immunol. 12:107,1982.

60. Bourne, J., and Cuirtis, J. The transfer of immunoglobulins IgG, IgA and IgM from serum to colostrum and milk in the sow. Immunology 24:157,1973.

61. Beh, K.J., Watson, D.L., and Lascelles, A.K. Concentrations of immunoglobulins and albumin in lymph collected from various regions of the body of the sheep. Aust. J. Exp. Med. Sci. 52:1974,1981.

62. Quin, TJ.W., Husband, A.J., and Lascelles, A.K. The origin of the immunoglobulins in intestinal lymph of sheep. Aust. J. Exp. Biol. Med. Sci. 53:205,1975.

63. Dhalgren, U.S., Ahlstedt, L., Hedman, C., Wadsworth, C., and Hanson, L. Scand. J. Immunol. 14:95-98,1981.

64. Montgomery, P.C., Rosner, B.R., and Cohn, J. The secretory antibody response. Anti-DNP antibodies induced by dinitrophenylated type III. Pneumococcus. Immunological Comm. 3:143-156,1974.

65. Montgomery, P.C., Connelly, K.M., Cohen, C., and Skandera, C.A. Remote site stimulation of secretory IgA antibodies following bronchial and gastric stimulation. Adv. Exp. Med. Biol. 107:113-122,1978.

66. Fishaut, M., Murphy, D., Neifert, M., McIntosh, K., and Ogra, P.L. Bronchomammary axis in the immune response to respiratory syncytial virus. J. Pediatrics 99:186-191,1981.

67. Peri, B.A., Theodore, C.M., Losonsky, G.A., Fishaut, J.M., Rothberg,

R.M., and Ogra, P.L. Antibody content of rabbit milk and serum following inhalation or injestion of respiratory syncytial virus and bovine serum albumin. Clin. Exp. immunol. 48:91-101,1982.

68. Losonsky, G.A., Fishaut, J.M., Strussenberg, J., and Ogra, P.L. Effect of immunization against rubella on lactation products. I. Development and characterization of specific immunologic reactivity in breast milk. J. Infectious Diseases 145:654,1982.

69. Losonsky, G.A., Fishaut, J.M., Strussenberg, J., and Ogra, P.L. Effect of immunization against rubella on lactation products. II. Maternal neonatal interactions. J. Infectious Diseases 145:661,199982.

70. Bienenstock, J., Befus,D.,McDermott, M., Mirski, S., and Rosenthal, K. Regulation of lymphoblast traffic and localization in mucosal tissues, with emphasis on IgA. Federation Proceedings. 42:3213,1983.

71. Bienenstock, J., Befus, D., McDermott, M., Mirski, S., Rosenthal, K., Taghabue. A. The mucosal immunological network in The Secretory Immune System Ed. by Jerry R. McGhee, and Jiri Mestecky NYAS 409,1983.

72. Weisz-Carrington, P., Roux, M.E., McWilliams, M., Phillips-Quagliata, J.M., Hamm, M.E. Hormonal induction of the secretory immune system in the mammary gland. Proc. BNatl. Acad. Sci. 75:2928,1978.

73. Drife, J.O., McClelland, D.B., Pryde, A, et. al. Immunoglobulin synthesis in the resting breast. Br. Med. J. 2:503-506,1976.

74. Bienenstock, J., McDermott, M., Befus, D. A common mucosal immune system in Immunology of Breast Milk Ed. by P.L. Ogra and D. Dayton. Raven Press, N.Y. 1979.

75. Hanson, L.A., Carlsson, B., Cruz, J.R., Garcia, B., et.al. Immune Response in the mammary gland. In Immunology of Breast Milk. Ed. by P.L. Ogra and D. Dayton, Raven Press, N.Y. 1979.

76. Wiman, K, Curman, B., Tragardh, L., Peterson, P.A., et. al. Demonstration of HLA-DR like antigens on milk fat globule membranes. Eur. J. Immunol. 9:190-195,1979.

77. Thomas, D.W., Yamashita, V., Sherach, E.M. The role of Ia antigens in T cell activation. Immunol. Rev. 35:95-120,1977.

78. Curtis, A.S.G. Clues, concepts and possible answers from other systems de Sousa med lymphocyte circulation. Experimental and Clinical Aspects, N.Y. Wiley p.162-196,1981.

79. Curtis, A.S., Davies, M.D. H2-D antigens released by thymocytes and cell adhesion. J. Immunogenet. 8:367-77,1981.

80. Strober, W. Regulation of mucosal immune system. J Allergy Clin. Immunol. p.225,1982.

81. Strober, W., Elso, C.O., Graeff, A., and Richman, L.K. Class specific T cell regulation of mucosal immune responses. In: Recent Advances in Mucosal Immunity p.121, 1982.

82. Kawanishi, H., Sallyman, L.E., and Strober, W. Characteristics and regulatory function of murine Con A induced cloned T cells obtained from peyer's patches and spleen. J. Immunol. 19:475,1982.

INVESTIGATIONS OF THE SECRETORY IMMUNE SYSTEM IN HUMAN MILK USING MONOCLONAL ANTIBODIES

Randall Goldblum, Steven Nothwehr, Jell Hsieh, Richard Denney and Alex Kurosky

Departments of Pediatrics and Human Biological Chemistry and Genetics
University of Texas Medical Branch
Galveston, Texas

INTRODUCTION

Secretory IgA (SIgA), the major immunoglobulin in human colostrum and milk, is a complex of glycopeptides. The pathway for the production of these molecules is complicated, since the peptide constituents of each molecule are the products of at least nine different genes and two different cell types. The major portion of the molecule is synthesized by specialized plasma cells which are part of the common mucosal immune system (1) and ultimately home to submucosal sites, including the lactating breast. Formation of an active immunoglobulin product within these plasma cells requires genetic rearrangements, post transcriptional modifications of the messenger RNA's, and post translational modification and assembly of the nascent peptides. The completed product, polymeric IgA (PIgA) consists of at least four alpha (heavy) chains, four kappa or lambda (light) chains, and a single J or joining chain. These glycopeptide subunits are held together by noncovalent forces as well as interchain disulfide bridges.

After release from the plasma cells near the mammary epithelium PIgA passively diffuses to the mammary secretory cell. There it binds to a transmembrane glycoprotein, the polymeric immunoglobulin receptor (PIgR). A major fragment of the PIgR was first recognized as a constituent of IgA molecules derived from human milk (2) and named secretory or transport piece and later secretory component (SC). Figure 1 represents a schematic model of the transport of PIgA into secretions such as milk.

It is now recognized that the PIgR is synthesized on the endoplasmic reticulum of epithelial cells as an integral membrane protein (3) and has four functional segments (4). Starting at the N-terminal end is a signal peptide which directs the newly formed protein into membranes, an extracellular segment which serves as the receptor site for PIgA and pentameric IgM binding, a transmembrane spanning segment, and a relatively large intracytoplasmic tail which is thought to mediate intracellular sorting of the receptor and its immunoglobulin ligands.

At an unidentified step in the transport of PIgA across the mammary secretory cell, the PIgR-PIgA complex is modified by the formation of two

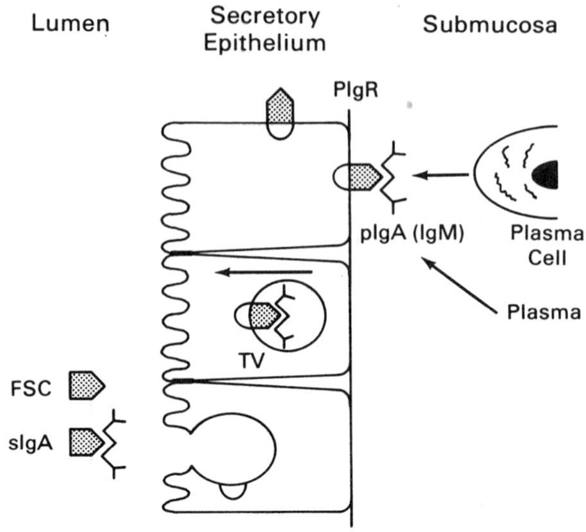

Figure 1. Transport of PIgA into milk by mammary secretory cells.

PIgR=Polymeric immunoglobulin receptor SIgA=Secretory IgA
FCS=Free secretory component TV=Transport vesicle PIgA=Polymeric IgA

interchain disulfide bridges between the extracellular segment of the PIgR (SC) and the constant region of one or two alpha chains of one of the IgA units (5). In addition, the PIgR is cleaved between the membrane spanning and extracellular segments, leaving a membrane-bound fragment and a soluable fragment (SC) attached to the PIgA which will be released as SIgA into the milk. The molecular site of this proteolytic cleavage may be somewhat variable, since Eiffert and coworkers found four different C-termini on secretory component isolated from human milk (6). The cellular site for formation of the disulfide bridges and for the proteolytic cleavage has not been defined. The cleavage may be mediated by a specific enzyme or it may be enhanced while the PIgA-PIgR complex is bound to the vesicle membrane, since the interaction of PIgA and SC conveys to SIgA unique resistance to a number of proteolytic enzymes (7,8).

The transcellular transport of PIgR-containing membrane can proceed independent of immunoglobulin, leading to the release into the milk of an unbound extracellular segment of PIgR, termed free secretory component (FSC). At present no specific function has been ascribed to FSC.

Table I. Variability in Human SIgA Structure

Demonstrated:	
Light chain classes	Kappa or Lambda
Heavy chain subclasses	Alpha 1 or Alpha 2
Allotypic variants	Am2 (+) or Am2 (-)
Antibody specificity	Variable region diversity
SC charge heterogeneity	Multiple isoelectric forms
Possible:	
SC size variants	
SC allotypes	
Variable glycosylation of SC or IgA	
Variable noncovalent and disulfide bonding	

The primary amino acid sequence of rabbit PIgR has been derived from analysis of complementary DNA from mammary and hepatic tissue (4), and the sequence of human extracellular segment (SC) was recently determined by peptide sequencing (6). These studies indicate that the PIgR consists of seven domains, defined primarily by intrachain disulfide bridges. The first five N-terminal domains, which make up most of the extracellular segment, share extensive regions of sequence homology with each other and with members of the immunoglobulin gene family, especially the immunoglobulin kappa variable region (4). The fifth domain is thought to contain the cysteines involved in the interchain bridge (4,6) with the alpha chain(s). The sixth domain, which shares some homology with the immunoglobulin kappa variable region but not with the first five SC domains, contains the membrane spanning segment (4). Even the cytoplasmic tail, or seventh domain of SC, contains some segments homologous with immunoglobulins (4).

The complexity of the synthetic and secretory mechanisms which lead to SIgA formation may reflect a system which is programmed for production of very diverse products. Table I shows a list of the identified variations in SIgA structure, and indicates others which might be anticipated, but have not yet been demonstrated. The finding that the gene or genes for PIgR are probably derived from an ancestral immunoglobulin gene (4), raises the question of whether PIgR might also participate in the generation of a variety of secretory molecules. However, very little diversity was noted in the primary sequence of human SC (6). Alternatively, there may be diversity in the covalent and noncovalent interaction between SC with PIgA.

The multi-step synthetic and transport process may also provide sites for regulatory mechanisms which control the output of SIgA. For instance, several steroid hormones appear to regulate the synthesis of PIgR (9) and subsequently the concentration of IgA in steroid sensitive tissue like the uterus (10). It may be feasible to manipulate this system to improve the function of the mammary gland and thereby enhance the protection of the

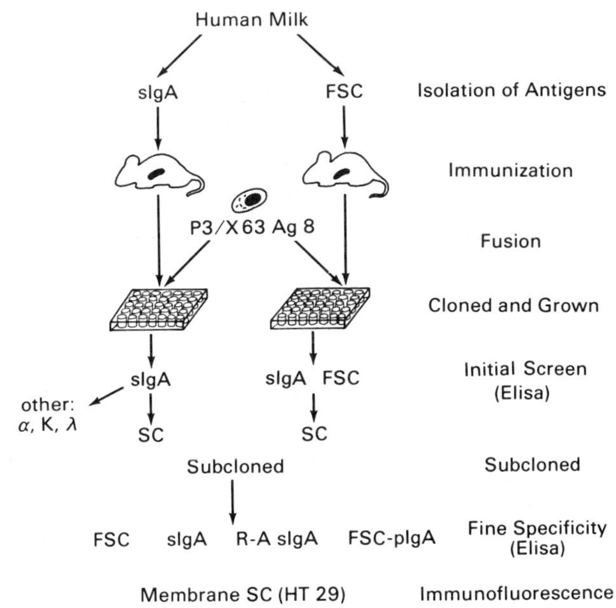

Figure 2. Production and Characterization of Monoclonal Antibodies to Secretory Component.

infant it supports. Hence this system offers interesting opportunities for basic studies of ultimate clinical significance.

As a step toward better understanding the critical steps in secretory immunoglobulin formation, we have prepared a panel of monoclonal antibodies (Mabs) against two different forms of human SC. We hoped that the exquisite specificity and homogeneity of such antibody reagents might allow us to dissect the steps in secretory immunoglobulin production and identify where diversity in the product may indicate the existence of alternate pathways which might be regulated independently.

METHODS

The details of our methods for antigen isolations, immunizations and production of Mabs have been described previously (11). Briefly, mice were immunized with either SIgA or FSC purified from human colostrum or milk, using classical salt precipitation, and ion exchange and molecular sieve chromatography. Spleen cells from these mice were fused with a secreting mouse myeloma line and the cloned hybrids were screened for the formation of antibodies to the immunizing preparations and other forms of SC by enzyme-linked immunosorbent assays. The forms of SC used for the screening included native SIgA and FSC isolated from human colostrum or milk, and SIgA which had been extensively reduced under denaturing conditions and alkylated with iodoacetamide. To define which antibodies were specific for the SC in SIgA, we also evaluated the binding of these antibodies to an isolated myeloma polymeric IgA (11). In addition, HT29 colon carcinoma cells, which are known to synthesize and display PIgR on their surface, were maintained in cell culture and used to examine the binding of the Mabs to membrane SC, using indirect immunofluorescence microscopy. The experimental protocol for production and characterization of the antibodies is summarized in Figure 2.

To determine which Mabs reacted with the same epitopes, selected Mabs were radiolabeled by incubating the subcloned hybridomas in media containing 35 S-methionine. These labeled antibodies were used in competitive binding assays in which they were mixed with ascites fluid (unlabeled antibody) produced from the same clones or from other clones which demonstrated predominant binding to the same form of SC. The mixture of labeled and unlabeled (competitor) antibodies was allowed to bind to microtiter wells coated with SC. After washing the microtiter plate, the bound Mabs were removed by alkali digestion and counted by scintillation spectrometry. The extent of inhibition was determined by comparing the counts from wells containing a mixture of labeled (test) and unlabeled (inhibitor) antibodies to counts from wells containing labeled antibody alone. Antibodies which produced over 50% inhibition of the labeled antibody binding were considered to bind to the same or closely associated sites on SC.

Table II. Results of Initial Screening of Hybridoma Clones from 4 Fusions

Immunogen and Fusion #	Viable cultures	ELISA positive	Antibody Specificity			
			SC	Alpha	Light	Unclassified
SIgA I	198	33%	22	24	8	13
SIgA II	51	ND	ND	ND	ND	ND
FSC I	300	34%	191	0	1	0
FSC II	240	73%	174	0	2	0

ND = not tested ELISA = Enzyme-linked immunosorbent assay

Table III. Fine Specificity of Subcloned Anti-SC Hybridomas

Immunogen	Clones Tested	Predominant Binding		
		SIgA	FSC	SIgA & FSC
SIgA	22	21	0	1
FSC	23	1	16	6

Predominant binding = Binding 10 times better than to alternative form

RESULTS

As previously described (11), a large number of antibody-producing clones were isolated. Table II shows the frequency of clones producing antibodies to the immunizing antigen used in four fusions. A number of clones from fusions SIgA I and FSC I and II were selected for subcloning and production of ascites fluids. This procedure assured that antibodies tested were from a single clone and could be tested at high enough concentrations to detect lower avidity interactions with alternative forms of SC. The data shown in Table III indicate that the majority of these clones produced antibodies which reacted only with the immunizing form of SC (either SIgA or FSC).

Very few of the SIgA antibodies reacted with SIgA which had been reduced and alkylated to disrupt the inter and intrachain disulfide bridges (Table IV). A number of antibodies which bound preferentially to FSC were capable of binding to SIgA which had been reduced and alkylated. Only three of the clones derived by immunization with SIgA or FSC reacted with the membrane form of SC displayed on a colon carcinoma cell line (Table V). However, the later reactivity was characteristic of antibodies which reacted with SIgA, FSC and reduced and alkylated SIgA in the enzyme-linked immunosorbent assay.

Competition assays using endogenously labeled antibodies indicated that our panel of antibodies could be divided into at least 7 competitive groups. Within each of these groups, each member effectively inhibited the binding of its radiolabeled partner to SC. However, members of different groups did not inhibit each other's binding. This result allowed us to define a minimum number of epitopes or closely apposed structural regions on the various forms of SC. These numbers represent minimum estimates, and are somewhat lower than the number calculated by Icsaki, on the basis of binding of radiolabeled Fab fragments of polyclonal antibodies to SC and SIgA (12).

Table IV. Reactions with Reduced and Alkylated (R-A) SIgA

Fine Specificity	Clones Tested	Reactions with R-A SIgA		
		+	+/-	-
SIgA	20	1	0	19
FSC	19	7	2	10
FSC & SIgA	8	2	0	6

Table V

Fine Specificity	Reaction with R-A SIgA	Clones Tested	Clones Positive
SIgA	-	11	Ø
FSC	- or +/-	8	Ø
FSC	+	4	3 Weak
SIgA & FSC	+	3	3 Strong

DISCUSSION

We concluded from these studies that SC is a relatively flexible structure. Many of the immunogenic sites are either modified or masked by interaction with IgA or cell membranes. The importance of interchain disulfide bonds in the tertiary structure of SIgA was indicated by the fact that only one of 2Ø characterized Mabs (representing four defined binding specificities) bound well to reduced and alkylated SIgA. Reduction of intrachain disulfide bonds within the SC chain did not appear to have such a devastating effect on the molecule's 3-dimensional structure, since several of the Mab groups which reacted with FSC also reacted, to varying extents, with reduced and alkylated SIgA.

These studies did not show whether all of the epitopes detected by our antibodies were on each FSC or SIgA molecule, or if our antibodies were distinguishing subtle subtypes of molecules. We are using affinity columns containing individual Mabs to approach this problem. Preliminary results indicate that two of the epitopes defined by our Mabs exist on distinct and separable molecular forms of human milk SIgA. These forms do not correspond to previously recognized subpopulations of IgA (i.e., IgA1/IgA2 or kappa/lambda light chains). We are currently evaluating the antibody activity in the two forms and using immunochemical and biochemical techniques to define the basis of this structural heterogeneity in SIgA.

In summary, SIgA is a complex of polypeptide chains, most of which are synthesized and assembled by cells of the immune system (IgA plasmacytes). An additional peptide chain, a major fragment of PIgR, is added during transport through the secretory epithelial cells of the breast and at other mucosal sites. Structural characterization of the PIgR from two species indicates a high degree of homology with members of the immunoglobulin gene family (immunoglobulins, T cell receptor, histocompatability antigens), suggesting that the PIgR evolved from a primordial immunoglobulin-like membrane protein. Since a major characteristic of this gene family is its ability to form diverse structures which recognize foreign molecules, it seems reasonable to search for diversity in PIgR structure as well.

We have begun this search by preparing Mabs to the major PIgR cleavage product, FSC, and its immunoglobulin complex, SIgA. These antibodies recognize at least seven different structural areas on SC, many of which are detectable on only the free or bound form of SC. Antibodies which recognize membrane-bound native PIgA were rare among the Mabs elicited to unbound SC. Using Mabs elicited to the different forms of SC, we have demonstrated that extensive changes in the 3-dimensional structure of this molecule also occur during transit through epithelial cells. Preliminary data suggest that Mabs recognize differences in the 3-dimensional structure of SIgA molecules in milk which are not related to previously described variations in this molecule. Further characterization of these isoforms may provide new insight into the structure of secretory immunoglobulins, regulation of their production, and the mechanisms by which they protect the recipient infant.

ACKNOWLEDGEMENTS

We Would like to acknowledge the assistance of Dr. Constance Denney and Stephanie Huery in the preparation of this manuscript. This work was supported by a grant from the National Institute of Allergy and Infectious Disease (AI-21412) and a contract from the National Institute of Child Health and Human Development (NØ1-HD-2-2812).

REFERENCES

1. M. E. Lamm, M. E. Roux, M. McWilliams, and Phillips-Quagliata, Differentiation and migration of mucosal cell precursors, in: "Recent Advances in Mucosal Immunity," W. W. Strober, L. A. Hanson and K. W. Sell ed., Raven Press, New York (1982).
2. L. A. Hanson, Comparative immunological studies of the immune globulins of human milk and of blood serum, Int. Arch. Allergy 18:241 (1961).
3. L. Huhn, and J. P. Kraehenbuhl, The Membrane Receptor for Polymeric Immunoglobulin is Structurally Related to secretory Component, J of Bio Chem 256:1249Ø-12495 (1981).
4. K. E. Mostov, M. Friedlander and G. Blobel, The receptor for tranepithelail transport of IgA and IgM contains multiple immunoglobulin-like domains, Nature 3Ø8:37-43 (1984).
5. B. Underdown, J. DeRose, and A. Plaut, Disulfide bonding of secretory component to a single monomer subunit in human secretory IgA, J of Immun 118:1816-1821 (1977).
6. H. Eiffert, E. Quentin, J. Decker, S. Hillermeir, Klingm, Die Primarystrucktur der menschlichen freien skeretkomponente und die Anodnung der disulfidbrucken, Hoppe-Seyler's Z. Physiol. Chem. 365:1489-95 (1984).
7. E. Lindh, Increased Resistance of Immunoglobulin A dimers to proteolytic degradation, J of Immun 114:284-286 (1875).
8. K. Kobayashi, J. Vaerman, and J. heramans, Studies of human secretory IgA (II). Comparative studies on a fragment obtained by enzymatic digestion in secretory component, Immunochem 1Ø:73-8Ø (1973).
9. C. R. Wira, and E. M. Colby, Regulation of secretory component by glucosteroids in primary cultures of rat hepatocytes, J Immunol. 134:1744-1788 (1973).
1Ø. C. R. Wira,and C. P. Sandoe, Hormonal regulation of immunoglobulins: Unfluence of extradiol on immunoglobulin A and G in rat uterus Endocrinology 1Ø6:1Ø2Ø (198Ø).
11. C. S. Woodard, J. B. Splawski, R. M. Goldblum, and R. M. Denney, Characterization of epitopes of human secretory component on free secretory component, secretory IgA, and membrane-associated secretory component, J of Immun 133:2116-2125 (1984).
12. C. Geneste, R. Magald, and S. Iscaki, Differences between the in vitro combination of secretory component (SC) and immunoglobulin polymers (Ig) by enumeration of SC epitopes, Immunol. letters 7:195-2Ø1 (1984).

FUNCTION OF LEUKOCYTES IN HUMAN MILK

H. Mandyla and M. Xanthou

Department of Immunology,First Pediatric Clinic Athens University and B'Neonatal Intensive Care Unit,"Aghia Sophia"Children's Hospital Athens Greece

A most important adaptation of the G.I. tract of the newborn to the extrauterine environment is its development of a mucosal barrier against the penetration of bacteria viruses and other environmental antigens i.e food proteins. The mechanisms of host defence at mucosal sites both immulogic and nonimmunologic are underdeveloped during the neonatal period and more so in prematures neonates (1).

The intestinal epithelial cells lack well defined brush border and retain a primitive transport mechanism for endocytosis of large molecular substances (2) (Fig.1).

It has been proved that the neonatal intestine may absorp larger antigenic quantities of ingested protein and proliferating micro-organisms than the adult intestine (3).

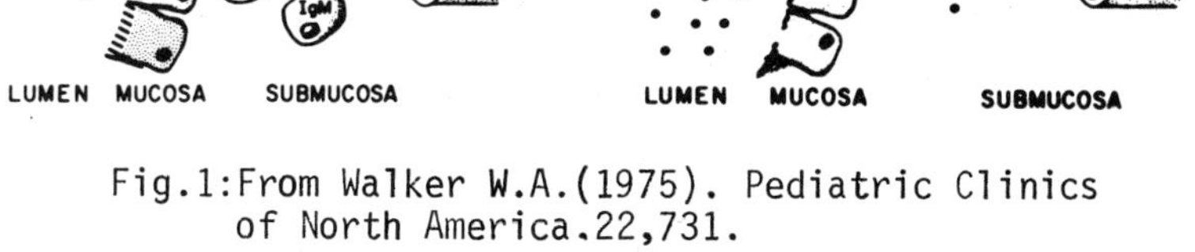

Fig.1:From Walker W.A.(1975). Pediatric Clinics of North America.22,731.

The number of the Payer patches is small in mammals during the neonatal period and although recent studies have described T-helper and T-suppressor lymphocytes,B-lymphocytes and macrophages on their lymphoid follicles (4) the functional ability of the cells seems to be immature until about one month of age (5).Furthermore plasma cells which are normally abundant in the mucosal lamina propria are not detected in utero and during the immediate neonatal period. SIgA is virtually absent during the early post-natal priod. By one month of age approximately all infants will start having some detactable SIgA (6).

The availability of immunological factors in the mammary gland exosecretions may represent an evulutionary event to compensate through breast feeding the transient deficiency of mucosal immunity in the neonate. And indeed the human colostrum and milk bear many similarities to the external body fluids bathing the mucosal surfaces of the G.I. and respiratory tracts. It is also very interesting that the evidence so far suggest that the immunoglobulin-producing cells observed in the mammary tissue during lactogenesis and in the colostrum and milk are of mucosal origin (7).

The contribution of human milk to neonatal immunity involves both humoral and cellular factors (8,9,10).

The white cells of human colostrum, although first observed in 1839 by the biologist-microscopist-photographer Alexander Donnee (11) have only quite recently attracted the attention of immunologist and neonatologists. Thus it was Smith in Goldman's laboratory who rediscovered then in 1966 (12). These cells were found to be present at concentrations of 0.5-10 million cells/ml in colostrum and comprise macrophages 30-85% polymorphonuclears 1-80% and lymphocytes 1-15% (13). Later on numerous epithelial cells and epithelial cell fragments are also seen in human colostrum. It is interesting that although the number of white cells/ml decreased significantly from colostrum to mature human milk we didn't find any change of the various white cell types during a breast-feeding time (14).

The lymphocytes in human milk appear to be quite significant in function and are the cells that have been most closely studied till now. Apart from T and B lymphocyte populations subpopulations of OKT4 (helper/inducer phenotype) and OKT8 (suppressor/cytotoxic phenotype) have been found in human milk (15,16).

Colostral and milk lymphocytes have been found to respond in vitro to a number of viral and microbial antigens (17). Several studies have shown, however, that colostral and milk lymphocytes often respond to different antigens from those that peripheral blood lymphocytes of the same persons do (18,19).

Antibody response in the milk appears to be the characteristic feature of antigenic exposure in the gut associated lymphoid tissue (GALT) or the bronchoepithelium associated lymphoid tissue (SALT) and strongly supports the concept of an enteromammary as well as a bronchomammary axis of immunologic reactivity in the breast. The more probable explanation for the appearance of milk antibodies after antigenic exposure on various mucosal sites is that specific IgA producing cells home to the mammary gland after they have been exposed to the antigen at these sites (20).

There is now substantial evidence that a major function of intestinal antibodies is the process of immune exclusion at the mucosal surface thus preventing infections and or allergies (2).

Milk lymphocytes have a decreased response to nonspecific mitogens, like PHA (18) and their cytotoxic potential is selectively deficient with its expression dependent on the particular stimulating or target antigens presented (21).

It has been found in rats that leukocytes may be transmitted through the milk from the mother's blood stream to the suckling's blood stream and this way may be beneficial causing adoptive immunity or very harmful causing graft-versus host disease (22).

We have no evidence so far that human milk lymphocytes can cross the human intestinal wall and enter neonatal blood circulation. However, the transfer of maternal T-cell reactivity to tuberculin protein (PPD) from the mother to the human neonate has been observed through breast feeding (23). It has also been suggested that partly digested cells or smaller molecules transported by the T cells, like transfer factor or migration inhibitory factor can be transferred to the breast fed baby (24). More studies are needed to elucidate the immunological benefits for the newborn transmitted through the immunocompetent cells in human milk.

Phagocytes, which represent the majority of cells found in human milk, have been studied far less. Morphologically the neutrophils are typical to those seen in the blood except that they contain numerous fat globules and fewer granules. The monocytic phagocytes are lipid laden motile cells which adhere to glass (12).Histochemically the milk macrophage differs from the blood monocyte as having increased numbers of lysosomes and somehow decreased peroxidase staining. Furthermore they contain significantly higher amounts of IgA in their cytoplasm. It has been suggested that these cells can function as a transport vehicle or storage for immunoglobulins in the breast milk (25). Recently using monoclonal antibodies they discovered different antigenic determinants on breast milk macrophages to those found on blood monocytes (26). Milk macrophages have been shown to posess Fc and C3b receptors (27). They are responsible for the synthesis of several host resistance factors of milk, including lysozyme, complement components and lactoferrin (27,28,29).

The origin of milk macrophages have not been clearly defined yet. Some investigators think that they come from blood monocytes which begin to home to the mammary gland during the last month of pregnancy. There, they defferentiate to activated - appearing macrophages (30).

Regarding the ability of human milk phagocytes (polymorphonuclear neutrophils and macrophages) to phagocytose and kill pathogenic organisms, two in vitro studies have given contradicting results. Robinson et al (31) found very good phagocytosis and killing of Staph aureus and E.coli after opsonization by the aqueous phase of milk. On the other hand Ho and Lawton (32) found good phagocytic power of colostral cells but poor killing activity of E.coli.

During the past few years we tried to further investigate the function of milk phagocytes by :a) estimating their ability to elicit antibody dependent cytotoxicity (ADCC) and b) by determining their oxidative metabolic response using the chemiluminescence assay.

a)Antibody dependent cytotoxicity of human Colostrum Phagocytes

Antibody dependent cytotoxicity involves the specific killing of antibody-coated target cells by non-immune effector cells which have in common the presence of a receptor for the Fc portion of IgG antibody (33). The type of target cell and the source of antibody appear to dictate the nature of the effector cells mediating cytolysis. Lysis of human erythrocytes in the presence of immune iso-antibody has been reported to be effected by monocytes and polymorphonuclear leucocytes only (34).

In our experiments human erythrocytes blood group A were used as target cells to which radioactive Cr^{51} was incorporated. Colostral leucocytes were cultured with them for 18 hours at $37^{o}C$ in the presence of anti-erythrocyte serum. After incubation the cytotoxic ability of milk leucocytes was estimated by measuring the release of isotope from the target cells they had killed.

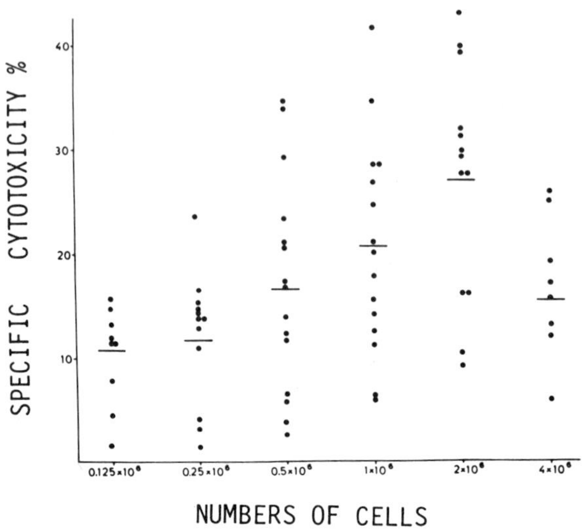

Fig.2:Antibody-dependent-cytotoxicity of colostral phagocytes (monocytes and polymorphonuclear neutrophils). Effector/target cells ratio ranging from 1:1 to 40:1. (From Mandyla et al (1982) Pediatr.Res. 16:995-999).

As shown in Figure 2 colostral phagocytes (monocytes and polymorphonuclear neutrophils) have the ability to function quite well in antibody-dependent cell-mediated cytotoxicity. The effector/target cells ratio's we used were 1:1, 2.5:1, 5:1, 10:1, 20:1, 40:1. The specific cytotoxicity of colostral phagocytes increased as the effector/target cells ratio rose from 1:1 to 20:1 ($p<0.001$). Further increase in effector cells (40:1) caused a significant fall in cytotoxicity ($p<0.05$).

We further separated colostral monocytes by incubating them for 4h in nonsiliconized glass flash and compared their cytotoxicity with **those elicited** from monocytes of adult and neonatal peripheral blood.

There was no difference in the ability of neonatal and adult peripheral blood monocytes to function in antibody-dependent cytotoxicity (Fig.3). Colostrum monocytes, however, showed a reduced cytotoxic capacity when compared to those of adult ($p<0.001$) or neonatal blood ($p<0.001$) at low effector/target cells ratio (1:1).

From our findings it is obvious that colostral monocytes and polymorphonuclear neutrophils have the ability to function in ADCC. The diminished cytotoxicity that colostral monocytes showed when compared to monocytes of adult or neonatal peripheral blood could be due to the extensive fat ingestion by these cells or other inhibitory factors found in colostrum (35).

b) Chemiluminescence of human colostrum phagocytes

In this part of our work we tried to investigate the metabolic response of milk phagocytes which is related to their killing abilities regarding pathogenic microorganisms. As we know bacterial killing involves a multiplicity of actions all of which are set into motion by two cellular events:degranulation and the initiation of the respiratory burst. The products of the respiratory burst oxidase the stimulating agent and during this process there is emission of light that can be detected as chemiluminescence (36).

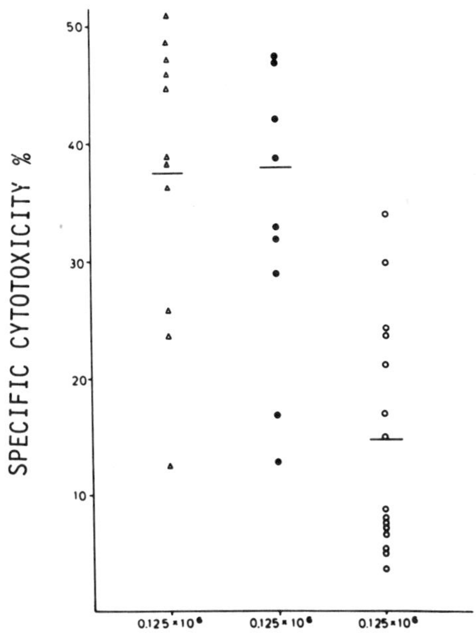

NUMBER OF CELLS

Fig.3:Antibody-dependent cytotoxicity of colostral and peripheral blood monocytes of adults and neonates.Effector/target cells ratio 1:1 Δ, adult monocytes,● neonatal monocytes and o colostral monocytes.

In this study we investigated Luminol-dependent chemiluminescence produced by human colostral cells on stimulation by opsonized Zymosan. Chemiluminescence of human blood monocytes and polymorphonuclears was also studied in the same experimental assay.

As shown in Fig.4 human blood polymorphs and monocytes give a very similar time curve of light emission. However blood monocytes gave a response that was much lower when compared to that of polymorphonuclear ($p<001$). The chemiluminescence elicited by human colostral cells was significantly lower to those elicited by either blood polymorphonuclears ($p<001$) or blood monocytes ($p<001$). The type of metabolic response of colostral cells appears to be similar to that observed in blood polymorphonuclears and monocytes (37).

From our findings we can assume that milk cells also generate bactericidal concentrations of superoxide intracellularly for ingested bacteria and extracellularly for "non associated" free bacteria.

The ability of milk cells to release oxygen radicals can be taken as a biochemical correlate of their level of antimicrobial function. The lower chemiluminescence response of colostral cells is in agreement with the results of our previous research in which we showed that colostral cells have a definite cytotoxic ability but lower than that observed in blood phagocytes.

The demonstration of killing abilities of human colostrum phagocytes in our studies gives further support to the biological importance of the cellular components of human milk.

In rats Pitt et al (27) have shown that a Klebsiella induced necrotizing enterocolitis could be prevented by feeding rat colostral macrophages but not by feeding soluble colostral factors. These findings are in agreement with the observation that necrotizing enterocolitis is a

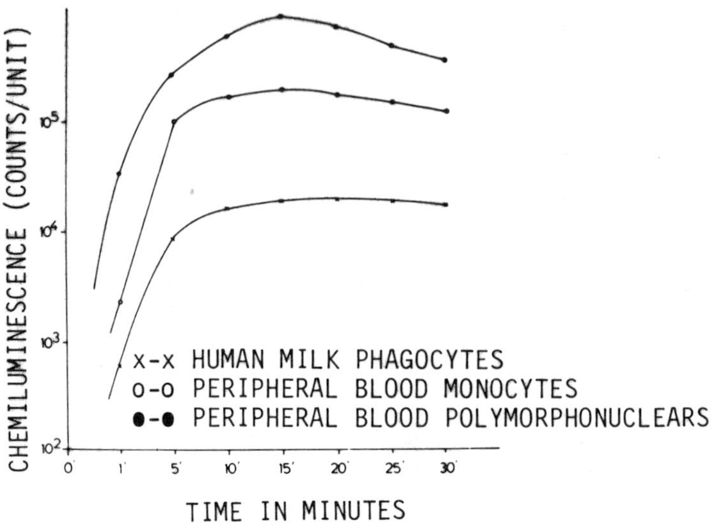

Fig.4:Luminol-dependent chemiluminescence of phagocytes of human milk and peripheral blood.

very rate disease of infants fed with untreated breast milk (38).

There is no doubt that human milk cells have various functional abilities that could enhance host defence mechanisms of the human neonate. However their exact role in vivo regarding either local intensinal immunity or systemic immunity of the human newborn remains to be elucidated.

REFERENCES

1. Ogra PL:Ontogeny of the local immune system. Pediatrics Supplement 64:765-774 (1979)
2. Walker WA and Isselbacher, JK:Uptake and transport of macromolecules by the intestine:possible role in clinical disorders. Gastroenterology 67:531-550 (1975)
3. Moxey PC and Trier JS:Structural features of the mucosa of human fetal small intestine , Gastroenterology 68, 1002-1007 (1975).
4. Richman LK, Graeff AS, Yorchoon R. et al:Simultaneous induction of antigen specific IgA helper, T cells and IgG-suppressor T-cells in the murine Peyer's partch after protein feeding J.Immunol.126: 2079-2087 (1981)
5. Reade JC:The development of bactericidal activity in rat peritoneal macrophages. Aust.J.Exp.Biol.Med.Sci.,46:231-236 (1968).
6. Losonsky GA and Ogra PL:Mucosal Immune System in Neonatal Infections ed PL Ogra Publ.Grume and Stratton Inc.,p.56 (1984).
7. Roux ME, McWilliams M.,Philips-Quagliate JM et al:Origin of IgA secreting plasma cells in the mammary gland. J.Exp.Med.146:1311-1321 (1977).
8. Goldman AS and Smith CW:Host resistance factors in human milk.J.Pediatr.82:1082 (1973).
9. Welch JK and May JT:Anti-infective properties of breast milk . J. Pediatrc. 94:1-9 (1979).
10. William WB:Breast milk immunology. Am.J.Dis.Child. 133, 83-87 (1979).
11. Donne A:Cours de microscopie. Vol.1 and Atlas No 1 Bailliere, Paris 1844-45.
12. Smith C.W.and Goldman AS:The cells of human colostrum I.In vitro studies of morphology and functions. Pediatr.Res.2:103-109 (1968).

13. Lawton JWM and Shortridge KF:Protective factors in human breast milk and colostrum. Lancet 1:253 (1977).
14. Mandyla H ,Xanthou M ,Baum JB and Matsaniotis N:Changes of human milk leucocytes during feeding time, pasteurization and various processes of milk storage. In Intensive Care in the Newborn IV,eds. L.Stern, H.Bard and B.Friis-Hansen Publ.Masson, New York p.51 (1983).
15. Richie ER, Bass R, Meistrich ML et al:Distribution of T-lymphocyte subsets in human colostrum. J.Immunol.129:1116-1119 (1982).
16. Bertotto A,Gentili F and Vaccaro R:Monoclonal antibody defined T-cell surface phenotypes in human breast milk. Boll 1st. Sieroter.Milan 62:370-371 (1983).
17. Ho FC, Wong RLC,Lawton YWM:Human colostral and breast milk cells. A light and electron microscopic study. Acta Paediatr.Scand. 68:389-396 (1979).
18. Parmely MJ, Beer AE, Billingham RE:In vitro studies of the T-lymphocyte population of human milk. J.Exp.Med.,144:358-370 (1976).
19. Ogra SS and Ogra PL:Immunologic aspects of human colostrum and milk. II Characteristics of lymphocytes reactivity and distribution of E-rosette forming cells at different times after the onset of lactation.J.Pediatr. 92:550-555 (1978).
20. Mellander L,Carlsson B, Dahlgren U. and Hauson LA:Humoral and cellular immunities transmitted by breastmilk in "Immunological Aspects of Infection in the Fetus and Newborn" Ed. H.P.Lambert and CBS Wood Publ.Academic Press, p.139-146 (1981).
21. Parmely MJ and Williams SB:Selective expression of Immunocompetence in Human Colostrum:Preliminary evidence for the control of Cytotoxic Lymphocytes including those specific for paternal Alloantigens in "Immunology of Breast Milk eds. PL Ogra and DH Dayton Publ.Raven Press . New York, p.173-180 (1979).
22. Beer AE and Billingham RE:Immunologic benefits and hazards of milk in maternal perinatal relationships. Ann.Int.Med.83:865-871 (1975).
23. Schlesinger JJ, Coveli HD:Evidence for transmission of lymphocyte response to tuberculin by breast feeding. Lancet,2:529-532(1977)
24. Diaz-Jonanen E and Williams JR.RC T and B-lymphocytes in human colostrum. Clinical Immunology and Immunopathology 3, 248-255.
25. Pittard WA, Polmar SH, and Fanaroff AA.The breast milk macrophage: a potential vehicle for immunoglobulin transport. J. of Reticuloendothelial Soc. 22:597-603 (1977).
26. Biondi A, Rossing TH, Bennett J and Todd RF:Surface membrane heterogeneity among human mononuclear phagocytes J.Immunol.132: 1237-43 (1984).
27. Pitt J, Barlow B, Heird WC:Protection against experimental necrotizing enterocolitis by maternal milk. I.Role of milk leukocytes Pediatr.Res.11:906-909 (1977).
28. Blan H, Passwell JH, Levanon M, Davidson J, Kohen F and Ramot B: Studies on human milk macrophages:effect of activation on phagocytosis and secretion of prostaglandin E2 and lysozyme. Pediatr. Res. 17:241-245 (1983).
29. Cole FS, Anerbach HS, Goldberger G and Colten HR:Tissue-specific pretranslational regulation of complement production in human mononuclear phagocytes. J.Immunol. 134:2610-2616 (1985).
30. Goldman AS and Smith CW:Host resistance factors in human milk of Pediatr. 82:1082-1090 (1973).
31. Robinson JE, Harvey BAM, Soothhill JF:Phagocytosis and killing of bacteria and yeast by human milk cells after opsonization in aqueous phase of milk. Br.Med.J.1:1443-1445 (1978).
32. Ho PC and Lawton JWM:Human colostral cells:Phagocytosis and killing of E.coli and C.albicans. J.Pediatrics 93:910-915 (1978).

33. Perlman P. and Holm G:Cytotoxic effects of lymphoid cells in vitro. Adv.Immunol.11:117-123 (1969).
34. MacDonald HR, Bonnard GD, Sordat B and Zawodnik SA:Antibody-dependent cell-mediated cytotoxicity. Heterogeneity of effector cells in human peripheral blood.Scand.J.Immunol.4:487-497 (1975).
35. Mandyla H, Xanthou M, Maravelias C, Baum D and Matsaniotis N.Antibody dependent cytotoxicity of human colostrum phagocytes. Pediatr. Res. 16:995-999 (1982).
36. Easmon CSF, Cole PJ, Williams AJ and Hastings M:The measurement of opsonic and phagocytic function by luminol-dependent chemiluminescence. Immunology 41, 67 (1980).
37. Mandyla H,Xanthou M. and Matsaniotis N.Luminol-pedendent chemiluminescence of colostral and mature human milk leucocytes. Abstract of International Neonatal Intensive Care Meeting, Spetses,Greece p.67 (1983).
38. Burnard ED, and Thomas DB:Fresh human milk in the prevention of necrotizing enterocolitis in very low birth weight infant. In Intensive Care in the Newborn III, eds.L.Stern, B.Salle and B. Friis-Hansen, Publ.Masson, New York (1981).

EFFECTS OF CHOLERA AND POLIOVIRUS IMMUNIZATIONS UPON SPECIFIC ANTIBODIES IN HUMAN MILK

L.Å. Hanson, S. Ahlstedt, B. Carlsson, U. Dahlgren, M. Hahn-Zoric, Fehmida Jalil, Shaukat R. Khan, L. Mellander, O. Porras and A. Wold

Dept. of Clinical Immunology, and Dept. of Pediatrics, University of Göteborg, Göteborg, Sweden. Dept. of Social and Preventive Pediatrics and Dept. of Pediatrics, King Edward Medical College, Lahore, Pakistan

IMMUNOLOGY OF MILK ANTIBODY RESPONSE

Human milk is rich in antibodies, primarily of the secretory IgA (SIgA) isotypes, which due to their stable structure, are specially adapted to protect mucous membranes. A number of studies,[1] have shown that SIgA antibody responses in milk originate from antigenic exposure in the gut. Lymphoid cells, primarily in the Peyer's patches, leave the intestine after antigen-presenting cells have brought them into contact with the antigen from the lumen of the intestine, and home to various sites of local SIgA production, including the mammary glands. This homing of cells from the gut to the mammary glands is called the enteromammaric pathway. Via a similar broncho-mammaric pathway, inhaled antigens also can cause transfer of committed lymphocytes to the mammary glands.[2]

It is not clear which signal is necessary to make these lymphocytes clone and produce IgA antibodies in the mammary gland. At other sites, such as in the intestinal mucosa, a "second signal", the antigen, makes the cells differentiate into antibody-producing plasma cells after homing to the mucosa. Mammary glands are remote from the many microbial and food antigens in the intestine or the microbes in the lungs and yet there are SIgA antibodies against many antigens in the milk.[1] It is possible, however, that the antigen in native or processed form is transported to the gland. For instance we and others have shown that protein in the mother's food, such as soy protein and egg albumin, can be found in low concentrations in the milk (Porras et al., unpublished data).[3] We also have demonstrated the transport of antigens from the gut to the milk in rats. Another possibility would be that anti-idiotypic antibodies, which are a normal constituent in the immune response, can reach the mammary gland via the circulation and function as the "second signal" for the SIgA response.[1]

It is difficult to induce local SIgA responses which provide long-lasting immunity. Such responses usually remain only for a few weeks or months since the immunologic memory often is weak, unless the antigen is cholera toxin, which has a special capacity to bind to cells via the GM1 ganglioside.[4]

Local immune responses have mostly been initiated by application of the antigen on the mucosa, but this does not seem easily applicable for the mammary gland. Injection in the gland of experimental animals has mainly given IgG antibody responses.[5,6,7]

VACCINATION OF LACTATING MOTHERS

Vaccination of lactating mothers in Pakistan with killed whole cell cholera vaccine given parenterally, produced a serum antibody response, as well as a striking increase of milk SIgA antibodies.[8] These women had been naturally exposed previously and this priming at the gut mucosal level, often inducing measurable prevaccination levels of milk SIgA antibodies to the V.cholerae endotoxin, provided the necessary basis for the response in the mammary gland. In contrast, Swedish women without previous natural exposure did not respond with milk SIgA antibodies, even after two vaccinations.[9]

Inactivated poliovirus vaccine given parenterally to Pakistani women also resulted in a boost of the milk SIgA antibodies.[8,10] The Swedish women who had not been exposed to wild poliovirus or live vaccine virus but only to the inactivated poliovirus vaccine, produced a small and shortlasting milk SIgA antibody response.[8] In contrast, when the live perorally poliovirus vaccine was given to Pakistani women, the prevaccination SIgA antibody levels often decreased (Fig. 1). This decrease of poliovirus antibodies became even more striking if the parenteral cholera vaccine was given simultaneously.[9] The explanation for this is not obvious and in a recent more extensive study we could not show any potentiated decrease of milk SIgA antibody responses to peroral live typhoid vaccine if the cholera vaccine was given at the same time. The typhoid vaccine alone decreased the specific milk SIgA antibody levels in five of ten Pakistani women.

The cause of the decrease of milk SIgA antibodies after vaccination with live poliovirus is not clear. After 2-4 weeks a booster response could be induced, however, using killed parenteral vaccine (Fig. 1). This might speak against immunologic tolerance as the mechanism and rather suggest a temporary suppressor effect. Another possibility is that the propagation of the live vaccine virus in the gut redistributes the specific IgA producing cells from the mammary gland to the gut. We have demonstrated that food protein given perorally in early lactation could decrease specific milk SIgA antibody levels.[12]

The most striking milk antibody responses were obtained with the new more antigen-rich inactivated poliovirus vaccine made by Dr. van Wezel in Holland.[11] This vaccine also produced the most longlasting antibody increases (Fig. 2).

THE MILK ANTIBODY RESPONSE IN ANIMAL MODELS

It has been suggested that milk SIgA antibodies may originate not only from local production in the mammary glands, but also from transport of IgA dimers from the serum, brought into the milk via the secretory component on the epithelial cells. Halsey et al.[14] found evidence for such transfer in mice, but we could not demonstrate that in rats.[13] Koertge was unable to detect more than traces of transfer from blood to milk in rats and mice.[15] In man only traces, or no transfer, has been shown.[16,17] It is important to determine the origin of milk antibodies since the origin may have relevance for the selection of the optimal mode of vaccination to induce such antibodies.

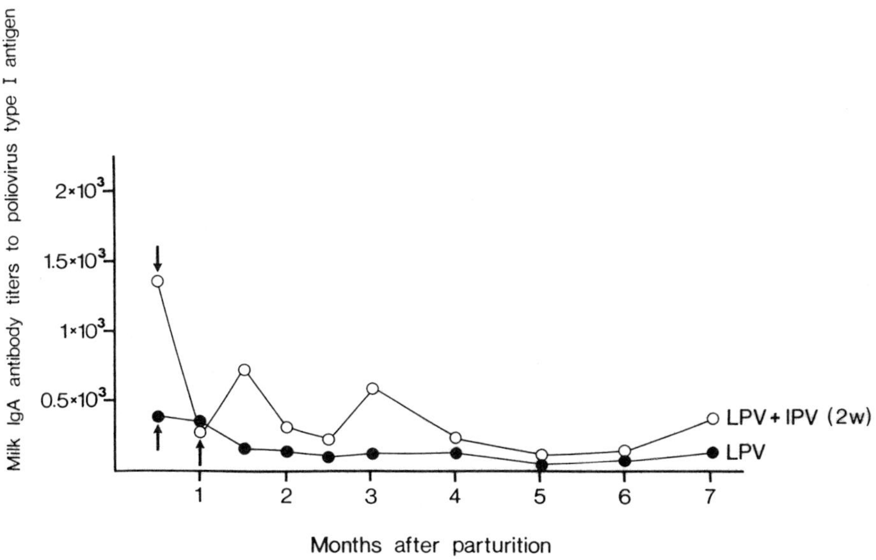

Fig. 1. Mean levels of milk IgA antibodies to poliovirus type I antigen after vaccination with one dose of oral vaccine given to Pakistani mothers (○), or one dose of oral vaccine followed by a booster dose, 2 weeks later, with inactivated Swedish vaccine (●).

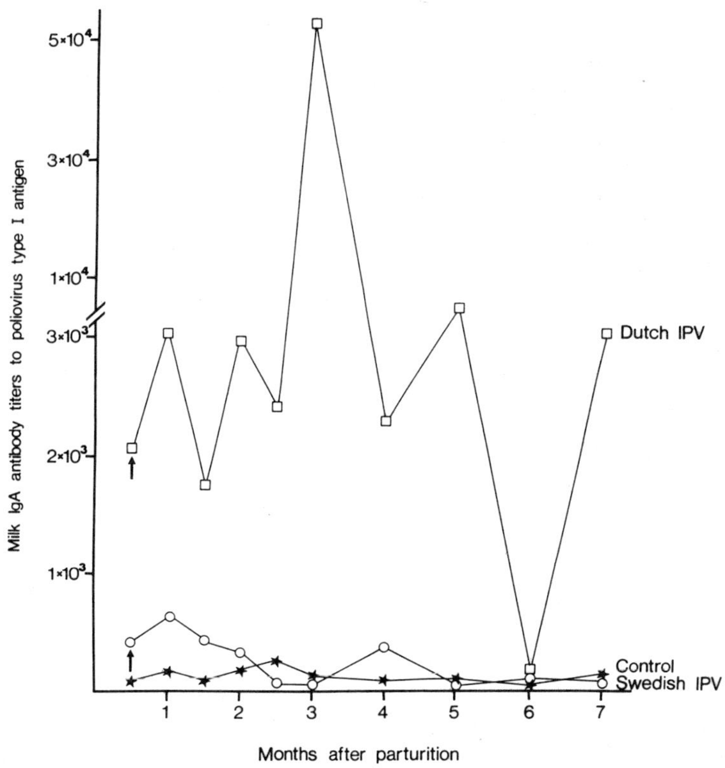

Fig. 2. Mean levels of milk IgA antibodies to poliovirus type I antigen after vaccination with one dose of Swedish inactivated vaccine (○), Dutch vaccine (□) or unvaccinated controls (*).

The response also may vary for different antigens. We recently noticed in rats immunized in the Peyer's patches with E.coli 06 bacteria carrying type 1 pili, that more of the IgA anti-06 antibodies came out in the bile than in the milk ($p<0.001$); the reverse took place for the IgA antibodies against the pili ($p<0.001$). The mechanism for this dichotomy is not known, but it may be necessary to test various antigens before they are assumed to induce or boost a milk SIgA antibody response.

CONCLUSION

It is evident that milk antibodies can be influenced by parenteral and peroral vaccination of the mother. Parenteral vaccination quite consistently enhances milk SIgA antibody levels, whereas certain perorally given vaccines and also foods can induce decreases of the milk SIgA antibody levels. The enhancement of the levels of certain milk antibodies may well result in improved protection of the breast-fed infant.

ACKNOWLEDGEMENT

These studies were supported by grants from the Swedish Medical Research Council (No. 215); the Swedish Agency for Research Cooperation with Developing Countries; the Ellen, Walter and Lennart Hesselman Foundation for Scientific Research; and the WHO Diarrheal Disease Program.

REFERENCES

1. L. Å. Hanson and P. Brandtzaeg, The mucosal defence system, in: "Immunologic disorders in infants and children", E. R. Stiehm, ed., Third edition, Saunders, Philadelphia, in press (1986).
2. P. L. Ogra, G. A. Losonsky and M. Fishaut, Colostrum derived immunity and maternal neonatal interaction, Ann. N.Y. Acad. Sci. 409:82 (1983).
3. P. J. Kilshaw and A. J. Cant, The passage of maternal dietary proteins into human breast milk, Int. Archs. Allergy appl. Immunol. 75:8 (1984).
4. J. Holmgren and N. Lycke, Immune mechanisms in enteric infections, in: "Nobel Conference II, Recent Advances in Vaccines and Drugs against Diarrhoeal Diseases", J. Holmgren, T. Holme and R. Möllby, eds., Svenska Förlags AB, Nordbok, Göteborg (1985).
5. E. H. Bohl and L. J. Saif, Passive immunity in transmissible gastroenteritis of swine: Immunoglobulin characteristics of antibodies in milk after inoculating virus by different routes, Infect. Immun. 11:23 (1975).
6. L. J. Saif and E. H. Bohl, Role of secretory IgA in passive immunity of swine to enteric viral infections, in: "Immunology of Breast Milk", P. L. Ogra, D. H. Dayton and L. Å. Hanson eds., Raven Press, N.Y. (1979).
7. U. I. H. Dahlgren, S. Ahlstedt and L. Å. Hanson, Origin and kinetics of IgA, IgG and IgM milk antibodies in primary and secondary responses of rats, Scand. J. Immunol., in press (1985).
8. A. M. Svennerholm, L. Å. Hanson, J. Holmgren, F. Jalil, B. S. Lindblad, S. Raza Khan, A. Nilsson and B. Svennerholm, Antibody response to live and killed poliovirus vaccines in the milk of Pakistani and Swedish women, J. Infect. Dis. 143:707 (1981).
9. A. M. Svennerholm, L. Å. Hanson, J. Holmgren, B. S. Lindblad, B. Nilsson and F. Quereshi, Different secretory immunoglobulin A antibody response to cholera vaccination in Swedish and Pakistani women, Infect. Immun. 30:427 (1980).

10. L. Å. Hanson, B. Carlsson, F. Jalil, B. S. Lindblad, S. R. Khan and A. L. van Wezel, Different secretory IgA antibody responses after immunization with inactivated and live polio virus vaccine, Rev. Inf. Dis. 6, suppl. 2:356 (1984).
11. B. Carlsson, F. Jalil, L. Å. Hanson and A. L. van Wezel, Secretory and serum antibody responses after immunization of lactating women with live and inactivated poliovirus (in manuscript).
12. J. R. Cruz and L. Å. Hanson, Specific milk immune response of rural and urban Guatemalan women, J. Pediatr. Gastroent. and Nutr., in press (1986).
13. U. Dahlgren, S. Ahlstedt, L. Hedman, C. Wadsworth and L. Å. Hanson, Dimeric IgA in the rat is transferred from serum into bile but not into milk, Scand. J. Immunol. 14:95 (1981).
14. J. F. Halsey, M. Craig and S. J. McKenzie, The origins of secretory IgA in milk: a shift during lactation from a serum origin to local synthesis in the mammary gland, Ann. N.Y. Acad. Science, 409:452 (1983).
15. T. E. Koertge, The quantitative capability of the enzyme-linked immunosorbent assay (ELISA) to study transport of antibodies into secretions, Thesis, University of Iowa, (1984).
16. S. S. Ogra and D. L. Ogra, Immunologic aspects of human colostrum and milk, I. Distribution, characteristics and concentration of immunoglobulin at different times after the onset of lactation, J. Pediatr., 92:546 (1978).
17. T. Klemola, E. Savilahti and P. Leinikki, Mumps IgA antibodies are not absorbed from human milk, Acta Pediatr. Scand., in press (1985).

POTENTIAL EFFECTS OF IMMUNIZATION ON THE HOST DEFENSE SYSTEMS IN HUMAN MILK

Larry K. Pickering and Guillermo Ruiz-Palacios

Program in Infectious Diseases and Clinical Microbiology and Department of Pediatrics, University of Texas Medical School at Houston, and Department of Infectious Diseases Institute of Nutrition, Mexico City, Mexico

INTRODUCTION

Diarrheal disease mortality data from the Pan American Health Organization (1,2) indicate that in 1976 in North America, diarrhea accounted for 1.4% and 0.9% of infant deaths in children less than 1 year of age and children 1 to 4 years of age, respectively. In tropical areas of America, diarrhea accounted for 15 to 23% of all infant deaths and 15 to 26% of deaths in children 1 to 4 years of age (table 1). In many areas of the world diarrhea remains the leading cause of death in infants and young children (2).

The number of enteric bacteria, viruses and parasites that are recognized as causing acute diarrheal disease has increased greatly since the early 1970's. Not only have new enteropathogens been described, but new pathophysiologic mechanisms of disease production have been defined (3). Table 2 shows the causes of acute infectious diarrhea in the United States and in tropical developing areas of the

Table 1. Diarrheal disease mortality in children four years of age and less in the Americas

	Age (years)			
	less than 1		1-4	
Area	Rate	%	Rate	%
North America	19	1.4	0.6	0.9
Central America	1078	22.8	154	25.8
South America (temperate)	496	10.9	20	9.1
South America (tropical)	1066	20.3	151	21.5

Modified from references 1 and 2.

Table 2. Causes of Acute Infectios Diarrhea

	Approximate Percentage	
	North America	Tropical Developing Areas
Bacteria		
Enterotoxigenic *E. coli*	5	25
Campylobacter	5	5-15
Shigella	1-5	5-10
Salmonella	1-5	1-5
Others	1-3	1-5
Viruses		
Rotavirus	10-50	5-20
Norwalk	10-20	Unknown
Enteric adenovirus	5-10	Unknown
Parasites		
Giardia lamblia	3-10	5
Cryptosporidium	Unknown	Unknown
E. histolytica	< 1	2-5

From references 3-8.

world (4-8). These enteropathogens produce diarrhea by enterotoxins released in the intestinal lumen or by mucosal invasion with or without release of proteolytic enzymes, cytotoxin or other humoral factors. Identification and characterization of these processes are important for the biologic control of enteric infection, particularly with respect to vaccine development. A brief description of various enteropathogens and their mechanisms of disease production will follow.

MECHANISMS OF DISEASE PRODUCED BY ENTEROPATHOGENS

Escherichia coli. Many new developments have occurred which have permitted clarification of the role of *E. coli* as a cause of diarrhea. *E. coli* that produce diarrhea can be divided into several categories based upon their mechanism of disease production and clinical manifestations (table 3). *E. coli* that produce diarrhea have been classified as enteropathogenic *E. coli* (EPEC), cytotoxin producing *E. coli*, enterotoxigenic *E. coli* (ETEC), and enteroinvasive *E. coli* (8,9).

For many years all *E. coli* that were associated with diarrhea were referred to as EPEC. Outbreaks of diarrheal disease in infants were recognized as being associated with a small number of *E. coli* serogroups defined by the O somatic antigen. These serogroups included O26, O55, O86, O111, O114, O119, O125, O126, O127, O128, and O142. However, with

Table 3. Categories of *Escherichia coli* that produce diarrhea

Category	Mechanism of disease
enteropathogenic	? adherence ? cytotoxin production
enterohemorrhagic	cytotoxin production
enterotoxigenic	adherence enterotoxin production
enteroinvasive	? invasion ? cytotoxin production

the recognition of invasiveness and production of heat stable (ST) and heat labile (LT) enterotoxins as important virulence properties of pathogenic *E. coli* (10), the role of EPEC as a cause of diarrhea became less clear. These EPEC have been shown to be non-invasive and ST^-/LT^-. With the demonstration that serogroup defined ST^-/LT^- EPEC can cause diarrhea in volunteers (11), there has been a resurgence of interest in EPEC (12). In some parts of the world EPEC are a frequent cause of endemic diarrhea in infants and young children (13). In Canada and Japan, EPEC occur more commonly in infants with endemic diarrhea than in well infants (14,15). EPEC are considered to be pathogenic because of epidemiologic studies as well as production of disease in volunteers (11,16).

Although the mechanism of production of gastroenteritis by EPEC is not known, both adherence and cytotoxin production have been suggested. The first involves factors that allow EPEC to adhere to enterocytes. Pathologically, these enterocyte adherent *E. coli* have been associated with morphologic changes on electron microscopy of small intestinal biopsies, including loss of microvilli with tightly adherent bacteria (18). The second potential mechanism that has been suggested is that EPEC produce a cytotoxin, variously referred to as Vero toxin (19) or Shiga-like cytotoxin (20), which damages cells by inhibition of peptide elongation during protein synthesis. Studies are being conducted to determine if either adherence or Shiga-like cytotoxin production is involved as the mechanism by which EPEC cause disease.

Both adherence and cytotoxin production appear to be important in *E. coli* diarrheal disease caused by serogroups not belonging to the classic EPEC. Non-EPEC enteroadherent *E. coli*, as defined by HEp-2 cell adherence, recently have been recognized as an important cause of travelers' diarrhea (21). In addition, high level Shiga-like cytotoxin production by *E. coli* is now recognized as the mechanism of a disease referred to as hemorrhagic colitis produced by *E. coli* O157:H7 (22). Although high level toxin-producing organisms can cause disease, the threshold for the amount of toxin production needed to produce symptoms remains to be defined.

As many as 25% of episodes of diarrhea in children in Mexico are caused by enterotoxigenic *E. coli* (ETEC) (5). In addition ETEC are responsible for approximately 40% of diarrhea in adults who travel from industrialized countries to developing countries. In North America enterotoxigenic *E. coli* have occasionally been recognized as a cause of diarrhea in children (4,5). Most enterotoxigenic *E. coli* produce ST only or ST plus LT (23). The genetic material that codes for production of enterotoxin may be located in plasmids (as is the case of *E. coli*) or in chromosomes (as in *V. cholerae*).

The initial step in production of disease by ETEC involves adherence of bacteria to intestinal mucosa, often mediated by fimbrial colonization factor antigens (CFA) (9). Although CFA-I and CFA-II are carried on the same plasmids that encode for ST and LT, many toxin producing strains do not possess these fimbrial antigens. LT works like cholera toxin through increased cyclic nucleotide (cAMP) levels in enterocytes. ST mediated fluid loss occurs through stimulation of guanylate cyclase with increased cGMP in enterocytes.

Invasive *E. coli* infrequently cause diarrheal disease, but when disease occurs, it clinically resembles shigellosis. Invasive *E. coli* have been shown to have a high molecular weight plasmid, similar to the high molecular weight plasmid that codes for invasiveness in Shigella species (25). Invasive *E. coli* are biochemically and serologically closely related to *Shigella* (49,50). These virulence factors can be transferred via plasmids between bacterial species (24). These similar properties may be useful in formulating vaccines that are effective against several organisms.

Shigella. There are four serogroups of shigella containing over 40 serotypes. *S. sonnei* is currently the most common cause of bacillary dysentery in the United States and Europe while *S. flexneri* serotypes account for a majority of the remaining cases. Shigellosis is currently believed to be a disease resulting from two major virulence properties, cytotoxin production and invasiveness. These factors determine clinical manifestations.

Salmonella. Currently, three species of Salmonella are differentiated on the basis of biochemical characteristics: *S. cholerae-suis*, *S. typhi*, and *S. enteritidis*. Nearly all of the 1700 serotypes of Salmonella are now grouped under *S. enteritidis*. Determining serotypes remains a useful epidemiologic tool for outbreak situations, although simple definition of one of the three species is still adequate for the vast majority of patients. The mechanism of Salmonella gastroenteritis is throught to involve penetration of organisms through the gut mucosa (26), a cholera-like enterotoxin (27) and a protein synthesis inhibiting cytotoxin. The enterotoxin appears to be more closely related to *E. coli* LT than to cholera toxin (28).

Campylobacter. *Campylobacter jejuni* and *C. coli* are enteric pathogens that are common causes of diarrhea world wide (29). A thermophilic strain of Campylobacter has been distinguished from *C. jejuni* by its nalidixic acid resistance and halotolerance. The species name *C. lardis* has been proposed because the great majority of isolates were from seagulls. It is a rare cause of diarrhea in humans. *C. fetus* produces fever and bacteremia in immunocompromised hosts. Clinically, *C. jejuni* frequently resembles bacillary dysentery; bloody diarrhea has been a common finding in this illness. This organism also may produce a heat labile enterotoxin (30). In many areas of the world Campylobacter is increasingly being recognized as the most commonly documented cause of bacterial diarrhea.

Vibrio cholerae. Cholera remains a public health problem primarily in Asia and Africa, although a focus of cholera is present in the Gulf Coast of the United States (31). Epidemic cholera is caused by 0-1 *V. cholerae*. However, non 01 or non agglutinating *V. cholerae* also can cause disease. *V. cholerae* 01 clinical isolates from the United States have been hemolytic, biotype El Tor, serotype Inaba and have had the same unique phage type and toxin gene sequence. The major mechanism by which this organism causes fluid loss is the production of a heat labile enterotoxin which has the ability to bind the terminal galactose of GM 1 receptors on intestinal epithelial cells with subsequent internalization of an active subunit capable of hydrolysing NAD to ADP ribosylate, a GTP binding regulatory protein of adenylate cyclase. This results in an increase in intracellular cAMP and fluid loss into the gut.

Clostridium difficile. Antimicrobial associated diarrhea (AAC) or pseudomembranous colitis represent the clinical spectrum of illness associated with *C. difficile* and its toxins (32). Many patients have diarrhea that is mild and self limited if antibiotics are discontinued. In others the illness is characterized by fever, bloody diarrhea, and pseudomembranes on protoscopy. Healthy infants can harbor this organism and its toxins in their stools and yet demostrate no illness (33). Healthy children also can be demonstrated to have serum antibodies to one or both toxins. The frequency of colonization with this organism (34) is higher in formula fed infants when compared to breast fed infants. There is evidence for both antibody and non antibody factors in milk that may be important in protecting infants from this organism (35,36). Two toxins, designated A and B, have been described. It is unclear which is more important in producing disease. Cytotoxin is usually demonstrated in tissue culture systems in which the neutralization of toxin by antiserum raised to *Clostridium sordellii* toxin (a toxin closely related to that made by *C. difficile*) is taken as demonstration of presence of this cytotoxin.

Viruses. Rotavirus, Norwalk-like virus and enteric adenovirus are recognized causes of acute infectious gastroenteritis (37). Other viruses which may cause infectious gastroenteritis include enteroviruses, astroviruses, calicivirus, coronavirus, and minirotavirus. These viruses exhibit different epidemiologic and clinical features, although most episodes are self limited and characterized by various combinations of diarrhea, nausea, vomiting, abdominal cramps, headache, myalgia and low grade fever. Rotavirus is the only one of these agents for which a vaccine is being developed.

Rotavirus is one of the most important enteric pathogens throughout the world, particularly in infants. The agent is a double stranded RNA virus. The precise significance of asymptomatic shedding of rotavirus is unclear at present, although it is a common event (38). Illness is particularly prevalent in temperate climates in winter months and may account for as much as 50-60% of diarrhea in infants and young children (37). In those symptomatic with rotavirus infection, nearly 100% have both diarrhea and vomiting. Because of increased insensible losses with fever, intestinal fluid losses, and emesis interferring with rehydration, it is common for rotavirus to be associated with significant dehydration. Because there are multiple serotypes, reinfection can occur (39). Circumstantial evidence suggests that human milk is useful in preventing rotavirus illness due to the presence of specific IgA. The data for prevention of rotavirus infection in animals by breast milk feeding is more convincing than that currently available from human studies. Rotavirus is the only enteropathogen against which vaccines are being developed.

Norwalk-like virus agents remain inaccessible to comprehensive study because of the difficulty in their diagnosis. They cannot be cultivated and therefore development of a vaccine is not yet possible. This same problem has skewed the epidemiologic data toward finding this agent only in outbreaks. Norwalk infection has been shown to be common in all age groups and has a worldwide distribution.

A group of fastidious adenoviruses with a distinct set of antigenic determinants and specific tissue culture growth characteristics has been linked with acute gastroenteritis. Illness is characterized by low grade fever, vomiting and watery stools in infants. These organisms fail to grow on conventional tissue culture cell lines, although they will grow on 293 cells, an adenovirus type 5 transformed line. These agents appear to be endemic in certain areas and infants may be especially susceptible. More information is needed on the epidemiology, extent of clinical involvement and immunology before vaccines can be considered.

Parasitic enteropathogens. Three parasites are the most frequent causes of parasitic diarrhea in persons in the United States. New information has become available about the pathogenic mechanisms and immunology of *Giardia lamblia* and *Entamoeba histolytica*. Another agent, Cryptosporidium, has been described as a cause of gastroenteritis in both immunocompromised and immunocompetent hosts. Immunization agents against these parasitic enteropathogens are not available.

G. lamblia is a flagellated protozoan that exists in trophozoite and cyst forms. Disease due to this organism is common in certain high risk populations and in persons who travel to hyperendemic areas. Children appear to be more susceptible to infection than adults. Infection with Giardia may range from asymptomatic excretion to acute explosive, watery, foul smelling diarrhea with abdominal distention, flatulence, nausea and anorexia. Chronic diarrhea with malabsorption and significant weight loss over many months also may occur. Asymptomatic colonization in young children is common.

Amebiasis is a major health problem in Asia, Latin America and Africa. Disease may remain localized to the intestine or may extend to other organs, most commonly the liver. *E. histolytica* adhere to the intestine by microfilament invasion and produce microabscesses, probably by production of enzymes and cytotoxin. The understanding of *Entamoeba histolytica* has improved with development of culture techniques for isolation and utilization of electrophoretic analysis of isoenzyme patterns. Multiple strains (zymodemes) have been identified on the basis of these characteristics. Identical zymodemes cause illness in different parts of the world and only pathogenic zymodemes elicit an immune reponse in infected patients. The vast majority of *E. histolytica* are nonpathogenic, although normal, healthy individuals can be asymptomatically infected with pathogenic zymodemes.

In 1976 the first human infections due to cryptosporidium were reported. With the onset of the AIDS epidemic, many patients with chronic malabsorption syndrome and severe protracted, watery diarrhea were recognized as having cryptosporidiosis; immunocompetent patients can also be infected. This pathogen probably accounts for less than 5% of diarrheal illness in most populations.

ENTERIC VACCINES

The prevention of infectious diarrhea by immunization is an attractive proposition, but is complicated by the number and diversity of enteropathogens that cause diarrhea. With regard to protection of infants from gastroenteritis by ingestion of milk containing specific antibodies, two methods of approach are available. One possible method is by oral administration of bovine milk containing immunoglobulins with specific antibody activity against infectious agents. Bovine milk immunoglobulin concentrations have been used in human infants against *E. coli* (40) and rotavirus (37). For bovine milk preparations to be effective, the antibody activity must be preserved during processing and during gastrointestinal passage, and it must be specific and show protective activity against the targeted enteropathgen. Current technology will provide the basis for development of effective, safe enteric vaccines. Table 4 shows potential vaccines against enteric disease producing organisms including cholera, *E. coli*, *S. typhi*, shigella and rotavirus. Oral rather than parenteral immunization is more likely to stimulate the protective intestinal immune response of secretory IgA antibodies.

Cholera. Natural infection with cholera is followed by solid, long-lasting immunity (41), stimulating the search for a vaccine. The search for a safe and protective vaccine against cholera began in 1885. Parenteral, killed whole-cell vaccines have been the most intensively evaluated in the past, but they have been found to give variable protection of only 3 to 6 months (42). In addition, the antigen reaches the intestinal lymphoid tissue inefficiently and stimulates suppressive mechanisms that interfere with subsequent attempts to prime or boost the immune response orally (43). Vaccination of lactating women in Pakistan with killed whole cell vaccine given parenterally, produced a serum response as well as an increase in milk secretory IgA antibodies. These women had been naturally exposed previously, priming the gut mucosa. Swedish women without previous natural exposure did not respond with milk secretory IgA antibodies (44,45). Oral rather than parenteral immunization is the route most likely to stimulate protective intestinal immune response of the secretory IgA type (46). The oral vaccines currently under development are inactivated *V. cholerae* strains combined with altered, nonreactogenic toxin or purified toxin subunits, and attenuated *V. cholerae* strains (47).

E. coli. Approaches to vaccine development for enterotoxigenic *E. coli* infections will involve vaccines that stimulate antitoxic or antiadhesion immunity. ETEC pathogens include strains with many cell

Table 4. Promising vaccines against enteric disease

Organisms	Candidates
Vibrio cholerae	Inactivated *V. cholerae* strains combined with altered, non-reactogenic toxin or purified toxin subunits Attenutated *V. cholerae* strains
Escherichia coli	Stimulate antitoxic or anti-adhesion immunity
Salmonella typhi	Live oral strain
Shigella	Recombinant vaccine
Rotavirus	Live virus (attenuated human strains, wild type animal strains, animal-human re-assortment strains and vaccine-rotavirus hybrid) Inactive or subunit (killed whole virus, subunit neutral-ization proteins)

wall lipopolysaccharides, capsular and flagellar serotypes, and several enterotoxin phenotypes. ST is the toxin most commonly produced by virulent strains, but ST is not antigenic. Moreover, although LT is antigenic, volunteer studies suggest that antitoxin immunity is not the principal protective mechanism in humans (48). Killed vaccines composed of purified ETEC pili have not provided satisfactory protection in volunteers (9). Future ETEC vaccine strains will replicate in the intestine and contain antigens intended to stimulate both antibacterial and antitoxic immunity (9).

Although antibodies to different O serogroups have been demonstrated in human milk, an understanding of the pathogenesis of EPEC in infants and children is necessary before a vaccine can be developed (22). It is known that unique entero-adhesive properties of some EPEC strains are associated with a plasmid (49), and it may be possible to identify the phenotypic gene products likely to be pili or outer membrane proteins and to prepare vaccines consisting of the purified gene products. The specific role that cytotoxin plays in the pathogenesis of EPEC diarrhea must be elucidated to determine if this aspect should be considered in vaccine strategy.

Typhoid. The available parenteral typhoid vaccines are neither entirely safe or fully protective (50). The development and successful trial of a live, oral S. typhi vaccine represents a major advance (51,52). In this vaccine a mutagenic strain of S. typhi (Ty2la) is incapable of utilizing galactose after galactose enters the bacterium. The strain proliferates in sufficient numbers to immunize the intestine before the galactose accumulates in the cell and kills it.

Shigella. Until recently oral, killed and attenuated vaccine candidates have lacked safety, stability or efficacy (53). Using genetic engineering plasmid genes coding for the protective antigen of S. sonnei have been inserted into the genome of the Ty2la vaccine strain of S. typhi. The resultant transconjugant strain manifested both S. sonnei and S. typhi antigens and was well tolerated and safe when fed to volunteers (54).

Rotavirus. Several types of rotavirus vaccine are being developed (47) (table 4). One type is an attenuated, otherwise virulent strain of human rotavirus. Attenuation was achieved by passing it repeatedly in gnotobiotic piglets and cell culture (55). This attenuated strain, referred to as WA, was fed to volunteers, but when questions of its safety arose, further trials were suspended. Cold-adapted human rotavirus also may provide future attenuated vaccine candidates. Strains obtained from newborn nurseries in which rotaviruses cause predominantly avirulent infection also may be potential vaccine strains since they may have become attenuated naturally (56).

A second strategy involves the use of rotavirus strains from animals. They need to infect humans and evoke cross-protective immunity without inducing illness. RIT 4237 is an attenuated animal strain that was derived from the Nebraska calf diarrhea virus strain of bovine rotavirus. It has been shown to be safe, immunogenic (57), and efficacious (58) in protecting infants against rotavirus diarrhea, but additional tests are necessary to substantiate effectiveness. Another oral candidate vaccine strain derived from animals has been isolated from a rhesus monkey with diarrhea. This rhesus strain of rotavirus has been safe and immunogenic in adult volunteers; tests in children and infants are underway. A third approach features fastidious human rotaviruses cultivated with less fastidious animal rotavirus strains in tissue culture to produce reassortment rotaviruses. The resulting virus progeny grow efficiently in cell culture, and have the neutralizing specificity of the human rotavirus parent. Gene reassortment techniques may produce useful rotavirus vaccine candidates.

Availability of cloned rotavirus genes and the protein sequences of important rotavirus antigens should permit additional approaches to vaccine development, such as incorporation into a expression vector (45). If rotavirus antigens can be synthesized in such systems, a large amount of rotavirus antigen could be produced for subunit vaccines and for structure analysis necessary for construction of a synthetic vaccine. In another novel scheme, rotavirus genes are inserted into vaccine virus to create an infectious hybrid virus vaccine. Recent reports of new, serologically distinct human rotavirus strains (59,60) demand that field trials be carried out over many years and in different locales because of the possible variation in rotaviruses and their periodic occurrence.

HUMAN MILD PROTECTIVE FACTORS

Diarrheal disease occurs less frequently in infants who are breast fed compared to those who are bottle fed (61,62). Protective factors in human milk that modify or prevent disease include cells, nonspecific factors including all nonantibody factors and antibodies (63,64). Breast milk protective factors that are protective against one enteropathogen or its toxin may not afford protection against others, further complicating breast milk immunity. The major immunoglobulin in human milk is secretory IgA. This immunoglobulin is not absorbed in significant quantity from the human intestine and therefore acts at the mucosal surface of the intestine. Total IgA as well as specific IgA to many respiratory and gastrointestinal pathogens have been reported in human milk (2); however, demonstration of protective affects of these antibodies is often lacking. Addition information about specific protection afforded by antibodies in human milk is needed.

SUMMARY

Control and prevention of acute diarrhea involves improvement in environmental conditions with regard to hygiene, continued use of oral rehydration solutions when diarrhea occurs, breast feeding, and development of vaccines against various enteropathogens. Recent knowledge about causes of diarrhea and methods of vaccine development has rapidly advanced. Use of vaccines to confer immunity against diarrheal disease via breast milk is a future consideration.

REFERENCES

1. Pan American Health Organization. 1980. Diarrheal diseases in the Americas. Epidemiol. Bull. (PAHO), 1:1.
2. Mata, L. 1982. Epidemiology of acute diarrhea in childhood. In Acute diarrhea: Its nutritional consequences in children. J.A. Bellanti ed. Raven Press, New York.
3. Cleary, T.G., Pickering, L.K.: 1986. Update on infectious diarrhea. In Advances in Pediatric Infectious Diseases. S. Aronoff, ed. Year Book Medical Publishers, Chicago, IL. 1:117.
4. Gurwith, M.J., Williams, T.W. 1977. Gastroenteritis in children: A two year review in Manitoba. I. Etiology. J. Infect. Dis. 136:239.
5. Pickering, L.K., Evans, D.J., Munoz, O., et al. 1978. Prospective study of enteropathogens in children with diarrhea in Houston and Mexico. J. Pediatr. 93:383.

6. Black, R.E., Merson, M.H., Huq, I., *et al*. 1981. Incidence and severity of rotavirus and *Escherichia coli* diarrhea in rural Bangladesh. Implications for vaccine development. Lancet 1:141.
7. Guerrant, R.L., Kirchoff, L.V., Shields, D.S., *et al*. 1983. Prospective study of diarrheal illness in North-eastern Brazil: Patterns of disease, nutritional impact, etiologies, and risk factors. J. Infect. Dis. 148:986.
8. Pickering, L.K., Cleary, T.C. Approach to patients with gastrointestinal infection and food poisoning. *In* Textbook of Pediatric Infectiou Disease. Ed. R.D. Feigin and J.D. Cherry. W.B. Saunders, Philadelphia, PA (in press).
9. Levine, M.M., Kaper, J.B., Black, R.E., *et al*. 1983. New knowledge on pathogenesis of bacterial enteric infections as applied to vaccine development. Microbiol. Rev. 47:510.
10. Guerrant, R.L., Moore, R.A., Kirschenfeld, P.M., *et al*. 1975. Role of toxigenic and invasive bacteria in acute diarrhea of childhood. N. Engl. J. Med. 293:567.
11. Levine, M.M., Bergquist, E.J., Nalin, D.R., *et al*. 1978. *Escherichia coli* strains that cause diarrhoea but do not produce heat-labile or heat-stabile enterotoxins and are non-invasive. Lancet 1:1119.
12. Edelman, R., Levine, M.M. 1983. Summary of a workshop on enteropathogenic *Escherichia coli*. J. Infect. Dis. 147:1108.
13. Toledo, M.R.F., Alvariza, M.C.B., Murahovschi, J., *et al*. 1983. Enteropathogenic *Escherichia coli* serotypes and endemic diarrhea in infants. Infect. Immun. 39:586.
14. Sakazaki, R., Tamura, K., Saito, M. 1967. Enteropathogenic *Escherichia coli* associated with diarrhea in children and adults. Jpn. J. Med. Sci. Biol. 20:387.
15. Gurwith, M., Hinde, D., Gross, R., *et al*. 1978. A prospective study of enteropathogenic *Escherichia coli* in endemic diarrheal disease. J. Infect. Dis. 137:292.
16. Levine, M.M., Edelman, R. 1984. EPEC of classic serotypes associated with infant diarrhea: Epidemiology and pathogenesis. Epidem. Rev. 6:31.
17. Clausen, C.R., Christie, D.L. 1982. Chronic diarrhea in infants caused by adherent enteropathogenic *Escherichia coli*. J. Pediatr. 100:358.
18. Rothbaum, R.J., Partin, J.C., Saalfield, K., *et al*. 1983. An ultrastructural study of enteropathogenic *Escherichia coli* infection in human infants. Ultrastruct. Pathol. 4:291.
19. Scotland, S.M., Day, N.P., Rowe, B. 1980. Production of a cytotoxin affecting Vero cells by strains of *Escherichia coli* belonging to traditional enteropathogenic serogroups. FEMS Micro. Let. 7:15.
20. Cleary, T.G., Mathewson, J.J., Faris, E., *et al*. 1985. Shiga-like cytotoxin production by enteropathogenic *Escherichia coli* serogroups. Infect. Immun. 47:335.
21. Mathewson, J.J., Johnson, P.C., DuPont, H.L., *et al*. 1985. A newly recognized cause of travelers' diarrhea: Enteroadherent *Escherichia coli*. J. Infect. Dis. 151:471.
22. Remis, R.S., MacDonald, K.L., Riley, L.W., *et al*. 1984. Sporadic cases of hemorrhagic colitis associated with *Escherichia coli* 0157:H7. Ann. Intern. Med. 101:624.
23. Reis, M.H.L., Guth, B.E.C., Gomes, T.A.T., *et al*. 1982. Frequency of *E. coli* strains producing LT, ST or both in children with and without diarrhea in Sao Paulo. J. Clin. Micro. 15:1062.
24. Yamamoto, T., Honda, T., Miwatani, T., *et al*. 1984. A virulence plasmid in *Escherichia coli* enterotoxogenic for humans. Intergenetic transfer and expression. J. Infect. Dis. 150:688.

25. Formal, S.B., Hale, T.L., Sansonetti, P.J. 1983. Invasive enteric pathogens. Rev. Infect. Dis. 5:S702.
26. Giannella, R.A., Formal, S.B., Dammin, G.J., *et al*. 1973. Pathogenesis of salmonellosis: Studies of fluid secretion, mucosal invasion, and morphologic reaction in the rabbit ileum. J. Clin. Invest. 52:441.
27. Jiwa, S.F. 1981. Probing for enterotoxigenicity among the salmonellae: An evaluation of biological assays. J. Clin. Micro. 14:463.
28. Finkelstein, R.A., Marchlewicz, B.A., McDonald, R.J., *et al*. 1983. Isolation and characterization of a cholera-related enterotoxin from *Salmonella typhimurium*. FEMS Microbio. Lett. 17:239.
29. Blaser, M.J., Wells, J.G., Feldman, R.A., *et al*. 1983. Campylobacter enteritis in the United States. Ann. Intern. Med. 98:360.
30. Ruiz-Palacios, G.M., Torres, J., Torres, N.I., *et al*. 1983. Cholera-like enterotoxin produced by *Campylobacter jejuni*. Characterization and significance. Lancet 2:250.
31. Kaper, J.B., Bradford, H.B., Roberts, N.C. *et al*. 1982. Molecular epidemiology of *Vibrio cholerae* in the U.S. Gulf Coast. J. Clin. Microbiol. 16:129.
32. Bartlett, J.G. 1979. Antibiotic-associated pseudomembranous colitis. Rev. Infect. Dis. 1:530.
33. Thompson, C.M., Gilligan, P.H., Fisher, M.C., *et al*. 1983. *C. difficile* cytotoxin in a pediatric population. Amer. J. Dis. Child. 137:271.
34. Cooperstock, M., Riegle, L., Woodruff, C.W., *et al*. 1983. Influence of age, sex and diet on asymptomatic colonization of infants with *Clostridium difficile*. J. Clin. Micro. 17:830.
35. Wada, N., Nishida, N., Iwaki, S., *et al*. 1980. Neutralizing activity against *C. difficile* toxin in the supernatants of cultured colostral cells. Infect. Immun. 29:545.
36. Kim, K., Pickering, L.K., DuPont, H.L., *et al*. 1984. *In vitro* and *in vivo* neutralizing activity of human colostrum and milk against purified toxins A and B of *Clostridium difficile*. J. Infect. Dis. 150:57.
37. Pickering, L.K. Keswick, B.H. Rotavirus and Norwalk virus. *In* Clinical Virology Manual. Edited by S. Spector, G. Lancz, and I. Lee. Elsevier Science Publishing Company, Inc., New York, New York (in press).
38. Champsaur, H., Questianx, E., Prevot, J., *et al*. 1984. Rotavirus carriage, asymptomatic infection, and disease in the first two years of life. I. Virus shedding. J. Infect. Dis. 149:667.
39. Yolken, R.H., Wyatt, R.G., Zissis, G., *et al*. 1978. Epidemiology of human rotavirus types 1 and 2 as studied by ELISA. N. Engl. J. Med. 299:1156.
40. Mietens, C., Kleinhorst, H., Hilpert, H., *et al*. 1976. Treatment of infantile *E. coli* gastroenteritis with specific bovine and *E. coli* milk immunoglobulins. Eur. J. Pediatr. 132:239.
41. Levine, M.M., Black, R.E., Clements, M.L., *et al*. 1981. Duration of infection derived immunity to cholera. J. Infect. Dis. 143:818.
42. Joo, I. 1974. Cholera vaccines. *In* Cholera. Ed. D. Barma and W. Burrows. W.B. Saunders, Philadelphia, PA.
43. Pierce, N.F. 1980. Suppression of the intestinal immune response to cholera toxin by specific serum antibody. Infect. Immun. 30:62.
44. Svennerholm, A.M., Holgren, J., Hanson, L.A., *et al*. 1977. Boosting of secretory IgA antibody response in man by parenteral cholera vaccination. Scand. J. Immunol. 6:1345.
45. Svennerholm, A.M, Hanson, L.A., Holgren, J., *et al*. 1980. Different secretory immunoglobulin A antibody response to cholera vaccination in Swedish and Pakistani women. Infect. Immun. 30:427.

46. Levine, M.M., Nalin, D.R., Craig, J.P., *et al*. 1979. Immunity to cholera in man: Relative role of antibacterial versus antitoxic immunity. Trans. R. Soc. Trop. Med Hyg. 73:3.
47. Edelman, R. 1985. Prevention and treatment of infectious diarrhea. Speculations on the next ten years. Am. J. Med. 785:99.
48. Levine, M.M., Nalin, D.R., Hooever,. D.L., *et al*. 1979. Immunity to enterotoxigenic *Escherichia coli*. Infect. Immun. 23:729.
49. Baldini, M.M., Kaper, J.B., Levine, M.M., *et al*. 1983. Plasmid-mediated adhesion in enteropathogenic *Escherichia coli*. J. Pediatr. Gastroenterol. Nutr. 2:534.
50. Woodward, W.E. 1980. Volunteer studies of typhoid fever and vaccines. Trans. R. Soc. Trop. Med. Hyg. 74:553.
51. Pierce, N.F., Sacci, J.B., Jr. 1984. Enhanced mucosal priming by cholera toxin and procholeragenoid with a lipoidal amine adjuvant (Avridine) delivered in liposomes. Infect. Immun. 44:469.
52. Wahdan, M.H., Serie, C., Cerisier, Y., *et al*. 1982. A controlled field trial of live *Salmonella typhi* strain Ty21a oral vaccine against typhoid: Three year results. J. Infect. Dis. 145:292.
53. Formal, S.B., Maenza, R.M., Austin, S., *et al*. 1967. Failure of parenteral vaccines to protect monkeys against experimental shigellosis. Proc. Soc. Exp. Biol. Med. 125:347.
54. Tramont, E.C., Chung, R., Berman, S., *et al*. 1984. Safety and antigenicity of typhoid-*Shigella sonnei* vaccine (strain 5076-1C). J. Infect. Dis. 149:133.
55. Wyatt, R.G., James, W.D., Bohl, E.H., *et al*. 1980. Human rotavirus type 2, cultivation *in vitro*. Science 207:189.
56. Bishop, R.F., Barnes, G.L., Cipriani, E., *et al*. 1983. Clinical immunity after neonatal rotavirus infection: A prospective longitudinal study in young children. N. Engl. J. Med. 309:72.
57. Vesikari, T., Isolauri, E., Delem, A., *et al*. 1983. Immunuogenicity and safety of live oral attenuated bovine rotavirus vaccine strain RIT 4237 in adults and young children. Lancet 11:807.
58. Vesikari, T., Isolauri, E., D'Hondt, E., *et al*. 1984. Protection of infants against rotavirus diarrhoea by RIT 4237 attenuated bovine rotavirus strain vaccine. Lancet 1:977.
59. Tao, H., Changan, W., Zhaoying, F., *et al*. 1984. Waterborne outbreak of rotavirus diarrhoea in adults in China caused by a novel rotavirus. Lancet 1:1139.
60. Dimitrov, D.H., Estes, M.K., Rangelova, S.M., *et al*. 1983. Detection of antigenically distinct rotaviruses from infants. Infect. Immun. 41:523.
61. Kovar, M.G., Serdula, M.K., Karks, J.S., *et al*. 1984. Review of the epidemiologic evidence for an association between infant feeding and infant health. Pediatrics 74(Suppl):615.
62. Feachem, R.G., Koblinsky, M.A. 1984. Interventions for the control of diarrhoeal diseases among young children: Promotion of breast feeding. Bull. W.H.O. 62:271.
63. Goldman, A.S., Goldblum, R.M. 1985. Protective properties of human milk in nutrition in pediatrics. *In* Walker W.A., ed., Basic Science and Clinical Application. Little Brown and Company.
64. Pickering, L.K., Kohl, S. Human milk humoral immunity and infant defense mechanisms. *In* Human Milk in Infant Nutrition and Health. Ed. R.R. Howell, F.H. Morriss, L.K. Pickering. Charles C. Thomas, Springfield, IL (in press).

INHIBITION OF ATTACHMENT OF <u>STREPTOCOCCUS PNEUMONIAE</u> AND <u>HAEMOPHILUS INFLUENZAE</u> BY HUMAN MILK

Oscar Porras, Bengt Andersson, Lars Å. Hanson, Teresa Lagergård and Catharina Svanborg Edén

National Children's Hospital, San José, Costa Rica and Departments of Clinical Immunology and Medical Microbiology, University of Göteborg Sweden

INTRODUCTION

Human milk contains several components with anti-microbial activity (1) and breast feeding is associated with decreased morbidity in infectious diseases (2-4).

Attachment to the epithelial surfaces has been suggested as the initial interaction between mucosal components and infectious agents (5). In several cases, the bacterial binding is specific, involving epithelial receptors. Such specific receptors have been defined on urinary tract epithelium for pyelonephritogenic *Escherichia coli* and on pharyngeal cells for *Streptococcus pneumoniae* (6,7). Soluble receptor molecules inhibit the attachment *in vitro* (6,7) and *in vivo* (8). *S.pneumoniae* and *Haemophilus influenzae* are the major bacterial agents associated with respiratory tract infections and acute otitis media. Both species attach to human oral mucosal cells *in vitro* (9,10).

Human milk contains immunoglobulins, specific antibodies, glycoconjugates and free oligosaccharides which interfere with bacterial adhesion to human epithelial cells (11-13).

In this study human milk was shown to inhibit the adhesion of *S.pneumoniae* and *H.influenzae* to pharyngeal and buccal epithelial cells. The inhibitory activity was only to a limited extent due to antibodies and was explained in part by the presence of receptor active oligosaccharides for the pneumococci and by a high molecular weight component for *H.influenzae* (14,15).

MATERIAL

Milk samples

Human milk was obtained on the 2-3 day and during the fourth week of lactation from 14 healthy women (labelled by capital letters). Samples were also given by two mothers with immunoglobulin A (IgA) levels of < 0.01 g/l in serum and 0.03 g/l in the milk from one and undetectable in the milk from the other mother.

The high and low molecular weight fractions (HMWF,LMWF) were obtained by filtration through a collodion-bag (Sartorious, Göttingen, FRG), retaining material of a molecular weight higher than 12.000 daltons.

Milk was centrifuged in the cold, and the fat removed. After precipitation of proteins and lactose in 67% ethanol, the supernatant was fractionated over Sephadex G-25 (Pharmacia, Uppsala, Sweden). The intermediate size fraction composed of tetra and hexa saccharides was used. Isolated milk oligosaccharides were obtained from Dr. D. Zopff, NIH, Bethesda, Md, USA and synthetic saccharides from the Swedish Sugar Company, Arlov, Sweden.

Fresh unpasteurized milk from cows and buffalos were also studied as were two infant formulas based on cow's milk (Semper AB, Stockholm, Sweden).

Bacteria

The four S.pneumoniae strains employed were isolated from the nasopharynx of three patients with acute otitis media and one healthy carrier. These strains were of the capsular types 6A (Culture Collection University of Göteborg (CCUG) 3114), 4 (CCUG 3296), 23F (CCUG 2987), 19F (CCUG 10175).

The four H.influenzae strains used were nontypeable, three of them isolates from the nasopharynx of three children with acute otitis media (Nos. 198, 3In, 23In) and the fourth was a noncapsulated mutant of H.influenzae type b (No. Sb).

METHODS

The adhesion and adhesion inhibition methods have been reported (14,15). Briefly, milk, milk fractions, oligosaccharides or phosphate saline buffer (pH 7.2) were mixed with a bacterial suspension. This was incubated at 37°C for 15 min for pneumococci and 30 min for H,influenzae. Subsequently, epithelial cells were added and the adherence mixture was incubated for 60 min. The adherence was estimated by interference contrast microscopy as the mean number of bacteria per cell, for 40 epithelial cells. The encoded samples were read by one person. Adhesion inhibition was given in per cent of the buffer control, or as the effective oligosaccharide dose required to reduce adhesion to 50% of the buffer control (9,10,14,15).

Immunoglobulins in serum were quantified with the Mancini technique (16). Milk secretory IgA was quantified by a modified enzyme-linked immunosorbent assay (ELISA) (17). Specific antibodies were determined in ELISA using the following antigens: phosphorylcholine prepared from pneumococci and coupled to bovine serum albumin (18,19), H.influenzae polysaccharide capsule b and outer membrane proteins (20).

Immunoglobulins were removed by immunoabsorption using Affigel-10 (Bio-Rad, Richmond, USA) coupled with rabbit anti-human immunoglobulin (Dakopatts, Copenhagen, Denmark).

RESULTS

Human milk efficiently inhibited the attachment of S.pneumoniae and H.influenzae to the epithelial cells (table 1).

Table 1
Effect of human milk on the adhesion of S.pneumoniae and H.influenzae to epithelial cells

Strain	Adhesion (% buffer control) mean	SD
S.pneumoniae		
CCUG 3114	4	7
CCUG 3296	0	0
CCUG 2987	0	0
CCUG 10175	1	1
H.influenzae		
3In	7	5
198	0	0
23IN	3	5
Sb	23	24

Milk from other species and the formulas reduced pneumococcal adherence less than human milk, but increased H.influenzae adhesion (table 2).

Inhibitory activity of the milk was retained after removal of the antibodies by immunoabsorption, although the elimination of the immunoglobulins resulted in a reduction in the inhibitory activity (table 3).

The inhibition of attachment did not correlate with the total immunoglobulin content of the milk samples. Specific antibodies to phosphorylcholine, H.influenzae polysaccharide type b and outer membrane antigens were present in the milk samples, but there was no correlation between adhesion inhibition and specific antibody activity.

Table 2
Effect of cow and buffalo milk and formula on the adhesion of *S.pneumoniae* and *H.influenzae* to epithelial cells

Strain	Adhesion (% buffer control) Cow mean	SD	Buffalo mean	SD	Formula mean	SD
S.pneumoniae						
CCUG 3114	19	17	37	25	9	8
CCUG 3296	24	32	49	9	27	38
CCUG 2987	66	2	53	11	23	32
CCUG 10175	39	18	44	21	14	19
H.influenzae						
3In	127	38	140	30	152	1
198	112	14	119	25	106	10
23In	255	21	200	28	165	23
Sb	148	78	178	60	173	47

Table 3
Inhibition of adhesion of *S.pneumoniae* and *H.influenzae* by immunoabsorbed milk

Tested material	Adhesion (% buffer control) mean	SD	Total SIgA g/l
S.pneumoniae			
HMWF (I)	9	2	1.09
Immunoabsorbed	31	8	0.00
H.influenzae			
Whole breast milk (N)	18	11	0.08
Immunoabsorbed	49	48	0.00
Whole breast milk (O)	35	13	0.12
Immunoabsorbed	29	6	0.00

Note: SIgA, secretory IgA; HMWF, high molecular weight fraction.

The samples from a few mothers were less inhibitory than those from others (table 4). The milk samples from the IgA deficient mothers blocked attachment as efficiently as the samples from mothers with normal IgA levels (table 4).

Table 4
Inhibition of adhesion of S.pneumoniae and H.influenzae by milk from various donors

Milk sample	Adhesion (% buffer control) S.pneumoniae mean	SD	H.influenzae mean	SD
Day 2-3				
Normal donors				
A	3	4	1	2
B	1	1	4	1
C	45	13	34	12
IgA deficient				
D	0	0	1	1
E	0	0	5	1
Week 4				
A	8	3	15	6
F	49	22	19	10

The HMWF of human milk inhibited the adhesion of H.influenzae and S.pneumoniae to epithelial cells (table 5).

Inhibitory activity of pneumococcal adhesion was also found in the LMWF. The LMWF of breast milk had no effect on the adhesion of H.influenzae (table 5). The LMWF did not contain detectable antibody activity.

Inhibition of S.pneumoniae adhesion was found in the human milk oligosaccharide fraction present in the LMWF. Milk oligosaccharides and purified and synthetic saccharides of the neolacto- and lactoseries inhibited in the same concentration range (table 6).

Table 5

Inhibition of adhesion of S.pneumoniae and H.influenzae by fractions of human milk

Tested material	Adhesion (% buffer control) S.pneumoniae* mean	SD	H.influenzae** mean	SD
Whole milk (G)	28	6	NT	
HMWF	6	4		
LMWF	31	6		
Whole milk (J)	NT		15	6
HMWF			1	1
LMWF			76	31
HMWF				
H	0	0	NT	
I	9	2	NT	
K	1	1	0	0
LMWF				
H	34	18	NT	
I	9	1	NT	
K	44	38	100	0
L	NT		100	0
M	NT		100	0

* CCUG 3114; ** 3In; HMWF high molecular weight fraction; LMWF low molecular weight fraction; NT not tested.

Table 6

Inhibition of adhesion of S.pneumoniae by human milk oligosaccharides

Structure	Source	EID50 (mg/ml)
Oligosaccharide fraction	human milk	6.0
Galβ1→4GlcNAcβ1→3Galβ1→4Glc	human milk	0.2
Galβ1→4GlcNAcβ1→3Galβ1→4Glc	synthetic	0.6
Galβ1→3GlcNAcβ1→3Galβ1→4Glc	human milk	1.3
Galβ1→4Glcβ1-O-Et	Synthetic	3.0
Galβ1→3GlcNAc	synthetic	1.0
Galβ1→3GlcNAcβ1-O-Me	synthetic	5.0

EID50 effective inhibitory dose reducing adherence to 50% of buffer control (50% inhibition).

DISCUSSION

Breast feeding decreases the incidence of infectious diseases e.g. diarrhoea and meningitis (21,22). Morbidity due to respiratory tract infections and otitis media is high in children (23). The incidence and course of these infections are affected by the use of breast milk (24). Breast feeding protects the infant by reducing the exposure to contaminated food and directly by the presence of specific and non-specific anti-microbial factors.

Breast feeding was reported to be less prevalent among cases with invasive *H,influenzae* type b disease (25). Children with invasive *H.influenzae* type b disease attending day care centers were less likely to have been breast fed (26).

Human milk was shown to abolish the attachment to pharyngeal epithelial cells both of *H.influenzae* and *S.pneumoniae*. The anti-adhesive capacity did not correlate with the level of secretory IgA in the milk or specific antibodies against pneumococcal phosphorylcholine or *H.influenzae* b polysaccharide or outer membrane proteins and milk without immunoglobulins after immunosorption retained inhibitory capacity.

The inhibitory effect on *H.influenzae* was restricted to the HMWF of breast milk whereas the adhesion inhibition of *S.pneumoniae* was found both in the HMWF and LMWF. Free oligosaccharides purified from the LMWF and synthetic as well as human milk derived saccharides blocked the adhesion of *S.pneumoniae*. Neolacto, lactotetraose and their fucosylated derivetives occur in human milk, in amounts of about 1.3 mg/dl which is within the range where they were active in the test employed (27).

The inhibitory effect of the HMWF on *H,influenzae* may be explained by the presence of receptor-active oligosaccharides determinants on milk glycoproteins or glycolipids. Inhibition of *Vibrio cholerae* haemagglutination has been reported associated to a fraction of human milk suggestive of glycoconjugates (28,29).

The adhesion inhibition activity provides a mechanism to explain at least part of an beneficial effect of breast feeding in diseases associated with H.influenzae and S.pneumoniae. Such inhibitory activity has been demonstrated to be poorly related to the antibody content of breast milk and in part explained by the presence of receptor-active oligosaccharides.

The inhibition of adhesion of *H.influenzae* and *S.pneumoniae* by breast milk provides a mechnism to explain the suggested beneficial effect of breast feeding on infections associated with those pathogens.

ACKNOWLEDGMENTS

This study was supported by grants from the Medical Faculty, University of Göteborg, the Swedish Medical Research Council and the Ellen, Walter and Lennart Hesselman Foundation for Scientific Research, the Swedish Board for Technical Development and SAREC.

REFERENCES

1. Hanson LÅ, Brandtzaeg P. Mucosal defence. In: Stiehm ER, Fulginiti VA, eds. Immunologic disorders in infants and children. 3rd ed. Philadelphia, WB Saunders, 1985 (in press)

2. Cunningham SS. Morbidity in breast-fed and artificially fed infants II. J Pediatr 1979; 95:685-9

3. Chandra RH. Prospective studies of the effect of breast-feeding on incidence of infection and allergy. Acta Paediatr Scand 1979; 68:691-4

4. Saarinen UM. Prolonged breast feeding as prophylaxis for recurrent otitis media. Acta Paediatr Scand 1982; 71:567-71

5. Beachey EH. Bacterial adherence: adhesin-receptor interactions mediating the attachment of bacteria to mucosal surfaces. J Infect Dis 1981; 143:325-45

6. Leffler H, Svanborg-Edén C. Chemical identificaction of a glycosphingolipid receptor for Escherichia coli attaching to human urinary tract epithelial cells and agglutnating human erythrocytes. FEMS Microbiol Lett 1980; 8:127-34

7. Andersson B, Dahmén J, Frejd T, Leffler H, Magnusson G, Noori G, Svanborg-Edén C. Identification of an active disaccharide unit of a glycoconjugate receptor for pneumococci attaching to human pharyngeal epithelial cells. J Exp Med 1983; 158:559-70

8. Leffler H, Svanborg-Edén C, Schoolnik G, Wadström T. Glycosphigolipids as receptors for bacterial adhesion. Host glycolipid diversity and other selected aspects. In: Boedekker EC, ed. Attachment of organisms to the gut mucosa II. CRC Press 1984; 177-87

9. Porras O, Svanborg-Edén C, Lagergård T, Hanson LÅ. Method for testing adherence of Haemophilus influenzae to human buccal epithelial cells. Eur J Clin Microbiol 1985; 51:480-7

10. Andersson B, Eriksson B, Falsen E, Fogh A, Hanson LÅ, Nylén O, Peterson H, Svanborg-Edén C. Adhesion of Streptococcus pneumoniae to human pharyngeal epithelial cells in vitro: differences in adhesive capacity among strains isolated from subjects with otitis media, septicemia, or meningitis or from healthy carriers. Infect Immun 1981; 32:311-7

11. Svanborg-Edén C, Svennerholm AM. Secretory immunoglobulin A and G antibodies prevent adhesion of Escherichia coli to human urinary tract epithelial cells. Infect Immun 1978; 22:790-7

12. Williams RC, Gibbons RJ. Inhibition of bacterial adherence by secretory immunoglobulin A: A mechanism of antigenic disposal. Science 1972; 177:697-9

13. Kobata A. Milk glycoproteins and oligosaccharides. In: Horowitz MI, Pigman W, eds. The Glycoconjugates. London, Academic Press, 1985: 423-40

14. Andersson B, Porras O, Hanson LÅ, Svanborg-Edén C, Leffler H. Non-antibody containing fractions of breast milk inhibit epithelial attachment of Streptococcus pneumoniae and Haemophilus influenzae. Lancet 1985; i:643

15. Andersson B, Porras O, Hanson LÅ, Lagergård T, Svanborg-Edén C. Inhibition of attachment of Streptococcus pneumoniae and Haemophilus influenzae by human milk and receptor oligosaccharides. J Infect Dis 1986;

16. Mancini G, Carbonara AO, Heremans JF. Immunochemical quantitation of antigens by single radial immunodiffusion. Immunochem 1965; 2:235-54

17. Sohl-Åkerlund A, Hanson LÅ, Ahlstedt S, Carlsson B. A Sensitive method for specific quantitation of secretory IgA. Scand J Immunol 1977; 6:1275-82

18.Briles DE, Nahm M, Schroer K, Davie J, Baker P, Kearney J, Barletta R. Antiphosphocholine antibodies found in normal mouse serum are protective against intravenous infection with type 3 Streptococcus pneumoniae. J Exp Med 1981; 153:694-705

19. Chesebro D, Matzger H. Affinity labeling of a phosphorylcholine-binding mouse myeloma protein. Biochem 1972; 2:766-71

20. Dahlberg T, Branefors P. Enzyme linked immunosorbent assay for titration of H.influenzae capsular and O antigen antibodies. J Clin Microbiol 1980; 12:185-92

21. Mata LJ, Urrutia JJ. Intestinal colonization of breast-fed children in a rural area of low socio-economic level. Ann N Y Acad Sci 1971; 176:93-109

22. Winberg J, Wessner G. Does breast milk protect against septicemia in the newborn? Lancet 1971; i:1091-4

23. Giebink GS, Quie PG. Otitis media: the spectrum of middle ear inflammation. Ann Rev Med 1978; 29:285-306

24. Saarinen UM. Prolonged breast-feeding as prophylaxis for recurrent otitis media. Acta Paediatr Scand 1982; 71:567-71

25. Jason JM, Nilburg P, Marks JS. Mortality and infectious disease associated with infant feeding patterns in developing countries. Pediatrics 1984; Supp:702-27

26. Istre GR, Conner JS, Broome CV, Hightower A, Hopkins RS. Risk factors for primary invasive H.influenzae disease: increased risk from day care attendance and school-aged household members. J Pediatr 1985; 106: 190-5

27. Kobata A, Ginsburg V, Tsuda M. Oligosaccharides of human milk. Isolation and characterization. Arch Biochem Biophys 1969; 130:509-13

28. Holmgren J, Svennerholm AM, Lindblad M. Receptors-like glycocompounds in human milk that inhibit classical and El Tor Vibrio cholera cell adherence (hemagglutination). Infect Immun 1983; 39:147-154

29. Holmgren J, Svennerholm AM, Åhrén C. Noninmmunoglobulin fraction of human milk inhibits bacterial adhesion (hemagglutination) and enterotoxin binding of E.coli and Vibrio cholerae. Infect Immun 1981; 33: 136-41

EFFECTS OF ETHNICITY ON IMMUNOLOGIC COMPONENTS IN HUMAN MILK

José Ramiro Cruz, Carolina Arevalo and Lars Å. Hanson

Chief, Nutrition Infection and Immunology Program INCAP

Scientist, Nutrition Infection and Immunology Program INCAP

Chief, Department of Clinical Immunology University of Göteborg

Human milk contains various defense components, such as bifidus and antistaphylococcal factors, lysozyme, lactoferrin, receptor analogues, and lipids, which have been shown to inhibit microbial adhesion to host cells, function, proliferation and/or expression in vitro.[1-5] The biologic significance of these substances in the gastrointestinal tract of the breast-fed infant needs further elucidation. In addition, human colostrum and milk contain large numbers of cells involved in immune reactions, such as macrophages, neutrophiles, B- and T- lymphocytes, and immunoglobulins G, M, and A.[6-9] The secretory immunoglobulin A (SIgA), is formed by two IgA monomers, a joining (J) chain, and a secretory component (SC); this particular arrangement makes the molecule of SIgA resistant to enzymatic degradation and, therefore, functional in the gastrointestinal tract.[10]

Glass and coworkers[11] have shown that high levels of milk specific SIgA antibodies are associated with protection against cholera in the breast-fed child, even in the presence of infection. Furthermore, feeding breast milk with SIgA antirotavirus antibodies to severely immune deficient children suffering from rotavirus-associated gastroenteritis stops viral shedding and symptomatology.[12] This information, coupled with that obtained experimentally, suggests that SIgA may be the most important single protective factor in human colostrum and milk. It is appropriate, therefore, to examine the concentration of SIgA and the content of specific antibodies of the SIgA class in colostrum and milk of women with different ethnic characteristics in order to estimate their protective capacity.

Several authors have approached the question by examining the content of total SIgA of colostrum and milk. Although the results may vary because of different methodologies employed, it is clear that human colostrum contains between 1.7 and 5.6 g of SIgA/l; the mean values fluctuate around 2.0 g (Table 1).[13-18] This figure seems to be independent from the nutritional status of the lactating woman, although one study[15] reported that deficient nutritional status resulted in the production of colostrum which was deficient in immune components. This detrimental effect of undernutrition was not seen in specimens collected two weeks postpartum. The concentration of SIgA is lower in mature milk than in colostrum. The concentrations reported in studies done in different locations vary from about 0.5 to 1.6 g/l one month after delivery (Table 1). These values persist for as long as one year, with no clear differences among groups of various ethnic backgrounds.

Table 1. SIgA Concentration (g/l) in Milk Samples from Women from Different Locations

Location	Time Postpartum						Reference
	2-3d	1m	3m	6m	9m	12m	
Texas, USA	2.0	1.0	0.5	0.5	0.8	1.0	13
The Gambia[a]			0.5	0.4	0.3	0.3	14
Cambridge, England			0.4	0.3			14
Colombia (WN)[b]	2.6		0.5	0.6			15
Colombia (UN)[c]	2.0		0.5	0.5			15
India (WN)	3.4		1.2				16
India (UN)	3.7		1.2				16
India	3.4		1.0	0.8	1.0	1.1	16
Ethiopia	1.7	0.4					17
Ethiopia	5.6	0.6					17
Sweden	2.5	0.7					17
Guatemala, rural		0.6	0.4	0.4	0.4	0.6	17
Guatemala, urban		0.8	0.6				17
Guatemala, urban		1.0	0.6				17
Guatemala, rural	3.0	1.6			1.5		18

[a] Estimated from the published curve.
[b] WN: well nourished.
[c] UN: undernourished.

Some authors have analyzed the amount of SIgA that a mother transfers to her infant in a day,[14, 17, 19] by determining SIgA concentration in colostrum and milk and by estimating the volume of milk that a breast-fed child ingests in a 24-h period. There may be some methodologic differences, but despite them, SIgA daily intake at one month of age is 0.2 to 0.6 g (Table 2). The amount of SIgA ingested tends to be lower as lactation progresses, probably due to a decrease in the volume of milk. An important consideration is the quantity of SIgA that a child ingests in relation to his body weight. Recently, Butte and colleagues[19] have shown that, during the first month of life, an infant may receive around 130 mg/kg/day of SIgA. There is a gradual decrease in the amount, to approximately 80 mg/kg/day four months postpartum. We have calculated the values for mother-infant pairs from Guatemala and found an identical pattern (Table 3). Moreover, the mean figures and the standard deviation for the urban, privileged group one month postpartum are almost identical to those observed among women from Texas. Goldman and coleagues (20) have shown that during weaning there is a decrease in the amount of milk that children ingest. There is, however, a concomitant increase in milk SIgA concentration. In our series of individuals, the volume of milk ingested correlated with the child's weight at the time of sampling; this variable also correlated with birth weight.

Table 2. Daily SIgA Intake (g) by Breast-fed Children from Different Locations

Location	Time Postpartum					Reference
	1m	3m	6m	9m	12m	
Tha Gambia[a,b]		0.3	0.2	0.2	0.2	14
Cambridge, England[b]		0.3	0.2			14
Texas, USA[b]	0.6	0.5				19
Sweden	0.5	0.4	0.3	0.3		17
Guatemala, rural	0.3	0.3	0.3	0.2	0.3	17
Guatemala, urban (poor)	0.4	0.3				17
Guatemala, urban (privileged)	0.5	0.3				17

[a] Original data given as mg/12h.
[b] Estimated from the published curve.

Table 3. Daily Milk SIga Intake (mg) per Kg of Body Weight by Children from Different Locations

Location		Time Postpartum						Reference
		1m	2m	3m	4m	9m	15-19m	
Texas, USA[a]	$\bar{x}$	132	103	82	78			19
	S.D.	60	45	38	35			
Guatemala, rural	$\bar{x}$	96		49	45	38	48	
	S.D.	28		18	26	16	23	
Guatemala, urban (poor)	$\bar{x}$	75		56	48			
	S.D.	32		28	13			
Guatemala, urban (privileged)	$\bar{x}$	122	74	55				
	S.D.	62	23	16				

[a] Estimated from the published curve.

In summary, the analysis of SIgA concentration in milk specimens collected from individuals of different ethnic groups indicates that ethnicity is not a determinant of the quantity of SIgA that women transfer via colostrum and milk to their infants.

Studies on specific antibodies in human milk are more difficult to interpret, since their presence in milk depends on maternal exposure to the antigens. Several investigators have determined milk SIgA antibodies specifically directed against Escherichia coli. Carlsson, et al. [21] have shown that women from Pakistan and Sweden have antibodies against somatic antigens of some serogroups of E. coli in similar concentrations. Another study (17) has provided information indicating that women from different ethnic groups have different levels of anti-*E. coli* antibodies. Milk specimens of women from a high socioeconomic group in Guatemala City have similar content of antibody to that of Swedish women, while women from lower socioeconomic urban and rural areas of Guatemala have similar titers between them, but lower than those seen in the other two population groups (Table 4).

Table 4. Anti-*E. coli* IgA Antibodies (% of Reference) in Milk Samples from Different Countries

Population Group		Time Postpartum					
		3d	5d	1m	3m	6m	9m
Ethiopian,							
underprivileged	$\bar{x}$	47	28	15			
	S.D.	30.9	26.5	13.3			
privileged	$\bar{x}$	121	47	34			
	S.D.	74.5	11.1	14.3			
Swedish	$\bar{x}$			48	50	72	92
	S.D.			46.3	28.8	56.9	62.0
Guatemalan,							
rural	$\bar{x}$			14	13	22	12
	S.D.			7.8	13.9	19.7	6.21
urban poor	$\bar{x}$			17	25		
	S.D.			12.5	13.9		
urban privileged	$\bar{x}$			37	55		
	S.D.			16.2	34.0		

Source: 17.

A similar observation has been made with regard to anti-*Salmonella* and anti-*Shigella* antibodies in the same population groups.[22] Obviously the variable of exposure and its timing cannot be controlled in these epidemiologic studies. Nevertheless, Holmgren and collaborators[23] have shown, with pathogens that have a more defined geographic distribution such as *Vibrio cholerae* and ETEC, that women who live in endemic areas have antibodies against cholera and coli entero toxin in their milk, while those women who have never traveled to those areas do not show antibody activity.

These facts have made it necessary to study the immune response of lactating women to a particular antigen, given under controlled conditions. We have studied the rate, magnitude and duration of the milk immune response of women from rural Guatemala in comparison with women from the capital city[24] after administrating a food protein antigen. There was no difference in the rate of lactoconversion (appearance of specific IgA antibodies in milk) between the two groups of women. The magnitude of the response and the duration of antibodies in milk were similar among the women in the two groups. Furthermore, when the women were classified according to their nutritional status, based on weight and height, there was no difference in the response of the well-nourished women when compared to women with deficit of weight-for-height. These results indicate that the milk SIgA response is not affected by either ethnicity or nutritional status.

Table 5. Correlation between SIgA Concentration and Specific Antibody Levels in Human Milk[a]

Subject No.	Observed correlation (r_s) value: *E. coli* LT	Shigella	Rotavirus	Critical r_s value (p = 0.975)
1	0.500	0.308	0.410	0.50
2	0.530	0.406	0.151	0.58
3	0.033	0.424	0.270	0.52
4	0.494	0.510	0.470	0.52
5	<u>0.810</u>	0.000	0.220	0.55
6	0.387	<u>0.620</u>	0.230	0.52
7	0.004	0.415		0.55
			0.058	0.61[b]
8	0.056	0.055	<u>0.699</u>	0.55
9	0.399	<u>0.580</u>	<u>0.587</u>	0.50
10	0.145	0.160	0.080	0.52

[a] Spearman correlation test.
[b] For RTV only.
When observed $r_s \leq$ critical r_s value IgA antibody levels are independent of total SIgA. Dependent levels are underlined.
Source: 26.

One factor that seems to be important in the persistence of specific antibodies in milk is the presence of antigen in the intestine of the lactating woman. Hanson and colleagues[25] have shown that a single dose of live, attenuated oral polio vaccine can induce a dramatic fall in the levels of preexisting milk anti-poliovirus antibodies. We have shown that specific antibodies tended to disappear in milk specimens from lactopositive women who were given a food protein antigen orally. Prospective studies in a group of rural women from Guatemala[26] have shown that levels of specific SIgA antibodies may fluctuate as lactation progresses. Fig. 1 summarizes the findings in one representative individual. This finding does not seem to be associated with ethnic factors, since Goldman, et al.,[13] and Cukor and coworkers[27] have made similar observations in women from two different communities in the United States. With the purpose of comparing these findings with those of Guatemalan women from urban settings, we analyzed milk specimens collected serially for the presence of anti-*E. coli* labile toxin (EcLT), anti-*Shigella* B6 and anti-rotaviruses antibodies. We were unable to demonstrate the same fluctuations as those observed in rural women (Fig. 2). Furthermore, when the relationships of the changes in specific antibodies found among rural women were analyzed in each of the subjects, it was clear that the fluctuations are independent from the titers of other specific antibodies as well as of the concentrations of total SIgA (Table 5).

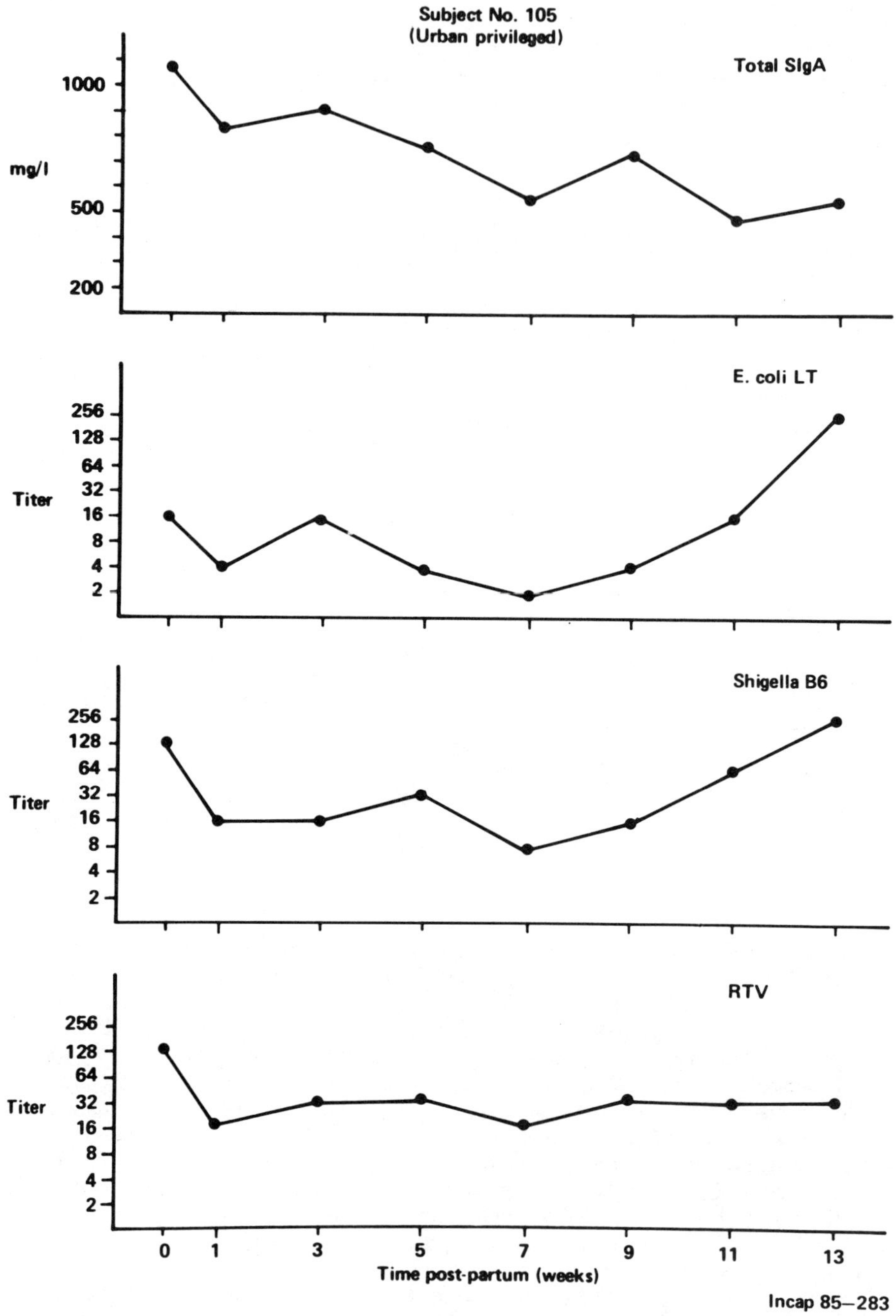

Fig. 1. Secretory IgA concentration (mg/l) and levels of specific anti-E. coli LT, Shigella B6 somatic and rotavirus antibodies in milk specimens of one representative rural woman.

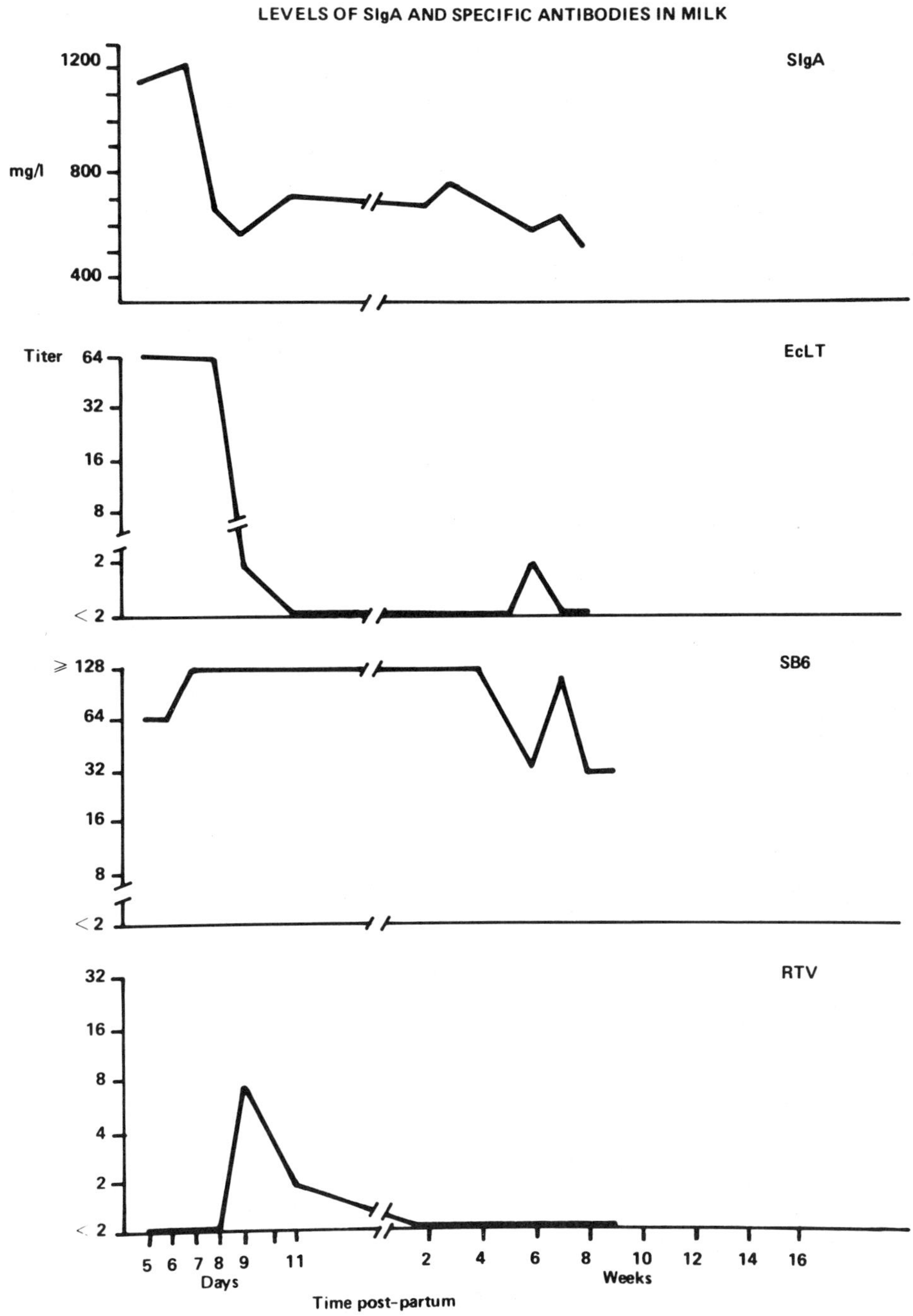

Fig. 2. Secretory IgA concentration (mg/l) and levels of specific anti-*E. coli* LT, *Shigella* B6 somatic and rotavirus antibodies in milk specimens of one representative urban woman.

These findings would explain why some authors have not demonstrated milk specific antibodies against pathogens, which are known to infect practically the totality of the population during the early stages of life, such as rotavirus.[28] Table 6 summarizes some of the findings, in terms of proportions of lactopositivity against rotaviruses in different population groups. Colostrum specimens tend to have high levels of specific anti-rotavirus antibodies; moreover, almost all samples tested (86-100%) contained measurable antibody activity. Samples of mature milk from the same locations not only have lower levels of antibody, but also the percent of those specimens with antibodies is not as high (36-94%) when compared to colostrum.[18, 27, 29-32]

Table 6. Presence of SIgA Anti-rotavirus Antibodies in Colostrum and Milk Specimens from Different Locations

Material	Location	Anti-rotavirus antibodies		Reference
		Number tested	Number (%) positive	
Colostrum	Guatemala	10	9(90)	29
	"	18	18(100)	18
	"	12	12(100)	30
	Costa Rica	21	18(86)	18
	"	21	19(90)	18
	"	32	32(100)	29
	"	43	43(100)	30
	Virginia, USA	12	11(92)	18
	Washington, DC, USA	12	12(100)	28
	Boston, USA	15	12(80)	27
	Norway	5	5(100)	32
Milk	Guatemala	25	21(84)	18
	"	25	22(88)	18
	"	95	89(94)	29
	"	38	28(74)	30
	Boston, USA	105	38(36)	27
	Bangladesh	39	35(90)	18
	"	39	34(87)	18

The practical implications of these findings are important Ethnicity and nutritional status do not seem to have a marked effect on the quantity of milk SIgA and on the levels of specific antibodies in milk. Infections and intestinal colonization in the lactating women, however, would be more important in the limitation of the enteromammaric traffic of IgA-committed lymphocytes and, therefore, in the appearance and/or persistence of specific antibodies in human milk. In this regard, infections in the mother, be they symptomatic or asymptomatic, may increase the likelihood of an infection in the breast-fed child resulting in diarrhea.

Other protective factors, including complement, also have been analyzed in breast milk. Various methodologies have been employed for measurement of complement in milk, but they do not seem to play an important role in the differences reported from different population groups. In one report from Colombia,[15] high levels (133-184 mg/dl of C3, and 23-31 mg/dl of C4) of different components of the complement system were detected, the values representing 50-75% of normal adult serum concentrations. Another study[33] from Japan has shown that colostrum has a lytic capacity of about 7% of normal serum. Women from other population groups do not have those high levels of complement components and, in fact, may show none. Only 18% of Brazilian women showed C1q and C3.[34] Mata and Wyatt[35] studied women from rural Guatemala and obtained similar results to those observed by us more recently (Table 7). The finding that the presence and concentration of C3 and C4 do not persist following delivery is of importance; specimens obtained serially from various women do not follow a particular pattern. The factors that induce the appearance of components of the complement system in milk still need further elucidation.

Table 7. C4 and C3c Concentration in Samples of Colostrum and Milk[a]

Age (years)	Colostrum C4 (mg/dl)	Colostrum C3c (mg/dl)	Milk C4 (mg/dl)	Milk C3c (mg/dl)
26 ± 5	4.4 ± 0.05	4.9 ± 2.3	4.6 ± 3.5	5.6 ± 3.0
	6/22[b]	8/22	2/22	3/22

[a] Mean ± S.D.
[b] Positive/tested

Since human milk is known to contain maturation factors, with the collaboration of Dr. Allan Goldstein (George Washington University) the content of thymosin in specimens obtained from rural and urban women from Guatemala was determined. The results show that these samples contain thymosin, although there are variations that seem to be associated with the time after delivery (Table 8) The presence of thymosin in milk may be important in the maturation of the gut immune response, both in terms of cell-mediated immunity, which is known to be functional in the intestine, and in terms of the SIgA response, which is known to be T-cell dependent.[37]

Table 8. Thymosin α_1 Levels in Mature Human Milk (>15 Days) from Urban and Rural Mothers in Guatemala

		Months Postpartum 1	2-3	6	9	15-18
Rural	-Not detectable	1	2	2	5	4
	-Trace	1		3	1	1
	-Quantifiable					
Urban	-Not detectable		6			
	-Trace	2	4			
	-Quantifiable	5[a]	3[b]			

[a] range 370-690 pg/ml [b] range 350-730 pg/ml

In summary, it is apparent that ethnicity and nutritional status do not seem to be important determinants of the quantity of immune factors in human milk. A more important variable is the level of intestinal exposure to antigens by the lactating woman, since exposure may determine the appearance, level and persistence of SIgA antibodies in milk.

Acknowledgment

Financial support for this research was provided by the Swedish Agency for Research Cooperation with Developing Countries (SAREC) and the Diarrheal Disease Control Program of the Pan American Health Organization.

REFERENCES

1. W. A. Falkler, Jr., A. R. Diwan and S. B. Halstead, A lipid inhibitor of dengue virus in human colostrum and milk; with a note on the absence of anti-dengue secretory antibody, Arch. Virol. 47:3 (1975).
2. A. S. Goldman and C. W. Smith, Host resistance factors in human milk, J. Pediatr. 82:1082 (1973).
3. W. B. Pittard III, Breast milk immunology. A frontier in infant nutrition, Am. J. Dis. Child. 133:83 (1979).
4. J. K. Welsh and J. T. May, Anti-infective properties of breast milk, J. Pediatr. 94:1 (1979).
5. J. Holmgren, A. M. Svennerholm and M. Lindblad, Receptor-like glycocompounds in human milk that inhibit Classical and El Tor Vibrio cholerae cell adherence (hemagglutination), Infect. Immunol. 39:147 (1983).
6. W. B. Pittard, S. H. Polmar and A. A. Fanaroff, The breast milk macrophage: A potential vehicle for immunoglobulin transport, J. Reticuloendothel. Soc. 22:597 (1977).
7. S. S. Ogra and P. L. Ogra, Immunologic aspects of human colostrum and milk. I. Distribution characteristics and concentrations of immunoglobulins at different times after the onset of lactation, J. Pediatr. 92:546 (1978).
8. S. S. Ogra and P. L. Ogra, Immunologic aspects of human colostrum and milk. II. Characteristics of lymphocyte reactivity and distribution of E-rosette forming cells at different times after the onset of lactation, J. Pediatr. 92:550 (1978).
9. L. K. Pickering, T. G. Cleary, S. Kohl and S. Getz, Polymorphonuclear leukocytes of human colostrum. I. Oxidative metabolism and kinetics of killing of radiolabeled Staphylococcus aureus, J. Infect. Dis. 142:685 (1980).
10. L. Å. Hanson and P. Brandtzaeq, The mucosal defense system, in: "Immunologic disorders in infants and children," Shehm and Fulginiti, eds., W. B. Saunders Co., Philadelphia, PA (1979).
11. R. I. Glass, A-M Svennerholm, B. J. Stoll, et al., Protection against cholera in breast-fed children by antibodies in breast milk, N. Engl. J. Med. 308:1389 (1983).
12. F. T. Saulsbury, J. A. Winkelstein and R. H. Yolken, Chronic rotavirus infection in immunodeficiency, J. Pediatr. 97:61 (1980).
13. A. S. Goldman, C. Garza, B. L. Nichols and R. M. Goldblum, Immunologic factors in human milk during the first year of lactation, J. Pediatr. 100:563 (1982).
14. A. Prentice, A. M. Prentice, T. J. Cole and R. G. Whitehead, Determinants of variations in breast milk protective factor concentrations of rural Gambian mothers, Arch. Dis. Child. 58:518 (1983).
15. R. Miranda, N. G. Saravia, R. Ackerman, et al., Effect of maternal nutritional status on immunological substances in human colostrum and milk, Am. J. Clin. Nutr. 37:632 (1983).

16. V. Reddy, C. Bhaskaram, N. Raghuvamulu and V. Jagadeesan, Antimicrobial factors in human milk, Acta. Paediatr. Scand. 66:229 (1977).
17. J. R. Cruz, B. Carlsson, B. García, et al., Studies on human milk. III. Secretory IgA quantity and antibody levels against Escherichia coli in colostrum and milk from underprivileged and privileged mothers, Pediatr. Res. 16:272 (1982).
18. R. H. Yolken, R. G. Wyatt, L. Mata, et al., Secretory antibody directed against rotavirus in human milk-measurement by means of the enzyme-linked immunosorbent assay, J. Pediatr. 93:916 (1978).
19. N. F. Butte, R. M. Goldblum, L. M. Fehl, et al., Daily ingestion of immunologic components in human milk during the first four months of life, Acta Paediatr. Scand. 73:296 (1984).
20. A. S. Goldman, R. M. Goldblum, C. Garza, et al., Immunologic components in human milk during weaning, Acta Paediatr. Scand. 72:133 (1983).
21. B. Carlsson, S. Ahlstedt, L. Å. Hanson, et al., Escherichia coli O antibody content in milk from healthy Swedish mothers and mothers from a very low socioeconomic group of a developing country, Acta Paediatr. Scand. 65:417 (1976).
22. J. R. Cruz, B. V. M. Carlsson, Y. Hofvander, et al., Studies of human milk. II. Concentration of antibodies against Salmonella and Shigella in milk of women from different populations and their daily intake by the breast-fed infants, Acta Paediatr. Scand. 74: 338 (1985).
23. J. Holmgren, L. Å. Hanson, B. Carlsson, et al., Neutralizing antibodies against E. coli and V. cholera enterotoxins in human milk from a developing country, Scand. J. Immunol. 5:867 (1976).
24. J. R. Cruz, and L. Å. Hanson, Specific milk immune response of rural and urban Guatemalan women to oral immunization with a food protein, J. Pediatr. Gastroenterol. Nutr. (in press).
25. L. Å. Hanson, B. Carlsson, F. Jalil, et al., Different secretory IgA antibody responses after immunization with inactivated and live poliovirus vaccines, Rev. Infect. Dis. 6:S356 (1984).
26. J. R. Cruz and C. Arévalo, Fluctuation of specific IgA antibodies in human milk, Acta Paediatr. Scand. 74:897 (1985).
27. G. Cukor, N. Blacklow, F. Capozza, et al., Secretory IgA antibody to rotavirus in human milk 6-9 months postpartum, Lancet 2:631 (1978).
28. A. Z. Kapikian and R. M. Chanock, Rotaviruses, in: "Virology," B. N. Fields, et al., eds., Raven Press, N. Y. (1985).
29. R. H. Yolken, R. G. Wyatt, G. Zissis, et al., Epidemiology of human rotavirus types 1 and 2 as studied by enzyme-linked immunosorbent assay, N. Engl. J. Med. 229:1156 (1978).
30. J. R. Cruz and C. Arevalo, Levels of human milk specific immunoglobulin A antibodies during lactation, Pediatr. Infect. Dis. 5:S148 (1986).
31. A. Simhon, R. H. Yolken, L. Mata, SIgA cholera toxin and rotavirus antibody in human colostrum, Acta Paediatr. Scand. 68:161 (1979).
32. A-B Otnaess and I. Orstavik, The effect of human milk fractions on rotavirus in relation to the secretory IgA content, Acta Pathol. Microbiol. Scand. Sect. C. 88:15 (1980).
33. S. Nakajima, A. S. Baba and N. Tamura, Complement system in human colostrum, Internat. Arch. Allergy Appl. Immunol. 54:428 (1977).
34. F. Santoro, R. Borojevic, D. Bout, et al., Mother-child relationship in human schistosomiasis mansoni. I. Parasitic antigens and antibodies in milk, Am. J. Trop. Med. Hyg. 26:1164 (1977).
35. L. J. Mata and R. G. Wyatt, Host resistance to infection, Am. J. Clin. Nutr. 24:976 (1971).
36. A. S. Goldman, R. M. Goldblum and C. Garza, Immunologic components in human milk during the second year of lactation, Acta Paediatr. Scand. 72:461 (1983).
37. T. B. Tomasi, Jr., Mechanisms of immune regulation at mucosal surfaces Rev. Infect. Dis. 5:S734 (1983).

HIGH PERFORMANCE LIQUID CHROMATOGRAPHY OF OLIGOSACCHARIDES FROM HUMAN MILK AND COLOSTRUM

David S. Newburg, Peter F. Daniel, Nancy E. O'Neil and Robert H. McCluer

Department of Biochemistry
E.K. Shriver Center for Mental Retardation
200 Trapelo Road
Waltham, MA 02254

INTRODUCTION

Human milk is unique with respect to the high concentration and complexity of its oligosaccharide fraction. Polonovsky and Lespagnol[1] isolated and studied a human milk fraction which they named gynolactose and reported that it contained mostly oligosaccharides. Montreuil and Mullet[2] determined that this fraction comprises 2.4% of human colostrum and between 1.2 and 1.3% of mature human milk. Thus, the oligosaccharide fraction is the fourth largest constituent of human milk, after water, lactose, and fat, and represents a significant portion of the non-protein nitrogen found therein. This fraction proved to be a rich source of a wide variety of oligosaccharides, in contrast to the analogous fraction from bovine milk which comprised only 0.1% and consisted of a limited number of oligosaccharide types[3]

Although no direct nutritional role has been reported for the oligosaccharides, several biological activities specific to human milk have been suggested for the oligosaccharide fraction, including the ability to stimulate the growth of Bifidobacterium bifidum ["bifidus activity"], the ability to protect the intestinal epithelium from the effects of heat stable enterotoxin, and the ability to inhibit colonization of the gut by enteropathic microorganisms.

Human milk is unique in its high oligosaccharide content and also in bifidus activity; bovine milk is much lower in both. The purported colonization of the infant's gut by B. bifidum would have at least two major effects: the anaerobic fermentation of sugars which lowers the pH considerably, and the exclusion of E. coli and other potentially enteropathic bacteria from the gut. The factors responsible for stimulating the growth of this bacterium were initially identified as components of the non-protein whey[4]. Gyorgy[5] reports that these factors are found in the nitrogen-containing oligosaccharides of human milk, and their structures contain N-acetylglucosamine, lactose, fucose, galactose, and sialic acid (N-acetylneuraminic acid). Bifidus activity of human milk has been identified with lacto-N-neotetraose[6] four of the five glycopeptide fractions of human colostrum[7], two glycoproteins in milk whey[8] and even simple acetylated amino sugars[9]. There have been two types of response to this aggregate of data. One is to suggest that the existence of bifidus factor in human milk has not yet been clearly demonstrated[10] because no compound with a bifidus activity could be clearly identified. Another is to assume that the several compounds with such activity may act synergistically[11]. We feel that if the structures of the molecular species having bifidus activity were known, they might demonstrate some structural commonality.

A second biological effect of human milk possibly associated with the oligosaccharide fraction is the protection of the gut against enteropathic bacteria. It is tragic that diarrheal disease is a major cause of death for children under 5 years of age in less developed areas of the world, and that these infections are especially frequent at weaning and in infants not receiving human milk[12,13]. Many of these bacteria are enterotoxinogenic, i.e., they produce enterotoxins which stimulate intestinal electrolyte and water secretion[14]. Oligosaccharide structures on a protein or lipid backbone seem to be the receptors for enterotoxins. If such oligosaccharide structures were present in the oligosaccharide fraction of milk, competitive binding could provide protection against these toxins. Cleary et al.[15] have shown that human milk contains a fraction which will protect young mice from the effects of orogastric administration of heat stable enterotoxin. Because this activity remained in a fraction of human colostrum which should have only contained neutral oligosaccharides, they concluded that this protective factor was a neutral oligosaccharide, but did not characterize it any further.

Over the past 30 years the combined efforts of several groups have led to the structural elucidation of more than 40 oligosaccharides from human milk[16-19]. These were shown to contain up to 11 sugar residues consisting of sialic acid, fucose, galactose, N-acetylglucosamine, and glucose. These oligosaccharides are derived from nine core oligosaccharides: lactose, lacto-N-tetraose, neo-lacto-N-tetraose, lacto-N-hexaose, neo-lacto-N-hexaose, para-lacto-N-hexaose, para-neo-lacto-N-hexaose, lacto-N-octaose, and neo-lacto-N-octaose[17,20]. Fucose and sialic acid occur in terminal positions. All oligosaccharides characterized from human milk have a lactose moiety at their reducing ends. However, N-acetyllactosamine and oligosaccharides derived from it have been isolated from bovine colostrum[21,22]. Four types of fucose linkages and three types of sialic acid linkages have been described on milk oligosaccharides, which can give rise to a vast array of possible structures. Recently, Egge et al.[23] reported the separation of neutral, fucose-containing milk oligosaccharides into at least 100 different components. Many of these neutral oligosaccharides probably also occur in sialylated form. The full characterization of this fraction in human colostrum and milk has been limited by the analytical techniques available and the complexity of the fraction.

Women can be classified into three groups based on the presence of fucosyl oligosaccharides in their milk[17]. Milk of the first group (blood type Le a^-b^+, secretors; approximately 75% of the population) contains all the major fucosyl oligosaccharides with 2-linked, 3-linked and 4-linked fucose residues. The second group (blood type Le a^+b^-; about 20% of the population) lacks oligosaccharides with 2-linked fucose residues. Women who belong to this group are non-secretors and lack a fucosyltransferase that forms a Fuc α1,2 Gal unit. As a result their milk lacks all of the oligosaccharides that have this unit as a partial structure. The third group (Le a^-b^-; 5% of the population) is lacking another fucosyltransferase that forms a Fuc α1,4 GlcNAc unit. The lack of certain fucosyloligosaccharides in these rare individuals led to the finding of minor components which are generally obscured by the major oligosaccharides.

It is obvious that much remains to be learned about the oligosaccharides of human milk. Only recently has the possibility emerged for developing the methodology necessary for the routine quantitation of the molecular species of the oligosaccharides in multiple samples of milk. Toward that end we have performed the following preliminary work.

METHODS

Milk was obtained from donor KN in the fourth week of lactation. Fresh milk was defatted by centrifugation followed by filtration through glass wool. Proteins were precipitated by acetone as described by Egge et al.[23] and the sediment was removed by centrifugation. The clear supernatant was applied to a charcoal-celite column. To remove monosaccharides the column was washed with water; much of the lactose was removed by elution with 5% aqueous ethanol[24]. Oligosaccharides were eluted with 50% aqueous ethanol and concentrated by rotary evaporation[25]. The oligosaccharide fraction was separated into neutral oligosaccharides and acidic oligosaccharides by ion-exchange chromatography on coupled Dowex 50 and Dowex 1 columns. Neutral oligosaccharides passed through the columns with a water rinse. Acidic oligosaccharides were eluted from Dowex 1 with 0.5 M pyridine acetate, pH 5.5. An aliquot of each fraction was separated by TLC on silica gel in n-butanol/acetic acid/water (3:3:2). Lactose was the sole component visible in the 5% ethanol eluate. Some 12 neutral oligosaccharide bands in addition to lactose were visualized by TLC of the 50% ethanol eluate. After reduction and perbenzoylation of an aliquot equivalent to 100 µl of milk, components were eluted from an octylsilica column by HPLC with a linear gradient from 80% aqueous acetonitrile to 100% acetonitrile and detected by UV absorption at 230 nm[26]. The major peaks were identified by comparison with authentic standards. The amount injected was equivalent to 0.2 µl of milk.

Colostrum samples were obtained from donor SK during postpartum days one through seven. A 200 µl aliquot of each sample was treated as above except that the acidic and neutral oligosaccharide fractions were first separated on a coupled Dowex 50/Dowex 1 column, and only the neutral oligosaccharides were run through the charcoal-celite column. Both fractions were then reduced and perbenzoylated. The equivalent of 0.08 µl of colostrum was applied to the HPLC column for each analysis of neutral oligosaccharides and 0.2 µl of colostrum for each analysis of acidic oligosaccharides. The major peaks were identified by their retention times relative to standards; however, authentic lacto-N-fucopentaose II was not available.

TLC analysis of acidic oligosaccharides revealed 8 bands; at least 30 peaks were obtained by HPLC. However, we observed evidence of some degradation of these compounds due to loss of sialic acid. We have now demonstrated that this loss occurred during the reduction step and the subsequent clean-up due to the use of strongly acidic Dowex 50 [H^+] at ambient temperature. Use of Dowex 50 in the pyridinium form eliminated this problem. When the acidic oligosaccharides are reduced at 4°C and Dowex 50 in the pyridinium form is utilized the absolute values can be accurately established.

RESULTS AND DISCUSSION

The chromatogram of neutral oligosaccharides from mature milk (4 weeks postpartum, KN) displays approximately 40 peaks (Fig. 1). Four of these were identified by comparing their retention times to those of authentic standards. The structures of the sugars identified in the chromatograms are given in Figure 3. Note that all of these milk oligosaccharides contain lactose at the reducing end.

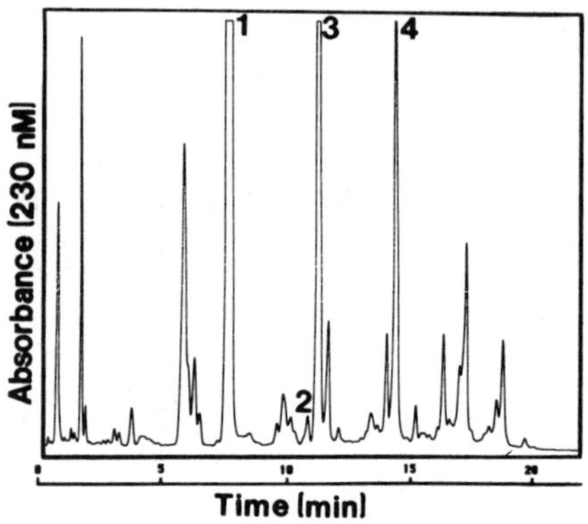

KEY

1 = Lactose

2 = Lacto-N-neotetraose

3 = Lacto-N-tetraose

4 = Lactodifucotetraose

5 = Lacto-N-fucopentaose II (in Fig. 2)

Figure 1. HPLC of Human (KN) Mature Milk Neutral Oligosaccharides

The presence of lactodifucotetraose in the milk of KN identifies this donor as a secretor. Secretors, who comprise approximately 75% of the population[17] are able to secrete blood group structures in various exocrine secretions. In non-secretors, such blood group activities are confined to cells.

In the chromatograms of neutral oligosaccharides from colostrum (days 1 and 2, SK) there are fewer major peaks than the more mature transitional milk (days 5 and 7) of the same donor (Fig 2), while the minor constituents of the colostrum display a more complex pattern. In addition, peak 5 (tentatively identified as lacto-N-fucopentaose II), increased linearly as a function of time ($r=0.879$, $P < 0.01$) in the colostrum of SK. The concentration of lacto-N-tetraose (peak 3), the precursor to lacto-N-fucopentaose II (peak 5), did not vary significantly, implying that the activity of 4-fucosyltransferase, the enzyme responsible for this conversion, may be increasing over the initial 7 days of lactation.

The pattern of the more mature transitional milk of SK (days 5 and 7) is less complex than that of mature milk of KN (Fig. 1). The lack of detectable lactodifucotetraose (peak 4) indicates that SK is a non-secretor of blood group substances. In addition to lactodifucotetraose, non-secretors also lack 2'-fucosyllactose, lacto-N-fucopentaose I and lacto-N-difucohexaose I in their milk, due to a lack of a fucosylα(1-2) transferase.

Acidic oligosaccharides likewise can be separated into at least 30 components and each of these quantitated. However, conditions must take into account the instability of sialo- and fuco-oligosaccharides under acidic conditions including exposure to Dowex 50 [H^+]. The ratio of 3'-sialyllactose to 6'-sialyllactose decreased dramatically (from 1.5 to 0.5) from the beginning to the 7th day of lactation in donor SK. This unanticipated finding must be confirmed using the improved isolation and reduction techniques.

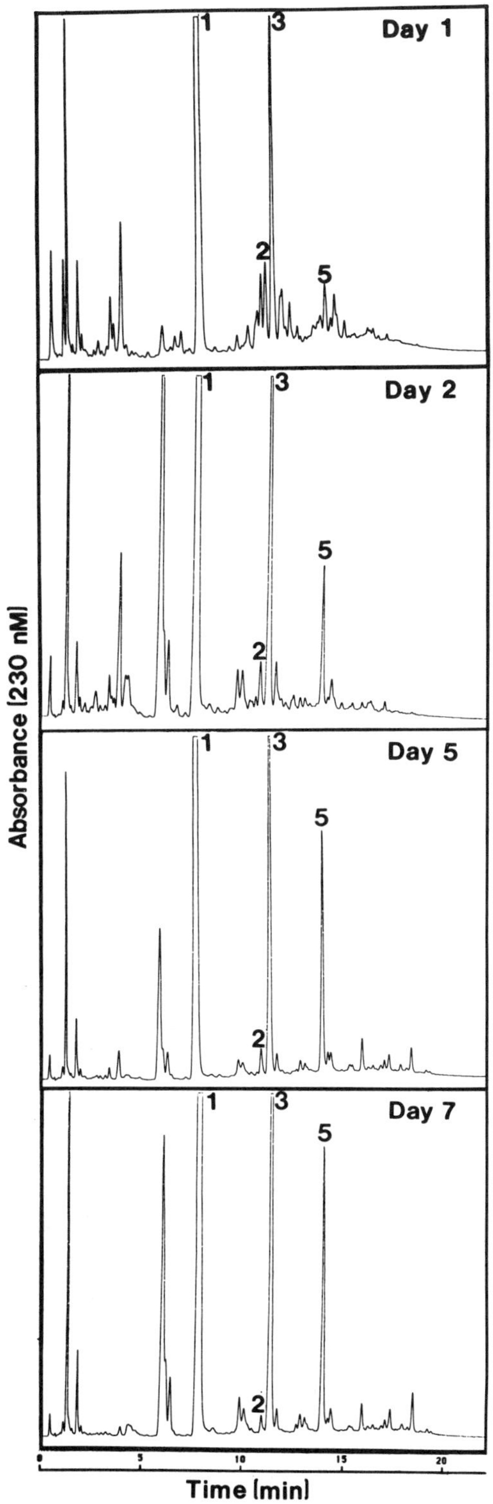

Figure 2. Human (SK) Milk Neutral Oligosaccharides

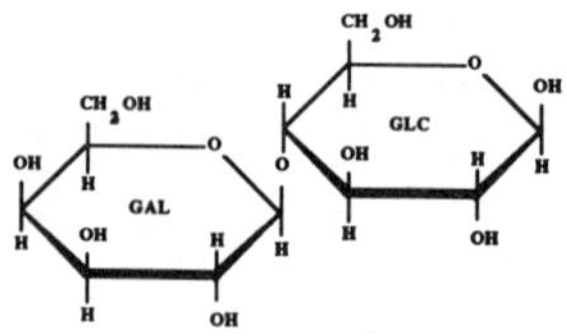

LACTOSE

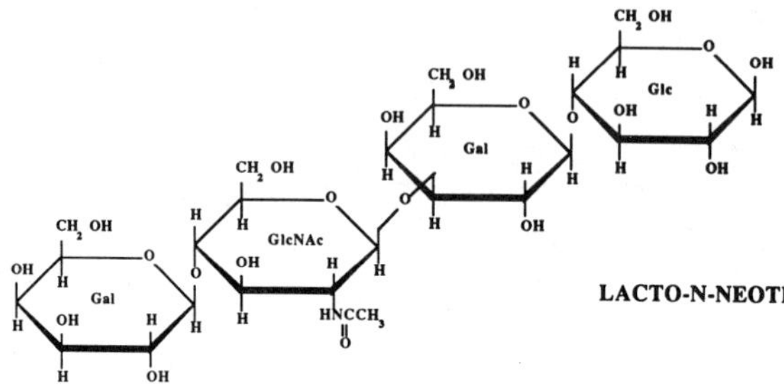

LACTO-N-NEOTETRAOSE

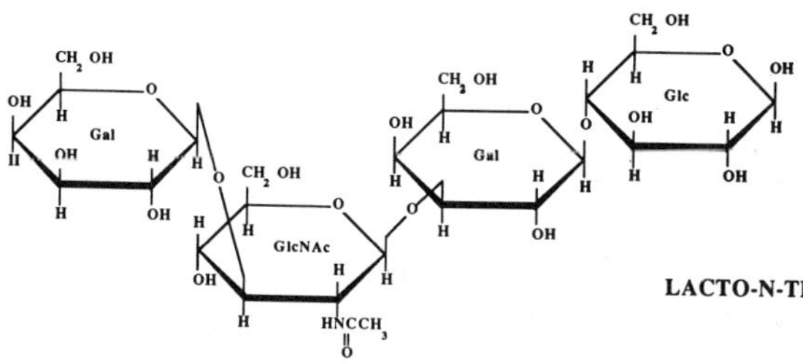

LACTO-N-TETRAOSE

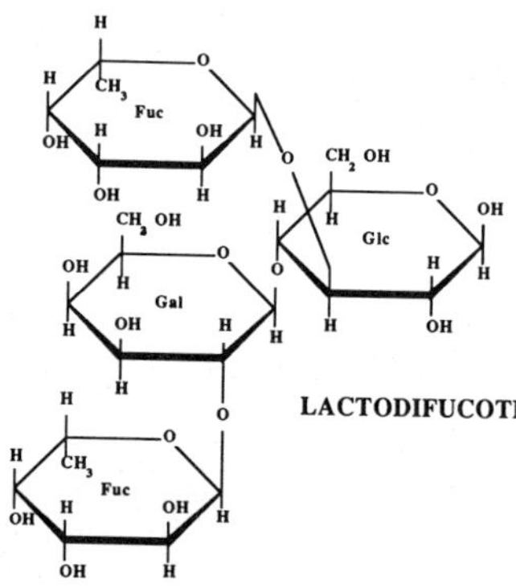

LACTODIFUCOTETRAOSE

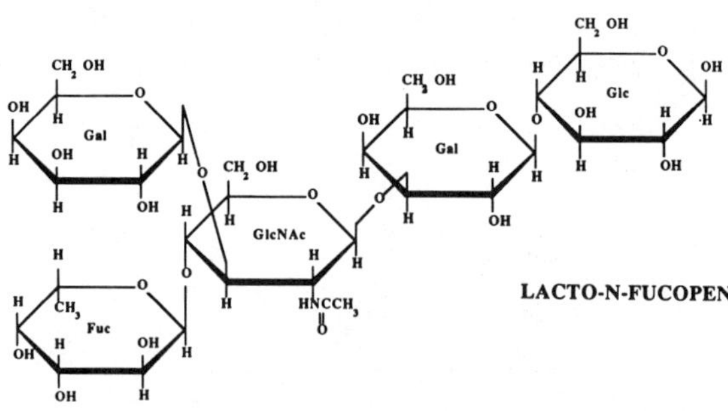

LACTO-N-FUCOPENTAOSE II

Figure 3. Structures of Neutral Oligosaccharides

CONCLUSION

These results indicate the feasibility of developing microanalytical methods by employing high performance liquid chromatography for the separation and quantitation of both neutral and acidic oligosaccharides from human milk and colostrum. High performance liquid chromatography can be used to separate neutral oligosaccharides from less than 1 µl of milk or colostrum into at least 40 components. However, each of these components must be purified and positively identified, and the chromatographic conditions optimized, for this technique to become useful for routine analysis. The ability to separate and quantitate these compounds routinely from human milk and colostrum will allow studies concerning the degree of individual variation of oligosaccharide production in lactating humans and changes in oligosaccharide composition as lactation proceeds. An increased understanding of the biological functions of milk oligosaccharides may also result.

REFERENCES

1. Polonovsky, M. et. Lespagnol, A., Nouvelles acquisitions sur les composes glucidiques du lait de femme, Bull. Soc. Chim. Biol. 15:320 (1933).
2. Montreuil, J. and Mullet, S., Etude des variations des constituents glucidiques du lait de femme au cours de la lactation, Bull. Soc. Chim. Biol., 42:365 (1960).
3. Montreuil, J. et Kobus, W., Variations des constituents glucidiques du lait de vache an cours de la lactation, C.R. Seanc. Soc. Biol., 154:2075 (1960).
4. Schonfeld, H., Uber die Beziehungen der eimzelnen bestandtelle der frauenmilch zur bifidus flora. Jb. Kinderhellk. Phys. Erzieh. 113:19 (1926).
5. Gyorgy, P., Biochemical aspects [of human milk], Am. J. Clin. Nutr. 24:970 (1971).
6. Grimmonprez, L., Les glucides du lait, Annls. Nutr. Aliment., 25:A39 (1971).
7. Hirano, S., Hayashi, H., Terabagashi, T. Onodera, K., Isoki, S., Kachibe, N., Nagai, Y., Yagi, N., Nakagaki, T. and Imagawa, T., Biologically active glycopeptides in human colostrum, J. Biochem. 64:563 (1968).
8. Bezkorovainy, A. and Nichols, J.H., Glycoproteins from human milk whey, Pediatr. Res., 10:1 (1976).
9. Jao, Y.C., Mikolajcik, E.M. and Hansen, P.M., Growth of Bifidobacterium bifidum var. pennsylvanicus in laboratory media supplemented with amino sugars and spent broth from Escherichia Coli, J. Food Sci. 43:1257 (1978).
10. Braun, O.H., Uber die infektionsverhutende Wirkung der Muttermilch und deren mogliche Ursachen, Klin. Padiat. 188:297 (1976).
11. Blanc, B., Biochemical aspects of human milk, World Review of Nutrition and Dietetics, 36:1 (1981).
12. Mata, L., Kronmal, R.A. and Villegas, H., Diarrheal diseases: a leading world health problem, in: "Cholera and related diarrheas," Ouchterlony and Holmgren, eds., S. Karger, Basel (1980).
13. Guerrant, R.L., Kirchhoff, L.V., Shields, D.S., Nations, M.K., Leslie, J., deSousa, M.A., Araujo, J.G., Correia, L.L., Sauer, K.T., McClelland, K.E., Trowbridge, F.L. and Hughes, J.M., Prospective study of diarrheal illness in Northeastern Brazil: Patterns of disease, nutritional impact, etiologies and risk factors, J. Infectious Diseases, 148:986 (1983).

14. Holmgren, J., Cellular action and pathophysiological effects of cholera toxin in: "The molecular basis of microbial pathogenicity," H. Smith, J.J. Skehel, and M.J. Turner eds., pp. 269-284 Dahlem Conferenzen. Verlag Chemie (1980).
15. Cleary, F.G., Chambers, J.P. and Pickering, L.K., Protection of suckling mice from the heat-stable enterotoxin of Escherichia coli by human milk, Journal of Infectious Diseases, 148:1114 (1983).
16. Kobata, A., Yamashita, K. and Tachibana, Y., Oligosaccharides from human milk, in: "Methods in Enzymology" Ginsburg, V., ed., Vol. 50, pp. 216-220 Academic Press, New York (1978).
17. Kobata, A., Milk glycoproteins and oligosaccharides, in: "The Glycoconjugates," Horowitz, M.S. and Pigman, W. eds., Vol. 1, pp 423-440, Academic Press, New York (1978).
18. Kobata, A., Isolation of oligosaccharides from human milk, in: "Methods in Enzymology," Ginsburg, V., ed., Vol. 28, pp. 262-271, Academic Press, New York (1972).
19. Smith, D.F., Zofp, D.A. and Ginsburg, V., Sialyloligosaccharides from milk, in: "Methods of Enzymology," Ginsburg, V., ed., Vol. 50, pp. 221-226, Academic Press, New York (1978).
20. Yamashita, K., Tachibana, Y. and Kobata, A., Oligosaccharides of Human Milk. Structural studies of two new octasaccharides, difucosyl derivatives of para-lacto-N-hexaose and para-lacto-N-neohexaose, J. Biol. Chem., 252:5408 (1977).
21. Saito, T., Itoh, T. and Adachi, S., Presence of two neutral disaccharides containing N-acetylhexosamine in bovine colostrum as free forms, Biochim. Biophys. Acta, 801:147 (1984).
22. Veh, R.W., Michalski, J.C., Corfield, A.P., Sander-Wewer, M., Gies, D. and Schauer, R., New chromatographic system for the rapid analysis and preparation of colostrum sialyloligosaccharides, J. Chromatogr., 212:313 (1981).
23. Egge, H., Dell, A. and Von Nicolai, H., Fucose containing oligosaccharides from human milk. Arch. Biochem. Biophys., 224:235 (1983).
24. Whistler, R.L. and BeMiller, J.N., Carbon column chromatography, in: "Methods in Carbohydrate Chemistry", Whistler, R.L. and BeMiller, J.N. eds., Vol. 1, pp. 42-44, Academic Press, New York (1962).
25. Strecker, G. and LeMaire-Poitau, A., Fractionation and characterization of acidic oligosaccharides and glycopeptides from normal and pathological urines, J. Chromatogr., 143:553 (1977).
26. Daniel, P.F., DeFeudis, D.F., Lott, I.T. and McCluer, R.H., Quantitative microanalysis of oligosaccharides by high performance liquid chromatography, Carbohydr. Res., 97:161 (1981).

FAT CONTENT AND CIS- AND TRANS-ISOMERIC FATTY ACIDS IN MATURE HUMAN FORE- AND HINDMILK

Bert Koletzko*, Maria Mrotzek and Hans Joachim Bremer

University Children's Hospital, Dept. of General Pediatrics, Metabolism, Nutrition and Nephrology Düsseldorf, West Germany

INTRODUCTION

Proper sampling is an essential prerequisite to obtain reliable data on composition of human milk. Already some 80 years ago it was known that lipid content and composition of breast milk varies within one feeding and during the course of the day (1), which has been confirmed in a number of later studies (2 - 7). Therefore as an ideal method for sample collection, complete pumping of the milk at the usual times of nursing over a period of 24 hours has been suggested (5, 8). This method is not only inconvenient, but it also implicates that the infant has to be bottle fed with a formula or previously pumped milk during the collection period, a procedure not acceptable to most breast feeding mothers.

The relative content of the major fatty acids of human milk lipids has been demonstrated not to differ in samples taken before and after one nursing (5, 9, 10) suggesting that samples of milk obtained at any time before, during of after nursing are adequate for measuring fatty acids. However, the published data does not show whether samples of fore- and hindmilk do also reliably reflect the content of a number of low concentrated long chain polyunsaturates, that may be of particular importance to the infant (11), and the contamination with the potentially harmful trans-isomeric fatty acids. Trans-fatty acids originating from ruminant fats and from partially hydrogenated vegetable oils are absorbed by the human being and incorporated in its body and milk lipids (12). There is concern about possible untoward effects of trans-fatty acids fed to the infant, mainly alteration of lipid metabolism and of membrane function (11). In the study described here we compared the fat content and the cis- and trans-fatty acid oomposition of fore- and hindmilk.

*Corresponding authors present address: Dr. B. Koletzko, The Hospital for Sick Children, Div. of Clinical Nutrition, 555 University Avenue, Toronto, Ontario, Canada, M5G 1X8

METHODS

Six healthy women from the area of Düsseldorf on ad libitum diets volunteered in donating milk samples. Each woman fully breastfed one infant born at term and all were in the third or fourth month of lactation. Over a period of 24 hours milk samples were manually expressed from the breast the infant nursed on before and after each feeding. Milk samples were immediately frozen at -20°C. Equal volumes of the fore- and hindmilk samples were pooled for each subject immediately prior to analysis. The use of human milk for this study was approved by the Ethics Commission of the Medical Faculty of the University of Düsseldorf.

Total milk lipids were extracted with methanol/chloroform (13) and quantified gravimetrically. After transesterification with methanolic HCl, fatty acid methyl esters were dissolved in hexane and analyzed on a Dani 6500 HR gas chromatograph equipped with a 50 m tm Sil 88 fused silica capillary column temperature programmed from 70 to 195°C with 28°C/min, and from 195°C to 220°C with 15°C/min (figure 1).

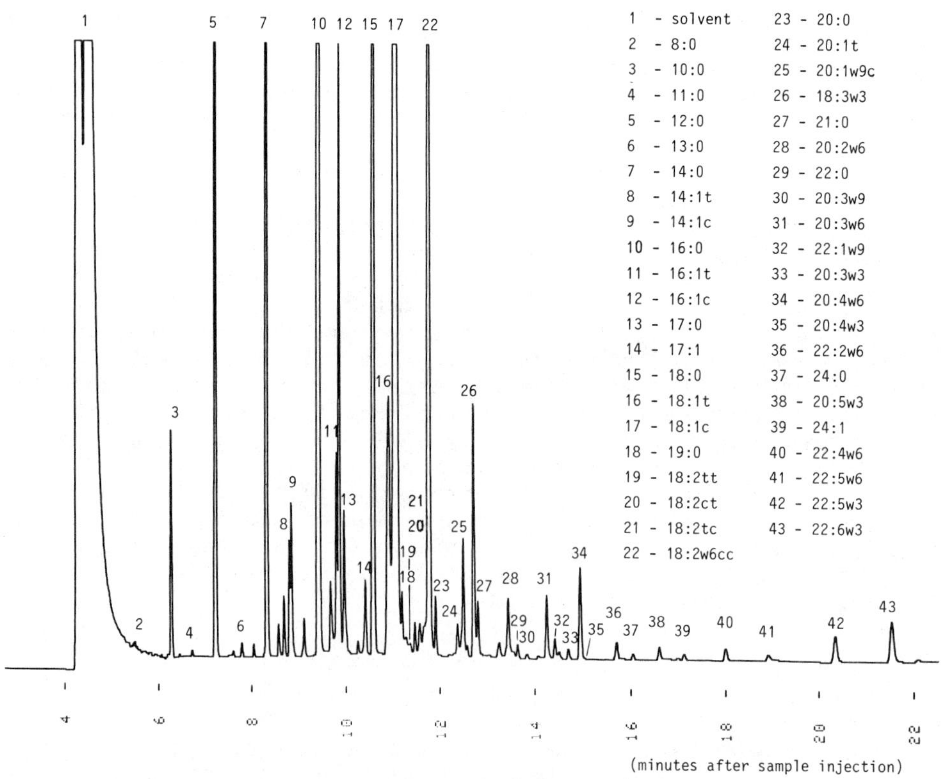

Figure 1: Chromatogram of fatty acids of human milk total lipids

Peaks were identified by comparison with appropriate standards and their areas were quantified with a Shimadzu CR 3 A digital integrator. Fatty acid concentrations were calculated using adaequate response factors and corrected for the differences in molecular weight between the fatty acids and their methyl esters. Results are expressed as weight % of all fatty acids detected with a chain length of C 12 to C 24.

RESULTS AND DISCUSSION:

The lipid content in hindmilk was 1.7-fold higher than in foremilk (cf. table 1). This increase is lower than some data in the literature, where a 2.1- to 3.6-fold increase of milk lipid concentration during nursing was reported (3, 5, 7, 9, 14). In

Table 1: Lipid content and fatty acid composition of pooled 24-hour collections of mature fore- and hindmilk from 6 mothers

		foremilk	hindmilk
Total lipid (g/dl, mean ± SD)		3.08 ± 0.35	5.30 ± 1.61
Fatty acids (weight %, mean ± SD)	12:0	5.47 ± 1.62	5.85 ± 1.63
	14:0	8.07 ± 0.77	8.12 ± 0.92
	14:1t	0.18 ± 0.08	0.21 ± 0.09
	14:1c	0.82 ± 0.34	0.82 ± 0.35
	16:0	23.94 ± 1.94	23.83 ± 2.10
	16:1t	0.59 ± 0.13	0.58 ± 0.14
	16:1c	2.97 ± 0.47	2.85 ± 0.47
	18:0	9.38 ± 0.77	9.57 ± 0.66
	18:1t	2.93 ± 0.81	2.98 ± 0.68
	18:1c	32.71 ± 1.91	32.37 ± 1.88
	18:2tt	0.11 ± 0.02	0.11 ± 0.01
	18:2ct	0.09 ± 0.02	0.09 ± 0.02
	18:2tc	0.07 ± 0.04	0.07 ± 0.03
	18:2cc	8.53 ± 2.01	8.42 ± 2.07
	18:3w6	0.24 ± 0.13	0.23 ± 0.15
	18:3w3	0.77 ± 0.22	0.76 ± 0.20
	20:0	0.32 ± 0.03	0.33 ± 0.06
	20:1w9	0.64 ± 0.16	0.65 ± 0.19
	20:2w6	0.44 ± 0.09	0.43 ± 0.12
	20:3w9	0.04 ± 0.03	0.04 ± 0.02
	20:3w6	0.35 ± 0.13	0.34 ± 0.17
	20:3w3	0.13 ± 0.09	0.09 ± 0.07
	20:4w6	0.47 ± 0.13	0.45 ± 0.13
	20:4w3	0.07 ± 0.04	0.07 ± 0.04
	20:5w3	0.05 ± 0.03	0.03 ± 0.01
	22:0	0.12 ± 0.05	0.14 ± 0.07
	22:1w9	0.09 ± 0.03	0.10 ± 0.05
	22:2w6	0.08 ± 0.05	0.07 ± 0.07
	22:4w6	0.10 ± 0.04	0.10 ± 0.04
	22:5w6	0.05 ± 0.01	0.05 ± 0.02
	22:5w3	0.17 ± 0.04	0.16 ± 0.04
	22:6w3	0.31 ± 0.17	0.30 ± 0.17
	24:0	0.04 ± 0.03	0.07 ± 0.02

these studies breast pumps were used for sampling, which tend to obtain greater volumes than the suckling infant. Pumping usually is continued as long as a fairly constant stream of milk can be obtained, whereas the amount of milk the infant takes depends on its satiation and in most cases is not limited by the milk supply (15). The lower increase of fat content during nursing in our study is presumably due to the frequent feeding (around 8 - 10 feedings per day) of relatively small portions of milk observed in our subjects, who were asked not to change their usual feeding habits during the study period. A similar factor of fat increase during nursing (1.95-fold) was found in milk samples collected with a nipple shield system (16).

There was no significant difference in the fatty acid composition of milk lipids between fore- and hindmilk (cf. table 1). During nursing the proportion of phospholipids, that are rich in long chain polyunsaturated fatty acids, decreases by about half reflecting an increase in size of the milk fat globule (7). This change, however, does not alter the fatty acid pattern of total lipids, because the phospholipid fraction contributes only less than 0.5 % of the lipids of mature milk (17). Therefore collection of either fore- or hindmilk samples is appropriate for studying fatty acid composition, including long chain polyunsaturates and trans-isomers.

It has been suggested that fatty acid composition of human milk lipids should be reported as gravimetric data (mg of each fatty acid per 100 ml milk) (18). Absolute amounts of fatty acids in milk show marked fluctuations and vary considerably with the sampling technique (6). We feel that the physiology of milk lipid secretion is better reflected by an expression of fatty acid data as relative amounts (weight or mole percentage of all fatty acids detected) being remarkably constant during a feeding. Moreover presentation of fatty acid data as relative amounts more easily allows to compare data from different studies and to draw conclusions on the effect of maternal diet (12, 19). However, the milk fat content should generally be stated (20).

CONCLUSIONS

1. The available data from milk samples collected with breast pumps seems not to reliably reflect the dietary intake of lipids by infants being brestfed on demand.

2. The relative fatty acid composition of mature human milk lipids, including long chain polyunsaturates and trans-isomers, does not differ between fore- and hindmilk.

3. Analysis results on fatty acid composition of human milk lipids should be expressed as relative proportions (weight or mole %).

ACKNOWLEDGEMENT

The authors wish to thank the mothers collecting milksamples. With support by the Ministry of Science and Research, Northrhine-Westphalia, Federal Republic of Germany (IV B5-FA 6) and the Deutsche Forschungsgemeinschaft (Ko 912/1-1).

REFERENCES

1. A. D. Czerny and A. Keller, "Des Kindes Ernährung, Ernährungsstörungen und Ernährungstherapie. Ein Handbuch für Ärzte. I. Theil: Ernährung des gesunden Kindes". Verlag von Franz Deuticke, Leipzig and Wien (1906)

2. M. Gunther and J. E. Stainer, Diurnal variation in the fat content of breast milk. Lancet II: 235 (1949)

3. F. E. Hytten, Clinical and chemical studies in human lactation. II. Variation in major constituents during a feeding. Br Med J I: 176 (1954)

4. F. E. Hytten, Clinical and chemical studies in human lactation. III. Diurnal variation in major constituents of milk. Br Med J I: 179 (1954)

5. B. Hall, Uniformity of human milk. Am J Clin Nutr 32: 404 (1979)

6. G. Harzer, M. Haug, I. Dieterich et al., Changing patterns of human milk lipids in the course of lactation and during the day. Am J Clin Nutr 37: 612 (1983)

7. G. Harzer and M. Haug, Abhängigkeit der Frauenmilchlipide von der Dauer der Stillperiode, der Tageszeit, dem Stillvorgang und der mütterlichen Ernährung. Z Ernährungswiss 23: 113 (1984)

8. A. N. Ferris and R. G. Jensen, Lipids in human milk: A review. 1: Sampling, determination and content. J Pediatr Gastroenterol Nutr 3: 108 (1984)

9. W. B. Emery, N. L. Canolty, J. M. Aitchison et al., Influence of sampling on fatty acid composition of human milk. Am J Clin Nutr 31: 1127 (1978)

10. R. A. Gibson and G. M. Kneebone, Effect of sampling on fatty acid composition of human colostrum. J Nutr 110: 1671 (1980)

11. B. Koletzko, Essentielle Fettsäuren: Bedeutung für Medizin und Ernährung. Aktuel Endokrinol Stoffwechsel 7: 18 (1986)

12. B. Koletzko, M. Gwosdz and H. J. Bremer, Trans isomeric fatty acids in human milk in West Germany. In: Composition and physiological properties of human milk, J. Schaub, ed., Elsevier Science Publishers, Amsterdam, 225 (1985)

13. E. G. Bligh and W. J. Dyer, A rapid method of total lipid extraction and purification. Can J Biochem Physiol 37: 911 (1959)

14. E. Forsum and B. Lönnerdal, Variation in the contents of nutrients of breast milk during one feeding. Nutr Rep Int 19: 815 (1979)

15. R. F. Drevett and M. Woolridge, Milk taken by human babies from the first and the second breast. Physiol Behav 26: 327 (1981)

16. A. Lucas, P. J. Lucas and J. D. Baum, The nipple-shield sampling system: A device for measuring the dietary intake of breast fed infants. Early Hum Dev 4: 365 (1980)

17. J. Bitman, D. L. Wood, N. R. Mehta et al., Comparison of the phospholipid composition of breast milk from mothers of term and preterm infants during lactation. Am J Clin Nutr 40: 1103 (1984)

18. R. G. Jensen, Effect of diet on lipid composition of human milk. Presentation at the International Workshop on Human Lactation, Maternal-Environmental Factors, Oaxaca, Mexico, January 15 - 19 (1986)

19. G. M. Kneebone, R. Kneebone and R. A. Gibson, Fatty acid composition of breast milk from three racial groups from Penang, Malaysia. Am J Clin Nutr 41: 765 (1984)

20. C. J. Lammi-Keefe and R. G. Jensen, Lipids in human milk: A review. 2: Composition ans fat soluble vitamins. J Pediatr Gastroenterol Nutr 3: 172 (1984)

BILE SALT STIMULATED LIPASE: THE ENZYME IS PRESENT IN NON PRIMATE MILK

Lois M. Freed*, Carla M. York*, Margit Hamosh*, N.R. Mehta*, John A. Sturman,** Olav T. Oftedal*** and Paul Hamosh*

*Departments of Pediatrics and Physiology and Biophysics Georgetown University Medical Center, Washington, D.C. ** Developmental Biochemistry, New York State Institute for Basic Research in Developmental Disabilities, Staten Island NY and ***National Zoological Park, Smithsonian Institution Washington, D.C.

INTRODUCTION

Freudenberg was the first to show that human milk contains a lipase that is stimulated by bile salts [1]. Presence of this enzyme in gorilla milk [2] and its absence in the milk of several other species (rat, guinea pig, rabbit, goat, cow, pig, dog, horse and rhesus monkey [2,3]) were subsequently reported. Dependency on bile salts was not characteristic of lipase activity identified in the milk of many species as lipoprotein lipase [4,5], an enzyme stimulated by a serum cofactor (apoprotein CII) and inhibited by bile salts [5]. However, while lipoprotein lipase has a key role in the mammary gland, where it regulates the uptake of long chain triglyceride-fatty acids from the circulation [6], and thereby controls their concentration in milk, the enzyme has no known function in milk. The bile salt stimulated lipase, on the other hand, may be an important compensatory digestive enzyme in the newborn infant [7-9]. Because of low pancreatic function at birth, the newborn depends on extrapancreatic lipases for the digestion of fat [8]. Several studies have measured bile salt stimulated lipase activity throughout lactation in human milk and have investigated the characteristics of the enzyme purified from human milk [8,10-12]. The lack of a convenient animal source of milk bile salt stimulated lipase has precluded the study of many important aspects of this enzyme such as ontogeny in the mammary gland and regulation of its synthesis and secretion before parturition and throughout lactation.

EXPERIMENTAL PROCEDURES

Preliminary experiments with milk specimens obtained at various times during lactation from 8 cats showed that each one had bile salt stimulted lipase activity. We have therefore conducted this study with serial milk specimens obtained throughout the entire lactation period from two common cats and two beagle dogs. Milk was expressed without prior injection of oxytocin. Milk was collected at room temperature and all specimens were stored at -70°C until analysis. Milk specimens from several other species (black bear, seal, rabbit, pig, gorilla, rhesus monkey and chimpanzee) were also collected for quantitation of bile salt stimulated lipase activity. For comparison of enzyme characteristics, milk specimens obtained from two women at mid lactation (with an Egnell breast pump) were also analyzed.

Assay System Bile salt stimulated lipase activity was quantitated in an assay system containing (in a final volume of 200 ul) 1.6 mM tri ^{3}H olein, 60 mM Tris-HCl buffer, pH 9.0, 150 mM NaCl, 12 mM sodium taurocholate, 2.8% bovine serum albumin and 50 ul milk diluted 1:100-1:1000 in 5 mM veronal buffer, pH 7.4 [13]. Incubation was for 15 minutes at 37°C. Lipase activity was quantitated by the amount of ^{3}H oleic acid released and is expressed in units/ml milk, 1U-1 umol FFA released/min.

Characterization of lipase. The milk lipase was characterized as bile salt stimulated lipase by the effects of pH, bile salts (structure and concentration) and specific inhibitors on enzyme activity.

RESULTS

The data presented in Fig. 1 show that bile salt stimulated lipase activity was present in all specimens of dog,cat and human milk. Activity levels were lower in cat than in human milk, while those in dog milk were

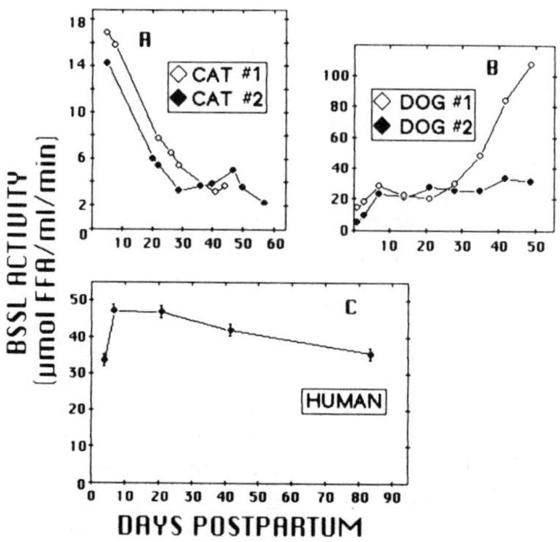

Figure 1 Bile salt stimulated lipase activity throughout lactation in cat (A) and dog (B) milk (lactation period is 8 wks in the cat and 6-7 wks in the dog) and throughout the first 3 months of lactation in human (C) milk. Note differences in scale of abscissas and ordinates for the three species.

higher than in human milk. Lipase activity levels throughout lactation differed among species, being highest during early lactation in the cat, and increasing from colostrum to mature milk in both human and dog. Lipoprotein lipase activity in the three species was 1-2 orders of magnitude lower than bile salt stimulated lipase activity (data not shown) [14]

Regardless of the source of lipase activity (cat, dog, or human milk) the pH optimum for the activity of bile salt stimulated lipase was between 7.3 and 8.5 (Fig. 2).

The lipase activity in the three species studied had an absolute requirement for bile salts (Fig. 3), no lipase activity being detected at concentrations under 5 mM.

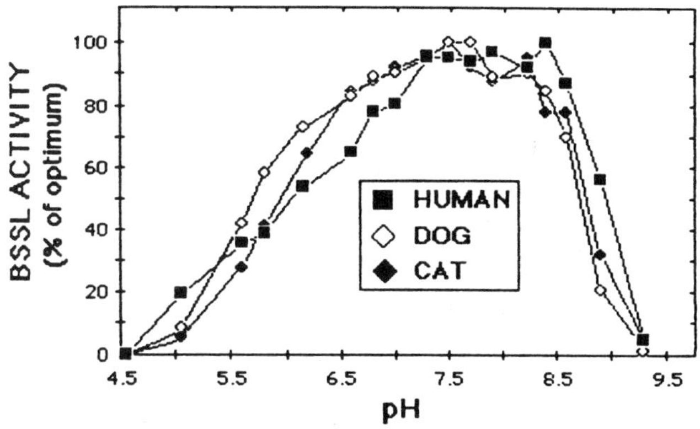

Figure 2 Effect of pH (4.6-9.3) on activity level of bile salt stimulated lipase in cat, dog and human milk. Buffers: sodium acetate-acetic acid (pH 4.6-5.6), MES (5.6-6.6), sodium phosphate (6.8-7.5), TRIS (7.1-8.6), glycine - NaOH (8.6-9.3). Bile salts, each at a final concentration of 12 mM.

In order to be active in fat digestion the lipase has to resist the low pH of the stomach. Although the presence of milk in the stomach raises the pH to 4.5-5.5, the empty stomach often has a pH of 1.5-2.5. Detailed studies (data not shown) indicate that bile salt stimulated lipase activity in human, cat and dog milk, is stable for at least 60 minutes of pH 3.0-8.0. Additional proof of similarity between the bile salt stimulated lipase in cat, dog, and human milk is complete inactivation by eserine (physostigmine) at concentrations above 0.4 mM (data now shown). Inhibition by eserine was previously used to characterize the enzyme in human [1] and gorilla [2] milk and to distinguish between pancreatic lipase and human milk bile salt stimulated lipase [9]. The search for bile salt stimulated lipase in the milk of other species showed that the enzyme is present only in bear and seal milk and that gorilla milk has very low activity levels (Table 1).

DISCUSSION

This study provides the first evidence for the presence of a bile salt stimulated lipase in the milk of non-primates. Cat and dog could thus serve as animal models for the study of the ontogeny and regulation

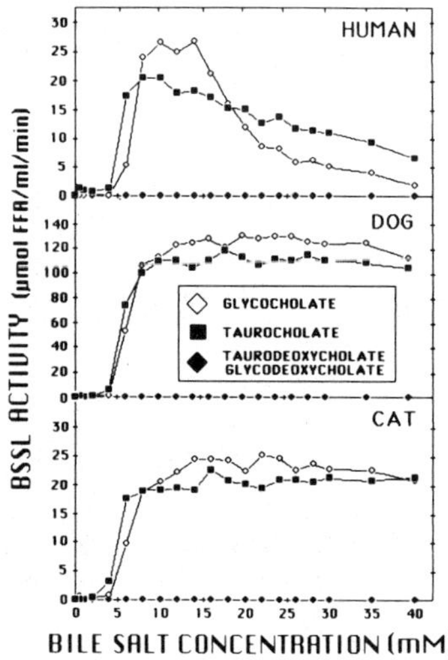

Figure 3 Effect of primary and secondary bile salts on the activity of bile salt stimulated lipase in cat, dog and human milk.

of enzyme synthesis and secretion in the mammary gland. Furthermore, animal studies will permit the quantitative evaluation of the role of this lipase in neonatal fat digestion.

In order to understand why carnivores and high primates are the only species with milk bile salt stimulated lipase we have examined the amount and composition of milk fat in species with and without this enzyme (Table 1). The amount of fat in milk is probably not related to the presence of lipase, because rabbit and sheep milk contains much higher concentrations of fat [16,17] than human milk [18]. A careful examination of the composition of milk fat (Table 1) shows a marked similarity between human milk [17] and that of carnivore species [18,19], all containing less than 1% short and medium chain fatty acids, whereas the other species studied contain high levels (24-69%) of short and medium chain fatty acids [18,19].

TABLE 1: Milk fat content and composition of species with and without milk bile salt stimulated lipase

Species	BSSL* U/ml	Fat+ %	Total Fatty Acids (mol %) C_4-C_{10}**	C_{12}-$C_{22:6}$**
Dog	32	10-12	1.0	99
Cat	7	8-10	1.0	99
Bear	12	18-30	?	?
Seal	77	35-50	0	100
Gorilla	3	?	?	?
Human	37	3.5-4.5	0.9	99
Rabbit	0	15-18	69	31
Donkey	0	0.6	?	?
Sheep	0	7.2-9.0	35	65
Pig	0	4.0-8.3	1.0	99
Chimpanzee	0	?	?	?
Rhesus monkey	0	?	24	76

* BSSL: bile salt stimulated lipase in milk. + Data from refs. # 15,16
** C_4-C_{10}: short and medium chain fatty acids, C_{12}-$C_{22:6}$: long chain fatty acids. Data from refs. #18,19

The data suggest that the short and medium chain triglyceride fatty acids in the milk of species without bile salt stimulated lipase can probably be adequately hydrolyzed by the newborn's endogenous lingual [18,20] and gastric [21, 22] lipases. However, while short and medium chain fatty acids are efficiently released from milk triglycerides by these preduodenal lipases [8, 20-22], the complete hydrolysis, of long chain triglycerides depends, in addition, upon the action of pancreatic lipase. The low activity of pancreatic lipase in the newborn suggests that milk bile salt stimulated lipase may be necessary for the efficient digestion of long chain triglycerides. The observation that pig milk contains no bile salt stimulated lipase, in spite of the high content of long chain fatty acids could be attributed to the fact that we have analyzed only colostrum specimens obtained during the immediate postpartum period. Analysis of the milk obtained throughout lactation will establish whether the enzyme is indeed absent from pig milk.

Milk bile salt stimulated lipase is closely related to the pancreatic non-specific lipase (also known as carboxyl ester hydrolase) [23]. The latter is phylogenetically old, being the only pancreatic digestive lipase in the leopard shark [24]. Furthermore, it is also the main pancreatic lipase in the newborn rat, before the rise in activity of the colipase-dependent lipase [25]. Thus, rather than being "an evolutionary newcomer" present only in the milk of high primates [3], we suggest that bile salt stimulated milk lipase is present in many species with milk fat containing predominantly long chain triglyceride. Because of lack of positional and fatty acid specificity, mammary gland (milk) and pancreas bile salt stimulated lipases might have a special function in neonatal fat digestion.

CONCLUSION

Our study is the first to show the presence of bile salt stimulated lipase in the milk of several non-primate species. This enzyme has previously been found only in the milk of human and gorilla. The data indicate that there is a relationship between milk bile salt stimulated lipase and milk fat composition, and suggest that the enzyme might have a special role in the digestion of milk long-chain triglyceride by the newborn.

ACKNOWLEDGEMENTS

The expert secretarial help of Ms. Barbara Runner is greatfully acknowledged. This study was supported by USDA Grant #85-CRCR-1-1825.

REFERENCES

1. E. Freudenberg, Die Frauenmilch Lipase. Karger, Basel (1953)
2. E. Freudenberg, A lipase in the milk of the gorilla Experientia 15:317 (1966)
3. L. Blackberg, O. Hernell, T. Olivecrona, L.Domellof and M.R. Malino. The bile salt stimulated lipase in human milk is a newcomer derived from a non-milk protein FEBS Lett. 112:51 (1980).
4. M. Hamosh, Physiological role of milk lipases. In "Textbook of Gastroenterology and Nutrition in Infancy". E. Lebenthal, ed. Raven Press, New York p 445 (1981).
5. T. Olivecrona and G. Bengtsson, Lipases in milk. In "Lipases", B. Borgstrom and H.L. Brockman, eds. Elsevier, Amsterdam p 205 (1984).
6. M. Hamosh, T.R. Clary, S.S. Chernick and R.O.Scow, Lipoprotein lipase activity of adipose and mammary tissue and plasma triglyceride in pregnant and lactating rats. Biochim. Biophys. Acta 210:473 (1970).
7. B. Alemi, M. Hamosh, J.W. Scanlon, C. Salzman-Mann and P. Hamosh, Fat digestion in very low birth weight infants: Effect of addition of human milk to low birth weight formula. Pediatrics 68:484 (1981)
8. M. Hamosh, Lingual and breast milk lipases. Adv. Pediatr. 29:33 (1982).
9. B. Fredrikzon, O. Hernell, L. Blackberg and T. Olivecrona, Bile salt stimulated lipase in human milk: evidence of activity in vitro and of a role in the digestion of retinol esters. Pediatr. Res. 12:1048, 1978.
10. N.R. Mehta, J.B. Jones and M. Hamosh, Lipases in preterm human milk: Ontogeny and physiologic significance. J. Pediatr. Gastroenterol. Nutr. 1:317 (1982).
11. L. Blackberg and O. Hernell, The bile salt stimulated lipase in human milk: purification and characterization. Eur. J. Biochem 16:221 (1981).
12. C.S. Wang, Purification of human milk bile salt-activated lipase by cholic acid coupled sepharose 4B affinity chromatography. Anal. Biochem. 105:398 (1980).
13. O. Hernell and T. Olivecrona, Human milk lipases II Bile salt stimulated lipase. Biochim. Biophys. Acta 369:234 (1974).
14. L.M. Freed, C.M. York, M. Hamosh, J.A. Sturman, O.T. Oftedal, and P. Hamosh, Bile salt stimulated lipase: enzyme activity in non-primate milk. Clin. Res. 34:796 (1986).
15. R. Jenness, Lactational performance of various mammalian species. J. Dairy Sci. 69:869 (1986).
16. O.T. Oftedal, Milk composition, milk yield and energy output at peak lactation: A comparative review. Symp. Zool. Soc. Lond. 51:33 (1984)

17. J. Bitman, D.L. Wood, M. Hamosh, P. Hamosh and N.R. Mehta, Comparison of the lipid composition of breast milk from mothers of term and pre-term infants. Am. J. Clin. Nutr. 38:300 (1983).
18. E.M. Widdowson, Feeding the newborn: comparative problems in man and animals. Proc. Nutr. Soc. 33:97 (1974).
19. R.R. Dils, Comparative aspects of milk fat synthesis. J. Dairy Sci. 69:904 (1986).
20. M. Hamosh, Lingual lipase In "Lipases" B.Borgstrom and H.L.Brockman, eds. Elsevier, Amsterdam p 49 (1984).
21. S.J. DeNigris, M. Hamosh, D.K. Kasbekar, C.S. Fink, T.C. Lee and P. Hamosh, Secretion of human gastric lipase from dispersed gastric glands. Biochim Biochys. Acta 835:67 (1985).
22. C.S. Fink, M. Hamosh, P. Hamosh, S.J. DeNigris and D.K. Kasbekar, Lipase secretion from dispersed rabbit gastric glands. Am. J. Physiol. 248:G68 (1985).
23. L. Blackberg, D. Lombardo, O. Hernell, O. Guy and T. Olivecrona, Bile salt stimulated lipase in human milk and carboxyl ester hydrolase in pancreatic juice. FEBS Lett. 136:294 (1981).
24. J.S. Patton, T.G. Warner and A.A. Benson, Partial characterization of the bile salt dependent triacylglycerol lipase from the leopard shark pancreas. Biochim. Biophys. Acta 486:322 (1977).
25. W.S. Bradshaw and W.J. Rutter, Multiple pancreatic lipases. Tissue distribution and pattern of accumulation during embriological development. Biochemistry 11:1517 (1972).

TOTAL NITROGEN AND NON-PROTEIN NITROGEN BALANCE IN PRETERM INFANTS FED PRETERM HUMAN MILK

S. M. Donovan, S. A. Atkinson[1] and B. Lonnerdal

Department of Nutrition
University of California
Davis, CA

[1]Department of Pediatrics
McMaster University
Hamilton, Ontario, Canada

INTRODUCTION

There has long been controversy over the optimal form of enteral feeding for the premature infant. It is generally accepted that human milk is the desired form of nutrition for the term infant, but it has been proposed that human milk, especially banked mature human milk, is not suitable for the premature infant[1,5]. Currently, attention has been focused on assessing the adequacy of feeding the preterm infant milk from his/her own mother[2-8]. Atkinson et al.[5] have suggested that the use of preterm milk supports significantly better nitrogen retention and protein nutritional status than pooled mature milk, especially during the first two weeks of life, due to its higher protein content. Therefore, it is thought that the use of "preterm milk" would more closely fulfill the needs of the preterm infant without causing the metabolic abnormalities that have been observed in infants fed formula with higher protein content[9]. Previous studies have all measured only total nitrogen of milk and excreta when determining nitrogen balance in premature infants. However, when assessing nitrogen utilization and protein requirements in infants fed human milk one has to consider the possible contribution of the non-protein nitrogen (NPN) fraction of human milk to the utilizable N pool provided to the recipient infant.

Human milk is unique in that the NPN fraction can account for up to 25% of the total nitrogen present[4,10,11]. The NPN components are low molecular weight nitrogen-containing compounds (usually <10,000 daltons) that are found in the soluble fraction following precipitation of protein with trichloroacetic acid (TCA). The NPN fraction of human milk is composed of a diverse group of nitrogen-containing compounds including urea, uric acid, ammonia, creatinine, creatine, free amino acids (with taurine and glutamic acid in highest concentration), carnitine, amino sugars (including N-acetylglucosamine and N-acetylneuraminic acid), nucleic acids, nucleotides, and polyamines[4,11,12]. Low-molecular-weight peptides also contribute to the NPN in human milk. The peptides include hormones, such as thyroxine, T_3, and insulin, in addition to other biologically active compounds such as epidermal growth factors[13]. Specific physiological roles have been proposed for many of these compounds[12].

Preterm milk NPN differs from mature milk in several respects (Table 1). First, the amount of NPN present in preterm milk is greater than in mature milk, with absolute amounts more similar to colostrum[4,11] (see also Atkinson, in this book). Although on a relative basis the amount is approximately the same, about 24% of the total nitrogen present. In addition, the composition of the preterm milk NPN appears different from mature milk. Urea nitrogen which constitutes approximately 50% of the NPN in mature milk, only accounts for approximately 21% of the total nitrogen in preterm milk, which is again similar to amounts found in colostrum[11] (see also Atkinson, in this book). The reasons for these differences are currently unknown.

Table 1. Comparison of Total Nitrogen, NPN, Urea Nitrogen in Mature Milk, Mature Milk Colostrum and Preterm Milk.

	Mature Milk	Colostrum[a]	Preterm Milk[b]
Total N (mg/100ml)	168 ± 19.5[c]	319 ± 7.1	250 ± 37.5
NPN (mg/100ml)	40.2 ± 3.1	61 ± 3.3	57.4 ± 9.5
NPN as % of TN	24%	19%	23%
Urea N/mg/100ml	21.7 ± 2.0	10.0 ± 2.6	12.0 ± 3.9
Urea as % of NPN	54%	16%	21%
	n=25	n=5	n=24

[a]days 1-3

[b]days 6-40

[c]mean ± SD

In a preliminary study of the utilization of preterm milk NPN as a nitrogen source in the preterm infant, we carried out metabolic balances to measure NPN and its components in preterm milk, and in urine and stool of infants receiving their own mothers' milk.

MATERIALS AND METHODS

Selection of Infants

Premature infants (n=7) were selected from the neonatal unit of McMaster University Medical Centre, Hamilton, Ontario, utilizing the following criteria: <1.8 kg birthweight, without congenital anomalies, not ventilated at the time the study was initiated, able to tolerate at least 150 ml/kg/day of human milk by 21 days of age. The infants were divided into two groups, one group receiving expressed breast milk (EBM) only, and the second group receiving 50% EBM and 50% standard infant formula. The infants in the two groups were matched for birthweight, gestational age, postnatal age at the time of study, and weight at the start of the balance period.

Two balance periods were carried out. During Balance Period 1, four infants received EBM ± infant formula only. During Balance Period 2, three infants received a calcium/phosphorus supplement (or placebo) and 800 IU of vitamin D in addition to the EBM ± infant formula.

Collection of Samples

Expressed human milk samples were obtained from each infant's mother and were fed fresh within 48 hours of pumping. During the 3-day metabolic balance study, a 24-hour collection of milk was pooled, warmed to 37°C and gently mixed. The milk samples were portioned into measured individual feedings, thus the amount of milk the infant received could be accurately quantified. An aliquot of each day's milk was taken for chemical analysis.

Urine and fecal samples were collected from the infants during the balance period as previously described[5]. All samples were frozen at -20°C after collection. Stool samples were homogenized and freeze-dried prior to analysis.

Analysis of Samples

Milk, urine and stool samples were analyzed for total nitrogen (TN) and non-protein nitrogen (NPN) by automated micro-Kjeldahl analysis[14]. NPN was determined in whey, urine and rehydrated stool samples following precipitation of proteins. To precipitate the proteins, an equal volume of 24% trichloroacetic acid was added to whey, urine and rehydrated stool samples, followed by centrifugation at 10,000 g for 20 minutes.

Urea nitrogen was determined using a modified urease-Berthelot reaction[15]. In this method, the amount of ammonia liberated by the action of urease on the urea present in the sample is measured colorimetrically.

Apparent absorption of total nitrogen, non-protein nitrogen and urea nitrogen was calculated by (intake - fecal output). Apparent retention of total nitrogen, non-protein nitrogen and urea nitrogen was calculated by (intake - fecal output - urinary output).

Statistical analysis was carried out on all samples using Student's t-test.

RESULTS

There were no significant differences in birthweight, gestational age, or weight at the start of the balance period. There was a significant difference (p=.005) in postnatal age of the infants in the two balance periods (Table 2). Responses of the infants in both balance periods were similar, therefore results from both studies were combined in the figures.

The infants readily absorbed the available nitrogen with an average absorption of 84 ± 0.9%*. All infants were in positive nitrogen balance, retaining an average of 267 ± 8.0 mg N/kg/d, or 68% of nitrogen intake.

*All results expressed as mean ± SEM.

There was no significant difference in the total nitrogen retention between the infants in Balance 1 or Balance 2, with retention equal to 249 ± 12.6 mg N/kg/d and 288.8 ± 70.6 mg N/kg/d respectively. The total nitrogen intake of the infants was significantly correlated with total nitrogen retention ($r=0.74$, $p<0.05$).

Table 2. Comparison of Infants in Balance Periods One and Two.

	Balance Period 1[a]	Balance Period 2[b]
Birthweight (grams)	1,310 ± 363[c]	1,150 ± 282
Gestational Age at Birth (weeks)	30.5 ± 1.0	30.3 ± 1.2
Postnatal Age (days)	24.5 ± 2.0	39.3 ± 3.1
Weight at Study (grams)	1,475 ± 455	1,510 ± 355

[a] n=4 infants

[b] n=3 infants

[c] Mean ± SD

Approximately 84% of the available non-protein nitrogen was absorbed by the infants, with a range of 57% to 98% between different infants (Figure 1). All infants but one were in positive NPN balance, retaining an average of 16 ± 3.5 mg N/kg/d (Figure 2) or 24% of the available NPN. Infants in Balance Period 2 (#3,4,7) did statistically better than infants in Balance Period 1 (#1,2,5,6), retaining an average of 29.1 ± 5.5 mg N/kg/d vs. 5.8 ± 6.6 mg N/kg/d ($p=.01$).

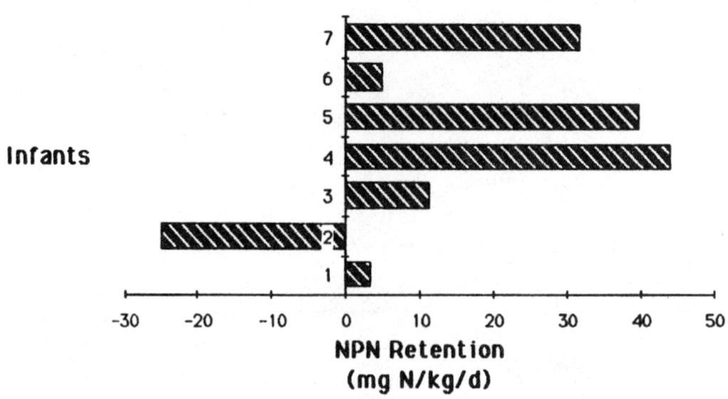

Figure 1. Apparent total non-protein nitrogen retention by infants studied. Results are expressed as mg N/kg/day.

As with total nitrogen and NPN, urea nitrogen was well absorbed by the infants (Figure 3). The infants absorbed an average of 90 ± 2.0% of the available urea. All infants but two were in negative urea nitrogen balance. This observation makes sense due to the contribution of endogenously produced urea as a result of protein metabolism. Therefore, estimation of urea nitrogen retention is most likely an underestimation of the true retention of urea from dietary sources.

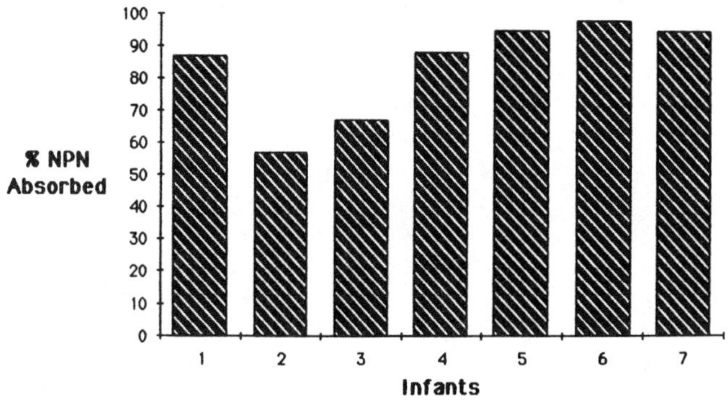

Figure 2. Apparent absorption of total non-protein nitrogen by premature infants. Results expressed as % of available milk non-protein nitrogen absorbed.

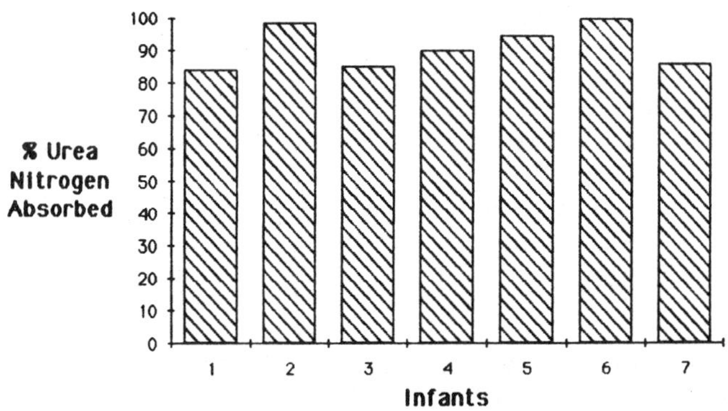

Figure 3. Apparent urea nitrogen absorption. Results are expressed as % of available milk urea nitrogen absorbed by the infant.

DISCUSSION

In this study we have demonstrated that preterm infants can be maintained in positive total nitrogen balance on expressed preterm milk. Our results are in close agreement with those of Atkinson et al.[5], Whyte et al.[16] and Brooke et al.[17] for nitrogen retention from human milk in premature infants. The total nitrogen retention from human milk is lower than retention values found in exclusively formula-fed infants[17]. This has caused many pediatricians to feel that feeding high protein formulas is desirable to maximize nitrogen retention and growth in the preterm infant.

We have also demonstrated in this study that preterm infants are apparently able to absorb and retain significant quantities of the non-protein nitrogen available in preterm milk. These observations may be supported by the study of Lindberg[18], who demonstrated that although protein digestion and absorption may be compromised in the premature infant, by 23 weeks of gestation, dipeptidase activity is comparable to that of the adult. In addition, Adibi[19] has shown that the ability of the newborn intestine to transport dipeptides and amino acids across the brush border membranes is parallel with the ability of the tissue to digest the peptide. Also, in the newborn transport velocity is higher than at any other time in life due to either the carrier substrate complex or the presence of more transport sites per unit of intestinal surface. Therefore it appears that the premature infant may be quite able physiologically to utilize the NPN that is available in human milk.

Although the direct metabolic fate of the absorbed NPN is currently not known, the fact that most of the infants were apparently maintained in positive NPN balance may support the work of previous investigators[20-22]. These investigators have demonstrated that both term and preterm infants are able to metabolize nitrogen (^{15}N) from various non-protein sources. The substrates used include ^{15}N-labeled urea[20], ^{15}N-labeled ammonium chloride[20,21] and ^{15}N-labeled amino acids[20,22]. Early work by Snyderman et al.[20] showed that infants maintained on "low-protein" diets could incorporate ^{15}N from labeled urea and ammonium chloride into plasma proteins and red blood cells. Later work in preterm infants by Nicholson[21] looked at the pattern of $^{15}NH_3$ and ^{15}N-urea excretion following ingestion of $^{15}NH_4Cl$. He concluded that the pattern of ^{15}N excretion was consistent with a sequence of metabolic events in which ingested ammonium was incorporated into a pool of metabolically active nitrogen that yielded both ammonia and urea. These results support the hypothesis that NPN compounds can be absorbed and utilized in vivo as a source of "unessential" nitrogen by the infant.

SUMMARY

In conclusion, although human milk-fed preterm infants receive less intact protein than their formula-fed counterparts, we feel that more research is necessary to further characterize the role that the non-protein nitrogen fraction is playing in the nutrition of the human-milk fed infant.

ACKNOWLEDGMENT

This research was supported in part by Ross Laboratories.

REFERENCES

1. D. P. Davies, Adequacy of expressed milk for early growth of preterm infants, Arch. Dis. Child. 51:296 (1977).
2. G. H. Anderson, S. A. Atkinson, and M. H. Bryan, Energy and macronutrient content of human milk during early lactation from mothers giving birth prematurely and at term, Am. J. Clin. Nutr. 34:258 (1981).
3. S. A. Atkinson, M. H. Bryan, and G. H. Anderson, Human milk: Difference in nitrogen concentration in milk from mothers of term and premature infants, J. Pediatr. 93:67 (1978).
4. S. A. Atkinson, G. H. Anderson, and M. H. Bryan, Human milk: Comparison of the nitrogen composition in milk from mothers of premature and full-term infants, Am. J. Clin. Nutr. 33:811 (1980).
5. S. A. Atkinson, H. M. Bryan, and G. H. Anderson, Human milk feeding in premature infants: protein, fat and carbohydrate balance in the first two weeks of life, J. Pediatr. 99:617 (1981).
6. P. Chessex, et al., Quality of growth in premature infants fed their own mothers' milk, J. Pediatr. 102:107 (1983).
7. C. M. Hibberd, O. G. Brookem, N. D. Carter, M. Haug, and G. Harzer, Variation in the composition of breast milk during the first 5 weeks of lactation: Implications for the feeding of preterm infants, Arch. Dis. Child. 57:658 (1982).
8. W. C. Heird, Feeding the premature infant. Human milk or an artificial formula?, Am. J. Dis. Child. 131:468 (1977).
9. N. C. R. Raiha, K. Heinonen, D. K. Rassin et al., Milk protein quantity and quality in low-birth-weight infants. I. Metabolic response and effects on growth, Pediatrics 57:659 (1976).
10. L. Hambraeus, B. Lonnerdal, E. Forsum, and M. Gebre-Medhin, Nitrogen and protein components of human milk, Acta Paediatr. Scand. 67:561 (1978).
11. S. M. Donovan and B. Lonnerdal, Non-protein nitrogen constituents in mature human milk and colostrum, Fed. Proc. 44:1676 (1985).
12. S. E. Carlson, Human milk nonprotein nitrogen: Occurrence and possible functions, in: "Advances in Pediatrics," L. A. Barness, ed., Year Book Medical Publishers, New York (1985).
13. J. R. Moran, M. E. Courtney, D. N. Orth et al., Epidermal Growth Factor in human milk: daily production and diurnal variation during early lactation in mothers delivering at term and at premature gestation, J. Pediatr. 107:402 (1983).
14. L. Hambraeus, E. Forsum, L. Abrahamsson, and B. Lonnerdal, Automatic total nitrogen analysis in nutritional evaluations using a block digestor, Anal. Biochem. 72:78 (1976).
15. A. P. Chaney and E. P. Marback, Modified reagents for determination of urea and ammonia, Clin. Chem. 8:130 (1962).
16. R. K. Whyte, R. Haslam, C. Vlainic, S. Shannon, K. Samulski, D. Campbell, H. S. Bayley, and J. C. Sinclair, Energy balance and nitrogen balance in growing low birthweight infants fed human milk or formula, Pediatr. Res. 17:891 (1983).
17. O. G. Brooke, C. Wood and J. Barley, Energy balance, nitrogen balance, and growth in preterm infants fed expressed breast milk, a premature infant formula and two low-solute adapted formulae, Arch. Dis. Child. 57:898 (1982).
18. T. Lindberg, Intestinal dipeptidases: characterization, development and distribution of intestinal dipeptidases of the human foetus, Clin. Sci. 30:505 (1966).
19. S. A. Adibi, Intestinal phase of protein assimilation in man, Am. J. Clin. Nutr. 29:205 (1976).

20. S. E. Snyderman, L. E. Holt, Jr., J. Dancis, E. Roitman, A. Boyer and M. E. Balis, "Unessential" nitrogen: a limiting factor for human growth, _J. Nutr._ 78:57 (1962).
21. J. F. Nicholson, Metabolism of ingested ammonium ^{15}N by premature infants, _Pediatr. Res._ 4:398 (1970).
22. J. F. Nicholson, Rate of protein synthesis in premature infants, _Pediatr. Res._ 4:389 (1970).

RECOVERY OF VITAMIN K FROM HUMAN MILK

Chun Por Lai, Ann F. Townsend-Blanton, and Louise M. Canfield*

Department of Biochemistry & Biophysics and Department of Animal Science, Texas Agricultural Experiment Station, and Texas A&M University, College Station, Texas 77843-2471

ABSTRACT

A rapid, sensitive and specific procedure for recovery and quantitation of vitamin K in human milk has been developed. Vitamin K was extracted from milk on dry columns, fractionated on TLC, eluted and resolved on an HPLC gradient using electrochemical detection. The entire procedure can be completed in four hours, can detect <20 nanograms of vitamin K, and is suitable for multiple assays. The unique redox properties of vitamin K have been utilized to define conditions which are highly selective for vitamin K and which avoid interference from other fat soluble vitamins. In addition, techniques for electrochemical detection of HPLC gradient chromatography have been developed; thus baseline resolution of the K vitamins is provided.

INTRODUCTION

Despite the importance of vitamin K in protecting against hemorrhage in infants, to date there has been very little effort devoted to the study of vitamin K in human milk. Thus there is poor agreement in the literature concerning both the forms and quantities of vitamin K in human milk (1-3). In major part this has been due to formidable technical problems introduced in quantitating the trace quantities of vitamin K estimated to be present. In addition, vitamins A and E, with similar chemical structures and thus similar chromatographic behaviors, are present in 100 to 1,000-fold molar excesses over vitamin K (1).

Electrochemical techniques offer the potential for greatly enhancing the detection of trace quantities of vitamin K. Due to its unique redox properties, vitamin K is easily detected at potentials which do not detect lipids with similar chromatographic properties which absorb in the UV, particularly vitamins A and E. In addition, sensitivity of electrochemical techniques is at least comparable to that of UV (4). To date, a major limitation has been the use of HPLC gradient elution with electrochemical detection due to the difficulty in maintaining a stable baseline. However, tetrabutylammonium perchlorate (TBAP) is freely soluble in our solvent systems and provides a constant electrochemical potential over our gradient.

In addition, we have substituted a "dry column" (5) extraction procedure for the commonly used organic extraction which is rapid, suitable for automation and avoids the biohazards commonly associated with organic solvents. In combination with TLC, this technique sufficiently removes contaminating lipids to allow HPLC determination of vitamin K in the extracts.

METHODS AND MATERIALS

^{3}H vitamin K_1 (50 μCi/μmol) was added to fresh milk, equilibrated at 37°C for 2 hours with gentle shaking and frozen at -70°C until use (6). Prior to extraction, samples were tempered at 37°C for 10 minutes.

Dry column extraction was performed by the method of Hundreiser et al. (5). Tritiated vitamin was added to 1 ml milk, 4 grams anhydrous sodium sulfate, 3 grams celite and ground with a porcelain mortar and pestle. The mixture was layered over 2 grams calcium phosphate:celite (1:9, w/w) in 0.14 X 19 cm glass columns and eluted with methylene chloride:methanol (90:10 v/v).

Thin Layer Chromatography of Vitamin K

Vitamins extracted by the dry column procedure were applied to 20 x 20 cm Kodak silica thin layer chromatograms pretreated with petroleum ether: paraffin oil (95:5, v/v). Chromatograms were developed for 1.5 hours at 25°C, with acetone:hexane:water (80:10:5, v/v/v) and regions containing vitamin K were scraped from the chromatograms, packed into disposable pipettes, eluted with 20 mls hexane and injected onto the HPLC column.

Gradient HPLC Elution and Electro-chemical Detection of Vitamin K

Vitamins were injected onto a Nova-Pak C_{18} reverse phase column using a Waters HPLC system equipped with Model 6000A and M45 pumps as previously described (7). Vitamins were eluted using a convex gradient generated by a model M45 solvent programmer (Curve 3) of ethanol: water (90:10 v/v) in 50 mM TBAP to ethanol: hexane (90:10 v/v) in 50 mM TBAP. Vitamins were detected using dual Bioanalytical Systems 4-B Ampometric Detectors at an applied voltage of -0.45V in the reductive mode and +0.25V in the oxidative mode.

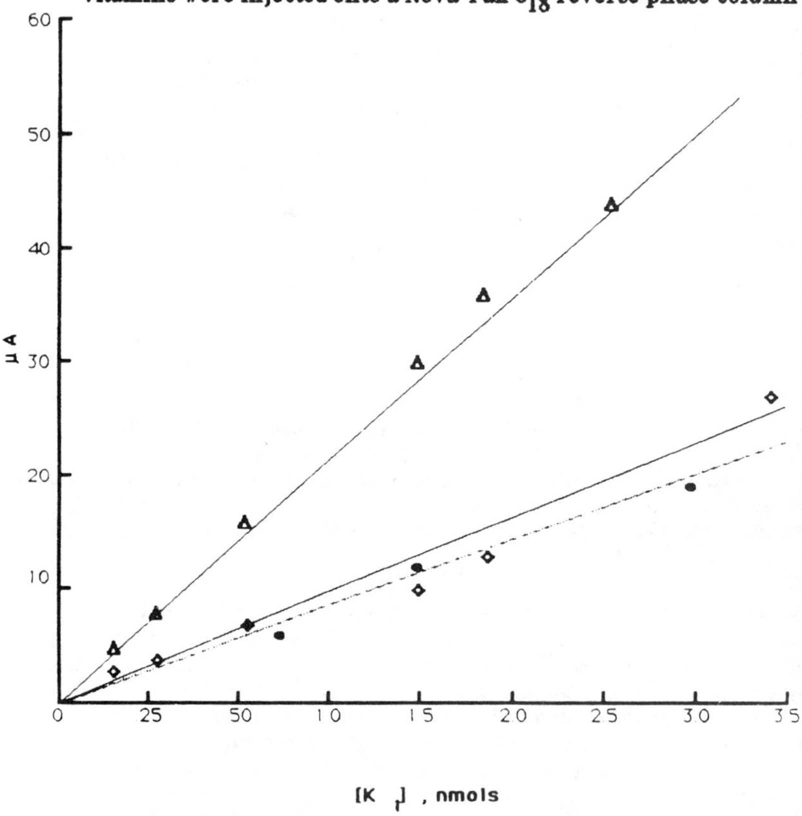

Figure 1. Linear relationship between vitamin K injected concentration and response of ampometric electrochemical detector of vitamin K.

△ Reductive mode, dual electrodes, -0.45V
◇ Oxidative mode, dual electrodes, +0.45V
● Reductive mode, single electrode, -0.45V

RESULTS AND DISCUSSION

Figure 1 shows the linear response of the

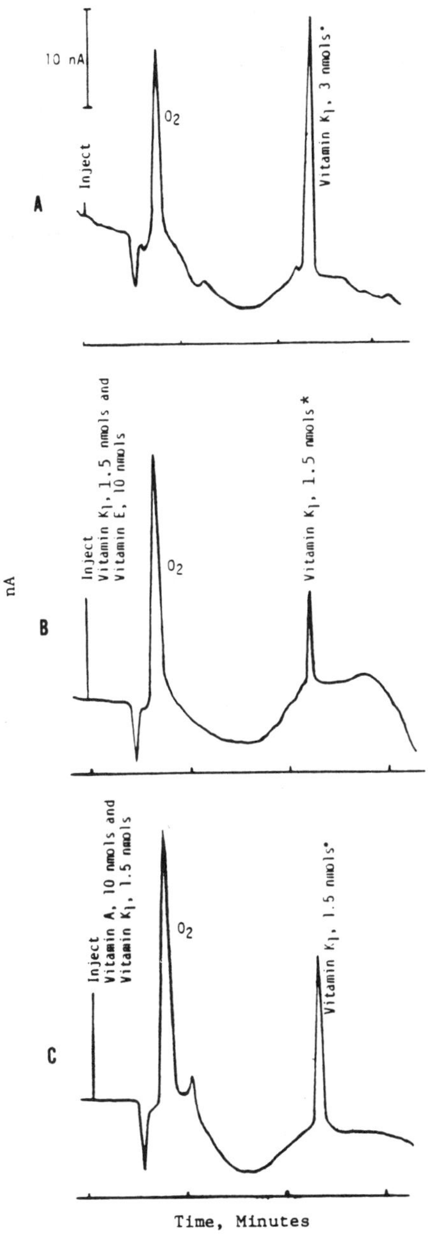

Figure 2. HPLC chromatograms showing electrochemical detection of fat soluble vitamins.

A. Vitamin K, 3 nmols
B. Vitamin K, 1.4 nmols and Vitamin E, 10 nmols, injected simultaneously
C. Vitamin K, .1.5 nmols and Vitamin A, 10 nmols, injected simultaneously
*single electrode mode
•dual electrode mode

ampometric detector to injection of vitamin K (0.15 to 3.5 nmols) in the reductive mode using a single electrode (-0.45V) and both oxidative and reductive modes using dual electrodes (+0.45V and -0.45V respectively). Note that a two-fold increase in sensitivity is achieved in the reductive mode using the dual electrode system compared to a single electrode. Similarly, using the dual electrode system, increased sensitivity is achieved in the reductive mode compared to the oxidative mode. Thus the most sensitive detection of vitamin K is achieved using the reductive mode in the dual electrode system. Unless otherwise indicated, all experiments were therefore conducted using the dual electrode system with a reductive electrode potential of -0.45V. The technique can easily detect 20 nanograms (~40 pmols) of vitamin K with minimum baseline instability.

The selectivity for vitamin K afforded by electrochemical detection is shown in Figure 2. Neither vitamins A nor E in 10-fold excess are seen using conditions in which vitamin K is readily detected. This selectivity offers a major improvement in techniques for quantitating vitamin K in milk, as vitamins A and E which have similar chromatographic properties are present in 100 to 1000 X molar excesses over vitamin K (1). A number of forms of vitamin K are known (7-9), and controversy exists over whether these are present in human milk (1-3). As fine resolution will be required to separate these vitamins if they are present, gradient elution will be necessary. As can be seen in Figure 2, the use of 50 mM TBAP in our solvents provided a sufficiently stable potential with only minimal baseline drift. Thus it should be possible to reproducibly resolve and quantitate the various vitamin K derivatives present in milk.

Figure 3 shows an HPLC chromatogram of ^3H vitamin K which was extracted from frozen milk. Tritiated vitamin was equilibrated with fresh milk prior to freezing, extracted on dry columns, fractionated on TLC and resolved on HPLC as described in Methods. Significant radioactivity was recovered only in the peak corresponding to vitamin K (Inset). Typical overall recoveries of ^3H vitamin for the entire procedure were 60-70%.

In summary, we have developed a three-step procedure for rapidly and efficiently extracting and quantitating vitamin K in human milk. Using this technique, picomolar quantitites of vitamin K can be detected, and interference from vitamins A, E, and other contaminating lipids is avoided. Only three fractionation steps are required, the procedure can be performed in half a day and the techniques are suitable for automation. Experiments are in progress to maximize recoveries, to refine the techniques for automation, and to determine the quantities of vitamin K and its derivatives in human milk.

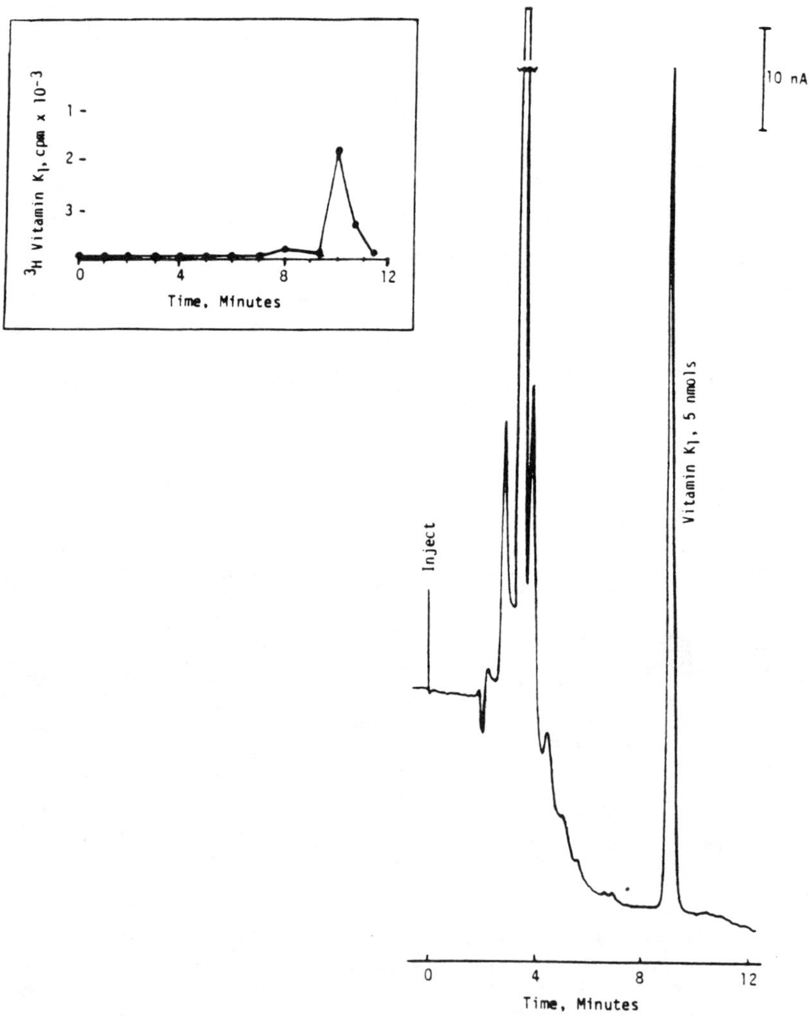

Figure 3. HPLC chromatogram of ^3H Vitamin K (5 nmols) extracted from human milk. Insert shows elution pattern of ^3H vitamin.

REFERENCES

1. C. J. Lammi-Keefe and R. G. Jensen, Lipids in human milk: a review. 2: Composition and fat-soluble vitamins, J. Ped. Gastr. and Nutr. 3:172 (1984).

2. Y. Haroon, M. J. Shearer, S. Rahim, W. G. Gunn, G. McEnery, and P. Barkan, The content of phylloquinone (vitamin K_1) in human milk, cows' milk and infant formula foods determined by high-performance liquid chromatography, J. Nutr. 112: 1105 (1982).

3. Y. Miyaji, Study on the idiopathic vitamin K deficiency of young infants. I. Vitamin K in human milk and formula milk, Acta Paedia. Japon. Overseas Ed. 24:506 (1982).

4. T. Ueno and J. W. Suttie, High-pressure liquid chromatographic-reductive electrochemical detection analysis of serum trans-phylloquinone, Anal. Bioch. 133:62 (1983).

5. K. E. Hundrieser, R. M. Clark, R. G. Jensen, and A. M. Ferris, A comparison of methods for determination of total lipids in human milk, Nutr. Res. 4: 21 (1984).

6. E. Forsum, Determination of α-lactalbumin in human milk, J. Dairy Sci. 59:14 (1975).

7. L. M. Canfield and R. B. Holzman, Reaction of vitamin K and dithiothreitol on reversed-phase C_{18} high-performance liquid chromatographic columns, J. Chrom. 299:225 (1984).

8. J. W. Suttie, Vitamin K, in: "Handbook of Lipid Research," Vol. 2, J.W. Suttie, ed., Plenum Press, New York, (1978).

9. L. M. Canfield, L. A. Davy, and K. B. Tomer, Photolytic production of vitamin K hydroperoxide: isolation, characterization and significance to vitamin K-dependent carboxylation, Photobiochem. and Photobiophys. 10:23 (1985).

SKIM MILK MEMBRANES IN HUMAN MILK

Charles E. Isaacs and Roger C. Moretz

Office of Mental Retardation and Developmental Disabilities
New York State Institute for Basic Research in Developmental Disabilities, Department of Developmental Biochemistry and Department of Pathological Neurobiology, 1050 Forest Hill Road
Staten Island, New York 10314

INTRODUCTION

Human milk contains biologically active proteins, e.g. enzymes and hormones, some of which have been shown to retain biological activity in the gastrointestinal tract[1,2,3]. It has been suggested that the binding of biologically active milk proteins to milk membranes may play a role in stabilizing them in the gastrointestinal tract. We have studied two enzymes, sulfhydryl oxidase (SOX) and γ-glutamyltranspeptidase (GGT), which have been shown to be membrane-bound in bovine milk[4], to both the milk fat globule membrane and to the skim milk membranes.

Bovine skim milk membranes are morphologically heterogeneous[5], but have been studied as if they are biochemically homogeneous[4]. However, when human milk was fractionated by differential centrifugation, SOX and GGT activities partitioned into a number of fractions with varying amounts of the two enzymes[6]. Significant amounts of GGT, but not SOX, were found in the milk fat globule membranes. A SOX-enriched fraction with little GGT activity was found following centrifugation at 150,000 g for 16 hours. Whether the 150,000 g pellet consisted of low density membranes or protein aggregates was not established. In the present work evidence is presented that following 100,000 g and 150,000 g sequential centrifugations of human milk, all fractions with significant amounts of SOX and GGT activity have membrane material.

MATERIALS AND METHODS

Human milk, previously stored at -70°C, was fractionated by sequential centrifugation. Milk was centrifuged at 4,000 g for 30 minutes at 4°C. The 4,000 g infranatant was then centrifuged at 100,000 g for 90 minutes. The 100,000 g supernatant was then centrifuged at 150,000 g for 16 hours, yielding a supernatant, a fluffy layer and a pellet.

Human milk samples were donated by the LaLeche League of Staten Island after informed consent was given.

SOX activity was measured as previously described using dithiothreitol as substrate[1]. GGT (EC 2.3.2.2) was measured by the method of Griffith and Tate[7].

RESULTS AND DISCUSSION

After centrifugation of human milk at 4,000 g, SOX is found primarily in the infranatant fraction (Table I). However, almost 50% of the GGT activity is concentrated in the lipid layer. The increase in total GGT activity may be due to a change in membrane configuration as a result of centrifugation. Based upon these results and on previous work [6], it appears that although a third of the SOX activity of bovine milk is bound to the cream membranes[4], human milk SOX is almost entirely a skim milk membrane enzyme. When the 4,000 g infranatant was centrifuged at 100,000 g, the remaining SOX and GGT again had a different distribution (Table I). Almost all of the recovered SOX is in the supernatant, whereas over 60% of the remaining GGT is in the fluffy layer at the bottom of the tube. Electron micrographs of the 100,000 g fluffy layer (Figure 1B) demonstrate the presence of membrane material, including densely stained vesicles. These results show that 70-75% of GGT activity in human milk is found in membrane fractions that have little SOX activity, including the skim milk fluffy fraction isolated at 100,000 g. Some membrane fragments were also found in the 100,000 g casein pellet (Figure 1A) but almost no SOX or GGT activity is present in this fraction (results not shown).

TABLE 1. Distribution of SOX and GGT in Human Milk *

Fraction	SOX u/ml	Total SOX units	% Yield	GGT u/ml	Total GGT units	% Yield
Whole milk	0.543	27.10	100	0.116	5.78	100
4,000 g lipid layer	0.214	0.96	3.5	0.832	3.74	64.7
4,000 g infranatant	0.628	21.70	80.1	0.125	4.30	74.4
100,000 g supernatant	0.431	13.13	48.4	0.064	1.56	27.0
100,000 g fluffy layer	0.747	1.34	4.9	1.42	2.56	44.3
150,000 g supernatant	0.037	0.73	2.7	0.003	0.06	1.0
150,000 g fluffy layer	2.67	4.8	17.7	0.43	0.78	13.5
150,000 g pellet	2.79	3.35	12.4	0.05	0.06	1.0

* One unit of SOX activity is expressed as umole SH oxidized/min. One unit of GGT activity is expressed as umole p-nitroaniline released/min.

Following centrifugation of the 100,000 g supernatant at 150,000 g, SOX was found in a fluffy layer and a pellet, whereas GGT was almost entirely in the fluffy layer (Table 1). The 150,000 g fluffy layer was the only membrane fraction isolated that had significant amounts of both SOX and GGT activity. The 150,000 pellet has SOX activity but almost no detectable GGT activity.

Electron micrographs show that there are similar membrane structures in the SOX and GGT fractions obtained by differential centrifugation (Figure 1b, c). Electron micrographs of the 150,000 g fluffy layer (not shown) indicate that there are similar structures in this fraction also.

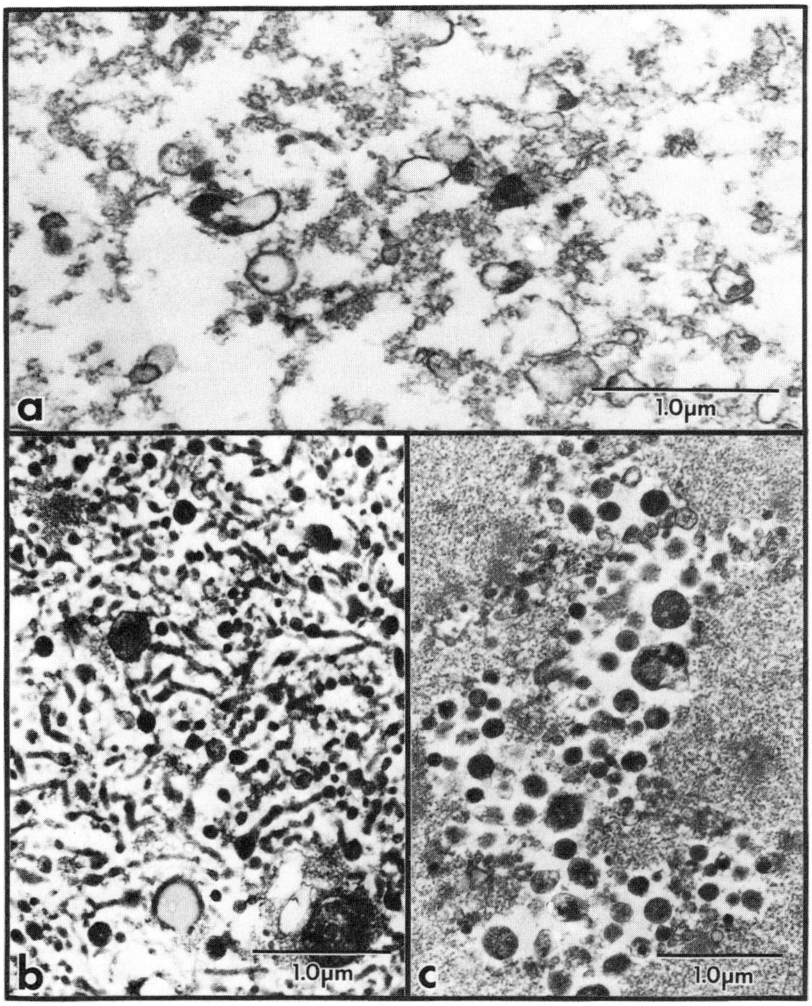

Figure 1. Electron micrographs of human milk membrane fractions.

a) 100,000 g pellet
b) 100,000 g fluffy layer
c) 150,000 g pellet.

The results presented in this paper indicate that human milk SOX and GGT are found in morphologically heterogeneous membrane fractions. However, the extent of heterogeneity within each fraction appears to be similar. The fractions differed biochemically with respect to SOX and GGT distribution and there was only one skim milk membrane fraction (150,000 g fluffy layer) with comparable yields of both SOX and GGT. The biochemical heterogeneity of human skim milk membranes is like that found for bovine milk fat globule membranes[8], which were shown to differ in their protein, carbohydrate and lipid composition. Future work is needed to determine the physiological significance of human milk membranes and whether the membrane distribution of enzymes and other proteins is altered by lactational stage or environmental influences.

SUMMARY

All human skim milk fractions with SOX and GGT activity have membrane material. Milk membranes within each fraction are morphologically heterogenous but there appear to be similar types of membrane fragments in each enzyme containing fraction. SOX and GGT are distributed differently not only between skim milk membranes and the milk fat globule membrane but also between different skim milk membrane fractions. Whether environmental influences can affect the relative abundance of morphologically different human skim milk membranes or the enzyme distribution between them remains to be determined.

REFERENCES

1. C.E. Isaacs, T. Pascal, C.E. Wright, and G.E. Gaull, Sulfhydryl oxidase in human milk: Stability of milk enzymes in the gastrointestinal tract. Ped. Res. 18:532 (1984).
2. A. Grueter, J. Lakshmanan, R. Tarris, J. Alm, and D.A. Fisher, Nerve growth factor in mouse milk during early lactation: Lack of dependency on submandibular salivary glands. Ped. Res. 19:934 (1985).
3. L. Aloe, P. Calissano, and R. Levi-Montalcini, Effects of oral administration of nerve growth factor and of its antiserum on sympathetic ganglia of neonatal mice. Devel. Br. Res. 4:31 (1982).
4. B.J. Kitchen, A comparison of the properties of membranes isolated from bovine skim milk and cream. Biochim. Biophys. Acta 356:257 (1974).
5. P.S. Stewart, D.L. Puppione, and S. Patton, The presence of microvilli and other membrane fragments in the non-fat phase of bovine milk. Z. Zellforsch 123:161 (1972).
6. C.E. Isaacs, Milk enzyme function: Effects of compartmentation and storage conditions on sulfhydryl oxidase and γ-glutamyltranspeptidase, in: Human Lactation, R.G. Jensen, M.C. Neville, eds. Plenum Publishing Corp., New York (1985).
7. O.W. Griffith, and S.S. Tate, The apparent glutathione oxidase activity of γ-glutamyltranspeptidase. J.Biol.Chem.255:5011 (1980).
8. B.J. Kitchen, Fractionation and characterization of the membranes from bovine milk fat globules. J. Dairy Res. 44:469 (1977).

BREASTFEEDING: CULTURAL PRACTICES AND VARIATIONS

Naomi Baumslag

Georgetown University Medical Schook, Washington, D.C.
7100 Oak Forest Lane, Bethesda, MD 20917

ABSTRACT

Throughout the centuries women have learned that foods, fears and even pregnancy affects their milk supply. Not surprisingly dietary restrictions in pregnancy abound. Food such as eggs, chicken, and milk are taboo for fear of hydrocephalus, abortions, convulsions. It is believed that if a nursing mother becomes pregnant her milk will be harmful to the infant on the breast. This belief may be related to the fact that mothers throw colostrum away, because of its yellow color, fearing it is "pus" or "poison", and purge the infant for 1-4 days with a variety of substances such as honey, rose water and hyssop. At the time of the delivery about one third of mothers with milk no longer have colostrum. Some societies provide or even prefer breast milk substitutes, others use wet nurses. Selection criteria for wet nurses have varied through the ages and with different cultures. At one stage "scientific studies" were used to justify the belief that the milk of a brunette was better than that of a redhead. Women with small breasts were not considered adequate, and it was seriously believed that mannerisms and racial characteristics were transmissable through milk. Some "authorities" even went as far as to profess that breast milk was so specific that women who had born infants of one sex could only nurse infants of the same sex. In different cultures certain causal associations with foods in pregnancy and lactation exist. To ensure an adequate milk supply prayers, witchcraft, herbs and special foods are advocated. Each culture has its own remedies for an "insufficient" milk supply. To promote lactation mothers in Latin American drink special teas made from "hot plants" called vervein: lactation soups in China are made from rooster or pig and in addition eggs are eaten in large quantities. In India drinks such as lassi are prescribed. Herb usage is universal; examples are sesame, abysinth and cumin. Heat is also thought to be beneficial. Special tests have been devised to ascertain the quality of the milk. Soratus used a nail test, later a rennet test was added. Truby King measured milk fat when the infant was not thriving. The Somoans have official milk testers. Recently, in the literature, a creamatocrit test was described to measure the fat content of the milk. Animals have also been fed on human breast milk and still are. Dogs have been put on the breasts of pregnant women to "draw them out" or on women with lumps in the breast, as treatment. Humans have also been nursed directly by animals such as goats, asses and pigs. Success stories however are few. Old incapacitated people too, have been nursed by lactating relatives. Nulliparous girls and old women have served as surrogate mothers. More amazingly, there are cases on record where men in desperate straights have suckled infants. Not only has breast milk served as a food, but since ancient times its medicinal qualities have been recognized. Apart from its known antibody content indispensable for infant health, it has been extensively used for eye infections, even in modern times, during epidemics of hemorrhagic conjunctivitis. Through their fads and fashionable treatments both traditional and Western practitioners have succeeded in confusing generations of mothers. History has much to teach about breast feeding and the variety of feeding patterns.

INTRODUCTION

Throughout the centuries women have had to rely on nursing for their infants to survive.[20] They have learned that foods, fears and even pregnancy affect their milk supply. They have developed techniques for ensuring an abundant milk supply, for stimulating lactation in cases of failure and for protecting the quality of the milk. Certain causal associations have been made in different cultures with foods and practices that they believe affects the infant, and as a result a wide variety of beliefs and practices exist during pregnancy and lactation. Interestingly there are many similarities in different parts of the world. The traditional practitioners and medical men of our times too have had their influence making certain routines, practices and foods into rituals and fashions. Nor have they been consistent. Often the fear of milk "drying up" has been added to by the practitioners own ignorance and prejudice. Both in developed and developing countries tests have been devised for checking on the milk quality throughout the ages and where no artificial substitute existed, wet nurses began to replace maternal breastfeeding, followed by "dry nursing" and finally "pocket-nursing." Unless we classify breastfeeding more scientifically comparisons will continue to be invalid.

Since biblical times man-made rules dictated breast feeding as a mother's sacred duty. Jeremiah addressing fashionable women who refused to nurse their young child, chided, "even the sea monsters draw out the breast for their young".[30] The bible refers to lactating breasts a "God's blessing". The Koran states that mothers should nurse their infants for two years. Furthermore it is at the fathers discretion not Allah's whether this period is to be shortened.[17]

Women through the ages have known that by expressing their breasts they can tell how soon the infant will be born from the color of their breast secretion[3] (Fig. 1). Until recently an infant lived or died depending on whether it was breastfed or not, and women in many cultures prayed that their breast milk would be bountiful. Votive paintings hung in Japanese temples show women praying for adequate breast milk and fulfillment of their prayers (Fig. 2).[29, 40] In addition to women praying for sufficient breastmilk, priests fasted and prayed on Thursdays that nursing women could go on feeding their offspring.[21] To ensure a good milk supply a number of precautionary measures evolved. For example, certain foods were to be eaten or avoided during pregnancy and lactation, and intercourse was to be avoided during lactation. Mothers were even expected to live away from the husband for 18-24 months and devote all their time to the infant. In many cultures there are special regimes for lactating mothers and culture specific galactogogues.

DIET AND PREGNANCY

It is not uncommon for pregnant women to be told that harm will come to

Table I: Analysis of a blonde and a brunette wet nurse (both age twenty-two) cited in ConeT.E. The history of American Pediatrics, Little Brown Publishers Boston 1979.

Constituents	Blonde		Brunette	
	Sample 1	Sample 2	Sample 1	Sample 2
Water	892	881.5	853.3	853
Solid constituents				
Butter	35.5	40.5	54.8	56.0
Casein	10	9.5	16.2	17.0
Sugar of milk	58.5	64.0	71.2	70.0
Salts	4.0	4.5	4.5	4.0
Total	1,000.0	1,000.0	1,000.0	1,000.0

Source: J. F. Simon. *Mother's Milk and Its Chemical and Physiological Properties.* Berlin, 1838.

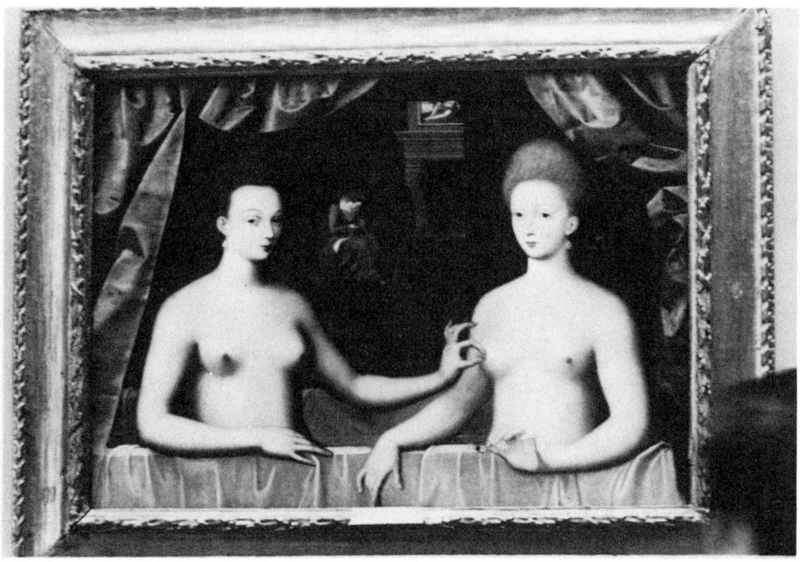

Figure 1

their infants if they eat foods that are taboo.[48, 1] These beliefs vary from country to country and sometimes even within the same region. Eggs are not eaten by mothers in one area of Tunis, while as many as six to eight eggs a day are eaten in another region.[45] In some African regions fruit, milk, meat and fish as well as eggs are taboo during pregnancy and the only foods eaten are watered down local staples such as maize, rice, sour porridge (maize fermented) or bread. These practices are often founded in age-old fears that some foods are responsible for inducing abortions or for bringing harm to mother or infant. For example in Sierra Leone, if the mother eats fish the baby will get worms or if eggs are eaten during pregnancy the baby may have a large head or dribble or have convulsions or even grow up to be a thief.[38] In Oman it is believed that the unborn child is located in the mothers stomach and that as the fetus grows more space must be left and less food eaten. Mothers in this region also believe that if they eat fish bones and scales the bones of their fetus will harden and lead to a difficult delivery.

Many believe that pregnancy alters digestion, so nutritious foods such as beans and lentils are avoided. Some dietary practices are beneficial, such as the consumption of liver by the pregnant Somali women (high of Vitamin A, B_{12}, iron.)

In the tropical forest of Zaire, such as Lake Tumba area, the Oto Bantu women and the Twa women refrain from having intercourse for 18 months after the birth of their first child to avoid a subsequent pregnancy as it is feared that pregnancy poisons the milk or nursing deprives the fetus. During this time the mother is covered with a red dye prepared from the bark of a tree (the "femme rouges"). She is separated from her husband and goes to live with her clan where she abstains from any type of heavy work. The nursing infant in this period never leaves the mother, but sleeps beside her and accompanies her at all times. At 18 months the infant is weaned and a party given when the mother rejoins her husband.[30, 32]

Fear of large babies has resulted in severe dietary restrictions manifesting as low birth weight infants. Sometimes mothers exhibit compulsive obsessive craving of non-food stuffs. This is called pica (magpie) and is found all over the world (Fig. 3). The eating of dirt or earth, known as geophagia, is one form and is common in poor women. In Sierra Leone it is called 'dotti'. Another is the eating of starch or clay known as amylophagia. Clay for pregnant women can be bought in markets such as Malawi, Sierra Leone, Zaire and until recently in the market in Atlanta, Georgia, USA. Pica is frequently associated with anemia and when the anemia is cured in some cases the pica may disappear.

DIETARY TABOOS DURING LACTATION

Among many sects in India, the mother is allowed cooked rice bread and coffee. Vegetables and fish are prohibited, as she is considered unable to digest food.

In one East African tribe chicken is thought to affect the milk and cause convulsions and fever in infancy. The restriction of animal protein obviously limits the mother's protein and iron intake. Common taboos may extend to fruits such as mango, papaya and coconut which are thought to reduce the mother's milk and cause diarrhoea.[45] Notably, many of the foods restricted in the diet of women in developing countries are recommended for U.S. mothers. While in some parts of the world foods are restricted, in others "strengthening" foods are given. In Ethiopia large amounts of butter are added to the mother's maize porridge and she is

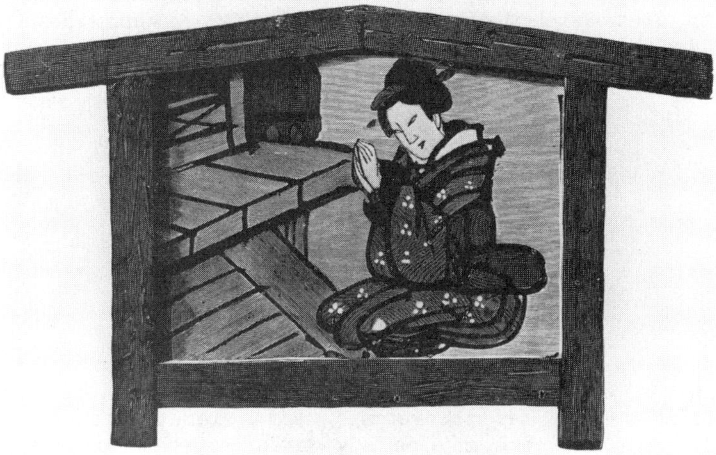

Figure 2a

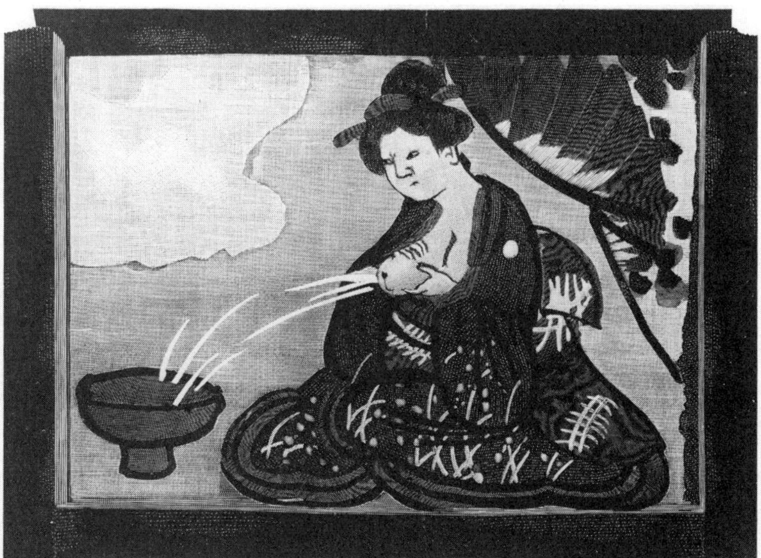

Figure 2b

often secluded for two months while all her domestic chores including food preparation are taken over by relatives. Desert Bedouin women of the Negev are not allowed to cook for a period of time. Women of the family may give the new mother meat, eggs and milk but this depends on the husband. The wife may be fed well if a son is born. Should the baby die while suckled, the mother or her breastmilk is blamed. Tanzanians give mothers a two month resting period and one tribe, the Watching, provides mothers with diets rich in milk, blood and fat. When the baby does not "thrive" a drop of milk is placed on a plate and if a fly settles on it, the breastmilk is blamed for the infant's condition. Among some Kenyan tribes if the infant dies, the unfortunate mother must have her breasts ritually purified before she can nurse again.[45]

GALACTOGOGUES

Each culture has milk producing (galactogenic) substances to ensure an abundant milk supply or to rectify milk insufficiency. In Western societies peanuts and coke may be advocated by some doctors and deplored by others. Galactogogues may improve the mother's diet and fluid content or they may be relaxing substances used to reduce anxiety and encourage the let down reflex. The medical literature abounds in treatments for lactation failure. For example, in the Papyrus Ebers (1550 BC), the earliest medical encyclopedia from Egypt, there is a short prescription for the promotion of breastfeeding.[47]

> "To get a supply of milk in a woman's breasts for suckling the child; warm the bones of a swordfish in oil and rub her back with it. Or, let the woman sit crosslegged and eat fragrant bread of soused durra. While rubbing her parts with the poppy plant."

In the sixteenth century, Phayer,[27] recommended in his "Remedie appropriate to ye encreasing of Mylke the Brestes" the following:

> "Parsneppe roots, fenelle roots sodden in broth of chicken and afterwards eaten with a little freshe butter rice soaked in cows milk, powder of earthworms dry and dronken in the broth of a neates tonge, the broth of an old cocke, with myntes, cynanon and maces."

If all that failed the local application of fennell plasters to the breasts was advocated. Arm exercises were also recommended.

Each present day culture has its own remedies and while some are spiritual, many are herbal and food related. In Pakistan foods that are considered to increase the milk supply include cumin, lassi, and cotton seeds as well as goat's stomach. In India fried ginger, jaggery, black pepper and ware may be given as a tonic for 10-30 days. Some remedies from Mexico include atoles (gruel) made from legumes, groundnut or chickpeas. Northern Mexicans make special teas from so called "hot plants" - sesame, abysinth and cotton seeds. In other parts of Latin America herb teas are drunk in the evening to stimulate milk for the next morning. In rural Tunisia a herb tea called "verveine" is made from caraway, fennelcreek and coriander seeds. Special foods such as wheat, barley and/or cous cous are eaten in the evening to stimulate the next morning's milk production. In the USA thistle tea is a known folk remedy

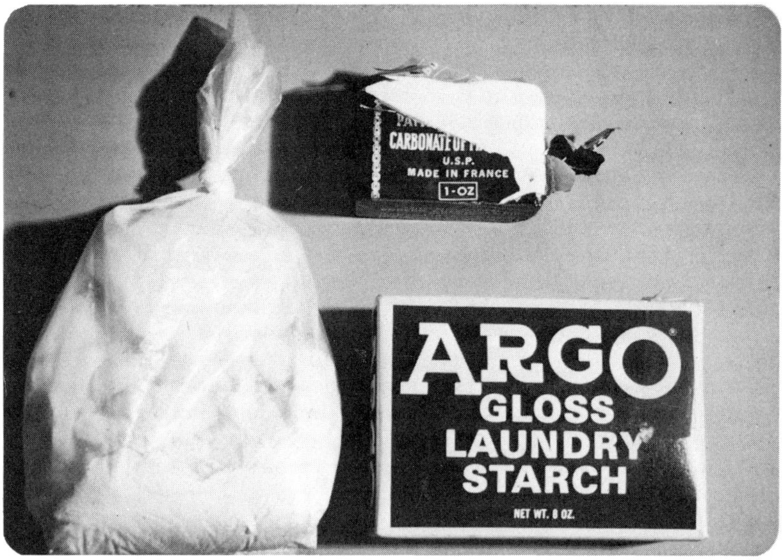

Figure 3

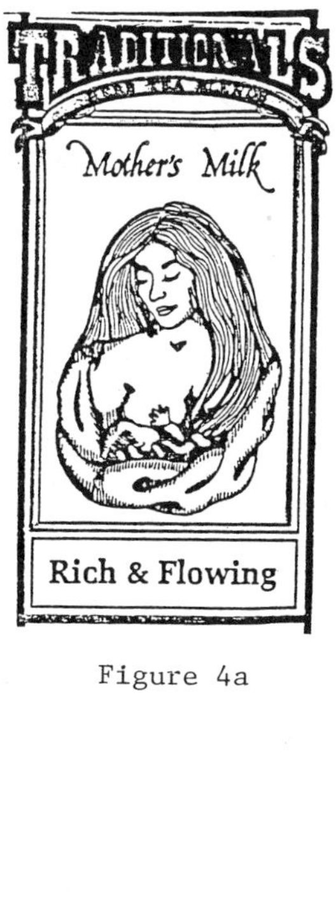

Figure 4a

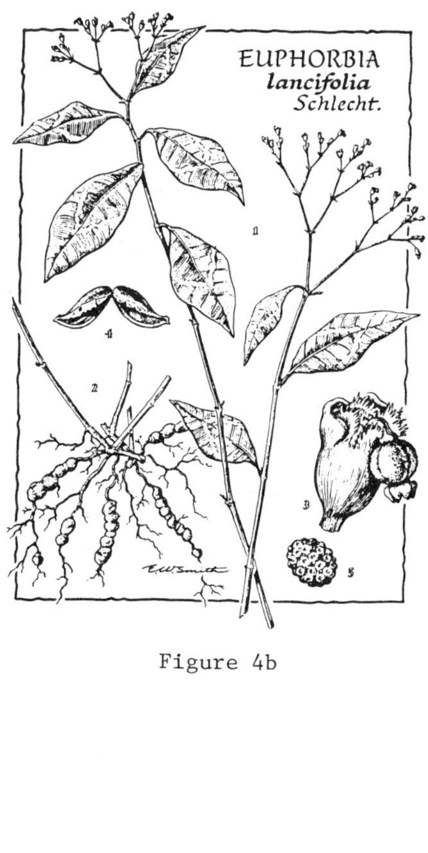

Figure 4b

(Fig. 4A). Plants such as comfrey and fenugreek have also been used. Guatemalan Indian women take steam baths in the belief that the heat applied to the back benefits milk production or drink ixbut tea (the leaves of Euphorbia lancifolia) (Fig. 4B).[45] In addition hot chocolate is usually drunk during the first week after the baby is born.

Continents apart, mothers have learned of herbs, fluids and foods for increasing their milk supply. Many of these remedies have not been "scientifically" tested but women swear by them. In the South China,[50] to improve the milk supply, soups made from pig's legs, tail bones cooked with beans or peanuts, or fish tails boiled with papya or coconut or chicken are common. A smaller percentage use salt-preserved marine fish eaten with the bones. In the North of China (Su Ging personal communication) chicken soup made from adult roosters is commonly used to promote lactation. This "lactation soup" is consumed from the first two weeks to two months after delivery. In parts of China the nursing mother is supposed to eat 5-10 eggs per day. For the city mothers many baskets of eggs may have to be collected from the countryside. Traditional herbs such as the seeds of the wolf berry, and shouwn tuber of the fleece flower, are also added. In addition to eggs and chicken, millet cooked in red sugar is prescribed. Many of these practices have not been scientifically examined.

ACTIVITY AND MOTHERING THE MOTHER

When mothers in traditional society are cared for in their own homes they often only have to feed the baby. The attendant cares for the baby, turns him to prevent "stiffness," and brings him to the mother when he cries or when the mother's breasts are full. A true two way demand feeding is established. During this important initial period rituals may be performed to keep away evil spirits, visitors are excluded, sometimes even husbands. In China in the rural areas as in many developing countries mother and infant are kept inside for 56 days and doors and windows kept closed. Often the mother is not allowed to do housework, sew, read or cook. The family does all the chores. Considering the high infant mortality, these practices have some basis. The isolation of infant and mother prevents the introduction of infectious disease at a very vulnerable period. It also helps the mother concentrate on the infant.

COLOSTRUM WITH OR WITHOUT

Long before the infant is born the breasts start producing secretions. Some women manually express this secretion to see how far along the pregnancy is. As many as a third of women no longer have colostrum but mature breastmilk in their breasts at the time their infant is born.[3, 23] This is particularly the case with women who have had a previous pregnancy. Some women are said to not stop lactating - 'permanent lactaters".[2] The mother may decide if her milk is good enough for the baby on the basis of color alone, although the color is not reflective of the content.

The first milk, called colostrum, is rich in antibodies which protect the infant against infections. Colostrum is increasingly being recognized as very important for infant health. In addition to all its wondrous antiinfective properties, it acts as a laxative for the infant and assists in the passage of meconium. In mothers who continue nursing while pregnant the milk changes in composition. Not much is known about nursing in tandem. Studies in Zaire[46] show that when the mother becomes pregnant while nursing the mature milk changes to colostrum. Nursing infants aged 3 or 4 have commented on the sour taste of the milk, and mothers have noticed these children develop "lactation diarrhoea", probably due to the laxative effect of colostrum. (Personal Communication from La Leche league mothers).

Looking back in history it appears keeping the newborn away from colostrum, was practiced almost universally by peasant societies save a few such as the Maoris who breast fed from day one.[10] For a long time people believed colostrum was harmful and infants were purged for 1-4 days and nursed by surrogate nurses for as many as 20 days.[9, 10]

As far back as 2 B.C. Indian Brahaminical Medicine recommended honey and clarified butter for the newborns first four days, while colostrum was expressed and discarded. In biblical times colostrum also was withheld while the infant was purged, to clean out the bowel, with honey till 'mature milk' was present in the mothers breasts. In the middle ages one of the purge was rose water. In Japan the elixir <u>jumi gokoto</u> was given to the newborn for the first 3 days. It was made from a variety of roots and herbs. The ingredients were determined by caste - high borns had 10 ingredients whereas infants of the poor only had 5. The Greeks, Romans, later French and English physicians unquestioningly continued this ritual until the eighteenth century when William Cadogan[7] wrote:

> "The mother's first milk is purgative and cleanses the child of its long hoarded excrement; no child can be deprived of it without manifest injury"

and he advocated breastfeeding from birth onwards. The neonatal mortality in the eighteenth century was very high in England and Wales. Changes about traditional beliefs about colostrum slowly began to be reflected in practice. One study showed that neonatal mortality in the UK at that time was reduced by sixteen percent and attributes this to colostrum[14]

In many developing countries even now mothers won't give their infants this first milk fearing it to be 'pus' or 'poison'. Strangely this belief exists in countries thousands of miles apart, for example among the Indians of Guatemala, Africans in Sierra Leone and in Lesotho.[23] If the mother eats a lot of foods containing vitamin A or carotene such as palm oil then the secretion may be very yellow. Still in Afganistan fela (colostrum) also is not given to newborns but a purge of bitter herbs, sweets and hyssop seeds instead.[26]

There is no question that colostrum is beneficial to the infant and that its anti-infective properties are protective. Even present day puppy dog food manufacturers are aware of this and insist that their product should not be used until the puppy has first had colostrum.

There is some difference in the composition of milk from mothers with premature infants compared to milk of mothers with full-term infants. Generally it is assumed that most mothers only start producing milk at the end of the pregnancy and have colostrum for the first three days. This gradually changes from transitional milk to mature milk over a five day period.

Concerned about the quality and quantity of the milk, since ancient times "milktests" were performed. In 2 A.D. Soranus[39] described a "nail test" for milk whereby a drop of milk was placed on the finger nail to judge its quality and consistence. He also realized that either the mother's or infant's health could be a cause of failure to thrive. The renowned physician Pauls Aegentica added rennet to milk, allowed the cheesy material to settle and compared the supernatant fluid with the sediment.[11] He was in fact precipitating the protein. The analysis and remedy suggested was as follows: they should be roughly equal in quantity. If the latter exceeds the former the milk will be indigestible; if the opposite occurred, then the milk is too weak. If on the other hand the milk was too thick the mother should be given emetics to evacuate the phleghm and if it was offensive it should be expressed and the mother fed on fragrant food and wines.

For a long time it was believed that breastmilk was white blood. For women who were not producing enough milk bloodletting was prescribed. Thomas Phayer,[26] urged that the milk be examined:

> "It is good to look upon the milk and see whether it be thicks and grosse or to muck thinne and watrye, blackyshe or bluse or chynge to redness or yellowe for all such is unnatural and evyll. Likewise why ye taste it in your mouth, it be ethyr bytter, salte or sour ye may well peceye it is unwholesome. The milk that is good is whyte and seate when you drop it on your nale and do move your finger neyther fleteth abrod at every stering wyll hanger faste upon your nale, when you turn downwards, but that which is between both is best."

Not only were the medical men of ancient civilizations concerned with assessing the quality of breastmilk. In Samoa there is an official milk tester usually an elderly woman, who puts samples of milk in a dish and adds water and two hot stones! If curdling occurs the milk is pronounced poisoned and suckling delayed.[47] Later the test is repeated usually with a favorable outcome.

The fears of 'bad milk' prey on women and affect their milk secretion. In the West the modern doctor neither looks at the milk nor the mother but religiously depends on the infants weight. If the infant fails to gain weight, by the standard based on formula fed infant's, too often it is assumed that the mother's milk is inadequate and formula is added as a supplement. Soranus, the Roman physician, realized that not only can there be a problem with the mother's milk, even though this is rare, but also with the mother's psyche or her health or her baby. The answer does not lie in blindly adding supplement to the infant's diet but in finding the cause; for each the treatment is different.

In the early 20th century Truby King,[19] a New Zealand physician farmer concerned with infant mortality, started training nurses to visit homes and encourage breastfeeding. Where mothers were having problems nursing or the infants' weight gain was less than expected, milk was collected and analyzed for fat content. If less than three percent of fat was present supplementary feeding was prescribed. The crematocrit has also been used for spinning down breastmilk and checking the amount of fat. In the U.S.A., a woman when told by her pediatrician, (who didn't even examine her breasts or milk), that her milk was not good, changed her doctor. The "new" physician sent a sample of her milk to a dairy for fat analysis. The note came back, "Dear Mrs.... if you were one of my herd I would keep you!" While the color of formula corresponds to its concentration, the color of breastmilk cannot be used to make any diagnosis of the quality of the milk. Nevertheless mothers do worry about the color of their milk.

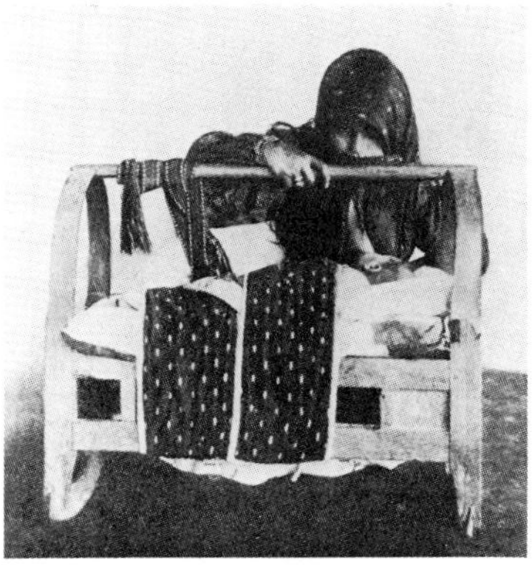

Figure 5a

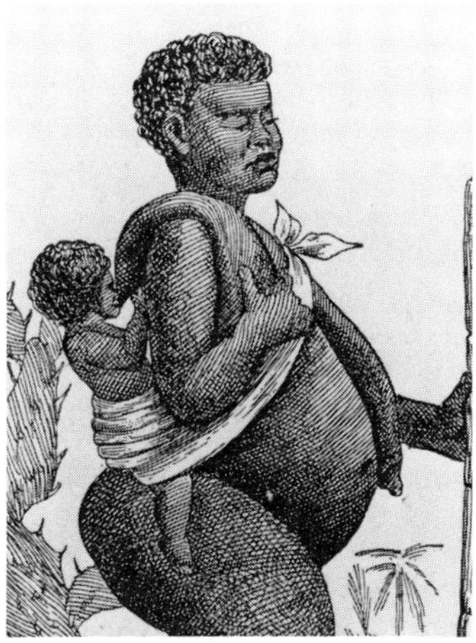

Figure 5b

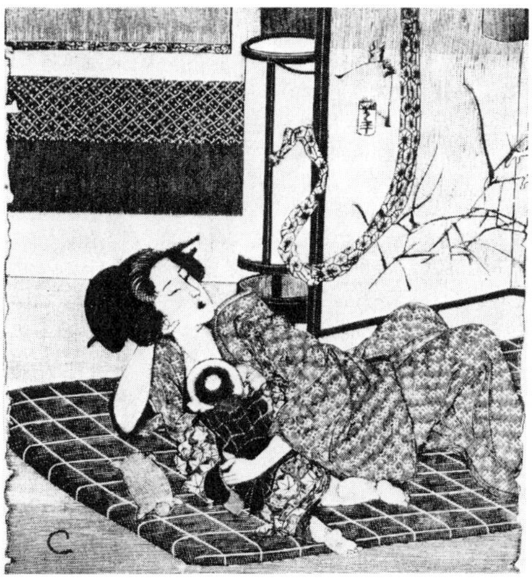

Figure 5c

FEEDING STYLES

Feeding styles also vary (Fig. 5A & B). In Asia, Africa, and Latin America, mothers carry their infants on their backs and swing them around for a feed "cafeteria style." The bushman women throw one of their pendulous breasts over their shoulders to provide the infants strapped on their backs with self service![40] Japanese women feed in a lying down position, as do most mothers that sleep with their infants next to them providing warmth, stimulation (touch, talk, ticking) the rhythmical beating of the mother's heart and milk on demand. Western infants early on sleep in isolettes. Toy teddy bears at $45 each for rhymical ticking are available. Some substitute! In Indonesia women feed their infants only on the left breast as they believe that the left breast has food and the right water.[35]

SURROGATE MOTHERS - WET NURSES

In peasant societies when a mother dies, is ill or cannot nurse, the infant is wet nursed by a close relative or at least someone within the clan. In biblical times the woman who did the feeding was considered the real mother even though she was not the biological mother. One of the well known examples in the Bible is Deborah who "gave suck" to Rebecca and acted as a surrogate mother. Sometimes the grandmother breastfed the infant as was the case when Naomi served as wet nurse to the infant of her daughther-in-law, Ruth. This practice of grandmothers breastfeeding is not uncommon in many part of Africa. They may take herbs orally or even apply them to the nipples in order to accelerate the onset of lactation. Though it may seem strange that a woman who has never been pregnant or a grandmother can produce milk[28] it is more surprising that there are case records of men who suckled their offspring and their siblings (Fig. 6).[11, 4]

Wet nurses have served as surrogate mothers since earliest times and ladies of high rank employed them.[15] Among the Greeks, for example, special slaves or bondwomen called duolas breastfed for 6 months and cared for their owners' infants. Ladies of high society afraid not only of ruining their health and their figures but also of neglecting "their duties", indulged in wet nurses, unfortunately at the expense of their infants many of whom died from neglect or inadequate nursing.[44, 33, 45] Also they lost the natural birth control effect of lactation and frequently had a large number of closely spaced infants also with high maternal and infant mortality.[24, 37]

In France wet nursing was well organized by the 12th century and continued into the 18th century.[10, 47] One of the most interesting and curious approaches to infant feeding had its origin in a foundling home. In the year 1204 Pope Pius III dedicated a large section of the hospital Santa Maria in Sassia (on the Tiber banks) to the care of unwanted infants who hitherto had been thrown into the river. A corp of wet nurses developed as the numbers of infants grew, and music of flutes and lutes were provided for all in a large room. The infants suckled peacefully and the nurses milk was found to flow more freely.[10]

Women who took jobs as wet nurses were usually of low social class, some even prostitutes. They neglected, abandoned, and even deliberately smothered their own infants to take on the lucrative job of breastfeeding someone else's child.[9] A 15th century painting by Francoise Clouet of "Diane de Pointier," allegedly the mistress of Henry the fourth, shows her having a bath while her wet nurse feeds the baby (Fig. 7). In the 17th century in France a law was finally passed which required registration of wet nurses, a medical examination and some proof that the wet nurse's own

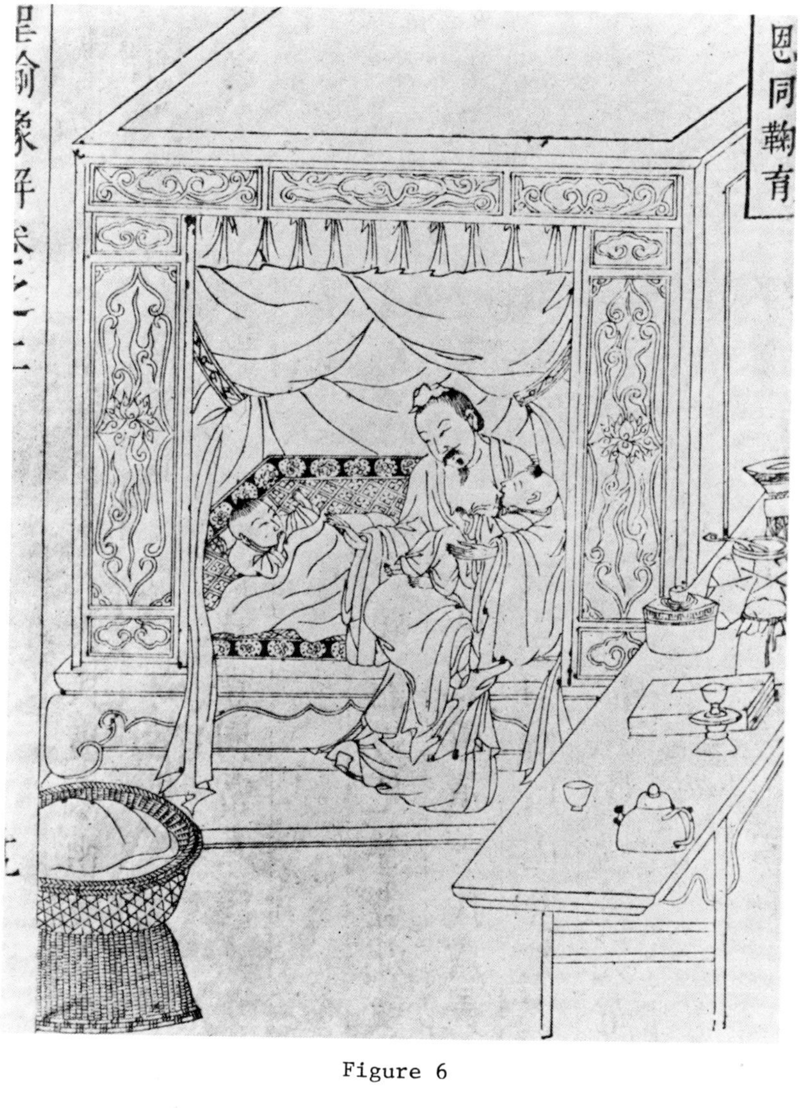

Figure 6

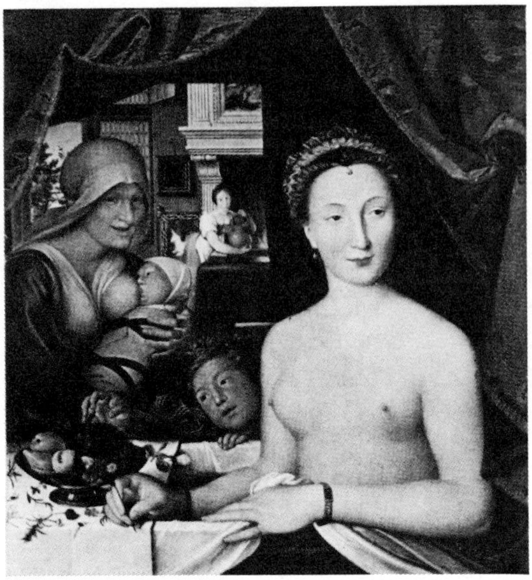

Figure 7

infant was at least nine months old before she could sell her services to someone else. Abandoning an infant became a punishable crime and the mother was imprisoned if she was found. However, the very law that aimed to keep mother and infant together in its execution often had the opposite effect. Nor was all wet nursing done in the home of the employer. Many infants were sent to wet nurses in the country, hence, the term "baby farm" or "farmed out".

WET NURSING FOUNDLINGS

Wet nurses served a vital function in foundling homes where they nursed "weaklings." They nursed not only their own infant but three or four others. In the Paris Maternite Hospital, Pierre Budin, an obstetrician, found that these women would nurse as often as 34 times a day. Forty times a day was the breaking point.[6] Usually women breastfeed four to six times a day but, this varies and recent evidence suggests that for successful lactation, mothers need to feed on the average 13 times a day. It was estimated that the wet nurses produced three to five pints of milk per day. The greater the demand for milk, the more they produced.[6] The milk volume was not only affected by suckling but also reduced with infection.

SLAVE MOTHERS

In the 18th century in Virginia for example slaves were used as breeders and feeders.[5] The directions given overseers for the protection of breeding women and their children were very explicit.

> "Sucklers are not required to leave their children at the childrens house before going to the field. The period of suckling is twelve months. Their work lies always within half a mile of their quarters.

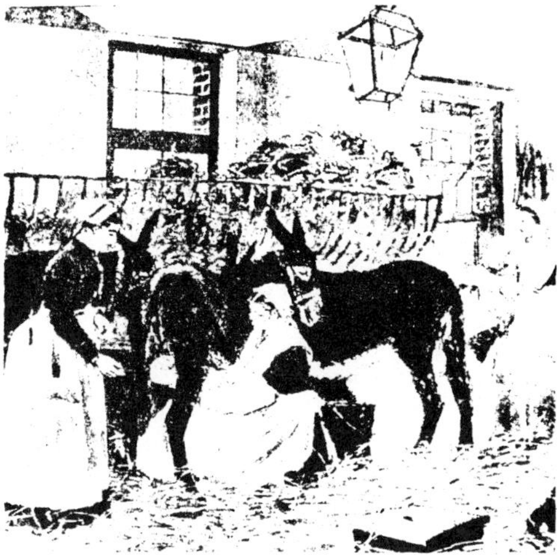

Figure 8a

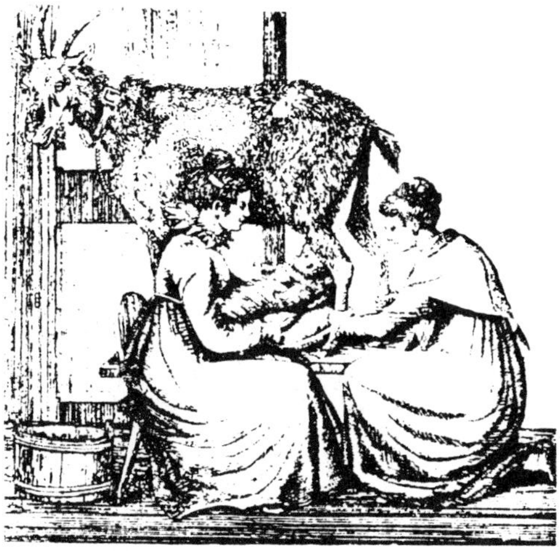

Figure 8b

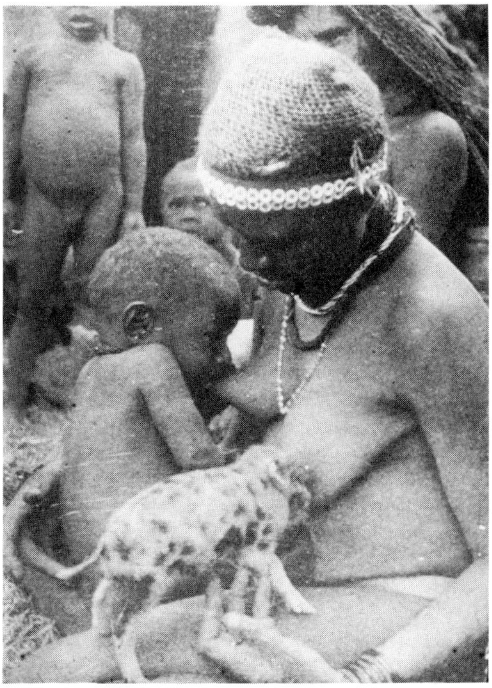

Figure 9

> They are required to cool before commencing to suckle - to wait 15 minutes at least in the summer, after reaching the children's house before nursing. They are allowed 45 minutes at each nursing to be with their children. They return three times a day until their children are 8 months old - in the middle of the morning, at noon and in the middle of the afternoon. The amount of work done by the suckler is about 3/5 of that done by a full hand, a little increased toward the last.... Pregnant women at 5 months are put on the sucklers gang. No ploughing or lifting must be required of them."[5]

Year after year "fruitful Virginia wives" gave birth to a long line of heirs and only a high mortality kept the household population within bounds. The strain of frequent pregnancies must have been very taxing. Early weaning and the pretty general use of wet nurses were doubtless responsible in part for the high birth rates, for here as elsewhere, in cutting short the period of lactation women sacrificed one of the best contraceptives.[24]

SELECTION OF WET NURSES

Wet nurses were selected according to certain criteria, many of them highly subjective, and some irrational such as: "Physically healthy with a pleasing countenance "rudis mouth" a rosy complexion "verie white teeth" and broad but not pendulous breasts with good nipples."[13, 18] The size of the breast incidentally is of no consequence. In addition one was cautioned not to employ redheads. A preposterous "study" cited as evidence for this attempted to show that the composition of brunette's milk was better than blondes (Table 1).[10, 34] No one knows how many poor red heads or blondes were deprived of a job on the basis of this research. Some women were even led to believe that personality traits were passed on in the milk as well.[41]

Medical examinations were useful and helped rule out chronic diseases such as tuberculosis and syphilis, which can be transmitted to the infant through the milk. In the American South, before the civil war, especially on the plantations, it was common for black "nannies" to feed white infants as well as their own. Nevertheless the racial prejudice of some whites was strong enough to preclude the use of black nannies as wet nurses as they feared that the accents and the mannerisms of the black nurse would be passed on through the milk.[41]

> Wet nurses were expected to eat and live "right" -- Warned against "bad air, bad smells, salty spiced foods, garlic mustard, stale cheese and also roast meat if the infant's complexion is moist and phylegmatic. .... Told to "spurn all raw fruit and drink only ale, beer, barley, water or wine, rest whenever, ... keep bowels open and shun all disquietness of mind...

Later smoking was added as a no no, and that was one of the few reasonable measures advocated. Were mothers so carefully screened and regimented today one wonders how many would be judged "fit" to care for their infants let alone breastfeed them.

Towards the end of the 19th century wet nurses fell into disrepute as they were promiscuous, expensive, socially problematic (interfered with family affairs), considered themselves a cut above servants. Many appear to have had difficulty nursing their charges and to fatten them they fed malt liquor; to quieten them they gave drops of opium either directly by mouth or applied to the nipple. This is not unique to wet nurses. Mothers too also been reported to use opium for their infants for their own peace. Many of the wet nurses however, were held in high esteem by their grown nurslings. The French physician Guillemeau in his book "Nursing of Young Children,"[16] tells of a boy who greeted his nurse with gold, but only gave silver to his mother because she had no alternative but to nourish him in her womb whereas the nurse carried him three years in her arms and "nourished me with her own bloude." Fear of the transmission of syphilis through the milk, although suspected as early as in the 15th century, increased significantly in the 17th century. Moralists, child advocates and the improvements in public health contributed to the move from "wet" to "dry" nursing. Artificial feeding made possible the replacement of the wet nurse by a nanny with a glass bottle and a rubber treat - a "pocket nurse."[36, 13]

INFANTS FED BY ANIMALS

When mother's milk was not available and artificial feeding a deadly risk, infants were fed by animals (Fig. 8A & B). This stems from Biblical times when some infants were fed off camel's teats. The story of Romulus and Remus who were given wolf's milk is a success story but many infants fed off animals directly didn't fare as well.

In the 17th century sick infants and foundlings were fed on asses' and goat's milk and the mortality was very high although the composition of these milks are closer to human milk than cow's milk. Alphonse Le Roy in 1775 instituted at his hospital direct suckling of foundlings by goats.

> "Each goat comes to feed enters bleating and goes to hunt the infant which has been given to it, pushes back the covering with its horns and straddles the crib to give suck to the infant. There is in milk besides different nutritious principles an invisible element, the element of life itself, a fugitive gas which is so volatile that it escapes as soon as the milk is in contact with the air. This is why it is impossible to rear infants with animal milk or milk which has been expressed from the breast."[10]

Goats as wet nurses have been used worldwide. Hottentots in Southern Africa tied their infants to goats' bellies so they could feed there. The Bedoins of Israel still resort to the use of a goat or sheep when a human nurse is not available. Goats were in some instances easier to obtain and cheaper than human wet nurses.

Asses too were used as wet nurses and some infants were fed directly with asses milk such as at the Hospice des Enfants Malades where the animal stalls were directly across from the wards and an elaborate procedure for this feeding. Using asses as wet nurses however was difficult. Pigs were also used as wet nurse but infrequently as they were socially persona non grata. In parts of Peru "children are fed milk from a black burro for a tonic and dog's milk for a good stomach."[31] Close to the turn of the 18th century milk was analyzed and asses milk was found to be closest in composition to human milk. Goat's milk was the next best. The Koran interestingly enough holds that children suckled by the same nurse are milk sisters and milk brothers since milk is considered altered blood, and they thus become blood relations. They are not permitted to marry because of the anathema of consanguinous marriages.[31]

LACTATING WOMEN FEED ANIMALS AND BABIES SIMULTANEOUSLY

Not only have animals fed humans but humans have and still do feed animals, extraordinary as it may seem. Animals were nursed by women for a variety of reasons including the survival of destitute young animals; to relieve the womans engorged breasts; to prevent conception; to promote lactation; to develop good nipples and even for other health reasons. Ancient Romans and Persians put animals to the breast and the custom is still found occurs among Neopolitans and roving gypsies of Transylvania, Germany, New Zealand, Australia, Sumatra, Thailand, Japan and South America. In parts of Africa, such as the Cameroons and in New Guinea and even among Amazon Indians, women suckle domestic puppies and piglets (Fig. 9). This evidentally was also practiced in Canada where Indian women often suckled young dogs and Puma Indians withdrew their breasts sooner from their own infants than from young dogs[31, 47].

In Persia and Turkey young dogs were put to the breasts to toughen the nipples and make them better for the infant to suck on. Wet nurses in Turkey used suckling puppies to maintain their milk supply if they had to travel by sea from distant villages to the capital. In Dauphine France where children were nursed 2-1/2 - 3 years to prevent another pregnancy, if the child died too soon, the mother suckled another child or puppy for the same purpose. There even is a report that young dogs were suckled by women to disperse obstinate breast nodules.[31] In America, Davies, (the first American pediatrician), recommended from the 7th month of pregnancy regular application of a strong puppy to harden and conform the nipples, improve breast secretion and prevent inflammation of the breasts. "The puppy's suckling efforts if started early enough prepared the nipples for future assaults of the child." For women too modest to make use of a puppy and so unfortunately organized as to lack nipples altogether or have them short or sunken in, he recommended drawing them out daily with a large tobacco pipe. It was also believed that "the dog laid on painful breasts could do good service."[11]

Strange that the societal norm in one country is offensive in another. And breastfeeding which was our societal norm up to the 1940's has become a rare and revolting practice for many Americans.

NURSING THE AGED

Women may nurse their own children, act as surrogate nurses, nurse animals or nurse the aged. This appears to be particularly so in cultures where the old are revered. Evidence of this is found in the old Chinese and Japanese literature[8, 22] and even American literature. One Chinese story indicates that on her deathbed an old lady blessed her dutiful daughther-in-law who had kept her alive for several years with her daily dose of breastmilk as a "health food". In Steinbeck's Grapes of Wrath, when the family reached California they were visited by an old sick, starving man. As they had no food or medicine to give him one of the daughters whose infant had recently died nursed him.[42]

THE DURATION OF BREASTFEEDING

Attitudes generally tend to dictate the duration of breastfeeding. In the Solomon Islands breastfeeding persisted until the children were 15 years of age! The duration in some cultures is related to the sex of infants. Among Iranians according to Moslem law it is traditional to breastfeed girls for two months longer than boys to compensate them for being born women (e.g. daughters inherit half of the property inherited by sons). Some compensation!

BREAST MILK AND ITS ANTI-INFECTIVE PROPERTIES

Human milk has had a long history of medical therapuetics particularly in the disorders of the human eye. In the Ebers Papyrus 1500BC reference is made to a lotion to improve sight which was prepared by combining the milk-of-a-woman who had borne a son. For eyes with a "flow of matter" a concoction was soaked first in water then in goose grease, then washed "in the milk of a woman who had borne a son and allowed to dry, and finally combined with myrrh and rubbed on the eye.[12, 43]

The milk of "a woman who had borne a son" was also used "to drive out blood from in the eyes" in combination with the fruit of the Dompalm.[12] Human milk was used as a cathartic, for sabs of the limbs" and for "uha disease" (hookworm,) Ancient Indians used it in eye operations and as a remedy for eye and ear infections. It was used as an antidote for henbane intoxication. For evacuating blood from the uterus wool soaked in breast milk was inserted into the vagina. According to Phiny, women's milk was useful for fevers, feeble stomachs, pimples, spots, freckles of the face, and disease of the ears. As early as the 11th century in Baghdad Ali ibn Isa described milk in the treatment of eye diseases including ophthalmia neonatorum.

The Chinese too were aware of its antiinfective properties. Among the 24 Chinese filial duties was the one where the son risked his life to get deer's milk and cured his old parents' sick eyes by applying the fresh milk to their eyes![8] Recently in Samoa there was an epidemic of hemorrhagic conjunctivitis.[25] Breast milk was squirted into the eyes of the affected patients when the supply of antibiotics ran out.

It is clear from some of the practices described that breastfeeding is not a simple measurable act like formula feeding. The wide range of practices that exists make it essential to classify breastfeeding on the age and weight of the infant; withholding of colostrum; use of pre or post lacteal feeds; frequency of feeding and duration of breastfeeding. The mothers nutritional status is another variable that should also be considered as well as her dietary intake and even her level of activity.

REFERENCES

1. Baumslag, N., Mothers and children -- Nutrition and health care in Kenya, Zimbabwe, Mozambique and Botswana, Ford Foundation report, New York, 1980.

2. Baumslag, N., Sierra Leone trip report Office of Nutrition USAID Washington, DC, 1981.

3. Baumslag, N., Perspectives in Nutrition in Africa, USAID Africa bureau, Washington, DC, 1984.

4. Baxandall, R., Gordon L. Reverby, S., Americas Women, Vintage Press, 1976.

5. Blanton, B.W., Medicine in Virginia in the Eighteenth Century, Richmond, Garrett and Massie, Inc., MCMXXXI, p. 163, 1931.

6. Budin, P., The nursling: the feeding and hygiene of premature and full term infants. Caxton, London, 1907.

7. Cadogan, W., Essay on Nursing and management of children from birth to three years of age... In a letter to one of the Governors of the Foundling Hospital: Published by general order of the general committee for transactions of the said hospital, London, 1773.

8. Chen, I., Wisdom of the East. The book of filial duty. Translated from the Chinese of Hsiao Ching by Ivan Chen, John Murray Albemarle Street, page 41, No. VII, 1908.

9. Cone, T.E., The history of American pediatrics, Little Brown publishers, Boston, 1979.

10. Davidson, W.D., A brief history of infant feeding, The Journal of Pediatrics, p.74-87, 1953.

11. Deaver, J.B., McFarland, J., The breast, its anomalies, its diseases and their treatment, Blakiston and son, Philadelphia, 1917.

12. Duke-Elder, S., The history of ocular therapeutics in System of Opthalmology: Heredity, Pathology, Diagnosis and Therapeutics. Mosby, St. Louis, 1962.

13. Ebrahim, G.J., Breastfeeding. The biological option, MacMillan Press, London, 1978.

14. Fildes, V., Neonatal feeding in practices and neonatal mortality during the 18th century. Journ. of Biosocial Sciences Vol. 12, p. 313-324, 1980.

15. Graham, H., The eternal Eve. The history of gynaecology and obstetrics, Doubleday and Co., Inc., Garden City, New York, 1951.

16. Guillemeau, J., Childbirth or, the Happy Delivery of Children, Amsterdam Theatrum Orbis Terrarum, 1972, (Facismile edition 1612).

17. Helsing, E., King, F.S., Breastfeeding in practice. A manual for health workers, Oxford University Press, Oxford, England, 1982.

18. Jelliffe, D.B., and E.F.P. Jelliffe, Human Milk in the modern world, Oxford University Press, Oxford, England, 1977.

19. King, T., The Man, London, England, 1948.

20. Kitzinger, S., Women as mothers, Fontana William Collins and Son, Great Britain, 1978.

21. Kottik, S.S., Breast feeding in ancient Jewish sources in Historical and legal aspects in human milk. Selected papers from the International Symposium on breast feeding. Tel Aviv February 24-28, 1980, Editors Freier S. And Eidelman, A.I.) Shaare Zadek Medical Centre Jerusalem Exerpta Medica Amsterdam, Oxford, Princeton, 1980.

22. Legend in Japanese art, Freer gallery, p.299, Washington, AISH.

23. Mata, L., The children of Santa Maria Cauque. A prospective field study of health and growth. MIT press, Boston, Massachusetts, 1978.

24. McClaren, D., Natures contraceptive, Wet-nursing and prolonged lactation: The Case of Chesham, Buckinghamshire, 1578-1601, Medical History, 23:426-441, 1979.

25. Morbidity and Mortality Report, Vol. 3, No. 31, 1982.

26. Pakmal, M.A., Afgan villages Kabul. Social attitudes, beliefs and practices that affect nutritional status of pregnant women lactating mothers and young children. APHA Clearinghouse.

27. Phayer, T., Regiment of life, 1546.

28. Phillips, V., Non-Puerperal Lactation among Australian Aboriginal Women. Current centres bulletin 47, 1971.

29. Ploss, H.H., Woman, Vols. I, II, III, Heineman publishers, Philadelphia, 1935.

30. Radbill, S., Pediatrics in the Bible, Clinical pediatrics, p. 199-212, 1963.

31. Radbill, S.X., The role of animals in infant feeding 21-30 in American Folk Medicine, A symposium, Editor Hand, W.D., University of California Press, Berkeley, 1976.

32. Read, M., Culture, health and disease, Tavistock publications, Great Britain, 1966.

33. Rousseau, J.J., Emile, Everymans library, 1977.

34. Routh, C.H.F., Infant feeding and its influence on life 3rd edition, New York, 1896.

35. Salubritas. Report from Java and Sumatra. Findings in the field change thinking in the capital, volume 4, number 1. p. 2, published by the APHA, 1980.

36. Schwab, M.G., The rise and fall of the baby bottle, Journal of Human Nutrition, 33, 276-282, 1979.

37. Schnucker, R.V., The English puritans and pregnancy, delivery and breastfeeding.

38. Scott, S., Food beliefs affecting the nutritional status of people in Sierra Leone. National School of Nursing, Freetown, Sierra Leone, 1978.

39. Soranus Ephesus Gynecology, Translated by Temkin O. and Eastman, N. et. al., Johns Hopkins Press Baltimore, 1956.

40. Speert, H., Iconographia Gyniartia. A pictorial history of gynecology and obstetrics. F.A. Davis Company, Philadelphia, 1945.

41. Spruill, J.C., Women's life and work in the Southern colonies, Chapel Hill, North Carolina, University of North Carolina Press, 1938.

42. Steinbeck, J., Grapes of Wrath.

43. Tomsak, R.L., The bulletin of the Cleveland Medical Library. A brief history of the use of mother's milk in occular therapeutics, 24(1):12-21, 1978.

44. Trollope, A., Doctor Thorne.

45. Vermury, M. Levine, H., Project on beliefs and practices that affect food habits. A literature review. Care, New York, 1978.

46. Vis, H.D., Hennart, P.H., Decline in breastfeeding, Acta pediatric Belg., 31, 195-206, 1978.

47. Wickes, I.G., A history of Infant feeding, Arch. Dis. in Child. 28; 151-158, 1953.

48. Williams, C.D., Baumslag, N. and Jelliffe, D.B., Mother and Child Health; Delivering the Services, 2nd edition, Oxford University Press, Oxford, England, 1985.

49. Zweirlein, C., The goat as the best and most agreeable wet nurse.

50. Zhi-chien Ho, Breastfeeding in Xinhui district in South China, Food and Nutrition bulletin, Vol. 3 no. 3, p. 42-48, 1978.

CONTRIBUTORS AND PARTICIPANTS

I. Adlerbert, University of Goteborg, Sweden

Jonathan C. Allen, Department of Physiology, University of Colorado School of Medicine, Denver, CO 80262

Lindsey Allen, Department of Nutritional Sciences U-17, University of Connecticut, Storrs, CT. 06268

Bengt Andersen, Department of Clinical Immunology, University of Goteborg, Sweden

Suniti Archarya, Ministry of Health, Kathmandu, Nepal

Philip Archer, Department of Preventive Medicine, University of Colorado, Medical Center, Denver, CO. 80262

Carolina Arevolo, Nutrition, Infection, and Immunology Program, INCAP, Guatemala City, Guatamala

David Armstrong, Department of Obstetrics and Gynecology, The University of Western Ontario, London, Canada

P.G. Arthur, Department of Biochemistry, University of Western Australia, Perth, WA 6009, Australia

Stephenia A. Atkinson, Department of Pediatrics, Faculty of Health Sciences, McMaster University,1200 Main St. West Hamilton,Ontario M9A 4RI

Tom Baranowski, Department of Preventive Medicine and Community Health, University of Texas Medical Branch, Galveston, Texas 77550

Naomi Baumslag, Department of Pediatrics, Georgetown University Medical School, Washington, D.C. 20007

John Benson, Ross Laboratories, 625 Cleveland Avenue, Columbus, OH 43216

Cheston M. Berlin, Jr., Department of Pediatrics, The Pennsylvania State University College of Medicine, The Milton S. Hershey Medical Center, Hershey, PA 17033

Joel Bitman, Milk Secretion and Mastitis Laboratory, USDA, Beltsville, Md. 20705

Alison Black, Dunn Nutrition Unit, University of Cambridge, Milton Road, Cambridge, UK

Peggy R. Borum, Department of Food Science and Human Nutrition, University of Florida, Gainesville, Florida 32611
Hans Joachim Bremer, Department of General Pediatrics, Metabolism and Nephrology, University Children's Hospital, Dusseldorf, West Germany

R. Don Brown, Department of Pharmacology, Louisiana State University Medical Center, Shreveport, LA 71140-33932

Nancy Butte, Department of Pediatrics, Baylor College of Medicine, 6608 Fannin, Houston, Texas 77030

Judy Canahuati, PROALMA, P.O. Box 512, San Pedro Sula, Honduras

Louis M. Canfield, Department of Biochemistry and Biophysics, and Department of Animal Science, Texas Agricultural Experiment Station, and Texas A&M University, College Station, Texas 77843-2471.

Barbro Carlsson, Department of Clinical Immunology, University of Goteborg, Sweden

Claire E. Casey, Department of Pediatrics, University of Colorado School of Medicine, Denver, CO 80262

J.J. Chapman, School of Nursing, Vanderbilt University, Nashville, TN

Janet E. Chappell, Medical Department, Bristol-Myers Pharmaceutical Group, Ottawa, Canada

Argentina de Chavez, PROALMA - Proyecto de Apoyo a Lactancia Materna Junta Nacional de Bienestar Social Tegucigalpa, Honduras, C.A.

M. Thomas Clandinin, Department of Foods and Nutrition, University of Alberta, Edmonton, Canada

Tim Cole, Dunn Nutrition Unit, University of Cambridge, Milton Road, Cambridge, UK

James C. Cumella, Department of Pediatrics and Microbiology, School of Medicine, State University of New York and Division of Infectious Diseases and Microbiology Laboratories, Children's Hospital, Buffalo, NY, 14222

U.Dahlgren, Department of Clinical Immunology, University of Goteborg, Sweden

Peter F. Daniel, E.K. Shriver Center for Mental Retardation, Waltham, MA 02254

Margarett K. Davis, University of North Carolina, 108 Laurel Hill Circle, Chapel Hill, NC 27514

Richard Denney, Department of Biological Chemistry, University of Texas Medical Branch, Galveston, Texas

Kay Dewey, Department of Nutrition, University of California, Davis, CA

S.M. Donovan, Department of Nutrition, University of California, Davis, CA 95616

Richard A. Ehrenkranz, Department of Pediatrics, Yale University School of Medicine 333 Cedar Street, New Haven, Connecticut 06510

Edward Emken, Department of Pediatrics, USDA/ARS Children's Nutrition Research Center, Baylor College of Medicine and Texas Children's Hospital, Houston, TX

Arlene Fanaroff, Fogarty International Center, NIH, Building 38A-610, Bethesda, Md. 20892

Ann M. Ferris, Department of Nutritional Sciences, University of Connecticut, U-17, Storrs, CT. 06268

Dorothy Ann Finley, Department of Nutrition, University of California, Davis, CA 95616

Thorsten A. Fjellstedt, NICHD, Room 7C17, Landow Building, 7910 Woodmont Avenue, Bethesda, MD. 20205

Samuel Flores-Huerta, Growth and Development Section, Unidad de Investigacion Biomedica, Apartdado Postal 73-197, Mexico, D.F. 03020 or Luz Savinon 214, Col. del Valle, Mexico, D.F. 03100

Debra Fraser, Department of Pediatrics, McMaster University, Hamilton, Ontario, Canada

Lois M. Freed, Department of Pediatrics, Georgetown University Medical Center, Washington, D.C. 20007

Cutberto Garza, Department of Pediatrics, Baylor College of Medicine, Children's Nutrition Research Center, Medical Towers Building, 6608 Fannin, Suite 601, Houston, TX 77030

Randall M. Goldblum, Department of Pediatrics, University of Texas, Medical Branch, Galveston, Texas 77550

Armond S. Goldman, Division of Immunology and Allergy, Department of Pediatrics, University of Texas Medical Branch, Galveston, TX 77550

Lynn Goldman, Epidemiological Studies and Surveillance Section, California Department of Health Services, 2151 Berkeley Way, Berkeley, CA 94706

Rae Greenberg, P.O. Box 46454, Philadelphia, PA 19160

M. Hahn-Zoric, Department of Pediatrics, University of Goteborg, Sweden

K. Michael Hambidge, Department of Pediatrics, School of Medicine, University of Colorado Health Sciences Center, 4200 East Ninth Avenue, Denver, CO 80262

Leif Hambraeus, Institute of Nutrition, University of Uppsala, Uppsala, Sweden

Margit Hamosh, Department of Pediatrics, Georgetown University Medical Center, Washington, D.C. 20007

Paul Hamosh, Department of Physiology and Biophysics, and Pediatrics, Georgetown University Medical Center, Washington, D.C. 20007

Lars A. Hanson, Department of Clinical Immunology, University of Goteborg, Sweden

Peter E. Hartmann, Department of Biochemistry, University of Western Australia, Perth, WA 6009 Australia

Rafia Hasan, Department of Psychology, Punjab University, Lahore, Pakistan

David Hatchey, Department of Pediatrics, USDA/ARS Children's Nutrition Research Center, Baylor College of Medicine and Texas Children's Hospital, Houston, TX

Homero Hernandez-Montes, Growth and Development Section, Unidad de Investigacion Biomedica, Apartado Postal 73-197, Mexico, D.F. 03020 or Luz Savinon 214, Col. del Valle, Mexico, D.F. 03100

James L. Hinson, Department of Pharmacology, Louisiana State University Medical Center, Shreveport, LA 71130-33932

Bruce W. Hollis, Department of Pediatrics, Medical University of South Carolina, 171 Ashley Avenue, Charleston, S.C. 29425

Judy Hopkinson, Department of Pediatrics, USDA/ARS Children's Nutrition Research Center, Baylor College of Medicine and Texas Children's Hospital, Houston, TX

Jell Hsieh, Department of Human Biological Chemistry and Genetics, University of Texas Medical Branch, Galveston, Texas

Gail E. Huston,School of Medicine, University of California, San Diego, La Jolla, CA 92093

Charles E. Isaacs, Office of Mental Retardation and Developmental Disabilities, New York State Institute for Basic Research in Developmental Disabilities, Department of Developmental Biochemistry, 1050 Forest Hill Road, Staten Island, NY 10314

Fehmida Jalil, Department of Social and Preventive Pediatrics, King Edward Medical College, Lahore, Pakistan

Robert G. Jensen, Department of Nutritional Sciences, University of Connecticut, Storrs, CT 06268

Virginia A. Johnson, Department of Pharmacology, Louisiana State University Medical Center, Shreveport, LA 71130-33932

Ronald V. Josephson, School of Family Studies and Consumer Sciences, San Diego, CA 92182

J. Karlberg, University of Goteborg, Sweden

Karyn J. Kaufman, Faculty of Health Sciences, McMaster University, Hamilton Ontario, Canada

M. Keegan, School of Nursing, Vanderbilt University, Nashville, TN

Marlyn Kefauver, Department of Health and Human Services, Office of International Health, Rm 18-75 Parklawn Bldg., Rockville, Md. 20857

Ronald P. Keller, Department of Physiology, University of Colorado School of Medicine, Denver, CO 80262

Shaukat R. Khan, Department of Pediatrics and of Social and Preventive Medicine, King Edward Medical College, Lahore, Pakistan

Avanelle Kirskey, Department Foods and Nutrition, Purdue University, West Lafayette, Indiana 47907

David Kittarns, Berkeley California

Bert Koletzko, Department of General Pediatrics, Metabolism and Nephrology, University Children's Hospital, Dusseldorf, West Germany

Nancy F. Krebs, Department of Pediatrics, School of Medicine, University of Colorado Health Sciences Center, 4200 East Ninth Avenue, Denver, CO 80262

Alex Kurosky, Department of Genetics, University of Texas Medical Branch, Galveston, Texas

Teresa Lagergard, Department of Medical Microbiology, University of Goteborg, Sweden

Chun Por Lai, Department of Biochemistry and Biophysics, and Department of Animal Science, Texas Agricultural Experimental Station and Texas A&M University, College Station, Texas 77843-2471

Ruth A. Lawrence, Division of Neonatology, University of Rochester School of Medicine, Rochester, NY

James E. Leklem, Oregan State University, Corvallis, Oregon 97331

Bo S. Lindblad, Department of Pediatrics, Karolinska Institute,Stockholm, Sweden

Bo Lonnerdal, Department of Nutrition, University of California, Davis, CA 95616

R.N. Macey, School of Nursing, Vanderbilt University, Nashville, TN

Helen Mandyla, Department of Immunology, First Pediatric Clinic, Athens University and B' Neonatal Intensive Care Unit, "Aghia Sophia" Children's Hospital, Athens, Greece

Robert H. McCluer, E.K. Shriver Center, 200 Trapelo Rd., Waltham, MA 02253, USA

Nitin R. Mehta, Department of Pediatrics, Georgetown University Medical Center, Washington, D.C. 20007

L. Mellander, University of Goteborg, Sweden

John A. Milner, Department of Food Science and Divison of Nutritional Sciences, University of Illinois, Urbana, IL 61801

Corinne Montandon, Department of Pediatrics, USDA/ARS Children's Nutrition Research Center, Baylor College of Medicine and Texas Children's Hospital, Houston, Texas

Pamela A. Montgomery, School of Family Studies and Consumer Sciences, San Diego, CA. 92182

Pamela A. Montgomery, School of Family Studies and Consumer Sciences, San Diego, CA 92182

Kathleen Motil, Department of Pediatrics, USDA/ARS Children's Nutrition Research Center, Baylor College of Medicine and Texas Children's Hospital, Houston, TX

Roger C. Moretz, Office of Mental Retardation and Developmental Disabilities, New York State Institute for Basic Research in Developmental Disabilities, Department of Pathological Neurobiology, 1050 Forest Hill Road, Staten Island, NY 10314

S.E.G. Morgan, Department of Biochemistry, University of Western Australia, Perth, WA 6009, Australia

Phyllis B. Moser, Department of Food and Nutrition, University of Maryland, College Park, MD.

Maria Mrotzek, Department of General Pediatrics, Metabolism and Nephrology, University Children's Hosptial Dusseldorf, West Germany

Audrey J. Naylor, Wellstart/The San Diego Lactation Program and UCSD School of Medicine, 4062 First Avenue, P.O. Box 87549, San Diego, CA 92138

Marianne R. Neifert, Lactation Program, Women's Hospital at AMI Saint Luke's and University of Colorado School of Medicine, Denver, Colorado

Margaret C. Neville, Department of Physiology, C240, University of Colorado School of Medicine, 4200 East Ninth Avenue, Denver, CO 80262

David S. Newburg, E.C. Shriver Center, 200 Trapelo Rd., Waltham, MA 02254

Steven Northwehr, Department of Pediatrics, University of Texas Medical Branch, Galveston, Texas

Linda V. Oberkotter, Department of Biological Sciences, Florida Institute of Technology, 150 W, University Boulevard, Melbourne, FL 32901

Olav T. Oftedal, National Zoological Park, Smithsonian Institution, Washington, D.C.

Pearay L. Ogra, Department of Pediatrics and Microbiology, School of Medicine State University of New York and Division of Infectious Diseases and Microbiology Laboratories, Children's Hospital, Buffalo, NY 14222

Nancy E. O'Neil, E.K. Shriver Center, 200 Trapelo Rd., Waltham, MA 02254

John S. Patton, Department of Pharmacological Sciences, Genentech, Inc. 460 Point San Bruno Boulevard, South San Francisco, CA 94080

Stuart Patton, School of Medicine, University of California, San Diego, La Jolla, CA 92093

Alison Paul, Dunn Nitrition Unit, University of Cambridge, Milton Road, Cambridge, UK

Gretel H. Pelto, Department of Nutritional Sciences, University of Connecticut, Storrs, CT

Mary Frances Picciano, Division of Foods and Nutrition, Division of Nutritional Sciences, College of Agriculture, the University of Illinois, 905 S. Goodwin Avenue, Urbana, IL 61801

Larry K. Pickering, Program in Infectious Diseases and Clinical Microbiology and Department of Pediatrics, University of Texas Medical School at Houston, Houton, TX 77225

Thomas A. Picone, Ross Laboratories, Pediatrics and Nutrition, 625 Cleveland Avenue, Columbus, OH 43216.

Oscar Porras, Hospital Nacional de Ninos, Immunology Branch, Apartado Postal 86010, 1000 San Jose, Costa Rica

Andrew Prentice, Dunn Nutrition Unit, University of Cambridge, Milton Road, Cambridge, UK

Anne Prentice, Dunn Nutrition Unit, University of Cambridge, Milton Road, Cambridge, UK

Jose Ramiro Cruz, Nutrition, Infection and Immunology Program, INCAP, P.O. Box 1188, Guatemala City, Guatemala

David K. Rassin, Division of Perinatal Pediatrics, Department of Pediatrics, University of Texas Medical Branch, Galveston, Texas 77550

Kathleen M. Rasmussen, Division of Nutritional Sciences, Cornell University,145 Savage Hall, Ithaca, NY 14853

Robert D. Reynolds, Human Nutrition Research Center, U.S. Department of Agriculture, Beltsville, MD. 20705

C. Joan Richardson, Division of Perinatal Pediatrics, Department of Pediatrics, University of Texas Medical Branch, Galveston, Texas 77550

Walter J. Rogan, Epidemiology Branch, National Institute of Environmental Health Sciences, Research Triangle Park, NC 27709

Guillermo Ruiz Palacios, Department of Infectious Diseases, Instituto Nacional de la Nutricion, Vasco de Quiroga 15, Mexico, D.F. 14000

Sylvia B. Rumball, Department of Chemistry, Biochemistry and Biophysics, Massey University, Palmerston North, New Zealand

Richard Schanler, Department of Peditrics, USDA/ARS Children's Nutrition Research Center, Baylor College of Medicine, Houston, Texas

Joy M. Seacat, Lactation Program, Women's Hospital at AMI, Saint Luke's and University of Colorado School of Medicine, Denver, Colorado

A. Kaleem Sheiku, Department of Psychology, Punjab University, Lahore, Pakistan.

L. Sherman-Martin, Department of Food Science and Division of Nutritional Sciences, University of Illinois, Urbana, Il 61801

Gary Silber, Department of Pediatrics, USDA/ARS Children's Nutrition Research Center, Baylor College of Medicine and Texas Children's Hospital, Houston, TX

Iain J. Smith, Department of Pharmacology, Louisiana State University Medical Center, Shreveport, LA 71130-33932

T. Soderstrom, Department of Pediatrics, Karolinska Institute, Stockholm, Sweden

Ruthann Stanhope, Department of Pediatrics, McMaster University, Hamilton, Ontario, Canada

Margaret Strode, Department of Nutrition, University of California, Davis, CA 95616

Janice Stuff, USDA/ARS Children's Nutrition Research Center, Department of Pediatrics, Baylor College of Medicine and Texas Children's Hospital, Houston, Texas

John A. Sturman, Department of Developmental Biochemistry, New York State Institute for Basic Research in Developmental Disabilities, Staten Island, NY 10314

Catharina Svanborg Eden, Medical Microbiology, University of Goteborg, Sweden

M. Rita Thomas, Mead Johnson Nutritional Group, Evansville, IN 47721

Ann F. Townsend-Blanton, Department of Biochemistry and Biophysics and Department of Animal Science, Texas Agricultural Experimental Station and Texas A&M University, College Station, Texas 77843-2471

Salvador Villalpando-Hernandez, Unidad de Investigacion Biomedica Growth, and Development Section, Apartado Postal 73-197, - Mexico, D.F. 03020 or Luz Savinon 214, Col. del Valle. Mexico, D.F. 03100

Carol L. Wade, Department of Pediatrics, McMaster University, Hamilton, Ontario, Canada.

Ruth A. Wester, Wellstart/San Diego Lactation Program, 4062 First Avenue, San Diego, CA 92138

Roger Whitehead, Dunn Nutrition Unit, University of Cambridge, Milton Road, Cambridge, UK

John T. Wilson, Department of Pharmacology, LSUMC, Shreveport, LA 73310

A. Wold, Department of Clinical Immunology, University of Goteborg, Sweden

D.L. Wood, Milk Secretion and Mastitis Laboratory, USDA/ARS, Beltsville, MD. 20705

Thomas W. Woods, Department of Pharmacology, Louisiana State Univesity Medical Center, Shreveport, LA 71130-33932

Marietta Xantou, Department of Immunology, First Pediatric Clinic, Athens University and B' Neonatal Intensive Care Unit, "Aghia Sophia" Children's Hospital, Athens, Greece

Sumner J. Yaffe, National Institutes of Health, Bethesda, MD. 20892

Carla M. York, Department of Pediatrics, Georgetown University Medical Center, Washington, D.C. 20007

INDEX